Pharmacotherapy Handbook

Tenth Edition

NOTICE

Medicine is an ever-changing science. As new research and clinical experience broaden our knowledge, changes in treatment and drug therapy are required. The authors of this work have checked with sources believed to be reliable in their efforts to provide information that is complete and generally in accord with the standards accepted at the time of publication. However, in view of the possibility of human error or changes in medical sciences, neither the authors nor the publisher nor any other party who has been involved in the preparation or publication of this work warrants that the information contained herein is in every respect accurate or complete, and they disclaim all responsibility for any errors or omissions or the results obtained from use of the information contained in this work. Readers are encouraged to confirm the information contained herein with other sources. For example and in particular, readers are advised to check the product information sheet included in the package of each drug they plan to administer to be certain that the information contained in this work is accurate and that changes have not been made in the recommended dose or in the contraindications for administration. This recommendation is of particular importance in connection with new or infrequently used drugs.

Pharmacotherapy Handbook

Tenth Edition

Barbara G. Wells, PharmD, FASHP, FCCP
Dean Emeritus and Professor Emeritus
Executive Director Emeritus, Research Institute of Pharmaceutical Sciences
School of Pharmacy, The University of Mississippi
Oxford, Mississippi

Joseph T. DiPiro, PharmD, FCCP
Professor and Dean
Archie O. McCalley Chair
School of Pharmacy
Virginia Commonwealth University
Richmond, Virginia

Terry L. Schwinghammer, PharmD, FCCP, FASHP, FAPhA, BCPS
Professor and Chair, Department of Clinical Pharmacy
School of Pharmacy, West Virginia University
Morgantown, West Virginia

Cecily V. DiPiro, PharmD, CDE
Consultant Pharmacist
Richmond, Virginia

New York   Chicago   San Francisco   Athens   London   Madrid   Mexico City
Milan   New Delhi   Singapore   Sydney   Toronto

Pharmacotherapy Handbook, Tenth Edition

Copyright © 2017 by McGraw-Hill Education. All rights reserved. Printed in the United States of America. Except as permitted under the United States Copyright Act of 1976, no part of this publication may be reproduced or distributed in any form or by any means, or stored in a data base or retrieval system, without the prior written permission of the publisher.

Previous edition copyright © 2015, 2012, 2009, 2006, 2003, 2000, by The McGraw-Hill Companies, Inc.; copyright © 1998 by Appleton & Lange.

2 3 4 5 6 7 8 9   LCR   22 21 20 19 18

ISBN 978-1-259-58643-9
MHID 1-259-58643-X

This book was set in Minion Pro by Cenveo® Publisher Services.
The editors were Michael Weitz and Brian Kearns.
The production supervisor was Catherine H. Saggese.
Project management was provided by Revathi Viswanathan, Cenveo Publisher Services.

Library of Congress Cataloging-in-Publication Data

Names: Wells, Barbara G., editor. | DiPiro, Joseph T., editor. |
   Schwinghammer, Terry L., editor. | DiPiro, Cecily V., editor.
Title: Pharmacotherapy handbook / [edited by] Barbara G. Wells, Joseph T.
   DiPiro, Terry L. Schwinghammer, Cecily V. DiPiro.
Description: Tenth edition. | New York : McGraw-Hill, 2017. | Includes index.
   Identifiers: LCCN 2017021244 (print) | LCCN 2017021685 (ebook) | ISBN
   9781259586415 (ebook) | ISBN 9781259586439 (pbk. : alk. paper)
Subjects: | MESH: Drug Therapy | Handbooks
Classification: LCC RM301.12 (ebook) | LCC RM301.12 (print) | NLM WB 39 | DDC
   615.5/8—dc23

International Edition ISBN 978-1-260-28816-2; MHID 1-260-28816-1.
Copyright © 2017. Exclusive rights by McGraw-Hill Education, for manufacture and export. This book cannot be re-exported from the country to which it is consigned by McGraw-Hill Education. The International Edition is not available in North America.

Contents

SECTION 1: BONE AND JOINT DISORDERS

Edited by Terry L. Schwinghammer

SECTION 2: CARDIOVASCULAR DISORDERS

Edited by Terry L. Schwinghammer

SECTION 3: DERMATOLOGIC DISORDERS

Edited by Terry L. Schwinghammer

SECTION 4: ENDOCRINOLOGIC DISORDERS

Edited by Terry L. Schwinghammer

SECTION 5: GASTROINTESTINAL DISORDERS

Edited by Joseph T. DiPiro and Terry L. Schwinghammer

Contents

SECTION 6: GYNECOLOGIC AND OBSTETRIC DISORDERS

Edited by Barbara G. Wells

SECTION 7: HEMATOLOGIC DISORDERS

Edited by Cecily V. DiPiro

SECTION 8: INFECTIOUS DISEASES

Edited by Joseph T. DiPiro

SECTION 9: NEUROLOGIC DISORDERS

Edited by Barbara G. Wells

Contents

Contents

APPENDICES

Edited by Barbara G. Wells

Preface

This 10th edition of the pocket companion to *Pharmacotherapy: A Pathophysiologic Approach* is designed to provide practitioners and students with critical information that can be easily used to guide drug therapy decision-making in the clinical setting. To ensure brevity and portability, the bulleted format provides the user with essential textual information, key tables and figures, and treatment algorithms. The authors make every effort to write as clearly and succinctly as possible.

Corresponding to the major sections in the main text, disorders are alphabetized within the following sections: Bone and Joint Disorders; Cardiovascular Disorders; Dermatologic Disorders; Endocrinologic Disorders; Gastrointestinal Disorders; Gynecologic and Obstetric Disorders; Hematologic Disorders; Infectious Diseases; Neurologic Disorders; Nutrition Support; Oncologic Disorders; Ophthalmic Disorders; Psychiatric Disorders; Renal Disorders; Respiratory Disorders; and Urologic Disorders. Drug-induced conditions associated with drug allergy, hematologic disorders, liver disease, pulmonary disease, and kidney disease appear in five tabular appendices. Tabular information on the management of pharmacotherapy in the elderly also appears as an appendix.

Each chapter is organized in a consistent format:

- Disease state definition
- Concise review of relevant pathophysiology
- Clinical presentation
- Diagnosis
- Treatment
- Evaluation of therapeutic outcomes

The treatment section may include goals of treatment, general approach to treatment, nonpharmacologic therapy, drug selection guidelines, dosing recommendations, adverse effects, pharmacokinetic considerations, and important drug-drug interactions. When more in-depth information is required, the reader is encouraged to refer to the primary text, *Pharmacotherapy: A Pathophysiologic Approach,* 10th edition.

It is our sincere hope that students and practitioners find this book helpful as they continuously strive to deliver highest quality patient-centered care. We invite your comments on how we may improve subsequent editions of this work.

Barbara G. Wells
Joseph T. DiPiro
Terry L. Schwinghammer
Cecily V. DiPiro

Please provide your comments about this book, Wells et al., *Pharmacotherapy Handbook,* 10th edition, to its authors and publisher by writing to pharmacotherapy@mcgraw-hill .com. Please indicate the author and title of this handbook in the subject line of your e-mail.

Acknowledgments

The editors wish to express their sincere appreciation to the authors whose chapters in the 10th edition of *Pharmacotherapy: A Pathophysiologic Approach* served as the basis for this book. The dedication and professionalism of these outstanding practitioners, teachers, and scientists are evident on every page of this work. These individuals are acknowledged at the end of each respective handbook chapter. We also appreciate the input of readers over the years who have helped us to make continuous improvements in this book.

SECTION 1
BONE AND JOINT DISORDERS

Edited by Terry L. Schwinghammer

CHAPTER 1

Gout and Hyperuricemia

- *Gout* involves hyperuricemia, recurrent attacks of acute arthritis with monosodium urate (MSU) crystals in synovial fluid leukocytes, deposits of MSU crystals in tissues in and around joints (tophi), interstitial renal disease, and uric acid nephrolithiasis.

PATHOPHYSIOLOGY

- Uric acid is the end product of purine degradation. An increased urate pool in individuals with gout may result from overproduction or underexcretion.
- Purines originate from dietary purine, conversion of tissue nucleic acid to purine nucleotides, and de novo synthesis of purine bases.
- Overproduction of uric acid may result from abnormalities in enzyme systems that regulate purine metabolism (eg, increased activity of phosphoribosyl pyrophosphate [PRPP] synthetase or deficiency of hypoxanthine-guanine phosphoribosyl transferase [HGPRT]).
- Uric acid may be overproduced because of increased breakdown of tissue nucleic acids, as with myeloproliferative and lymphoproliferative disorders. Cytotoxic drugs can result in overproduction of uric acid due to lysis and the breakdown of cellular matter.
- Dietary purines are insignificant in generation of hyperuricemia without some derangement in purine metabolism or elimination.
- Two thirds of uric acid produced daily is excreted in urine. The remainder is eliminated through gastrointestinal (GI) tract after degradation by colonic bacteria. Decline in urinary excretion to a level below rate of production leads to hyperuricemia and increased pool of sodium urate.
- Drugs that decrease renal uric acid clearance include diuretics, nicotinic acid, salicylates (<2 g/day), ethanol, pyrazinamide, levodopa, ethambutol, cyclosporine, and cytotoxic drugs.
- Deposition of urate crystals in synovial fluid results in inflammation, vasodilation, increased vascular permeability, complement activation, and chemotactic activity for polymorphonuclear leukocytes. Phagocytosis of urate crystals by leukocytes results in rapid lysis of cells and discharge of proteolytic enzymes into cytoplasm. The ensuing inflammatory reaction causes intense joint pain, erythema, warmth, and swelling.
- Uric acid nephrolithiasis occurs in 10% to 25% of patients with gout. Predisposing factors include excessive urinary excretion of uric acid, acidic urine, and highly concentrated urine.
- In acute uric acid nephropathy, acute renal failure occurs because of blockage of urine flow from massive precipitation of uric acid crystals in collecting ducts and ureters. Chronic urate nephropathy is caused by long-term deposition of urate crystals in the renal parenchyma.
- Tophi (urate deposits) are uncommon and are a late complication of hyperuricemia. Most common sites are the base of the fingers, olecranon bursae, ulnar aspect of forearm, Achilles tendon, knees, wrists, and hands.

CLINICAL PRESENTATION

- Acute gout attacks are characterized by rapid onset of excruciating pain, swelling, and inflammation. The attack is typically monoarticular, most often affecting the first metatarsophalangeal joint (podagra), and then, in order of frequency, the insteps, ankles, heels, knees, wrists, fingers, and elbows. Attacks commonly begin at night, with the patient awakening with excruciating pain. Affected joints are erythematous, warm, and swollen. Fever and leukocytosis are common. Untreated attacks last from 3 to 14 days before spontaneous recovery.
- Acute attacks may occur without provocation or be precipitated by stress, trauma, alcohol ingestion, infection, surgery, rapid lowering of serum uric acid by uric acid–lowering agents, and ingestion of drugs known to elevate serum uric acid concentrations.

DIAGNOSIS

- Definitive diagnosis requires aspiration of synovial fluid from the affected joint and identification of intracellular crystals of MSU monohydrate in synovial fluid leukocytes.
- When joint aspiration is not feasible, a presumptive diagnosis is based on presence of characteristic signs and symptoms as well as the response to treatment.

TREATMENT

- <u>Goals of Treatment</u>: Terminate the acute attack, prevent recurrent attacks, and prevent complications associated with chronic deposition of urate crystals in tissues.

ACUTE GOUTY ARTHRITIS (FIG. 1–1)

Nonpharmacologic Therapy

- Local ice application is the most effective adjunctive treatment. Dietary supplements (eg, flaxseed and celery root) are not recommended.

Pharmacologic Therapy

- Most patients may be treated successfully with nonsteroidal anti-inflammatory drugs (NSAIDs), corticosteroids, or colchicine.

NSAIDS

- NSAIDs have excellent efficacy and minimal toxicity with short-term use. Indomethacin, naproxen, and sulindac have Food and Drug Administration (FDA) approval for gout, but others are likely to be effective (Table 1–1).
- Start therapy within 24 hours of attack onset and continue until complete resolution (usually 5–8 days). Tapering may be considered after resolution, especially if comorbidities such as hepatic or renal insufficiency make prolonged therapy undesirable.
- The most common adverse effects involve the GI tract (gastritis, bleeding, and perforation), kidneys (renal papillary necrosis and reduced creatinine clearance [CL_{cr}]), cardiovascular system (increased blood pressure, sodium and fluid retention), and central nervous system (impaired cognitive function, headache, and dizziness).
- Selective cyclooxygenase-2 inhibitors (eg, celecoxib) may be an option for patients unable to take nonselective NSAIDs, but the risk-to-benefit ratio in acute gout is unclear, and cardiovascular risk must be considered.

CORTICOSTEROIDS

- Corticosteroid efficacy is equivalent to NSAIDs; they can be used systemically or by intra-articular (IA) injection. Systemic therapy is necessary if an attack is polyarticular.

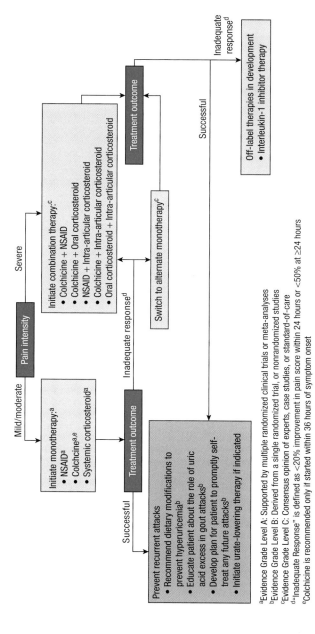

FIGURE 1–1. Algorithm for management of an acute gout attack.

[a] Evidence Grade Level A: Supported by multiple randomized clinical trials or meta-analyses
[b] Evidence Grade Level B: Derived from a single randomized trial, or nonrandomized studies
[c] Evidence Grade Level C: Consensus opinion of experts, case studies, or standard-of-care
[d] "Inadequate Response" is defined as <20% improvement in pain score within 24 hours or <50% at ≥24 hours
[e] Colchicine is recommended only if started within 36 hours of symptom onset

TABLE 1-1	Dosage Regimens of Oral Nonsteroidal Anti-Inflammatory Drugs for Treatment of Acute Gout	
Generic Name	**Initial Dose**	**Usual Range**
Etodolac	300 mg twice daily	300–500 mg twice daily
Fenoprofen	400 mg three times daily	400–600 mg three to four times daily
Ibuprofen	400 mg three times daily	400–800 mg three to four times daily
Indomethacin	50 mg three times daily	50 mg three times daily initially until pain is tolerable then rapidly reduce to complete cessation
Ketoprofen	75 mg three times daily or 50 mg four times daily	50–75 mg three to four times daily
Naproxen	750 mg followed by 250 mg every 8 hours until the attack has subsided	—
Piroxicam	20 mg once daily or 10 mg twice daily	—
Sulindac	200 mg twice daily	150–200 mg twice daily for 7–10 days
Celecoxib	800 mg followed by 400 mg on day one, then 400 mg twice daily for 1 week	—

- **Prednisone** or **prednisolone** oral dosing strategies: (1) 0.5 mg/kg daily for 5 to 10 days followed by abrupt discontinuation; or (2) 0.5 mg/kg daily for 2 to 5 days followed by tapering for 7 to 10 days. Tapering is often used to reduce the hypothetical risk of a rebound attack upon steroid withdrawal.
- **Methylprednisolone dose pack** is a 6-day regimen starting with 24 mg on day 1 and decreasing by 4 mg each day.
- **Triamcinolone acetonide** 20 to 40 mg given by IA injection may be used if gout is limited to one or two joints. IA corticosteroids should generally be used with oral NSAID, colchicine, or corticosteroid therapy.
- **Methylprednisolone** (a long-acting corticosteroid) given by a single intramuscular (IM) injection followed by oral corticosteroid therapy is another reasonable approach. Alternatively, IM corticosteroid monotherapy may be considered in patients with multiple affected joints who cannot take oral therapy.
- Short-term corticosteroid use is generally well tolerated. Use with caution in patients with diabetes, GI problems, bleeding disorders, cardiovascular disease, and psychiatric disorders. Avoid long-term use because of risk for osteoporosis, hypothalamic–pituitary–adrenal axis suppression, cataracts, and muscle deconditioning.
- **Adrenocorticotropic hormone (ACTH)** gel 40 to 80 USP units may be given IM every 6 to 8 hours for 2 or 3 days and then discontinued. Limit use for patients with contraindications to first-line therapies (eg, heart failure, chronic renal failure, and history of GI bleeding) or patients unable to take oral medications.

COLCHICINE

- **Colchicine** is highly effective in relieving acute gout attacks; when it is started within the first 24 hours of onset, about two thirds of patients respond within hours. Use only within 36 hours of attack onset because the likelihood of success decreases substantially if treatment is delayed.

- Colchicine causes dose-dependent GI adverse effects (nausea, vomiting, and diarrhea). Non-GI effects include neutropenia and axonal neuromyopathy, which may be worsened in patients taking other myopathic drugs (eg, statins) or in renal insufficiency. Do not use concurrently with P-glycoprotein or strong CYP450 3A4 inhibitors (eg, clarithromycin) because reduced biliary excretion may lead to increased plasma colchicine levels and toxicity. Use with caution in renal or hepatic insufficiency.
- **Colcrys** is an FDA-approved colchicine product available in 0.6 mg oral tablets. The recommended dose is 1.2 mg (two tablets) initially, followed by 0.6 mg (one tablet) 1 hour later. Although not an FDA-approved regimen, the American College of Rheumatology (ACR) gout treatment guidelines suggest that colchicine 0.6 mg once or twice daily can be started 12 hours after the initial 1.2-mg dose and continued until the attack resolves.

HYPERURICEMIA IN GOUT

- Recurrent gout attacks can be prevented by maintaining low uric acid levels, but adherence with nonpharmacologic and pharmacologic therapies is poor.

Nonpharmacologic Therapy

- Patient education should address the recurrent nature of gout and the objective of each lifestyle/dietary modification and medication.
- Promote weight loss through caloric restriction and exercise in all patients to enhance renal urate excretion.
- Alcohol restriction is important because consumption correlates with gout attacks. ACR guidelines recommend limiting alcohol use in all gout patients and avoidance of any alcohol during periods of frequent gout attacks and in patients with advanced gout under poor control.
- Dietary recommendations include limiting consumption of high-fructose corn syrup and purine-rich foods (organ meats and some seafood) and encouraging consumption of vegetables and low-fat dairy products.
- Evaluate the medication list for potentially unnecessary drugs that may elevate uric acid levels. Gout is not necessarily a contraindication to use of thiazide diuretics in hypertensive patients. Low-dose aspirin for cardiovascular prevention should be continued in patients with gout because aspirin has a negligible effect on elevating serum uric acid.

Pharmacologic Therapy (Fig. 1–2)

- After the first attack of acute gout, prophylactic pharmacotherapy is recommended if patients have two or more attacks per year, even if serum uric acid is normal or only minimally elevated. Other indications include presence of tophi, chronic kidney disease, or history of urolithiasis.
- Urate-lowering therapy can be started during an acute attack if anti-inflammatory prophylaxis has been initiated.
- The goal of urate-lowering therapy is to achieve and maintain serum uric acid less than 6 mg/dL (357 μmol/L), and preferably less than 5 mg/dL (297 μmol/L) if signs and symptoms of gout persist.
- Urate lowering should be prescribed for long-term use. Serum urate can be reduced by decreasing synthesis of uric acid (xanthine oxidase inhibitors) or by increasing renal excretion of uric acid (uricosurics).
- Apply a step-wise approach to hyperuricemia (see Fig. 1–2). Xanthine oxidase inhibitors are recommended first-line therapy; the uricosuric agent probenecid is recommended as alternative therapy in patients with a contraindication or intolerance to xanthine oxidase inhibitors. In refractory cases, combination therapy with a xanthine oxidase inhibitor plus a drug with uricosuric properties (probenecid, losartan, or fenofibrate) is suggested. Pegloticase may be used in severe cases in which the patient cannot tolerate or is not responding to other therapies.

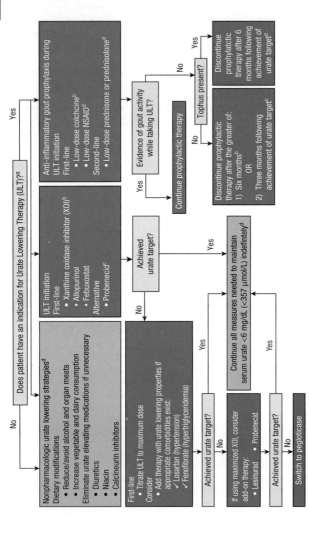

FIGURE 1–2. Algorithm for management of hyperuricemia in gout.

aIndications for ULT include: (1) presence of tophus, (2) ≥2 gout attacks per year, (3) CKD stage 2 or worse, and (4) past urolithiasis
bEvidence Grade Level A: Supported by multiple randomized clinical trials or meta-analyses
cEvidence Grade Level B: Derived from a single randomized trial, or nonrandomized studies
cEvidence Grade Level C: Consensus opinion of experts, case studies, or standard-of-care

XANTHINE OXIDASE INHIBITORS

- Xanthine oxidase inhibitors reduce uric acid by impairing conversion of hypoxanthine to xanthine and xanthine to uric acid. Because they are effective in both overproducers and underexcretors of uric acid, they are the most widely prescribed agents for long-term prevention of recurrent gout attacks.
- **Allopurinol** lowers uric acid levels in a dose-dependent manner. ACR guidelines recommend a starting dose no greater than 100 mg daily in patients with normal renal function and no more than 50 mg/day in patients with chronic kidney disease (stage 4 or worse) to avoid allopurinol hypersensitivity syndrome and prevent acute gout attacks common during initiation of urate-lowering therapy. The dose should be titrated gradually every 2 to 5 weeks up to a maximum dose of 800 mg/day until the serum urate target is achieved.
- Mild adverse effects of allopurinol include skin rash, leukopenia, GI problems, headache, and urticaria. More severe adverse reactions include severe rash (toxic epidermal necrolysis, erythema multiforme, or exfoliative dermatitis) and allopurinol hypersensitivity syndrome characterized by fever, eosinophilia, dermatitis, vasculitis, and renal and hepatic dysfunction that occurs rarely but is associated with a 20% mortality rate.
- **Febuxostat** (Uloric) also lowers serum uric acid in a dose-dependent manner. The recommended starting dose is 40 mg once daily. Increase the dose to 80 mg once daily for patients who do not achieve target serum uric acid concentrations after 2 weeks of therapy. Febuxostat is well tolerated, with adverse events of nausea, arthralgias, and minor hepatic transaminase elevations. Febuxostat does not require dose adjustment in mild to moderate hepatic or renal dysfunction. Due to rapid mobilization of urate deposits during initiation, give concomitant therapy with colchicine or an NSAID for at least the first 8 weeks of therapy to prevent acute gout flares.

URICOSURICS

- **Probenecid** increases renal clearance of uric acid by inhibiting the postsecretory renal proximal tubular reabsorption of uric acid. Patients with a history of urolithiasis should not receive uricosurics. Start therapy with uricosurics at a low dose to avoid marked uricosuria and possible stone formation. Maintaining adequate urine flow and alkalinization of the urine during the first several days of therapy may also decrease likelihood of uric acid stone formation.
- Initial probenecid dose is 250 mg twice daily for 1 to 2 weeks, then 500 mg twice daily for 2 weeks. Increase the daily dose thereafter by 500-mg increments every 1 to 2 weeks until satisfactory control is achieved or a maximum dose of 2 g/day is reached.
- Major side effects of probenecid include GI irritation, rash and hypersensitivity, precipitation of acute gouty arthritis, and stone formation. Contraindications include impaired renal function (CL_{cr} <50 mL/min or <0.84 mL/s) and overproduction of uric acid.
- **Lesinurad** (Zurampic) is a selective uric acid reabsorption inhibitor that inhibits urate transporter 1, a transporter in proximal renal tubules, thereby increasing uric acid excretion. It is approved as combination therapy with a xanthine oxidase inhibitor for treatment of hyperuricemia associated with gout in patients who have not achieved target serum uric acid levels with xanthine oxidase inhibitor monotherapy.
- The only approved dose of lesinurad dose is 200 mg once daily in the morning with food and water in combination with a xanthine oxidase inhibitor. The drug should not be used in patients with creatinine clearance below 45 mL/min.
- Adverse effects of lesinurad include urticaria and elevated levels of serum creatinine, lipase, and creatine kinase. It carries a black box warning about increased risk of acute renal failure when used in the absence of xanthine oxidase inhibitor therapy.

PEGLOTICASE

- **Pegloticase** (Krystexxa) is a pegylated recombinant uricase that reduces serum uric acid by converting uric acid to allantoin, which is water soluble. Pegloticase is indicated for antihyperuricemic therapy in adults refractory to conventional therapy.

- The dose is 8 mg by IV infusion over at least 2 hours every 2 weeks. Because of potential infusion-related allergic reactions, patients must be pretreated with antihistamines and corticosteroids. Pegloticase is substantially more expensive than first-line urate-lowering therapies.
- The ideal duration of pegloticase therapy is unknown. Development of pegloticase antibodies resulting in loss of efficacy may limit the duration of effective therapy.
- Because of its limitations, reserve pegloticase for patients with refractory gout who are unable to take or have failed all other urate-lowering therapies.

ANTI-INFLAMMATORY PROPHYLAXIS DURING INITIATION OF URATE-LOWERING THERAPY

- Initiation of urate-lowering therapy can precipitate an acute gout attack due to remodeling of urate crystal deposits in joints after rapid lowering of urate concentrations. Prophylactic anti-inflammatory therapy is often used to prevent such gout attacks.
- The ACR guidelines recommend low-dose oral colchicine (0.6 mg twice daily) and low-dose NSAIDs (eg, naproxen 250 mg twice daily) as first-line prophylactic therapies, with stronger evidence supporting use of colchicine. For patients on long-term NSAID prophylaxis, a proton pump inhibitor or other acid-suppressing therapy is indicated to protect from NSAID-induced gastric problems.
- Low-dose corticosteroid therapy (eg, prednisone ≤10 mg/day) is an alternative for patients with intolerance, contraindication, or lack of response to first-line therapy. The potential severe adverse effects of prolonged corticosteroid therapy preclude their use as first-line therapy.
- Continue prophylaxis for at least 6 months or 3 months after achieving target serum uric acid, whichever is longer. For patients with one or more tophi, continue prophylactic therapy for 6 months after achieving the serum urate target (see Fig. 1–2).

EVALUATION OF THERAPEUTIC OUTCOMES

- Check the serum uric acid level in patients suspected of having an acute gout attack, particularly if it is not the first attack, and a decision is to be made about starting prophylaxis. However, acute gout can occur with normal serum uric acid concentrations.
- Monitor patients with acute gout for symptomatic relief of joint pain as well as potential adverse effects and drug interactions related to drug therapy. Acute pain of an initial gout attack should begin to ease within about 8 hours of treatment initiation. Complete resolution of pain, erythema, and inflammation usually occurs within 48 to 72 hours.
- For patients receiving urate-lowering therapy, obtain baseline assessment of renal function, hepatic enzymes, complete blood count, and electrolytes. Recheck the tests every 6 to 12 months in patients receiving long-term treatment.
- During titration of urate-lowering therapy, monitor serum uric acid every 2 to 5 weeks; after the urate target is achieved, monitor uric acid every 6 months.
- Because of the high rates of comorbidities associated with gout (diabetes, chronic kidney disease, hypertension, obesity, myocardial infarction, heart failure, and stroke), elevated serum uric acid levels or gout should prompt evaluation for cardiovascular disease and the need for appropriate risk reduction measures. Clinicians should also look for possible correctable causes of hyperuricemia (eg, medications, obesity, malignancy, and alcohol abuse).

See Chapter 93, Gout and Hyperuricemia, authored by Michelle A. Fravel and Michael E. Ernst, for a more detailed discussion of this topic.

2 Osteoarthritis

- *Osteoarthritis* (OA) is a common, progressive disorder affecting primarily weight-bearing diarthrodial joints, characterized by progressive destruction of articular cartilage, osteophyte formation, pain, limitation of motion, deformity, and disability.

PATHOPHYSIOLOGY

- *Primary* (*idiopathic*) *OA*, the most common type, has no known cause.
- *Secondary OA* is associated with a known cause, such as trauma, metabolic or endocrine disorders, and congenital factors.
- OA usually begins with damage to articular cartilage through injury, excessive joint loading from obesity or other reasons, or joint instability or injury. Damage to cartilage increases activity of chondrocytes in attempt to repair damage, leading to increased synthesis of matrix constituents with cartilage swelling. Normal balance between cartilage breakdown and resynthesis is lost, with increasing destruction and cartilage loss.
- Subchondral bone adjacent to articular cartilage undergoes pathologic changes and releases vasoactive peptides and matrix metalloproteinases. Neovascularization and increased permeability of adjacent cartilage occur, which contribute to cartilage loss and chondrocyte apoptosis.
- Cartilage loss causes joint space narrowing and painful, deformed joints. Remaining cartilage softens and develops fibrillations, followed by further cartilage loss and exposure of underlying bone. New bone formations (osteophytes) at joint margins distant from cartilage destruction are thought to help stabilize affected joints.
- Inflammatory changes can occur in the joint capsule and synovium. Crystals or cartilage shards in synovial fluid may contribute to inflammation. Interleukin-1, prostaglandin E_2, tumor necrosis factor-α, and nitric oxide in synovial fluid may also play a role. Inflammatory changes result in synovial effusions and thickening.
- Pain may result from distention of the synovial capsule by increased joint fluid; microfracture; periosteal irritation; or damage to ligaments, synovium, or the meniscus.

CLINICAL PRESENTATION

- Risk factors include increasing age, obesity, sex, certain occupations and sports activities, history of joint injury or surgery, and genetic predisposition.
- The predominant symptom is deep, aching pain in affected joints. Pain accompanies joint activity and decreases with rest.
- Joints most commonly affected are the distal interphalangeal (DIP) and proximal interphalangeal (PIP) joints of the hand, first carpometacarpal joint, knees, hips, cervical and lumbar spine, and first metatarsophalangeal (MTP) joint of the toe.
- Limitation of motion, stiffness, crepitus, and deformities may occur. Patients with lower extremity involvement may report weakness or instability.
- Upon arising, joint stiffness typically lasts less than 30 minutes and resolves with motion.
- Presence of warm, red, and tender joints suggests inflammatory synovitis.
- Physical examination of affected joints reveals tenderness, crepitus, and possibly enlargement. Heberden and Bouchard nodes are bony enlargements (osteophytes) of the DIP and PIP joints, respectively.

DIAGNOSIS

- Diagnosis is made through patient history, physician examination, radiologic findings, and laboratory testing.

- American College of Rheumatology criteria for classification of OA of the hips, knees, and hands include presence of pain, bony changes on examination, normal erythrocyte sedimentation rate (ESR), and radiographs showing osteophytes or joint space narrowing.
- For hip OA, patient must have hip pain and two of the following: (1) ESR less than 20 mm/h (<5.6 μm/s), (2) radiographic femoral or acetabular osteophytes, and/or (3) radiographic joint space narrowing.
- For knee OA, patient must have knee pain and radiographic osteophytes in addition to one or more of the following: (1) age more than 50 years, (2) morning stiffness lasting 30 minutes or less, (3) crepitus on motion, (4) bony enlargement, (6) bony tenderness, and/or (7) palpable joint warmth.
- ESR may be slightly elevated if inflammation is present. Rheumatoid factor is negative. Analysis of synovial fluid reveals high viscosity and mild leukocytosis (<2000 white blood cells/mm³ [<2 × 10⁹/L]) with predominantly mononuclear cells.

TREATMENT

- Goals of Treatment: (1) educate the patient, family members, and caregivers; (2) relieve pain and stiffness; (3) maintain or improve joint mobility; (4) limit functional impairment; and (5) maintain or improve quality of life.

NONPHARMACOLOGIC THERAPY

- Educate the patient about the disease process and extent, prognosis, and treatment options. Promote dietary counseling, exercise, and weight loss program for overweight patients.
- Physical therapy—with heat or cold treatments and an exercise program—helps maintain range of motion and reduce pain and need for analgesics.
- Assistive and orthotic devices (canes, walkers, braces, heel cups, and insoles) can be used during exercise or daily activities.
- Surgical procedures (eg, osteotomy, arthroplasty, and joint fusion) are indicated for functional disability and/or severe pain unresponsive to conservative therapy.

PHARMACOLOGIC THERAPY (TABLE 2–1)

General Approach

- Drug therapy is targeted at relief of pain. A conservative approach is warranted because OA often occurs in older individuals with other medical conditions.
- Apply an individualized approach (Figs. 2–1 and 2–2). Continue appropriate non-drug therapies when initiating drug therapy.

Knee and Hip OA

- **Acetaminophen** is a preferred first-line treatment; it may be less effective than oral nonsteroidal anti-inflammatory drugs (NSAIDs) but has less risk of serious gastrointestinal (GI) and cardiovascular events. Acetaminophen is usually well tolerated, but potentially fatal hepatotoxicity with overdose is well documented. It should be avoided in chronic alcohol users or patients with liver disease.
- **Nonselective NSAIDs** or **cyclooxygenase-2 (COX-2) selective inhibitors** (eg, **celecoxib**) are recommended if a patient fails acetaminophen. Nonselective NSAIDs cause minor GI complaints such as nausea, dyspepsia, anorexia, abdominal pain, flatulence, and diarrhea in 10% to 60% of patients. They may cause gastric and duodenal ulcers and bleeding through direct (topical) or indirect (systemic) mechanisms. Risk factors for NSAID-associated ulcers and ulcer complications (perforation, gastric outlet obstruction, and GI bleeding) include longer duration of NSAID use, higher dosage, age older than 60, past history of peptic ulcer disease of any cause, history of alcohol use, and concomitant use of glucocorticoids or anticoagulants. Options for reducing the GI risk of nonselective NSAIDs include using (1) the lowest dose possible and only when needed, (2) misoprostol four times daily with the NSAID, (3) a PPI or full-dose H$_2$-receptor antagonist daily with the NSAID.

TABLE 2–1	Medications for the Treatment of Osteoarthritis	
Drug	**Starting Dose**	**Usual Range**
Oral analgesics		
Acetaminophen	325–500 mg three times a day	325–650 mg every 4–6 h or 1 g three to four times/day
Tramadol	25 mg in the morning	Titrate dose in 25-mg increments to reach a maintenance dose of 50–100 mg three times a day
Tramadol ER	100 mg daily	Titrate to 200–300 mg daily
Hydrocodone/ acetaminophen	5 mg/325 mg three times daily	2.5–10 mg/325–650 mg three to five times daily
Oxycodone/ acetaminophen	5 mg/325 mg three times daily	2.5–10 mg/325–650 mg three to five times daily
Topical analgesics		
Capsaicin 0.025% or 0.075%		Apply to affected joint three to four times per day
Diclofenac 1% gel		Apply 2 or 4 g per site as prescribed, four times daily
Diclofenac 1.3% patch		Apply one patch twice daily to the site to be treated, as directed
Diclofenac 1.5% solution		Apply 40 drops to the affected knee, applying and rubbing in 10 drops at a time. Repeat for a total of four times daily.
Intra-articular corticosteroids		
Triamcinolone	5–15 mg per joint	10–40 mg per large joint (knee, hip, shoulder)
Methylprednisolone acetate	10–20 mg per joint	20–80 mg per large joint (knee, hip, shoulder)
NSAIDs		
Aspirin (plain, buffered, or enteric-coated)	325 mg three times a day	325–650 mg four times a day
Celecoxib	100 mg daily	100 mg twice daily or 200 mg daily
Diclofenac IR	50 mg twice a day	50–75 mg twice a day
Diclofenac XR	100 mg daily	100–200 mg daily
Diflunisal	250 mg twice a day	500–750 mg twice a day
Etodolac	300 mg twice a day	400–500 mg twice a day
Fenoprofen	400 mg three times a day	400–600 mg three to four times a day
Flurbiprofen	100 mg twice a day	200–300 mg/day in two to four divided doses
Ibuprofen	200 mg three times a day	1200–3200 mg/day in three to four divided doses

(continued)

TABLE 2-1	Medications for the Treatment of Osteoarthritis *(Continued)*	
Drug	**Starting Dose**	**Usual Range**
Indomethacin	25 mg twice a day	Titrate dose by 25–50 mg/day until pain controlled or maximum dose of 50 mg three times a day
Indomethacin SR	75 mg SR once daily	Can titrate to 75 mg SR twice daily if needed
Ketoprofen	50 mg three times a day	50–75 mg three to four times a day
Meclofenamate	50 mg three times a day	50–100 mg three to four times a day
Mefenamic acid	250 mg three times a day	250 mg four times a day
Meloxicam	7.5 mg daily	15 mg daily
Nabumetone	500 mg daily	500–1000 mg one to two times a day
Naproxen	250 mg twice a day	500 mg twice a day
Naproxen sodium	220 mg twice a day	220–550 mg twice a day
Naproxen sodium CR	750–1000 mg once daily	500–1500 mg once daily
Oxaprozin	600 mg daily	600–1200 mg daily
Piroxicam	10 mg daily	20 mg daily
Salsalate	500 mg twice a day	500–1000 mg two to three times a day

(CR, controlled-release; ER, extended-release; IR, immediate-release; SR, sustained-release; XR, extended-release.)

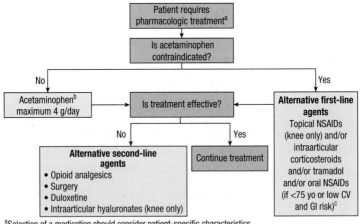

[a]Selection of a medication should consider patient-specific characteristics.
[b]The patient must be counseled regarding all acetaminophen-containing products.
[c]When used for chronic management of OA, consider addition of a proton-pump inhibitor.

(CV, cardiovascular; GI, gastrointestinal; NSAID, nonsteroidal anti-inflammatory drug.)

FIGURE 2-1. Treatment recommendations for hip and knee osteoarthritis.

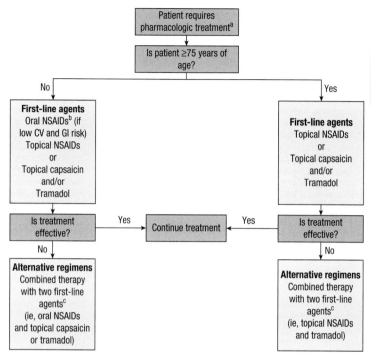

aSelection of a medication should consider patient-specific characteristics.
bWhen used for chronic management of OA, consider addition of a proton-pump inhibitor.
cShould not combine topical NSAIDs and oral NSAIDs.

(CV, cardiovascular; GI, gastrointestinal; NSAID, nonsteroidal anti-inflammatory drug.)

FIGURE 2–2. Treatment recommendations for hand osteoarthritis.

- COX-2 inhibitors pose less risk for adverse GI events than nonselective NSAIDs, but this advantage may not be sustained beyond 6 months and is substantially reduced for patients taking aspirin. Both nonselective and selective NSAIDs are associated with an increased risk for cardiovascular events (hypertension, stroke, myocardial infarction, and death).
- NSAIDs may also cause kidney diseases, hepatitis, hypersensitivity reactions, rash, and CNS complaints of drowsiness, dizziness, headaches, depression, confusion, and tinnitus. All nonselective NSAIDs inhibit COX-1–dependent thromboxane production in platelets, thereby increasing bleeding risk. Avoid NSAIDs in late pregnancy because of risk of premature closure of the ductus arteriosus. The most potentially serious drug interactions include use of NSAIDs with lithium, warfarin, oral hypoglycemics, methotrexate, antihypertensives, angiotensin-converting enzyme inhibitors, β-blockers, and diuretics.
- **Topical NSAIDs** are recommended for knee OA if acetaminophen fails, and they are preferred over oral NSAIDs in patients older than 75 years. Topical NSAIDs provide similar pain relief with fewer adverse GI events than oral NSAIDs but may be associated with adverse events at the application site (eg, dry skin, pruritus, and rash). Patients using topical products should avoid oral NSAIDs to minimize the potential for additive side effects.

- **Intra-articular (IA) corticosteroid injections** are recommended for both hip and knee OA when analgesia with acetaminophen or NSAIDs is suboptimal. They can provide excellent pain relief, particularly when joint effusion is present. Injections can be given with concomitant oral analgesics for additional pain control. After aseptic aspiration of the effusion and corticosteroid injection, initial pain relief may occur within 24 to 72 hours, with peak relief occurring after 7 to 10 days and lasting for 4 to 8 weeks. Local adverse effects can include infection, osteonecrosis, tendon rupture, and skin atrophy at the injection site. Do not administer injections more frequently than once every 3 months to minimize systemic adverse effects. Systemic corticosteroid therapy is not recommended in OA, given lack of proven benefit and well-known adverse effects with long-term use.
- **Tramadol** is recommended for hip and knee OA in patients who have failed scheduled full-dose acetaminophen and topical NSAIDs, who are not appropriate candidates for oral NSAIDs, and who are not able to receive IA corticosteroids. Tramadol can be added to partially effective acetaminophen or oral NSAID therapy. Tramadol is associated with opioid-like adverse effects such as nausea, vomiting, dizziness, constipation, headache, and somnolence. However, tramadol is not associated with life-threatening GI bleeding, cardiovascular events, or renal failure. The most serious adverse event is seizures. Tramadol is classified as a Schedule IV controlled substance due to its potential for dependence, addiction, and diversion. There is increased risk of serotonin syndrome when tramadol is used with other serotonergic medications, including duloxetine.
- **Opioids** should be considered in patients not responding adequately to non-pharmacologic and first-line pharmacologic therapies. Patients who are at high surgical risk and cannot undergo joint arthroplasty are also candidates for opioid therapy. Opioid analgesics should be used in the lowest effective dose and the smallest quantity needed. Combinations of opioids and sedating medications should be avoided whenever possible. Patients should be informed on how to use, store, and dispose of opioid medications. Sustained-release compounds usually offer better pain control throughout the day. Common adverse effects include nausea, somnolence, constipation, dry mouth, and dizziness. Opioid dependence, addiction, tolerance, hyperalgesia, and issues surrounding drug diversion may be associated with long-term treatment.
- **Duloxetine** can be used as adjunctive treatment in patients with partial response to first-line analgesics (acetaminophen, oral NSAIDs). It may be a preferred second-line medication in patients with both neuropathic and musculoskeletal OA pain. Pain reduction occurs after about 4 weeks of therapy. Duloxetine may cause nausea, dry mouth, constipation, anorexia, fatigue, somnolence, and dizziness. Serious rare events include Stevens-Johnson syndrome and liver failure. Concomitant use with other medications that increase serotonin concentration (including tramadol) increases risk of serotonin syndrome.
- **IA hyaluronic acid** (sodium hyaluronate) is not routinely recommended because injections have shown limited benefit for knee OA and have not been shown to benefit hip OA. Injections are usually well tolerated, but acute joint swelling, effusion, stiffness, and local skin reactions (eg, rash, ecchymoses, or pruritus) have been reported. Intra-articular preparations and regimens for OA knee pain include:

  ✓ **Cross-linked hyaluronate 30 mg/3 mL** (Gel-One) single injection
  ✓ **Hyaluronan 30 mg/2 mL** (Orthovisc) once weekly for three injections
  ✓ **Hyaluronan 88 mg/4 mL** (Monovisc) single injection
  ✓ **Hylan polymers 16 mg/2 mL** (Synvisc) once weekly for three injections
  ✓ **Hylan polymers 48 mg/6 mL** (Synvisc-One) single injection
  ✓ **Sodium hyaluronate 20 mg/2 mL** (Hyalgan) once weekly for five injections
  ✓ **Sodium hyaluronate 20 mg/2 mL** (Euflexxa) once weekly for three injections
  ✓ **Sodium hyaluronate 25 mg/2.5 mL** (Supartz FX) once weekly for five injections
  ✓ **Sodium hyaluronate 25 mg/2.5 mL** (GenVisc 850) once weekly for five injections

- **Glucosamine and/or chondroitin** and **topical rubefacients** (eg, **methyl salicylate, trolamine salicylate**) lack uniform efficacy for hip and knee pain and are not preferred treatment options. Glucosamine adverse effects are mild and include flatulence, bloating, and abdominal cramps; do not use in patients with shellfish allergies. The most common adverse effect of chondroitin is nausea.

Hand OA

- **Topical NSAIDs** are a first-line option for hand OA. Diclofenac has efficacy similar to oral ibuprofen and oral diclofenac with fewer adverse GI events, albeit with some local application site events.
- **Oral NSAIDs** are an alternative first-line treatment for patients who cannot tolerate the local skin reactions or who received inadequate relief from topical NSAIDs.
- **Capsaicin cream** is an alternative first-line treatment and demonstrates modest improvement in pain scores. It is a reasonable option for patients unable to take oral NSAIDs. Capsaicin must be used regularly to be effective, and it may require up to 2 weeks to take effect. Adverse effects are primarily local with one third of patients experiencing burning, stinging, and/or erythema that usually subsides with repeated application. Warn patients not to get cream in their eyes or mouth and to wash hands after application. Application of the cream, gel, or lotion is recommended four times daily, but twice-daily application may enhance long-term adherence with adequate pain relief.
- **Tramadol** is an alternative first-line treatment and is a reasonable choice for patients who do not respond to topical therapy and are not candidates for oral NSAIDs because of high GI, cardiovascular, or renal risks. Tramadol may also be used in combination with partially effective acetaminophen, topical therapy, or oral NSAIDs.

EVALUATION OF THERAPEUTIC OUTCOMES

- To monitor efficacy, assess baseline pain with a visual analog scale, and assess range of motion for affected joints with flexion, extension, abduction, or adduction.
- Depending on the joint(s) affected, measurement of grip strength and 50-ft walking time can help assess hand and hip/knee OA, respectively.
- Baseline radiographs can document extent of joint involvement and follow disease progression with therapy.
- Other measures include the clinician's global assessment based on patient's history of activities and limitations caused by OA, the Western Ontario and McMaster Universities Arthrosis Index, Stanford Health Assessment Questionnaire, and documentation of analgesic or NSAID use.
- Ask patients about adverse effects from medications. Monitor for signs of drug-related effects, such as skin rash, headaches, drowsiness, weight gain, or hypertension from NSAIDs.
- Obtain baseline serum creatinine, hematology profile, and serum transaminases with repeat levels at 6- to 12-month intervals to identify specific toxicities to the kidney, liver, GI tract, or bone marrow.

See Chapter 90, Osteoarthritis, authored by Lucinda M. Buys and Sara A. Wiedenfeld, for a more detailed discussion of this topic.

Osteoporosis

3 CHAPTER

- *Osteoporosis* is a bone disorder characterized by low bone density, impaired bone architecture, and compromised bone strength predisposing to fracture.

PATHOPHYSIOLOGY

- Bone loss occurs when resorption exceeds formation, usually from high bone turnover when the number or depth of bone resorption sites greatly exceeds the ability of osteoblasts to form new bone. Accelerated bone turnover can increase the amount of immature bone that is not adequately mineralized.
- Men and women begin to lose bone mass starting in the third or fourth decade because of reduced bone formation. Estrogen deficiency during menopause increases osteoclast activity, increasing bone resorption more than formation. Men are at a lower risk for developing osteoporosis and osteoporotic fractures because of larger bone size, greater peak bone mass, increase in bone width with aging, fewer falls, and shorter life expectancy. Male osteoporosis results from aging or secondary causes.
- Age-related osteoporosis results from hormone, calcium, and vitamin D deficiencies leading to accelerated bone turnover and reduced osteoblast formation.
- Drug-induced osteoporosis may result from systemic corticosteroids, thyroid hormone replacement, antiepileptic drugs (eg, phenytoin and phenobarbital), depot medroxyprogesterone acetate, and other agents.

CLINICAL PRESENTATION

- Many patients are unaware that they have osteoporosis and only present after fracture. Fractures can occur after bending, lifting, or falling or independent of any activity.
- The most common fractures involve vertebrae, proximal femur, and distal radius (wrist or Colles fracture). Vertebral fractures may be asymptomatic or present with moderate to severe back pain that radiates down a leg. Pain usually subsides after 2 to 4 weeks, but residual back pain may persist. Multiple vertebral fractures decrease height and sometimes curve the spine (kyphosis or lordosis).
- Patients with a nonvertebral fracture frequently present with severe pain, swelling, and reduced function and mobility at the fracture site.

DIAGNOSIS

- The World Health Organization (WHO) created the FRAX tool, which uses these risk factors to predict the percent probability of fracture in the next 10 years: age, race/ethnicity, sex, previous fragility fracture, parent history of hip fracture, body mass index, glucocorticoid use, current smoking, alcohol (three or more drinks per day), rheumatoid arthritis, and select secondary causes with femoral neck or total hip bone mineral density (BMD) data optional.
- The Garvan calculator uses four risk factors (age, sex, low-trauma fracture, and falls) with the option to also use BMD. It calculates 5- and 10-year risk estimates of any major osteoporotic and hip fracture. This tool corrects some disadvantages of FRAX because it includes falls and number of previous fractures, but it does not use as many other risk factors.
- Physical examination findings: bone pain, postural changes (ie, kyphosis), and loss of height (>1.5 in [3.8 cm]).
- Laboratory testing: complete blood count, creatinine, blood urea nitrogen, calcium, phosphorus, electrolytes, alkaline phosphatase, albumin, thyroid-stimulating hormone, total testosterone (for men), 25-hydroxyvitamin D, and 24-hour urine concentrations of calcium and phosphorus.

- Measurement of central (hip and spine) BMD with dual-energy x-ray absorptiometry (DXA) is the diagnostic standard. Measurement at peripheral sites (forearm, heel, and finger) with DXA or quantitative ultrasonography is used only for screening and for determining need for further testing.
- A T-score compares the patient's BMD to the mean BMD of a healthy, young (20- to 29-year-old), sex-matched, white reference population. The T-score is the number of standard deviations from the mean of the reference population.
- Diagnosis of osteoporosis is based on low-trauma fracture or femoral neck, total hip, and/or spine DXA using WHO T-score thresholds. Normal bone mass is T-score above −1, low bone mass (osteopenia) is T-score between −1 and −2.4, and osteoporosis is T-score at or below −2.5.

TREATMENT

- Goals of Treatment: The primary goal of osteoporosis care is prevention. Optimizing peak bone mass when young reduces the future incidence of osteoporosis. After low bone mass or osteoporosis develops, the objective is to stabilize or improve bone mass and strength and prevent fractures. Goals in patients with osteoporotic fractures include reducing pain and deformity, improving function, reducing falls and fractures, and improving quality of life.
- Figure 3–1 provides an osteoporosis management algorithm for postmenopausal women and men ages 50 and older.

NONPHARMACOLOGIC THERAPY

- All individuals should have a balanced diet with adequate intake of **calcium** and **vitamin D** (Table 3–1). Achieving daily calcium requirements from calcium-containing foods is preferred.
  - ✔ Consumers can calculate the amount of calcium in a food serving by adding a zero to the percentage of the daily value on food labels. One serving of milk (8 oz or 240 mL) has 30% of the daily value of calcium; this converts to 300 mg of calcium per serving.
  - ✔ To calculate the amount of vitamin D in a food serving, multiply the percent daily value of vitamin D listed on the food label by 4. For example, 20% vitamin D = 80 units.
- Alcohol consumption should not exceed 1 to 2 drinks per day for women and 2 to 3 drinks per day for men.
- Ideally, caffeine intake should be limited to two or fewer servings per day.
- Smoking cessation helps optimize peak bone mass, minimize bone loss, and ultimately reduce fracture risk.
- Weight-bearing aerobic and strengthening exercises can decrease risk of falls and fractures by improving muscle strength, coordination, balance, and mobility.
- Fall prevention programs that are multifactorial can decrease falls, fractures, other injuries, and nursing home and hospital admissions.
- Vertebroplasty and kyphoplasty involve injection of cement into fractured vertebra(e) for patients with debilitating pain from compression fractures. The procedures may reduce pain for some patients but may also be associated with complications.

PHARMACOLOGIC THERAPY

ANTIRESORPTIVE THERAPY

Calcium Supplementation

- **Calcium** generally maintains or increases BMD, but its effects are less than those of other therapies. Fracture prevention is only documented with concomitant vitamin D therapy. Because the fraction of calcium absorbed decreases with increasing dose, maximum single doses of 600 mg or less of elemental calcium are recommended.

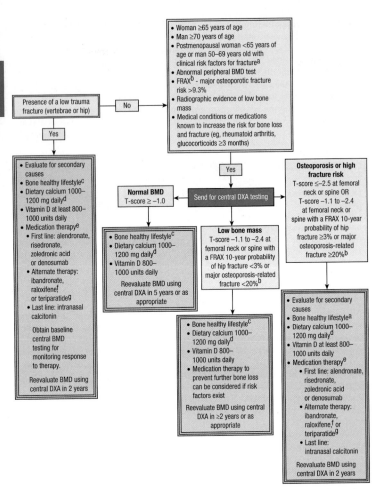

aMajor clinical risk factors for fracture: current smoker, low body weight or body mass index, history of osteoporosis/low trauma fracture in a first-degree relative, personal history of fracture as an adult (after age 50 years), excessive alcohol intake.

bFRAX = World Health Organization fracture risk assessment tool.

cBone-healthy lifestyle includes smoking cessation, limited alcohol intake, well-balanced diet with adequate calcium and vitamin D intakes, weight-bearing/resistance exercises, and fall prevention.

dDietary calcium preferred. If diet is inadequate, supplement as necessary.

eSometimes men with hypogonadism also receive testosterone replacement; sometimes women with menopausal symptoms receive low dose hormone therapy for a short time.

fRaloxifene can be a good option in women at high risk for breast cancer.

gTeriparatide can be considered a first-line option in patients with a very high risk of fracture (eg, T-score <−3.5 or multiple low trauma fractures) or intolerant to other medications

(BMD, bone mineral density; DXA, dual-energy x-ray absorptiometry.)

FIGURE 3–1. Algorithm for management of osteoporosis in postmenopausal women and men aged 50 and older.

| TABLE 3-1 | Calcium and Vitamin D Recommended Dietary Allowances and Upper Limits |

Group and Ages	Elemental Calcium (mg)	Calcium Upper Limit (mg)	Vitamin D (Units)[a]	Vitamin D Upper Limit (Units)
Infants				
Birth to 6 months	200	1000	400	1000
6–12 months	260	1500	400	1500
Children				
1–3 years	700	2500	600	2500
4–8 years	1000	2500	600	3000
9–18 years	1300	3000	600	4000
Adults				
19–50 years	1000	2500	600[b]	4000
51–70 years (men)	1000	2000	600[b]	4000
51–70 years (women)	1200	2000	600[b]	4000
>70 years	1200	2000	800[b]	4000

[a]Other guidelines recommend intake to achieve a 25(OH) vitamin D concentration of more than 30 ng/mL (mcg/L; > 75 nmol/L), which is higher than the Institute of Medicine goal of more than 20 ng/mL (mcg/L; > 50 nmol/L).
[b]2014 National Osteoporosis Foundation Guidelines recommend 400 to 800 units for adults under 50 years old and 800 to 1000 units for adults 50 years and older.

- **Calcium carbonate** is the salt of choice because it contains the highest concentration of elemental calcium (40%) and is least expensive. It should be ingested with meals to enhance absorption in an acidic environment.
- **Calcium citrate** (21% calcium) has acid-independent absorption and need not be taken with meals. It may have fewer GI side effects (eg, flatulence) than calcium carbonate.
- **Tricalcium phosphate** contains 38% calcium, but calcium-phosphate complexes could limit overall calcium absorption. It might be helpful in patients with hypophosphatemia that cannot be resolved with increased dietary intake.
- Constipation is the most common adverse reaction; treat with increased water intake, dietary fiber (given separately from calcium), and exercise. Calcium carbonate can sometimes cause flatulence or upset stomach. Calcium causes kidney stones rarely.
- Calcium can decrease the oral absorption of some drugs including iron, tetracyclines, quinolones, bisphosphonates, and thyroid supplements.

Vitamin D Supplementation

- **Vitamin D** supplementation maximizes intestinal calcium absorption and BMD; it may also reduce fractures and falls.
- Supplementation is usually provided with daily nonprescription cholecalciferol (vitamin D_3) products. Higher-dose prescription ergocalciferol (vitamin D_2) regimens given weekly, monthly, or quarterly may be used for replacement and maintenance therapy.
- The recommended dietary allowances in **Table 3–1** should be achieved through food and supplementation with a goal to achieve a 25 (OH) vitamin D concentration of 20 to 30 ng/mL (50–75 nmol/L).
- Because the half-life of vitamin D is about 1 month, recheck the vitamin D concentration after about 3 months of therapy.

Bisphosphonates

- Bisphosphonates (**Table 3–2**) inhibit bone resorption and become incorporated into the bones, giving them long biologic half-lives of up to 10 years.
- Of the antiresorptive agents available, bisphosphonates provide some of the higher BMD increases and fracture risk reductions.

TABLE 3–2   Medications Used to Prevent and Treat Osteoporosis

Drug	Brand Name	Dose	Comments
Antiresorptive Medications—Nutritional Supplements			
Calcium	Various	*Adequate daily intake:* IOM: 200–1200 mg/day, varies per age); Supplement dose is difference between required adequate intake and dietary intake. Immediate-release doses should be <500–600 mg.	Recommend food first to achieve goal intake. Available in different salts including carbonate and citrate, absorption of other salts not fully quantified. Different formulations including chewable, liquid, gummy, softgel, drink, and wafer; different combination products. Review package to determine number of units to create a serving size and desired amount of elemental calcium. Give calcium carbonate with meals to improve absorption.
Vitamin D D3 (cholecalciferol) D$_2$ (ergocalciferol)	Over the counter, Tablets, 400, 1000, and 2000 units Capsule, 400, 1000, 2000, 5000, and 10,000 units Gummies, 300, 500, 1000 units Drops 300, 400, 1000 and 2000 units/mL or drop Solution, 400 and 5000 units/mL Spray 1000 and 5000 units/spray Creams and lotions 500 and 1000 units per ¼ teaspoonful. Prescription, Capsule, 50,000 units Solution, 8000 units/mL	Adequate daily intake: IOM: 400–800 units/day to achieve adequate intake; NOF: 800–1000 units orally daily; if low 25(OH) vitamin D concentrations, malabsorption, or altered metabolism higher doses (>2000 units daily) might be required. *Vitamin D deficiency:* 50,000 units orally once to twice weekly for 8–12 weeks; repeat as needed until therapeutic concentrations.	Vegetarians and vegans need to read label to determine if a plant-based product. Slight advantage of D3 over D2 for increasing serum 25(OH) vitamin D concentrations. For drops, make sure measurement is correct for desired dose. Ability of sprays, lotions, and creams to resolve deficiencies or maintain adequate intakes is unknown.

Antiresorptive Prescription Medications

Bisphosphonates

Alendronate	Fosamax Fosamax Plus D Binosto (effervescent tab)	Treatment: 10 mg orally daily or 70 mg orally weekly Prevention: 5 mg orally daily or 35 mg orally weekly	Generic available for weekly tablet product. 70 mg dose is available as a tablet, effervescent tablet, oral liquid or combination tablet with 2800 or 5600 units of vitamin D3. Administered in the morning on an empty stomach with 6–8 ounces of plain water. Do not eat and remain upright for at least 30 minutes following administration. Do not coadminister with any other medication or supplements, including calcium and vitamin D.
Ibandronate	Boniva	Treatment: 150 mg orally monthly, 3 mg intravenous quarterly Prevention: 150 mg orally monthly	Generic available for oral product. Administration instructions same as for alendronate, except must delay eating and remain upright for at least 60 minutes.
Risedronate	Actonel Atelvia (delayed-release)	Treatment and Prevention: 5 mg orally daily, 35 mg orally weekly, 150 mg orally monthly	Generic available for immediate-release product. 35 mg dose is also available as a delayed-release product. Administration instructions same as for alendronate, except delayed-release product is taken immediately following breakfast.
Zoledronic acid	Reclast	Treatment: 5 mg intravenous infusion yearly Prevention: 5 mg intravenous infusion every 2 years	Can premedicate with acetaminophen to decrease infusion reactions. Contraindicated if CrCl <35 mL/min Also marketed under the brand name Zometa (4 mg) for treatment of hypercalcemia and prevention of skeletal-related events from bone metastases from solid tumors with different dosing.

(continued)

TABLE 3–2	Medications Used to Prevent and Treat Osteoporosis (Continued)		
Drug	Brand Name	Dose	Comments
RANK Ligand Inhibitor			
Denosumab	Prolia	Treatment: 60 mg subcutaneously every 6 months	Administered by a healthcare practitioner. Correct hypocalcemia before administration. Also marketed under the brand name Xgeva (70 mg/mL) for treatment of hypercalcemia and prevention of skeletal-related events from bone metastases from solid tumors with different dosing.
Estrogen Agonist/Antagonist and Tissue Selective Estrogen Complex			
Raloxifene	Evista	60 mg daily	Generic available
Bazedoxifene with conjugated equine estrogens (CEE)	Duavee	20 mg plus 0.45 mg CEE daily	For postmenopausal women with an uterus; no progestogen needed. Bazedoxifene monotherapy available in some countries.
Calcitonin			
Calcitonin (salmon)	Fortical	200 units (1 spray) intranasally daily, alternating nares every other day.	Generic available. Refrigerate nasal spray until opened for daily use, then room temperature.
		100 units subcutaneously daily	Prime with first use.
Formation Medications			
Recombinant human parathyroid hormone (PTH 1–34 units)			
Teriparatide	Forteo	20 mcg subcutaneously daily for up to 2 years	First dose at night. Refrigerate before and after use. Use new needle with each dose. Inject thigh or stomach. Discard after 28 days or if cloudy.

(IOM, Institute of Medicine; NOF, National Osteoporosis Foundation; NSAID, nonsteroidal anti-inflammatory drug.)

- BMD increases are dose dependent and greatest in the first 12 months of therapy. After discontinuation, the increased BMD is sustained for a prolonged period that varies per bisphosphonate.
- **Alendronate**, **risedronate**, and **IV zoledronic acid** are Food and Drug Administration (FDA) indicated for postmenopausal, male, and glucocorticoid-induced osteoporosis. **IV and oral ibandronate** are indicated only for postmenopausal osteoporosis. Weekly alendronate, weekly and monthly risedronate, and monthly oral and quarterly IV ibandronate therapy produce equivalent BMD changes to their respective daily regimens.
- Bisphosphonates must be administered carefully to optimize clinical benefit and minimize adverse GI effects. Each oral tablet should be taken in the morning with at least 6 oz (180 mL) of plain water (not coffee, juice, mineral water, or milk) at least 30 minutes (60 minutes for oral ibandronate) before consuming any food, supplements, or medications. An exception is delayed-release risedronate, which is administered immediately after breakfast with at least 4 oz (120 mL) of plain water. The patient should remain upright (sitting or standing) for at least 30 minutes after alendronate and risedronate and 1 hour after ibandronate administration to prevent esophageal irritation and ulceration.
- If a patient misses a weekly dose, it can be taken the next day. If more than 1 day has elapsed, that dose is skipped until the next scheduled ingestion. If a patient misses a monthly dose, it can be taken up to 7 days before the next scheduled dose.
- The most common bisphosphonate adverse effects include nausea, abdominal pain, and dyspepsia. Esophageal, gastric, or duodenal irritation, perforation, ulceration, or bleeding may occur. The most common adverse effects of IV bisphosphonates include fever, flu-like symptoms, and local injection-site reactions.
- Rare adverse effects include osteonecrosis of the jaw (ONJ) and subtrochanteric femoral (atypical) fractures. ONJ occurs more commonly in patients with cancer receiving higher-dose IV bisphosphonate therapy and other risk factors including glucocorticoid therapy and diabetes mellitus.

Denosumab

- **Denosumab** (Prolia) is a RANK ligand inhibitor that inhibits osteoclast formation and increases osteoclast apoptosis. It is indicated for treatment of osteoporosis in women and men at high risk for fracture. It is also approved to increase bone mass in men receiving androgen-deprivation therapy for nonmetastatic prostate cancer and in women receiving adjuvant aromatase inhibitor therapy for breast cancer who are at high risk for fracture.
- Denosumab is administered as a 60-mg subcutaneous injection in the upper arm, upper thigh, or abdomen once every 6 months.
- Adverse reactions not associated with the injection site include back pain, arthralgia, eczema, cellulitis, and infection. Osteonecrosis of the jaw and atypical femoral shaft fracture occur rarely. Denosumab is contraindicated in patients with hypocalcemia until the condition is corrected.

Mixed Estrogen Agonists/Antagonists and Tissue-Selective Estrogen Complexes

- **Raloxifene** (Evista) is an estrogen agonist on bone receptors but an antagonist at breast receptors, with minimal effects on the uterus. It is approved for prevention and treatment of postmenopausal osteoporosis.
- **Bazedoxifene** is an estrogen agonist/antagonist that is combined with **conjugated equine estrogens** (CEE), making it a tissue-selective estrogen complex (proprietary product DUAVEE). It is approved for prevention of postmenopausal osteoporosis and vasomotor menstrual symptoms.
- Raloxifene and bazedoxifene decrease vertebral but not hip fractures. The drugs increase spine and hip BMD, but to a lesser extent than bisphosphonates. The fracture-prevention effects of bazedoxifene combined with CEE are unknown. After raloxifene discontinuation, the beneficial effect is lost, and bone loss returns to age- or disease-related rates.

- Hot flushes are common with raloxifene but decreased with bazedoxifene/CEE. Raloxifene rarely causes endometrial thickening and bleeding; bazedoxifene decreases these events making progestogen therapy unnecessary when combined with CEE. Leg cramps and muscle spasms are common with these agents. Thrombo-embolic events are uncommon but can be fatal. Bazedoxifene with CEE has all the contraindications and precautions for estrogens as a class.

Calcitonin

- **Calcitonin** is an endogenous hormone released from the thyroid gland when serum calcium is elevated. Salmon calcitonin is used clinically because it is more potent and longer lasting than the mammalian form.
- Calcitonin is indicated for osteoporosis treatment for women at least 5 years past menopause. An FDA Advisory Committee Panel voted against use for postmeno-pausal osteoporosis, but it can be used if alternative therapies are not appropriate.
- Only vertebral fractures have been documented to decrease with intranasal calcitonin therapy. Calcitonin does not consistently affect hip BMD. No data exist for men. Intra-nasal calcitonin may provide some pain relief in patients with acute vertebral fractures. If used for this purpose, calcitonin should be prescribed for short-term (4 weeks) treatment and should not be used in place of other more effective and less expensive analgesics nor should it preclude use of more appropriate osteoporosis therapy.

Hormone Therapies

- Hormone therapies are not recommended solely for osteoporosis but have positive bone effects when used for other indications. Estrogens are FDA-indicated for pre-vention of osteoporosis in women at significant risk and for whom other osteoporosis medications cannot be used. Estrogens are an option for women in early menopause when positive bone effects are needed in addition to vasomotor symptom reduction.
- Estrogen with or without a progestogen significantly decreases fracture risk and bone loss in women. Oral and transdermal estrogens at equivalent doses and continuous or cyclic regimens have similar BMD effects. Effect on BMD is dose dependent, with some benefit seen with lower estrogen doses. When estrogen therapy is discontinued, bone loss accelerates and fracture protection is lost.

Testosterone

- Testosterone is not FDA indicated for osteoporosis. No fracture data are available, but some data support minor bone loss prevention for testosterone use in men and women.

ANABOLIC THERAPIES

Teriparatide

- **Teriparatide** (Forteo) is a recombinant human product representing the first 34 amino acids in human parathyroid hormone. Teriparatide increases bone formation, bone remodeling rate, and osteoblast number and activity.
- Teriparatide is indicated for postmenopausal women at high risk for fracture, men with idiopathic or hypogonadal osteoporosis at high fracture risk, men or women intolerant to other osteoporosis medications, and patients with glucocorticoid-induced osteoporosis.
- Two years of teriparatide therapy reduces fracture risk in postmenopausal women, but no fracture data are available in men or patients taking corticosteroids. Lumbar spine BMD increases are higher than with other osteoporosis medications. Although wrist BMD is decreased, wrist fractures are not increased. Discontinuation of therapy results in decreased BMD, which can be alleviated with subsequent antiresorptive therapy.
- Transient hypercalcemia rarely occurs. Teriparatide is contraindicated in patients at increased risk for osteosarcoma and should not be used in patients with hypercalce-mia, metabolic bone diseases other than osteoporosis, metastatic or skeletal cancers, premenopausal women of childbearing potential, or men who received previous radiation therapy.

GLUCOCORTICOID-INDUCED OSTEOPOROSIS

- Glucocorticoids decrease bone formation through decreased proliferation and differentiation as well as enhanced apoptosis of osteoblasts. They also increase bone resorption, decrease calcium absorption, and increase renal calcium excretion.
- Bone losses are rapid, with up to 12% to 15% loss over the first year, the greatest decrease occurs in the first 6 months of therapy. Bone loss is about 2% to 3% per year after the first year.
- Measure baseline BMD using central DXA for all patients starting on prednisone 5 mg or more daily (or equivalent) for at least 6 months. Consider BMD testing at baseline in patients being started on shorter durations of systemic glucocorticoids if they are at high risk for low bone mass and fractures. Because bone loss can occur rapidly, central DXA can be repeated yearly or more often if needed.
- All patients starting or receiving systemic glucocorticoid therapy (any dose or duration) should practice a bone-healthy lifestyle and ingest 1200 to 1500 mg elemental calcium and 800 to 1200 units of vitamin D daily to achieve therapeutic 25(OH) vitamin D concentrations. Use the lowest possible corticosteroid dose and duration.
- Treatment guidelines divide recommendations for prescription medication use by fracture risk, age, menopause and childbearing status, glucocorticoid dose and duration, and fragility fracture. Alendronate, risedronate, zoledronic acid, and teriparatide are FDA approved for glucocorticoid-induced osteoporosis. Standard osteoporosis therapy doses are used. Raloxifene and denosumab do not have FDA indications but have some clinical data documenting decreased bone loss.

EVALUATION OF THERAPEUTIC OUTCOMES

- To evaluate efficacy, obtain a central DXA BMD measurement 2 years after initiating medication therapy. Central DXAs are repeated every 2 years until BMD is stable, at which time the reassessment interval can be expanded. More frequent monitoring may be warranted in patients with conditions associated with high rates of bone loss (eg, glucocorticoid use).
- Assess medication adherence and tolerance at each visit.
- Ask patients about possible fracture symptoms (eg, bone pain or disability) at each visit. Assessment of fracture, back pain, and height loss can help identify worsening osteoporosis.

See Chapter 92, Osteoporosis and Osteomalacia, authored by Mary Beth O'Connell and Jill S. Borchert, for a more detailed discussion of this topic.

Rheumatoid Arthritis

- *Rheumatoid arthritis* (RA) is a chronic, progressive inflammatory disorder of unknown etiology characterized by polyarticular symmetric joint involvement and systemic manifestations.

PATHOPHYSIOLOGY

- RA results from dysregulation of humoral and cell-mediated immunity. Most patients produce antibodies called *rheumatoid factors*; these seropositive patients tend to have a more aggressive course than seronegative patients.
- Immunoglobulins (Ig) activate the complement system, which amplifies the immune response by enhancing chemotaxis, phagocytosis, and release of lymphokines by mononuclear cells that are then presented to T lymphocytes. Processed antigen is recognized by the major histocompatibility complex proteins on the lymphocyte surface, resulting in activation of T and B cells.
- Tumor necrosis factor-α (TNF-α), interleukin-1 (IL-1), and IL-6 are proinflammatory cytokines important in initiation and continuance of inflammation.
- Activated T cells produce cytotoxins and cytokines, which stimulate further activation of inflammatory processes and attract cells to areas of inflammation. Macrophages are stimulated to release prostaglandins and cytotoxins. T-cell activation requires both stimulation by proinflammatory cytokines as well as interaction between cell surface receptors, called *costimulation*. One such costimulation interaction is between CD28 and CD80/86.
- Activated B cells produce plasma cells, which form antibodies that, in combination with the complement system, result in accumulation of polymorphonuclear leukocytes. These leukocytes release cytotoxins, oxygen-free radicals, and hydroxyl radicals that promote damage to synovium and bone.
- Signaling molecules are important for activating and maintaining inflammation. Janus kinase (JAK) is a tyrosine kinase responsible for regulating leukocyte maturation and activation. JAK also has effects on production of cytokines and immunoglobulins.
- Vasoactive substances (histamine, kinins, and prostaglandins) are released at sites of inflammation, increasing blood flow and vascular permeability. This causes edema, warmth, erythema, and pain, and facilitates granulocyte passage from blood vessels to sites of inflammation.
- Chronic inflammation of synovial tissue lining the joint capsule results in tissue proliferation (pannus formation). Pannus invades cartilage and eventually the bone surface, producing erosions of bone and cartilage and leading to joint destruction. End results may be loss of joint space and joint motion, bony fusion (ankylosis), joint subluxation, tendon contractures, and chronic deformity.

CLINICAL PRESENTATION

- Nonspecific prodromal symptoms developing over weeks to months include fatigue, weakness, low-grade fever, anorexia, and joint pain. Stiffness and myalgias may precede development of synovitis.
- Joint involvement tends to be symmetric and affect small joints of the hands, wrists, and feet; elbows, shoulders, hips, knees, and ankles may also be affected.
- Joint stiffness typically is worse in the morning, usually exceeds 30 minutes, and may persist all day.
- On examination, joint swelling may be visible or apparent only by palpation. Tissue is soft, spongy, warm, and may be erythematous. Joint deformities may involve subluxations of wrists, metacarpophalangeal joints, and proximal interphalangeal joints (swan neck deformity, boutonnière deformity, and ulnar deviation).

- Extra-articular involvement may include rheumatoid nodules, vasculitis, pleural effusions, pulmonary fibrosis, ocular manifestations, pericarditis, cardiac conduction abnormalities, bone marrow suppression, and lymphadenopathy.

DIAGNOSIS

- The American College of Rheumatology (ACR) and the European League Against Rheumatism (EULAR) revised criteria for diagnosis of RA in 2010. These criteria are intended for patients early in their disease and emphasize early manifestations. Late manifestations (bone erosions, subcutaneous nodules) are no longer in the diagnostic criteria. Patients with synovitis of at least one joint and no other explanation for the finding are candidates for assessment. The criteria use a scoring system with a combined score of 6 or more out of 10 indicating that the patient has definite RA.
- Laboratory abnormalities include normocytic, normochromic anemia; thrombocytosis or thrombocytopenia; leukopenia; elevated erythrocyte sedimentation rate and C-reactive protein; positive rheumatoid factor (60%–70% of patients); positive anticitrullinated protein antibody (ACPA) (50%–85% of patients); and positive antinuclear antibodies (25% of patients).
- Aspirated synovial fluid may reveal turbidity, leukocytosis, reduced viscosity, and normal or low glucose relative to serum concentrations.
- Early radiologic findings include soft tissue swelling and osteoporosis near the joint (periarticular osteoporosis). Erosions later in the disease course are usually seen first in the metacarpophalangeal and proximal interphalangeal joints of the hands and metatarsophalangeal joints of the feet.

TREATMENT

- <u>Goals of Treatment</u>: The ultimate goal is to induce complete remission or low disease activity (referred to as "treat to target"). Additional goals are to control disease activity and joint pain, maintain ability to function in daily activities, slow destructive joint changes, and delay disability.

NONPHARMACOLOGIC THERAPY

- Adequate rest, weight reduction if obese, occupational therapy, physical therapy, and use of assistive devices may improve symptoms and help maintain joint function.
- Patients with severe disease may benefit from surgical procedures such as tenosynovectomy, tendon repair, and joint replacements.
- Patient education about the disease and the benefits and limitations of drug therapy is important.

PHARMACOLOGIC THERAPY
General Approach

- Pharmacologic agents that reduce RA symptoms and impede radiographic joint damage are categorized as either conventional synthetic disease-modifying antirheumatic drugs (referred to simply as *DMARDs*) or biologic disease-modifying drugs (referred to as *biologics*). The 2015 American College of Rheumatology (ACR) guideline considers **tofacitinib** (a synthetic small molecule) separately.
- Common DMARDs include **methotrexate (MTX)**, **leflunomide**, **hydroxychloroquine**, and **sulfasalazine**.
- Biologics include the anti-TNF agents **etanercept**, **infliximab**, **adalimumab**, **certolizumab**, and **golimumab**; the costimulation modulator **abatacept**; the IL-6 receptor antagonist **tocilizumab**; and **rituximab**, which depletes peripheral B cells. Biologics have proven effective for patients failing treatment with DMARDs.

27

- Agents used infrequently because of less efficacy and/or greater toxicity include **anakinra** (IL-1 receptor antagonist), **azathioprine**, **penicillamine**, **gold** (including **auranofin**), **minocycline**, **cyclosporine**, and **cyclophosphamide**.
- DMARDs should be started as soon as possible after disease onset because they slow disease progression, and early treatment results in more favorable outcomes, including lower mortality rates.
- Treatment guidelines recommend initial therapy with a DMARD, preferably methotrexate (MTX), for most patients regardless of clinical disease activity (Fig. 4–1). Patients with moderate-to-severe disease activity despite initial treatment should be switched to another DMARD, a biologic agent, or combination DMARD therapy. Recommended DMARD combinations include (1) MTX plus hydroxychloroquine, (2) MTX plus leflunomide, (3) MTX plus sulfasalazine, and (4) MTX plus hydroxychloroquine plus sulfasalazine.
- The ACR guideline endorses use of anti-TNF biologics as monotherapy or in combination with DMARDs in patients with moderate-to-high disease activity after treatment with DMARD therapy. Use of biologics in combination with MTX is more effective than biologic monotherapy. Dual biologic use is not recommended due to the risk of infection associated with immunosuppression.

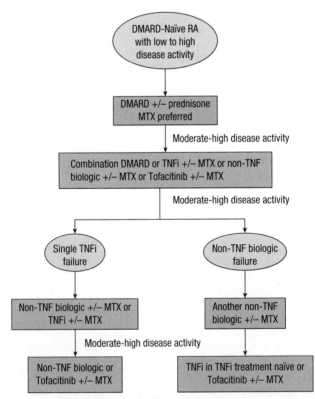

(DMARD, disease-modifying antirheumatic drug; MTX, methotrexate; TNFi, tumor necrosis factor inhibitor.)

FIGURE 4–1. **Algorithm for treatment of rheumatoid arthritis (RA) in early (<6 months) or established (≥ 6 months) RA with low to high disease activity.**

- Nonsteroidal anti-inflammatory drugs (NSAIDs) and/or corticosteroids may be used for symptomatic relief if needed. They provide relatively rapid improvement compared with DMARDs, which may take weeks to months to take effect. However, NSAIDs have no impact on disease progression, and corticosteroids have potential for long-term complications.
- Because DMARDs, biologics, and some corticosteroid regimens result in immuno-suppression, vaccination status should be assessed and updated before therapy is started to protect against vaccine-preventable infections. Some biologics are contraindicated in the setting of hepatitis C or malignancies because of immunosuppression.
- Patients who achieve remission can be considered for tapering but not discontinuation of all RA therapies. Patients who achieve low disease activity should continue RA treatment.
- See Tables 4–1 and 4–2 for usual dosages and monitoring parameters for DMARDs, biologics, and NSAIDs used in RA.

Nonsteroidal Anti-inflammatory Drugs

- NSAIDs inhibit prostaglandin synthesis, which is only a small portion of the inflammatory cascade. They possess both analgesic and anti-inflammatory properties and reduce stiffness, but they do not slow disease progression or prevent bony erosions or joint deformity. Common NSAID dosage regimens are shown in Table 4–3.

Corticosteroids

- Corticosteroids have anti-inflammatory and immunosuppressive properties but should not be used as monotherapy. They interfere with antigen presentation to T lymphocytes, inhibit prostaglandin and leukotriene synthesis, and inhibit neutrophil and monocyte superoxide radical generation.
- Oral corticosteroids (eg, **prednisone**, **methylprednisolone**) can be used to control pain and synovitis while DMARDs are taking effect ("bridging therapy").
- Low-dose, long-term corticosteroid therapy may be used to control symptoms in patients with difficult-to-control disease. Prednisone doses below 7.5 mg/day (or equivalent) are well tolerated but are not devoid of long-term adverse effects. Use the lowest dose that controls symptoms. Alternate-day dosing of low-dose oral corticosteroids is usually ineffective in RA.
- High-dose oral or IV bursts may be used for several days to suppress disease flares. After symptoms are controlled, taper the drug to the lowest effective dose.
- The intramuscular route is preferable in nonadherent patients. Depot forms (**triamcinolone acetonide**, **triamcinolone hexacetonide**, and **methylprednisolone acetate**) provide 2 to 6 weeks of symptomatic control. Onset of effect may be delayed for several days. The depot effect provides a physiologic taper, avoiding hypothalamic-pituitary axis suppression.
- Intra-articular injections of depot forms may be useful when only a few joints are involved. If effective, injections may be repeated every 3 months. Do not inject any one joint more than two or three times per year.
- Adverse effects of systemic glucocorticoids limit long-term use. Consider dosage tapering and eventual discontinuation at some point during chronic therapy.

DMARDs

Methotrexate

- **Methotrexate (MTX)** inhibits cytokine production and purine biosynthesis, and may stimulate adenosine release, all of which may lead to anti-inflammatory properties. Onset is as early as 2 to 3 weeks, and 45% to 67% of patients remained on it in studies ranging from 5 to 7 years.
- Concomitant folic acid may reduce some adverse effects without loss of efficacy. Monitor liver injury tests periodically, but a liver biopsy is recommended during therapy only in patients with persistently elevated hepatic enzymes. MTX is teratogenic, and patients should use contraception and discontinue the drug if conception is planned.

TABLE 4–1	Usual Doses and Monitoring Parameters for Antirheumatic Drugs		
Drug	**Usual Dose**	**Initial Monitoring Tests**	**Maintenance Monitoring Tests**
NSAIDs	See **Table 4–3**	S_{cr} or BUN, CBC every 2–4 weeks after starting therapy for 1–2 months; salicylates: serum salicylate levels if therapeutic dose and no response	Same as initial plus stool guaiac every 6–12 months
Corticosteroids	Oral, IV, IM, IA, and soft-tissue injections: variable	Glucose; blood pressure every 3–6 months	Same as initial
Methotrexate	Oral or IM: 7.5–15 mg/week	Baseline: AST, ALT, ALK-P, albumin, total bilirubin, hepatitis B and C studies, CBC with platelets, S_{cr}	CBC with platelets, AST, albumin every 1–2 months
Leflunomide	Oral: 100 mg daily for 3 days, then 10–20 mg daily, or 10–20 mg daily without loading dose	Baseline: ALT, CBC with platelets	CBC with platelets and ALT monthly initially, then every 6–8 weeks
Hydroxychloroquine	Oral: 200–300 mg twice daily; after 1–2 months may decrease to 200 mg once or twice daily	Baseline: color fundus photography and automated central perimetric analysis	Ophthalmoscopy every 9–12 months and Amsler grid at home every 2 weeks
Sulfasalazine	Oral: 500 mg twice daily, then increase to 1 g twice daily	Baseline: CBC with platelets, then every week for 1 month	Same as initial every 1–2 months
Minocycline	Oral: 100–200 mg daily	None	None
Etanercept	50 mg SC once weekly or 25 mg twice weekly	Tuberculin skin test	None
Infliximab	3 mg/kg IV at 0, 2, 6 weeks, then every 8 weeks	Tuberculin skin test	None
Adalimumab	40 mg SC every 2 weeks	Tuberculin skin test	None
Certolizumab	400 mg (2 doses of 200 mg) SC at weeks 0, 2, 4, then 200 mg every 2 weeks	Tuberculin skin test	None
Golimumab	50 mg SC once monthly	Tuberculin skin test	None
Rituximab	1000-mg IV infusion given twice, 2 weeks apart	Tuberculin skin test	None

Drug	Dose/Administration	Baseline Monitoring	Follow-up Monitoring
Abatacept	IV infusion: 30-min weight-based infusion: <60 kg = 500 mg; 60–100 kg = 750 mg; >100 kg = 1000 mg. SC injection: 125 mg SC within 24 h after a single IV infusion loading dose of ~10 mg/kg; then 125 mg SC every 7 days	Tuberculin skin test	None
Tocilizumab	4–8 mg/kg IV every 4 weeks	Tuberculin skin test, AST/ALT, CBC with platelets, lipids	AST/ALT, CBC with platelets, lipids every 4–8 weeks
Anakinra	100 mg SC daily	Tuberculin skin test, neutrophil count	Neutrophil count monthly for 3 months, then quarterly for up to 1 year
Tofacitinib	Oral: 5 mg twice daily; Oral XR: 11 mg once daily	Tuberculin skin test, CBC with differential; hepatic enzymes, lipids	CBC with differential after 4–8 weeks and every 3 months thereafter
Auranofin	Oral: 3 mg once or twice daily	Baseline: UA, CBC with platelets	Same as initial every 1–2 months
Gold thiomalate	IM: 10 mg test dose, then weekly dosing 25–50 mg; after response may increase dosing interval	Baseline and until stable: UA, CBC with platelets preinjection	Same as initial every other dose
Azathioprine	Oral: 50–150 mg daily	CBC with platelets, AST every 2 weeks for 1–2 months	Same as initial every 1–2 months
Penicillamine	Oral: 125–250 mg daily, may increase by 125–250 mg every 1–2 months; max 750 mg/day	Baseline: UA, CBC with platelets, then every week for 1 month	Same as initial every 1–2 months, but every 2 weeks if dose changes
Cyclophosphamide	Oral: 1–2 mg/kg/day	UA, CBC with platelets every week for 1 month	Same tests as initial but every 2–4 weeks
Cyclosporine	Oral: 2.5 mg/kg/day divided twice daily	S_{cr}, blood pressure every month	Same as initial

(ALK-P, alkaline phosphatase; ALT, alanine aminotransferase; AST, aspartate aminotransferase; BUN, blood urea nitrogen; CBC, complete blood cell count; IA, intra-articular; IM, intramuscular; IV, intravenous; NSAIDs, nonsteroidal anti-inflammatory drugs; SC, subcutaneous; Scr, serum creatinine; UA, urinalysis.)

TABLE 4–2	Clinical Monitoring of Drug Therapy in Rheumatoid Arthritis	
Drug	**Toxicities Requiring Monitoring**	**Symptoms to Inquire About[a]**
NSAIDs and salicylates	GI ulceration and bleeding, renal damage	Blood in stool, black stool, dyspepsia, nausea/vomiting, weakness, dizziness, abdominal pain, edema, weight gain, shortness of breath
Corticosteroids	Hypertension, hyperglycemia, osteoporosis[b]	Blood pressure, polyuria, poly-dipsia, edema, shortness of breath, visual changes, weight gain, headaches, broken bones or bone pain
Methotrexate	GI (stomatitis, nausea/vomiting, diarrhea), myelosuppression (thrombocytopenia, leukopenia), hepatic (elevated enzymes, rarely cirrhosis), pulmonary (fibrosis, pneumonitis), rash	Symptoms of myelosuppression, shortness of breath, nausea/vomiting, lymph node swelling, coughing, mouth sores, diarrhea, jaundice
Leflunomide	Hepatotoxicity, myelosuppression, GI distress, alopecia	Nausea/vomiting, gastritis, diarrhea, hair loss, jaundice
Hydroxychloroquine	GI (nausea/vomiting, diarrhea), ocular (benign corneal deposits, blurred vision, scotomas, night blindness, preretinopathy), dermatologic (rash, alopecia, pigmentation), neurologic (headache, vertigo, insomnia)	Visual changes, including a decrease in night or peripheral vision, rash, diarrhea
Sulfasalazine	GI (anorexia, nausea/vomiting, diarrhea), dermatologic (rash, urticaria), myelosuppression (leukopenia, rarely agranulocytosis), elevated hepatic enzymes	Symptoms of myelosuppression, photosensitivity, rash, nausea/vomiting
Etanercept, adalimumab, certolizumab, golimumab, tocilizumab, anakinra	Local injection site reactions, infection	Symptoms of infection
Infliximab, rituximab, abatacept	Immune reactions, infection	Postinfusion reactions, symptoms of infection
Tofacitinib	Infection, malignancy, GI perforation, upper respiratory tract infection, headache, diarrhea, nasopharyngitis, elevated hepatic enzymes and lipids	Symptoms of infection or myelosuppression, shortness of breath, blood in stool, black stool, dyspepsia
Gold (intramuscular or oral)	Myelosuppression, proteinuria, rash, stomatitis	Symptoms of myelosuppression, edema, rash, oral ulcers, diarrhea
Azathioprine	Myelosuppression, hepatotoxicity, lymphoproliferative disorders	Symptoms of myelosuppression (extreme fatigue, easy bleeding or bruising, infection), jaundice

(continued)

TABLE 4–2	Clinical Monitoring of Drug Therapy in Rheumatoid Arthritis (Continued)	
Drug	**Toxicities Requiring Monitoring**	**Symptoms to Inquire About[a]**
Penicillamine	Myelosuppression, proteinuria, stomatitis, rash, dysgeusia	Symptoms of myelosuppression, edema, rash, diarrhea, altered taste perception, oral ulcers
Cyclophosphamide	Alopecia, infertility, GI distress, hemorrhagic cystitis, myelo-suppression, nephrotoxicity, cardiotoxicity	Nausea/vomiting, gastritis, diarrhea, hair loss, urination difficulties, chest pain, rash, respiratory difficulties
Cyclosporine	Hepatotoxicity, nephrotoxicity, hypertension, headache, malig-nancy, infections, GI distress	Nausea/vomiting, diarrhea, symptoms of infection, symptoms of elevated blood pressure

(GI, gastrointestinal; NSAIDs, nonsteroidal anti-inflammatory drugs.)
[a]Altered immune function increases infection, which should be considered particularly in patients taking azathioprine, methotrexate, corticosteroids, or other drugs that may produce myelosuppression.
[b]Osteoporosis is not likely to manifest early in treatment, but all patients should be taking appropriate steps to prevent bone loss.

- MTX is contraindicated in pregnant and nursing women, chronic liver disease, immunodeficiency, pleural or peritoneal effusions, leukopenia, thrombocytopenia, preexisting blood disorders, and creatinine clearance of less than 40 mL/min (0.67 mL/s).

Leflunomide

- **Leflunomide** (Arava) inhibits pyrimidine synthesis, which reduces lymphocyte proliferation and modulation of inflammation. Efficacy for RA is similar to that of MTX.
- A loading dose of 100 mg/day for 3 days may result in therapeutic response within the first month. The usual maintenance dose of 20 mg/day may be lowered to 10 mg/day in cases of GI intolerance, alopecia, or other dose-related toxicity.
- Leflunomide is contraindicated in patients with preexisting liver disease. It is teratogenic and must be avoided during pregnancy.

Hydroxychloroquine

- **Hydroxychloroquine** is often used in mild RA or as an adjuvant in combination DMARD therapy. It lacks the myelosuppressive, hepatic, and renal toxicities seen with some other DMARDs, which simplifies monitoring. Onset may be delayed for up to 6 weeks, but the drug should not be considered a therapeutic failure until after 6 months of therapy with no response.
- Periodic ophthalmologic examinations are necessary for early detection of reversible retinal toxicity.

Sulfasalazine

- **Sulfasalazine** use is often limited by adverse effects. Antirheumatic effects should be seen within 2 months.
- GI symptoms may be minimized by starting with low doses, dividing the dose evenly throughout the day, and taking it with food.

Minocycline

- Minocycline may inhibit metalloproteinases active in damaging articular cartilage. It may be an alternative for patients with mild disease and without features of poor prognosis.

TABLE 4-3	Dosage Regimens for Nonsteroidal Anti-inflammatory Drugs		
	Recommended Total Daily Anti-inflammatory Dosage		
Drug	**Adult**	**Children**	**Dosing Schedule**
Aspirin	2.6–5.2 g	60–100 mg/kg	4 times daily
Celecoxib	200–400 mg	–	Once or twice daily
Diclofenac	150–200 mg	–	3 or 4 times daily; extended release: twice daily
Diflunisal	0.5–1.5 g	–	Twice daily
Etodolac	0.2–1.2 g (max 20 mg/kg)	–	2–4 times daily
Fenoprofen	0.9–3 g	–	4 times daily
Flurbiprofen	200–300 mg	–	2–4 times daily
Ibuprofen	1.2–3.2 g	20–40 mg/kg	3 or 4 times daily
Indomethacin	50–200 mg	2–4 mg/kg (max 200 mg)	2–4 times daily; extended release: once daily
Meclofenamate	200–400 mg	–	3–4 times daily
Meloxicam	7.5–15 mg	–	Once daily
Nabumetone	1–2 g	–	Once or twice daily
Naproxen	0.5–1 g	10 mg/kg	Twice daily; extended release: once daily
Naproxen sodium	0.55–1.1 g	–	Twice daily
Nonacetylated salicylates	1.2–4.8 g	–	2–6 times daily
Oxaprozin	0.6–1.8 g (max 26 mg/kg)	–	1–3 times daily
Piroxicam	10–20 mg	–	Once daily
Sulindac	300–400 mg	–	Twice daily
Tolmetin	0.6–1.8 g	15–30 mg/kg	2–4 times daily

Tofacitinib

- **Tofacitinib** (Xeljanz) is a nonbiologic JAK inhibitor indicated for patients with moderate to severe RA who have failed or have intolerance to MTX.
- The recommended dose is 5 mg twice daily (or extended-release 11 mg once daily) as monotherapy or in combination with other DMARDs. It should not be given with biologic agents.
- Labeling includes black-box warnings about serious infections, lymphomas, and other malignancies. Live vaccinations should not be given during treatment. Patients should be tested and treated for latent tuberculosis before starting therapy. Elevated liver enzymes and lipids and gastrointestinal perforations have been reported.

BIOLOGIC AGENTS

- Biologic may be effective when DMARDs fail to achieve adequate responses but are considerably more expensive.
- These agents have no toxicities requiring laboratory monitoring, but they do carry a small increased risk for infection, including tuberculosis. Tuberculin skin testing or interferon gamma release assay (IGRA) blood test should be performed before treatment to detect latent tuberculosis.

- Biologics should be at least temporarily discontinued in patients who develop infections while on therapy until the infection is cured. Live vaccines should not be given to patients taking biologic agents.

TNF-α Inhibitors

- Inhibitors of TNF-α are generally the first biologics used. About 30% of patients eventually discontinue use owing to inadequate efficacy or adverse effects. In such situations, addition of a DMARD may be beneficial if the patient is not already taking one. Choosing an alternative TNF inhibitor may benefit some patients; treatment with rituximab or abatacept may also be effective in patients failing TNF inhibitors.
- Congestive heart failure (HF) is a relative contraindication for anti-TNF agents due to reports of increased cardiac mortality and HF exacerbations. Patients with New York Heart Association class III or IV and an ejection fraction of 50% or less should not use anti-TNF therapy. Discontinue the drugs if HF worsens during treatment.
- Anti-TNF therapy has been reported to induce a multiple sclerosis (MS)–like illness or exacerbate MS in patients with the disease. Discontinue therapy if patients develop neurologic symptoms suggestive of MS.
- TNF inhibitors are associated with increased risk of cancer, especially lymphoproliferative cancers. The drugs contain a black-box warning about increased risk of lymphoproliferative and other cancers in children and adolescents treated with these drugs.
- See Tables 4–1 and 4–2 for dosing and monitoring information.
    - ✓ **Etanercept** (Enbrel) is a fusion protein consisting of two p75-soluble TNF receptors linked to an Fc fragment of human IgG_1. It binds to and inactivates TNF, preventing it from interacting with the cell-surface TNF receptors and thereby activating cells. Clinical trials using etanercept in patients who failed DMARDs demonstrated responses in 60% to 75% of patients. It slows erosive disease progression more than oral MTX in patients with inadequate response to MTX monotherapy.
    - ✓ **Infliximab** (Remicade) is a chimeric anti-TNF antibody fused to a human constant-region IgG_1. It binds to TNF and prevents its interaction with TNF receptors on inflammatory cells. To prevent formation of an antibody response to this foreign protein, MTX must be given orally in doses used to treat RA for as long as the patient continues infliximab. In clinical trials, the combination of infliximab and MTX halted progression of joint damage and was superior to MTX monotherapy. An acute infusion reaction with fever, chills, pruritus, and rash may occur within 1 to 2 hours after administration. Autoantibodies and lupus-like syndrome have also been reported.
    - ✓ **Adalimumab** (Humira) is a human IgG_1 antibody to TNF-α that is less antigenic than infliximab. It has response rates similar to other TNF inhibitors.
    - ✓ **Golimumab** (Simponi) is a human antibody to TNF-α with activity and precautions similar to other TNF-α inhibitors.
    - ✓ **Certolizumab** (Cimzia) is a humanized antibody specific for TNF-α with precautions and side effects similar to other TNF-α inhibitors.

Abatacept

- **Abatacept** (Orencia) is a costimulation modulator approved for patients with moderate to severe disease who fail to achieve an adequate response from one or more DMARDs. By binding to CD80/CD86 receptors on antigen-presenting cells, abatacept inhibits interactions between the antigen-presenting cells and T cells, preventing T cells from activating to promote the inflammatory process.

Rituximab

- **Rituximab** (Rituxan) is a monoclonal chimeric antibody consisting of human protein with the antigen-binding region derived from a mouse antibody to CD20 protein found on the cell surface of mature B lymphocytes. Binding of rituximab to B cells results in nearly complete depletion of peripheral B cells, with a gradual recovery over several months.

• Rituximab is useful in patients who failed MTX or TNF inhibitors. Give methyl-prednisolone 100 mg 30 minutes prior to rituximab to reduce incidence and severity of infusion reactions. Acetaminophen and antihistamines may also benefit patients who have a history of reactions. MTX should be given concurrently in the usual doses for RA to achieve optimal therapeutic outcomes.

Tocilizumab

• **Tocilizumab** (Actemra) is a humanized monoclonal antibody that attaches to IL-6 receptors, preventing the cytokine from interacting with IL-6 receptors. It is approved for adults with moderately to severely active RA who have failed to respond to one or more DMARDs. It is used as either monotherapy or in combination with MTX or another DMARD.

Anakinra

• **Anakinra** (Kineret) is an IL-1 receptor antagonist; it is less effective than other bio-logics and is not included in the current ACR treatment recommendations. However, select patients with refractory disease may benefit. It can be used alone or in combi-nation with any of the other DMARDs except TNF-α inhibitors.

EVALUATION OF THERAPEUTIC OUTCOMES

• Clinical signs of improvement include reduction in joint swelling, decreased warmth over actively involved joints, and decreased tenderness to joint palpation.
• Symptom improvement includes reduction in joint pain and morning stiffness, longer time to onset of afternoon fatigue, and improvement in ability to perform daily activities.
• Periodic joint radiographs may be useful in assessing disease progression.
• Laboratory monitoring is of little value in assessing response to therapy but is essential for detecting and preventing adverse drug effects (see **Table 4–2**).
• Ask patients about the presence of symptoms that may be related to adverse drug effects (see **Table 4–3**).

See Chapter 91, Rheumatoid Arthritis, authored by Kimberly Wahl and Arthur A. Schuna, for a detailed discussion of this topic.

CHAPTER 5 Acute Coronary Syndromes

- *Acute coronary syndrome* (ACS) includes all syndromes compatible with acute myocardial ischemia resulting from imbalance between myocardial oxygen demand and supply.
- ACS is classified according to electrocardiographic (ECG) changes into: (1) ST-segment-elevation myocardial infarction (STEMI) or (2) non–ST-segment-elevation ACS (NSTE-ACS), which includes non–ST-segment-elevation MI (NSTEMI) and unstable angina (UA).

PATHOPHYSIOLOGY

- Endothelial dysfunction, inflammation, and formation of fatty streaks contribute to development of atherosclerotic coronary artery plaques.
- With rupture of an atherosclerotic plaque, exposure of collagen and tissue factor induces platelet adhesion and activation, promoting release of adenosine diphosphate (ADP) and thromboxane A_2 from platelets, leading to vasoconstriction and platelet activation. A change in the conformation of the glycoprotein IIb/IIIa surface receptors of platelets occurs that cross-links platelets to each other through fibrinogen bridges.
- Simultaneously, activation of the extrinsic coagulation cascade occurs as a result of exposure of blood to the thrombogenic lipid core and endothelium, which are rich in tissue factor. This leads to formation of a fibrin clot composed of fibrin strands, cross-linked platelets, and trapped red blood cells.
- Subtypes of MI are based on etiology:
  ✓ Type 1: Rupture, fissure, or erosion of an atherosclerotic plaque (90% of cases);
  ✓ Type 2: Reduced myocardial oxygen supply or increased demand in the absence of a coronary artery process;
  ✓ Type 3: MI resulting in death without the possibility of measuring biomarkers;
  ✓ Type 4: MI associated with percutaneous coronary intervention (PCI; Type 4a) or stent thrombosis (Type 4b); and
  ✓ Type 5: MI associated with coronary artery bypass graft (CABG) surgery.
- Ventricular remodeling after MI is characterized by left ventricular (LV) dilation and reduced pumping function, leading to heart failure (HF).
- Complications of MI include cardiogenic shock, HF, valvular dysfunction, arrhythmias, pericarditis, stroke secondary to LV thrombus embolization, venous thromboembolism, LV free-wall or septal rupture, aneurysm formation, and ventricular and atrial tachyarrhythmias.

CLINICAL PRESENTATION

- The predominant symptom is midline anterior chest pain (usually at rest), severe new-onset angina, or increasing angina that lasts at least 20 minutes. Discomfort may radiate to the shoulder, down the left arm, to the back, or to the jaw. Accompanying symptoms may include nausea, vomiting, diaphoresis, and shortness of breath.
- No specific features indicate ACS on physical examination. However, patients with ACS may present with signs of acute decompensated HF or arrhythmias.

DIAGNOSIS

- Obtain 12-lead ECG within 10 minutes of presentation. Key findings indicating myo-cardial ischemia or MI are STE, ST-segment depression, and T-wave inversion. Appear-ance of a new left bundle-branch block with chest discomfort is highly specific for acute MI. Some patients with myocardial ischemia have no ECG changes, so biochemical markers and other risk factors for coronary artery disease (CAD) should be assessed.
- Diagnosis of MI is confirmed with detection of rise and/or fall of cardiac biomarkers (mainly troponin T or I) with at least one value above the 99th percentile of the upper reference limit and at least one of the following: (1) symptoms of ischemia; (2) new significant ST-segment–T-wave changes or new left bundle-branch block; (3) pathological Q waves; or (4) imaging evidence of new loss of viable myocardium or new regional wall motion abnormality. Typically, a blood sample is obtained once in the emergency department, then 3 to 6 hours after symptom onset.
- Patient symptoms, past medical history, ECG, and biomarkers are used to stratify patients into low, medium, or high risk of death, MI, or likelihood of failing pharma-cotherapy and needing urgent coronary angiography and PCI.

TREATMENT

- Goals of Treatment: Short-term goals include: (1) early restoration of blood flow to the infarct-related artery to prevent infarct expansion (in the case of MI) or prevent complete occlusion and MI (in UA), (2) prevention of death and other complications, (3) prevention of coronary artery reocclusion, (4) relief of ischemic chest discomfort, and (5) resolution of ST-segment and T-wave changes on ECG. Long-term goals include control of cardiovascu-lar (CV) risk factors, prevention of additional CV events, and improvement in quality of life.

GENERAL APPROACH

- General measures include hospital admission, oxygen if saturation is low, continuous multilead ST-segment monitoring for arrhythmias and ischemia, frequent measure-ment of vital signs, bed rest for 12 hours in hemodynamically stable patients, use of stool softeners to avoid Valsalva maneuver, and pain relief.
- Assess kidney function (serum creatinine, creatinine clearance) to identify patients who may need dosing adjustments and those at high risk of morbidity and mortality.
- Obtain complete blood cell count (CBC) and coagulation tests (aPTT, INR) because most patients will receive antithrombotic therapy.
- Fasting lipid panel is optional.
- Triage and treat patients according to their risk category (Fig. 5–1).
- Patients with STEMI are at high risk of death, so initiate immediate efforts to reestab-lish coronary perfusion and adjunctive pharmacotherapy.

NONPHARMACOLOGIC THERAPY

- For patients with STEMI presenting within 12 hours of symptom onset, early reperfu-sion with primary PCI of the infarct artery within 90 minutes of first medical contact is the reperfusion treatment of choice.
- For patients with NSTE-ACS, practice guidelines recommend an early (within 24 hours) invasive strategy with left heart catheterization, coronary angiography, and revascu-larization with either PCI or CABG surgery as early treatment for high-risk patients; such an approach may also be considered for patients not at high risk.

EARLY PHARMACOTHERAPY FOR STEMI (FIG. 5–2)

- In addition to reperfusion therapy, all patients with STEMI and without contra-indications should receive within the first day of hospitalization and preferably in the emergency department: (1) intranasal oxygen (if oxygen saturation is low), (2) sublingual (SL) nitroglycerin (NTG), (3) aspirin, (4) a $P2Y_{12}$ platelet inhibitor, and (5) anticoagulation with bivalirudin, unfractionated heparin (UFH), enoxaparin, or fondaparinux (depending on reperfusion strategy).

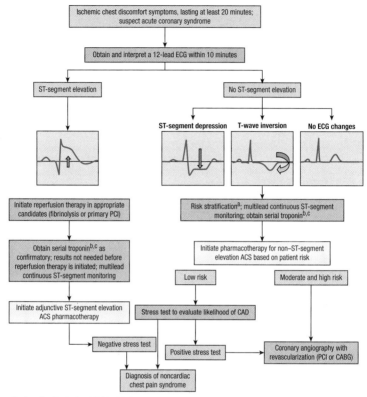

[a]As described in textbook Table 17–1.
[b]"Positive": Above the myocardial infarction decision limit.
[c]"Negative": Below the myocardial infarction decision limit.
(ACS, acute coronary syndrome; CABG, coronary artery bypass graft; CAD, coronary artery disease; ECG, electrocardiogram; PCI, percutaneous coronary intervention.)

FIGURE 5–1. Evaluation of the acute coronary syndrome patient. (Modified from Rogers KC, de Denus S, Finks SW. Acute Coronary Syndromes. In: Chisholm-Burns MA, Schwinghammer TL, Wells BG, et al, eds. *Pharmacotherapy: Principles and Practice.* 4th ed. New York: McGraw-Hill Companies; 2016:111-136.)

- A glycoprotein IIb/IIIa receptor inhibitor (GPI) may be administered with UFH to patients undergoing primary PCI.
- Intravenous NTG may be given to select patients.
- β-Blockers are reasonable at the time of presentation for patients with hypertension and ongoing ischemia but without cardiogenic shock or other contraindications.
- Morphine may be given for refractory angina as an analgesic and venodilator to lower preload, but its use should be limited.
- An angiotensin-converting enzyme (ACE) inhibitor is recommended within 24 hours in patients who have either anterior wall MI or LV ejection fraction (LVEF) of 40% or less and no contraindications.

Fibrinolytic Therapy

- A fibrinolytic agent is indicated in patients with STEMI who present within 12 hours of the onset of chest discomfort to a hospital not capable of primary PCI and have at least

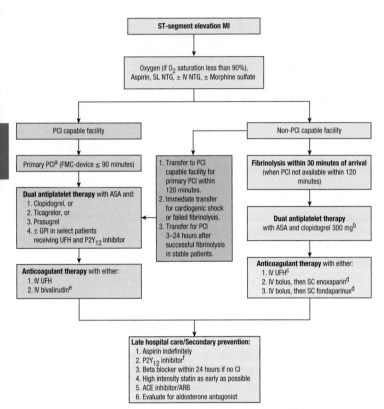

ST-segment elevation MI

Oxygen (if O$_2$ saturation less than 90%), Aspirin, SL NTG, ± IV NTG, ± Morphine sulfate

PCI capable facility

Primary PCI^a (FMC-device ≤ 90 minutes)

Dual antiplatelet therapy with ASA and:
1. Clopidogrel, or
2. Ticagrelor, or
3. Prasugrel
4. ± GPI in select patients receiving UFH and P2Y$_{12}$ inhibitor

Anticoagulant therapy with either:
1. IV UFH
2. IV bivalirudin^e

1. Transfer to PCI capable facility for primary PCI within 120 minutes.
2. Immediate transfer for cardiogenic shock or failed fibrinolysis.
3. Transfer for PCI 3–24 hours after successful fibrinolysis in stable patients.

Non-PCI capable facility

Fibrinolysis within 30 minutes of arrival (when PCI not available within 120 minutes)

Dual antiplatelet therapy with ASA and clopidogrel 300 mg^b

Anticoagulant therapy with either:
1. IV UFH^c
2. IV bolus, then SC enoxaparin^d
3. IV bolus, then SC fondaparinux^d

Late hospital care/Secondary prevention:
1. Aspirin indefinitely
2. P2Y$_{12}$ inhibitor^f
3. Beta blocker within 24 hours if no CI
4. High intensity statin as early as possible
5. ACE inhibitor/ARB
6. Evaluate for aldosterone antagonist

^{a}Options after coronary angiography also include medical management alone or CABG surgery.
^{b}Clopidogrel preferred P2Y$_{12}$ inhibitor when fibrinolytic therapy is utilized. No loading dose recommended if age older than 75 years.
^{c}Given for up to 48 hours or until revascularization.
^{d}Given for the duration of hospitalization, up to 8 days or until revascularization.
^{e}If pretreated with UFH, stop UFH infusion for 30 minutes prior to administration of bivalirudin (bolus plus infusion).
^{f}In patients with STEMI receiving a fibrinolytic or who do not receive reperfusion therapy, administer clopidogrel for at least 14 days and ideally up to 1 year.

(ACE, angiotensin-converting enzyme; ARB, angiotensin receptor blocker; ASA, aspirin; CI, contraindication; FMC, first medical contact; GPI, glycoprotein IIb/IIIa inhibitor; IV, intravenous; MI, myocardial infarction; NTG, nitroglycerin; PCI, percutaneous coronary intervention; SC, subcutaneous; SL, sublingual; UFH, unfractionated heparin.)

FIGURE 5–2. Initial pharmacotherapy for ST-segment elevation myocardial infarction. (Reproduced with permission from Rogers KC, de Denus S, Finks SW. Acute Coronary Syndromes. In: Chisholm-Burns MA, et al, eds. *Pharmacotherapy: Principles and Practice.* 4th ed. New York: McGraw-Hill; 2016:111-136.)

a 1-mm STE in two or more contiguous ECG leads, have no absolute contraindications to fibrinolytic therapy and cannot be transferred and undergo primary PCI within 120 minutes of medical contact. Fibrinolytic use between 12 and 24 hours after symptom onset should be limited to patients with ongoing ischemia.

- It is not necessary to obtain the troponin result before initiating fibrinolytic therapy.
- Contraindications to fibrinolytic therapy include: any prior intracranial hemorrhage, known structural cerebrovascular lesion (eg, AV malformation), known intracranial neoplasm, ischemic stroke within 3 months, active bleeding (excluding menses), and significant closed head or facial trauma within 3 months. Primary PCI is preferred in these situations.

- A fibrin-specific agent (alteplase, reteplase, or tenecteplase) is preferred over the non–fibrin-specific agent streptokinase.
- Treat eligible patients as soon as possible, but preferably within 30 minutes from the time they present to the emergency department, with one of the following regimens:
  - ✓ **Alteplase:** 15-mg intravenous (IV) bolus followed by 0.75 mg/kg infusion (maximum 50 mg) over 30 minutes, followed by 0.5 mg/kg infusion (maximum 35 mg) over 60 minutes (maximum dose 100 mg)
  - ✓ **Reteplase:** 10 units IV over 2 minutes, followed 30 minutes later with another 10 units IV over 2 minutes
  - ✓ **Tenecteplase:** A single IV bolus dose given over 5 seconds based on patient weight: 30 mg if less than 60 kg; 35 mg if 60 to 69.9 kg; 40 mg if 70 to 79.9 kg; 45 mg if 80 to 89.9 kg; and 50 mg if 90 kg or greater
  - ✓ **Streptokinase:** 1.5 million units in 50 mL of normal saline or 5% dextrose in water IV over 60 minutes
- Intracranial hemorrhage (ICH) and major bleeding are the most serious side effects of fibrinolytics. The risk of ICH is higher with fibrin-specific agents than with streptokinase. However, the risk of systemic bleeding other than ICH is higher with streptokinase than with fibrin-specific agents.

Aspirin

- Administer **aspirin** to all patients without contraindications within 24 hours before or after hospital arrival. It provides additional mortality benefit in patients receiving fibrinolytic therapy.
- Give non–enteric-coated aspirin (which may be chewed for more rapid effect) 162 to 325 mg regardless of the reperfusion strategy being considered. Patients undergoing PCI not previously taking aspirin should receive 325-mg non–enteric-coated aspirin.
- A daily maintenance dose of 75 to 162 mg is recommended thereafter and should be continued indefinitely. Because of increased bleeding risk in patients receiving aspirin plus a $P2Y_{12}$ inhibitor, low-dose aspirin (81 mg daily) is preferred following PCI.
- Discontinue other nonsteroidal anti-inflammatory drugs (NSAIDs) and cyclooxygenase-2 (COX-2) selective inhibitors at the time of STEMI due to increased risk of death, reinfarction, HF, and myocardial rupture.
- The most frequent side effects of aspirin include dyspepsia and nausea. Inform patients about the risk of GI bleeding.

Platelet $P2Y_{12}$ Inhibitors

- Clopidogrel, prasugrel, and ticagrelor are oral agents that block a subtype of ADP receptor (the $P2Y_{12}$ receptor) on platelets, preventing binding of ADP to the receptor and subsequent expression of platelet GP IIb/IIIa receptors, reducing platelet aggregation. Doses are as follows:
  - ✓ **Clopidogrel:** 300-mg oral loading dose followed by 75 mg orally daily in patients receiving a fibrinolytic or who do not receive reperfusion therapy. Avoid loading dose in patients aged 75 years or more. A 600-mg oral loading dose is recommended before primary PCI, except that 300 mg should be given if within 24 hours of fibrinolytic therapy.
  - ✓ **Prasugrel:** 60-mg oral loading dose followed by 10 mg orally once daily for patients weighing 60 kg (132 lb) or more. Consider 5 mg once daily for patients weighing less than 60 kg.
  - ✓ **Ticagrelor:** 180-mg oral loading dose in patients undergoing PCI, followed by 90 mg orally twice daily.
- **Cangrelor** is an IV drug indicated as an adjunct to PCI to reduce periprocedural MI, repeat revascularization, and stent thrombosis in patients not receiving oral $P2Y_{12}$ inhibitors or planned GPIs. The dose is 30 mcg/kg IV bolus prior to PCI followed by 4 mcg/kg/min infusion for duration of PCI or 2 hours, whichever is longer.

- A P2Y$_{12}$ receptor inhibitor in addition to aspirin is recommended for all patients with STEMI. For patients undergoing primary PCI, clopidogrel, prasugrel, ticagrelor, or IV cangrelor should be given in addition to aspirin to prevent subacute stent thrombosis and longer-term CV events.
- The recommended duration of P2Y$_{12}$ inhibitors for a patient undergoing PCI (either STEMI or NSTE-ACS) is at least 12 months for patients receiving either a bare metal or drug-eluting stent.
- If elective CABG surgery is planned, withhold clopidogrel and ticagrelor for 5 days prior, and prasugrel at least 7 days prior, to reduce risk of postoperative bleeding, unless the need for revascularization outweighs the bleeding risk. The hold time for urgent surgery is 24 hours.
- The most frequent side effects of clopidogrel and prasugrel are nausea, vomiting, and diarrhea, (2%–5% of patients). Clopidogrel hypersensitivity (usually a rash) develops in up to 6% of patients. Thrombotic thrombocytopenic purpura has been reported rarely with clopidogrel. Ticagrelor is associated with nausea (4%), diarrhea (3%), dyspnea (up to 19%), and, rarely, ventricular pauses, and bradyarrhythmias.
- In STEMI patients receiving fibrinolysis, early therapy with clopidogrel 75 mg once daily during hospitalization and up to 28 days reduces mortality and reinfarction without increasing risk of major bleeding. In adults younger than 75 years receiving fibrinolytics, the first dose of clopidogrel can be a 300-mg loading dose.
- For patients with STEMI who do not undergo reperfusion therapy with either primary PCI or fibrinolysis, clopidogrel (added to aspirin) is the preferred P2Y$_{12}$ inhibitor and should be continued for at least 14 days (and up to 1 year). Ticagrelor may also be an option in medically managed patients with ACS not receiving fibrinolytics.

Glycoprotein IIb/IIIa Receptor Inhibitors

- GPIs block the final common pathway of platelet aggregation, namely, cross-linking of platelets by fibrinogen bridges between the GP IIb and IIIa receptors on the platelet surface.
- Abciximab (IV or intracoronary administration), eptifibatide, or tirofiban may be administered in patients with STEMI undergoing primary PCI who are treated with UFH. Do not administer GPIs to patients with STEMI who will not be undergoing PCI.
- **Abciximab:** 0.25-mg/kg IV bolus given 10 to 60 minutes before the start of PCI, followed by 0.125 mcg/kg/min (maximum 10 mcg/min) for 12 hours.
- **Eptifibatide:** 180-mcg/kg IV bolus, repeated in 10 minutes, followed by infusion of 2 mcg/kg/min for 18 to 24 hours after PCI.
- **Tirofiban:** 25-mcg/kg IV bolus, then 0.15 mcg/kg/min up to 18 to 24 hours after PCI.
- Routine use of a GPI is not recommended in patients who have received fibrinolytics or in those receiving bivalirudin because of increased bleeding risk.
- Bleeding is the most significant adverse effect of GPIs. Do not use GPIs in patients with a history of hemorrhagic stroke or recent ischemic stroke. Risk of bleeding is increased in patients with chronic kidney disease; reduce the dose of eptifibatide and tirofiban in renal impairment. An immune-mediated thrombocytopenia occurs in approximately 5% of patients with abciximab and fewer than 2% of patients receiving eptifibatide or tirofiban.

Anticoagulants

- Either UFH or bivalirudin is preferred for patients undergoing primary PCI, whereas for fibrinolysis, either UFH, enoxaparin, or fondaparinux may be used.
- **UFH** initial dose for primary PCI is 50 to 70 units/kg IV bolus if a GPI is planned and 70 to 100 units IV bolus if no GPI is planned; give supplemental IV bolus doses to maintain the target activated clotting time. UFH initial dose with fibrinolytics is 60 units IV bolus (maximum 4000 units), followed by constant IV infusion of 12 units/kg/h (maximum 1000 units/h). Titrate to maintain a target activated partial

thromboplastin time (aPTT) of 1.5 to 2 times control (50–70 seconds) for STE-ACS with fibrinolytics. Measure the first aPTT at 3 hours in patients with STE-ACS who are treated with fibrinolytics and at 4 to 6 hours in patients not receiving thrombolytics or undergoing primary PCI. Continue for 48 hours or until the end of PCI.

- **Enoxaparin** dose is 1 mg/kg subcutaneous (SC) every 12 hours (creatinine clearance $[Cl_{cr}] \geq 30$ mL/min) or once every 24 hours if impaired renal function (Cl_{cr} 15–29 mL/min). For patients with STEMI receiving fibrinolytics, enoxaparin 30-mg IV bolus is followed immediately by 1 mg/kg SC every 12 hours if younger than 75 years. In patients 75 years and older, give enoxaparin 0.75 mg/kg SC every 12 hours. Continue enoxaparin throughout hospitalization or up to 8 days.
- **Bivalirudin** dose for PCI in STEMI is 0.75 mg/kg IV bolus, followed by 1.75 mg/kg/h infusion. Discontinue at the end of PCI or continue at 0.25 mg/kg/h if prolonged anticoagulation is necessary.
- **Fondaparinux** dose is 2.5 mg IV bolus followed by 2.5 mg SC once daily starting on hospital day 2.
- For patients undergoing PCI, discontinue anticoagulation immediately after the procedure. In patients receiving an anticoagulant plus a fibrinolytic, continue UFH for a minimum of 48 hours and enoxaparin and fondaparinux for the duration of hospitalization, up to 8 days. In patients who do not undergo reperfusion therapy, anticoagulant therapy may be administered for up to 48 hours for UFH or for the duration of hospitalization for enoxaparin or fondaparinux.

β-Adrenergic Blockers

- Benefits result from blockade of β_1 receptors in the myocardium, which reduces heart rate, myocardial contractility, and BP, thereby decreasing myocardial oxygen demand. Reduced heart rate increases diastolic time, thus improving ventricular filling and coronary artery perfusion.
- β-Blockers reduce risk for recurrent ischemia, infarct size, reinfarction, and ventricular arrhythmias in the hours and days after an MI.
- Because of an early risk of cardiogenic shock in susceptible patients, β-blockers (particularly when given IV) should be limited to patients who present with hypertension or signs of myocardial ischemia and do not have signs or symptoms of acute HF. Patients already taking β-blockers can continue taking them.
- Usual doses of β-blockers, with target resting heart rate of 50 to 60 beats/min:
  ✓ **Metoprolol:** 5 mg by slow (over 1–2 minutes) IV bolus, repeated every 5 minutes for total initial dose of 15 mg, followed in 1 to 2 hours by 25 to 50 mg orally every 6 hours. If a very conservative regimen is desired, reduce initial doses to 1 to 2 mg. If appropriate, initial IV therapy may be omitted and treatment started with oral dosing.
  ✓ **Propranolol:** 0.5- to 1-mg slow IV push, followed in 1 to 2 hours by 40 to 80 mg orally every 6 to 8 hours. If appropriate, the initial IV therapy may be omitted.
  ✓ **Atenolol:** 5 mg IV dose, followed 5 minutes later by a second 5 mg IV dose, then 50 to 100 mg orally once daily beginning 1 to 2 hours after the IV dose. The initial IV therapy may be omitted.
- The most serious side effects early in ACS include hypotension, acute HF, bradycardia, and heart block. Initial acute administration of β-blockers is not appropriate for patients presenting with acute HF but may be attempted in most patients before discharge after treatment of acute HF.
- Continue β-blockers for at least 3 years in patients with normal LV function and indefinitely in patients with LV systolic dysfunction and LVEF of 40% or less.

Statins

- Administer a high-intensity statin (**atorvastatin** 80 mg or **rosuvastatin** 40 mg) to all patients prior to PCI (regardless of prior lipid-lowering therapy) to reduce the frequency of periprocedural MI (Type IVa MI) following PCI.

Nitrates

- NTG causes venodilation, which lowers preload and myocardial oxygen demand. In addition, arterial vasodilation may lower BP, thereby reducing myocardial oxygen demand. Arterial dilation also relieves coronary artery vasospasm and improves myocardial blood flow and oxygenation.
- Immediately upon presentation, administer one **SL NTG** tablet (0.4 mg) every 5 minutes for up to three doses to relieve chest pain and myocardial ischemia.
- **Intravenous NTG** is indicated for patients with an ACS who do not have a contra-indication and who have persistent ischemic discomfort, HF, or uncontrolled high BP. The usual dose is 5 to 10 mcg/min by continuous infusion, titrated up to 75 to 100 mcg/min until relief of symptoms or limiting side effects (eg, headache or hypotension). Discontinue IV infusion after 24 to 48 hours.
- Oral nitrates play a limited role in ACS because clinical trials have failed to show a mortality benefit for IV followed by oral nitrate therapy in acute MI.
- The most significant adverse effects of nitrates include tachycardia, flushing, head-ache, and hypotension. Nitrates are contraindicated in patients who have taken the oral phosphodiesterase-5 inhibitors sildenafil or vardenafil within the prior 24 hours or tadalafil within the prior 48 hours.

Calcium Channel Blockers

- After STEMI, calcium channel blockers (CCBs) are used for relief of ischemic symp-toms in patients who have contraindications to β-blockers. There is little clinical benefit beyond symptom relief, so avoid CCBs in acute management of ACS unless there is a clear symptomatic need or contraindication to β-blockers.
- A CCB that lowers heart rate (diltiazem or verapamil) is preferred unless the patient has LV systolic dysfunction, bradycardia, or heart block. In those cases, either amlo-dipine or felodipine is preferred. Avoid nifedipine because it causes reflex sympa-thetic activation, tachycardia, and worsened myocardial ischemia.
  - ✓ **Diltiazem:** 120 to 360 mg sustained release orally once daily
  - ✓ **Verapamil:** 180 to 480 mg sustained release orally once daily
  - ✓ **Amlodipine:** 5 to 10 mg orally once daily

EARLY PHARMACOTHERAPY FOR NSTE-ACS (FIG. 5–3)

- Early pharmacotherapy for NSTE-ACS is similar to that for STEMI.
- In absence of contraindications, treat all patients in the emergency department with intranasal oxygen (if oxygen saturation is low), SL NTG, aspirin, and an anticoagu-lant (UFH, enoxaparin, fondaparinux, or bivalirudin).
- High-risk patients should proceed to early angiography and may receive a GPI (optional with either UFH or enoxaparin but should be avoided with bivalirudin).
- Administer a $P2Y_{12}$ inhibitor to all patients; choice and timing depend on the inter-ventional approach selected.
- Give IV β-blockers and IV NTG to select patients.
- Initiate oral β-blockers within the first 24 hours in patients without cardiogenic shock.
- Give morphine to patients with refractory angina, as described previously.
- Never administer fibrinolytic therapy in NSTE-ACS.

Aspirin

- **Aspirin** reduces risk of death or MI by approximately 50% compared with no anti-platelet therapy in patients with NSTE-ACS. Dosing of aspirin is the same as for STE-ACS, and aspirin is continued indefinitely.

Anticoagulants

- For patients treated by an early invasive approach with early coronary angiography and PCI, administer **UFH**, **enoxaparin**, **fondaparinux**, or **bivalirudin**.

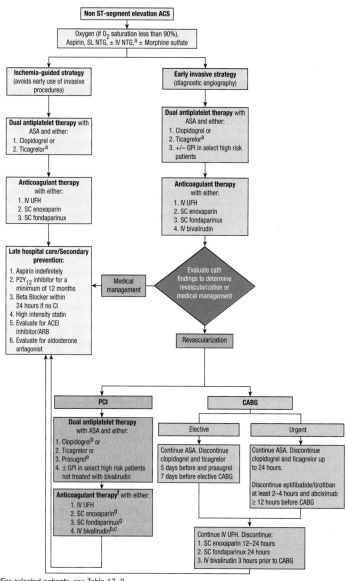

Non ST-segment elevation ACS

Oxygen (if O_2 saturation less than 90%),
Aspirin, SL NTG, ± IV NTG,[a] ± Morphine sulfate

Ischemia-guided strategy
(avoids early use of invasive
procedures)

Early invasive strategy
(diagnostic angiography)

Dual antiplatelet therapy with
ASA and either:
1. Clopidogrel or
2. Ticagrelor[a]

Dual antiplatelet therapy with
ASA and either:
1. Clopidogrel or
2. Ticagrelor[a]
3. +/– GPI in select high risk
patients

Anticoagulant therapy
with either:
1. IV UFH
2. SC enoxaparin
3. SC fondaparinux

Anticoagulant therapy
with either:
1. IV UFH
2. SC enoxaparin
3. SC fondaparinux
4. IV bivalirudin

**Late hospital care/Secondary
prevention:**
1. Aspirin indefinitely
2. P2Y$_{12}$ inhibitor for a
minimum of 12 months
3. Beta Blocker within
24 hours if no CI
4. High intensity statin
5. Evaluate for ACEI
inhibitor/ARB
6. Evaluate for aldosterone
antagonist

Medical
management

Evaluate cath
findings to determine
revascularization or
medical management

Revascularization

PCI

Dual antiplatelet therapy
with ASA and either:
1. Clopidogrel[b] or
2. Ticagrelor or
3. Prasugrel[e]
4. ± GPI in select high risk patients
not treated with bivalirudin

Anticoagulant therapy[f] with either:
1. IV UFH
2. SC enoxaparin[d]
3. SC fondaparinux[g]
4. IV bivalirudin[b,c]

CABG

Elective

Continue ASA. Discontinue
clopidogrel and ticagrelor
5 days before and prasugrel
7 days before elective CABG

Urgent

Continue ASA. Discontinue
clopidogrel and ticagrelor up
to 24 hours.

Discontinue eptifibatide/tirofiban
at least 2–4 hours and abciximab
≥ 12 hours before CABG

Continue IV UFH. Discontinue:
1. SC enoxaparin 12–24 hours
2. SC fondaparinux 24 hours
3. IV bivalirudin 3 hours prior to CABG

[a]For selected patients, see Table 17–2.
[b]Preferred in patients at high risk for bleeding.
[c]If pretreated with UFH, stop UFH infusion for 30 minutes prior to administration of bivalirudin bolus plus infusion.
[d]May require IV supplemental dose of enoxaparin; see textbook Table 17–2.
[e]Do not use if prior history of stroke/transient ischemic attack (TIA), age older than 75 years, or body weight less than or equal to 60 kg.
[f]SC enoxaparin or UFH can be continued at a lower dose for venous thromboembolism prophylaxis.

(ACE, angiotensin-converting enzyme; ACS, acute coronary syndrome; ARB, angiotensin receptor blocker; CABG, coronary artery bypass graft; CAD, coronary artery disease; CHD, coronary heart disease; GP, glycoprotein; NTG, nitroglycerin; PCI, percutaneous coronary intervention; SC, subcutaneous; SL, sublingual; UFH, unfractionated heparin.)

FIGURE 5–3. Initial pharmacotherapy for non–ST-segment elevation ACS. (Reproduced with permission from Rogers KC, de Denus S, Finks SW. Acute Coronary Syndromes. In: Chisholm-Burns MA, et al, eds. *Pharmacotherapy: Principles and Practice.* 4th ed. New York: McGraw-Hill; 2016:111-136.)

- If an initial ischemia-guided strategy is planned (no coronary angiography or revascularization), enoxaparin, UFH, or low-dose fondaparinux is recommended.
- Continue therapy for at least 48 hours for UFH, until the patient is discharged from the hospital (or 8 days, whichever is shorter) for either enoxaparin or fondaparinux, and until the end of the PCI or angiography procedure (or up to 72 hours after PCI) for bivalirudin.
- For NSTE-ACS, the dose of UFH is 60 units IV bolus (maximum 4000 units), followed by a continuous IV infusion of 12 units/kg/h (maximum 1000 units/h). Titrate the dose to maintain aPTT between 1.5 and 2 times control.

P2Y$_{12}$ Inhibitors

- A P2Y$_{12}$ receptor inhibitor (plus aspirin) is recommended for most patients with NSTE-ACS. They are the preferred antiplatelet agents because of efficacy and ease of use, resulting in decreased use of IV antiplatelet agents such as GPIs.
- With an ischemia-guided approach, either **ticagrelor** (preferred) or **clopidogrel** (300–600 mg loading dose followed by 75 mg daily) can be used with low-dose aspirin and continued for up to 12 months.
- If an invasive management strategy is selected, either ticagrelor (preferred) or clopidogrel can be used either prehospital or in the ED. After PCI in patients not already treated with a P2Y$_{12}$ inhibitor, clopidogrel, prasugrel or ticagrelor can be used and should be initiated at the time of or within 1 hour after PCI and continued for at least 12 months.
- Following PCI, continue dual oral antiplatelet therapy for at least 12 months.
- For patients receiving an initial conservative strategy, either clopidogrel or ticagrelor can be administered in addition to aspirin. Continue dual antiplatelet therapy for at least 12 months.

Glycoprotein IIb/IIIa Receptor Inhibitors

- The role of GPIs in NSTE-ACS is diminishing as P2Y$_{12}$ inhibitors are used earlier, and **bivalirudin** is often selected for early interventional approaches.
- Routine administration of **eptifibatide** (added to aspirin and clopidogrel) prior to angiography and PCI in NSTE-ACS does not reduce ischemic events and increases bleeding risk. Therefore, the two antiplatelet initial therapy options described in the previous section are preferred.
- For low-risk patients receiving a conservative management strategy, there is no role for routine GPIs because bleeding risk exceeds the benefit.

Nitrates

- Administer **SL NTG** followed by **IV NTG** to patients with NSTE-ACS and ongoing ischemia, HF, or uncontrolled high BP. Continue IV NTG for approximately 24 hours after ischemia relief.

β-Blockers

- In the absence of contraindications, administer oral β-blockers to patients with NSTE-ACS within 24 hours of hospital admission. Benefits are assumed to be similar to those seen in patients with STEMI.
- Continue β-blockers indefinitely in patients with LVEF of 40% or less and for at least 3 years in patients with normal LV function.

Calcium Channel Blockers

- As for STE-ACS, CCBs should be limited to patients with certain contraindications to β-blockers and those with continued ischemia despite β-blocker and nitrate therapy.
- **Diltiazem** and **verapamil** are preferred unless the patient has LV dysfunction, bradycardia, or heart block; **amlodipine** or **felodipine** is preferred in those situations. Immediate-release nifedipine is contraindicated.

SECONDARY PREVENTION FOLLOWING MI

- <u>Goals of Treatment</u>: The long-term goals after MI are to: (1) control modifiable coronary heart disease (CHD) risk factors; (2) prevent development of systolic HF; (3) prevent recurrent MI and stroke; (4) prevent death, including sudden cardiac death; and (5) prevent stent thrombosis after PCI.

PHARMACOTHERAPY

- For all ACS patients, treat and control modifiable risk factors such as hypertension, dyslipidemia, obesity, smoking, and diabetes mellitus (DM).
- Start pharmacotherapy that has been proven to decrease mortality, HF, reinfarction or stroke, and stent thrombosis prior to hospital discharge for secondary prevention.
- After an ACS, all patients (in the absence of contraindications) should receive indefinite treatment with **aspirin** (or **clopidogrel** if aspirin contraindications), an ACE inhibitor, and a high-intensity statin for secondary prevention of death, stroke, or recurrent infarction.
- Chronic aspirin doses should not exceed 81 mg/day.
- Start an oral ACE inhibitor early (within 24 hours) and continue indefinitely in all patients after MI to reduce mortality, decrease reinfarction, and prevent HF. Use a low initial dose and titrate to the dose used in clinical trials if tolerated. For example:
  - ✓ **Captopril:** 6.25 to 12.5 mg initially; target dose 50 mg two or three times daily
  - ✓ **Enalapril:** 2.5 to 5 mg initially; target dose 10 mg twice daily
  - ✓ **Lisinopril:** 2.5 to 5 mg initially; target dose 10 to 20 mg once daily
  - ✓ **Ramipril:** 1.25 to 2.5 mg initially; target dose 5 mg twice daily or 10 mg once daily
  - ✓ **Trandolapril:** 1 mg initially; target dose 4 mg once daily
- An angiotensin receptor blocker may be prescribed for patients with ACE inhibitor cough and a low LVEF and HF after MI:
  - ✓ **Candesartan:** 4 to 8 mg initially; target dose 32 mg once daily
  - ✓ **Valsartan:** 40 mg initially; target dose 160 mg twice daily
  - ✓ **Losartan:** 12.5 to 25 mg initially; target dose 100 mg once daily
- All patients, regardless of LDL-cholesterol level, should ideally be prescribed a high-intensity statin. Patients over 75 years of age may be prescribed a moderate-intensity statin.
- Continue a β-blocker for at least 3 years in patients with normal LV function and indefinitely in patients with LVEF of 40% or less.
- A CCB can be used to prevent anginal symptoms in patients who cannot tolerate or have contraindications to β-blockers but should not be used routinely in the absence of such findings.
- Continue a P2Y$_{12}$ inhibitor for at least 1 year in most patients with STEMI or NSTE-ACS. For patients with STEMI managed with fibrinolytics, continue clopidogrel for at least 14 days and ideally 1 year. New guidelines indicate that it is reasonable to continue dual antiplatelet therapy after 12 months in patients with STEMI and NSTE-ACS who were medically treated, who received fibrinolytics, or who had a PCI if they are not at high risk of bleeding and have not had overt bleeding.
- To reduce mortality, consider an aldosterone antagonist (eplerenone or spironolactone) within the first 7 days after MI in all patients already receiving an ACE inhibitor (or angiotensin receptor blocker) and a β-blocker and have an LVEF of 40% or less and either HF symptoms or DM. The drugs are continued indefinitely.
  - ✓ **Eplerenone:** 25 mg initially; target dose 50 mg once daily
  - ✓ **Spironolactone:** 12.5 mg initially; target dose 25 to 50 mg once daily
- Prescribe a short-acting SL NTG or lingual NTG spray for all patients to relieve anginal symptoms when necessary. Chronic long-acting nitrates have not been shown to reduce CHD events after MI and are not used in ACS patients who have undergone revascularization unless the patient has stable ischemic heart disease or significant coronary stenoses that were not revascularized.

EVALUATION OF THERAPEUTIC OUTCOMES

- Monitoring parameters for efficacy for both STEMI and NSTE-ACS include: (1) relief of ischemic discomfort, (2) return of ECG changes to baseline, and (3) absence or resolution of HF signs and symptoms.
- Monitoring parameters for adverse effects are dependent on the individual drugs used. In general, the most common adverse reactions from ACS therapies include hypotension and bleeding.

See Chapter 17, Acute Coronary Syndromes, authored by Kelly C. Rogers, Simon de Denus, Shannon W. Finks, and Sarah A. Spinler for a more detailed discussion of this topic.

6 Arrhythmias

- *Arrhythmia* is loss of cardiac rhythm, especially irregularity of heartbeat.

PATHOPHYSIOLOGY

SUPRAVENTRICULAR ARRHYTHMIAS

- Common supraventricular tachycardias requiring drug treatment are atrial fibrillation (AF), atrial flutter, and paroxysmal supraventricular tachycardia (PSVT). Other arrhythmias that usually do not require drug therapy are not discussed here (eg, premature atrial complexes, sinus arrhythmia, and sinus tachycardia).

Atrial Fibrillation and Atrial Flutter

- AF has extremely rapid (400–600 atrial beats/min) and disorganized atrial activation. There is loss of atrial contraction (atrial kick), and supraventricular impulses penetrate the atrioventricular (AV) conduction system to variable degrees, resulting in irregular ventricular activation and irregularly irregular pulse (120–180 beats/min).
- Atrial flutter has rapid (270–330 atrial beats/min) but regular atrial activation. Ventricular response usually has a regular pattern and a pulse of 300 beats/min. This arrhythmia occurs less frequently than AF but has similar precipitating factors, consequences, and drug therapy.
- The predominant mechanism of AF and atrial flutter is reentry, which is usually associated with organic heart disease that causes left atrial distention (eg, ischemia or infarction, hypertensive heart disease, and valvular disorders). Additional associated disorders include acute pulmonary embolus and chronic lung disease, resulting in pulmonary hypertension and cor pulmonale, and states of high adrenergic tone such as thyrotoxicosis, alcohol withdrawal, sepsis, and excessive physical exertion.

Paroxysmal Supraventricular Tachycardia Caused by Reentry

- PSVT arising by reentrant mechanisms includes arrhythmias caused by AV nodal reentry, AV reentry incorporating an anomalous AV pathway, sinoatrial (SA) nodal reentry, and intraatrial reentry.

VENTRICULAR ARRHYTHMIAS

Premature Ventricular Complexes

- Premature ventricular complexes (PVCs) can occur in patients with or without heart disease.

Ventricular Tachycardia

- Ventricular tachycardia (VT) is defined by three or more repetitive PVCs occurring at a rate greater than 100 beats/min. It is a wide QRS tachycardia that may result acutely from severe electrolyte abnormalities (hypokalemia or hypomagnesemia), hypoxia, drug toxicity (eg, digoxin), or (most commonly) during an acute myocardial infarction (MI) or ischemia complicated by heart failure (HF). The chronic recurrent form is almost always associated with organic heart disease (eg, idiopathic dilated cardiomyopathy or remote MI with left ventricular [LV] aneurysm).
- Sustained VT is that which requires intervention to restore a stable rhythm or persists a relatively long time (usually >30 s). Nonsustained VT self-terminates after a brief duration (usually <30 s). *Incessant VT* refers to VT occurring more frequently than sinus rhythm, so that VT becomes the dominant rhythm. Monomorphic VT has a consistent QRS configuration, whereas polymorphic VT has varying QRS complexes. TdP is a polymorphic VT in which the QRS complexes appear to undulate around a central axis.

Ventricular Proarrhythmia

- *Proarrhythmia* refers to the development of a significant new arrhythmia, such as VT, ventricular fibrillation (VF), or TdP, or worsening of an existing arrhythmia. Proarrhythmia results from the same mechanisms that cause other arrhythmias or from an alteration in the underlying substrate due to the antiarrhythmic agent. TdP is a rapid form of polymorphic VT associated with evidence of delayed ventricular repolarization due to blockade of potassium conductance. TdP may be hereditary or acquired. Acquired forms are associated with many clinical conditions and drugs, especially class Ia and class III I_{Kr} blockers.

Ventricular Fibrillation

- VF is electrical anarchy of the ventricle resulting in no cardiac output and cardiovascular collapse. Sudden cardiac death occurs most commonly in patients with coronary artery disease and those with LV dysfunction. VF associated with acute MI may be classified as either (1) primary (an uncomplicated MI not associated with HF) or (2) secondary or complicated (an MI complicated by HF).

BRADYARRHYTHMIAS

- Sinus bradyarrhythmias (heart rate <60 beats/min) are common, especially in young, athletically active individuals, and are usually asymptomatic and do not require intervention. However, some patients have sinus node dysfunction (sick sinus syndrome) because of underlying structural heart disease (SHD) and the normal aging process, which attenuates SA nodal function. Sinus node dysfunction is usually representative of diffuse conduction disease, which may be accompanied by AV block and by paroxysmal tachycardias such as AF. Alternating bradyarrhythmias and tachyarrhythmias are referred to as the tachy–brady syndrome.
- AV block or conduction delay may occur in any area of the AV conduction system. AV block may be found in patients without underlying heart disease (eg, trained athletes) or during sleep when vagal tone is high. It may be transient when the underlying etiology is reversible (eg, myocarditis, myocardial ischemia, after cardiovascular surgery, or during drug therapy). β-Blockers, digoxin, or nondihydropyridine calcium blockers (CCBs) may cause AV block, primarily in the AV nodal area. Class I antiarrhythmics may exacerbate conduction delays below the level of the AV node. AV block may be irreversible if the cause is acute MI, rare degenerative diseases, primary myocardial disease, or congenital heart disease.

CLINICAL PRESENTATION

- Supraventricular tachycardias may cause clinical manifestations ranging from no symptoms to minor palpitations or irregular pulse to severe and even life-threatening symptoms. Patients may experience dizziness or acute syncopal episodes, symptoms of HF, anginal chest pain, or, more often, a choking or pressure sensation during the tachycardia episode.
- AF or atrial flutter may be manifested by the entire range of symptoms associated with other supraventricular tachycardias, but syncope is uncommon. Arterial embolization from atrial stasis and poorly adherent mural thrombi may result in embolic stroke.
- PVCs often cause no symptoms or only mild palpitations. The presentation of VT may vary from totally asymptomatic to pulseless hemodynamic collapse. Consequences of proarrhythmia range from no symptoms to worsening of symptoms to sudden death. VF results in hemodynamic collapse, syncope, and cardiac arrest.
- Patients with bradyarrhythmias experience symptoms associated with hypotension, such as dizziness, syncope, fatigue, and confusion. If LV dysfunction exists, patients may experience worsening HF symptoms.

DIAGNOSIS

- Electrocardiogram (ECG) is the cornerstone of diagnosis for cardiac rhythm disturbances.
- Cardiac auscultation can reveal the irregularly irregular pulse characteristic of AF.

- Proarrhythmia can be difficult to diagnose because of the variable nature of underlying arrhythmias.
- TdP is characterized by long QT intervals or prominent U waves on the surface ECG.
- Specific maneuvers may be required to delineate the etiology of syncope associated with bradyarrhythmias. Diagnosis of carotid sinus hypersensitivity can be confirmed by performing carotid sinus massage with ECG and blood pressure monitoring. Vasovagal syncope can be diagnosed using the upright body-tilt test.
- Based on ECG findings, AV block is usually categorized as first-, second-, or third-degree AV block.

TREATMENT

- <u>Goals of Treatment</u>: The desired outcome depends on the underlying arrhythmia. For example, the goals of treating AF or atrial flutter are restoring sinus rhythm, preventing thromboembolic complications, and preventing further recurrences.

GENERAL APPROACH

- Use of antiarrhythmic drugs has declined because major trials showed increased mortality with use in several situations, the realization of proarrhythmia as a significant side effect, and the advancing technology of nondrug therapies, such as ablation and the implantable cardioverter-defibrillator (ICD).

CLASSIFICATION OF ANTIARRHYTHMIC DRUGS

- Drugs may depress the automatic properties of abnormal pacemaker cells by decreasing the slope of phase 4 depolarization and/or by elevating threshold potential. Drugs may alter conduction characteristics of the pathways of a reentrant loop.
- The Vaughan Williams classification is most frequently used (**Table 6–1**). Class Ia drugs slow conduction velocity, prolong refractoriness, and decrease the automatic properties of sodium-dependent (normal and diseased) conduction tissue. Class Ia drugs are effective for both supraventricular and ventricular arrhythmias.

TABLE 6–1 Classification of Antiarrhythmic Drugs

Class	Drug	Conduction Velocity[a]	Refractory Period	Automaticity	Ion Block
Ia	Quinidine Procainamide Disopyramide	↓	↑	↓	Sodium (intermediate) Potassium
Ib	Lidocaine Mexiletine	0/↓	↓	↓	Sodium (fast on–off)
Ic	Flecainide Propafenone[b]	↓↓	0	↓	Sodium (slow on–off)
II[c]	β-Blockers	↓	↑	↓	Calcium (indirect)
III	Amiodarone[d] Dofetilide Dronedarone[d] Sotalol[b] Ibutilide	0	↑↑	0	Potassium
IV[c]	Verapamil Diltiazem	↓	↑	↓	Calcium

0, no change; ↑, increased; ↓, decreased.
[a]Variables for normal tissue models in ventricular tissue.
[b]Also has β-blocking actions.
[c]Variables for sinoatrial (SA) and atrioventricular (AV) nodal tissue only.
[d]Also has sodium, calcium, and β-blocking actions.

- Although categorized separately, class Ib drugs probably act similarly to class Ia drugs, except that class Ib agents are considerably more effective in ventricular than supraventricular arrhythmias.
- Class Ic drugs slow conduction velocity while leaving refractoriness relatively unaltered. Although effective for both ventricular and supraventricular arrhythmias, their use for ventricular arrhythmias has been limited by the risk of proarrhythmia.
- Class I drugs are sodium channel blockers. Antiarrhythmic sodium channel receptor principles account for drug combinations that are additive (eg, **quinidine** and **mexiletine**) and antagonistic (eg, **flecainide** and **lidocaine**) as well as potential antidotes to excess sodium channel blockade (sodium bicarbonate).
- Class II drugs include **β-adrenergic antagonists**; effects result from antiadrenergic actions. β-Blockers are most useful in tachycardias in which nodal tissues are abnormally automatic or are a portion of a reentrant loop. These agents are also helpful in slowing ventricular response in atrial tachycardias (eg, AF) by effects on the AV node.
- Class III drugs prolong refractoriness in atrial and ventricular tissue and include very different drugs that share the common effect of delaying repolarization by blocking potassium channels.
  ✓ **Amiodarone** and **sotalol** are effective in most supraventricular and VTs. Amiodarone displays electrophysiologic characteristics consistent with each type of antiarrhythmic drug. It is a sodium channel blocker with relatively fast on-off kinetics, has nonselective β-blocking actions, blocks potassium channels, and has slight calcium-blocking activity. Sotalol inhibits outward potassium movement during repolarization and also possesses nonselective β-blocking actions.
  ✓ **Dronedarone**, **ibutilide**, and **dofetilide** are indicated only for treatment of supraventricular arrhythmias.
- Class IV drugs inhibit calcium entry into cells, which slows conduction, prolongs refractoriness, and decreases SA and AV nodal automaticity. **Calcium channel antagonists** are effective for automatic or reentrant tachycardias that arise from or use the SA or AV nodes.
- See Table 6–2 for recommended doses of oral antiarrhythmic drugs, Table 6–3 for usual IV antiarrhythmic doses, and Table 6–4 for common side effects.

TABLE 6–2	Typical Maintenance Doses of Oral Antiarrhythmic Drugs	
Drug	**Dose**	**Dose Adjusted**
Disopyramide	100–150 mg every 6 hours 200–300 mg every 12 hours (SR form)	HEP, REN
Quinidine	200–300 mg sulfate salt every 6 hours 324–648 gluconate salt every 8–12 hours	HEP
Mexiletine	200–300 mg every 8 hours	HEP
Flecainide	50–200 mg every 12 hours	HEP, REN
Propafenone	150–300 mg every 8 hours 225–425 mg every 12 hours (SR form)	HEP
Amiodarone	400 mg 2 or 3 times daily until 10 g total, and then 200–400 mg daily[a]	
Dofetilide	500 mcg every 12 hours	REN[b]
Dronedarone	400 mg twice daily (with meals)[c]	
Sotalol	80–160 mg every 12 hours	REN[d]

HEP, hepatic disease; REN, renal impairment; SR, sustained release.
[a]Usual maintenance dose for atrial fibrillation is 200 mg/day (may further decrease dose to 100 mg/day with long-term use if patient clinically stable in order to decrease risk of toxicity); usual maintenance dose for ventricular arrhythmias is 300–400 mg/day.
[b]Dose should be based on creatinine clearance; should not be used when creatinine clearance <20 mL/min.
[c]Should not be used in severe hepatic impairment.
[d]Should not be used for atrial fibrillation when creatinine clearance <40 mL/min.

TABLE 6–3	Intravenous Antiarrhythmic Dosing	
Drug	**Clinical Situation**	**Dose**
Amiodarone	Pulseless VT/VF	300 mg IV/IO push (can give additional 150 mg IV/IO push if persistent VT/VF or if VT/VF recurs), followed by infusion of 1 mg/min for 6 hours, and then 0.5 mg/min
	Stable VT (with a pulse)	150 mg IV over 10 min, followed by infusion of 1 mg/min for 6 hours, and then 0.5 mg/min
	AF (termination)	5 mg/kg IV over 30 min, followed by infusion of 1 mg/min for 6 hours, and then 0.5 mg/min
Diltiazem	PSVT; AF (rate control)	0.25 mg/kg IV over 2 min (may repeat with 0.35 mg/kg IV over 2 min), followed by infusion of 5–15 mg/h
Ibutilide	AF (termination)	1 mg IV over 10 min (may repeat if needed)
Lidocaine	Pulseless VT/VF	1–1.5 mg/kg IV/IO push (can give additional 0.5–0.75 mg/kg IV/IO push every 5–10 min if persistent VT/VF [maximum cumulative dose = 3 mg/kg]), followed by infusion of 1–4 mg/min (1–2 mg/min if liver disease or HF)
	Stable VT (with a pulse)	1–1.5 mg/kg IV push (can give additional 0.5–0.75 mg/kg IV push every 5–10 min if persistent VT [maximum cumulative dose = 3 mg/kg]), followed by infusion of 1–4 mg/min (1–2 mg/min if liver disease or HF)
Procainamide	AF (termination); stable VT (with a pulse)	15–18 mg/kg IV over 60 min, followed by infusion of 1–4 mg/min
Verapamil	PSVT; AF (rate control)	2.5–5 mg IV over 2 min (may repeat up to maximum cumulative dose of 20 mg); can follow with infusion of 2.5–10 mg/h

(AF, atrial fibrillation; HF, heart failure; IO, intraosseous; IV, intravenous; PSVT, paroxysmal supraventricular tachycardia; VF, ventricular fibrillation; VT, ventricular tachycardia.)

ATRIAL FIBRILLATION OR ATRIAL FLUTTER

• Treatment of AF involves several sequential goals. First, evaluate need for acute treatment (usually with drugs that slow ventricular rate). Next, consider methods to restore sinus rhythm, considering risks involved (eg, thromboembolism). Lastly, consider ways to prevent long-term complications, such as recurrent arrhythmia and thromboembolism (Fig. 6–1).

• In patients with new-onset AF or atrial flutter with signs and/or symptoms of hemodynamic instability (eg, severe hypotension, angina, and/or pulmonary edema), direct-current cardioversion (DCC) is indicated to restore sinus rhythm immediately (without regard to the risk of thromboembolism).

• If patients are hemodynamically stable, the focus should be directed toward controlling ventricular rate. Use drugs that slow conduction and increase refractoriness in the AV node as initial therapy. In patients with normal LV function (left ventricular ejection fraction [LVEF] >40%), an IV β-blocker (**propranolol**, **metoprolol**, or **esmolol**) or nondihydropyridine CCB (**diltiazem** or **verapamil**) are recommended as first-line therapy. If a high adrenergic state is the precipitating factor, IV β-blockers can be highly effective and should be considered first. In patients with LVEF 40% or less, avoid IV diltiazem and verapamil, and use IV β-blockers with caution. In patients having an exacerbation of HF symptoms, use IV **digoxin** or **amiodarone** as first-line therapy for

TABLE 6–4	Side Effects of Antiarrhythmic Drugs
Disopyramide	Anticholinergic symptoms (dry mouth, urinary retention, constipation, blurred vision), nausea, anorexia, TdP, HF, conduction disturbances, ventricular arrhythmias
Procainamide[a]	Hypotension, TdP, worsening HF, conduction disturbances, ventricular arrhythmias
Quinidine	Cinchonism, diarrhea, abdominal cramps, nausea, vomiting, hypotension, TdP, worsening HF, conduction disturbances, ventricular arrhythmias, fever
Lidocaine	Dizziness, sedation, slurred speech, blurred vision, paresthesia, muscle twitching, confusion, nausea, vomiting, seizures, psychosis, sinus arrest, conduction disturbances
Mexiletine	Dizziness, sedation, anxiety, confusion, paresthesia, tremor, ataxia, blurred vision, nausea, vomiting, anorexia, conduction disturbances, ventricular arrhythmias
Flecainide	Blurred vision, dizziness, dyspnea, headache, tremor, nausea, worsening HF, conduction disturbances, ventricular arrhythmias
Propafenone	Dizziness, fatigue, blurred vision, bronchospasm, headache, taste disturbances, nausea, vomiting, bradycardia or AV block, worsening HF, ventricular arrhythmias
Amiodarone	Tremor, ataxia, paresthesia, insomnia, corneal microdeposits, optic neuropathy/neuritis, nausea, vomiting, anorexia, constipation, TdP (<1%), bradycardia or AV block (IV and oral use), pulmonary fibrosis, liver function test abnormalities, hypothyroidism, hyperthyroidism, photosensitivity, blue-gray skin discoloration, hypotension (IV use), phlebitis (IV use)
Dofetilide	Headache, dizziness, TdP
Dronedarone	Nausea, vomiting, diarrhea, serum creatinine elevations, bradycardia, worsening HF, hepatotoxicity, pulmonary fibrosis, acute renal failure, TdP (<1%)
Ibutilide	Headache, TdP, bradycardia or AV block, hypotension
Sotalol	Dizziness, weakness, fatigue, nausea, vomiting, diarrhea, bradycardia or AV block, TdP, bronchospasm, worsening HF

(AV, atrioventricular; HF, heart failure; IV, intravenous; TdP, torsade de pointes.)
[a]Side effects listed are for the IV formulation only; oral formulations are no longer available.

ventricular rate control. IV amiodarone can also be used in patients who are refractory or have contraindications to β-blockers, nondihydropyridine CCBs, and digoxin.

- After treatment with AV nodal blocking agents and a subsequent decrease in ventricular response, assess the patient for the possibility of restoring sinus rhythm if AF persists.
- If sinus rhythm is to be restored, initiate anticoagulation prior to cardioversion because return of atrial contraction increases risk of thromboembolism. Patients become at increased risk of thrombus formation and a subsequent embolic event if the duration of AF exceeds 48 hours.
  ✓ Patients with AF for longer than 48 hours or an unknown duration should receive warfarin (target international normalized ratio [INR] 2–3), apixaban, dabigatran, or rivaroxaban for at least 3 weeks prior to cardioversion. If cardioversion is successful, continue anticoagulation for at least 4 weeks.
  ✓ Patients with AF less than 48 hours in duration do not require anticoagulation prior to cardioversion. Patients at high risk for stroke should receive IV unfractionated heparin (target aPTT 60 s), low-molecular-weight heparin (subcutaneously at treatment doses), apixaban, dabigatran, or rivaroxaban as soon as possible either before or after cardioversion. If cardioversion is successful in these high-risk patients, continue anticoagulation with warfarin (target INR 2–3), apixaban, dabigatran, or rivaroxaban for at least 4 weeks.

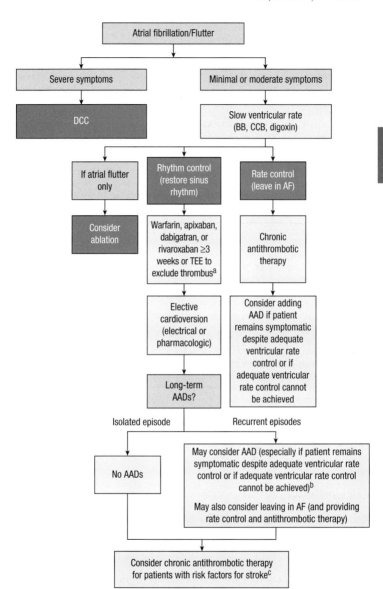

a If AF is less than 48 hours in duration, anticoagulation prior to cardioversion is unnecessary; initiate anticoagulation with unfractionated heparin, a low-molecular-weight heparin, apixaban, dabigatran, or rivaroxaban as soon as possible either before or after cardioversion for patients at high risk for stroke (this anticoagulant regimen or no antithrombotic therapy may be considered in low-risk patients).

b Ablation may be considered for patients who fail or do not tolerate at least 1 AAD or as first-line therapy (before AAD therapy) for select patients with recurrent symptomatic paroxysmal AF.

c Chronic antithrombotic therapy should be considered in all patients with AF and risk factors for stroke regardless of whether or not they remain in sinus rhythm.

(AAD, antiarrhythmic drug; AF, atrial fibrillation; AFl, atrial flutter; BB, β-blocker; CCB, calcium channel blocker [ie, verapamil or diltiazem]; DCC, direct current cardioversion; TEE, transesophageal echocardiogram.)

FIGURE 6–1. Algorithm for the treatment of AF and atrial flutter.

- After prior anticoagulation (or after transesophageal echocardiography demonstrated absence of a thrombus, obviating need for warfarin), methods for restoring sinus rhythm are pharmacologic cardioversion and DCC. DCC is quick and more often successful, but it requires prior sedation or anesthesia and has a small risk of serious complications, such as sinus arrest or ventricular arrhythmias. Advantages of initial drug therapy are that an effective agent may be determined in case long-term therapy is required. Disadvantages are significant side effects, such as drug-induced TdP, drug–drug interactions, and lower cardioversion rate for drugs compared with DCC. There is good evidence for efficacy of class III pure Ik blockers (**ibutilide** and **dofetilide**), class Ic drugs (eg, **flecainide** and **propafenone**), and **amiodarone** (oral or IV). With the "pill in the pocket" approach, outpatient, patient-controlled self-administration of a single, oral loading dose of either flecainide or propafenone can be relatively safe and effective for termination of recent-onset AF in select patients without sinus or AV node dysfunction, bundle-branch block, QT interval prolongation, Brugada's syndrome, or SHD. It should only be considered for patients who have been successfully cardioverted with these drugs on an inpatient basis.
- When initiating chronic antithrombotic therapy to prevent stroke in patients with AF, selection of the appropriate regimen is based on the patient's stroke risk as determined by the CHA_2DS_2-Vasc risk scoring system. Patients are given 2 points each if they have a history of a previous stroke, transient ischemic attack, or thromboembolism, or if they are at least 75 years old. Patients are given 1 point each for age 65 to 74 years; having hypertension, diabetes, HF, or vascular disease; and being female.
  - ✓ Patients with a total score of 2 or higher are considered to be at high stroke risk; oral anticoagulant therapy with warfarin (target INR 2.5; range 2–3), apixaban, dabigatran, edoxaban, or rivaroxaban is preferred over aspirin.
  - ✓ Patients with a score of 1 are considered to be at intermediate stroke risk; oral anticoagulant therapy (warfarin [target INR 2.5; range 2–3], apixaban, dabigatran, edoxaban, or rivaroxaban), aspirin 75 to 325 mg/day, or no antithrombotic therapy can be selected.
  - ✓ Patients with a CHA_2DS_2-VASc score of 0 are at low stroke risk, and it is reasonable to not give any antithrombotic therapy to these patients.
- In patients with nonvalvular AF, current practice guidelines recommend warfarin, dabigatran, rivaroxaban, and apixaban for prevention of initial and recurrent strokes. The guidelines were published prior to FDA approval of edoxaban. If a patient is unable to maintain a therapeutic INR on warfarin, therapy with one of the other agents is recommended.
- In patients with mechanical heart valves, warfarin is the anticoagulant of choice; the target INR should be based on the type and location of the valve placed. Dabigatran, edoxaban, and rivaroxaban should be avoided in patients with a creatinine clearance less than 15 mL/min.
- Decisions regarding chronic antithrombotic therapy should be based on a patient's risk for stroke using the CHA_2DS_2-VASc scoring system.
- Selection of an antiarrhythmic drug to maintain sinus rhythm should be based primarily on whether the patient has SHD. Dofetilide, dronedarone, flecainide, propafenone, or sotalol should be considered initially for patients with no underlying SHD. Amiodarone is an alternative if the patient fails or does not tolerate one of these drugs. In the presence of SHD, flecainide and propafenone should be avoided because of the risk of proarrhythmia. For patients with HF with reduced ejection fraction (HFrEF; LVEF 40% or less), amiodarone, or dofetilide are the drugs of choice. Dronedarone and sotalol should be avoided in patients with HFrEF because of the risk for increased mortality (dronedarone) or worsening HF (sotalol).

PAROXYSMAL SUPRAVENTRICULAR TACHYCARDIA

- The choice between pharmacologic and nonpharmacologic methods for treating PSVT depends on symptom severity (**Fig. 6–2**). Treatment measures are directed first at terminating the acute episode and then at preventing recurrences. For patients with severe symptoms (eg, syncope, near syncope, anginal chest pain, or severe HF), synchronized DCC is the treatment of choice. If symptoms are mild to moderate, nondrug measures

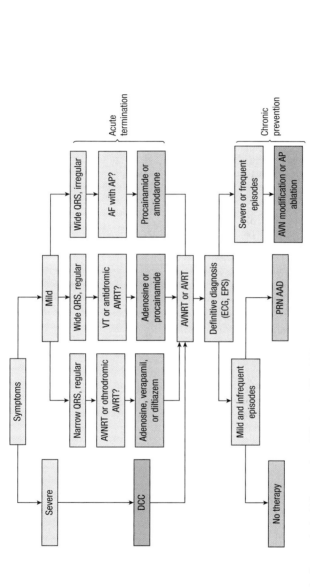

Note: For empiric bridge therapy prior to ablation procedures, CCBs (or other AV nodal blockers) should not be used if the patient has AV reentry with an accessory pathway. (AAD, antiarrhythmic drug; AF, atrial fibrillation; AP, accessory pathway; AV, atrioventricular; AVN, atrioventricular nodal; AVNRT, atrioventricular nodal reentrant tachycardia; AVRT, atrioventricular reentrant tachycardia; CCBs, calcium channel blockers; DCC, direct current cardioversion; ECG, electrocardiogram; EPS, electrophysiologic studies; PRN, as needed; PSVT, paroxysmal supraventricular tachycardia; VT, ventricular tachycardia.)

FIGURE 6–2. Algorithm for the treatment of acute (*top portion*) PSVT and chronic prevention of recurrences (*bottom portion*).

that increase vagal tone to the AV node (eg, unilateral carotid sinus massage and Valsalva maneuver) can be used initially. If these methods fail, drug therapy is the next option.

- The choice among drugs is based on the QRS complex (see **Fig. 6–2**). Drugs can be divided into three broad categories: (1) those that directly or indirectly increase vagal tone to the AV node (eg, **digoxin**); (2) those that depress conduction through slow, calcium-dependent tissue (eg, **adenosine**, **β-blockers**, and **nondihydropyridine calcium channel blockers**); and (3) those that depress conduction through fast, sodium-dependent tissue (eg, **quinidine**, **procainamide**, **disopyramide**, and **flecainide**).
- **Adenosine** has been recommended as the drug of first choice for patients with PSVT because its short duration of action will not cause prolonged hemodynamic compromise in patients with wide QRS complexes who actually have VT rather than PSVT.
- After acute PSVT is terminated, long-term prophylaxis is indicated if frequent episodes necessitate therapeutic intervention or if episodes are infrequent but severely symptomatic. Serial testing of antiarrhythmic agents can be performed via ambulatory ECG recordings (Holter monitors) or telephonic transmissions of cardiac rhythm (event monitors) or by invasive electrophysiologic techniques in the laboratory.
- Catheter ablation using radiofrequency current on the PSVT substrate is now the preferred treatment strategy (over antiarrhythmic drugs) for patients with symptomatic PSVT. It is highly effective and curative, rarely results in complications, obviates need for chronic antiarrhythmic drug therapy, and is cost effective.

PREMATURE VENTRICULAR COMPLEXES

- In apparently healthy individuals, drug therapy is unnecessary because PVCs without associated SHD carry little or no risk. In patients with symptomatic PVCs who have risk factors for arrhythmic death (recent MI, LV dysfunction, or complex PVCs), limit chronic therapy to **β-blockers**. β-Blockers can also be used to suppress symptomatic PVCs in patients without underlying heart disease.

VENTRICULAR TACHYCARDIA

Acute Ventricular Tachycardia

- If severe symptoms are present, institute synchronized DCC immediately to restore sinus rhythm and correct precipitating factors if possible. If VT is an isolated electrical event associated with a transient initiating factor (eg, acute myocardial ischemia or digitalis toxicity), there is no need for long-term antiarrhythmic therapy after precipitating factors are corrected.
- Patients with mild or no symptoms can be treated initially with antiarrhythmic drugs. IV **procainamide**, **amiodarone**, or **sotalol** may be considered in this situation; **lidocaine** is an alternative agent. Deliver synchronized DCC if the patient's status deteriorates, VT degenerates to VF, or drug therapy fails.

Sustained Ventricular Tachycardia

- Patients with chronic recurrent sustained VT are at high risk for death; trial-and-error attempts to find effective therapy are unwarranted. Neither electrophysiologic studies nor serial Holter monitoring with drug testing is ideal. These findings and the side effect profiles of antiarrhythmic agents have led to nondrug approaches.
- The automatic ICD is a highly effective method for preventing sudden death due to recurrent VT or VF.

Ventricular Proarrhythmia

- The typical form of proarrhythmia caused by the class Ic antiarrhythmic drugs is a rapid, sustained, monomorphic VT with a characteristic sinusoidal QRS pattern that is often resistant to resuscitation with cardioversion or overdrive pacing. IV **lidocaine** (competes for the sodium channel receptor) or **sodium bicarbonate** (reverses the excessive sodium channel blockade) have been used successfully by some clinicians.

Torsade de Pointes

- For an acute episode of torsade de pointes (TdP), most patients require and respond to DCC. However, TdP tends to be paroxysmal and often recurs rapidly after DCC.
- IV **magnesium sulfate** is the drug of choice for preventing recurrences of TdP. If ineffective, institute strategies to increase heart rate and shorten ventricular repolarization (ie, temporary transvenous pacing at 105 to 120 beats/min or pharmacologic pacing with **isoproterenol** or **epinephrine** infusion). Discontinue agents that prolong the QT interval and correct exacerbating factors (eg, hypokalemia and hypomagnesemia). Drugs that further prolong repolarization (eg, IV procainamide) are contraindicated. Lidocaine is usually ineffective.

Ventricular Fibrillation

- Manage patients with pulseless VT or VF (with or without associated myocardial ischemia) according to American Heart Association guidelines for cardiopulmonary resuscitation and emergency cardiovascular care (see Chapter 7).

BRADYARRHYTHMIAS

- Treatment of sinus node dysfunction involves elimination of symptomatic bradycardia and possibly managing alternating tachycardias such as AF. Asymptomatic sinus bradyarrhythmias usually do not require therapeutic intervention.
- In general, a permanent ventricular pacemaker is the long-term therapy of choice for patients with significant symptoms.
- Drugs commonly employed to treat supraventricular tachycardias should be used with caution, if at all, in the absence of a functioning pacemaker.
- Symptomatic carotid sinus hypersensitivity also should be treated with permanent pacemaker therapy. Patients who remain symptomatic may benefit from adding an α-adrenergic stimulant such as **midodrine**.
- Vasovagal syncope has traditionally been treated successfully with oral β-blockers (eg, **metoprolol**) to inhibit the sympathetic surge that causes forceful ventricular contraction and precedes the onset of hypotension and bradycardia. Other drugs that have been used successfully (with or without β-blockers) include fludrocortisone, anticholinergics (**scopolamine patches** and **disopyramide**), α-adrenergic agonists (**midodrine**), adenosine analogues (**theophylline** and **dipyridamole**), and selective serotonin reuptake inhibitors (**sertraline** and **paroxetine**).

Atrioventricular Block

- If patients with Mobitz II or third-degree AV block develop signs or symptoms of poor perfusion (eg, altered mental status, chest pain, hypotension, and/or shock) administer **atropine** (0.5 mg IV given every 3–5 minutes, up to 3 mg total dose). Transcutaneous pacing can be initiated in patients unresponsive to atropine. Infusions of **epinephrine** (2–10 mcg/min) or **dopamine** (2–10 mcg/kg/min) can also be used in the event of atropine failure. These agents usually do not help if the site of the AV block is below the AV node (Mobitz II or trifascicular AV block).
- Chronic symptomatic AV block warrants insertion of a permanent pacemaker. Patients without symptoms can sometimes be followed closely without the need for a pacemaker.

EVALUATION OF THERAPEUTIC OUTCOMES

- The most important monitoring parameters include: (1) mortality (total and due to arrhythmic death), (2) arrhythmia recurrence (duration, frequency, and symptoms), (3) hemodynamic consequences (rate, blood pressure, and symptoms), and (4) treatment complications (side effects or need for alternative or additional drugs, devices, or surgery).

See Chapter 18, The Arrhythmias, authored by Cynthia A. Sanoski and Jerry L. Bauman, for a more detailed discussion of this topic.

Cardiac Arrest

- *Cardiac arrest* involves cessation of cardiac mechanical activity as confirmed by absence of signs of circulation (eg, detectable pulse, unresponsiveness, and apnea).

PATHOPHYSIOLOGY

- Coronary artery disease is the most common finding in adults with cardiac arrest and causes ~80% of sudden cardiac deaths. In pediatric patients, cardiac arrest typically results from respiratory failure, asphyxiation, or progressive shock.
- Two different pathophysiologic conditions are associated with cardiac arrest:
  ✓ Primary: arterial blood is typically fully oxygenated at the time of arrest.
  ✓ Secondary: results from respiratory failure in which lack of ventilation leads to severe hypoxemia, hypotension, and cardiac arrest.
- Cardiac arrest in adults usually results from arrhythmias. Historically, ventricular fibrillation (VF) and pulseless ventricular tachycardia (PVT) were most common. The incidence of VF in out-of-hospital arrests is declining, which is of concern because survival rates are higher after VF/PVT than with cardiac arrest resulting from nonshockable rhythms like asystole or pulseless electrical activity (PEA).
- Because in-hospital cardiac arrest is typically preceded by hypoxia or hypotension, asystole or PEA occurs more commonly than VF or PVT.

CLINICAL PRESENTATION

- Cardiac arrest may be preceded by anxiety, shortness of breath, chest pain, nausea, vomiting, and diaphoresis.
- After an arrest, individuals are unresponsive, apneic, and hypotensive without a detectable pulse. Extremities are cold and clammy, and cyanosis is common.

DIAGNOSIS

- Rapid diagnosis is vital to success of cardiopulmonary resuscitation (CPR). Patients must receive early intervention to prevent cardiac rhythms from degenerating into less treatable arrhythmias.
- Diagnosis is made by observation of clinical manifestations consistent with cardiac arrest. Diagnosis is confirmed by vital signs, especially heart rate and respirations.
- Electrocardiography (ECG) identifies the cardiac rhythm, which in turn determines drug therapy.
  ✓ VF is electrical anarchy of the ventricle resulting in no cardiac output and cardiovascular collapse.
  ✓ PEA is absence of a detectable pulse and presence of some type of electrical activity other than VF or PVT.
  ✓ Asystole is presence of a flat line on the ECG.

TREATMENT

- <u>Goals of Treatment</u>: Resuscitation goals are to preserve life, restore health, relieve suffering, limit disability, and respect the individual's decisions, rights, and privacy. This can be accomplished via CPR by return of spontaneous circulation (ROSC) with effective ventilation and perfusion as quickly as possible to minimize hypoxic damage to vital organs. After successful resuscitation, primary goals include optimizing tissue oxygenation, identifying precipitating cause(s) of arrest, and preventing subsequent episodes.

GENERAL APPROACH

- The 2015 American Heart Association (AHA) guidelines for CPR and emergency cardiovascular care (ECC) emphasize timely implementation of the "chain of survival" for out-of-hospital and in-hospital arrests:
  - ✓ Out-of-Hospital Arrests: (1) recognition and activation of the emergency response system, (2) immediate high-quality CPR, (3) rapid defibrillation, (4) basic and advanced emergency medical services, and (5) advanced life support and post-arrest care.
  - ✓ In-Hospital Arrests: (1) surveillance and prevention, (2) recognition and activation of the emergency response system, (3) immediate high-quality CPR, (4) rapid defibrillation, and (5) advanced life support and post-arrest care.
- Basic life support *given by healthcare providers trained in CPR* includes the following actions performed in this order:
  - ✓ First, determine patient responsiveness. If unresponsive with no breathing or no normal breathing (ie, only gasping), activate the emergency medical response team and obtain an automated external defibrillator (AED) if available.
  - ✓ Check for pulse, but if not definitely felt within 10 seconds, begin CPR and use the AED when available.
  - ✓ Begin CPR with 30 chest compressions at a rate of 100 to 120/min and a compression depth of at least 2 in (5 cm) in adults and at least one third of the anteroposterior chest diameter in infants and children (~1.5 in [4 cm] in infants and 2 in [5 cm] in children).
  - ✓ Open the airway and deliver two rescue breaths, then repeat chest compressions. Follow each cycle of 30 chest compressions by two rescue breaths.
  - ✓ Continue cycles of 30 compressions/2 breaths until an AED arrives and is ready for use or emergency medical service (EMS) providers take over care.
  - ✓ If AED is available, check rhythm to determine if defibrillation is advised. If so, deliver one shock with immediate resumption of chest compressions/rescue breaths. After five cycles, reevaluate the rhythm to determine need for further defibrillation. Repeat this sequence until help arrives or the rhythm is no longer shockable.
  - ✓ If rhythm is not shockable, continue chest compressions/rescue breath cycles until help arrives or spontaneous circulation returns. If rhythm is not shockable, it is likely to be either asystole or PEA.
- Once ACLS providers arrive, further definitive therapy is given following the ACLS algorithm shown in Fig. 7–1.
- Central venous catheter access results in faster and higher peak drug concentrations than peripheral venous administration, but central line access is not needed in most resuscitation attempts. However, if a central line is already present, it is the access site of choice. If IV access (either central or peripheral) has not been established, insert a large peripheral venous catheter. If this is not successful, insert an intraosseous (IO) device.
- If neither IV nor IO access can be established, lidocaine, epinephrine, naloxone, and vasopressin may be administered endotracheally. The endotracheal dose should generally be 2 to 2.5 times larger than the IV/IO dose. Medications should be diluted in 5 to 10 mL of either sterile water (preferred) or normal saline.

TREATMENT OF VENTRICULAR FIBRILLATION AND PULSELESS VENTRICULAR TACHYCARDIA

Nonpharmacologic Therapy

- Administer electrical defibrillation with one shock using 360 J (monophasic defibrillator) or 120 to 200 J (biphasic defibrillator). After defibrillation is attempted, restart CPR immediately and continue for about five cycles (~2 min) before analyzing the rhythm or checking a pulse. If there is still evidence of VF/PVT after 2 minutes, then give pharmacologic therapy with repeat attempts at single-discharge defibrillation.

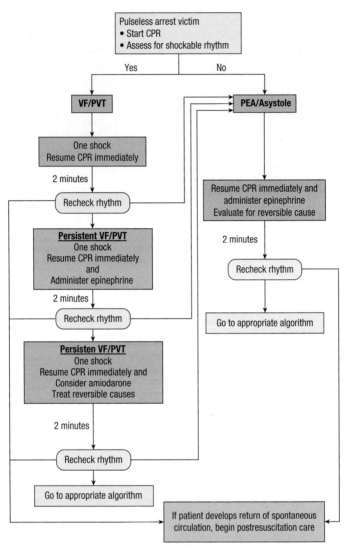

FIGURE 7-1. Treatment algorithm for adult cardiac arrest: Advanced cardiac life support (ACLS).

• Obtain endotracheal intubation and IV access when feasible, but not at the expense of stopping chest compressions. Once an airway is achieved, ventilate patients with 100% oxygen.

Pharmacologic Therapy

EPINEPHRINE

• **Epinephrine** is a drug of first choice for treating VF, PVT, asystole, and PEA. It is an agonist of both α and β receptors, but effectiveness is primarily due to α effects.

It increases systemic arteriolar vasoconstriction, thereby improving coronary and cerebral perfusion pressure during the low-flow state associated with CPR.

- The recommended adult dose of epinephrine is 1 mg administered by IV or IO injection every 3 to 5 minutes. Although higher doses have been studied, they are not recommended for routine use in cardiac arrest.

VASOPRESSIN

- **Vasopressin** (40 units IV/IO) is a potent nonadrenergic vasoconstrictor that increases blood pressure (BP) and systemic vascular resistance. Despite some theoretical advantages, it appears to offer no benefit as a substitute for epinephrine, and vasopressin coadministered with epinephrine offers no benefit over standard-dose epinephrine alone. For these reasons, vasopressin was removed from the 2015 AHA cardiac arrest algorithm.

ANTIARRHYTHMICS

- The purpose of antiarrhythmic drug therapy after unsuccessful defibrillation and vasopressor administration is to prevent development or recurrence of VF and PVT by raising the fibrillation threshold. However, clinical evidence demonstrating improved survival to hospital discharge is lacking.
- **Amiodarone** is the recommended antiarrhythmic in patients with VF/VT unresponsive to CPR, defibrillation, and vasopressors. The dose is 300 mg IV/IO followed by a second dose of 150 mg.
- **Lidocaine** may be used if amiodarone is unavailable, but it has not been shown to improve rates of ROSC, admission to the hospital, or survival to discharge compared with amiodarone. The initial dose is 1 to 1.5 mg/kg IV. Additional doses of 0.5 to 0.75 mg/kg can be administered at 5- to 10-minute intervals to a maximum dose of 3 mg/kg if VF/PVT persists.

MAGNESIUM

- Severe hypomagnesemia has been associated with VF/PVT, but routine administration of magnesium during cardiac has not improved clinical outcomes. Two trials showed improved ROSC in cardiac arrests associated with torsades de pointes. Therefore, limit magnesium administration to these patients. The dose is 1 to 2 g diluted in 10 mL of 5% dextrose in water administered IV/IO push over 15 minutes.

THROMBOLYTICS

- Thrombolytic use during CPR has been investigated because most cardiac arrests are related to either myocardial infarction (MI) or pulmonary embolism (PE). Although several studies demonstrated successful use, few have shown improvements to hospital discharge, and an increase in intracranial hemorrhage was noted. Therefore, fibrinolytic therapy should not be used routinely in cardiac arrest but can be considered when PE is the presumed or known cause of the arrest.

TREATMENT OF PULSELESS ELECTRICAL ACTIVITY AND ASYSTOLE

Nonpharmacologic Therapy

- Successful treatment of PEA and asystole depends on diagnosis of the underlying cause. Potentially reversible causes include: (1) hypovolemia, (2) hypoxia, (3) acidosis, (4) hyper- or hypokalemia, (5) hypothermia, (6) hypoglycemia, (7) drug overdose, (8) cardiac tamponade, (9) tension pneumothorax, (10) coronary thrombosis, (11) pulmonary thrombosis, and (12) trauma.
- PEA and asystole are treated the same way. Both conditions require CPR, airway control, and IV access. Avoid defibrillation in asystole because the resulting parasympathetic discharge can reduce the chance of ROSC and decrease the likelihood of survival. If available, transcutaneous pacing can be attempted.

Pharmacologic Therapy

- **Epinephrine** (1 mg by IV or IO injection every 3–5 minutes) is the primary pharmacologic agent used; vasopressin is no longer recommended.
- Atropine is no longer recommended for treatment of asystole or PEA because there are no prospective controlled trials showing benefit and there is conflicting evidence from retrospective and observational reports.

ACID–BASE MANAGEMENT

- Acidosis occurs during cardiac arrest because of decreased blood flow or inadequate ventilation. Chest compressions generate only about 25% of normal cardiac output, leading to inadequate organ perfusion, tissue hypoxia, and metabolic acidosis. Lack of ventilation causes CO_2 retention, leading to respiratory acidosis. The combined acidosis reduces myocardial contractility and may cause arrhythmias.
- Routine use of sodium bicarbonate in cardiac arrest is not recommended because there are few clinical data supporting its use, and it may have detrimental effects. It can be used in special circumstances (eg, preexisting metabolic acidosis, hyperkalemia, and tricyclic antidepressant overdose). The dosage should be guided by laboratory analysis if possible.

POSTRESUSCITATIVE CARE

- ROSC from a cardiac arrest may be followed by a post-cardiac arrest syndrome characterized by brain injury, myocardial dysfunction, systemic ischemia/reperfusion response, and persistent precipitating pathology.
- It is imperative to ensure adequate airway and oxygenation. Raise the head of the bed to 30 degrees to reduce risk for aspiration, ventilator-associated pneumonia, and cerebral edema. After use of 100% oxygen during the resuscitation effort, titrate the oxygen fraction down as tolerated to avoid oxygen toxicity. Overventilation can be avoided by using end-tidal (ET) CO_2 measurements targeting an $ETCO_2$ of 40 to 45 mm Hg.
- Evaluate for ECG changes consistent with acute myocardial infarction as soon as possible and perform revascularization as appropriate.
- Therapeutic hypothermia or targeted temperature management is an integral component of postresuscitative care. Hypothermia can protect from cerebral injury by suppressing chemical reactions that occur after restoration of blood flow. Current guidelines recommend targeted temperature management for all comatose adults patients after ROSC, with a target temperature between 32 and 36°C maintained for at least 24 hours. A rewarming phase should consist of slow and controlled warming at a rate of 0.2 to 0.5°C per hour. It is also reasonable to actively prevent fever after targeted temperature management. Potential complications of hypothermia include coagulopathy, dysrhythmias, hyperglycemia, electrolyte disorders, infection risks, and profound effects on drug distribution and clearance.

EVALUATION OF THERAPEUTIC OUTCOMES

- Monitoring should occur both during the resuscitation attempt and in the postresuscitation phase. The optimal outcome following CPR is an awake, responsive, spontaneously breathing patient. Ideally, patients must remain neurologically intact with minimal morbidity after the resuscitation.
- Assess and document heart rate, cardiac rhythm, and BP throughout the resuscitation attempt and after each intervention. Determination of the presence or absence of a pulse is paramount to deciding which interventions are appropriate.
- Avoid and immediately correct hypotension (mean arterial pressure [MAP] < 65 mmHg or SBP < 90 mmHg), but a specific target MAP remains unknown.

- Coronary perfusion pressure (CPP) and central venous oxygen saturation ($ScvO_2$) can provide useful information on the patient's response to therapy. Thresholds associated with poor achievement of ROSC include CPP < 15 mmHg and $ScvO_2$ < 30%. If CPP is not available during CPR, arterial diastolic pressure can be used instead; values <20 mm Hg are considered suboptimal.
- $ETCO_2$ monitoring is a safe and effective method to assess cardiac output during CPR and has been associated with ROSC. Persistently low $ETCO_2$ values (< 10 mm Hg) during CPR in intubated patients suggest that ROSC is unlikely.
- Consider the precipitating cause of the cardiac arrest (eg, MI, electrolyte imbalance, primary arrhythmia). Review prearrest status carefully, particularly if the patient was receiving drug therapy.
- Address any altered cardiac, hepatic, and renal function resulting from ischemic damage during the arrest.
- Assess neurologic function by the Cerebral Performance Category and the Glasgow Coma Scale.

See Chapter 12, Cardiac Arrest, authored by Jeffrey F. Barletta, for a more detailed discussion of this topic.

Dyslipidemia

- *Dyslipidemia* is defined as elevated total cholesterol, low-density lipoprotein (LDL) cholesterol, or triglycerides; low high-density lipoprotein (HDL) cholesterol; or a combination of these abnormalities.

PATHOPHYSIOLOGY

- Cholesterol, triglycerides, and phospholipids are transported in blood as complexes of lipids and proteins (lipoproteins). Elevated total and LDL cholesterol and reduced HDL cholesterol are associated with development of coronary heart disease (CHD).
- Risk factors such as oxidized LDL, mechanical injury to endothelium, and excessive homocysteine can lead to endothelial dysfunction and cellular interactions culminating in atherosclerosis. Eventual clinical outcomes may include angina, myocardial infarction (MI), arrhythmias, stroke, peripheral arterial disease, abdominal aortic aneurysm, and sudden death.
- Atherosclerotic lesions arise from transport and retention of plasma LDL through the endothelial cell layer into the extracellular matrix of the subendothelial space. Once in the artery wall, LDL is chemically modified through oxidation and nonenzymatic glycation. Mildly oxidized LDL recruits monocytes into the artery wall, which transform into macrophages that accelerate LDL oxidation. Oxidized LDL provokes an inflammatory response mediated by chemoattractants and cytokines.
- Repeated injury and repair within an atherosclerotic plaque eventually lead to a fibrous cap protecting the underlying core of lipids, collagen, calcium, and inflammatory cells. Maintenance of the fibrous plaque is critical to prevent plaque rupture and coronary thrombosis.
- Primary or genetic lipoprotein disorders are classified into six categories: I (chylomicrons), IIa (LDL), IIb (LDL + very-low-density lipoprotein [VLDL]), III (intermediate-density lipoprotein), IV (VLDL), and V (VLDL + chylomicrons). Secondary forms of dyslipidemia also exist, and several drug classes may elevate cholesterol levels (eg, progestins, thiazide diuretics, glucocorticoids, β-blockers, isotretinoin, protease inhibitors, cyclosporine, mirtazapine, and sirolimus).
- The primary defect in familial hypercholesterolemia is inability to bind LDL to the LDL receptor (LDL-R). This leads to a lack of LDL degradation by cells and unregulated biosynthesis of cholesterol.

CLINICAL PRESENTATION

- Most patients are asymptomatic for many years. Symptomatic patients may complain of chest pain, palpitations, sweating, anxiety, shortness of breath, or abdominal pain. They may also experience difficulty with speech or movement or loss of consciousness.
- Depending on the lipoprotein abnormality, signs on physical examination may include cutaneous xanthomas, peripheral polyneuropathy, high blood pressure, and increased body mass index or waist size.

DIAGNOSIS

- Measure fasting (preferred) lipoprotein profile (total cholesterol, LDL, HDL, and triglycerides) in all adults 20 years of age or older at least once every 5 years.
- Measure plasma cholesterol, triglyceride, and HDL levels after a 12-hour fast because triglycerides may be elevated in nonfasting individuals; total cholesterol is only modestly affected by fasting.

- Two determinations, 1 to 8 weeks apart are recommended to minimize variability and obtain a reliable baseline. If the total cholesterol is greater than 200 mg/dL (>5.17 mmol/L), a second determination is recommended, and if the values are greater than 30 mg/dL (>0.78 mmol/L) apart, use the average of three values.
- History and physical examination should assess: (1) presence or absence of cardiovascular risk factors or definite cardiovascular disease; (2) family history of premature cardiovascular disease or lipid disorders; (3) presence or absence of secondary causes of dyslipidemia, including concurrent medications; and (4) presence or absence of xanthomas, abdominal pain, or history of pancreatitis, renal or liver disease, peripheral vascular disease, abdominal aortic aneurysm, or cerebral vascular disease (carotid bruits, stroke, or transient ischemic attack).
- Diabetes mellitus is a CHD risk equivalent; its presence in patients without known CHD is associated with the same level of risk as patients without diabetes but having confirmed CHD.
- Lipoprotein electrophoresis is sometimes performed to determine which class of lipoproteins is involved. If the triglycerides are less than 400 mg/dL (4.52 mmol/L), and neither type III dyslipidemia nor chylomicrons are detected by electrophoresis, then one can calculate VLDL and LDL concentrations: $VLDL = triglycerides \div 5$; $LDL = total cholesterol - (VLDL + HDL)$.
- Pooled cohort equations are recommended to predict an individual's risk of ASCVD (see http://tools.acc.org/ASCVD-Risk-Estimator/).

TREATMENT

- Goals of Treatment: Lower total and LDL cholesterol to reduce the risk of first or recurrent events such as MI, angina, heart failure, ischemic stroke, or peripheral arterial disease.

GENERAL APPROACH

- In 2013, the American College of Cardiology/American Heart Association (ACC/AHA) published revised treatment guidelines that supersede the National Cholesterol Education Program Adult Treatment Panel III (NCEP ATP III). Rather than recommending specific lipid level targets, the guidelines identify four patient groups who quality for treatment with statins to reduce the 10-year risk of atherosclerotic cardiovascular disease (ASCVD) in secondary and primary intervention; see **Fig. 8–1** for an algorithm for statin initiation.
- The ACC/AHA guidelines established categories of statin intensity including high, moderate, and low intensity (**Table 8–1**) based on evidence from randomized clinical trials and package insert information.

NONPHARMACOLOGIC THERAPY

- Begin therapeutic lifestyle changes (TLCs) on the first visit, including dietary therapy, weight reduction, and increased physical activity. Advise overweight patients to lose 10% of body weight. Encourage physical activity of moderate intensity 30 minutes a day for most days of the week. Assist patients with smoking cessation and control of hypertension.
- The objectives of dietary therapy are to progressively decrease intake of total fat, saturated fat, and cholesterol and to achieve a desirable body weight (**Table 8–2**).
- Increased intake of soluble fiber (oat bran, pectins, and psyllium) can reduce total and LDL cholesterol by 5% to 20%. However, they have little effect on HDL-C or triglycerides. Fiber products may also be useful in managing constipation associated with bile acid resins (BARs).
- Fish oil supplementation reduces triglycerides and VLDL-C, but it either has no effect on total and LDL-C or may elevate these fractions. Other actions of fish oil may account for any cardioprotective effects.

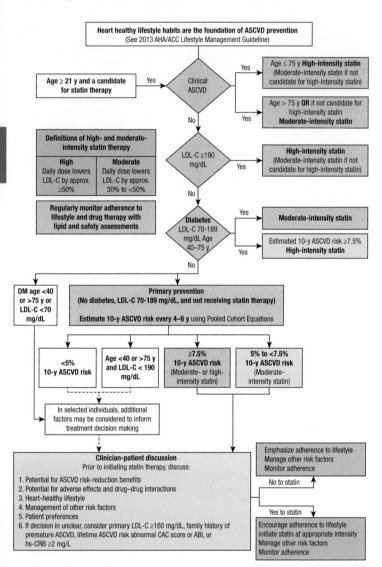

FIGURE 8-1. Statin initiation.

- Ingestion of 2 to 3 g daily of plant sterols reduces LDL by 6% to 15%. They are usually available in commercial margarines.
- If all recommended dietary changes were instituted, the estimated average reduction in LDL would range from 20% to 30%.

PHARMACOLOGIC THERAPY

- The effect of drug therapy on lipids and lipoproteins is shown in Table 8-3.
- Recommended drugs of choice for each lipoprotein phenotype are given in Table 8-4.
- Available products and their doses are provided in Table 8-5.

TABLE 8–1	Intensity of Statin Therapy by Drug and Dose	
High-Intensity Statin Therapy	**Moderate-Intensity Statin Therapy**	**Low-Intensity Statin Therapy**
Daily dose lowers LDL on average by ≥50%	Daily dose lowers LDL on average by 30 to <50%	Daily dose lowers LDL on average by <30%
Atorvastatin (40) 80 mg **Rosuvstatin (20) 40 mg**	**Atorvastatin 10 (20) mg** **Rosuvastatin (5) 20 mg** **Simvastatin 20–40 mg**[a] **Pravastatin 40 (80) mg** **Lovastatin 40 mg** Fluvastin XL 80 mg **Fluvastatin 40 mg twice daily** Pitavastatin 2–4 mg	Simvastatin 10 mg **Pravastatin 10–20 mg** **Lovastatin 20 mg** Fluvastatin 20–40 mg Pitavastin 1 mg

[a]Simvastatin is not recommended by the U.S. Food and Drug Administration to be started at 80 mg/day due to increased risk of myopathy and rarely rhabdomyolysis.
Boldface type indicates specific doses that have been tested in randomized controlled trials.

TABLE 8–2	Macronutrient Recommendations for the Therapeutic Lifestyle Change (TLC) Diet
Component[a]	**Recommended Intake**
Total fat	25%–35% of total calories
Saturated fat	Less than 7% of total calories
Polyunsaturated fat	Up to 10% of total calories
Monounsaturated fat	Up to 20% of total calories
Carbohydrates[b]	50%–60% of total calories
Cholesterol	<200 mg/day
Dietary Fiber	20–30 g/day
Plant sterols	2 g/day
Protein	Approximately 15% of total calories
Total calories	To achieve and maintain desirable body weight

[a]Calories from alcohol not included.
[b]Carbohydrates should derive from foods rich in complex carbohydrates such as whole grains, fruits, and vegetables.

Bile Acid Resins

- BARs (**cholestyramine**, **colestipol**, and **colesevelam**) bind bile acids in the intestinal lumen, with a concurrent interruption of enterohepatic circulation of bile acids, which decreases the bile acid pool size and stimulates hepatic synthesis of bile acids from cholesterol. Depletion of the hepatic cholesterol pool increases cholesterol biosynthesis and the number of LDL-Rs on hepatocyte membranes, which enhances the rate of catabolism from plasma and lowers LDL levels. Increased hepatic cholesterol biosynthesis may be paralleled by increased hepatic VLDL production; consequently, BARs may aggravate hypertriglyceridemia in patients with combined dyslipidemia.
- BARs are useful in treating primary hypercholesterolemia (familial hypercholesterolemia, familial combined dyslipidemia, and type IIa hyperlipoproteinemia).

TABLE 8-3	Effects of Drug Therapy on Lipids and Lipoproteins		
Drug	**Mechanism of Action**	**Effects on Lipids**	**Effects on Lipoproteins**
Cholestyramine, colestipol, and colesevelam	↑ LDL catabolism ↓ Cholesterol absorption	↓ Cholesterol	↓ LDL ↑ VLDL
Niacin	↓ LDL and VLDL synthesis	↓ Triglyceride ↓ cholesterol	↓ VLDL, ↓ LDL, ↑ HDL
Gemfibrozil, fenofibrate, clofibrate	↑ VLDL clearance ↓ VLDL synthesis	↓ Triglyceride ↓ Cholesterol	↓ VLDL, ↓ LDL, ↑ HDL
Lovastatin, pravastatin, simvastatin, fluvastatin, atorvastatin rosuvastatin	↑ LDL catabolism ↓ LDL synthesis	↓ Cholesterol	↓ LDL
Ezetimibe	Blocks cholesterol absorption across the intestinal border	↓ Cholesterol	↓ LDL
Mipomerson	Inhibits apolipoprotein B-100 synthesis	↓ Cholesterol	↓ LDL, non-HDL
Lomitapide	Inhibits microsomal triglyceride transfer protein	↓ Cholesterol	↓ LDL, non-HDL
Alirocumab	PCSK9 inhibitor	↓ Cholesterol, ↓ Lpa	↓ Cholesterol and LDL
Evolocumab	PCSK9 inhibitor	↓ Cholesterol, ↓ Lpa	↓ Cholesterol and LDL

- Common GI complaints include constipation, bloating, epigastric fullness, nausea, and flatulence. They can be managed by increasing fluid intake, increasing dietary bulk, and using stool softeners.
- The gritty texture and bulk may be minimized by mixing the powder with orange drink or juice. Colestipol may have better palatability than cholestyramine because it is odorless and tasteless. Tablet forms may help improve adherence.
- Other potential adverse effects include impaired absorption of fat-soluble vitamins A, D, E, and K; hypernatremia and hyperchloremia; GI obstruction; and reduced bioavailability of acidic drugs such as warfarin, nicotinic acid, thyroxine, acetaminophen, hydrocortisone, hydrochlorothiazide, loperamide, and possibly iron. Drug interactions may be avoided by alternating administration times with an interval of 6 hours or more between the BARs and other drugs.

Niacin

- **Niacin** (nicotinic acid) reduces hepatic synthesis of VLDL, which in turn reduces synthesis of LDL. Niacin also increases HDL by reducing its catabolism.
- The principal use of niacin is for mixed dyslipidemia or as a second-line agent in combination therapy for hypercholesterolemia. It is a first-line agent or alternative for treatment of hypertriglyceridemia and diabetic dyslipidemia.
- Cutaneous flushing and itching appear to be prostaglandin mediated and can be reduced by taking aspirin 325 mg shortly before niacin ingestion. Taking the niacin dose with meals and slowly titrating the dose upward may minimize these effects. Concomitant alcohol and hot drinks may magnify the flushing and pruritus from niacin, and they should be avoided at the time of ingestion. GI intolerance is also a common problem.

TABLE 8–4	Lipoprotein Phenotype and Recommended Drug Treatment	
Lipoprotein Type	**Drug of Choice**	**Combination Therapy**
I	Not indicated	–
II[a]	Statins	Niacin or BAR
	Cholestyramine or colestipol	Statins or niacin
	Niacin	Statins or BAR
		Ezetimibe
		Mipomersen, lomitapide[b]
II[b]	Statins	BAR or fibrates or niacin
	Fibrates	Statins or niacin or BAR[a]
	Niacin	Statins or fibrates
		Ezetimibe
III	Fibrates	Statins or niacin
	Niacin	Statins or fibrates
		Ezetimibe
IV	Fibrates	Niacin
	Niacin	Fibrates
V	Fibrates	Niacin
	Niacin	Fish oils

(BAR, bile acid resins; fibrates includes gemfibrozil or fenofibrate.)
[a]BAR are not used as first-line therapy if triglycerides are elevated at baseline since hypertriglyceridemia may be worsen with BAR alone.
[b]Mipomersen and lomitapide are used in combinations with other lipid lowering therapy, in particular, statins for patients with familial hypercholestermia (homozygotes or heterzygotes) and in patient who cannot be managed adequately with maximally tolerated statin therapy.

- Laboratory abnormalities may include elevated liver function tests, hyperuricemia, and hyperglycemia. Niacin-associated hepatitis is more common with sustained-release preparations, and their use should be restricted to patients intolerant of regular-release products. Niacin is contraindicated in patients with active liver disease, and it may exacerbate preexisting gout and diabetes.
- **Niaspan** is a prescription-only, extended-release niacin formulation with pharmaco-kinetics intermediate between prompt- and sustained-release products. It has fewer dermatologic reactions and a low risk of hepatotoxicity. Combination with statins can produce large reductions in LDL and increases in HDL.
- Nicotinamide should not be used in the treatment of dyslipidemia because it does not effectively lower cholesterol or triglyceride levels.

HMG-CoA Reductase Inhibitors

- Statins (**atorvastatin**, **fluvastatin**, **lovastatin**, **pitavastatin**, **pravastatin**, **rosuvastatin**, and **simvastatin**) inhibit 3-hydroxy-3-methylglutaryl coenzyme A (HMG-CoA) reductase, interrupting conversion of HMG-CoA to mevalonate, the rate-limiting step in cholesterol biosynthesis. Reduced LD synthesis and enhanced LDL catabolism mediated through LDL-Rs appear to be the principal mechanisms for lipid-lowering effects.
- When used as monotherapy, statins are the most potent total and LDL cholesterol–lowering agents and among the best tolerated. Total and LDL cholesterol are reduced in a dose-related fashion by 30% or more when added to dietary therapy.
- Combination therapy with a statin and a BAR is rational because the numbers of LDL-Rs are increased, leading to greater degradation of LDL cholesterol; intra-cellular synthesis of cholesterol is inhibited; and enterohepatic recycling of bile acids is interrupted.

TABLE 8–5 Comparison of Drugs Used in the Treatment of Dyslipidemia

Drug	Dosage Forms	Usual Daily Dose	Maximum Daily Dose
Cholestyramine (Questran) Cholestyramine (Questran Light) Cholestyramine (Cholybar)	Bulk powder/4-g packets Bulk powder/4-g packets 4-g resin per bar	8 g 3 times daily	32 g
Colestipol hydrochloride (Colestid)	Bulk powder/5-g packets	10 g twice daily	30 g
Colesevelam (Welchol)	625 mg tablets	1875 mg twice daily	4375 mg
Niacin	50-, 100-, 250-, and 500-mg tablets; 125-, 250-, and 500-mg capsules	2 g 3 times daily	9 g
Extended release niacin (Niaspan)	500, 750 and 1000 mg tablets	500 mg	2000 mg
Extended release niacin + lovastatin (Advicor)[a]	Niacin/lovastatin 500 mg/20 mg tablets Niacin/lovastatin 750 mg/20 mg tablets Niacin/lovastatin 1000 mg/20 mg tablets	Niacin/lovastatin 500 mg/20 mg	Niacin/lovastatin 1000 mg/20 mg
Fenofibrate (Tricor and others)	67, 134 and 200 mg capsules (micronized); 54 and 160 mg tablets; 40, 120 mg tablets; 50, 160 mg tablets	54 mg or 67 mg	201 mg
Gemfibrozil (Lopid)	300-mg capsules	600 mg twice daily	1.5 g
Lovastatin (Mevacor)	20- and 40-mg tablets	20–40 mg	80 mg
Pravastatin (Pravachol)	10- and 20-mg tablets	10–20 mg	40 mg
Simvastatin (Zocor)	5, 10, 20, 40, and 80-mg tablets	10–20 mg	80 mg
Atorvastatin (Lipitor)	10 mg tablets	10 mg	80 mg
Rosuvastatin (Crestor)	5- and 10-mg tablets	5 mg	40 mg
Pitavastatin (Livalo)	1, 2, and 4 mg tablets	2 mg	4 mg
Ezetimibe (Zetia)	10 mg tablet	10 mg	10 mg

Atorvastatin/amlodipine (Caduet)	Atorvastatin/amlodipine 10 mg/5 mg Atorvastatin/amlodipine 20 mg/5 mg Atorvastatin/amlodipine 40 mg/5 mg Atorvastatin/amlodipine 80 mg/5 mg Atorvastatin/amlodipine 10 mg/10 mg Atorvastatin/amlodipine 20 mg/10 mg Atorvastatin/amlodipine 40 mg/10 mg Atorvastatin/amlodipine 80 mg/10 mg	Atorvastatin/amlodipine 10 mg/5 mg	Atorvastatin/amlodipine 80 mg/10 mg
Pravastatin/aspirin (Pravigard PAC)	Pravastatin/aspirin 20 mg/81 mg Pravastatin/aspirin 20 mg/325 mg Pravastatin/aspirin 40 mg/81 mg Pravastatin/aspirin 40 mg/325 mg Pravastatin/aspirin 80 mg/81 mg Pravastatin/aspirin 80 mg/325 mg		
Simvastatin/ezetimibe (Vytorin)	Simvastatin/ezetimibe 10 mg/10 mg Simvastatin/ezetimibe 20 mg/10 mg Simvastatin/ezetimibe 40 mg/10 mg	Simvastatin/ezetimibe 20 mg/10 mg	Simvastatin/ezetimibe 40 mg/10 mg
Omega-3 acid ethyl esters (Lovaza)	Eicosapentaenoic acid (EPA) 465 mg, docosahexaenoic acid (DHA) 375 mg	41 gram capsules once daily or 21 gram capsules twice daily	41 gram capsules once daily or 21 gram capsules twice daily
Lomitapide	5, 10, 20 mg capsules	5 mg once daily increasing at 2 week intervals to response or maximum dose; dose 2 hours after evening meal	60 mg once daily
Mipomersen	200 mg/mL for SC injection	200 mg SC once weekly	200 mg SC once weekly
Alirocumab	75 or 150 mg	SC every 2 weeks	150 mg
Evolocumab	140 mg or 420 mg	SC 140 mg every 2 weeks or 420 mg once a month	420 mg

(SC, subcutaneously.)

[a]The manufacturer does not recommend use of the fixed combination as initial therapy of primary hypercholesterolemia or mixed dyslipidemia. It is specifically indicated in patients receiving lovastatin alone plus diet who require an additional reduction in triglyceride levels or increase in HDL-cholesterol levels; it is also indicated in those treated with niacin alone who require additional decreases in LDL cholesterol. Lomitapide and mipomersen can be hepatotoxic and close monitoring is recommended for both.

73

- Combination therapy with a statin and ezetimibe is also rational because ezetimibe inhibits cholesterol absorption across the gut border and adds 12% to 20% further reduction when combined with a statin or other drug.
- Constipation occurs in less than 10% of patients taking statins. Other adverse effects include elevated alanine aminotransferase, elevated creatine kinase levels, myopathy, and, rarely, rhabdomyolysis.

Fibric Acids

- Fibrate monotherapy (**gemfibrozil**, **fenofibrate**, and **clofibrate**) is effective in reducing VLDL, but a reciprocal rise in LDL may occur, and total cholesterol values may remain relatively unchanged. Plasma HDL concentrations may rise 10% to 15% or more with fibrates.
- Gemfibrozil reduces synthesis of VLDL and, to a lesser extent, apolipoprotein B with a concurrent increase in the rate of removal of triglyceride-rich lipoproteins from plasma. Clofibrate is less effective than gemfibrozil or niacin in reducing VLDL production.
- GI complaints occur in 3% to 5% of patients. Rash, dizziness, and transient elevations in transaminase levels and alkaline phosphatase may also occur. Gemfibrozil and probably fenofibrate enhance gallstone formation rarely.
- A myositis syndrome of myalgia, weakness, stiffness, malaise, and elevations in creatine kinase and aspartate aminotransferase may occur and may be more common in patients with renal insufficiency.
- Fibrates may potentiate the effects of oral anticoagulants, and the international normalized ratio (INR) should be monitored very closely with this combination.

Ezetimibe

- **Ezetimibe** interferes with absorption of cholesterol from the brush border of the intestine, making it a good choice for adjunctive therapy. It is approved as monotherapy and for use with a statin. The dose is 10 mg once daily, given with or without food. When used alone, it results in ~18% reduction in LDL cholesterol. When added to a statin, ezetimibe lowers LDL by an additional 12% to 20%. A combination product (Vytorin) containing ezetimibe 10 mg and simvastatin 10, 20, 40, or 80 mg is available. Ezetimibe is well tolerated; ~4% of patients experience GI upset. Because cardiovascular outcomes with ezetimibe have not been evaluated, it should be reserved for patients unable to tolerate statin therapy or those who do not achieve satisfactory lipid lowering with a statin alone.

Fish Oil Supplementation

- Diets high in omega-3 polyunsaturated fatty acids (from fish oil), most commonly eicosapentaenoic acid (EPA), reduce cholesterol, triglycerides, LDL, and VLDL and may elevate HDL cholesterol.
- Fish oil supplementation may be most useful in patients with hypertriglyceridemia, but its role in treatment is not well defined.
- **LOVAZA (omega-3-acid ethyl esters)** is a prescription form of concentrated fish oil EPA 465 mg and docosahexaenoic acid 375 mg. The daily dose is 4 g, which can be taken as four 1-g capsules once daily or two 1-g capsules twice daily. This product lowers triglycerides by 14% to 30% and raises HDL by ~10%.
- Complications of fish oil supplementation such as thrombocytopenia and bleeding disorders have been noted, especially with high doses (EPA 15–30 g/day).

Mipomersen

- **Mipomersen** (Kynamro) is an antisense oligonucleotide inhibitor of apolipoprotein B-100 synthesis. It is indicated as an adjunct to lipid-lowering medications and diet to reduce LDL-cholesterol, apolipoprotein B, total cholesterol, and non-HDL cholesterol in patients with homozygous familial hypercholesterolemia. The dose is 200 mg once weekly given by subcutaneous (SC) injection. When given in combination with maximum tolerated doses of lipid-lowering therapy, mipomersen can produce an additional

25% reduction in LDL cholesterol. Adverse reactions include injection site reactions, flu-like symptoms, nausea, headache, and elevations in serum transaminases.

Lomitapide

- **Lomitapide** (Juxtapid) is a microsomal triglyceride transfer protein (MTP) inhibitor that reduces the amount of cholesterol that the liver and intestines assemble and secrete into the circulation. It is indicated as an adjunct to diet and other lipid-lowering treatments to reduce LDL cholesterol, total cholesterol, apolipoprotein B, and non-HDL cholesterol in patients with homozygous familial hypercholesterolemia. Lomitapide may reduce LDL cholesterol by about 40% in patients on maximum tolerated lipid-lowering therapy and LDL apheresis. The initial dose is 5 mg orally once daily, which may be increased as tolerated to 10 mg daily after at least 2 weeks. The dose may be further increased at 4-week intervals to 20 mg, 40 mg, and then the maximum of 60 mg daily. Because of the risk of hepatotoxicity, lomitapide is available only through the Risk Evaluation and Mitigation Strategy (REMS) program.

Proprotein Convertase Subtilisin/Kexin Type 9 (PCSK9) Inhibitors

- PCSK9 promotes intracellular degradation of hepatic LDL, prevents LDL recycling to the cell surface, and reduces LDL clearance from the circulation; inhibiting PCSK9 substantially lowers LDL cholesterol. These drugs are indicated as an adjunct to diet and maximally tolerated lipid-lowering therapy for adults with heterozygous familial hypercholesterolemia or ASCVD who require additional lowering of LDL cholesterol. The typical LDL reduction ranges from 40% to over 60%. The most common adverse effect reported in clinical trials was injection site pain. The drugs are administered by SC injection into the thigh, abdomen, or upper arm as follows:
  ✓ **Alirocumab** (Praluent) 75 mg SC every 2 weeks; if the response is inadequate, the dose may be increased to 150 mg SC every 2 weeks
  ✓ **Evolocumab** (Repatha) 140 mg SC every 2 weeks or 420 mg once monthly

TREATMENT RECOMMENDATIONS

- Treatment of type I hyperlipoproteinemia is directed toward reduction of chylomicrons derived from dietary fat with the subsequent reduction in plasma triglycerides. Total daily fat intake should be no more than 10 to 25 g, or ~15% of total calories. Secondary causes of hypertriglyceridemia should be excluded, and, if present, the underlying disorder should be treated appropriately.
- Primary hypercholesterolemia (familial hypercholesterolemia, familial combined dyslipidemia, and type IIa hyperlipoproteinemia) is treated with **BARs**, **statins**, **niacin**, or **ezetimibe**.
- Combined hyperlipoproteinemia (type IIb) may be treated with **statins**, **niacin**, or **gemfibrozil** to lower LDL-C without elevating VLDL and triglycerides. Niacin is the most effective agent and may be combined with a BAR. A BAR alone in this disorder may elevate VLDL and triglycerides, and their use as single agents for treating combined hyperlipoproteinemia should be avoided.
- Type III hyperlipoproteinemia may be treated with **fibrates** or **niacin**. Although fibrates have been suggested as the drugs of choice, niacin is a reasonable alternative because of the lack of data supporting a cardiovascular mortality benefit from fibrates and because of potentially serious adverse effects. Fish oil supplementation may be an alternative therapy.
- Type V hyperlipoproteinemia requires stringent restriction of dietary fat intake. Drug therapy with **fibrates** or **niacin** is indicated if the response to diet alone is inadequate. **Medium-chain triglycerides**, which are absorbed without chylomicron formation may be used as a dietary supplement for caloric intake if needed for both types I and V.

Combination Drug Therapy

- Combination therapy may be considered after adequate trials of monotherapy and for patients documented to be adherent to the prescribed regimen. Two or three lipoprotein profiles at 6-week intervals should confirm the lack of response prior to initiation of combination therapy.

- Screen carefully for contraindications and drug interactions with combined therapy, and consider the extra cost of drug product and monitoring.
- In general, a **statin** plus a **BAR** or **niacin** plus a **BAR** provides the greatest reduction in total and LDL cholesterol.
- Regimens intended to increase HDL levels should include either **gemfibrozil** or **niacin**, bearing in mind that **statins** combined with either of these drugs may result in a greater incidence of hepatotoxicity or myositis.
- Familial combined dyslipidemia may respond better to a fibrate and a statin than to a fibrate and a BAR.

TREATMENT OF HYPERTRIGLYCERIDEMIA

- Lipoprotein pattern types I, III, IV, and V are associated with hypertriglyceridemia, and these primary lipoprotein disorders should be excluded prior to implementing therapy.
- A family history positive for CHD is important in identifying patients at risk for premature atherosclerosis. If a patient with CHD has elevated triglycerides, the associated abnormality is probably a contributing factor to CHD and should be treated.
- High serum triglycerides should be treated by achieving desirable body weight, consumption of a low saturated fat and cholesterol diet, regular exercise, smoking cessation, and restriction of alcohol (in select patients).
- Drug therapy with **niacin** should be considered in patients with borderline-high triglycerides but with risk factors of established CHD, family history of premature CHD, concomitant LDL elevation or low HDL, and genetic forms of hypertriglyceridemia associated with CHD. Alternative therapies include **gemfibrozil** or **fenofibrate**, **statins**, and **fish oil**. The goal of therapy is to lower triglycerides and VLDL particles that may be atherogenic, increase HDL, and reduce LDL.
- Very high triglycerides are associated with pancreatitis and other adverse consequences. Management includes dietary fat restriction (10–20% of calories as fat), weight loss, alcohol restriction, and treatment of coexisting disorders (eg, diabetes). Drug therapy includes **gemfibrozil** or **fenofibrate**, **niacin**, and higher-potency statins (**atorvastatin**, **pitavastatin**, **rosuvastatin**, and **simvastatin**). Successful treatment is defined as reduction in triglycerides to less than 500 mg/dL (5.65 mmol/L).

TREATMENT OF LOW HDL CHOLESTEROL

- Low HDL cholesterol is a strong independent risk predictor of CHD. ATP III redefined low HDL cholesterol as less than 40 mg/dL (<1.03 mmol/L) but specified no goal for HDL raising. In low HDL, the primary target remains LDL, but treatment emphasis shifts to weight reduction, increased physical activity, and smoking cessation, and to **fibrates** and **niacin** if drug therapy is required.

TREATMENT OF DIABETIC DYSLIPIDEMIA

- Diabetic dyslipidemia is characterized by hypertriglyceridemia, low HDL, and minimally elevated LDL. Small, dense LDL (pattern B) in diabetes is more atherogenic than larger, more buoyant forms of LDL (pattern A).
- ATP III considers diabetes to be a CHD risk equivalent, and the primary target is to lower the LDL to less than 100 mg/dL (<2.59 mmol/L). When LDL is greater than 130 mg/dL (>3.36 mmol/L), most patients require simultaneous TLCs and drug therapy. When LDL is between 100 and 129 mg/dL (2.59 and 3.34 mmol/L), intensifying glycemic control, adding drugs for atherogenic dyslipidemia (**fibrates** and **niacin**) and intensifying LDL-lowering therapy are options. **Statins** are considered by many to be the drugs of choice because the primary target is LDL.

EVALUATION OF THERAPEUTIC OUTCOMES

- Short-term evaluation of therapy for dyslipidemia is based on response to diet and drug treatment as measured by total cholesterol, LDL-C, HDL-C, and triglycerides.

- Many patients treated for primary dyslipidemia have no symptoms or clinical manifestations of a genetic lipid disorder (eg, xanthomas), and monitoring may be solely laboratory based.
- In patients treated for secondary intervention, symptoms of atherosclerotic cardiovascular disease, such as angina and intermittent claudication, may improve over months to years. Xanthomas or other external manifestations of dyslipidemia should regress with therapy.
- Obtain lipid measurements in the fasting state to minimize interference from chylomicrons. Monitoring is needed every few months during dosage titration. Once the patient is stable, monitoring at intervals of 6 months to 1 year is sufficient.
- Patients on BAR therapy should have a fasting panel checked every 4 to 8 weeks until a stable dose is reached; check triglycerides at a stable dose to ensure they have not increased.
- Niacin requires baseline tests of liver function (alanine aminotransferase), uric acid, and glucose. Repeat tests are appropriate at doses of 1000 to 1500 mg/day. Symptoms of myopathy or diabetes should be investigated and may require creatine kinase or glucose determinations. Patients with diabetes may require more frequent monitoring.
- Patients receiving statins should have a fasting lipid panel 4 to 8 weeks after the initial dose or dose changes. Obtain liver function tests at baseline and periodically thereafter. Some experts believe that monitoring for hepatotoxicity and myopathy should be triggered by symptoms.
- For patients with multiple risk factors and established CHD, evaluate for progress in managing other risk factors such as BP control, smoking cessation, exercise and weight control, and glycemic control (if diabetic).
- Evaluation of dietary therapy with diet diaries and recall survey instruments allows information about diet to be collected in a systematic fashion and may improve patient adherence to dietary recommendations.

See Chapter 11, Dyslipidemia, authored by Robert L. Talbert, for a more detailed discussion of this topic.

Heart Failure

- *Heart failure* (HF) is a progressive clinical syndrome caused by inability of the heart to pump sufficient blood to meet the body's metabolic needs. HF can result from any disorder that affects the ability of the heart to contract (systolic dysfunction) and/or relax (diastolic dysfunction). HF with reduced systolic function (ie, reduced left ventricular ejection fraction, LVEF) is referred to as HF with reduced ejection fraction (HFrEF). Preserved LV systolic function (ie, normal LVEF) with presumed diastolic dysfunction is termed HF with preserved ejection fraction (HFpEF).

PATHOPHYSIOLOGY

- Causes of systolic dysfunction (decreased contractility) are reduced muscle mass (eg, myocardial infarction [MI]), dilated cardiomyopathies, and ventricular hypertrophy. Ventricular hypertrophy can be caused by pressure overload (eg, systemic or pulmonary hypertension and aortic or pulmonic valve stenosis) or volume overload (eg, valvular regurgitation, shunts, and high-output states).
- Causes of diastolic dysfunction (restriction in ventricular filling) are increased ventricular stiffness, ventricular hypertrophy, infiltrative myocardial diseases, myocardial ischemia and MI, mitral or tricuspid valve stenosis, and pericardial disease (eg, pericarditis and pericardial tamponade).
- The leading causes of HF are coronary artery disease and hypertension.
- Regardless of the index event, decreased cardiac output results in activation of compensatory responses to maintain circulation: (1) tachycardia and increased contractility through sympathetic nervous system activation; (2) the Frank–Starling mechanism, whereby increased preload (through sodium and water retention) increases stroke volume; (3) vasoconstriction; and (4) ventricular hypertrophy and remodeling. Although these compensatory mechanisms initially maintain cardiac function, they are responsible for the symptoms of HF and contribute to disease progression.
- In the *neurohormonal model* of HF, an initiating event (eg, acute MI) leads to decreased cardiac output; the HF state then becomes a systemic disease whose progression is mediated largely by neurohormones and autocrine/paracrine factors that drive myocyte injury, oxidative stress, inflammation, and extracellular matrix remodeling. These substances include angiotensin II, norepinephrine, aldosterone, natriuretic peptides, and arginine vasopressin.
- Common precipitating factors that may cause a previously compensated HF patient to decompensate include myocardial ischemia and MI, atrial fibrillation, pulmonary infections, nonadherence with diet or drug therapy, and inappropriate medication use. Drugs may precipitate or exacerbate HF through negative inotropic effects, direct cardiotoxicity, or increased sodium and water retention.

CLINICAL PRESENTATION

- Patient presentation may range from asymptomatic to cardiogenic shock.
- Primary symptoms are dyspnea (especially on exertion) and fatigue, which lead to exercise intolerance. Other pulmonary symptoms include orthopnea, paroxysmal nocturnal dyspnea, tachypnea, and cough.
- Fluid overload can result in pulmonary congestion and peripheral edema.
- Nonspecific symptoms may include fatigue, nocturia, hemoptysis, abdominal pain, anorexia, nausea, bloating, ascites, poor appetite or early satiety, mental status changes, and weight gain.
- Physical examination findings may include pulmonary crackles, S_3 gallop, cool extremities, Cheyne–Stokes respiration, tachycardia, narrow pulse pressure, cardiomegaly,

symptoms of pulmonary edema (extreme breathlessness and anxiety, sometimes with coughing and pink, frothy sputum), peripheral edema, jugular venous distention, hepatojugular reflux, and hepatomegaly.

DIAGNOSIS

- Consider diagnosis of HF in patients with characteristic signs and symptoms. A complete history and physical examination with appropriate laboratory testing are essential in evaluating patients with suspected HF.
- Laboratory tests for identifying disorders that may cause or worsen HF include complete blood cell count; serum electrolytes (including calcium and magnesium); renal, hepatic, and thyroid function tests; urinalysis; lipid profile; and A1C. B-type natriuretic peptide (BNP) will generally be greater than 100 pg/mL.
- Ventricular hypertrophy can be demonstrated on chest radiograph or electrocardiogram (ECG). Chest radiograph may also show pleural effusions or pulmonary edema.
- Echocardiogram can identify abnormalities of the pericardium, myocardium, or heart valves and quantify LVEF to determine if systolic or diastolic dysfunction is present.
- The New York Heart Association Functional Classification System is intended primarily to classify symptoms according to the physician's subjective evaluation. Functional class (FC)-I patients have no limitation of physical activity, FC-II patients have slight limitation, FC-III patients have marked limitation, and FC-IV patients are unable to carry on physical activity without discomfort.
- The American College of Cardiology/American Heart Association (ACC/AHA) staging system provides a more comprehensive framework for evaluating, preventing, and treating HF (see further discussion below).

TREATMENT OF CHRONIC HEART FAILURE

- <u>Goals of Treatment</u>: Improve quality of life, relieve or reduce symptoms, prevent or minimize hospitalizations, slow disease progression, and prolong survival.

GENERAL APPROACH

- The first step is to determine the etiology or precipitating factors. Treatment of underlying disorders (eg, hyperthyroidism) may obviate the need for treating HF.
- Nonpharmacologic interventions include cardiac rehabilitation and restriction of fluid intake (maximum 2 L/day from all sources) and dietary sodium (<2–3 g of sodium/day). Drugs that aggravate HF should be discontinued if possible.
- **ACC/AHA Stage A:** These are patients at high risk for developing heart failure. The emphasis is on identifying and modifying risk factors to prevent development of structural heart disease and subsequent HF. Strategies include smoking cessation and control of hypertension, diabetes mellitus, and dyslipidemia. Although treatment must be individualized, angiotensin-converting enzyme (ACE) inhibitors or angiotensin receptor blockers (ARBs) are recommended for HF prevention in patients with multiple vascular risk factors.
- **ACC/AHA Stage B:** In these patients with structural heart disease but no HF signs or symptoms, treatment is targeted at minimizing additional injury and preventing or slowing the remodeling process. In addition to treatment measures outlined for stage A, patients with reduced LVEF should receive an ACE inhibitor (or ARB) and a β-blocker to prevent development of HF, regardless of whether they have had an MI. Patients with a previous MI and reduced LVEF should also receive an ACE inhibitor or ARB, evidence-based β-blockers, and a statin.
- **ACC/AHA Stage C:** These patients have structural heart disease and previous or current HF symptoms and include both HFrEF and HFpEF. In addition to treatments for stages A and B, patients with HFrEF should be treated with guideline-directed medical therapy (GDMT) that includes an ACE inhibitor or ARB and an evidence-based β-blocker (Fig. 9–1). Loop diuretics, aldosterone antagonists, and hydralazine–isosorbide dinitrate (ISDN) are also used routinely. Digoxin, ivabradine,

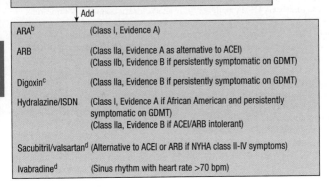

| GDMT for HFrEF Stage C |

Initiate and titrate ACEI or ARB and β-blocker[a] (Class I, Evidence A)
Initiate loop diuretic if fluid retention (Class I, Evidence C)

↓ Add

ARA[b]	(Class I, Evidence A)
ARB	(Class IIa, Evidence A as alternative to ACEI) (Class IIb, Evidence B if persistently symptomatic on GDMT)
Digoxin[c]	(Class IIa, Evidence B if persistently symptomatic on GDMT)
Hydralazine/ISDN	(Class I, Evidence A if African American and persistently symptomatic on GDMT) (Class IIa, Evidence B if ACEI/ARB intolerant)
Sacubitril/valsartan[d]	(Alternative to ACEI or ARB if NYHA class II-IV symptoms)
Ivabradine[d]	(Sinus rhythm with heart rate >70 bpm)

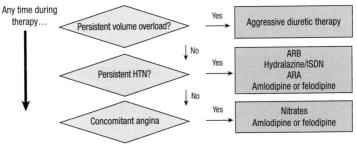

Any time during therapy...

Persistent volume overload? → Yes → Aggressive diuretic therapy
↓ No
Persistent HTN? → Yes → ARB / Hydralazine/ISDN / ARA / Amlodipine or felodipine
↓ No
Concomitant angina → Yes → Nitrates / Amlodipine or felodipine

[a]If not already receiving this therapy for previous MI, LV dysfunction, or other indication.
[b]If NYHA class II-IV symptoms, estimated creatinine clearance >30 mL/min, and K+ <5.0 mEq/L.
[c]Indication is to reduce hospitalization.
[d]Not included in current guidelines.
(ACEI, angiotensin-converting enzyme inhibitor; ARA, aldosterone receptor antagonist; ARB, angiotensin receptor blocker; bpm, beats per minute; GDMT, guideline-directed medical therapy; HTN, hypertension; ISDN, isosorbide dinitrate; LV, left ventricular; MI, myocardial infarction.)

FIGURE 9–1. Guideline-directed treatment algorithms for patients with ACC/AHA stage C heart failure with reduced ejection fraction. (*Adapted from Yancy CW, Jessup M, Bozkurt B, et al. 2013 ACCF/AHA guideline for the management of heart failure: A report of the American College of Cardiology Foundation/American Heart Association Task Force on Practice Guidelines. J Am Coll Cardiol 2013;62:e147–239.*)

and sacubitril/valsartan can be considered in select patients. Other general measures include moderate sodium restriction, daily weight measurement, immunization against influenza and pneumococcus, modest physical activity, and avoidance of medications that can exacerbate HF.

• **ACC/AHA Stage D HFrEF:** These are patients with persistent HF symptoms despite maximally tolerated GDMT. They should be considered for specialized interventions, including mechanical circulatory support, continuous IV positive inotropic therapy, cardiac transplantation, or hospice care (when no additional treatments are appropriate). Restriction of sodium and fluid intake may be beneficial. High doses of diuretics, combination therapy with a loop and thiazide diuretic, or mechanical fluid removal methods such as ultrafiltration may be required. Patients may be less tolerant to ACE inhibitors and β-blockers, so low starting doses, slow upward dose titration, and close monitoring are essential.

- **Management of HFpEF:** Treatment includes controlling heart rate (HR) and blood pressure (BP), alleviating causes of myocardial ischemia, reducing volume, and restoring and maintaining sinus rhythm in patients with atrial fibrillation. Many of the drugs are the same as those used to treat HFrEF (eg, β-blockers and diuretics), but the rationale and dosing may be different. Calcium channel blockers (eg, diltiazem, amlodipine, and verapamil) may be useful in HFpEF but have little utility in treating HFrEF.

PHARMACOLOGIC THERAPY

Drug Therapies for Routine Use in Stage C HFrEF (Fig. 9–1)

DIURETICS

- Compensatory mechanisms in HF stimulate excessive sodium and water retention, often leading to systemic and pulmonary congestion. Consequently, diuretic therapy (in addition to sodium restriction) is recommended for all patients with clinical evidence of fluid retention. However, because they do not alter disease progression or prolong survival, diuretics are not required for patients without fluid retention. In patients with HFpEF, diuretic treatment should be initiated at low doses to avoid hypotension and fatigue.
- Thiazide diuretics (eg, **hydrochlorothiazide**) are relatively weak and are infrequently used alone in HF. However, thiazides or the thiazide-like diuretic **metolazone** can be used in combination with a loop diuretic to promote very effective diuresis. Thiazides may be preferred over loop diuretics in patients with only mild fluid retention and elevated BP because of their more persistent antihypertensive effects.
- Loop diuretics (**furosemide, bumetanide**, and **torsemide**) are usually necessary to restore and maintain euvolemia in HF. In addition to acting in the thick ascending limb of the loop of Henle, they induce a prostaglandin-mediated increase in renal blood flow that contributes to their natriuretic effect. Unlike thiazides, loop diuretics maintain their effectiveness in the presence of impaired renal function, although higher doses may be necessary. See Table 9–1 for initial doses and usual dose ranges.

ANGIOTENSIN-CONVERTING ENZYME INHIBITORS

- ACE inhibitors decrease angiotensin II and aldosterone, attenuating many of their deleterious effects, including reducing ventricular remodeling, myocardial fibrosis, myocyte apoptosis, cardiac hypertrophy, norepinephrine release, vasoconstriction, and sodium and water retention.
- Clinical trials have documented favorable effects of ACE inhibitors on symptoms, NYHA functional classification, clinical status, HF progression, hospitalizations, and quality of life. ACE inhibitors improve survival by 20% to 30% compared with placebo. All patients with HFrEF should receive ACE inhibitors unless contraindications are present. Post-MI patients without HF symptoms or reduced LVEF (Stage B) should also receive ACE inhibitors to prevent development of HF and to reduce mortality.
- Therapy should be started with low doses followed by gradual titration as tolerated to target doses to minimize the risk of hypotension and renal insufficiency (**Table 9–1**). Renal function and serum potassium should be evaluated at baseline and within 1 to 2 weeks after the start of therapy with periodic assessments thereafter. Initiation of β-blocker therapy should not be delayed while the ACE inhibitor is titrated to the target dose because low–intermediate ACE inhibitor doses are equally effective as higher doses for improving symptoms and survival.

TABLE 9-1	Drug Dosing Table			
Drug	Brand Name	Initial Dose	Usual Range	Special Population Dose
Loop Diuretics				
Furosemide	Lasix	20–40 mg once or twice daily	20–160 mg once or twice daily	Cl_{cr} 20–50 mL/min: 160 mg once or twice daily Cl_{cr}<20 mL/min: 400 mg daily
Bumetanide	Bumex	0.5–1.0 mg once or twice daily	1–2 mg once or twice daily	Cl_{cr} 20–50 mL/min: 2 mg once or twice daily Cl_{cr}<20 mL/min: 8–10 mg daily
Torsemide	Demadex	10–20 mg once daily	10–80 mg once daily	Cl_{cr} 20–50 mL/min: 40 mg once daily Cl_{cr}<20 mL/min: 200 mg daily
ACE Inhibitors				
Captopril	Capoten	6.25 mg three times daily	50 mg three times daily[a]	
Enalapril	Vasotec	2.5 mg twice daily	10–20 mg twice daily[a]	
Lisinopril	Zestril, Prinivil	2.5–5 mg once daily	20–40 mg once daily[a]	
Quinapril	Accupril	5 mg twice daily	20–40 mg twice daily	
Ramipril	Altace	1.25–2.5 mg	5 mg twice daily[a]	
Fosinopril	Monopril	5–10 mg once daily	40 mg once daily	
Trandolapril	Mavik	0.5–1 mg once daily	4 mg once daily[a]	
Perindopril	Aceon	2 mg once daily	8–16 mg once daily	
Angiotensin Receptor Blockers				
Candesartan	Atacand	4 mg once daily	32 mg once daily[a]	
Valsartan	Diovan	20–40 mg twice daily	160 mg twice daily[a]	
Losartan	Cozaar	25–50 mg once daily	150 mg once daily[a]	
Beta-Blockers				
Bisoprolol	Zebeta	1.25 mg once daily	10 mg once daily[a]	
Carvedilol	Coreg	3.125 mg twice daily	25 mg twice daily[a]	Target dose for patients weighing >85 kg is 50 mg twice daily
Carvedilol phosphate	Coreg CR	10 mg once daily	80 mg once daily	
Metoprolol succinate CR/XL	Toprol-XL	12.5–25 mg once daily	200 mg once daily[a]	

TABLE 9–1	Drug Dosing Table (*Continued*)			
Drug	Brand Name	Initial Dose	Usual Range	Special Population Dose
Aldosterone Antagonists				
Spironolac- tone	Aldactone	eGFR ≥50 mL/min/1.73m²: 12.5–25 mg once daily	25–50 mg once daily[a]	eGFR 30–49 mL/min/1.73m²: 12.5 mg once daily or every other day
Eplerenone	Inspra	eGFR ≥50 mL/min/1.73m²: 25 mg once daily	50 mg once daily[a]	eGFR 30–49 mL/min/1.73m²: 25 mg every other day
Other				
Hydralazine- Isosor- bide Dinitrate	Bidil	Hydralazine 37.5 mg three times daily Isosorbide dinitrate 20 mg three times daily	Hydralazine 75 mg three times daily[a] Isosorbide dinitrate 40 mg three times daily[a]	
Digoxin	Lanoxin	0.125–0.25 mg once daily	0.125–0.25 mg once daily	Reduce dose in elderly, patients with low lean body mass, and patients with impaired renal function
Ivabradine	Corlanor	5 mg twice daily	5–7.5 mg twice daily	Avoid if resting heart rate <60 BPM before treatment
Sacubitril/ valsartan	Entresto	49/51 mg sacubitril/ valsartan twice daily	97/103 mg sacubitril/ valsartan twice daily[a]	For patients taking a low dose of or not taking an ACEI or ARB or if eGFR is <30 mL/min/1.73m², the starting dose is 24/26 mg sacubitril/ valsartan twice daily

[a]Regimens proven in large clinical trials to reduce mortality.
ACEI, angiotensin-converting enzyme inhibitor; ARB, angiotensin receptor blocker; Cl_{cr}, creatinine clearance; eGFR, estimated glomerular filtration rate; HFrEF, heart failure with reduced ejection fraction.
(*Data from Brater DC. Pharmacology of diuretics. Am J Med Sci 2000;319:38-50; Yancy CW, Jessup M, Bozkurt B, et al. 2013 ACCF/AHA guideline for the management of heart failure: A report of the American College of Cardiology Foundation/American Heart Association Task Force on Practice Guidelines. J Am Coll Cardiol 2013;62:e147–e239.*)

ANGIOTENSIN RECEPTOR BLOCKERS

- The ARBs block the angiotensin II receptor subtype AT_1, preventing the deleterious effects of angiotensin II, regardless of its origin. Because they do not affect the ACE enzyme, ARBs do not affect bradykinin, which is linked to ACE inhibitor cough and angioedema.
- Although ACE inhibitors remain first-line therapy in patients with Stage C HFrEF, current guidelines recommend use of ARBs in patients unable to tolerate (usually due to cough) ACE inhibitors. Combined use of ACE inhibitors, ARBs, and aldosterone antagonists is not recommended because of an increased risk of renal dysfunction and hyperkalemia. Current guidelines recommend that addition of an ARB can

be considered in patients with HFrEF who remain symptomatic despite treatment with an ACE inhibitor and a β-blocker if an aldosterone antagonist cannot be used. Although a number of ARBs are available, only candesartan, losartan, and valsartan are recommended because efficacy has been demonstrated in clinical trials. As with ACE inhibitors, initial doses should be low with titration to targets achieved in clinical trials (see **Table 9–1**).

- Assess BP, renal function, and serum potassium within 1 to 2 weeks after therapy initiation and dose increases, with these endpoints used to guide subsequent dose changes. It is not necessary to reach target ARB doses before adding a β-blocker.

- Caution should be exercised when ARBs are used in patients with angioedema from ACE inhibitors because cross reactivity has been reported. ARBs are not alternatives in patients with hypotension, hyperkalemia, or renal insufficiency due to ACE inhibitors because they are just as likely to cause these adverse effects.

β-BLOCKERS

- There is overwhelming clinical trial evidence that certain β-blockers slow disease progression, decrease hospitalizations, and reduce mortality in patients with systolic HF.

- The ACC/AHA guidelines recommend use of β-blockers in all stable patients with HF and a reduced LVEF in the absence of contraindications or a clear history of β-blocker intolerance. Patients should receive a β-blocker even if symptoms are mild or well controlled with ACE inhibitor and diuretic therapy. It is not essential that ACE inhibitor doses be optimized before a β-blocker is started because the addition of a β-blocker is likely to be of greater benefit than an increase in ACE inhibitor dose.

- β-Blockers are also recommended for asymptomatic patients with a reduced LVEF (stage B) to decrease the risk of progression to HF.

- Initiate β-blockers in stable patients who have no or minimal evidence of fluid overload. Because of their negative inotropic effects, start β-blockers in very low doses with slow upward dose titration to avoid symptomatic worsening or acute decompensation. Titrate to target doses when possible to provide maximal survival benefits.

- Carvedilol, metoprolol succinate (CR/XL), and bisoprolol are the only β-blockers shown to reduce mortality in large HF trials. Because bisoprolol is not available in the necessary starting dose of 1.25 mg, the choice is typically limited to either carvedilol or metoprolol succinate. Initial and target doses are those associated with reductions in mortality in placebo-controlled clinical trials (see **Table 9–1**).

- Doses should be doubled no more often than every 2 weeks, as tolerated, until the target dose or the maximally tolerated dose is reached. Patients should understand that dose up-titration is a long, gradual process and that achieving the target dose is important to maximize benefits. Further, the response to therapy may be delayed, and HF symptoms may actually worsen during the initiation period.

ALDOSTERONE ANTAGONISTS

- **Spironolactone** and **eplerenone** block the mineralocorticoid receptor, the target site for aldosterone. In the kidney, aldosterone antagonists inhibit sodium reabsorption and potassium excretion. However, diuretic effects are minimal, suggesting that their therapeutic benefits result from other actions. In the heart, aldosterone antagonists inhibit cardiac extracellular matrix and collagen deposition, thereby attenuating cardiac fibrosis and ventricular remodeling. Aldosterone antagonists also attenuate the systemic proinflammatory state, atherogenesis, and oxidative stress caused by aldosterone.

- Based on clinical trial results demonstrating reduced mortality, low-dose aldosterone antagonists may be appropriate for: (1) patients with mild to moderately severe HFrEF (NYHA class II–IV) who are receiving standard therapy, and (2) those with LV dysfunction and either acute HF or diabetes early after MI.

- Aldosterone antagonists must be used cautiously and with careful monitoring of renal function and potassium concentration. They should be avoided in patients with renal impairment, recent worsening of renal function, serum potassium greater than 5 mEq/L, or a history of severe hyperkalemia. Spironolactone also interacts with androgen and progesterone receptors, which may lead to gynecomastia, impotence, and menstrual irregularities in some patients.

- Initial doses should be low, and doses should be limited to those associated with beneficial effects to decrease the risk for hyperkalemia (see **Table 9–1**).

Drugs to Consider for Select Patients with HFrEF

NITRATES AND HYDRALAZINE

- Nitrates (eg, **ISDN**) and **hydralazine** have complementary hemodynamic actions. Nitrates are primarily venodilators, producing reductions in preload. Hydralazine is a direct arterial vasodilator that reduces systemic vascular resistance (SVR) and increases stroke volume and cardiac output. The mechanism for the beneficial effects of hydralazine/ISDN in HF remains uncertain but is likely related to normalization of the increased oxidative stress and reduced nitric oxide signaling that contributes to HF progression.
- Guidelines recommend addition of hydralazine/ISDN to self-described African Americans with HFrEF and NYHA class III–IV symptoms treated with ACE inhibitors and β-blockers. The combination can also be useful in patients unable to tolerate either an ACE inhibitor or ARB because of renal insufficiency, hyperkalemia, or possibly hypotension.
- Obstacles to successful therapy with this drug combination include the need for frequent dosing (ie, three times daily with the fixed-dose combination product), high frequency of adverse effects (eg, headache, dizziness, and GI distress), and increased cost for the fixed-dose combination product.

ARB/NEPRILYSIN INHIBITOR (ARNI)

- Valsartan/sacubitril is an angiotensin receptor/neprilysin inhibitor approved for treatment of HFrEF. The drug product is a crystalline complex composed of both drugs. Neprilysin is one of the enzymes that break down endogenous natriuretic peptides. The peptides are beneficial because they cause vasodilation, increased glomerular filtration, natriuresis, and diuresis. Sacubitril is a neprilysin inhibitor prodrug that is cleaved into its active form, which inhibits neprilysin thereby promoting vasodilation through a different mechanism than the ARB. Combination with valsartan negates the elevated levels of AT_2 that would result from use of neprilysin alone.
- The combination product is indicated to reduce the risk of cardiovascular death and hospitalization for HF in patients with NYHA Class II–IV HF and reduced LVEF. When titrated to a target dose of 200 mg (sacubitril 97 mg/valsartan 103 mg) twice daily, the combination reduced the combined endpoint of cardiovascular death and hospitalization for HF by 20% compared to enalapril 10 mg twice daily in patients with symptomatic HF and reduced LVEF. Its use will likely be incorporated into future HF guidelines.

IVABRADINE

- Ivabradine blocks the I_f current in the sinoatrial node that is responsible for controlling heart rate, thereby slowing spontaneous depolarization of the sinus node and resulting in a dose-dependent slowing of the heart rate.
- It is indicated to reduce the risk of hospitalization for worsening HF in patients with LVEF ≤ 35% who are in sinus rhythm with resting heart rate ≥ 70 bpm and either are on maximally tolerated doses of β-blockers or have a contraindication to β-blocker use. The most common adverse effects are bradycardia, atrial fibrillation, and visual disturbances.

DIGOXIN

- Although digoxin has positive inotropic effects, its benefits in HF are related to its neurohormonal effects. Digoxin improves cardiac function, quality of life, exercise tolerance, and HF symptoms in patients with HFrEF but does not improve survival.

- Based on available data, digoxin is not considered a first-line agent in HF, but a trial may be considered in conjunction with GDMT including ACE inhibitors, β-blockers, and diuretics in patients with symptomatic HFrEF to improve symptoms and reduce hospitalizations. Digoxin may also be considered to help control ventricular response rate in patients with HFrEF and supraventricular arrhythmias, although β-blockers are generally more effective rate control agents, especially during exercise.
- In the absence of digoxin toxicity or serious adverse effects, digoxin should be continued in most patients. Digoxin withdrawal may be considered for asymptomatic patients who have significant improvement in systolic function with optimal ACE inhibitor and β-blocker treatment.
- The target serum digoxin concentration for most patients is 0.5 to 0.9 ng/mL (0.6–1.2 nmol/L). Most patients with normal renal function can achieve this level with a dose of 0.125 mg/day. Patients with decreased renal function, the elderly, or those receiving interacting drugs (eg, amiodarone) should receive 0.125 mg every other day.

TREATMENT OF ACUTE DECOMPENSATED HEART FAILURE

GENERAL APPROACH

- *Acute decompensated heart failure (ADHF)* involves patients with new or worsening signs or symptoms (often resulting from volume overload and/or low cardiac output) requiring medical intervention, such as emergency department visit or hospitalization.
- Goals of Treatment: The overall goal is to relieve symptoms while optimizing volume status and cardiac output so the patient can be discharged in a stable compensated state on oral drug therapy.
- Hospitalization should be considered based on clinical findings. Most patients may be admitted to a monitored unit or general medical floor. Admission to an intensive care unit (ICU) may be required if the patient experiences hemodynamic instability requiring frequent monitoring of vital signs, invasive hemodynamic monitoring, or rapid titration of IV medications with close monitoring.
- History and physical exam should focus on potential etiologies of ADHF; presence of precipitating factors (eg, arrhythmias, hypertension, myocardial infarction, anemia, and thyroid disorders); onset, duration, and severity of symptoms; and a careful medication history. Laboratory tests that may be obtained include BNP or N-terminal pro-BNP, thyroid function tests, complete blood count, cardiac enzymes, and routine serum chemistries.
- Ascertain hemodynamic status to guide initial therapy. Patients may be categorized into one of four hemodynamic subsets based on volume status (euvolemic or "dry" vs volume overloaded or "wet") and cardiac output (adequate cardiac output or "warm" vs hypoperfusion or "cold") (**Fig. 9–2**).
- Reserve invasive hemodynamic monitoring for patients who are refractory to initial therapy, whose volume status is unclear, or who have significant hypotension or worsening renal function despite appropriate initial therapy.
- Address and correct reversible or treatable causes of decompensation.
- Assess medications being taken prior to admission and determine whether adjustment or discontinuation is required.
- If fluid retention is evident on physical exam, pursue aggressive diuresis, often with IV diuretics.
- In the absence of cardiogenic shock or symptomatic hypotension, strive to continue all GDMT for HF. β-blockers may be temporarily held or dose-reduced if recent changes are responsible for acute decompensation. Other GDMT (ACE inhibitors, ARBs, neprilysin inhibitors, and aldosterone antagonists) may also need to be temporarily held in the presence of renal dysfunction, with close monitoring of serum potassium. Most patients may continue to receive digoxin at doses targeting a trough serum concentration of 0.5 to 0.9 ng/mL (0.6–1.2 nmol/L).

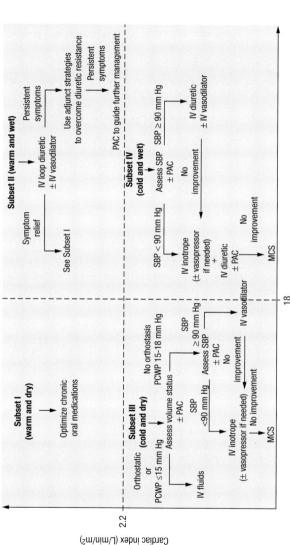

Cardiac index (L/min/m²)

Pulmonary capillary wedge pressure (mm Hg)

Subset I (warm and dry)
→ Optimize chronic oral medications

Subset II (warm and wet)
Symptom relief ← IV loop diuretic ± IV vasodilator → Persistent symptoms → Use adjunct strategies to overcome diuretic resistance → Persistent symptoms → PAC to guide further management
See Subset I

Subset III (cold and dry)
Orthostatic or PCWP ≤15 mm Hg → IV fluids
No orthostasis PCWP 15-18 mm Hg → Assess volume status ± PAC
SBP ≥ 90 mm Hg → Assess SBP ± PAC → No improvement → IV vasodilator
SBP <90 mm Hg → IV inotrope (± vasopressor if needed) → No improvement → MCS

Subset IV (cold and wet)
Assess SBP ± PAC
SBP ≥ 90 mm Hg → IV diuretic ± IV vasodilator
SBP < 90 mm Hg → IV inotrope (± vasopressor if needed) + IV diuretic ± PAC → No improvement → MCS

18

2.2

(IV, intravenous; MCS, mechanical circulatory support; PAC, pulmonary artery catheter; PCWP, pulmonary capillary wedge pressure; SBP, systolic BP.)

FIGURE 9-2. General management algorithm for acute decompensated heart failure based on clinical presentation. Patients may be categorized into a hemodynamic subset based on signs and symptoms or invasive hemodynamic monitoring. Adjunct strategies for overcoming diuretic resistance include increasing the dose of loop diuretic; switching to a continuous infusion; adding a diuretic with an alternative mechanism of action, an IV vasodilator, or an IV inotrope; and in select patients, ultrafiltration or a vasopressin antagonist.

PHARMACOTHERAPY OF ACUTE DECOMPENSATED HEART FAILURE

Diuretics

- IV loop diuretics, including **furosemide, bumetanide**, and **torsemide**, are used for ADHF, with furosemide being the most widely studied and used agent.
- Bolus administration reduces preload by functional venodilation within 5 to 15 minutes and later (>20 min) via sodium and water excretion, thereby improving pulmonary congestion. However, acute reductions in venous return may severely compromise effective preload in patients with significant diastolic dysfunction or intravascular depletion.
- Because diuretics can cause excessive preload reduction, they must be used judiciously to obtain the desired improvement in congestive symptoms while avoiding a reduction in cardiac output, symptomatic hypotension, or worsening renal function.
- Diuretic resistance may be overcome by administering larger IV bolus doses or continuous IV infusions of loop diuretics. Diuresis may also be improved by adding a second diuretic with a different mechanism of action (eg, combining a loop diuretic with a distal tubule blocker such as **metolazone** or **hydrochlorothiazide**). The loop diuretic–thiazide combination should generally be reserved for inpatients who can be monitored closely for development of severe electrolyte and intravascular volume depletion. In the outpatient setting, very low doses of the thiazide-type diuretic or infrequent administration (eg, 1–3 times weekly) are recommended.

Vasodilators

- Venodilators reduce preload by increasing venous capacitance, improving symptoms of pulmonary congestion in patients with high ventricular filling pressures. Arterial vasodilators reduce afterload and cause a reflex increase in cardiac output, which may promote diuresis via improved renal perfusion. Mixed vasodilators act on both arterial resistance and venous capacitance vessels, reducing congestive symptoms while increasing cardiac output.

NITROGLYCERIN

- IV **nitroglycerin** is often preferred for preload reduction in ADHF, especially in patients with pulmonary congestion. It reduces preload and pulmonary capillary wedge pressure (PCWP) via functional venodilation and mild arterial vasodilation. In higher doses, nitroglycerin displays potent coronary vasodilating properties and beneficial effects on myocardial oxygen demand and supply, making it the vasodilator of choice for patients with severe HF and ischemic heart disease.
- Initiate nitroglycerin at 5 to 10 mcg/min (0.1 mcg/kg/min) and increase every 5 to 10 minutes as necessary and tolerated. Maintenance doses usually range from 35 to 200 mcg/min (0.5–3 mcg/kg/min). Hypotension and an excessive decrease in PCWP are important dose-limiting side effects. Tolerance to the hemodynamic effects may develop over 12 to 72 hours of continuous administration.

NESIRITIDE

- **Nesiritide** is a recombinant form of endogenous BNP, which is secreted by the myocardium in response to volume overload. Nesiritide mimics the vasodilatory and natriuretic actions of BNP, resulting in venous and arterial vasodilation; increased cardiac output; natriuresis and diuresis; and decreased cardiac filling pressures, sympathetic nervous system activity, and renin–angiotensin–aldosterone system activity. In contrast to nitroglycerin or dobutamine, tolerance to its pharmacologic effects does not develop.
- Evidence from clinical trials indicates a limited role for nesiritide beyond relief of congestive symptoms in patients with acute dyspnea. Its use for management of ADHF has declined because it produces marginal improvement in clinical outcomes and is substantially more expensive than other IV vasodilators.

NITROPRUSSIDE

- **Sodium nitroprusside** is a mixed arteriovenous vasodilator that acts directly on vascular smooth muscle to increase cardiac index and decrease venous pressure to a similar degree as dobutamine and milrinone despite having no direct inotropic activity. However, nitroprusside generally produces greater decreases in PCWP, SVR, and BP.
- Hypotension is an important dose-limiting adverse effect of nitroprusside, and its use should be primarily reserved for patients with elevated SVR. Close monitoring is required because even modest heart rate increases can have adverse consequences in patients with underlying ischemic heart disease or resting tachycardia.
- Nitroprusside is effective in the short-term management of severe HF in a variety of settings (eg, acute MI, valvular regurgitation, after coronary bypass surgery, and ADHF). Generally, it does not worsen, and may improve, the balance between myocardial oxygen demand and supply. However, an excessive decrease in systemic arterial pressure can decrease coronary perfusion and worsen ischemia.
- Nitroprusside has a rapid onset and a duration of action less than 10 minutes, necessitating continuous IV infusions. Initiate therapy with a low dose (0.1–0.2 mcg/kg/min) to avoid excessive hypotension, and increase by small increments (0.1–0.2 mcg/kg/min) every 5 to 10 minutes as tolerated. Usual effective doses range from 0.5 to 3 mcg/kg/min. Taper nitroprusside slowly when stopping therapy because of possible rebound after abrupt withdrawal. Nitroprusside-induced cyanide and thiocyanate toxicity are unlikely when doses less than 3 mcg/kg/min are administered for less than 3 days, except in patients with significant renal impairment (ie, serum creatinine > 3 mg/dL [>265 μmol/L]).

Vasopressin Antagonists

- The vasopressin receptor antagonists currently available affect one or two arginine vasopressin (AVP; antidiuretic hormone) receptors, V_{1A} or V_2. Stimulation of V_{1A} receptors (located in vascular smooth muscle cells and myocardium) results in vasoconstriction, myocyte hypertrophy, coronary vasoconstriction, and positive inotropic effects. V_2 receptors are located in renal tubules, where they regulate water reabsorption.

  - ✓ **Tolvaptan** selectively binds to and inhibits the V_2 receptor. It is an oral agent indicated for hypervolemic and euvolemic hyponatremia in patients with syndrome of inappropriate antidiuretic hormone (SIADH), cirrhosis, and HF. Tolvaptan is typically initiated at 15 mg orally daily and then titrated to 30 or 60 mg daily as needed to resolve hyponatremia. It is a substrate of cytochrome P450-3A4 and is contraindicated with potent inhibitors of this enzyme. The most common side effects are dry mouth, thirst, urinary frequency, constipation, and hyperglycemia.
  - ✓ **Conivaptan** nonselectively inhibits both the V_{1A} and V_2 receptors. It is an IV agent indicated for hypervolemic and euvolemic hyponatremia due to a variety of causes; however, it is not indicated for hyponatremia associated with HF.

- Monitor patients closely to avoid an excessively rapid rise in serum sodium that could cause hypotension or hypovolemia; discontinue therapy if that occurs. Therapy may be restarted at a lower dose if hyponatremia recurs or persists and/or these side effects resolve.
- The role of vasopressin receptor antagonists in the long-term management of HF is unclear. In clinical trials, tolvaptan improved hyponatremia, diuresis, and signs/symptoms of congestion. However, one study failed to demonstrate improvement in global clinical status at discharge or a reduction in 2-year all-cause mortality, cardiovascular mortality, or HF rehospitalization.

Inotropes

- Low cardiac output in ADHF may worsen renal perfusion, resulting in resistance to diuretic therapy. IV inotropes may improve peripheral hypoperfusion and diuresis by improving central hemodynamics. However, because of their adverse effect profile they should generally be reserved for patients not responding to other modalities or those with clear evidence of low cardiac output.

- Guidelines recommend that inotropes be considered only as a temporizing measure for maintaining end-organ perfusion in patients with cardiogenic shock or evidence of severely depressed cardiac output and low systolic BP (ie, ineligible for IV vasodilators) until definitive therapy can be initiated, as a "bridge" for patients with advanced HF who are eligible for mechanical circulatory support (MCS) or cardiac transplantation, or for palliation of symptoms in patients with advanced HF who are not eligible for MCS or cardiac transplantation.
- Dobutamine and milrinone produce similar hemodynamic effects, but dobutamine is usually associated with more pronounced increases in heart rate.

DOBUTAMINE

- **Dobutamine** is a β_1- and β_2-receptor agonist with some α_1-agonist effects. It does not result in norepinephrine release from nerve terminals, so the positive inotropic effects are attributed to effects on β_1-receptors. Stimulation of cardiac β_1-receptors does not generally produce a significant increase in heart rate. Modest peripheral β_2-receptor-mediated vasodilation tends to offset minor α_1-receptor-mediated vasoconstriction; the net vascular effect is usually vasodilation.
- The initial dose for ADHF is 1 to 2 mcg/kg/min, titrated by 1 to 2 mcg/kg/min every 10 to 20 minutes to a maximum of 20 mcg/kg/min on the basis of clinical and hemodynamic responses.
- Cardiac index is increased because of inotropic stimulation, arterial vasodilation, and a variable increase in heart rate. It causes relatively little change in mean arterial pressure compared with the more consistent increases observed with dopamine.
- Although attenuation of dobutamine's hemodynamic effects may occur with prolonged administration, the dobutamine dose should be tapered rather than abruptly discontinued.

MILRINONE

- **Milrinone** inhibits phosphodiesterase III and produces positive inotropic and arterial and venous vasodilating effects (an inodilator). It has supplanted use of amrinone, which has a higher rate of thrombocytopenia.
- During IV administration, milrinone increases stroke volume and cardiac output with minimal change in heart rate. However, the venodilating effects may predominate, leading to decreased BP and a reflex tachycardia. Milrinone also lowers pulmonary PCWP by venodilation and is particularly useful in patients with a low cardiac index and elevated LV filling pressure. However, this decrease in preload can be hazardous for patients without excessive filling pressure, thus blunting the improvement in cardiac output.
- Use milrinone cautiously in severely hypotensive HF patients because it does not increase, and may even decrease, arterial BP.
- Most patients are started on a continuous IV infusion of 0.1 to 0.3 mcg/kg/min, titrated to a maximum of 0.75 mcg/kg/min. A loading dose of 50 mcg/kg over 10 minutes can be given if rapid hemodynamic changes are required, but it should generally be avoided because of the risk of hypotension.
- The most notable adverse events are arrhythmia, hypotension, and, rarely, thrombocytopenia. Measure the platelet count before and during therapy.

DOPAMINE

- **Dopamine** should generally be avoided in ADHF, but its pharmacologic actions may be preferable to dobutamine or milrinone in patients with marked systemic hypotension or cardiogenic shock in the face of elevated ventricular filling pressures, where dopamine in doses greater than 5 mcg/kg/min may be necessary to raise central aortic pressure.
- Dopamine produces dose-dependent hemodynamic effects because of its relative affinity for α_1-, β_1-, β_2-, and D_1- (vascular dopaminergic) receptors. Positive

inotropic effects mediated primarily by β_1-receptors become more prominent with doses of 2 to 5 mcg/kg/min. At doses between 5 and 10 mcg/kg/min, chronotropic and α_1-mediated vasoconstricting effects become more prominent.

- Evidence supporting use of low-dose dopamine (2–5 mcg/kg/min) to enhance diuresis is controversial. Most studies indicate little if any improvement in urine output, renal protection, or symptom relief, but increased rates of tachycardia. Thus, it may not provide any advantage over traditional inotropes in this setting.

MECHANICAL CIRCULATORY SUPPORT

- For patients with refractory ADHF, temporary MCS may be considered for hemodynamic stabilization until the underlying etiology of cardiac dysfunction resolves or has been corrected ("bridge to recovery") or until evaluation for definitive therapy (eg, durable MCS or cardiac transplantation) can be completed ("bridge to decision").
- Because of its invasive nature and potential complications, MCS should be reserved for patients refractory to maximally tolerated pharmacologic therapy.
- IV vasodilators and inotropes may be used with temporary MCS to maximize hemodynamic and clinical benefits or facilitate device removal.
- Systemic anticoagulant therapy is generally required to prevent device thrombosis, regardless of the method selected.
- The **intraaortic balloon pump (IABP)** is most commonly employed due to ease of use; however, it only increases cardiac output by about 1 L/min. It may be particularly useful for patients with myocardial ischemia complicated by cardiogenic shock, but it has not been shown to improve mortality in this setting.
- **Ventricular assist devices** (VADs) are surgically implanted and assist, or in some cases replace, the pumping functions of the right and/or left ventricles. Compared to an IABP, VADs confer greater hemodynamic improvements but no differences in long-term survival.
- **Extracorporeal membrane oxygenation** (ECMO) may be venoarterial or venovenous in nature. In venoarterial ECMO, deoxygenated blood is transported from the venous circulation to an extracorporeal oxygenator and returned as oxygenated blood to the arterial circulation. Venovenous ECMO consists of only extracorporeal oxygenation; hemodynamic support is provided by native cardiac function. Venoarterial ECMO is more commonly employed in the management of ADHF.

SURGICAL THERAPY

- Orthotopic cardiac transplantation is the best therapeutic option for patients with irreversible advanced HF, as 10-year survival rates approach 60% in patients transplanted after 2001.

EVALUATION OF THERAPEUTIC OUTCOMES

CHRONIC HEART FAILURE

- Ask patients about the presence and severity of symptoms and how symptoms affect daily activities.
- Evaluate efficacy of diuretic treatment by disappearance of the signs and symptoms of excess fluid retention. Physical examination should focus on body weight, extent of jugular venous distention, presence of hepatojugular reflux, and presence and severity of pulmonary congestion (rales, dyspnea on exertion, orthopnea, and paroxysmal nocturnal dyspnea) and peripheral edema.
- Other outcomes are improvement in exercise tolerance and fatigue, decreased nocturia, and a decrease in heart rate.
- Monitor BP to ensure that symptomatic hypotension does not develop as a result of drug therapy.
- Body weight is a sensitive marker of fluid loss or retention, and patients should weigh themselves daily and report changes to their healthcare provider so that adjustments can be made in diuretic doses.

- Symptoms may worsen initially on β-blocker therapy, and it may take weeks to months before patients notice symptomatic improvement.
- Routine monitoring of serum electrolytes and renal function is mandatory in patients with HF.

ACUTE DECOMPENSATED HEART FAILURE

- Initial stabilization requires adequate arterial oxygen saturation, cardiac index, and BP. Functional end-organ perfusion may be assessed by mental status, renal function sufficient to prevent metabolic complications, hepatic function adequate to maintain synthetic and excretory functions, stable heart rate and rhythm, absence of ongoing myocardial ischemia or MI, skeletal muscle and skin blood flow sufficient to prevent ischemic injury, and normal arterial pH (7.34–7.47) and serum lactate concentration. These goals are most often achieved with a cardiac index greater than 2.2 L/min/m^2, mean arterial BP greater than 60 mm Hg, and PCWP 15 mm Hg or greater.
- Daily monitoring should include weight, strict fluid intake and output measurements, and HF signs/symptoms to assess the efficacy of drug therapy. Monitoring for electrolyte depletion, symptomatic hypotension, and renal dysfunction should be performed frequently. Vital signs should be assessed frequently throughout the day.
- Patients should not be discharged until optimal volume status is achieved and the patient is successfully transitioned from IV to oral diuretics, GDMT is stable, and IV inotropes and vasodilators have been discontinued for at least 24 hours.

See Chapter 14, Chronic Heart Failure, authored by Robert B. Parker, Jean M. Nappi, and Larisa H. Cavallari, and Chapter 15, Acute Decompensated Heart Failure, authored by Jo E. Rodgers and Brent N. Reed, for a more detailed discussion of this topic.

10 Hypertension

- *Hypertension* is defined as persistently elevated arterial blood pressure (BP). The classification of BP in adults (age 18 years and older) is shown in Table 10–1.
- Isolated systolic hypertension is diastolic blood pressure (DBP) values less than 90 mm Hg and systolic blood pressure (SBP) values of 140 mm Hg or more.
- Hypertensive crisis (BP >180/120 mm Hg) may be categorized as hypertensive emergency (extreme BP elevation with acute or progressing end-organ damage) or hypertensive urgency (high BP elevation without acute or progressing end-organ injury).

PATHOPHYSIOLOGY

- Hypertension may result from an unknown etiology (primary or essential hypertension) or from a specific cause (secondary hypertension). Secondary hypertension (<10% of cases) is usually caused by chronic kidney disease (CKD) or renovascular disease. Other conditions are Cushing syndrome, coarctation of the aorta, obstructive sleep apnea, hyperparathyroidism, pheochromocytoma, primary aldosteronism, and hyperthyroidism. Some drugs that may increase BP include corticosteroids, estrogens, nonsteroidal anti-inflammatory drugs (NSAIDs), amphetamines, sibutramine, cyclosporine, tacrolimus, erythropoietin, and venlafaxine.
- Factors contributing to development of primary hypertension include:
  ✓ Humoral abnormalities involving the renin–angiotensin–aldosterone system (RAAS) or natriuretic hormone;
  ✓ Disturbance in the CNS, autonomic nerve fibers, adrenergic receptors, or baroreceptors;
  ✓ Abnormalities in renal or tissue autoregulatory processes for sodium excretion, plasma volume, and arteriolar constriction;
  ✓ Deficiency in synthesis of vasodilating substances in vascular endothelium (prostacyclin, bradykinin, and nitric oxide) or excess vasoconstricting substances (angiotensin II, endothelin I); and
  ✓ High sodium intake or lack of dietary calcium.
- Main causes of death are cerebrovascular events, cardiovascular (CV) events, and renal failure. Probability of premature death correlates with the severity of BP elevation.

CLINICAL PRESENTATION

- Patients with uncomplicated primary hypertension are usually asymptomatic initially.
- Patients with secondary hypertension may have symptoms of the underlying disorder. Patients with pheochromocytoma may have headaches, sweating, tachycardia, palpitations, and orthostatic hypotension. In primary aldosteronism, hypokalemic symptoms of muscle cramps and weakness may be present. Patients with Cushing syndrome may have weight gain, polyuria, edema, menstrual irregularities, recurrent acne, or muscular weakness in addition to classic features (moon face, buffalo hump, and hirsutism).

DIAGNOSIS

- Elevated BP may be the only sign of primary hypertension on physical examination. Diagnosis should be based on the average of two or more readings taken at each of two or more clinical encounters.
- Signs of end-organ damage occur primarily in the eye, brain, heart, kidneys, and peripheral blood vessels.
- Funduscopic examination may reveal arteriolar narrowing, focal arteriolar constrictions, arteriovenous nicking, retinal hemorrhages and exudates, and disk edema.

TABLE 10–1	Classification of Blood Pressure in Adults		
Classification	**Systolic (mm Hg)**		**Diastolic (mm Hg)**
Normal	<120	and	<80
Prehypertension	120–139	or	80–89
Stage 1 hypertension	140–159	or	90–99
Stage 2 hypertension	≥160	or	≥100

Presence of papilledema usually indicates a hypertensive emergency requiring rapid treatment.
- Cardiopulmonary examination may reveal abnormal heart rate or rhythm, left ventricular (LV) hypertrophy, coronary heart disease, or heart failure (HF).
- Peripheral vascular examination may reveal aortic or abdominal bruits, distended veins, diminished or absent peripheral pulses, or lower extremity edema.
- Patients with renal artery stenosis may have an abdominal systolic-diastolic bruit.
- Baseline hypokalemia may suggest mineralocorticoid-induced hypertension. Protein, blood cells, and casts in the urine may indicate renovascular disease.
- *Laboratory tests*: Blood urea nitrogen (BUN)/serum creatinine, fasting lipid panel, fasting blood glucose, serum electrolytes (sodium and potassium), hemoglobin and hematocrit, spot urine albumin-to-creatinine ratio, and estimated glomerular filtration rate (eGFR, using the Modification of Diet in Renal Disease [MDRD] equation). A 12-lead electrocardiogram (ECG) should also be obtained.
- *Laboratory tests to diagnose secondary hypertension*: Plasma norepinephrine and urinary metanephrine levels for pheochromocytoma, plasma and urinary aldosterone concentrations for primary aldosteronism, plasma renin activity, captopril stimulation test, renal vein renin, and renal artery angiography for renovascular disease.

TREATMENT

- Goals of Treatment: The overall goal is to reduce morbidity and mortality by the least intrusive means possible. The goal BP for most patients, including those with diabetes or CKD (nondialysis), is less than 140/90 mm Hg. Lower goals may be an option in certain populations. The goal for patients 80 years of age or older without diabetes or CKD is less than 150/90 mm Hg.

NONPHARMACOLOGIC THERAPY

- Lifestyle modifications: (1) weight loss if overweight or obese, (2) adoption of the Dietary Approaches to Stop Hypertension (DASH) eating plan, (3) dietary sodium restriction ideally to 1.5 g/day (3.8 g/day sodium chloride), (4) regular aerobic physical activity, (5) moderation of alcohol consumption (two or fewer drinks per day), and (6) smoking cessation.
- Lifestyle modification alone is sufficient for most patients with prehypertension but inadequate for patients with hypertension and additional CV risk factors or target-organ damage.

PHARMACOLOGIC THERAPY

- Initial drug selection depends on the degree of BP elevation and presence of compelling indications for selected drugs.
- **Angiotensin-converting enzyme (ACE) inhibitors, angiotensin II receptor blockers (ARBs), calcium channel blockers (CCBs),** and **thiazide diuretics** are acceptable first-line options.
- **β-Blockers** are used to either treat a specific compelling indication or as combination therapy with a first-line antihypertensive agent for patients without a compelling indication (**Table 10–2**).

TABLE 10–2 First-Line and Other Common Antihypertensive Agents

Class	Subclass	Drug (Brand Name)	Usual Dose Range (mg/day)	Daily Frequency
ACEi		Benazepril (Lotensin)	10–40	1 or 2
		Captopril (Capoten)	12.5–150	2 or 3
		Enalapril (Vasotec)	5–40	1 or 2
		Fosinopril (Monopril)	10–40	1
		Lisinopril (Prinivil, Zestril)	10–40	1
		Moexipril (Univasc)	7.5–30	1 or 2
		Perindopril (Aceon)	4–16	1
		Quinapril (Accupril)	10–80	1 or 2
		Ramipril (Altace)	2.5–10	1 or 2
		Trandolapril (Mavik)	1–4	1
ARB		Azilsartan (Edarbi)	40–80	1
		Candesartan (Atacand)	8–32	1 or 2
		Eprosartan (Teveten)	600–800	1 or 2
		Irbesartan (Avapro)	150–300	1
		Losartan (Cozaar)	50–100	1 or 2
		Olmesartan (Benicar)	20–40	1
		Telmisartan (Micardis)	20–80	1
		Valsartan (Diovan)	80–320	1
Calcium channel blocker	Dihydropyridine	Amlodipine (Norvasc)	2.5–10	1
		Felodipine (Plendil)	5–20	1
		Isradipine (DynaCirc)	5–10	2
		Isradipine SR (DynaCirc SR)	5–20	1
		Nicardipine sustained release (Cardene SR)	60–120	2
		Nifedipine long-acting (Adalat CC, Nifedical XL, Procardia XL)	30–90	1
		Nisoldipine (Sular)	10–40	1
	Nondihydropyridine	Diltiazem sustained release (Cardizem SR)	180–360	2
		Diltiazem sustained release (Cardizem CD, Cartia XT, Dilacor XR, Diltia XT, Tiazac, Taztia XT)	120–480	1
		Diltiazem extended release (Cardizem LA)	120–540	1 (morning or evening)
		Verapamil sustained release (Calan SR, Isoptin SR, Verelan)	180–480	1 or 2
		Verapamil controlled onset, extended release (Covera-HS)	180–420	1 (in the evening)
		Verapamil chrono-therapeutic oral drug absorption system (Verelan PM)	100–400	1 (in the evening)

(continued)

TABLE 10-2	First-Line and Other Common Antihypertensive Agents *(Continued)*		
Class	**Subclass**	**Drug (Brand Name)**	**Usual Dose Range (mg/day)**	**Daily Frequency**
Diuretic	Thiazide	Chlorthalidone (Hygroton)	12.5–25	1
		Hydrochlorothiazide (Esidrix, HydroDiuril, Microzide, Oretic)	12.5–50	1
		Indapamide (Lozol)	1.25–2.5	1
		Metolazone (Zaroxolyn)	2.5–10	1
	Loop	Bumetanide (Bumex)	0.5–4	2
		Furosemide (Lasix)	20–80	2
		Torsemide (Demadex)	5–10	1
	Potassium sparing	Amiloride (Midamor)	5–10	1 or 2
		Amiloride/ hydrochlorothiazide (Moduretic)	5–10/50–100	1
		Triamterene (Dyrenium)	50–100	1 or 2
		Triamterene/ hydrochlorothiazide (Dyazide)	37.5–75/25–50	1
	Aldosterone antagonist	Eplerenone (Inspra)	50–100	1 or 2
		Spironolactone (Aldactone)	25–50	1 or 2
		Spironolactone/ hydrochlorothiazide (Aldactazide)	25–50/25–50	1
β-Blocker	Cardioselective	Atenolol (Tenormin)	25–100	1
		Betaxolol (Kerlone)	5–20	1
		Bisoprolol (Zebeta)	2.5–10	1
		Metoprolol tartrate (Lopressor)	100–400	2
		Metoprolol succinate extended release (Toprol XL)	50–200	1
	Nonselective	Nadolol (Corgard)	40–120	1
		Propranolol (Inderal)	160–480	2
		Propranolol long acting (Inderal LA, Inderal XL, InnoPran XL)	80–320	1
		Timolol (Blocadren)	10–40	1
	Intrinsic sympatho- mimetic activity	Acebutolol (Sectral)	200–800	2
		Carteolol (Cartrol)	2.5–10	1
		Pindolol (Visken)	10–60	2
	Mixed α- and β-blockers	Carvedilol (Coreg)	12.5–50	2
		Carvedilol phosphate (Coreg CR)	20–80	1
		Labetalol (Normodyne, Trandate)	200–800	2
	Cardioselective and vasodilatory	Nebivolol (Bystolic)	5–20	1

- Most patients with stage 1 hypertension should be treated initially with a first-line antihypertensive drug or a two-drug combination (Fig. 10–1). Combination therapy is recommended for patients with stage 2 hypertension, preferably with two first-line agents.
- There are six compelling indications where specific antihypertensive drug classes provide unique benefits (Fig. 10–2).
- Other antihypertensive drug classes (α_1-blockers, **direct renin inhibitors**, **central** α_2-agonists, **adrenergic inhibitors**, and **direct arterial vasodilators**) are alternatives that may be used for select patients after first-line agents (Table 10–3). However, there is no compelling outcome data showing reduced morbidity and mortality in hypertension.

Angiotensin-Converting Enzyme Inhibitors

- ACE inhibitors are a first-line option, and if they are not the first agent used, they should be the second agent tried in most patients.
- ACE inhibitors block conversion of angiotensin I to angiotensin II, a potent vasoconstrictor and stimulator of aldosterone secretion. ACE inhibitors also block degradation of bradykinin and stimulate synthesis of other vasodilating substances, including prostaglandin E_2 and prostacyclin.

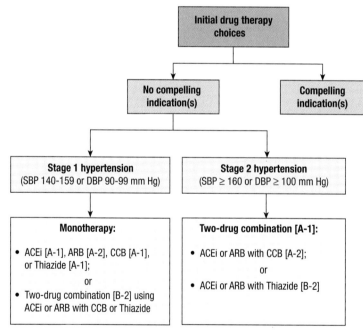

FIGURE 10–1. Algorithm for treatment of hypertension. Drug therapy recommendations are graded with strength of recommendation and quality of evidence in brackets. Strength of recommendations: A, B, and C are good, moderate, and poor evidence to support recommendation, respectively. Quality of evidence: (1) evidence from more than one properly randomized controlled trial; (2) evidence from at least one well-designed clinical trial with randomization, from cohort or case-controlled studies, or dramatic results from uncontrolled experiments or subgroup analyses; and (3) evidence from opinions of respected authorities, based on clinical experience, descriptive studies, or reports of expert communities.

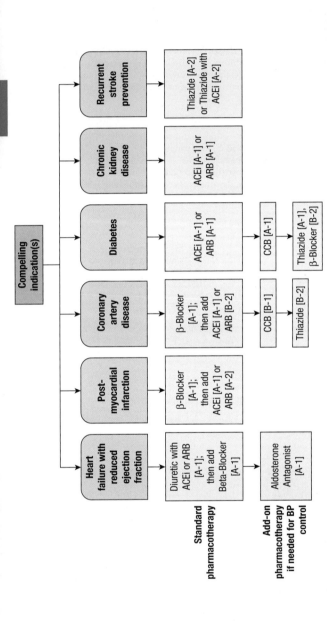

FIGURE 10–2. Compelling indications for individual drug classes. Compelling indications for specific drugs are evidenced-based recommendations from outcome studies or existing clinical guidelines. The order of drug therapies serves as a general guidance that should be balanced with clinical judgment and patient response. Add-on pharmacotherapy recommendations are when additional agents are needed to lower BP to goal values. Blood pressure control should be managed concurrently with the compelling indication. Drug therapy recommendations are graded with strength of recommendation and quality of evidence in brackets. Strength of recommendations: A, B, and C are good, moderate, and poor evidence to support recommendation, respectively. Quality of evidence: (1) evidence from more than one properly randomized controlled trial; (2) evidence from at least one well-designed clinical trial with randomization, from cohort or case-controlled analytic studies or multiple time series, or dramatic results from uncontrolled experiments or subgroup analyses; and (3) evidence from opinions of respected authorities, based on clinical experience, descriptive studies, or reports of expert communities.

TABLE 10–3 Alternative Antihypertensive Agents

Class Drug (Brand Name)	Usual Dose Range (mg/day)	Daily Frequency
α_1-Blockers		
Doxazosin (Cardura)	1–8	1
Prazosin (Minipress)	2–20	2 or 3
Terazosin (Hytrin)	1–20	1 or 2
Direct renin inhibitor		
Aliskiren (Tekturna)	150–300	1
Central α_2-agonists		
Clonidine (Catapres)	0.1–0.8	2
Clonidine patch (Catapres-TTS)	0.1–0.3	1 weekly
Methyldopa (Aldomet)	250–1,000	2
Peripheral adrenergic antagonist		
Reserpine (generic only)	0.05–0.25	1
Direct arterial vasodilators		
Minoxidil (Loniten)	10–40	1 or 2
Hydralazine (Apresoline)	20–100	2 to 4

- Starting doses should be low with slow dose titration. Acute hypotension may occur at the onset of therapy, especially in patients who are sodium or volume depleted, in HF exacerbation, very elderly, or on concurrent vasodilators or diuretics. Start administering doses in such patients, using half the normal dose followed by slow dose titration.
- ACE inhibitors decrease aldosterone and can increase serum potassium concentrations. Hyperkalemia occurs primarily in patients with CKD or those also taking potassium supplements, potassium-sparing diuretics, ARBs, or a direct renin inhibitor.
- Acute renal failure is a rare but serious side effect; preexisting kidney disease increases risk. Bilateral renal artery stenosis or unilateral stenosis of a solitary functioning kidney renders patients dependent on the vasoconstrictive effect of angiotensin II on efferent arterioles, making these patients particularly susceptible to acute renal failure.
- GFR declines in patients receiving ACE inhibitors because of inhibition of angiotensin II vasoconstriction on efferent arterioles. Serum creatinine concentrations often increase, but modest elevations (eg, absolute increases <1 mg/dL [88 μmol/L]) do not warrant treatment changes. Discontinue therapy or reduce dose if larger increases occur.
- Angioedema occurs in fewer than 1% of patients. Drug withdrawal is necessary, and some patients may require drug treatment and/or emergent intubation. An ARB can generally be used in patients with a history of ACE inhibitor–induced angioedema, with careful monitoring.
- A persistent dry cough occurs in up to 20% of patients and is thought to be due to inhibition of bradykinin breakdown.
- ACE inhibitors (as well as ARBs and direct renin inhibitors) are contraindicated in pregnancy.

Angiotensin II Receptor Blockers

- ARBs are a first-line therapy option in most patients with hypertension and reduce CV events similar to ACE inhibitors. The combination of an ACE inhibitor and ARB has no additional CV event lowering but is associated with a higher risk of side effects (renal dysfunction, hypotension).
- Angiotensin II is generated by the renin–angiotensin pathway (which involves ACE) and an alternative pathway that uses other enzymes such as chymases. ACE inhibitors block only the renin–angiotensin pathway, whereas ARBs antagonize angiotensin II

generated by either pathway. The ARBs directly block the angiotensin II type 1 receptor that mediates the effects of angiotensin II.

- Unlike ACE inhibitors, ARBs do not block bradykinin breakdown. Although this accounts for the lack of cough as a side effect, there may be negative consequences because some of the antihypertensive effect of ACE inhibitors may be due to increased levels of bradykinin.
- All ARBs have similar antihypertensive efficacy and fairly flat dose-response curves. Addition of a CCB or thiazide diuretic significantly increases antihypertensive efficacy.
- ARBs have a low incidence of side effects. Like ACE inhibitors, they may cause renal insufficiency, hyperkalemia, and orthostatic hypotension. ARBs are contraindicated in pregnancy.

Calcium Channel Blockers

- Calcium channel blockers (CCBs), including both dihydropyridine and nondihydropyridine types, are first-line therapy options. They are also used in addition to or instead of other first-line antihypertensives for the compelling indications of coronary artery disease and diabetes.
- CCBs cause relaxation of cardiac and smooth muscle by blocking voltage-sensitive calcium channels, thereby reducing entry of extracellular calcium into cells. This leads to vasodilation and a corresponding reduction in BP. Dihydropyridine calcium channel antagonists may cause reflex sympathetic activation, and all agents (except amlodipine and felodipine) may have negative inotropic effects.
- **Verapamil** decreases heart rate, slows atrioventricular (AV) nodal conduction, and produces a negative inotropic effect that may precipitate HF in patients with borderline cardiac reserve. **Diltiazem** decreases AV conduction and heart rate to a lesser extent than verapamil.
- Diltiazem and verapamil can cause cardiac conduction abnormalities such as bradycardia, AV block, and HF. Both can cause anorexia, nausea, peripheral edema, and hypotension. Verapamil causes constipation in about 8% of patients.
- Dihydropyridines cause a baroreceptor-mediated reflex increase in heart rate because of potent peripheral vasodilating effects. Dihydropyridines do not decrease AV node conduction and are not effective for treating supraventricular tachyarrhythmias.
- Short-acting nifedipine may rarely increase frequency, intensity, and duration of angina in association with acute hypotension. This effect may be obviated by using sustained-release formulations of nifedipine or other dihydropyridines. Other side effects of dihydropyridines are dizziness, flushing, headache, gingival hyperplasia, and peripheral edema.

Diuretics

- **Thiazides** are the preferred type of diuretic and are considered a first-line option for most patients with hypertension.
- **Loop diuretics** are more potent for inducing diuresis but are not ideal antihypertensives unless relief of edema is also needed. Loops are sometimes preferred over thiazides in patients with CKD when estimated GFR is less than 30 mL/min/1.73 m^2, especially when edema is present.
- **Potassium-sparing diuretics** are weak antihypertensives when used alone and provide minimal additive effect when combined with a thiazide or loop diuretic. Their primary use is in combination with another diuretic to counteract potassium-wasting properties.
- **Aldosterone antagonists (spironolactone** and **eplerenone)** are also potassium-sparing diuretics but are more potent antihypertensives with a slow onset of action (up to 6 weeks with spironolactone).
- Acutely, diuretics lower BP by causing diuresis. The reduction in plasma volume and stroke volume associated with diuresis decreases cardiac output and BP. The initial drop in cardiac output causes a compensatory increase in peripheral vascular resistance.

With chronic therapy, extracellular fluid volume and plasma volume return to near pretreatment levels, and peripheral vascular resistance falls below baseline. Reduced peripheral vascular resistance is responsible for the long-term hypotensive effects. Thiazides also mobilize sodium and water from arteriolar walls, which may contribute to decreased peripheral vascular resistance and lowered BP.

- When diuretics are combined with other antihypertensive agents, an additive hypotensive effect is usually observed because of independent mechanisms of action. Furthermore, many nondiuretic antihypertensive agents induce sodium and water retention, which is counteracted by concurrent diuretic use.
- Side effects of thiazides include hypokalemia, hypomagnesemia, hypercalcemia, hyperuricemia, hyperglycemia, dyslipidemia, and sexual dysfunction. Loop diuretics have less effect on serum lipids and glucose, but hypokalemia is more pronounced, and hypocalcemia may occur.
- Hypokalemia and hypomagnesemia may result in cardiac arrhythmias, especially in patients receiving digoxin, patients with LV hypertrophy, and those with ischemic heart disease. Low-dose therapy (eg, 25 mg hydrochlorothiazide or 12.5 mg chlorthalidone daily) causes small electrolyte disturbances.
- Potassium-sparing diuretics may cause hyperkalemia, especially in patients with CKD or diabetes and in patients receiving concurrent treatment with an ACE inhibitor, ARB, direct renin inhibitor, or potassium supplement. Eplerenone has an increased risk for hyperkalemia and is contraindicated in patients with impaired renal function or type 2 diabetes with proteinuria. Spironolactone may cause gynecomastia in up to 10% of patients; this effect occurs rarely with eplerenone.

β-Blockers

- β-Blockers are only considered appropriate first-line agents to treat specific compelling indications (eg, post-MI and coronary artery disease). Their hypotensive mechanism may involve decreased cardiac output through negative chronotropic and inotropic effects on the heart and inhibition of renin release from the kidney.
- **Atenolol, betaxolol, bisoprolol, metoprolol,** and **nebivolol** are cardioselective at low doses and bind more avidly to β_1-receptors than to β_2-receptors. As a result, they are less likely to provoke bronchospasm and vasoconstriction and may be safer than nonselective β-blockers in patients with asthma, chronic obstructive pulmonary disease (COPD), diabetes, and peripheral arterial disease (PAD). Cardioselectivity is a dose-dependent phenomenon, and the effect is lost at higher doses.
- **Acebutolol, carteolol,** and **pindolol** possess intrinsic sympathomimetic activity (ISA) or partial β-receptor agonist activity. When sympathetic tone is low, as in resting states, β-receptors are partially stimulated, so resting heart rate, cardiac output, and peripheral blood flow are not reduced when receptors are blocked. Theoretically, these drugs may have advantages in patients with HF or sinus bradycardia. Unfortunately, they do not reduce CV events as well as other β-blockers and may increase risk after MI or in those with high coronary disease risk. Thus, agents with ISA are rarely needed.
- **Atenolol** and **nadolol** have relatively long half-lives and are excreted renally; the dosage may need to be reduced in patients with renal insufficiency. Even though the half-lives of other β-blockers are shorter, once-daily administration still may be effective.
- Myocardial side effects include bradycardia, AV conduction abnormalities, and acute HF. Blocking β_2-receptors in arteriolar smooth muscle may cause cold extremities and aggravate PAD or Raynaud phenomenon because of decreased peripheral blood flow. Increases in serum lipids and glucose appear to be transient and of little clinical importance.
- Abrupt cessation of β-blocker therapy may produce unstable angina, MI, or even death in patients with coronary disease. In patients without heart disease, abrupt discontinuation of β-blockers may be associated with tachycardia, sweating, and generalized malaise in addition to increased BP. For these reasons, the dose should always be tapered gradually over 1 to 2 weeks before discontinuation.

α$_1$-Receptor Blockers

- **Prazosin**, **terazosin**, and **doxazosin** are selective α$_1$-receptor blockers that inhibit catecholamine uptake in smooth muscle cells of peripheral vasculature, resulting in vasodilation and BP lowering.
- A first-dose phenomenon characterized by orthostatic hypotension accompanied by transient dizziness or faintness, palpitations, and even syncope may occur within 1 to 3 hours of the first dose or after later dosage increases. The patient should take the first dose (and subsequent first increased doses) at bedtime. Occasionally, orthostatic hypotension and dizziness persist with chronic administration.
- Sodium and water retention can occur; these agents are most effective when given with a thiazide to maintain antihypertensive efficacy and minimize edema.
- Because doxazosin (and probably other α$_1$-receptor blockers) may not be as protective against CV events as other therapies, they should be reserved as alternative agents for unique situations, such as men with benign prostatic hyperplasia. If used to lower BP in this situation, they should only be used in combination with first-line antihypertensives.

Direct Renin Inhibitor

- **Aliskiren** blocks the RAAS at its point of activation, resulting in reduced plasma renin activity and BP. BP reductions are comparable to an ACE inhibitor, ARB, or CCB. Aliskiren is approved for monotherapy or in combination with other agents. It should not be used in combination with an ACE inhibitor or an ARB because of a higher risk of adverse effects without additional reduction in CV events. Aliskiren is an alternative therapy because of lack of long-term studies evaluating CV event reduction and its significant cost compared with generic agents that have outcomes data.
- Many of the cautions and adverse effects seen with ACE inhibitors and ARBs apply to aliskiren. It is contraindicated in pregnancy due to known teratogenic effects.

Central α$_2$-Agonists

- **Clonidine**, **guanabenz**, **guanfacine**, and **methyldopa** lower BP primarily by stimulating α$_2$-adrenergic receptors in the brain, which reduces sympathetic outflow from the vasomotor center and increases vagal tone. Stimulation of presynaptic α$_2$-receptors peripherally may contribute to reduced sympathetic tone. Consequently, there may be decreases in heart rate, cardiac output, total peripheral resistance, plasma renin activity, and baroreceptor reflexes.
- Chronic use results in sodium and fluid retention. Other side effects include depression, orthostatic hypotension, dizziness, and anticholinergic effects.
- Abrupt cessation may lead to rebound hypertension, perhaps from a compensatory increase in norepinephrine release that follows discontinuation of presynaptic α-receptor stimulation.
- Methyldopa rarely causes hepatitis or hemolytic anemia. A transient elevation in hepatic transaminases occasionally occurs. Discontinue therapy if persistent increases in liver function tests occur, because this may herald onset of fulminant, life-threatening hepatitis. Coombs-positive hemolytic anemia occurs rarely, and 20% of patients exhibit a positive direct Coombs test without anemia. For these reasons, methyldopa has limited usefulness except in pregnancy.

Reserpine

- **Reserpine** depletes norepinephrine from sympathetic nerve endings and blocks transport of norepinephrine into storage granules. When the nerve is stimulated, less than the usual amount of norepinephrine is released into the synapse. This reduces sympathetic tone, decreasing peripheral vascular resistance and BP.
- Reserpine has a long half-life that allows for once-daily dosing, but it may take 2 to 6 weeks before the maximal antihypertensive effect is seen.
- Reserpine can cause significant sodium and fluid retention and therefore should be given with a thiazide.

- Reserpine's strong inhibition of sympathetic activity results in parasympathetic activity, which is responsible for side effects of nasal stuffiness, increased gastric acid secretion, diarrhea, and bradycardia. Dose-related depression can be minimized by not exceeding 0.25 mg daily.

Direct Arterial Vasodilators

- **Hydralazine** and **minoxidil** cause direct arteriolar smooth muscle relaxation. Compensatory activation of baroreceptor reflexes results in increased sympathetic outflow from the vasomotor center, increasing heart rate, cardiac output, and renin release. Consequently, hypotensive effectiveness of direct vasodilators diminishes over time unless the patient is also taking a sympathetic inhibitor and a diuretic.
- Patients taking these drugs for long-term hypertension therapy should first receive both a thiazide and a β-blocker. The diuretic minimizes the side effect of sodium and water retention. Direct vasodilators can precipitate angina in patients with underlying coronary artery disease unless the baroreceptor reflex mechanism is blocked with a β-blocker. Nondihydropyridine CCBs can be used as an alternative to β-blockers in patients with contraindications to β-blockers.
- Hydralazine may cause dose-related, reversible lupus-like syndrome, which is more common in slow acetylators. Lupus-like reactions can usually be avoided by using total daily doses less than 200 mg. Because of side effects, hydralazine has limited usefulness for chronic hypertension management.
- Minoxidil is a more potent vasodilator than hydralazine, and compensatory increases in heart rate, cardiac output, renin release, and sodium retention are more dramatic. Due to significant water retention, a loop diuretic is often more effective than a thiazide in patients treated with minoxidil. Reversible hypertrichosis on the face, arms, back, and chest may be a troublesome. Reserve minoxidil for very difficult to control hypertension and for patients requiring hydralazine who experience drug-induced lupus.

COMPELLING INDICATIONS

- Six compelling indications represent specific comorbid conditions for which clinical trial data support using specific antihypertensive drug classes to treat both hypertension and the compelling indication (see **Fig. 10–2**).

Heart Failure with Reduced Ejection Fraction (HFrEF)

- Standard pharmacotherapy consists of three to four drugs: ACE inhibitor or ARB plus diuretic therapy, followed by addition of an evidence-based β-blocker (ie, bisoprolol, carvedilol, and metoprolol succinate) and possibly an aldosterone receptor antagonist.
- Start an ACE inhibitor or ARB in low doses to avoid orthostatic hypotension because of the high renin state in HF.
- Diuretics provide symptomatic relief of edema by inducing diuresis. Loop diuretics are often needed, especially in patients with more advanced heart failure.
- β-Blocker therapy is appropriate to further modify disease in HFrEF and is a component of standard therapy. Because of the risk of exacerbating HF, β-blockers must be started in very low doses and titrated slowly to high doses based on tolerability. Bisoprolol, carvedilol, and sustained-release metoprolol succinate are the only β-blockers proven to be beneficial in HFrEF.
- After implementation of a standard three-drug regimen, an aldosterone antagonist (spironolactone and eplerenone) may be considered.

Postmyocardial Infarction

- β-Blockers (without ISA) and ACE inhibitors (or ARBs) are recommended. β-Blockers decrease cardiac adrenergic stimulation and reduce risk of subsequent MI or sudden cardiac death. ACE inhibitors improve cardiac function and reduce CV events after MI. These two drug classes, with β-blockers first, are the drugs of first choice for post-MI patients.

Coronary Artery Disease

- β-Blockers (without ISA) are first-line therapy in chronic stable angina; they reduce BP and decrease myocardial oxygen consumption and demand. Long-acting CCBs (the nondihydropyridine CCBs diltiazem and verapamil) may be either alternatives or add-on therapy (dihydropyridines) to β-blockers in chronic stable angina. Once ischemic symptoms are controlled with β-blocker and/or CCB therapy, other antihypertensives (eg, ACE inhibitor or ARB) can be added to provide additional CV risk reduction. Thiazide diuretics may be added thereafter to provide additional BP lowering and further reduce CV risk.
- For acute coronary syndromes, first-line therapy includes a β-blocker and ACE inhibitor (or ARB); the combination lowers BP, controls acute ischemia, and reduces CV risk.

Diabetes Mellitus

- Treat all patients with diabetes and hypertension with an ACE inhibitor or ARB. Both classes provide nephroprotection and reduced CV risk.
- CCBs are the most appropriate add-on agents for BP control in patients with diabetes. The combination of an ACE inhibitor with a CCB is more effective in reducing CV events than an ACE inhibitor plus a thiazide diuretic.
- A thiazide diuretic is recommended add-on therapy to lower BP and provide additional CV risk reduction.
- β-Blockers, similar to CCBs, are useful add-on agents for BP control in patients with diabetes. They should also be used to treat another compelling indication (eg, post-MI). However, they may mask symptoms of hypoglycemia (tremor, tachycardia, and palpitations but not sweating) in tightly controlled patients, delay recovery from hypoglycemia, and produce elevations in BP due to vasoconstriction caused by unopposed β-receptor stimulation during the hypoglycemic recovery phase. Despite these potential problems, β-blockers can be used safely in patients with diabetes.

Chronic Kidney Disease

- In addition to lowering BP, ACE inhibitors and ARBs reduce intraglomerular pressure, which may further slow CKD progression.
- Start with low doses and evaluate the serum creatinine soon after starting therapy to minimize the risk of rapid and profound BP drops that could precipitate acute kidney failure.

Recurrent Stroke Prevention

- A thiazide diuretic, either as monotherapy or combined with an ACE inhibitor, is recommended for patients with history of stroke or transient ischemic attack. Implement antihypertensive drug therapy only after patients have stabilized after an acute cerebrovascular event.

SPECIAL POPULATIONS

Older People

- Elderly patients may present with either isolated systolic hypertension or elevation in both SBP and DBP. CV morbidity and mortality are more closely related to SBP than to DBP in patients 50 years of age and older.
- Diuretics, ACE inhibitors, and ARBs provide significant benefits and can be used safely in the elderly, but smaller-than-usual initial doses must be used for initial therapy.

Children and Adolescents

- Secondary hypertension is more common in children and adolescents than in adults. Medical or surgical management of the underlying disorder usually normalizes BP.
- Nonpharmacologic treatment (particularly weight loss in obese children) is the cornerstone of therapy of primary hypertension.
- ACE inhibitors, ARBs, β-blockers, CCBs, and thiazide diuretics are all acceptable drug therapy choices.

- ACE inhibitors, ARBs, and direct renin inhibitors are contraindicated in sexually active girls because of potential teratogenic effects.

Pregnancy

- *Preeclampsia* is defined as hypertension (elevated BP ≥140/90 mm Hg on more than 2 occasions at least 4 hours apart after 20 weeks' gestation or ≥160/110 mm Hg confirmed within a short interval) in association with thrombocytopenia, impaired liver function, new development of renal insufficiency, pulmonary edema, or new-onset cerebral or visual disturbances. It can lead to life-threatening complications for both mother and fetus.
- *Eclampsia*, the onset of convulsions in preeclampsia, is a medical emergency.
- Definitive treatment of preeclampsia is delivery, and this is indicated if pending or frank eclampsia is present. Otherwise, management consists of restricting activity, bedrest, and close monitoring. Salt restriction or other measures that contract blood volume should be avoided. Antihypertensives are used prior to induction of labor if the DBP is greater than 105 mm Hg, with a target DBP of 95 to 105 mm Hg. IV hydralazine is most commonly used; IV labetalol is also effective.
- *Chronic hypertension* is hypertension that predates pregnancy. Labetalol, nifedipine, or methyldopa is recommended as first-line therapy due to favorable safety profiles. β-Blockers (other than atenolol) and CCBs are also reasonable alternatives. ACE inhibitors, ARBs, and the direct renin inhibitor aliskiren are contraindicated in pregnancy.

African Americans

- Hypertension is more common and more severe in African Americans than in those of other races. Differences in electrolyte homeostasis, glomerular filtration rate, sodium excretion and transport mechanisms, plasma renin activity, and BP response to plasma volume expansion have been noted. African Americans tend to have a low-renin pattern of hypertension.
- CCBs and thiazides are most effective in African Americans. Antihypertensive response is significantly increased when either class is combined with a β-blocker, ACE inhibitor, or ARB.
- Appropriate drug therapies should be used for compelling indications, even if the antihypertensive effect may not be as great as with another drug class (eg, a β-blocker is first-line for BP control in post-MI African Americans).

Pulmonary Disease and Peripheral Arterial Disease

- Although β-blockers (especially nonselective agents) have generally been avoided in hypertensive patients with asthma and COPD because of fear of inducing bronchospasm, data suggest that cardioselective β-blockers can be used safely. Consequently, cardioselective agents should be used to treat a compelling indication (ie, post-MI, coronary disease, or HF) in patients with reactive airway disease.
- PAD is considered a noncoronary form of atherosclerotic vascular disease. β-Blockers can theoretically be problematic because of possible decreased peripheral blood flow secondary to unopposed stimulation of α-receptors that results in vasoconstriction. This can be mitigated by using a β-blocker with α-blocking properties (eg, carvedilol). However, β-blockers are not contraindicated in PAD and have not been shown to adversely affect walking capacity.

HYPERTENSIVE URGENCIES AND EMERGENCIES

- **Hypertensive urgencies** are ideally managed by adjusting maintenance therapy, adding a new antihypertensive, and/or increasing the dose of a present medication.
- Acute administration of a short-acting oral drug (**captopril**, **clonidine**, or **labetalol**) followed by careful observation for several hours to ensure a gradual BP reduction is an option.
  ✓ Oral captopril doses of 25 to 50 mg may be given at 1- to 2-hour intervals. The onset of action is 15 to 30 minutes.

✓ For treatment of hypertensive rebound after withdrawal of clonidine, 0.2 mg is given initially, followed by 0.2 mg hourly until the DBP falls below 110 mm Hg or a total of 0.7 mg has been administered; a single dose may be sufficient.

✓ Labetalol can be given in a dose of 200 to 400 mg, followed by additional doses every 2 to 3 hours.

• **Hypertensive emergencies** require immediate BP reduction to limit new or progressing end-organ damage. The goal is not to lower BP to less than 140/90 mm Hg; instead, the initial target is a reduction in mean arterial pressure of up to 25% within

TABLE 10–4	Parenteral Antihypertensive Agents for Hypertensive Emergency			
Drug	**Dose**	**Onset (min)**	**Duration (min)**	**Adverse Effects**
Clevidipine	1–2 mg/h (32 mg/h max)	2–4	5–15	Headache, nausea, tachycardia, hypertriglyceridemia
Enalaprilat	1.25–5 mg IV every 6 h	15–30	360–720	Precipitous fall in BP in high-renin states; variable response
Esmolol hydrochloride	250–500 mcg/kg/min IV bolus, then 50–100 mcg/kg/min IV infusion; may repeat bolus after 5 min or increase infusion to 300 mcg/min	1–2	10–20	Hypotension, nausea, asthma, first-degree heart block, heart failure
Fenoldopam mesylate	0.1–0.3 mcg/kg/min IV infusion	<5	30	Tachycardia, headache, nausea, flushing
Hydralazine hydrochloride	12–20 mg IV 10–50 mg IM	10–20 20–30	60–240 240–360	Tachycardia, flushing, headache, vomiting, aggravation of angina
Labetalol hydrochloride	20–80 mg IV bolus every 10 min; 0.5–2 mg/min IV infusion	5–10	180–360	Vomiting, scalp tingling, bronchoconstriction, dizziness, nausea, heart block, orthostatic hypotension
Nicardipine hydrochloride	5–15 mg/h IV	5–10	15–30; may exceed 240	Tachycardia, headache, flushing, local phlebitis
Nitroglycerin	5–100 mcg/min IV infusion	2–5	5–10	Headache, vomiting, methemoglobinemia, tolerance with prolonged use
Sodium nitroprusside	0.25–10 mcg/kg/min IV infusion (requires special delivery system)	Immediate	1–2	Nausea, vomiting, muscle twitching, sweating, thiocyanate and cyanide intoxication

(BP, blood pressure; IM, intramuscular; IV, intravenous.)

minutes to hours. If BP is then stable, it can be reduced toward 160/100 to 110 mm Hg within the next 2 to 6 hours. Precipitous drops in BP may cause end-organ ischemia or infarction. If BP reduction is well tolerated, additional gradual decrease toward the goal BP can be attempted after 24 to 48 hours.

✓ Nitroprusside is the agent of choice for minute-to-minute control in most cases. It is usually given as a continuous IV infusion at a rate of 0.25 to 10 mcg/kg/min. Onset of hypotensive action is immediate and disappears within 1 to 2 minutes of discontinuation. When the infusion must be continued longer than 72 hours, measure serum thiocyanate levels, and discontinue the infusion if the level exceeds 12 mg/dL (~2.0 mmol/L). The risk of thiocyanate toxicity is increased in patients with impaired kidney function. Other adverse effects are nausea, vomiting, muscle twitching, and sweating.

✓ Dosing guidelines and adverse effects of parenteral agents for treating hypertensive emergency are listed in Table 10–4.

EVALUATION OF THERAPEUTIC OUTCOMES

• Evaluate BP response 2 to 4 weeks after initiating or making changes in therapy. Once goals BP values are obtained, monitor BP every 3 to 6 months, assuming no signs or symptoms of acute end-organ damage. Evaluate more frequently in patients with a history of poor control, nonadherence, progressive end-organ damage, or symptoms of adverse drug effects.

• Self-measurements of BP or automatic ambulatory BP monitoring can be useful to establish effective 24-hour control. These techniques are currently recommended only for select situations such as suspected white coat hypertension.

• Monitor patients for signs and symptoms of progressive hypertension-associated complications. Take a careful history for chest pain (or pressure), palpitations, dizziness, dyspnea, orthopnea, headache, sudden change in vision, one-sided weakness, slurred speech, and loss of balance.

• Monitor funduscopic changes on eye examination, LV hypertrophy on ECG, proteinuria, and changes in kidney function periodically.

• Monitor for adverse drug effects 2 to 4 weeks after starting a new agent or dose increases, then every 6 to 12 months in stable patients. For patients taking aldosterone antagonists, assess potassium concentration and kidney function within 3 days and again at 1 week after initiation to detect potential hyperkalemia.

• Assess patient adherence with the regimen regularly. Ask patients about changes in their general health perception, energy level, physical functioning, and overall satisfaction with treatment.

See Chapter 13, Hypertension, authored by Joseph J. Saseen and Eric J. MacLaughlin, for a more detailed discussion of this topic.

Ischemic Heart Disease

11

- *Ischemic heart disease* (IHD) is defined as lack of oxygen and decreased or no blood flow to the myocardium resulting from coronary artery narrowing or obstruction. It may present as acute coronary syndrome (ACS), which includes unstable angina and non–ST-segment elevation (NSTE) or ST-segment elevation (STE) myocardial infarction (MI), chronic stable exertional angina, ischemia without symptoms, microvascular angina, or ischemia due to coronary artery vasospasm (variant or Prinzmetal angina). The focus of this chapter is stable IHD.

PATHOPHYSIOLOGY

- Angina pectoris usually results from increased myocardial oxygen demand (MVo_2) in the setting of a fixed decrease in myocardial oxygen supply because of atherosclerotic plaque.
- Major determinants of MVo_2 are heart rate (HR), contractility, and intramyocardial wall tension during systole. A doubling in any of these individual parameters requires a 50% increase in coronary flow to maintain myocardial supply.
- The rate–pressure product, or double product (DP), is the heart rate multiplied by the systolic blood pressure: DP = HR × SBP. This is a common, noninvasive measure of MVo_2 but has limitations.
- Coronary atherosclerotic plaques typically develop in larger epicardial (R_1 or conductance) vessels, which normally offer little resistance to myocardial flow. As plaques grow and narrow the lumen, the affected vessel begins to provide considerable resistance to blood flow. Smaller endocardial (R_2 or resistance) vessels provide most resistance to flow in normal coronary arteries and can contract and dilate to maintain blood flow based on metabolic demands of the myocardium (referred to as autoregulation). As a result, coronary plaques that occupy less than 50% to 70% of the vessel luminal diameter rarely produce ischemia or angina. However, smaller plaques have a lipid-rich core and thin fibrous cap and are prone to rupture and cause acute thrombosis. When the luminal diameter of epicardial vessels is reduced by 70% or more, endocardial vessels are maximally dilated, coronary flow reserve has been exhausted, and even low levels of exertion may result in a flow deficit with myocardial ischemia and often angina. When epicardial stenosis exceeds 90%, endocardial flow reserve is completely exhausted at rest (referred to as critical stenosis).
- When coronary stenosis exceeds 70%, ischemic episodes lead to production of growth factors (eg, vascular endothelial growth factor and fibroblast growth factor) that, combined with endogenous vasodilators (eg, nitrous oxide and prostacyclin), cause native collateral vessels to increase in diameter (arteriogenesis) to maintain perfusion. New collateral vessels can also develop (angiogenesis).
- Inflammation also plays a role in IHD; macrophages and T-lymphocytes produce cytokines, chemokines, and growth factors that activate endothelial cells, increase vasoreactivity, and cause proliferation of vascular smooth muscle cells. C-reactive protein may be elevated and correlates with adverse cardiovascular events.
- Some patients have plaque that causes a fixed decrease in supply but also have reduced myocardial oxygen supply transiently due to vasospasm at the site of the plaque. Vasospasm is typically caused by endothelial damage induced by the plaque. Patient symptoms depend on the extent of the fixed obstruction and the degree of dynamic change in arterial tone. The pattern of ischemic symptoms can change due to a variable amount of vasospasm under certain conditions (referred to as *variable threshold angina*). Ischemic episodes may be more common in the morning hours (due to circadian release of vasoconstrictors) and be precipitated by cold exposure, and emotional or mental stress.
- Patients with *variant (Prinzmetal) angina* usually do not have a coronary flow-obstructing plaque but instead have significant reduction in myocardial oxygen supply due to vasospasm in epicardial vessels.

CLINICAL PRESENTATION

- Patients typically complain of chest pain precipitated by exertion or activities of daily living that is described as squeezing, crushing, heaviness, or chest tightness. It can also be more vague and described as a numbness or burning in the chest. The location is substernal and may radiate to the right or left shoulder or arm (left more commonly), neck, back, or abdomen. Ischemic symptoms may be associated with diaphoresis, nausea, vomiting, and dyspnea. Chest pain generally lasts from 5 to 20 minutes and is usually relieved by rest or sublingual nitroglycerin (SL NTG).
- Some patients (especially women and older individuals) present with atypical chest pain, characterized by midepigastric discomfort, effort intolerance, dyspnea, and excessive fatigue. Patients with diabetes mellitus may have decreased pain sensation due to neuropathy.
- Patients with variant (Prinzmetal) angina are typically younger and may present with chest pain at rest, often early in the morning, and may have ST-segment elevation.

DIAGNOSIS

- Obtain the medical history to identify the quality and severity of chest pain, precipitating factors, location, duration, pain radiation, and response to nitroglycerin or rest. Ischemic chest pain may resemble pain from noncardiac sources, and diagnosis of anginal pain may be difficult based on history alone.
- Assess nonmodifiable risk factors for coronary artery disease (CAD): age, sex, and family history of atherosclerotic disease in first-degree relatives (male onset before age 55 or female before age 65). Identify the presence of modifiable CAD risk factors: hypertension, diabetes mellitus, dyslipidemia, and cigarette smoking.
- Physical exam findings are usually nonspecific, but patients having an ischemic episode may present with tachycardia, diaphoresis, shortness of breath, and nausea. Other findings related to CAD risk factors may include increased blood pressure (BP) and a fourth heart sound reflecting longstanding hypertension. Other positive findings may include pulmonary crackles, displaced point of maximal impulse, or a third heart sound in patients with heart failure.
- Resting ECG is normal in at least half of patients with angina who are not experiencing acute ischemia. About 50% of patients develop ischemic ST-T wave changes during an episode of angina, which can be observed on the ECG during an exercise stress test. Patients who cannot endure stress testing can have the myocardium stressed pharmacologically with adenosine, dipyridamole, or dobutamine.
- Coronary angiography is the most accurate test for confirming CAD but is invasive and requires arterial access.
- Cardiac troponin concentrations are not typically elevated in IHD.

TREATMENT

- <u>Goals of Treatment</u>: A primary goal of therapy is complete (or nearly complete) elimination of angina chest pain and return to normal activities. Long-term goals are to slow progression of atherosclerosis and prevent complications such as myocardial infarction (MI), heart failure, stroke, and death.

NONPHARMACOLOGIC THERAPY

- Risk factor modification is the primary nondrug approach for primary and secondary prevention of CAD events. Lifestyle modifications include daily physical activity, weight management, dietary therapy (reduced intake of saturated fats to <7% of total calories, trans-fatty acids to <1% of total calories, and cholesterol to <200 mg/day), smoking cessation, psychological interventions, and limitation of alcohol intake.

- Surgical revascularization options for select patients include coronary artery bypass grafting (CABG) or percutaneous coronary intervention (PCI) with or without stent placement.

PHARMACOLOGIC THERAPY

- Guideline-directed medical therapy (GDMT) reduces the rates of death and MI similar to revascularization therapy. The most recent American College of Cardiology/American Heart Association (ACC/AHA) recommendations for management of stable IHD were published in 2012.
- Figure 11–1 is a treatment algorithm containing evidence-based drug therapy recommendations from the ACC/AHA.
- Refer to the guidelines or textbook Chapter 16, Stable Ischemic Heart Disease, for pharmacologic approaches to risk factor modification, which include the following recommendations:
  - ✓ Dyslipidemia: Use moderate- or high-dose statin therapy in the absence of contraindications or adverse effects, in addition to lifestyle changes. A bile acid sequestrant, niacin, or both is reasonable for patients who do not tolerate statins.
  - ✓ Blood pressure: If BP is 140/90 mm Hg or higher, institute drug therapy in addition to or after lifestyle modifications.
  - ✓ Diabetes mellitus: Pharmacotherapy to achieve a target A1C might be reasonable.

Antiplatelet Therapy

- Aspirin almost completely blocks cyclooxygenase-1 (COX-1) activity and subsequent thromboxane A_2 production, leading to reduced platelet activation and aggregation for the life of the platelet. Nonsteroidal anti-inflammatory drugs (NSAIDs) may interfere with aspirin's antiplatelet effect when coadministered due to competition for the site of action in the COX-1 enzyme. The ACC/AHA guidelines contain the following recommendations for stable IHD:
  - ✓ Aspirin 75 to 162 mg daily should be continued indefinitely in the absence of contraindications.
  - ✓ Clopidogrel 75 mg daily is an alternative for patients unable to take aspirin due to allergy or intolerance. Some studies have suggested that patients receiving a proton pump inhibitor (mainly omeprazole) have reduced antiplatelet activity because the drugs inhibit cytochrome P450 enzymes, which are involved in the conversion of clopidogrel to its active metabolite. However, other studies do not support the clinical significance of the interaction.
  - ✓ The combination of aspirin (75–162 mg daily) and clopidogrel 75 mg daily may be reasonable in certain high-risk patients.
  - ✓ Dipyridamole therapy is not recommended.

Angiotensin-Converting Enzyme Inhibitors and Angiotensin Receptor Blockers

- In the setting of IHD, angiotensin-converting enzyme (ACE) inhibitors can stabilize coronary plaque, restore or improve endothelial function, inhibit vascular smooth muscle cell growth, decrease macrophage migration, and perhaps provide antioxidant activity. However, ACE inhibitors have not been shown to improve symptomatic ischemia. Two trials demonstrated reductions in cardiovascular death, MI, or stroke compared to placebo in patients at high risk for such events, but a third trial did not show these benefits. The ACC/AHA guidelines for stable IHD recommend the following strategies:
  - ✓ Use of ACE inhibitors in patients who also have hypertension, diabetes, left ventricular dysfunction (ejection fraction 40% or less), or chronic kidney disease, unless contraindicated.
  - ✓ Angiotensin receptor blockers (ARBs) are recommended for the same populations if patients are intolerant to ACE inhibitors. Combination ACE inhibitor/ARB therapy is not justified.
  - ✓ Usual dosage ranges for ACE inhibitors and ARBs in stable IHD are provided in Table 11–1.

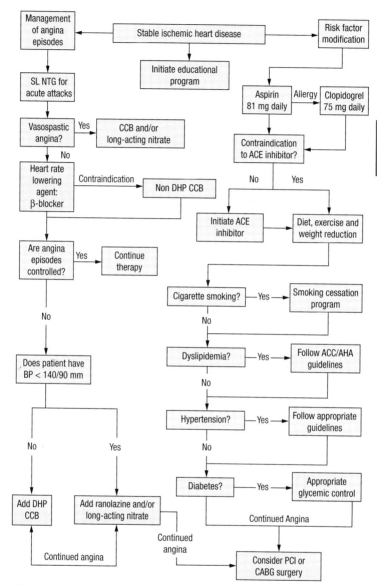

(ACC/AHA, American College of Cardiology/American Heart Association; ACE, angiotensin-converting enzyme; CABG, coronary artery bypass graft; CCB, calcium channel blocker; DHP, dihydropyridine; NTG, nitroglycerin; PCI, percutaneous coronary intervention; SL, sublingual.)

FIGURE 11–1. Algorithm for treatment of stable ischemic heart disease (guideline-directed medical therapy).

TABLE 11–1	Drugs and Regimens for Stable Ischemic Heart Disease
Drug Class and Generic Names	**Usual Dosage Range[a]**
Angiotensin-Converting Enzyme Inhibitors	
Captopril	6.25–50 mg 3 times daily
Enalapril	2.5–40 mg daily in 1–2 divided doses
Fosinopril	10–80 mg daily in 1–2 divided doses
Lisinopril	2.5–40 mg once daily
Perindopril	4–8 mg once daily
Quinapril	5–20 mg twice daily
Ramipril	2.5–10 mg daily in 1–2 divided doses
Trandolapril	1–4 mg once daily
Angiotensin Receptor Blockers	
Candesartan	4–32 mg once daily
Valsartan	80–320 mg daily in 1–2 divided doses
Telmisartan	20–80 mg once daily
β-Adrenergic Blockers	
Atenolol[b]	25–200 mg once daily
Betaxolol[b]	5–20 mg once daily
Bisoprolol[b]	2.5–10 mg once daily
Carvedilol[c]	3.125–25 mg twice daily
Carvedilol phosphate[c]	10-80 mg once daily
Labetalol[c]	100–400 mg twice daily
Metoprolol[b]	50–200 mg twice daily (once daily for extended release)
Nadolol[d]	40–120 mg once daily
Propranolol[d]	20–120 mg twice daily (60–240 mg once daily for long-acting formulation)
Timolol[d]	10–20 mg twice daily
Calcium Channel Blockers: Nondihydropyridine Type	
Diltiazem, extended release	120–360 mg once daily
Verapamil, extended release	180–480 mg once daily
Calcium Channel Blockers: Dihydropyridine Type	
Amlodipine	5–10 mg once daily
Felodipine	5–10 mg once daily
Nifedipine, extended release	30–90 mg once daily
Nicardipine	20–40 mg three times daily
Nitrates	
Nitroglycerin extended-release capsules	2.5 mg three times daily initially, with up-titration according to symptoms and tolerance; allow a 10- to 12-hour nitrate-free interval
Isosorbide dinitrate tablets	5–20 mg two to three times daily, with a daily nitrate-free interval of at least 14 hours (eg, dose at 7 AM, noon, and 5 PM)
Isosorbide dinitrate slow-release capsules	40 mg one to two times daily, with a daily nitrate-free interval of at least 18 hours (eg, dose at 8 AM and 2 PM)
Isosorbide mononitrate tablets	5–20 mg two times daily initially, with up-titration according to symptoms and tolerance; doses should be taken 7 hours apart (eg, 8 AM and 3 PM)

TABLE 11-1	Drugs and Regimens for Stable Ischemic Heart Disease (*Continued*)
Drug Class and Generic Names	**Usual Dosage Range[a]**
Isosorbide mononitrate extended-release tablets	30–120 mg once daily
Nitroglycerin transdermal extended-release film	0.2–0.8 mg/h, on for 12–14 hours, off for 10–12 hours

[a]Consult official prescribing information. In patients with renal and hepatic dysfunction, adjust initial and maintenance doses for all agents as appropriate based on FDA-approved labeling.
[b]Relatively β_1-selective (selectively is lost at higher doses).
[c]Blocks α_1, β_1, and β_2 receptors.
[d]Nonselective (blocks both β_1 and β_2 receptors).
(*Data from DiDomenico RJ, Cavallari L. Ischemic heart disease. In: Chisholm-Burns MA, et al., eds. Pharmacotherapy Principles & Practice, 4th ed. New York: McGraw-Hill Education, 2016*).

β-Adrenergic Blockers

- β-Blockers competitively inhibit the effects of neuronally released and circulating catecholamines on β-adrenoceptors. Blockade of β_1-receptors in the heart and kidney reduces HR, contractility, and BP, thereby decreasing MVo_2.
- β-Blockers should be prescribed as initial therapy for relief of symptoms in patients with stable IHD. An initial goal is to lower the resting HR to as low as the patient can tolerate above 60 beats per minute. β-Blockers may be combined with calcium channel blockers or long-acting nitrates when initial treatment with β-blockers alone is unsuccessful.
- After MI or acute coronary syndrome, β-blocker therapy should be started and continued for 3 years in patients with normal LV function.
- Only the β-blockers carvedilol, metoprolol succinate, and bisoprolol should be used in patients with LV systolic dysfunction (ejection fraction 40% or less) and heart failure or MI; they should be employed for these IHD patients unless contraindicated.
- Selection of a particular agent depends on the presence of comorbid states, preferred dosing frequency, and cost. β_1-Selective agents are preferred in patients with chronic obstructive pulmonary disease, peripheral arterial disease (PAD), diabetes, dyslipidemia, and sexual dysfunction. Drugs with combined α_1- and β-blockade are effective for IHD, but agents with intrinsic sympathomimetic activity provide little to no reduction in resting HR and are not preferred except perhaps in patients with PAD or dyslipidemia.
- Common adverse effects include bradycardia, hypotension, heart block, impaired glucose metabolism, altered serum lipids (transiently increased triglycerides, decreased HDL-C, and no change in LDL-C), fatigue, depression, insomnia, and malaise. β-Blockers are contraindicated in patients with existing bradycardia, hypotension, 2nd- or 3rd-degree atrioventricular (AV) block, asthma, severe PAD, LV dysfunction with unstable fluid status, and diabetes associated with frequent episodes of hypoglycemia.
- If β-blocker therapy needs to be discontinued, doses should be tapered over 2 to 3 weeks to prevent abrupt withdrawal, which can significantly increase in MVo_2 and induce ischemia and even MI because of up-regulation of β-receptors in the myocardium.
- See **Table 11-1** for the usual dosage ranges of β-blockers in stable IHD.

Calcium Channel Blockers

- CCBs modulate calcium entry into the myocardium, vascular smooth muscle, and other tissues, which reduces the cytosolic concentration of calcium responsible for activation of the actin–myosin complex and contraction of vascular smooth muscle and myocardium. All CCBs reduce MVo_2 due to reduced wall tension secondary to decreased arterial pressure and (to a minor extent) depressed contractility.

- Calcium channel blockers (CCBs) or long-acting nitrates should be prescribed for relief of symptoms when β-blockers are contraindicated or cause unacceptable side effects.
- Dihydropyridine CCBs (eg, **nifedipine**, **amlodipine**, **isradipine**, and **felodipine**) primarily affect vascular smooth muscle with little effect on the myocardium. These drugs produce minimal reduction in contractility and either no change or increased HR due to reflex tachycardia from direct arterial dilation. Nifedipine produces more impairment of LV function than amlodipine and felodipine. Short-acting agents should not be used because of their greater propensity to cause reflex tachycardia. Other side effects of these CCBs include hypotension, headache, gingival hyperplasia, and peripheral edema. Although most CCBs are contraindicated in systolic heart failure, amlodipine and felodipine are considered safe options in these patients.
- Nondihydropyridine CCBs (**verapamil** and **diltiazem**) mostly affect the myocardium with minimal effects on vascular smooth muscle. They reduce HR and contractility and reduce all components of MVo_2. Initial therapy for relief of symptoms with a long-acting nondihydropyridine CCB instead of a β-blocker is a reasonable approach. Common side effects of these CCBs include bradycardia, hypotension, AV block, and symptoms of LV depression. These agents should be avoided in patients with LV dysfunction (especially if receiving concomitant β-blocker therapy) due to negative inotropic effects. Verapamil may cause significant constipation in up 8% of patients. Verapamil and diltiazem inhibit clearance of drugs that utilize the cytochrome P450 3A4 isoenzyme such as carbamazepine, cyclosporine, lovastatin, simvastatin, and benzodiazepines. Verapamil, and to a lesser extent diltiazem, also inhibit P-glycoprotein–mediated drug transport, which can increase concentrations of digoxin and cyclosporine. Verapamil also decreases digoxin clearance. Agents that induce the 3A4 isoenzyme can reduce the effectiveness of all CCBs.
- See **Table 11–1** for the usual dosage ranges of CCBs in stable IHD.

Nitrates

- Nitrates increase concentrations of cyclic guanosine monophosphate in vascular endothelium, leading to reduced cytoplasmic calcium and vasodilation. Most vasodilation occurs on the venous side, leading to reduced preload, myocardial wall tension, and MVo_2. Arterial vasodilation increases as doses are escalated, which can produce reflex tachycardia that counters some of the antianginal benefits. This effect can be mitigated with concomitant β-blocker therapy. Nitrates also produce vasodilation of stenotic epicardial vessels and intracoronary collateral vessels, increasing oxygen supply to the ischemic myocardium.
- All patients should have access to sublingual (SL) NTG 0.3 or 0.4 mg tablets or spray to treat acute angina episodes. Relief typically occurs within 5 minutes of administration.
- SL nitrates can also be used to prevent acute episodes if given 2 to 5 minutes prior to activities known to produce angina; protection can last for up to 30 minutes with SL NTG and up to 1 hour with SL isosorbide dinitrate (ISDN).
- Long-acting nitrates (or CCBs) should be prescribed for relief of symptoms when β-blockers are contraindicated or cause unacceptable side effects. Various nitrate formulations are available for acute and chronic use (**Table 11–1**).
- Transdermal patches and isosorbide mononitrate (ISMN) are most commonly prescribed for long-term prevention of angina episodes. ISDN is also effective, but the three times daily regimen requires dosing every 4 to 5 hours during the day to provide a nitrate-free interval. Chronic nitrate use should incorporate a 10- to 14-hour nitrate-free interval each day to reduce nitrate tolerance. Because this approach places the patient at risk for angina episodes, the nitrate-free interval is usually provided during the nighttime hours when the patient has a reduced MVo_2 while sleeping. The extended-release ISMN products that are dosed twice daily should be given 7 hours apart (eg, 7:00 AM and 2:00 PM). An extended-release, once-daily ISMN product is

available that provides 12 hours of nitrate exposure followed by a 12-hour nitrate-free interval. Transdermal NTG patches are typically prescribed as "on in the a.m. and off in the p.m." but patients should be given specific application and removal times.

- Nitrates should not be used routinely as monotherapy for stable IHD because of the lack of angina coverage during the nitrate-free interval, lack of protection against circadian rhythm (nocturnal) ischemic events, and potential for reflex tachycardia. Concomitant β-blocker or diltiazem therapy can prevent rebound ischemia during the nitrate-free interval.
- Common nitrate side effects include headache, flushing, nausea, postural hypotension, and syncope. Headache can be treated with acetaminophen and usually resolves after about two weeks of continued therapy. Transdermal NTG may cause skin erythema and inflammation. Initiating therapy with smaller doses and/or rotating the application site can minimize transdermal nitroglycerin side effects.
- See **Table 11–1** for the usual dosage ranges of nitrates in stable IHD.

Ranolazine

- Ranolazine reduces ischemic episodes by selective inhibition of late sodium current (I_{Na}), which reduces intracellular sodium concentration and improves myocardial function and perfusion. It does not impact HR, BP, the inotropic state, or increase coronary blood flow.
- Ranolazine (Ranexa) is effective as monotherapy for relief of angina symptoms but should only be used if patients cannot tolerate traditional agents due to hemodynamic or other adverse effects. Because it does not substantially affect HR and BP, it is recommended as add-on therapy for patients who achieve goal HR and BP and still have exertional angina symptoms, patients who cannot achieve these hemodynamic goals due to adverse effects, and patients who reach maximum doses of traditional agents but still have angina symptoms.
- The initial ranolazine dose is 500 mg twice daily, increased to 1000 mg twice daily within the next 1 to 2 weeks if tolerated. It can be combined with a β-blocker when initial treatment with β-blockers alone is unsuccessful.
- Adverse effects include constipation, nausea, dizziness, and headache. Ranolazine can prolong the QTc interval and should be used with caution in patients receiving concomitant QTc-prolonging agents.
- Potent inhibitors of CYP3A4 and P-glycoprotein (ketoconazole, itraconazole, protease inhibitors, clarithromycin, and nefazodone) or potent inducers of CYP3A4 and P-glycoprotein (phenytoin, phenobarbital, carbamazepine, rifampin, rifabutin, rifapentine, St. John's wort) are contraindicated with ranolazine due to significant increases and decreases in ranolazine drug concentrations, respectively. Moderate CYP3A4 inhibitors (eg, diltiazem, verapamil, erythromycin, and fluconazole) can be used with ranolazine, but the maximum dose should not exceed 500 mg twice daily.

TREATMENT OF VARIABLE THRESHOLD ANGINA AND PRINZMETAL ANGINA

- Patients with variable threshold angina require pharmacotherapy for vasospasm. Most patients respond well to SL NTG for acute attacks.
- Both CCBs and nitrates are effective for chronic therapy. CCBs may be preferred because they are dosed less frequently. Nifedipine, verapamil, and diltiazem are equally effective as single agents for initial management of vasospasm; dose titration is important to maximize the response. Patients unresponsive to CCBs alone may have nitrates added.
- β-blockers are not appropriate therapy for vasospasm because they may induce coronary vasoconstriction and prolong ischemia.

EVALUATION OF THERAPEUTIC OUTCOMES

- Improvement of symptoms can be assessed by number of angina episodes, weekly SL NTG use, and increased exercise capacity or duration of exertion needed to induce angina.
- Use of statins for dyslipidemia, achieving BP and A1C goals, and achievement of the lifestyle modification goals of smoking cessation, weight loss, and regular exercise regimens are important targets.
- Once patients have been optimized on medical therapy, symptoms should improve over 2 to 4 weeks and remain stable until the disease progresses. Patients may require evaluation every 1 to 2 months until target endpoints are achieved; follow-up every 6 to 12 months thereafter is appropriate.
- The Seattle Angina Questionnaire, Specific Activity Scale, and Canadian Cardiovascular Society classification system can be used to improve reproducibility of symptom assessment.
- If the patient is doing well, no other assessment may be necessary. Although follow-up exercise tolerance testing with or without cardiac imaging can be performed to objectively assess control of ischemic episodes, this is rarely done if patients are doing well because of the expense involved.
- Monitor for adverse drug effects such as headache and dizziness with nitrates; fatigue and lassitude with β-blockers; and peripheral edema, constipation, and dizziness with CCBs.

See Chapter 16, Stable Ischemic Heart Disease, authored by Paul P. Dobesh, for a more detailed discussion of this topic.

CHAPTER 12

Shock

- *Shock* is an acute state of inadequate perfusion of critical organs that can lead to death if therapy is not optimal. Shock is defined as systolic blood pressure (SBP) less than 90 mm Hg or reduction of at least 40 mm Hg from baseline with perfusion abnormalities despite adequate fluid resuscitation.

PATHOPHYSIOLOGY

- Shock results in failure of the circulatory system to deliver sufficient oxygen (O_2) to tissues despite normal or reduced O_2 consumption. Shock may be caused by intravascular volume deficit (hypovolemic shock), myocardial pump failure (cardiogenic shock), or peripheral vasodilation (septic, anaphylactic, or neurogenic shock).
- Hypovolemic shock is characterized by acute intravascular volume deficiency due to external losses or internal redistribution of extracellular water. It can be precipitated by hemorrhage; burns; trauma; surgery; intestinal obstruction; and dehydration from considerable insensible fluid loss, overaggressive diuretic administration, and severe vomiting or diarrhea. Relative hypovolemia leading to hypovolemic shock occurs during significant vasodilation, which accompanies anaphylaxis, sepsis, and neurogenic shock.
- Fall in blood pressure (BP) is compensated by increased sympathetic outflow, activation of the renin–angiotensin system, and other factors that stimulate peripheral vasoconstriction. Compensatory vasoconstriction redistributes blood away from skin, skeletal muscles, kidneys, and gastrointestinal (GI) tract toward vital organs (eg, heart and brain) in attempt to maintain oxygenation, nutrition, and organ function.
- Severe lactic acidosis often develops secondary to tissue ischemia and causes localized vasodilation, which further exacerbates the impaired cardiovascular state.

CLINICAL PRESENTATION

- Patients with hypovolemic shock may have thirst, anxiousness, weakness, light-headedness, dizziness, scanty urine output, and dark yellow urine.
- Signs of more severe volume loss include tachycardia (>120 beats/min), tachypnea (>30 breaths/min), hypotension (SBP <90 mm Hg), mental status changes or unconsciousness, agitation, and normal or low body temperature (in the absence of infection) with cold extremities and decreased capillary refill.
- Serum sodium and chloride concentrations are usually high with acute volume depletion. The blood urea nitrogen (BUN):creatinine ratio may be elevated initially, but the creatinine increases with renal dysfunction. Metabolic acidosis results in elevated base deficit and lactate concentrations with decreased bicarbonate and pH.
- Complete blood cell count (CBC) is normal in absence of infection. In hemorrhagic shock, the red cell count, hemoglobin, and hematocrit will decrease.
- Urine output is decreased to less than 0.5 to 1 mL/h. With more severe volume depletion, dysfunction of other organs may be reflected in laboratory testing (eg, elevated serum transaminases levels with hepatic dysfunction).

DIAGNOSIS AND MONITORING

- Noninvasive and invasive monitoring (Table 12–1) and evaluation of medical history, clinical presentation, and laboratory findings are important in establishing the diagnosis and assessing mechanisms responsible for shock. Findings include hypotension (SBP <90 mm Hg), depressed cardiac index (CI <2.2 L/min/m²), tachycardia (heart rate >100 beats/min), and low urine output (<20 mL/h).

TABLE 12–1	Hemodynamic and Oxygen-Transport Monitoring Parameters
Parameter	**Normal Value[a]**
Blood pressure (systolic/diastolic)	100–130/70–85 mm Hg
Mean arterial pressure (MAP)	80–100 mm Hg
Pulmonary artery pressure (PAP)	25/10 mm Hg
Mean pulmonary artery pressure (MPAP)	12–15 mm Hg
Central venous pressure (CVP)	8–12 mm Hg
Pulmonary artery occlusion pressure (PAOP)	12–15 mm Hg
Heart rate (HR)	60–80 beats/min
Cardiac output (CO)	4–7 L/min
Cardiac index (CI)	2.8–3.6 L/min/m²
Stroke volume index (SVI)	30–50 mL/m²
Systemic vascular resistance index (SVRI)	1300–2100 dyne · s/m² · cm⁵
Pulmonary vascular resistance index (PVRI)	45–225 dyne · s/m² · cm⁵
Arterial oxygen saturation (Sao_2)	97% (range, 95%–100%)
Mixed venous oxygen saturation (Svo_2)	70%–75%
Arterial oxygen content (Cao_2)	20.1 vol% (range, 19–21)
Venous oxygen content (Cvo_2)	15.5 vol% (range, 11.5–16.5)
Oxygen content difference ($C[a\text{-}v]O_2$)	5 vol% (range, 4–6)
Oxygen consumption index (Vo_2)	131 mL/min/m² (range, 100–180)
Oxygen delivery index (Do_2)	578 mL/min/m² (range, 370–730)
Oxygen extraction ratio (O_2ER)	25% (range, 22–30)
Intramucosal pH (pHi)	7.40 (range, 7.35–7.45)
Index (I)	Parameter indexed to body surface area

[a]Normal values may not be the same as values needed to optimize the management of a critically ill patient.

- Pulmonary artery (Swan–Ganz) catheter can be used to determine central venous pressure (CVP), pulmonary artery pressure (PAP), cardiac output (CO), and pulmonary artery occlusion pressure (PAOP).
- Renal function can be assessed grossly by hourly measurements of urine output, but estimation of creatinine clearance based on isolated serum creatinine values may be inaccurate. Decreased renal perfusion and aldosterone release result in sodium retention and thus low urinary sodium (<30 mEq/L).
- In normal individuals, O_2 consumption (Vo_2) is dependent on O_2 delivery (Do_2) up to a certain critical level (Vo_2 flow dependency). At this point, tissue O_2 requirements have been satisfied, and further increases in Do_2 will not alter Vo_2 (flow independency). However, studies in critically ill patients show a continuous, pathologic dependence relationship of Vo_2 with Do_2. These indexed parameters are calculated as

$$Do_2 = CI \times (Cao_2) \text{ and } Vo_2 = CI \times (Cao_2 - Cvo_2)$$

where CI = cardiac index, Cao_2 = arterial oxygen content determined by hemoglobin concentration and SaO_2, and Cvo_2 = mixed venous oxygen content determined by hemoglobin concentration and Svo_2.

- The Vo_2:Do_2 ratio (O_2 extraction ratio) can be used to assess adequacy of perfusion and metabolic response. Patients who can increase Vo_2 when Do_2 is increased are more likely to survive. However, low Vo_2 and O_2 extraction ratio values indicate poor O_2 utilization and lead to greater mortality.

TREATMENT

- <u>Goals of Treatment</u>: The goal during resuscitation from shock is to achieve and maintain mean arterial pressure (MAP) consistently above 65 mm Hg while ensuring adequate perfusion to critical organs. The ultimate goals are to prevent further disease progression with subsequent organ damage and, if possible, to reverse organ dysfunction that has already occurred.

GENERAL APPROACH

- **Figures 12–1** and **12–2** contain algorithms for acute and ongoing management of adults with hypovolemia.
- Initiate supplemental O_2 at the earliest signs of shock, beginning with 4 to 6 L/min via nasal cannula or 6 to 10 L/min by face mask.
- Fluid resuscitation to maintain circulating blood volume is essential (see next section). If fluid administration does not achieve desired end points, pharmacologic support is necessary with inotropic and vasoactive drugs.
- Supportive care measures include assessment and management of pain, anxiety, agitation, and delirium.

FLUID RESUSCITATION FOR HYPOVOLEMIC SHOCK

- *Crystalloids*: Isotonic (or near isotonic) crystalloid solutions (**0.9% sodium chloride** or **lactated Ringer solution**) are the initial fluids of choice. The choice between normal saline and lactated Ringer solution is based on clinician preference and adverse effect concerns. Crystalloids can be rapidly and easily administered, are compatible with most drugs, and have low cost. Their disadvantages include the need to use large fluid volumes and the possibility that dilution of oncotic pressure may lead to pulmonary edema. Crystalloids are administered at a rate of 500 to 2000 mL/h, depending on severity of the deficit, degree of ongoing fluid loss, and tolerance to infusion volume. Usually 2 to 4 L of crystalloid normalizes intravascular volume.
- *Colloids*: **Albumin**, **hydroxyethyl starch**, and **dextran** possess the theoretical advantage of prolonged intravascular retention time compared with crystalloid solutions. However, colloids are expensive and have been associated with fluid overload, renal dysfunction, and bleeding. In 2013, the U.S. Food and Drug Administration (FDA) analyzed data from randomized controlled trials, meta-analyses, and observational studies and concluded that hydroxyethyl starch is associated with increased mortality and renal injury requiring renal replacement therapy in critically ill adult patients, including patients with sepsis and those admitted to the intensive care unit (ICU). The FDA concluded that the solutions should not be used in these patient populations and added a boxed warning to the labeling describing the risk of mortality and severe renal injury.
- *Blood products*: Some patients require blood products (**whole blood**, **packed red blood cells**, **fresh frozen plasma**, or **platelets**) to ensure maintenance of O_2-carrying capacity, as well as clotting factors and platelets for blood hemostasis. Blood products may be associated with transfusion-related reactions, virus transmission (rare), hypocalcemia resulting from added citrate, increased blood viscosity from supranormal hematocrit elevations, and hypothermia from failure to appropriately warm solutions before administration.

PHARMACOLOGIC THERAPY FOR SHOCK

- *Hypovolemic shock*: Inotropic agents and vasopressors are generally not indicated in initial treatment of hypovolemic shock (if fluid therapy is adequate), because the body's compensatory response is to increase CO and peripheral resistance to maintain BP. Use of vasopressors in lieu of fluids may exacerbate this resistance to the point that circulation is stopped. Therefore, vasoactive agents that dilate peripheral vasculature such as dobutamine are preferred if blood pressure is stable and high enough to tolerate the vasodilation. Vasopressors are only used as a temporizing measure or last resort when other measures fail to maintain perfusion.
- *Septic shock*: An algorithm for use of fluid resuscitation, vasopressors, and inotropes in septic shock is shown in **Fig. 12–3**. Initial hemodynamic therapy for septic shock

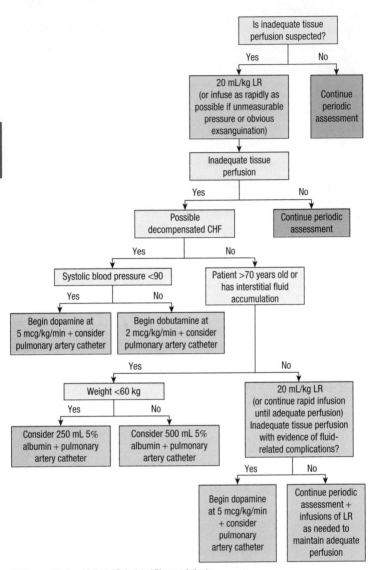

(CHF, congestive heart failure; LR, lactated Ringer solution.)

FIGURE 12-1. Hypovolemia protocol for adults. Normal saline (or a lower chloride-containing isotonic crystalloid) may be used instead of lactated Ringer solution. This protocol is not intended to replace or delay therapies such as surgical intervention or blood products for restoring oxygen-carrying capacity or hemostasis. For the resuscitation of patients with trauma prior to bleeding control, usually no more than 1 L of crystalloid should be given initially in an attempt to use the minimal amount of fluid necessary to maintain perfusion and not exacerbate bleeding. If available, some measurements can be used in addition to those listed in the algorithm, such as mean arterial pressure or pulmonary artery catheter recordings. The latter can be used to assist in medication choices (eg, agents with primary pressor effects may be desirable in patients with normal cardiac outputs, whereas dopamine or dobutamine may be indicated in patients with suboptimal cardiac outputs). Lower maximal doses of the medications in this algorithm should be considered when pulmonary artery catheterization is not available.

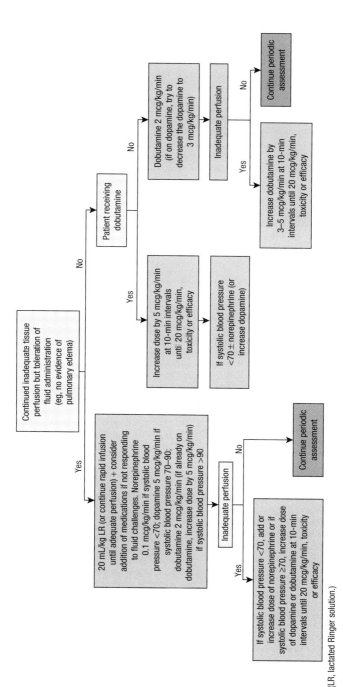

FIGURE 12-2. Ongoing management of inadequate tissue perfusion. Normal saline (or a lower chloride-containing isotonic crystalloid) may be substituted for lactated Ringer solution in this figure.

(LR, lactated Ringer solution.)

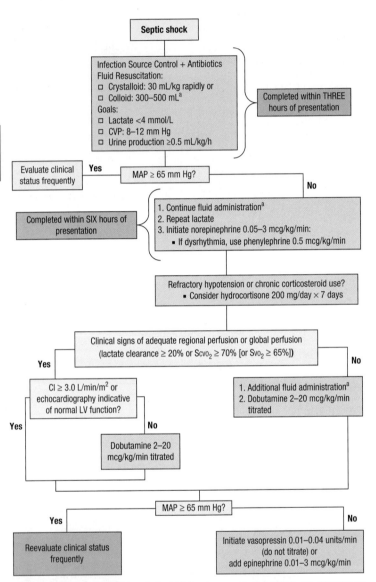

^aColloid (albumin) may be initiated in patients at risk for adverse events from redistribution of intravenous fluids to extravascular tissues (eg, patients with renal dysfunction, decompensated heart failure, and ascites compromising diaphragmatic function), those that are fluid restricted, or those not responding to crystalloid therapy.

(CI, cardiac index; CVP, central venous pressure; echo, echocardiography; Hct, hematocrit; MAP, mean arterial pressure; Scvo₂, central venous oxygen saturation; Svo₂, mixed venous oxygen saturation.)

FIGURE 12–3. Algorithm for resuscitative management of septic shock. Intended to be used in conjunction with clinical judgment, hemodynamic monitoring parameters, global and regional perfusion goals, and therapy end points.

is administration of IV fluid (30 mL/kg of crystalloid), with the aim of using the least amount of fluid and lowest CVP to achieve end-organ perfusion (recommended goal CVP = 8 to 12 mm Hg or 15 mm Hg in mechanically ventilated patients or patients with abdominal distention or preexisting ventricular dysfunction). More than 30 mL/kg of crystalloid fluids may be needed to obtain goal MAP, reverse global hypoperfusion (lactate clearance, SCVO2 ≥70%), or achieve clinical indication of regional organ-specific perfusion (eg, urine production). Therefore, dynamic fluid response and clinical assessment should occur frequently after each fluid challenge. Current recommendations are to measure serum lactate and administer 30 mL/kg of crystalloid for hypotension within 3 hours of presentation and obtain MAP ≥65 mm Hg with vasopressors, reassess volume status, and re-measure serum lactate if the initial lactate was elevated within 6 hours of presentation. Although crystalloids and colloids are arguably considered equivalent for shock resuscitation, crystalloids are generally preferred over colloids (because of ready availability and lower cost) unless patients are at risk for adverse events from redistribution of IV fluids to extravascular tissues or are fluid restricted.

- ✓ **Norepinephrine** is the preferred initial vasopressor in septic shock not responding to fluid administration.
- ✓ **Epinephrine** may be added in cases where there is suboptimal hemodynamic response to norepinephrine.
- ✓ **Phenylephrine** may be tried as the initial vasopressor in cases of severe tachydysrhythmias, when CO is known to be high, or as salvage therapy when combination vasopressors including low-dose vasopressin fail to achieve goals
- ✓ **Dobutamine** is used in low CO states despite adequate fluid resuscitation pressures or ongoing signs of global or regional hypoperfusion despite adequate resuscitation.
- ✓ **Vasopressin** 0.03 units/min may be considered as adjunctive therapy in patients who are refractory to catecholamine vasopressors despite adequate fluid resuscitation. Doses of 0.04 units/min or less increase SVR and arterial BP to reduce the dose requirement of catecholamine adrenergic agents.

- Dosage titration and monitoring of vasopressor and inotropic therapy should be guided by clinical response, the goals of early goal-directed therapy, and lactate clearance. Vasopressor/inotrope therapy is continued until myocardial depression and vascular hyporesponsiveness (ie, blood pressure) of septic shock improve, usually measured in hours to days. Discontinuation of therapy should be executed slowly with careful monitoring.
- Receptor selectivities of vasopressors and inotropes are listed in Table 12–2. In general, these drugs act rapidly with short durations of action and are given as continuous infusions. Potent vasoconstrictors such as norepinephrine and phenylephrine should be given through central veins because of possibility of extravasation and tissue damage with peripheral administration. Careful monitoring and calculation of infusion rates are advised because dosing adjustments are made frequently, and varying admixture concentrations are used in volume-restricted patients.
- **Norepinephrine** is first-line therapy for septic shock because it effectively increases MAP. It has strong α_1-agonist activity and less potent β_1-agonist effects while maintaining weak vasodilatory effects of β_2-receptor stimulation. Norepinephrine infusions are initiated at 0.05 to 0.1 mcg/kg/min and rapidly titrated to preset goals of MAP (usually at least 65 mm Hg), improvement in peripheral perfusion (to restore urine production or decrease blood lactate), and/or achievement of desired oxygen-transport variables while not compromising cardiac index. Norepinephrine 0.01 to 2 mcg/kg/min improves hemodynamic parameters to "normal" values in most patients with septic shock. As with other vasopressors, norepinephrine dosages exceeding those recommended by most references frequently are needed in critically ill patients with septic shock to achieve predetermined goals.
- **Phenylephrine** is a pure α_1-agonist; in sepsis, it improves MAP by increasing cardiac index through enhanced venous return to the heart (increase in CVP and stroke index) and by acting as a positive inotrope. Phenylephrine 0.5 to 9 mcg/kg/min, used

TABLE 12–2	Receptor Pharmacology and Adverse Events of Selected Inotropic and Vasopressor Agents Used in Septic Shock[a]						
Agent (Adverse Events)	α_1	α_2	β_1	β_2	D	V_1	V_2
Dobutamine (0.5–4 mg/mL D_5W or NS)	Tachycardia, dysrhythmias, hypotension						
2–10 mcg/kg/min	+	0	++++	++	0	0	0
>10–20 mcg/kg/min	++	0	++++	+++	0	0	0
Dopamine (0.8–3.2 mg/mL D_5W or NS)	Tachycardia, dysrhythmias, decreased PaO₂, mesenteric hypoperfusion, gastrointestinal motility inhibition, T-cell inhibition						
1–3 mcg/kg/min	0	0	+	0	++++	0	0
3–10 mcg/kg/min	0/+	0	++++	+	++++	0	0
>10–20 mcg/kg/min	+++	0	++++	+	0	0	0
Epinephrine (0.008–0.016 mg/mL D_5W or NS)	Tachycardia, dysrhythmias, decreased PaO₂, mesenteric hypoperfusion, increased lactate, hyperglycemia, immunomodulation						
0.01–0.05 mcg/kg/min	++	++	++++	+++	0	0	0
0.05–3 mcg/kg/min	++++	++++	+++	+	0	0	0
Norepinephrine (0.016–0.064 mg/mL D_5W)	Mixed effects on myocardial performance and mesenteric perfusion, peripheral ischemia						
0.02–3 mcg/kg/min	+++	+++	+++	+/++	0	0	0
Phenylephrine (0.1–0.4 mg/mL D_5W or NS)	Mixed effects on myocardial performance, peripheral ischemia						
0.5–9 mcg/kg/min	+++	+	+	0	0	0	0
Vasopressin (0.8 units/mL D_5W or NS)	Mixed effects on myocardial performance, mesenteric hypoperfusion, peripheral ischemia, hyponatremia, thrombocytopenia						
0.01–0.04 units/min	0	0	0	0	0	+++	+++

(D, dopamine; D_5W, dextrose 5% in water; NS, normal saline; PaO₂, partial pressure of arterial oxygen; V, vasopressin.)
[a]Activity ranges from no activity (0) to maximal (++++) activity.

alone or in combination with dobutamine or low doses of dopamine, improves blood pressure and myocardial performance in fluid-resuscitated septic patients. Adverse effects, such as tachydysrhythmias, are infrequent, particularly when it is used as a single agent or at higher doses, because it does not have β_1-adrenergic agonist activity. Phenylephrine may be a useful alternative in patients who cannot tolerate tachycardia or tachydysrhythmias from dopamine or norepinephrine and in patients who are refractory to dopamine or norepinephrine.

- **Epinephrine** has combined α- and β-agonist effects; it is an acceptable choice for hemodynamic support of septic shock because of its combined vasoconstrictor and inotropic effects, but it is associated with tachydysrhythmias and lactate elevation. As a result, it is considered second-line or as adjunctive therapy to norepinephrine. Infusion rates of 0.04 to 1 mcg/kg/min alone increase hemodynamic and oxygen-transport variables to supranormal values without adverse effects in septic patients without coronary artery disease. Large dosages (0.5–3 mcg/ kg/min) often are required. Smaller dosages (0.10–0.50 mcg/kg/min) are effective when epinephrine is added to other vasopressors and inotropes. Younger patients appear to respond better to epinephrine, possibly because of greater β-adrenergic reactivity. Based on current evidence, epinephrine may be used as a second-line vasopressor as added on to norepinephrine in patients with septic shock refractory to fluid administration. Although it effectively increases CO and Do_2, it has deleterious effects on the splanchnic circulation.

- **Dopamine** is generally not as effective as norepinephrine and epinephrine for achieving goal MAP in patients with septic shock. Dopamine doses of 5 to 10 mcg/kg/min increase cardiac index by improving contractility and heart rate, primarily from its β_1 effects. It increases MAP and SVR as a result of both increased CO and, at higher doses (>10 mcg/kg/min), its α_1 agonist effects. The clinical utility of dopamine is limited because large dosages are frequently necessary to maintain CO and MAP. At dosages exceeding 20 mcg/kg/min, further improvement in cardiac performance and regional hemodynamics is limited. Its clinical use frequently is hampered by tachycardia and tachydysrhythmias, which may lead to myocardial ischemia. Use dopamine with caution in patients with elevated preload because it may worsen pulmonary edema.

- **Dobutamine** is an inotrope with vasodilatory properties (an "inodilator"). It is used to increase the cardiac index, typically by 25% to 50%. Dobutamine should be started at dosages ranging from 2.5 to 5 mcg/kg/min. Although a dose response may be seen, dosages greater than 5 mcg/kg/min may provide limited beneficial effects on oxygen transport values and hemodynamics and may increase adverse cardiac effects. If given to patients who are intravascularly depleted, dobutamine will result in hypotension and a reflexive tachycardia.

- **Vasopressin** produces rapid and sustained improvement in hemodynamic parameters at dosages not exceeding 0.04 units/min. Doses above 0.04 units/min are associated with negative changes in CO and mesenteric mucosal perfusion. It should be used with extreme caution in septic shock patients with cardiac dysfunction. Cardiac ischemia appears to be a rare occurrence when low doses are used; therefore, use of higher doses in septic shock patients with cardiac dysfunction warrants extreme caution. In order to minimize adverse events and maximize beneficial effects, use vasopressin as add-on therapy to catecholamine adrenergic agents rather than as first-line therapy or salvage therapy, and limit dosages to 0.03 to 0.04 units/min. Vasopressin should be used when response to one or two adrenergic agents is inadequate or as a method for reducing the dosage of those therapies. Increased arterial pressure should be evident within the first hour of vasopressin therapy, at which time the dose(s) of adrenergic agent(s) should be reduced while maintaining goal MAP. Attempt to discontinue vasopressin when the dosage(s) of adrenergic agent(s) has been minimized (dopamine ≤5 mcg/kg/min, norepinephrine ≤0.1 mcg/kg/min, phenylephrine ≤1 mcg/kg/min, epinephrine ≤0.15 mcg/kg/min).

- **Corticosteroids** can be initiated in septic shock when adrenal insufficiency is suspected (eg, patients receiving long-term corticosteroid therapy for other indications prior to the onset of shock), when vasopressor dosages are escalating, or when weaning of vasopressor therapy proves futile. Assessment of adrenal function to guide therapy is not recommended. Adverse events are few because corticosteroids are administered for a short time, usually 7 days. Acutely, elevated BUN, white blood cell count, glucose, and sodium may occur. In general, treatment of septic shock with corticosteroids improves hemodynamic variables and lowers catecholamine vasopressor dosages with minimal to no adverse effect on patient safety.

EVALUATION OF THERAPEUTIC OUTCOMES

- Monitor patients with suspected volume depletion initially by vital signs, urine output, mental status, and physical examination.
- Placement of a CVP line provides a useful (although indirect and insensitive) estimate of the relationship between increased right atrial pressure and CO.
- Reserve pulmonary artery catheterization for complicated cases of shock not responding to conventional fluid and medication therapies. Complications related to catheter insertion, maintenance, and removal include damage to vessels and organs during insertion, arrhythmias, infections, and thromboembolic damage.

- Laboratory tests for ongoing monitoring of shock include electrolytes and renal function tests (BUN and serum creatinine); CBC to assess possible infection, O_2-carrying capacity of the blood, and ongoing bleeding; PT and aPTT to assess clotting ability; and lactate concentration and base deficit to detect inadequate tissue perfusion.
- Monitor cardiovascular and respiratory parameters continuously (see Table 12–1). Watch for trends, rather than specific CVP or PAOP numbers, because of interpatient variability in response.
- Successful fluid resuscitation should increase SBP (>90 mm Hg), CI (>2.2 L/min/m²), and urine output (0.5–1 mL/kg/h) while decreasing SVR to the normal range. MAP of greater than 65 mm Hg should be achieved to ensure adequate cerebral and coronary perfusion pressure.
- Intravascular volume overload is characterized by high filling pressures (CVP >12–15 mm Hg, PAOP >20–24 mm Hg) and decreased CO (<3.5 L/min). If volume overload occurs, administer furosemide, 20 to 40 mg, by slow IV push to produce rapid diuresis of intravascular volume and "unload" the heart through venous dilation.
- Coagulation problems are primarily associated with low levels of clotting factors in stored blood, as well as dilution of endogenous clotting factors and platelets following administration of the blood. As a result, check a coagulation panel (PT, international normalized ratio [INR], and aPTT) in patients undergoing replacement of 50% to 100% of blood volume in 12 to 24 hours.

See Chapter 23, Use of Vasopressors and Inotropes in the Pharmacotherapy of Shock, authored by Robert MacLaren, Scott Mueller, and Joseph F. Dasta, and Chapter 24, Hypovolemic Shock, authored by Brian L. Erstad, for a more detailed discussion of this topic.

13 Stroke

- *Stroke* involves abrupt onset of focal neurologic deficit that lasts at least 24 hours and is presumed to be of vascular origin. Stroke can be either ischemic or hemorrhagic. Transient ischemic attacks (TIAs) are focal ischemic neurologic deficits lasting less than 24 hours and usually less than 30 minutes.

PATHOPHYSIOLOGY

ISCHEMIC STROKE

- Ischemic strokes (87% of all strokes) are due either to local thrombus formation or emboli occluding a cerebral artery. Cerebral atherosclerosis is a cause in most cases, but 30% are of unknown etiology. Emboli arise either from intra- or extracranial arteries. Twenty percent of ischemic strokes arise from the heart.
- Carotid atherosclerotic plaques may rupture, resulting in collagen exposure, platelet aggregation, and thrombus formation. The clot may cause local occlusion or dislodge and travel distally, eventually occluding a cerebral vessel.
- In cardiogenic embolism, stasis of blood flow in the atria or ventricles leads to formation of local clots that can dislodge and travel through the aorta to the cerebral circulation.
- Thrombus formation and embolism result in arterial occlusion, decreasing cerebral blood flow and causing ischemia and ultimately infarction distal to the occlusion.

HEMORRHAGIC STROKE

- Hemorrhagic strokes (13% of strokes) include subarachnoid hemorrhage (SAH) and intracerebral hemorrhage. SAH may result from trauma or rupture of an intracranial aneurysm or arteriovenous malformation (AVM). Intracerebral hemorrhage occurs when a ruptured blood vessel within the brain causes a hematoma.
- Blood in the brain parenchyma causes mechanical compression of vulnerable tissue and subsequent activation of inflammation and neurotoxins.

CLINICAL PRESENTATION

- Patients may be unable to provide a reliable history because of neurologic deficits. Family members or other witnesses may need to provide this information.
- Symptoms include unilateral weakness, inability to speak, loss of vision, vertigo, or falling. Ischemic stroke is not usually painful, but headache may occur in hemorrhagic stroke.
- Neurologic deficits on physical examination depend on the brain area involved. Hemi- or monoparesis and hemisensory deficits are common. Patients with posterior circulation involvement may have vertigo and diplopia. Anterior circulation strokes commonly result in aphasia. Patients may experience dysarthria, visual field defects, and altered levels of consciousness.

DIAGNOSIS

- Laboratory tests for hypercoagulable states should be done only when the cause cannot be determined based on presence of risk factors. Protein C, protein S, and antithrombin III are best measured in steady state rather than in the acute stage. Antiphospholipid antibodies are of higher yield but should be reserved for patients younger than 50 years and those who have had multiple venous or arterial thrombotic events or livedo reticularis.
- Computed tomography (CT) and magnetic resonance imaging (MRI) head scans can reveal areas of hemorrhage and infarction.
- Carotid Doppler (CD), electrocardiogram (ECG), transthoracic echocardiogram (TTE), and transcranial Doppler (TCD) studies can each provide valuable diagnostic information.

TREATMENT

- <u>Goals of Treatment</u>: The goals are to: (1) reduce ongoing neurologic injury and decrease mortality and long-term disability; (2) prevent complications secondary to immobility and neurologic dysfunction; and (3) prevent stroke recurrence.

GENERAL APPROACH

- Ensure adequate respiratory and cardiac support and determine quickly from CT scan whether the lesion is ischemic or hemorrhagic.
- Evaluate ischemic stroke patients presenting within hours of symptom onset for reperfusion therapy.
- Elevated blood pressure (BP) should remain untreated in the acute period (first 7 days) after ischemic stroke to avoid decreasing cerebral blood flow and worsening symptoms. BP should be lowered if it exceeds 220/120 mm Hg or there is evidence of aortic dissection, acute myocardial infarction (MI), pulmonary edema, or hypertensive encephalopathy. If BP is treated, short-acting parenteral agents (eg, labetalol and nicardipine) are preferred.
- Assess patients with hemorrhagic stroke to determine whether they are candidates for surgical intervention.
- After the hyperacute phase, focus on preventing progressive deficits, minimizing complications, and instituting secondary prevention strategies.

NONPHARMACOLOGIC THERAPY

- *Acute ischemic stroke*: Endovascular thrombectomy with a stent retriever (done within 6 hours of symptom onset and after IV tPA) improves outcomes in select patients with proximal large artery occlusion and salvageable tissue on imaging. Surgical decompression (performed within 48 hours of stroke onset in patients less than age 60) is sometimes necessary to reduce intracranial pressure. An interprofessional team approach that includes early rehabilitation can reduce long-term disability. In secondary prevention, carotid endarterectomy and stenting may be effective in reducing stroke incidence and recurrence in appropriate patients.
- *Hemorrhagic stroke*: In SAH from ruptured intracranial aneurysm or arteriovenous malformation, surgical intervention to clip or ablate the vascular abnormality reduces mortality from rebleeding. After primary intracerebral hemorrhage, surgical evacuation may be beneficial in some situations, but this remains under investigation. Insertion of an external ventricular drain with monitoring of intracranial pressure is commonly performed in these patients.

PHARMACOLOGIC THERAPY OF ISCHEMIC STROKE

- Evidence-based recommendations for pharmacotherapy of ischemic stroke are given in **Table 13–1**.
- **Alteplase** (t-PA, tissue plasminogen activator) initiated within 4.5 hours of symptom onset reduces disability from ischemic stroke. Adherence to a strict protocol is essential to achieving positive outcomes: (1) activate the stroke team; (2) treat as early as possible within 4.5 hours of onset; (3) obtain CT scan to rule out hemorrhage; (4) meet all inclusion and no exclusion criteria (**Table 13–2**); (5) administer alteplase 0.9 mg/kg (maximum 90 mg) infused IV over 1 hour, with 10% given as initial bolus over 1 minute; (6) avoid anticoagulant and antiplatelet therapy for 24 hours; and (7) monitor the patient closely for elevated BP, response, and hemorrhage.
- **Aspirin** 160 to 325 mg/day started between 24 and 48 hours after completion of alteplase also reduces long-term death and disability.
- Secondary prevention of ischemic stroke:
  - ✓ Use antiplatelet therapy in noncardioembolic stroke. **Aspirin**, **clopidogrel**, and **extended-release dipyridamole plus aspirin** are all first-line agents (see **Table 13–1**). Limit the combination of clopidogrel and ASA to select patients

TABLE 13–1	Recommendations for Pharmacotherapy of Ischemic Stroke	
	Recommendation	**Evidence**[a]
Acute treatment	tPA 0.9 mg/kg IV (maximum 90 mg) over 1 hour in selected patients within 3 hours of onset	IA
	tPA 0.9 mg/kg IV (maximum 90 mg) over 1 hour between 3 and 4.5 hours of onset	IB
	ASA 160–325 mg daily started within 48 hours of onset	IA
Secondary prevention		
Noncardioembolic	Antiplatelet therapy	IA
	Aspirin 50–325 mg daily	IB
	Aspirin 25 mg + extended-release dipyridamole 200 mg twice daily	IB
	Clopidogrel 75 mg daily	IIaB
Cardioembolic (especially atrial fibrillation)	VKA (INR = 2.5)	IA
	Apixaban 5 mg twice daily	IA
	Dabigatran 150 mg twice daily	IB
	Rivaroxaban 20 mg daily	IIaB
Atherosclerosis + LDL > 100 mg/dL	High intensity statin therapy	IB
BP > 140/90 mm Hg	BP reduction	IB

(ASA, acetylsalicylic acid; INR, international normalized ratio; IV, intravenous; LDL, low-density lipoprotein; tPA, tissue plasminogen activator; VKA, vitamin K antagonist.)
[a]Classes: I, evidence or general agreement about usefulness and effectiveness; II, conflicting evidence about the usefulness; IIa, weight of evidence in favor of the treatment; IIb, usefulness less well established; III, not useful and maybe harmful. Levels of evidence: A, multiple randomized clinical trials; B, a single randomized trial or nonrandomized studies; C, expert opinion or case studies.

with a recent MI history or intracranial stenosis and only with ultra–low-dose ASA to minimize bleeding risk.
✓ For patients with atrial fibrillation and a presumed cardiac source of embolism, oral anticoagulation with a vitamin K antagonist (**warfarin**), **apixaban**, **dabigatran**, or **rivaroxaban** is recommended.
• Treatment of elevated BP after ischemic stroke reduces risk of stroke recurrence. Treatment guidelines recommend reduction of BP greater than 140/90 mm Hg in patients with stroke or TIA after the acute period (first 7 days).
• **Statins** reduce risk of stroke by approximately 30% in patients with coronary artery disease and elevated plasma lipids. Patients experiencing ischemic stroke of presumed atherosclerotic origin who have low-density lipoprotein (LDL) cholesterol above 100 mg/dL should be treated with high-intensity statin therapy for secondary stroke prevention.
• **Low-molecular-weight heparin** or **low-dose subcutaneous unfractionated heparin** (5000 units three times daily) is recommended for prevention of deep vein thrombosis in hospitalized patients with decreased mobility due to stroke and should be used in all but the most minor strokes.

TABLE 13–2	Inclusion and Exclusion Criteria for tPA Use in Acute Ischemic Stroke

Inclusion criteria
- Age 18 years or older
- Clinical diagnosis of ischemic stroke causing a measurable neurologic deficit
- Time of symptom onset well established to be <4.5 hours before treatment would begin

Exclusion criteria
- History of previous intracranial hemorrhage
- Symptoms suggestive of SAH
- Active internal bleeding
- Acute bleeding diathesis, including but not limited to a platelet count <100,000/mm³ (<100 × 10¹²/L)
- Patient has received heparin within 48 hours, resulting in an elevated aPTT
- Recent anticoagulant use and elevated INR (>1.7) or PT (>15 seconds)
- Current use of direct thrombin inhibitors or direct factor Xa inhibitors with elevated sensitive laboratory tests (such as aPTT, INR, platelet count, and ECT; TT; or appropriate factor Xa activity assays)
- Significant head trauma or previous stroke within 3 months
- Arterial puncture at noncompressible site within 7 days
- Intracranial neoplasm, arteriovenous malformation, or aneurysm
- SBP >185 mm Hg or DBP >110 mm Hg
- Blood glucose <50 mg/dL (2.7 mmol/L)
- CT demonstrates multilobar infarction (hypodensity >1/3 cerebral hemisphere)

Relative exclusion criteria (considering risk to benefit in individual patients, may be wise to administer tPA despite 1 or more of the following:)
- Only minor or rapidly improving symptoms
- Pregnancy
- Seizure at onset with postictal residual impairments
- Major surgery or serious trauma within 14 days
- Gastrointestinal or urinary tract hemorrhage within 21 days
- Acute myocardial infarction within 3 months

Additional exclusion criteria if within 3–4.5 hours of onset:
- Age greater than 80 years
- Current treatment with oral anticoagulants
- NIH Stroke Scale Score >25 (severe stroke)
- Imaging evidence of large infarct (>1/3 MCA territory)
- History of both stroke and diabetes

(aPTT, activated partial thromboplastin time; CT, computed tomography; DBP, diastolic blood pressure; ECT, Ecarin clotting time; INR, international normalized ratio; MCA, middle cerebral artery; NIH, National Institutes of Health; PT, prothrombin time; SBP, systolic blood pressure; SAH, subarachnoid hemorrhage; TT, thrombin time.)

PHARMACOLOGIC THERAPY OF HEMORRHAGIC STROKE

- There are no standard pharmacologic strategies for treating intracerebral hemorrhage. Follow medical guidelines for managing BP, increased intracranial pressure, and other medical complications in acutely ill patients in neurointensive care units.
- All patients with warfarin-associated ICH should receive intravenous vitamin K and therapy to replace the affected clotting factors. Prothrombin complex concentrate (PCC) has advantages over fresh frozen plasma (FFP) alone because it results in a faster normalization of the INR and less chance of fluid overload.
- SAH due to aneurysm rupture is often associated with delayed cerebral ischemia in the 2 weeks after the bleeding episode. Vasospasm of the cerebral vasculature is thought to be responsible for the delayed ischemia and occurs between 4 and 21 days after the bleed. The calcium channel blocker **nimodipine** 60 mg every 4 hours for

21 days, along with maintenance of intravascular volume with pressor therapy, is recommended to reduce the incidence and severity of neurologic deficits resulting from delayed ischemia.

EVALUATION OF THERAPEUTIC OUTCOMES

- Monitor patients with acute stroke intensely for development of neurologic worsening (recurrence or extension), complications (thromboembolism, infection), and adverse treatment effects.
- The most common reasons for clinical deterioration in stroke patients include: (1) extension of the original lesion in the brain; (2) development of cerebral edema and raised intracranial pressure; (3) hypertensive emergency; (4) infection (eg, urinary and respiratory tract); (5) venous thromboembolism; (6) electrolyte abnormalities and rhythm disturbances; and (7) recurrent stroke.
- For patients receiving alteplase therapy, monitor for bleeding with neurologic examination every 15 minutes for 1 hour, then every half-hour for 6 hours, then every hour for 17 hours, then once every shift thereafter.
- For aspirin, clopidogrel, extended-release dipyridamole plus aspirin, warfarin, and other oral anticoagulants, monitor for bleeding daily.
- For patients receiving warfarin, check the INR and hemoglobin/hematocrit daily.

See Chapter 20, Stroke, authored by Susan C. Fagan and David C. Hess, for a more detailed discussion of this topic.

- *Venous thromboembolism* (VTE) results from clot formation in the venous circulation and is manifested as deep vein thrombosis (DVT) and pulmonary embolism (PE).

PATHOPHYSIOLOGY

- Risk factors for VTE include increasing age, history of VTE, and aspects related to Virchow's triad: (1) blood stasis (eg, immobility and obesity); (2) vascular injury (eg, surgery, trauma, and venous catheters); and (3) hypercoagulability (eg, malignancy, coagulation factor abnormalities, antiphospholipid antibodies, and certain drugs).
- The most common inherited hypercoagulability disorder is activated protein C (aPC) resistance (Caucasian prevalence 2%–7%), which increases the risk of VTE threefold. Most aPC resistance results from a factor V gene mutation (known as factor V Leiden) that renders it resistant to degradation by aPC.
- The prothrombin G20210A mutation is the second most frequent inherited hyper-coagulability disorder (Caucasian prevalence 2%–4%) and imparts a threefold increased risk of VTE. The mutation increases circulating prothrombin and may enhance thrombin generation.
- Inherited deficiencies of protein C, protein S, and antithrombin occur in less than 1% of the population and may increase the lifetime VTE risk by as much as sevenfold.
- Normal hemostasis maintains integrity of the circulatory system after blood vessel damage. Disruption of the endothelial cell lining with injury results in platelet activation and tissue-factor–mediated initiation of the clotting factor cascade, culminating in formation of thrombin and ultimately a fibrin clot. In contrast to physiologic hemostasis, pathologic VTE occurs in the absence of gross vessel wall damage and may be triggered by tissue factor (TF) brought to the clot formation site by circulating microparticles. Clots causing VTE impair blood flow and often cause complete vessel occlusion.
- Exposure of blood to damaged vessel endothelium causes platelets to become activated after binding to adhesion proteins (eg, von Willebrand factor and collagen). Activated platelets recruit additional platelets, causing formation of a platelet thrombus. Activated platelets change shape and release components that sustain further thrombus formation at the site. Activated platelets accumulating in the thrombus express the adhesion molecule P-selectin, which facilitates capture of blood-borne microparticles bearing tissue-factor, thereby triggering fibrin clot formation via the coagulation cascade.
- The conceptual model for the coagulation cascade involves reactions that occur on cell surfaces in three overlapping phases (Fig. 14–1):
  ✓ *Initiation*: A TF/VIIa complex (known as extrinsic tenase or X-ase) on cells bearing TF that have been exposed after vessel injury or captured via P-selectin activates limited amounts of factors IX and X. The resulting factor Xa then associates with factor Va to form the prothrombinase complex, which cleaves prothrombin (factor II) to generate a small amount of thrombin (factor IIa). Factor IXa moves to the surface of activated platelets in the growing platelet thrombus. Tissue factor pathway inhibitor (TFPI) regulates TF/VIIa-induced coagulation, rapidly terminating the initiation phase.
  ✓ *Amplification:* Thrombin produced during initiation activates factors V and VIII, which bind to platelet surfaces and support the large-scale thrombin generation occurring during the propagation phase. Platelet-bound factor XI is also activated by thrombin during amplification.
  ✓ *Propagation:* Factor VIIIa/IXa (known as intrinsic tenase) and prothrombinase complexes assemble on the surface of activated platelets and accelerate the generation of factor Xa and thrombin, respectively, causing a burst of thrombin production. Thrombin generation is further supported by factor XIa bound to platelet surfaces, which activates factor IX to form additional intrinsic tenase.

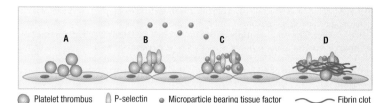

Platelet thrombus   P-selectin   Microparticle bearing tissue factor   Fibrin clot

FIGURE 14–1. Model of pathologic thrombus formation: (*A*) activated platelets adhere to vascular endothelium; (*B*) activated platelets express P-selectin; (*C*) pathologic microparticles express active tissue factor and are present at a high concentration in the circulation—these microparticles accumulate, perhaps by binding to activated platelets expressing P-selectin; and (*D*) tissue factor can lead to thrombin generation, and thrombin generation leads to platelet thrombus formation and fibrin generation.

- Thrombin then converts fibrinogen to fibrin monomers that precipitate and polymerize to form fibrin strands. Factor XIIIa (also activated by the action of thrombin) covalently bonds these strands to form an extensive meshwork that encases the aggregated platelet thrombus and red cells to form a stabilized fibrin clot.
- Hemostasis is controlled by antithrombotic substances secreted by intact endothelium adjacent to damaged tissue. Thrombomodulin modulates thrombin activity by converting protein C to its activated form (aPC), which joins with protein S to inactivate factors Va and VIIIa. This prevents coagulation reactions from spreading to uninjured vessel walls. In addition, circulating antithrombin inhibits thrombin and factor Xa. Heparan sulfate is secreted by endothelial cells and accelerates antithrombin activity. These self-regulatory mechanisms limit fibrin clot formation to the zone of vessel injury.
- The fibrinolytic system dissolves formed blood clots; inactive plasminogen is converted to plasmin by tissue plasminogen activator (tPA). Plasmin is an enzyme that degrades the fibrin mesh into soluble end products (known as fibrin degradation products including D-dimer).
- Thrombi can form in any part of the venous circulation but usually begin in the leg(s). Isolated calf vein thrombi seldom embolize; those involving the popliteal and larger veins above it are more likely to embolize and lodge in the pulmonary artery or one of its branches, occluding blood flow to the lung and impairing gas exchange. Without treatment, the affected lung area becomes necrotic and oxygen delivery to other vital organs may decrease, potentially resulting in fatal circulatory collapse.

CLINICAL PRESENTATION

- Many patients never develop symptoms from the acute event.
- Symptoms of DVT may include unilateral leg swelling, pain, tenderness, erythema, and warmth. Physical signs may include a palpable cord and a positive Homan sign.
- Symptoms of PE may include cough, chest pain or tightness, shortness of breath, palpitations, hemoptysis, dizziness, or lightheadedness. Signs of PE include tachypnea, tachycardia, diaphoresis, cyanosis, hypotension, shock, and cardiovascular collapse.
- Postthrombotic syndrome may produce chronic lower extremity swelling, pain, tenderness, skin discoloration, and ulceration.

DIAGNOSIS

- Assessment should focus on identifying risk factors (see Pathophysiology section).
- Compression ultrasound (CUS) and computed tomography pulmonary angiography (CTPA) are used most often for initial evaluation of suspected VTE.

- Radiographic contrast studies (venography, pulmonary angiography) are the most accurate and reliable diagnostic methods but are expensive, invasive, and difficult to perform and evaluate. The ventilation-perfusion (V/Q) scan is an alternative PE diagnostic test.
- Serum concentration of D-dimer is nearly always elevated; values less than 500 ng/mL (mcg/L) combined with clinical decision rules are useful in ruling out VTE.
- Clinical assessment checklists (eg, Wells score) can be used to determine whether a patient is likely or unlikely to have DVT or PE.

TREATMENT

- Goals of Treatment: The initial goal is to prevent VTE in at-risk populations. Treatment of VTE is aimed at preventing thrombus extension and embolization, reducing recurrence risk, and preventing long-term complications (eg, postthrombotic syndrome and chronic thromboembolic pulmonary hypertension).

PREVENTION OF VTE

- Nonpharmacologic methods improve venous blood flow by mechanical means and include early ambulation, graduated compression stockings, intermittent pneumatic compression (IPC) devices, and inferior vena cava filters.
- Hospitalized and acutely ill medical patients at high VTE risk and low bleeding risk should receive pharmacologic prophylaxis with low-dose unfractionated heparin (LDUH), low-molecular-weight heparin (LMWH), or fondaparinux during hospitalization or until fully ambulatory.
- In general, nonorthopedic surgery patients at high VTE risk but low bleeding risk should receive LDUH or LMWH prophylaxis plus graduated compression stockings or IPC.
- Recommended VTE prophylaxis following joint replacement surgery may include aspirin, adjusted-dose warfarin, unfractionated heparin (UFH), LMWH, fondaparinux, dabigatran, apixaban, or rivaroxaban for at least 10 days postsurgery. Clinical trials support prophylaxis for 21 to 35 days after total hip replacement and hip fracture repair surgeries.
- Refer to *Antithrombotic Therapy and Prevention of Thrombosis, 9th edition: Evidence-Based Clinical Practice Guidelines* published by the American College of Chest Physicians for detailed information on prophylaxis strategies based on the clinical situation and level of risk for VTE.

GENERAL APPROACH TO TREATMENT OF VTE

- Anticoagulation is the primary treatment for VTE; DVT and PE are treated similarly (Fig. 14–2).
- After VTE is confirmed objectively, therapy with a rapid-acting anticoagulant should be instituted as soon as possible. Anticoagulants can be administered in the outpatient setting in most patients with DVT and in carefully selected hemodynamically stable patients with PE.
- Three months is the appropriate initial duration of anticoagulation therapy for the acute first episode of VTE for all patients. This duration is also recommended when the initial thrombotic event was associated with a major transient or reversible risk factor (eg, surgery, hospitalization).
- Continuing anticoagulation is required to prevent new VTE episodes not directly related to the preceding episode. Extended therapy beyond 3 months should be considered for patients with a first unprovoked (idiopathic) VTE when feasible because of a relatively high recurrence rate. In patients with VTE and active cancer, extended therapy is rarely stopped because of a high recurrence risk.

NONPHARMACOLOGIC THERAPY

- Encourage patients to ambulate as much as symptoms permit.
- Ambulation in conjunction with graduated compression stockings results in faster reduction in pain and swelling than strict bedrest with no increase in embolization rate.

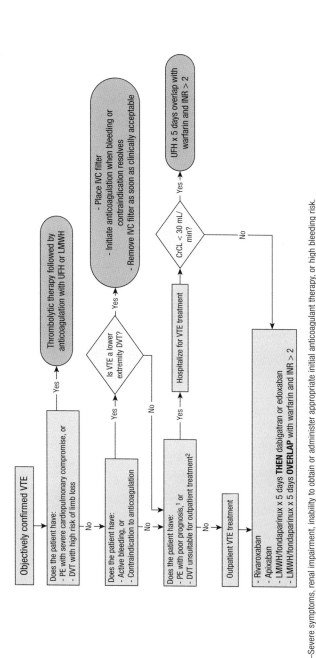

FIGURE 14–2. Treatment of venous thromboembolism (VTE).

[1]–Severe symptoms, renal impairment, inability to obtain or administer appropriate initial anticoagulant therapy, or high bleeding risk.

[2]–PESI score ≥ 86 points: age (1 pt for each year); male sex (10 pts); cancer (30 pts); heart failure (10 pts); COPD (10 pts); heart rate > 110 bpm (20 pts); respiratory rate > 30 bpm (20 pts); temperature < 36°C (20 pts); altered mental status (60 pts); O₂ sat < 90% (20 pts).

(CrCl, creatinine clearance; DVT, deep vein thrombosis; IV, intravenous; IVC, inferior vena cava; LMWH, low-molecular-weight heparin; PE, pulmonary embolism; PESI, pulmonary embolism severity index; SC, subcutaneous; UFH, unfractionated heparin.)

The flowchart reads as follows:

Objectively confirmed VTE
→ Does the patient have: PE with severe cardiopulmonary compromise, or DVT with high risk of limb loss
— Yes → Thrombolytic therapy followed by anticoagulation with UFH or LMWH
— No →

Does the patient have: Active bleeding, or Contraindication to anticoagulation
— Yes → Is VTE a lower extremity DVT?
  — Yes → Place IVC filter; Initiate anticoagulation when bleeding or contraindication resolves; Remove IVC filter as soon as clinically acceptable
  — No →
— No →

Does the patient have: PE with poor prognosis,[1] or DVT unsuitable for outpatient treatment[2]
— Yes → Hospitalize for VTE treatment → CrCl < 30 mL/min?
  — Yes → UFH x 5 days overlap with warfarin and INR > 2
  — No →
— No → Outpatient VTE treatment

- Rivaroxaban
- Apixaban
- LMWH/fondaparinux x 5 days THEN dabigatran or edoxaban
- LMWH/fondaparinux x 5 days OVERLAP with warfarin and INR > 2

- Inferior vena cava filters should only be used when anticoagulants are contraindicated due to active bleeding.
- Elimination of the obstructing thrombus via thrombolysis or thrombectomy may be warranted in life- or limb-threatening DVT.

PHARMACOLOGIC THERAPY

Direct Oral Anticoagulants (DOACs)

- **Rivaroxaban** (Xarelto), **apixaban** (Eliquis), and **edoxaban** (Savaysa) are oral selective inhibitors of both free and clot-bound factor Xa and do not require antithrombin to exert their anticoagulant effect. **Dabigatran** (Pradaxa) is an oral selective, reversible, direct factor IIa inhibitor.
- See Table 14–1 for DOAC indications and dosing. DOACs should be used with caution in patients with renal dysfunction.
- Single-drug oral therapy with rivaroxaban or apixaban is noninferior to traditional therapy with warfarin overlapped with enoxaparin for acute DVT and PE with similar rates of recurrent VTE and perhaps less major bleeding. Both drugs are initiated with a higher dose with eventual transition to maintenance dosing. Until further data are available, these drugs should not be used in patients with creatinine clearance (CrCl) less than 25 mL/min (0.42 mL/s), active cancer, and patients requiring thrombolytic therapy. Neither drug requires routine anticoagulation monitoring. Both drugs have a high acquisition cost and lack effective reversal agents.

TABLE 14–1	Approved Indications and Dosing for the Direct Oral Anticoagulants		
	VTE Prophylaxis Following Orthopedic Surgery	**Acute VTE Treatment**	**Extended VTE Treatment (after the first 6 months of anticoagulant therapy)**
Dabigatran	Not approved for use	150 mg PO twice daily with or without food FOLLOWING at least 5 days of parenteral anticoagulant therapy	150 mg PO twice daily with or without food
Rivaroxaban	10 mg PO once daily with or without food beginning 6–10 hours after surgery as soon as hemostasis is achieved and continuing for 12–35 days postoperatively	15 mg PO twice daily with food for Days 1–21, then 20 mg PO once daily with food beginning on Day 22	20 mg PO once daily with food
Apixaban	2.5 mg PO twice daily with or without food beginning 12–24 hours after surgery and continuing for 12–35 days postoperatively	10 mg PO twice daily with or without food for Days 1–7, then 5 mg PO twice daily with or without food beginning on Day 8	2.5 mg PO twice daily with or without food
Edoxaban	Not approved for use	60 mg PO once daily with or without food FOLLOWING at least 5 days of parenteral anticoagulant therapy	Not approved for use

(PO, by mouth; VTE, venous thromboembolism.)

- Edoxaban and dabigatran must be given only after at least 5 days of subcutaneous (SC) anticoagulation with UFH, LMWH, or fondaparinux. These regimens were noninferior to warfarin in patients with acute VTE for the outcome of recurrent VTE. Compared to warfarin, dabigatran caused similar major bleeding and edoxaban caused significantly less bleeding. Until further data are available, these agents should not be given to patients with hemodynamically unstable PE or at high bleeding risk.
- Bleeding is the most common adverse effect with DOAC therapy. Patients experiencing significant bleeding should receive routine supportive care and discontinuation of anticoagulant therapy. **Idarucizumab** (Praxbind) 5 g IV rapidly reverses the dabigatran anticoagulant effect when needed during emergency situations (eg, life-threatening bleeding) and need for urgent surgical intervention. Adding aspirin to DOAC therapy nearly doubles bleeding rates and should be avoided in most patients with VTE. Rivaroxaban and apixaban are subject to interactions involving inhibitors or inducers of CYP 3A4.

Low-Molecular-Weight Heparin

- LMWH fragments produced by either chemical or enzymatic depolymerization of UFH are heterogeneous mixtures of sulfated glycosaminoglycans with approximately one-third the mean UFH molecular weight. LMWH prevents thrombus propagation by accelerating the activity of antithrombin similar to UFH.
- LMWH given SC in fixed, weight-based doses is at least as effective as UFH given IV for VTE treatment. LMWH has largely replaced UFH for initial VTE treatment due to improved pharmacokinetic and pharmacodynamic profiles and ease of use. Advantages of LMWH over UFH include: (1) predictable anticoagulation dose response; (2) improved SC bioavailability; (3) dose-independent clearance; (4) longer biologic half-life; (5) lower incidence of thrombocytopenia; and (6) less need for routine laboratory monitoring.
- Stable patients with DVT or PE who have normal vital signs, low bleeding risk, and no other uncontrolled comorbid conditions requiring hospitalization can be discharged early or treated entirely on an outpatient basis (if considered appropriate candidates). Hemodynamically unstable patients with PE should generally be admitted for initiation of anticoagulation therapy.
- Recommended doses (based on actual body weight) include:
  - ✓ **Enoxaparin** (Lovenox): For acute DVT treatment with or without PE, 1 mg/kg SC every 12 hours or 1.5 mg/kg every 24 hours
  - ✓ **Dalteparin** (Fragmin): For acute DVT treatment, 200 units/kg SC every 24 hours (not FDA approved in the U.S. for this indication). For VTE in patients with cancer, 200 units/kg SC every 24 hours for 30 days, followed by 150 units SC every 24 hours. The maximum total daily dose is 18,000 units.
- In patients without cancer, acute LMWH treatment is generally transitioned to long-term warfarin therapy after 5 to 10 days.
- Routine laboratory monitoring is unnecessary because LMWH anticoagulant response is predictable when given SC. Prior to initiating therapy, obtain a baseline complete blood cell count (CBC) with platelet count and serum creatinine. Check the CBC every 5 to 10 days during the first 2 weeks of LMWH therapy and every 2 to 4 weeks thereafter to monitor for occult bleeding. Measuring anti–factor Xa activity is the most widely used method to monitor LMWH; routine measurement is unnecessary in stable and uncomplicated patients. Monitoring may be helpful in patients who have significant renal impairment, weigh less than 50 kg, are morbidly obese, or require therapy longer than 14 days.
- As with other anticoagulants, bleeding is the most common adverse effect of LMWH therapy, but major bleeding may be less common than with UFH. If major bleeding occurs, IV **protamine sulfate** can be administered, but it cannot neutralize the anticoagulant effect completely. The recommended protamine sulfate dose is 1 mg per 1 mg of enoxaparin or 1 mg per 100 anti–factor Xa units of dalteparin administered in the previous 8 hours. A second dose of 0.5 mg per 1 mg or 100 anti–factor Xa units can be given if bleeding continues. Smaller protamine doses can be used if the

LMWH dose was given in the previous 8 to 12 hours. Protamine sulfate is not recommended if the LMWH was given more than 12 hours earlier.

- Thrombocytopenia can occur with LMWHs, but the incidence of heparin-induced thrombocytopenia (HIT) is three times lower than with UFH. LMWH has been associated with osteopenia, but the risk of osteoporosis appears to be lower with LMWH than with UFH.

Fondaparinux

- **Fondaparinux** (Arixtra) prevents thrombus generation and clot formation by indirectly inhibiting factor Xa activity through its interaction with antithrombin. Unlike UFH or LMWH, fondaparinux inhibits only factor Xa activity.
- Fondaparinux is a safe and effective alternative to LMWH for acute VTE treatment and is likewise followed by long-term warfarin therapy.
- Fondaparinux is dosed once daily via weight-based SC injection: 5 mg if less than 50 kg, 7.5 mg if 50 to 100 kg, and 10 mg if more than 100 kg.
- Patients receiving fondaparinux do not require routine coagulation testing. Determine baseline kidney function before starting therapy because fondaparinux is contraindicated if CrCl is less than 30 mL/min (0.5 mL/s).
- Bleeding is the primary adverse effect associated with fondaparinux therapy. Measure CBC at baseline and periodically thereafter to detect occult bleeding. Monitor for signs and symptoms of bleeding daily. There is no specific antidote to reverse the antithrombotic activity of fondaparinux.

Unfractionated Heparin

- **Unfractionated heparin** binds to antithrombin, provoking a conformation change that makes it much more potent in inhibiting the activity of factors IXa, Xa, XIIa, and IIa. This prevents thrombus growth and propagation allowing endogenous thrombolytic systems to lyse the clot. Because some patients fail to achieve an adequate response, IV UFH has largely been replaced by LMWH or fondaparinux. UFH continues to have a role in patients with CrCl less than 30 mL/min (0.5 mL/s).
- When immediate and full anticoagulation is required, a weight-based IV loading dose followed by a continuous IV infusion is preferred (Table 14–2). Fixed dosing

TABLE 14–2	Weight-Based[a] Dosing for Unfractionated Heparin Administered by Continuous IV Infusion	
Indication	**Initial Loading Dose**	**Initial Infusion Rate**
Deep venous thrombosis/ pulmonary embolism	80–100 units/kg Maximum = 10,000 units	17–20 units/kg/h Maximum = 2,300 units/h
Activated Partial Thromboplastin Time (seconds)	**Maintenance Infusion Rate**	
	Dose Adjustment	
<37 (or anti–factor Xa <0.20 unit/mL [kU/L])	80 units/kg bolus, and then increase infusion by 4 units/kg/h	
37–47 (or anti–factor Xa 0.20–0.29 unit/mL [kU/L])	40 units/kg bolus, and then increase infusion by 2 units/kg/h	
48–71 (or anti–factor Xa 0.30–0.70 unit/mL [kU/L])	No change	
72–93 (or anti–factor Xa 0.71–1 unit/mL [kU/L])	Decrease infusion by 1–2 units/kg/h	
>93 (or anti–factor Xa >1 unit/mL [kU/L])	Hold infusion for 1 hour, and then decrease by 3 units/kg/h	

[a]Use actual body weight for all calculations. Adjusted body weight may be used for obese patients (>130% of ideal body weight).

(eg, 5000-unit bolus followed by 1000-units/h continuous infusion) produces similar clinical outcomes.

- Weight-based SC UFH (initial dose 333 units/kg SC followed by 250 units/kg every 12 hours) without coagulation monitoring also provides adequate anticoagulation and is a less costly option for select patients.

- The activated partial thromboplastin time (aPTT) is generally recommended for monitoring UFH, provided that institution-specific therapeutic ranges are defined. Measure aPTT prior to initiation of therapy and 6 hours after the start of therapy or a dose change. Adjust the UFH dose based on patient response and the institution-specific aPTT therapeutic range.

- Monitor patients closely for bleeding signs and symptoms during UFH therapy. If major bleeding occurs, discontinue UFH immediately, identify and treat the underlying bleeding source, and give **protamine sulfate** by slow IV infusion over 10 minutes (1 mg/100 units of UFH infused during the previous 4 hours; maximum 50 mg).

- Heparin-induced thrombocytopenia (HIT) is a rare immunologic reaction requiring immediate intervention and that may be fatal. The most common complication of HIT is VTE; arterial thrombosis occurs less frequently. Thrombocytopenia is the most common clinical manifestation, but serologic confirmation of heparin antibodies is required to diagnose HIT. Use of a clinical prediction rule, such as the 4Ts score (*T*hrombocytopenia, *T*iming of platelet count fall or thrombosis, *T*hrombosis, o*T*her explanation for thrombocytopenia), can improve the predictive value of platelet count monitoring and heparin antibody testing. Discontinue all heparin if new thrombosis occurs in the setting of falling platelets in conjunction with a moderate or high 4Ts score. Alternative anticoagulation with a direct thrombin inhibitor should then be initiated.

- Using UFH doses of 20,000 units/day or more for longer than 6 months, especially during pregnancy, is associated with significant bone loss and may lead to osteoporosis.

Warfarin

- **Warfarin** inhibits enzymes responsible for cyclic interconversion of vitamin K in the liver. Reduced vitamin K is a cofactor required for carboxylation of the vitamin K–dependent coagulation factors II (prothrombin), VII, IX, and X and the endogenous anticoagulant proteins C and S. By inhibiting the reduced vitamin K supply needed for production of these proteins, warfarin therapy produces coagulation proteins with less activity. By suppressing fully functional clotting factor production, warfarin prevents initial thrombus formation and propagation. The time required to achieve its anticoagulant effect depends on the elimination half-lives of the coagulation proteins (6 hours for factor VII and 72 hours for prothrombin). Full antithrombotic effect is not achieved for at least 6 days after warfarin therapy initiation.

- Because of its slow onset of effect, warfarin must be started concurrently with injectable anticoagulant therapy (UFH, LMWH, or fondaparinux) with an overlap of at least 5 days and until an INR of 2 or greater has been achieved for at least 24 hours.

- Guidelines for initiating warfarin therapy are given in Fig. 14–3. The initial warfarin dose should be 5 to 10 mg for most patients and periodically adjusted to achieve and maintain an INR between 2 and 3. Lower starting doses may be acceptable in patients with advanced age, malnutrition, liver disease, or heart failure. Starting doses more than 10 mg should be avoided.

- Monitor warfarin therapy by the INR; the recommended target INR for treatment of VTE is 2.5, with an acceptable range of 2 to 3. After an acute thromboembolic event, obtain a baseline INR and CBC prior to initiating warfarin therapy and at least every 3 days during the first week of therapy. Once the patient's dose response is established, obtain an INR every 7 to 14 days until it stabilizes, then ideally every 4 to 12 weeks thereafter.

- In general, maintenance doe changes should not be made more frequently than every 3 days. Adjust maintenance doses by calculating the weekly dose and reducing or increasing it by 5% to 25%. The full effect of a dose changes may not become evident for 5 to 7 days.

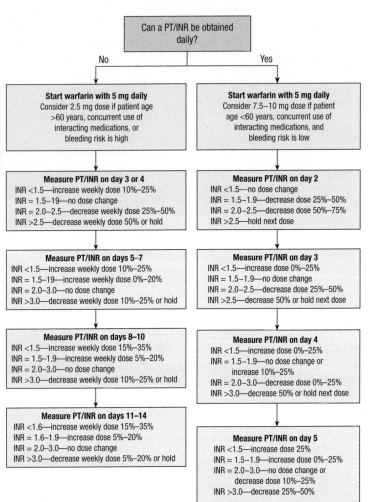

(INR, international normalized ratio; PT, prothrombin time.)

FIGURE 14-3. Initiation of warfarin therapy.

- Warfarin's primary adverse effect is bleeding that can range from mild to life threatening. It does not cause bleeding per se, but it exacerbates bleeding from existing lesions and enables massive bleeding from ordinarily minor sources. The likelihood of bleeding rises with increased intensity of anticoagulation therapy; therefore, correcting high INR values is important to reduce bleeding risk:
  ✓ When the INR is greater than 4.5 without evidence of bleeding, the INR can be lowered by withholding warfarin, adjusting the dose of warfarin, and/or providing a small dose of vitamin K to shorten the time to return to normal INR. Although vitamin K can be given parenterally or orally, the oral route is preferred in the absence of serious bleeding.
  ✓ If the INR is between 5 and 10 and no bleeding is present, routine vitamin K use is not recommended because it has not been shown to affect the risk of

developing subsequent bleeding or thromboembolism compared to simply withholding warfarin alone.

✓ For INR greater than 10 without evidence of bleeding, oral vitamin K (**phytonadione** 2.5 mg) is suggested. Use vitamin K with caution in patients at high risk of recurrent thromboembolism because of the possibility of INR overcorrection.

- Patients with warfarin-associated major bleeding require supportive care. Rapid reversal of anticoagulation with a four-factor prothrombin complex concentrate and 5 to 10 mg of vitamin K given by slow IV injection are also recommended.
- Nonhemorrhagic adverse effects of warfarin include the rare "purple toe" syndrome and skin necrosis.
- Because of the large number of food–drug and drug–drug interactions with warfarin, close monitoring and additional INR determinations may be indicated whenever other medications are initiated, discontinued, or an alteration in consumption of vitamin K–containing foods is noted.

Thrombolytics

- Thrombolytic agents are proteolytic enzymes that enhance conversion of plasminogen to plasmin, which subsequently degrades the fibrin matrix.
- The majority of patients with VTE do not require thrombolytic therapy. Treatment should be reserved for patients who present with extensive proximal (eg, ileofemoral) DVT within 14 days of symptom onset, have good functional status, and are at low risk of bleeding.
- Patients with massive PE and evidence of hemodynamic compromise (hypotension or shock) should receive thrombolytic therapy unless contraindicated by bleeding risk.
- For DVT, catheter-directed thrombolysis is preferred if appropriate expertise and resources are available. The same duration and intensity of anticoagulation therapy is recommended as for DVT patients who do not receive thrombolysis. Patients with DVT involving the iliac and common femoral veins are at highest risk for post-thrombotic syndrome and may receive the greatest benefit from thrombus removal strategies.
- For patients with massive PE manifested by shock and cardiovascular collapse (~5% of patients with PE), thrombolytic therapy is considered necessary in addition to aggressive interventions such as volume expansion, vasopressor therapy, intubation, and mechanical ventilation. Administer thrombolytic therapy in these patients without delay to reduce the risk of progression to multisystem organ failure and death. However, the risk of death from PE should outweigh the risk of serious bleeding associated with thrombolytic therapy.
- **Alteplase** (Activase) 100 mg by IV infusion over 2 hours is the most commonly used thrombolytic therapy for patients with PE.
- Before giving thrombolytic therapy for PE, IV UFH should be administered in full therapeutic doses. During thrombolytic therapy, IV UFH may be either continued or suspended; the most common practice in the United States is to suspend UFH.
- Measure the aPTT after completion of thrombolytic therapy. If the aPTT is less than 80 seconds, start UFH infusion and adjust to maintain the aPTT in the therapeutic range. If the posttreatment aPTT is longer than 80 seconds, remeasure it every 2 to 4 hours and start UFH infusion when the aPTT is less than 80 seconds.

EVALUATION OF THERAPEUTIC OUTCOMES

- Monitor patients for resolution of symptoms, development of recurrent thrombosis, symptoms of the postthrombotic syndrome, and adverse effects from anticoagulants.
- Monitor hemoglobin, hematocrit, and blood pressure carefully to detect bleeding from anticoagulant therapy.
- Perform coagulation tests (aPTT, PT, and INR) prior to initiating therapy to establish the patient's baseline values and guide later anticoagulation.

- Ask outpatients taking warfarin about medication adherence to prior dosing instructions, other medication use, changes in health status, and symptoms related to bleeding and thromboembolic complications. Any changes in concurrent medications should be carefully explored, and dietary intake of vitamin K-rich foods should be assessed.

See Chapter 19, Venous Thromboembolism, authored by Daniel M. Witt, Nathan P. Clark, and Sara R. Vazquez for a more detailed discussion of this topic.

CHAPTER 15 — Acne Vulgaris

- *Acne* is a common, usually self-limiting disease involving inflammation of the sebaceous follicles of the face and upper trunk.

PATHOPHYSIOLOGY

- Acne usually begins in the prepubertal period and progresses as androgen production and sebaceous gland activity increase with gonad development.
- Acne progresses through four stages: (1) increased sebum production by sebaceous glands, (2) *Propionibacterium acnes* follicular colonization (and bacterial lipolysis of sebum triglycerides to free fatty acids), (3) release of inflammatory mediators, and (4) increased follicular keratinization.
- Circulating androgens cause sebaceous glands to increase their size and activity. There is increased keratinization of epidermal cells and development of an obstructed sebaceous follicle, called a *microcomedone*. Cells adhere to each other, forming a dense keratinous plug. Sebum, produced in increasing amounts, becomes trapped behind the keratin plug and solidifies, contributing to open or closed comedone formation.
- Pooling of sebum in the follicle facilitates proliferation of the anaerobic bacterium *Propionibacterium acnes*, which generates a T-cell response resulting in inflammation. *P. acnes* produces a lipase that hydrolyzes sebum triglycerides into free fatty acids that may increase keratinization and lead to microcomedone formation.
- The closed comedone (whitehead) is the first visible lesion of acne. It is almost completely obstructed to drainage and has a tendency to rupture.
- An open comedone (blackhead) is formed as the plug extends to the upper canal and dilates its opening. Acne characterized by open and closed comedones is termed *noninflammatory acne*.
- Pus formation occurs due to recruitment of neutrophils into the follicle during the inflammatory process and release of *P. acnes*–generated chemokines. *P. acnes* also produces enzymes that increase permeability of the follicular wall, causing it to rupture, thereby releasing keratin, lipids, and irritating free fatty acids into the dermis. Inflammatory lesions that may form and lead to scarring include pustules, nodules, and cysts.

CLINICAL PRESENTATION

- Lesions usually occur on the face, back, upper chest, and shoulders. Severity varies from a mild comedonal form to severe inflammatory acne. The disease is categorized as mild, moderate, or severe, depending on the type and severity of lesions.
- Lesions may take months to heal completely, and fibrosis associated with healing may lead to permanent scarring.

DIAGNOSIS

- Diagnosis is established by patient assessment, which includes observation of lesions and excluding other potential causes (eg, drug-induced acne). Several different systems are in use to grade acne severity.

TREATMENT

- <u>Goals of Treatment</u>: The goals are to reduce the number and severity of lesions, improve appearance, slow progression, limit duration and recurrence, prevent disfigurement associated with scarring and hyperpigmentation, and avoid psychologic suffering.

GENERAL APPROACH (FIG. 15–1)

- Acne is treated as a chronic disease that warrants early and aggressive treatment. Maintenance therapy is often needed for optimal outcomes. Patient adherence to lengthy treatment regimens is crucial to long-term disease control.
- Eliminating follicular occlusion will arrest the acne cascade. Nondrug and pharmacologic measures should be directed toward cleansing, reducing triggers, and combination therapy targeting all four pathogenic mechanisms.
- Combination therapy is often more effective than single therapy and may decrease side effects and minimize resistance or tolerance to individual treatments.
- Topical therapy is standard treatment for mild-to-moderate acne, whereas systemic therapy is required for moderate-to-severe acne.
- First-, second-, and third-line therapies should be selected and altered as appropriate for the severity and staging of the disease. Treatment is directed at control, not cure. Regimens should be tapered over time, adjusting to response.
- Combine the smallest number of agents at the lowest possible dosages to ensure efficacy, safety, avoidance of resistance, and patient adherence. Once control is achieved, simplify the regimen but continue with some suppressive therapy.

NONPHARMACOLOGIC THERAPY

- Encourage patients to avoid aggravating factors, maintain a balanced diet, and control stress.
- Patients should wash no more than twice daily with a mild, nonfragranced opaque or glycerin soap or a soapless cleanser. Scrubbing should be minimized to prevent follicular rupture.
- Comedone extraction results in immediate cosmetic improvement but has not been widely tested in clinical trials.

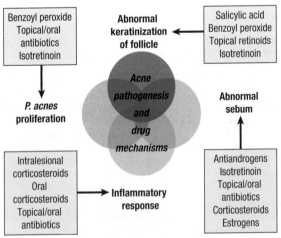

© Debra Sibbald

FIGURE 15–1. **Acne pathogenesis and drug mechanisms.**

PHARMACOLOGIC THERAPY

- *Comedonal noninflammatory acne*: Select topical agents that target the increased keratinization by producing exfoliation. Topical retinoids (especially adapalene) are drugs of choice. Benzoyl peroxide or azelaic acid can be considered.
- *Mild to moderate papulopustular inflammatory acne*: It is important to reduce the population of *P. acnes*. Either the fixed-dose combination of adapalene and benzoyl peroxide or the fixed-dose combination of topical clindamycin and benzoyl peroxide is first choice therapy. As alternatives, a different topical retinoid used with a different topical antimicrobial agent could be used, with or without benzoyl peroxide. Azelaic acid or benzoyl peroxide can also be recommended. In more widespread disease, combination of a systemic antibiotic with adapalene is recommended for moderate papulopustular acne. If there are limitations in use of first-choice agents, alternatives include fixed-dose combination of erythromycin and tretinoin, fixed-dose combination of isotretinoin and erythromycin, or oral zinc. In cases of widespread disease, a combination of a systemic antibiotic with either benzoyl peroxide or adapalene in fixed combination with benzoyl peroxide can be considered.
- *Severe papulopustular or moderate nodular acne*: Oral isotretinoin monotherapy is first choice. Alternatives include systemic antibiotics in combination with adapalene, with the fixed-dose combination of adapalene and benzoyl peroxide or in combination with azelaic acid. If there are limitations to use of these agents, consider oral antiandrogens in combination with oral antibiotics or topical treatments, or systemic antibiotics in combination with benzoyl peroxide.
- *Nodular or conglobate acne*: Monotherapy with oral isotretinoin is first choice. An alternative is systemic antibiotics in combination with azelaic acid. If limitations exist to these agents, consider oral antiandrogens in combination with oral antibiotics, systemic antibiotics in combination with adapalene, benzoyl peroxide, or the adapalene-benzoyl peroxide fixed-dose combination.
- *Maintenance therapy for acne*: Topical retinoids are most commonly recommended (adapalene, tazarotene, or tretinoin). Topical azelaic acid is an alternative. Maintenance is usually begun after a 12-week induction period and continues for 3 to 4 months. A longer duration may be necessary to prevent relapse upon discontinuation. Long-term therapy with antibiotics is not recommended to minimize antibiotic resistance.

Exfoliants (Peeling Agents)

- Exfoliants induce continuous mild drying and peeling by irritation, damaging superficial skin layers and inciting inflammation. This stimulates mitosis, thickening the epidermis and increasing horny cells, scaling, and erythema. Decreased sweating results in a dry, less oily surface and may resolve pustular lesions.
- **Resorcinol** is less keratolytic than salicylic acid and, when used alone, is classified as the Food and Drug Administration (FDA) category II (not generally recognized as safe and effective). The FDA considers resorcinol 2% and resorcinol monoacetate 3% to be safe and effective when used in combination with sulfur 3% to 8%. Resorcinol is an irritant and sensitizer and should not be applied to large areas or on broken skin. It produces a reversible dark brown scale on some dark-skinned individuals.
- **Salicylic acid** is keratolytic, has mild antibacterial activity against *P. acnes*, and offers slight anti-inflammatory activity at concentrations up to 5%. Salicylic acid is recognized by the FDA as safe and effective, but it may be less potent than benzoyl peroxide or topical retinoids. Salicylic acid products are often used as first-line therapy for mild acne because of their availability in concentrations up to 2% without a prescription. Concentrations of 5% to 10% can also be used by prescription, beginning with a low concentration and increasing as tolerance develops to the irritation. Salicylic acid is often used when patients cannot tolerate topical retinoids because of skin irritation.
- **Sulfur** is keratolytic and has antibacterial activity. It can quickly resolve pustules and papules, mask lesions, and produce irritation that leads to skin peeling. Sulfur is used

in the precipitated or colloidal form in concentrations of 2% to 10%. Although it is often combined with salicylic acid or resorcinol to increase effect, use is limited by offensive odor and availability of more effective agents.

Topical Retinoids

- Retinoids reduce obstruction within the follicle and are useful for both comedonal and inflammatory acne. They reverse abnormal keratinocyte desquamation and are active keratolytics. They inhibit microcomedone formation, decreasing the number of mature comedones and inflammatory lesions.
- Topical retinoids are safe, effective, and economical for treating all but the most severe cases of acne. They should be the first step in moderate acne, alone or in combination with antibiotics and benzoyl peroxide, reverting to retinoids alone for maintenance once adequate results are achieved. Side effects include erythema, xerosis, burning, and peeling.
- Retinoids should be applied at night, a half hour after cleansing, starting with every other night for 1 to 2 weeks to adjust to irritation. Doses can be increased only after beginning with 4 to 6 weeks of the lowest concentration and least irritating vehicle.
- **Tretinoin** (retinoic acid and vitamin A acid) is available as 0.05% solution (most irritating); 0.01% and 0.025% gels; and 0.025%, 0.05%, and 0.1% creams (least irritating). Tretinoin should not be used in pregnant women because of risk to the fetus.
- **Adapalene** (Differin) is the topical retinoid of first choice for both treatment and maintenance therapy because it is as effective but less irritating than other topical retinoids. Adapalene is available as 0.1% gel, cream, alcoholic solution, and pledgets. A 0.3% gel formulation is also available.
- **Tazarotene** (Tazorac) is as effective as adapalene in reducing noninflammatory and inflammatory lesion counts when applied half as frequently. Compared with tretinoin, it is as effective for comedonal and more effective for inflammatory lesions when applied once daily. The product is available as a 0.05% and 0.1% gel or cream.

Topical Antibacterial Agents

- **Benzoyl peroxide** is bactericidal and also suppresses sebum production and reduces free fatty acids, which are comedogenic and inflammatory triggers. It is useful for both noninflammatory and inflammatory acne. It has a rapid onset and may decrease the number of inflamed lesions within 5 days. Used alone or in combination, benzoyl peroxide is the standard of care for mild to moderate papulopustular acne. It is an agent of first choice when combined with adapalene for most patients with mild-to-moderate inflammatory acne vulgaris and a second-line choice for patients with noninflammatory comedonal acne. It is often combined with topical retinoids or an antimicrobial. For maintenance therapy, benzoyl peroxide can be added to a topical retinoid.
- Soaps, lotions, creams, washes, and gels are available in concentrations of 1% to 10%. All single-agent preparations are available without prescription. Gel formulations are usually most potent, whereas lotions, creams, and soaps have weaker potency. Alcohol-based gel preparations generally cause more dryness and irritation.
- Therapy should be initiated with the weakest concentration (2.5%) in a water-based formulation or the 4% hydrophase gel. Once tolerance is achieved, the strength may be increased to 5% or the base changed to the acetone or alcohol gels, or to paste. It is important to wash the product off in the morning. A sunscreen should be applied during the day.
- Side effects of benzoyl peroxide include dryness, irritation, and, rarely, allergic contact dermatitis. It may bleach hair and clothing.
- **Topical erythromycin** and **clindamycin** have become less effective due to resistance by *P. acnes*. Addition of benzoyl peroxide or topical retinoids to the macrolide is more effective than antibiotic monotherapy. Clindamycin is preferred because of potent action and lack of systemic absorption. It is available as a single-ingredient topical preparation or in combination with benzoyl peroxide. Erythromycin is available alone and in combination with retinoic acid or benzoyl peroxide.

- **Azelaic acid** (Azelex) has antibacterial, anti-inflammatory, and comedolytic activity. It is used for mild to moderate inflammatory acne but has limited efficacy compared with other therapies. It is an alternative to first-choice therapy for comedonal and all types inflammatory acne, particularly in combination. It is also an alternative to topical retinoids for maintenance therapy. Azelaic acid is well tolerated, with adverse effects of pruritus, burning, stinging, and tingling occurring in 1% to 5% of patients. Erythema, dryness, peeling, and irritation occur in fewer than 1% of patients. Azelaic acid is available in 20% cream and 15% gel formulations, which are usually applied twice daily (morning and evening) on clean, dry skin. Most patients experience improvement within 4 weeks, but treatment may be continued over several months if necessary.
- **Dapsone** 5% topical gel (Aczone) is a sulfone that has anti-inflammatory and antibacterial properties that improve both inflammatory and noninflammatory acne. It may be useful for patients with sensitivities or intolerance to conventional antiacne agents and may be used in sulfonamide-allergic patients. Topical dapsone 5% gel has been used alone or in combination with adapalene or benzoyl peroxide but may be more irritating than other topical agents.

Oral Antibacterials

- Systemic antibiotics are standard therapy for moderate and severe acne and treatment-resistant inflammatory acne. Because of increasing bacterial resistance, patients with less severe forms should not be treated with oral antibiotics, and where possible duration of therapy should be limited (eg, 6–8 weeks).
- **Erythromycin** is effective, but because of bacterial resistance, its use should be limited to patients who cannot use a tetracycline derivative (eg, pregnant women and children <8 years old).
- **Ciprofloxacin**, **trimethoprim-sulfamethoxazole**, and **trimethoprim** alone are also effective in cases where other antibiotics cannot be used or are ineffective.
- **Tetracyclines** (**minocycline** and **doxycycline**) have antibacterial and anti-inflammatory effects. Tetracycline itself is no longer the drug of choice in this family due to diet-related effects on absorption and lower antibacterial and anti-inflammatory efficacy. Minocycline has been associated with pigment deposition in the skin, mucous membranes, and teeth; it may also cause dose-related dizziness, urticaria, hypersensitivity syndrome, autoimmune hepatitis, a systemic lupus erythematosus–like syndrome, and serum sickness–like reactions. Doxycycline is a photosensitizer, especially at higher doses.

Antisebum Agents

- **Isotretinoin** decreases sebum production, inhibits *P. acnes* growth, and reduces inflammation. It is approved for treatment of severe recalcitrant nodular acne. It is also useful for less severe acne that is treatment resistant or that produces either physical or psychological scarring. Isotretinoin is the only drug treatment for acne that produces prolonged remission.
- The approved dose is 0.5 to 2 mg/kg/day, usually given over a 20-week course. Drug absorption is greater when taken with food. Initial flaring can be minimized by starting with 0.5 mg/kg/day or less. Alternatively, lower doses can be used for longer periods, with a total cumulative dose of 120 to 150 mg/kg.
- Adverse effects are frequent and often dose related. Approximately 90% of patients experience mucocutaneous effects; drying of the mouth, nose, and eyes is most common. Cheilitis and skin desquamation occur in more than 80% of patients. Systemic effects include transient increases in serum cholesterol and triglycerides, increased creatine kinase, hyperglycemia, photosensitivity, pseudotumor cerebri, abnormal liver injury tests, bone abnormalities, arthralgias, muscle stiffness, headache, and a high incidence of teratogenicity. Patients should be counseled about and screened for depression during therapy, although a causal relationship to isotretinoin therapy is controversial.

- Because of teratogenicity, two different forms of contraception must be started in female patients of childbearing potential beginning 1 month before therapy, continuing throughout treatment, and for up to 4 months after discontinuation of therapy. All patients receiving isotretinoin must participate in the iPLEDGE program, which requires pregnancy tests and assurances by prescribers and pharmacists that they will follow required procedures.
- **Oral contraceptives** containing estrogen can be useful for acne in some women. Agents with FDA approval for this indication include **norgestimate with ethinyl estradiol** and **norethindrone acetate with ethinyl estradiol**; other estrogen-containing products may also be effective.
- **Spironolactone** in higher doses is an antiandrogenic compound. Doses of 50 to 200 mg have been shown to be effective in acne.
- **Cyproterone acetate** is an antiandrogen that may be effective for acne in females when combined with ethinyl estradiol (in the form of an oral contraceptive). No cyproterone/estrogen–containing oral contraceptives are available in the United States.
- **Oral corticosteroids** in high doses used for short courses may be of temporary benefit in patients with severe inflammatory acne.

EVALUATION OF THERAPEUTIC OUTCOMES

- Provide patients with acne with a monitoring framework that includes specific parameters and frequency of monitoring. They should record the objective response to treatment in a diary. Contact patients within 2 to 3 weeks after the start of therapy to assess progress.
- Lesion counts should decrease by 10% to 15% within 4 to 8 weeks or by more than 50% within 2 to 4 months. Inflammatory lesions should resolve within a few weeks, and comedones should resolve by 3 to 4 months. If anxiety or depression is present at the outset, control or improvement should be achieved within 2 to 4 months.
- Long-term parameters should include no progression of severity, lengthening of acne-free periods throughout therapy, and no further scarring or pigmentation throughout therapy.
- Monitor patients regularly for adverse treatment effects, with appropriate dose reduction, alternative treatments, or drug discontinuation considered if these effects become intolerable.

See Chapter 96, Acne Vulgaris, authored by Debra J. Sibbald, for a more detailed discussion of this topic.

- *Drug-induced skin reactions* can be irritant or allergic in origin. Allergic drug reactions are classified into exanthematous, urticarial, blistering, and pustular eruptions.
- Severe cutaneous adverse reactions to drugs (SCARs) include Stevens-Johnson syndrome (SJS), toxic epidermal necrolysis (TEN), and drug reaction with eosinophilia and systemic symptoms (DRESS).
- Skin disorders discussed in this chapter include contact dermatitis, diaper dermatitis, and atopic dermatitis.

PATHOPHYSIOLOGY

- **Exanthematous** drug reactions include maculopapular rashes and drug hypersensitivity syndrome. **Urticarial** reactions include urticaria, angioedema, and serum sickness-like reactions. **Blistering** reactions include fixed drug eruptions, Stevens–Johnson syndrome, and toxic epidermal necrolysis. **Pustular** eruptions include acneiform drug reactions and acute generalized exanthematous pustulosis (AGEP) (**Fig. 16–1**).
- Drug-induced **hyperpigmentation** may be related to increased melanin (eg, hydantoins), direct deposition (eg, silver, mercury, tetracyclines, and antimalarials), or other mechanisms (eg, fluorouracil).
- Drug-induced photosensitivity reactions may be **phototoxic** (a nonimmunologic reaction) or **photoallergic** (an immunologic reaction). Medications associated with phototoxicity include amiodarone, tetracyclines, sulfonamides, psoralens, and coal tar. Common causes of photoallergic reactions include sulfonamides, sulfonylureas, thiazides, nonsteroidal anti-inflammatory drugs (NSAIDs), chloroquine, and carbamazepine.
- **Contact dermatitis** is skin inflammation caused by irritants or allergic sensitizers. In **allergic contact dermatitis (ACD)**, an antigenic substance triggers an immunologic response, sometimes several days later. **Irritant contact dermatitis (ICD)** is caused by an organic substance that usually results in a reaction within a few hours of exposure.
- **Diaper dermatitis** (diaper rash) is an acute, inflammatory dermatitis of the buttocks, genitalia, and perineal region. It is a type of contact dermatitis resulting from direct fecal and moisture contact with the skin in an occlusive environment.
- **Atopic dermatitis** is an inflammatory condition with genetic, environmental, and immunologic mechanisms. Neuropeptides, irritation, or pruritus-induced scratching may cause release of proinflammatory cytokines from keratinocytes.

CLINICAL PRESENTATION

- **Maculopapular skin reaction** presents with erythematous macules and papules that may be pruritic. Lesions usually begin within 7 to 10 days after starting the offending medication and generally resolve within 7 to 14 days after drug discontinuation. Because of the delayed reaction, the offending agent could be discontinued (eg, a 7-day antibiotic treatment course) before the lesions appear. Lesions may spread and become confluent. Common culprits include penicillins, cephalosporins, sulfonamides, and some anticonvulsants.
- **Drug hypersensitivity syndrome** (also known as drug reaction with eosinophilia and systemic symptoms or DRESS) is an exanthematous eruption accompanied by fever, lymphadenopathy, and multiorgan involvement (kidneys, liver, lung, bone marrow, heart, and brain). Signs and symptoms begin 1 to 4 weeks after starting the offending drug, and the reaction may be fatal if not promptly treated. Drugs implicated include allopurinol, sulfonamides, some anticonvulsants (barbiturates, phenytoin, carbamazepine, and lamotrigine), and dapsone.

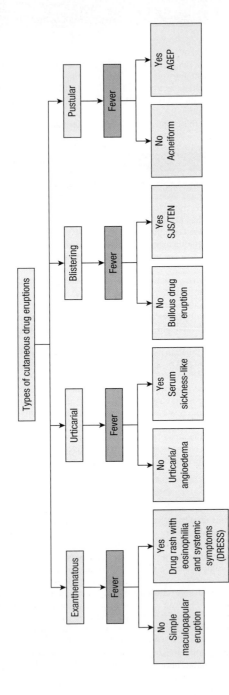

(AGEP, acute generalized exanthematous pustulosis; SJS, Stevens-Johnson syndrome; TEN, toxic epidermal necrolysis.)
(Adapted from Knowles, S. Drug-Induced Skin Reactions, Table 3, Description of Drug Eruptions. In: Compendium of Therapeutic Choices for Minor Ailments, 2nd ed. Ottawa (ON): Canadian Pharmacists Association; © 2016.)

FIGURE 16–1. Types of cutaneous drug eruptions.

- **Urticaria** and **angioedema** are simple eruptions that are caused by drugs in 5% to 10% of cases. Other causes are foods (most common) and physical factors such as cold or pressure, infections, and latex exposure. Urticaria may be the first sign of an emerging anaphylactic reaction characterized by hives, extremely pruritic red raised wheals, angioedema, and mucous membrane swelling that typically occurs within minutes to hours. Offending drugs include penicillins and related antibiotics, aspirin, sulfonamides, radiograph contrast media, and opioids.
- **Serum sickness-like reactions** are complex urticarial eruptions presenting with fever, rash (usually urticarial), and arthralgias usually within 1 to 3 weeks after starting the offending drug.
- **Fixed drug eruptions** present as pruritic, red, raised lesions that may blister. Symptoms can include burning or stinging. Lesions may evolve into plaques. These so-called fixed eruptions recur in the same area each time the offending drug is given. Lesions appear and disappear within minutes to days, leaving hyperpigmented skin for months. Usual offenders include tetracyclines, barbiturates, sulfonamides, codeine, phenolphthalein, and NSAIDs.
- **Stevens–Johnson syndrome (SJS)** and **toxic epidermal necrolysis (TEN)** are blistering eruptions that are rare but severe and life-threatening. They are considered variants of the same disorder and are often discussed together as SJS/TEN. Onset occurs within 7 to 14 days after drug exposure. Patients present with generalized tender/painful bullous formation with fever, headache, and respiratory symptoms leading to rapid clinical deterioration. Lesions show rapid confluence and spread, resulting in extensive epidermal detachment and sloughing. This may result in marked fluid loss, hypotension, electrolyte imbalances, and secondary infections. Usual offending drugs include sulfonamides, penicillins, some anticonvulsants (hydantoins, carbamazepine, barbiturates, and lamotrigine), NSAIDs, and allopurinol.
- **Acneiform drug reactions** are pustular eruptions that induce acne. Onset is within 1 to 3 weeks. Common culprits include corticosteroids, androgenic hormones, some anticonvulsants, isoniazid, and lithium.
- **Acute generalized exanthematous pustulosis (AGEP)** has an acute onset (within days after starting the offending drug), fever, diffuse erythema, and many pustules. Generalized desquamation occurs 2 weeks later. Usual offending drugs include β-lactam antibiotics, macrolides, and calcium channel blockers.
- **Sun-induced skin reactions** appear similar to a sunburn and present with erythema, papules, edema, and sometimes vesicles. They appear in areas exposed to sunlight (eg, ears, nose, cheeks, forearms, and hands).
- **Diaper dermatitis** results in an erythematous rash, and severe cases may have vesicles and oozing erosions. The rash may be infected by *Candida* species and present with confluent red plaques, papules, and pustules.
- **Atopic dermatitis** presents differently depending on age. In infancy, an erythematous, patchy, pruritic, papular skin rash may first appear on the cheeks and chin and progress to red, scaling, oozing lesions. The rash affects the malar region of the cheeks, forehead, scalp, chin, and behind the ears while sparing the nose and paranasal creases. Over several weeks, lesions may spread to extensor surfaces of the lower legs (due to the infant's crawling), and eventually the entire body may be involved except for the diaper area and nose. In childhood, the skin is often dry, flaky, rough, and cracked. Pruritus is a quintessential feature, and a diagnosis cannot be made if there is no history of itching. Scratching and rubbing itchy skin may result in bleeding and lichenification. In adulthood, lesions are more diffuse with underlying erythema. The face is commonly involved and may be dry and scaly. Lichenification may be seen.

DIAGNOSIS

- A comprehensive patient history is important to obtain the following information:
  ✓ Signs and symptoms (onset, progression, timeframe, lesion location and description, presenting symptoms, and previous occurrence)

✓ Urgency (severity, area, and extent of skin involvement; signs of a systemic/generalized reaction or disease condition)

✓ Medication history (temporal correlation, previous exposure, and nonprescribed products)

✓ Differential diagnosis

- Lesion assessment includes identifying macules, papules, nodules, blisters, plaques, and lichenification. Some skin conditions cause more than one type of lesion.
- Inspect lesions for color, texture, size, and temperature. Areas that are oozing, erythematous, and warm to the touch may be infected.

TREATMENT

- <u>Goals of Treatment</u>: Relieve bothersome symptoms, remove precipitating factors, prevent recurrences, avoid adverse treatment effects, and improve quality of life.

DRUG-INDUCED SKIN REACTIONS

- If a drug-induced skin reaction is suspected, the most important treatment is discontinuing the suspected drug as quickly as possible and avoiding use of potential cross-sensitizers.
- The next step is to control symptoms (eg, pruritus). Signs or symptoms of a systemic or generalized reaction may require additional supportive therapy. For high fevers, acetaminophen is more appropriate than aspirin or another NSAID, which may exacerbate some skin lesions.
- Most maculopapular reactions disappear within a few days after discontinuing the agent, so symptomatic control of the affected area is the primary intervention. **Topical corticosteroids** and **oral antihistamines** can relieve pruritus. In severe cases, a short course of **systemic corticosteroids** may be warranted.
- Treatment of fixed drug reactions involves removal of the offending agent. Other therapeutic measures include **topical corticosteroids, oral antihistamines** to relieve itching, and perhaps cool water compresses on the affected area.
- Photosensitivity reactions typically resolve with drug discontinuation. Some patients benefit from **topical corticosteroids** and **oral antihistamines,** but these are relatively ineffective. **Systemic corticosteroids** (eg, **oral prednisone** 1 mg/kg/day tapered over 3 weeks) are more effective.
- For life-threatening SJS/TEN, supportive measures such as maintenance of adequate blood pressure, fluid and electrolyte balance, broad-spectrum antibiotics and vancomycin for secondary infections, and IV immunoglobulin (IVIG) may be appropriate. Corticosteroid use is controversial; if used, employ relatively high doses initially, followed by rapid tapering as soon as disease progression stops.
- Inform patients about the suspected drug, potential drugs to avoid in the future, and which drugs may be used instead. Give patients with photosensitivity reactions information about preventive measures, such as use of sunscreens and sun avoidance.

CONTACT DERMATITIS

- The first intervention involves identification, withdrawal, and avoidance of the offending agent.
- The second treatment is symptomatic relief while decreasing skin lesions. **Cold compresses** help soothe and cleanse the skin; they are applied to wet or oozing lesions, removed, remoistened, and reapplied every few minutes for a 20- to 30-minute period. If affected areas are already dry or hardened, wet dressings applied as soaks (without removal for up to 20–30 minutes) will soften and hydrate the skin; soaks should not be used on acute exudating lesions. **Calamine lotion** or **Burow solution (aluminum acetate)** may also be soothing.
- **Topical corticosteroids** help resolve the inflammatory process and are the mainstay of treatment. ACD responds better to topical corticosteroids than does ICD. Generally, use higher potency corticosteroids initially, switching to medium or lower

potency corticosteroids as the condition improves (see Chapter 17, Table 17–1, for topical corticosteroid potencies).
- **Oatmeal baths** or oral **first-generation antihistamines** may provide relief for excessive itching.
- **Moisturizers** may be used to prevent dryness and skin fissuring.

DIAPER DERMATITIS

- Management involves frequent diaper changes, air drying (removing the diaper for as long as practical), gentle cleansing (preferably with nonsoap cleansers and lukewarm water), and use of barrier products. **Zinc oxide** has astringent and absorbent properties and provides an effective barrier. **Petrolatum** also provides a water-impermeable barrier but has no absorbent ability and may trap moisture.
- Candidal (yeast) diaper rash should be treated with a topical antifungal agent and then covered by a barrier product. **Imidazoles** are the treatment of choice. The antifungal agents should be stopped once the rash subsides and the barrier product continued.
- In severe inflammatory diaper rashes, a very low potency topical corticosteroid (**hydrocortisone 0.5%–1%**) may be used for short periods (1–2 weeks).

ATOPIC DERMATITIS

- Nonpharmacologic measures for infants and children include the following:
  ✓ Apply moisturizers frequently throughout the day
  ✓ Give lukewarm baths
  ✓ Apply lubricants/moisturizers immediately after bathing
  ✓ Use nonsoap cleansers (which are neutral to low pH, hypoallergenic, fragrance free)
  ✓ Use wet-wrap therapy (with or without topical corticosteroid) during flare-ups for patients with moderate to severe disease. Wet-wrap involves applying damp tubular elasticized bandages and occlusive dressing to the limbs to promote skin hydration and absorption of emollients and topical corticosteroids.
  ✓ Keep fingernails filed short
  ✓ Select clothing made of soft cotton fabrics
  ✓ Consider sedating oral antihistamines to reduce scratching at night
  ✓ Keep the child cool; avoid situations that cause overheating
  ✓ Learn to recognize skin infections and seek treatment promptly
  ✓ Identify and remove irritants and allergens
- Topical corticosteroids are the drug treatment of choice. Low-potency agents (eg, **hydrocortisone 1%**) are suitable for the face, and medium-potency products (eg, **betamethasone valerate 0.1%**) may be used for the body. For longer-duration maintenance therapy, low-potency corticosteroids are recommended. Use midstrength and high-potency corticosteroids for short-term management of exacerbations. Reserve ultra-high and high-potency agents (eg, **betamethasone dipropionate 0.05%** and **clobetasone propionate 0.05%**) for short-term treatment (1–2 weeks) of lichenified lesions in adults. After lesions have improved significantly, use a lower-potency corticosteroid for maintenance when necessary. Avoid potent fluorinated corticosteroids on the face, genitalia, and intertriginous areas and in infants.
- The topical immunomodulators **tacrolimus** (Protopic) and **pimecrolimus** (Elidel) inhibit calcineurin, which normally initiates T-cell activation. Both agents are approved for atopic dermatitis in adults and children older than age 2. They can be used on all parts of the body for prolonged periods without producing corticosteroid-induced adverse effects. Tacrolimus ointment 0.03% (for moderate to severe atopic dermatitis in patients ages 2 and older) and 0.1% (for ages 16 and older) is applied twice daily. Pimecrolimus cream 1% is applied twice daily for mild to moderate atopic dermatitis in patients older than age 2. The most common adverse effect is transient burning at the site of application. Both drugs are recommended as second-line

treatments due to concerns about a possible risk of cancer. For this reason, sun protection factor (SPF) 30 or higher is recommended on all exposed skin areas.
- Phototherapy may be recommended when the disease is not controlled by topical corticosteroids and calcineurin inhibitors. It may also be steroid sparing, allowing for use of lower-potency corticosteroids, or even eliminating the need for corticosteroids in some cases.
- Coal tar preparations reduce itching and skin inflammation and are available as **crude coal tar** (1%–3%) or **liquor carbonis detergens** (5%–20%). They have been used in combination with topical corticosteroids, as adjuncts to permit effective use of lower corticosteroid strengths, and in conjunction with ultraviolet light therapies. Patients can apply the product at bedtime and wash it off in the morning. Factors limiting coal tar use include its strong odor and staining of clothing. Coal tar preparations should not be used on acute oozing lesions, which would result in stinging and irritation.
- Systemic therapies that have been used (but not FDA approved) for atopic dermatitis include corticosteroids, cyclosporine, interferon-γ, azathioprine, methotrexate, mycophenolate mofetil, IVIG, and biologic agents.

EVALUATION OF THERAPEUTIC OUTCOMES

- Provide patients with information regarding causative factors, avoidance of substances that trigger skin reactions, and potential benefits and limitations of nondrug and drug therapy.
- Evaluate patients with chronic skin conditions periodically to assess disease control, the efficacy of current therapy, and the presence of possible adverse effects.

See Chapter e99, Dermatologic Drug Reactions and Common Skin Conditions, by Rebecca M. Law and David T.S. Law; and Chapter 98, Atopic Dermatitis, by Rebecca M. Law and Po Gin Kwa, for a more detailed discussion of these topics.

CHAPTER 17

Psoriasis

- *Psoriasis* is a chronic T-lymphocyte–mediated systemic inflammatory disease characterized by recurrent exacerbations and remissions of thickened, erythematous, and scaling plaques and multiple comorbidities.

PATHOPHYSIOLOGY

- Genetic predisposition coupled with an unknown precipitating factor triggers an abnormal immune response mediated via T-lymphocytes, resulting in keratinocyte proliferation and the initial psoriatic skin lesions.
- Psoriasis susceptibility genes and variants reside on various chromosomes. The psoriasis susceptibility locus 1 (*PSORS1*) on chromosome 6p is a key gene locus, accounting for up to 50% of disease heritability. The major histocompatibility complex antigen HLA-Cw6 and tumor necrosis factor (TNF)-α are major psoriasis susceptibility genes, along with interleukin (IL)-23 and many other loci. Genes corresponding to these loci are involved in pathogenesis pathways in the immune system. There appears to be a general role for T lymphocytes and a specific role for TH17 lymphocytes in psoriasis pathogenesis and as indicators of psoriasis risk.
- Interactions between dermal dendritic cells and activated Th-1 and Th-17 cells in concert with numerous growth factors and cytokines (eg, TNF-α, interferon gamma, interleukin-1) cause epidermal hyperplasia and dermal inflammation.
- Precipitating factors implicated in the development of psoriasis include skin injury, infection, drugs, smoking, alcohol consumption, obesity, and psychogenic stress.

CLINICAL PRESENTATION

- Plaque psoriasis (psoriasis vulgaris) is seen in about 90% of psoriasis patients. Lesions are erythematous, red-violet in color, at least 0.5 cm in diameter, well demarcated, and typically covered with silver flaking scales. They may appear as single lesions at predisposed areas (eg, knees and elbows) or generalized over a wide body surface area (BSA).
- Pruritus may be severe and require treatment to minimize excoriations from frequent scratching. Lesions may be physically debilitating or socially isolating.
- Preexisting psoriasis can be exacerbated by drugs (eg, lithium, nonsteroidal anti-inflammatory drugs [NSAIDs], antimalarials such as chloroquine, β-adrenergic blockers, fluoxetine, and withdrawal of corticosteroids), times of stress, and seasonal changes.
- Potential comorbidities resulting from the systemic immune response include psoriatic arthritis, heart disease, diabetes, metabolic syndrome, and other immune-mediated disorders such as Crohn disease and multiple sclerosis.
- Psoriatic arthritis involves both psoriatic lesions and inflammatory arthritis-like symptoms. Distal interphalangeal joints and adjacent nails are most commonly involved, but knees, elbows, wrists, and ankles may be affected.

DIAGNOSIS

- Diagnosis is based on physical examination findings of characteristic lesions. Skin biopsies are not diagnostic of psoriasis.
- Classification of psoriasis as mild, moderate, or severe is based on BSA and Psoriasis Area and Severity Index (PASI) measurements. A 2011 European classification system defines severity of plaque psoriasis as either mild or moderate-to-severe.

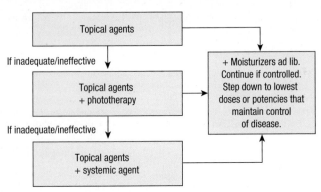

FIGURE 17–1. Treatment algorithm for mild to moderate psoriasis.

TREATMENT

- <u>Goals of Treatment</u>: Minimize or eliminate skin lesions, alleviate pruritus, reduce frequency of flare-ups, treat comorbid conditions, screen for and manage lifestyle factors that may trigger exacerbations, avoid adverse treatment effects, provide cost-effective treatment, provide appropriate counseling (eg, stress reduction), and maintain or improve quality of life.
- See Figs. 17–1 and 17–2 for psoriasis treatment algorithms based on disease severity.

NONPHARMACOLOGIC THERAPY

- Stress reduction using guided imagery and stress management can improve extent and severity of psoriasis.
- Nonmedicated moisturizers help maintain skin moisture, reduce skin shedding, control scaling, and reduce pruritus.
- Oatmeal baths further reduce pruritus, and regular use may reduce need for systemic antipruritic drugs. Harsh soaps and detergents should be avoided. Cleansing should involve tepid water, preferably with lipid- and fragrance-free cleansers.

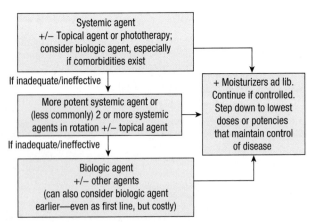

FIGURE 17–2. Treatment algorithm for moderate to severe psoriasis.

- Sunscreens (preferably sun protection factor [SPF] 30 or higher) should be used when outdoors.

PHARMACOLOGIC THERAPY
Topical Therapies

- **Corticosteroids** (Table 17–1) have anti-inflammatory, antiproliferative, immunosuppressive, and vasoconstrictive effects.
- Lower-potency products should be used for infants and for lesions on the face, intertriginous areas, and areas with thin skin. Mid- to high-potency agents are recommended as initial therapy for other areas of the body in adults. Reserve the highest potency corticosteroids for patients with very thick plaques or recalcitrant disease, such as plaques on the palms and soles. Use potency class I corticosteroids for only 2 to 4 weeks.
- Ointments are the most occlusive and most potent formulations because of enhanced penetration into the dermis. Patients may prefer the less greasy creams or lotions for daytime use.
- Cutaneous adverse effects include skin atrophy, acne, contact dermatitis, hypertrichosis, folliculitis, hypopigmentation, perioral dermatitis, striae, telangiectasias, and traumatic purpura. Systemic adverse effects may occur with superpotent agents or with extended or widespread use of midpotency agents. Such effects include hypothalamic-pituitary-adrenal axis suppression and less commonly Cushing's syndrome, osteonecrosis of the femoral head, cataracts, and glaucoma. All topical corticosteroids are pregnancy category C.
- **Calcipotriene** (Dovonex) is a synthetic vitamin D_3 analogue that binds to vitamin D receptors, which inhibits keratinocyte proliferation and enhances keratinocyte differentiation. Vitamin D_3 analogues also inhibit T-lymphocyte activity.
- For mild psoriasis, calcipotriene is more effective than anthralin and comparable to or slightly more effective than class 3 (upper mid-strength) topical corticosteroid ointments. Calcipotriene 0.005% cream, ointment, or solution is applied one or two times daily (no more than 100 g/week).
- Adverse effects of calcipotriene include mild irritant contact dermatitis, burning, pruritus, edema, peeling, dryness, and erythema. Calcipotriene is pregnancy category C.
- **Tazarotene** (Tazorac) is a topical retinoid that normalizes keratinocyte differentiation, diminishes keratinocyte hyperproliferation, and clears the inflammatory infiltrate in psoriatic plaques. It is available as a 0.05% or 0.1% gel and cream and is applied once daily (usually in the evening).
- Adverse effects of tazarotene include a high incidence of dose-dependent irritation at application sites, resulting in burning, stinging, and erythema. Irritation may be reduced by using the cream formulation, lower concentration, alternate-day applications, or short-contact (30–60 minutes) treatment. Tazarotene is pregnancy category X and should not be used in women of childbearing potential unless effective contraception is being used.
- **Anthralin** has a direct anti-proliferative effect on epidermal keratinocytes, normalizing keratinocyte differentiation. Short-contact anthralin therapy (SCAT) is the preferred regimen, with ointment applied only to the thick plaque lesions for 2 hours or less and then wiped off. Zinc oxide ointment or nonmedicated stiff paste should be applied to the surrounding normal skin to protect it from irritation. Use anthralin with caution, if at all, on the face and intertriginous areas due to potential for severe irritation.
- Anthralin concentrations for SCAT range from 1% to 4% or as tolerated. Concentrations for continuous therapy vary from 0.05% to 0.4%.
- Anthralin may cause severe skin irritation, folliculitis, and allergic contact dermatitis. Anthralin is pregnancy category C.
- **Coal tar** is keratolytic and may have anti-proliferative and anti-inflammatory effects. Formulations include crude coal tar and tar distillates (liquor carbonis detergens) in ointments, creams, and shampoos. Coal tar is used infrequently due to limited efficacy and poor patient adherence and acceptance. It has a slower onset of action than calcipotriene, has an unpleasant odor, and stains clothing.

TABLE 17–1	Topical Corticosteroid Potency Chart
Potency Rating	**Corticosteroid—Topical Preparations**
Class 1: Superpotent	Betamethasone dipropionate 0.05% ointment (Diprolene and Diprosone ointment) Clobetasol propionate 0.05% lotion/spray/shampoo/foam (Clobex lotion/spray/shampoo, OLUX-E foam) Clobetasol propionate 0.05% cream and ointment (Cormax, Temovate, Dermovate) Desoximetasone 0.25% spray (Topicort) Fluocinonide 0.1% cream (Vanos) Halobetasol propionate 0.05% cream, lotion, and ointment (Ultravate) Flurandrenolide tape 4 mcg/cm² (Cordran)
Class 2: Potent	Amcinonide 0.1% ointment (Cyclocort ointment) Betamethasone dipropionate 0.05% cream/gel (Diprolene cream, gel, and Diprosone cream) Desoximetasone 0.25% cream, ointment (Topicort) Diflorasone diacetate 0.05% ointment (Florone, Psorcon) Fluocinonide 0.05% cream, gel, ointment (Lidex) Halonide 0.1% cream (Halog)
Class 3: Upper mid-strength	Amcinonide 0.1% cream (Cyclocort cream) Betamethasone valerate 0.1% ointment (Betnovate/Valisone ointment) Diflorasone diacetate 0.05% cream (Psorcon cream) Fluticasone propionate 0.005% ointment (Cutivate ointment) Mometasone furoate 0.1% ointment (Elocon ointment) Triamcinolone acetonide 0.5% cream and ointment (Aristocort)
Class 4: Mid-strength	Betamethasone valerate 0.12% foam (Luxiq) Clocortolone pivalate 0.1% cream (Cloderm) Desoximetasone 0.05% cream, ointment, and gel (Topicort LP) Fluocinolone acetonide 0.025% ointment (Synalar ointment) Fluocinolone acetonide 0.2% cream (Synalar-HP) Flurandrenolide 0.05% ointment (Cordran) Hydrocortisone valerate 0.2% ointment (Westcort ointment) Mometasone furoate 0.1% cream (Elocon cream) Triamcinolone acetonide 0.1% ointment (Kenalog)
Class 5: Lower mid-strength	Betamethasone dipropionate 0.05% lotion (Diprosone lotion) Betamethasone valerate 0.1% cream and lotion (Betnovate/Valisone cream & lotion) Desonide 0.05% lotion (DesOwen) Fluocinolone acetonide 0.01% shampoo (Capex shampoo) Fluocinolone acetonide 0.025%, 0.03% cream (Synalar cream) Flurandrenolide 0.05% cream and lotion (Cordran) Fluticasone propionate 0.05% cream and lotion (Cutivate cream and lotion) Hydrocortisone butyrate 0.1% cream (Locoid) Hydrocortisone valerate 0.2% cream (Westcort cream) Prednicarbate 0.1% cream (Dermatop) Triamcinolone acetonide 0.1% cream and lotion (Kenalog cream and lotion)
Class 6: Mild	Alclometasone dipropionate 0.05% cream and ointment (Aclovate) Betamethasone valerate 0.05% cream and ointment Desonide 0.05% cream, ointment, gel (DesOwen, Desonate, Tridesilon) Desonide 0.05% foam (Verdeso) Fluocinolone acetonide 0.01% cream and solution (Synalar) Fluocinolone acetonide 0.01% FS oil (Derma-Smoothe)
Class 7: Least Potent	Hydrocortisone 0.5%, 1%, 2%, 2.5% cream, lotion, spray, and ointment (various brands)

Data from The National Psoriasis Foundation—Mild Psoriasis: Steroid potency chart, https://www.psoriasis.org/about-psoriasis/treatments/topicals/steroids/potency-chart; Rosso JD, Friedlander SF. Corticosteroids: Options in the era of steroid-sparing therapy. J Am Acad Dermatol 2005;53:S50–S58; Leung DYM, Nicklas RA, Li JT, et al. Disease management of atopic dermatitis: An updated practice parameter. Ann Allergy Asthma Immunol 2004;93:S1–S17.

- Adverse effects include folliculitis, acne, local irritation, and phototoxicity. Risk of teratogenicity when used in pregnancy is low.
- **Salicylic acid** has keratolytic properties and has been used in shampoos or bath oils for scalp psoriasis. It enhances penetration of topical corticosteroids, thereby increasing corticosteroid efficacy. Systemic absorption and toxicity can occur, especially when applied to greater than 20% BSA or in patients with renal impairment. Salicylic acid should not be used in children. It may be used for limited and localized plaque psoriasis in pregnancy.
- **Pimecrolimus** 1% cream (Elidel) is a calcineurin inhibitor shown to be effective for plaque psoriasis when used under occlusion and for patients with moderate-to-severe inverse psoriasis (involving intertriginous areas). It may be a useful alternative for patients with intertriginous or facial lesions because it is less irritating than calcipotriene and does not have the topical adverse effects of corticosteroids (eg, skin atrophy).

Phototherapy and Photochemotherapy

- Phototherapy consists of nonionizing electromagnetic radiation, either ultraviolet A (UVA) or ultraviolet B (UVB), as light therapy for psoriatic lesions. UVB is given alone as either broadband or narrowband (NB-UVB). UVB is also given as photochemotherapy with topical agents such as crude coal tar (Goeckerman regimen) or anthralin (Ingram regimen) for enhanced efficacy. UVA is generally given with a photosensitizer such as an oral psoralen to enhance efficacy; this regimen is called PUVA (psoralen + UVA treatment).
- Adverse effects of phototherapy include erythema, pruritus, xerosis, hyperpigmentation, and blistering. Patients must be provided with eye protection during and for 24 hours after PUVA treatments. PUVA therapy may also cause nausea or vomiting, which may be minimized by taking the oral psoralens with food or milk. Long-term PUVA use can lead to photoaging and cataracts. PUVA is also associated with a dose-related risk of carcinogenesis.

Systemic Therapies

- **Acitretin** (Soriatane) is a retinoic acid derivative and the active metabolite of etretinate. Retinoids may be less effective than methotrexate or cyclosporine when used as monotherapy. Acitretin is more commonly used in combination with topical calcipotriene or phototherapy. The initial recommended dose is 25 or 50 mg; therapy is continued until lesions have resolved. It is better tolerated when taken with meals. Adverse effects include hypertriglyceridemia and mucocutaneous effects such as dryness of the eyes, nasal and oral mucosa, chapped lips, cheilitis, epistaxis, xerosis, brittle nails, and burning skin. Ophthalmologic changes include photosensitivity, decreased color vision and impaired night vision. Hepatitis and jaundice are rare and liver enzyme elevations are usually transient. All retinoids are teratogenic and are pregnancy category X. Acitretin should not be used in women of childbearing potential unless they use effective contraception for the duration of therapy and for at least 2 years after drug discontinuation. Blood donation (men and women) is not permitted during and for at least 1 year after treatment.
- **Cyclosporine** is a systemic calcineurin inhibitor that is effective for inducing remission and for maintenance therapy of moderate to severe plaque psoriasis. It is also effective for pustular, erythrodermic, and nail psoriasis. Intermittent short-course therapy (less than 12 weeks) is preferable because this appears to reduce the risk of nephrotoxicity compared with continuous therapy. Cyclosporine is significantly more effective than etretinate and has similar or slightly better efficacy than methotrexate. The usual dose is between 2.5 and 5 mg/kg/day given in two divided doses. After inducing remission, maintenance therapy using low doses (1.25–3 mg/kg/day) may prevent relapse. When discontinuing cyclosporine, a gradual taper of 1 mg/kg/day each week may prolong the time before relapse when compared with abrupt discontinuation. Because more than half of patients stopping cyclosporine relapse within 4 months, patients should be given appropriate alternative treatments shortly

before or after discontinuing cyclosporine. Adverse effects include nephrotoxicity, hypertension, hypomagnesemia, hyperkalemia, hypertriglyceridemia, hypertrichosis, and gingival hyperplasia. The risk of skin cancer increases with the duration of treatment and with prior PUVA treatments.

- **Methotrexate** has anti-inflammatory effects due to its effects on T-cell gene expression and also has cytostatic effects. It is more effective than acitretin and has similar or slightly less efficacy than cyclosporine. Methotrexate can be administered orally, subcutaneously, or intramuscularly. The starting dose is 7.5 to 15 mg once weekly, increased incrementally by 2.5 mg every 2 to 4 weeks until response; maximal doses are 25 mg weekly. Adverse effects include nausea, vomiting, stomatitis, macrocytic anemia, and hepatic and pulmonary toxicity. Nausea and macrocytic anemia may be reduced by giving oral folic acid 1 to 5 mg daily. Methotrexate should be avoided in patients with active infections and in those with liver disease. It is an abortifacient and teratogenic and is contraindicated in pregnancy (pregnancy category X).

Systemic Therapy with Biologic Agents

- Biologic agents are considered for moderate to severe psoriasis when other systemic agents are inadequate or contraindicated. Cost considerations tend to limit their use as first-line therapy.
- **Adalimumab** (Humira) is a monoclonal TNF-α antibody that provides rapid control of psoriasis. It is indicated for psoriatic arthritis and treatment of adults with moderate to severe chronic plaque psoriasis who are candidates for systemic therapy or phototherapy. The recommended dose for psoriatic arthritis is 40 mg subcutaneously every other week. The recommended dose for adults with plaque psoriasis is an initial dose of 80 mg, followed by 40 mg every other week starting 1 week after the initial dose. The most common adverse reactions are infections (eg, upper respiratory and sinusitis), injection site reactions, headache, and rash.
- **Etanercept** (Enbrel) is a fusion protein that binds TNF-α, competitively interfering with its interaction with cell-bound receptors. Unlike the chimeric infliximab, etanercept is fully humanized, minimizing the risk of immunogenicity. Etanercept is FDA approved for reducing signs and symptoms and inhibiting the progression of joint damage in patients with psoriatic arthritis. It can be used in combination with methotrexate in patients who do not respond adequately to methotrexate alone. It is also indicated for adults with chronic moderate to severe plaque psoriasis. The recommended dose for psoriatic arthritis is 50 mg subcutaneously once per week. For plaque psoriasis, the dose is 50 mg subcutaneously twice weekly (administered 3 or 4 days apart) for 3 months, followed by a maintenance dose of 50 mg once weekly. Adverse effects include local reactions at the injection site (20% of patients), respiratory tract and GI infections, abdominal pain, nausea and vomiting, headaches, and rash. Serious infections (including tuberculosis) and malignancies are rare.
- **Infliximab** (Remicade) is a chimeric monoclonal antibody directed against TNF-α. It is indicated for psoriatic arthritis and chronic severe plaque psoriasis. The recommended dose is 5 mg/kg as an IV infusion at weeks 0, 2, and 6, then every 8 weeks thereafter. For psoriatic arthritis, it may be used with or without methotrexate. Adverse effects include headaches, fever, chills, fatigue, diarrhea, pharyngitis, and upper respiratory and urinary tract infections. Hypersensitivity reactions (urticaria, dyspnea, and hypotension) and lymphoproliferative disorders have been reported.
- **Alefacept** (Amevive) is a dimeric fusion protein that binds to CD2 on T cells to inhibit cutaneous T-cell activation and proliferation. It also produces a dose-dependent decrease in circulating total lymphocytes. Alefacept is approved for treatment of moderate to severe plaque psoriasis and is also effective for treatment of psoriatic arthritis. Significant response is usually achieved after about 3 months of therapy. The recommended dose is 15 mg intramuscularly once weekly for 12 weeks. Repeat courses (up to 2 more courses per year) may be given for unacceptable loss of disease control. Adverse effects are mild and include pharyngitis, flu-like symptoms, chills, dizziness, nausea, headache, injection site pain and inflammation, and nonspecific infection.

- **Ustekinumab** (Stelara) is an IL-12/23 monoclonal antibody approved for the treatment of psoriasis in adults 18 years or older with moderate to severe plaque psoriasis. The recommended dose for patients weighing 100 kg or less is 45 mg initially and 4 weeks later, followed by 45 mg every 12 weeks. For patients weighing 100 kg or more, the dose is 90 mg initially and 4 weeks later, followed by 90 mg every 12 weeks. Common adverse effects include upper respiratory infections, headache, and tiredness. Serious adverse effects include those seen with other biologics, including tubercular, fungal, and viral infections and cancers. One case of reversible posterior leukoencephalopathy syndrome (RPLS) has been reported.
- **Secukinumab** (Cosentyx) is a fully human IgG1κ monoclonal antibody that selectively binds and inhibits IL-17A, a proinflammatory cytokine, thus inhibiting release of chemokines and other proinflammatory mediators. It is FDA approved for treatment of moderate-to-severe plaque psoriasis in adults who are candidates for systemic therapy or phototherapy. It is also approved for psoriatic arthritis. Recommended dosing for plaque psoriasis is 300 mg by subcutaneous (SC) injection at weeks 0, 1, 2, 3, and 4 followed by 300 mg SC every 4 weeks. The most common adverse effects are nasopharyngitis, diarrhea, and upper respiratory tract infections.

Combination Therapies

- Combination therapy may be used to enhance efficacy or minimize toxicity. Combinations can include two topical agents, a topical agent plus phototherapy, a systemic agent plus topical therapy, a systemic agent plus phototherapy, two systemic agents used in rotation, or a systemic agent and a biologic agent (see **Figs. 17–1** and **17–2**).
- The combination of a topical corticosteroid and a topical vitamin D_3 analogue is effective and safe with less skin irritation than monotherapy with either agent. The combination product containing calcipotriene and betamethasone dipropionate ointment (Taclonex) is effective for relatively severe psoriasis and may also be steroid sparing.
- The combination of retinoids with phototherapy (eg, tazarotene plus broadband UVB, acitretin plus broadband UVB or NB-UVB) also increases efficacy. Because retinoids may be photosensitizing and increase the risk of burning after UV exposure, doses of phototherapy should be reduced to minimize adverse effects. The combination of acitretin and PUVA (RE-PUVA) may be more effective than monotherapy with either treatment.
- Phototherapy has also been used with other topical agents, such as UVB with coal tar (Goeckerman regimen) to increase treatment response, because coal tar is also photosensitizing.
- Cyclosporine in combination with calcipotriol or betamethasone dipropionate is superior to cyclosporine alone. Cyclosporine may also be used with SCAT, but it should not be used with PUVA due to reduced efficacy and an increased risk of cutaneous malignancies.
- The combination of methotrexate and UVB appears to be synergistic. Methotrexate in combination with a TNF inhibitor (adalimumab, etanercept, infliximab) may be beneficial.

Alternative Drug Treatments

- **Mycophenolate mofetil** (CellCept) inhibits DNA and RNA synthesis and may have a lymphocyte antiproliferative effect. Although not FDA approved for this indication, oral mycophenolate mofetil may be effective in some cases of moderate to severe plaque psoriasis. The dosage used is 500 mg orally four times daily, up to a maximum of 4 g daily. Common adverse effects include GI toxicity (diarrhea, nausea, and vomiting), hematologic effects (anemia, neutropenia, and thrombocytopenia), and viral and bacterial infections. Lymphoproliferative disease or lymphoma has been reported.
- **Hydroxyurea** inhibits cell synthesis in the S phase of the DNA cycle. It is sometimes used for patients with recalcitrant severe psoriasis, but biologic agents may be a better option in these patients. The typical dose is 1 g daily, with a gradual increase to 2 g daily as needed and as tolerated. Adverse effects include bone marrow suppression, lesional erythema, localized tenderness, and reversible hyperpigmentation.

EVALUATION OF THERAPEUTIC OUTCOMES

- Help patients understand the general principles of therapy and the importance of adherence.
- A positive response involves normalization of involved areas of skin, as measured by reduced erythema and scaling, as well as reduction of plaque elevation.
- PASI is a uniform method to determine the extent of BSA affected, along with the degree of erythema, induration, and scaling. Severity scores are rated as less than 12 (mild), 12 to 18 (moderate), and more than 18 (severe).
- The Physician Global Assessment can also be used to summarize erythema, induration, scaling, and extent of plaques relative to baseline assessment.
- The National Psoriasis Foundation Psoriasis Score incorporates quality of life and the patient's perception of well-being, as well as induration, extent of involvement, the physician's static global assessment, and pruritus.
- Achievement of efficacy by any therapeutic regimen requires days to weeks. Initial dramatic response may be achieved with some agents, such as corticosteroids. However, sustained benefit with pharmacologically specific antipsoriatic therapy may require 2 to 8 weeks or longer for clinically meaningful response.

See Chapter 98, Psoriasis, authored by Rebecca M. Law and Wayne P. Gulliver, for a more detailed discussion of this topic.

CHAPTER 18 — Adrenal Gland Disorders

- Hyperfunction of the adrenal glands involves excess production of the adrenal hormones cortisol (resulting in Cushing syndrome) or aldosterone (resulting in hyperaldosteronism).
- Adrenal gland hypofunction is associated with primary (Addison disease) or secondary adrenal insufficiency.

CUSHING SYNDROME

PATHOPHYSIOLOGY

- Cushing syndrome results from effects of supraphysiologic glucocorticoid levels originating from either exogenous administration or endogenous overproduction by the adrenal gland (adrenocorticotropic hormone [ACTH] dependent) or by abnormal adrenocortical tissues (ACTH independent).
- ACTH-dependent Cushing syndrome (80% of all Cushing syndrome cases) is usually caused by overproduction of ACTH by the pituitary gland, causing adrenal hyperplasia. Pituitary adenomas account for about 85% of these cases (Cushing disease). Ectopic ACTH-secreting tumors and nonneoplastic corticotropin hypersecretion cause the remaining 20% of ACTH-dependent cases.
- Ectopic ACTH syndrome refers to excessive ACTH production resulting from an endocrine or nonendocrine tumor, usually of the pancreas, thyroid, or lung (eg, small-cell lung cancer).
- ACTH-independent Cushing syndrome is usually caused by adrenal adenomas and carcinomas.

CLINICAL PRESENTATION

- The most common findings in Cushing syndrome are central obesity and facial rounding (90% of patients). Peripheral obesity and fat accumulation occur in 50% of patients. Fat accumulation in the dorsocervical area (buffalo hump) is nonspecific, but increased supraclavicular fat pads are more specific for Cushing syndrome. Patients are often described as having moon facies and a buffalo hump.
- Other findings may include myopathy or muscular weakness, abdominal striae, hypertension, glucose intolerance, psychiatric changes, gonadal dysfunction, facial plethora (a reddish complexion), and amenorrhea and hirsutism in women.
- Up to 60% of patients develop Cushing-induced osteoporosis; about 40% present with back pain, and 20% progress to spinal compression fractures.

DIAGNOSIS

- Hypercortisolism can be established with one or more of the following tests: 24-hour urinary free cortisol (UFC), midnight plasma cortisol, late-night (11 PM) salivary cortisol, and/or low-dose dexamethasone suppression test (DST).
- Other tests to determine etiology are plasma ACTH test; adrenal vein catheterization; metyrapone stimulation test; adrenal, chest, or abdominal computed tomography (CT); corticotropin-releasing hormone (CRH) stimulation test; inferior petrosal sinus sampling; and pituitary magnetic resonance imaging (MRI).

- Adrenal nodules and masses are identified using high-resolution CT scanning or MRI.

TREATMENT

- <u>Goals of Treatment</u>: Limit morbidity and mortality and return the patient to a normal functional state by removing the source of hypercortisolism while minimizing pituitary or adrenal deficiencies.
- Treatment plans in Cushing syndrome based on etiology are included in Table 18–1.

Nonpharmacologic Therapy

- Treatment of choice for both ACTH-dependent and ACTH-independent Cushing syndrome is surgical resection of offending tumors. Transsphenoidal resection of the pituitary tumor is the treatment of choice for Cushing disease.
- Pituitary irradiation provides clinical improvement in ~50% of patients within 3 to 5 years, but improvement may not be seen for 6 to 12 months, and pituitary-dependent hormone deficiencies (hypopituitarism) can occur.
- Laparoscopic adrenalectomy may be preferred in patients with unilateral adrenal adenomas or for whom transsphenoidal surgery and pituitary radiotherapy have failed or cannot be used.

Pharmacologic Therapy (See Table 18–1)

- Pharmacotherapy is generally used as second-line treatments in patients who are not surgical candidates and may also be used for preoperative patients or as adjunctive therapy in postoperative patients awaiting response. Rarely, monotherapy is used as a palliative treatment when surgery is not indicated.

STEROIDOGENESIS INHIBITORS

- **Metyrapone** inhibits 11 β-hydroxylase, thereby inhibiting cortisol synthesis. Initially, patients can demonstrate increased plasma ACTH concentrations because of a sudden drop in cortisol. This can increase androgenic and mineralocorticoid hormones, resulting in hypertension, acne, and hirsutism. Nausea, vomiting, vertigo, headache, dizziness, abdominal discomfort, and allergic rash have been reported after oral administration. Metyrapone is currently available through the manufacturer only for compassionate use.
- **Ketoconazole** inhibits cytochrome P-450 enzymes, including 11 β-hydroxylase and 17 α-hydroxylase. It is effective in lowering serum cortisol levels after several weeks of therapy. It also has antiandrogenic activity, which may be beneficial in women but can cause gynecomastia and hypogonadism in men. The most common adverse effects are reversible elevation of hepatic transaminases, GI discomfort, and dermatologic reactions. Because of the risk of severe hepatotoxicity, monitoring should include liver function tests at baseline followed by weekly monitoring of serum ALT throughout therapy. Ketoconazole may be used concomitantly with metyrapone to achieve synergistic reduction in cortisol levels; in addition, ketoconazole's antiandrogenic actions may offset the androgenic potential of metyrapone.
- **Etomidate** is an imidazole derivative similar to ketoconazole that inhibits 11 β-hydroxylase and may have other mechanisms. Because it is only available in a parenteral formulation, use is limited to patients with acute hypercortisolemia requiring emergency treatment or in preparation for surgery. Frequent monitoring of serum cortisol is advised to prevent hypocortisolemia. The initial dose is 0.03 mg/kg by IV bolus followed by a continuous infusion of 0.1 to 0.3 mg/kg/h.

ADRENOLYTIC AGENTS

- **Mitotane** is a cytotoxic drug that inhibits the 11-hydroxylation of 11-deoxycortisol and 11-desoxycorticosterone in the adrenal cortex, reducing synthesis of cortisol and corticosterone. Similar to ketoconazole, mitotane takes weeks to months to exert beneficial effects. Sustained cortisol suppression occurs in most patients and may

TABLE 18-1 Treatment Options in Cushing Syndrome Based on Etiology

Etiology	Nondrug	Generic (Brand) Drug Name	Dosing		
			Initial Dose	Usual Range	Maximum
Ectopic ACTH syndrome	Surgery, chemotherapy, irradiation	Metyrapone (Metopirone) 250 mg capsules	0.5-1 g/day, divided every 4 to 6 hours	1-2 g/day, divided every 4-6 hours	6 g/day
		Ketoconazole (Nizoral) 200 mg tablets	200 mg once or twice a day	200-1200 mg/day, divided twice daily	1600 mg/day divided four times daily
Pituitary dependent	Surgery, irradiation	Mitotane (Lysodren) 500 mg tablets	0.5-1 g/day, increased by 0.5-1 g/day every 1-4 weeks	1-4 g daily, with food to decrease GI effects	12 g/day
		Metyrapone	See above	See above	See above
		Mifepristone (Korlym) 300 mg tablets	300 mg once daily, increased by 300 mg/day every 2-4 weeks	600-1200 mg/day	1200 mg/day or 20 mg/kg/day
		Cabergoline (Dostinex) 0.5 mg tablets	0.5 mg once weekly	0.5-7 mg once weekly	7 mg/week
		Pasireotide (Signifor) 0.3, 0.6, and 0.9 mg/mL solution	0.6-0.9 mg twice daily	0.3-0.9 mg twice daily	1.8 mg/day
Adrenal adenoma	Surgery, postoperative replacement	Ketoconazole	See above	See above	See above
Adrenal carcinoma	Surgery	Mitotane	See above	See above	See above

(ACTH, adrenocorticotropic hormone.)

persist after drug discontinuation in up to one third of patients. Mitotane degenerates cells within the zona fasciculata and reticularis; the zona glomerulosa is minimally affected during acute therapy but can be damaged during long-term treatment. Mitotane can cause significant neurologic and GI side effects, and patients should be monitored carefully or hospitalized when initiating therapy. Nausea and diarrhea are common at doses greater than 2 g/day and can be avoided by gradually increasing the dose and/or administering it with food. Lethargy, somnolence, and other CNS effects are also common. Reversible hypercholesterolemia and prolonged bleeding times can occur.

NEUROMODULATORS OF ACTH RELEASE

- Pituitary secretion of ACTH is normally mediated by neurotransmitters such as serotonin, γ-aminobutyric acid (GABA), acetylcholine, and catecholamines. Although ACTH-secreting pituitary tumors (Cushing disease) self-regulate ACTH production to some degree, these neurotransmitters can still promote pituitary ACTH production. Consequently, agents that target these transmitters have been proposed for treatment of Cushing disease, including cyproheptadine, bromocriptine, cabergoline, valproic acid, octreotide, lanreotide, pasireotide, rosiglitazone, and tretinoin. With the exception of pasireotide, none of these drugs have demonstrated consistent clinical efficacy for treating Cushing syndrome.
- **Cyproheptadine**, a nonselective serotonin receptor antagonist and anticholinergic drug, can decrease ACTH secretion in some patients with Cushing disease. However, side effects such as sedation and weight gain significantly limit its use.
- **Pasireotide** (Signifor) is a somatostatin analogue that binds and activates somatostatin receptors, thereby inhibiting ACTH secretion, leading to decreased cortisol secretion. It is approved for treatment of adults with Cushing disease for whom pituitary surgery is not an option or has not been curative.

GLUCOCORTICOID-RECEPTOR BLOCKING AGENTS

- **Mifepristone** (Korlym) is a progesterone- and glucocorticoid-receptor antagonist that inhibits dexamethasone suppression and increases endogenous cortisol and ACTH levels in normal subjects. Evidence suggests that mifepristone is highly effective in reversing the manifestations of hypercortisolism (hyperglycemia, hypertension, and weight gain). It is FDA approved for treatment of endogenous Cushing's syndrome in patients who have type 2 diabetes or glucose intolerance and who are not eligible for, or have had poor response to, surgery. Common adverse effects include fatigue, nausea, headache, arthralgia, peripheral edema, endometrial thickening (with or without vaginal bleeding), and reductions in serum potassium.

EVALUATION OF THERAPEUTIC OUTCOMES

- Close monitoring of 24-hour UFC and serum cortisol is essential to identify adrenal insufficiency in patients with Cushing syndrome. Monitor steroid secretion with all drug therapy (except mifepristone) and give corticosteroid replacement if needed.

HYPERALDOSTERONISM

PATHOPHYSIOLOGY

- Hyperaldosteronism involves excess aldosterone secretion and is categorized as either primary (stimulus arising from within the adrenal gland) or secondary (stimulus from extraadrenal etiologies).
- *Primary hyperaldosteronism* is usually caused by bilateral adrenal hyperplasia and aldosterone-producing adenoma (Conn syndrome). Rare causes include unilateral (primary) adrenal hyperplasia, adrenal cortex carcinoma, renin-responsive adrenocortical adenoma, and three forms of familial hyperaldosteronism (FH): Type I

(glucocorticoid-remediable aldosteronism); Type II (familial occurrence of adenoma or hyperplasia type II); and Type III.

- *Secondary hyperaldosteronism* results from excessive stimulation of the zona glomerulosa by an extra-adrenal factor, usually the renin–angiotensin system. Elevated aldosterone secretion can result from excessive potassium intake, oral contraceptives, pregnancy, and menses. Heart failure, cirrhosis, renal artery stenosis, and Bartter syndrome also can lead to elevated aldosterone concentrations.

CLINICAL PRESENTATION

- Patients may complain of muscle weakness, fatigue, paresthesias, headache, polydipsia, and nocturnal polyuria.
- Signs may include hypertension and tetany/paralysis.
- Laboratory findings include suppressed renin activity, elevated plasma aldosterone, hypernatremia (>142 mEq/L), hypokalemia, hypomagnesemia, elevated serum bicarbonate (>31 mEq/L), and glucose intolerance.

DIAGNOSIS

- Patients with suspected hyperaldosteronism (e.g., resistant hypertension) should receive screening, usually by the plasma-aldosterone-concentration–to–plasma-renin-activity (PAC-to-PRA) ratio (also called the aldosterone-to-renin ratio, ARR). An elevated ARR is highly suggestive of primary hyperaldosteronism.
- If the ARR is positive, confirmatory tests to exclude false-positives include the oral sodium-loading test, saline infusion test, fludrocortisone suppression test (FST), and captopril challenge test. A positive test indicates autonomous aldosterone secretion under inhibitory pressures and is diagnostic for primary hyperaldosteronism.

TREATMENT

Nonpharmacologic Therapy

- Aldosterone-producing adenomas are treated by laparoscopic resection of the tumor, leading to permanent cures in up to 72% of patients. Medical management can be effective if surgery is contraindicated.

Pharmacologic Therapy

- Bilateral adrenal hyperplasia is treated primarily with aldosterone receptor antagonists, but several other drug classes have been used.
  - ✓ **Spironolactone** (Aldactone) is a nonselective aldosterone receptor antagonist that competes with aldosterone for binding at aldosterone receptors, thus preventing the negative effects of aldosterone receptor activation. The initial dose is 25 mg once daily titrated upward at 4- to 8-week intervals. Most patients respond to doses between 25 and 400 mg/day given in single or divided doses. Adverse effects include GI discomfort, impotence, gynecomastia, menstrual irregularities, and hyperkalemia.
  - ✓ **Eplerenone** (Inspra) is a selective aldosterone receptor antagonist with high affinity for aldosterone receptors and low affinity for androgen and progesterone receptors. Consequently, it elicits fewer sex-steroid–dependent effects than spironolactone. Dosing starts at 50 mg daily, with titration at 4- to 8-week intervals to 50 mg twice a day; some patients may require total daily doses as high as 200 to 300 mg.
  - ✓ **Amiloride** (Amiloride), a potassium-sparing diuretic, is less effective than spironolactone, and patients often require additional therapy to adequately control blood pressure. The initial dose is 5 mg twice daily, with a usual range of 20 mg/day given in two divided doses; doses up to 30 mg/day may be necessary.
  - ✓ Additional second-line options include calcium channel blockers, ACE inhibitors, and diuretics such as chlorthalidone, although all of these lack outcome data.
- Treatment of secondary aldosteronism is dictated by etiology. Control or correction of the extra-adrenal stimulation of aldosterone secretion should resolve the disorder. Medical therapy with spironolactone is undertaken until the etiology is identified.

ADRENAL INSUFFICIENCY

PATHOPHYSIOLOGY

- Primary adrenal insufficiency (Addison disease) usually involves destruction of all regions of the adrenal cortex. There are deficiencies of cortisol, aldosterone, and the various androgens, and levels of CRH and ACTH increase in a compensatory manner.
- Autoimmune dysfunction is responsible for 80% to 90% of cases in developed countries, whereas tuberculosis is the predominant cause in developing countries.
- Medications that inhibit cortisol synthesis (eg, ketoconazole) or accelerate cortisol metabolism (eg, phenytoin, rifampin, and phenobarbital) can also cause primary adrenal insufficiency.
- Secondary adrenal insufficiency most commonly results from exogenous corticosteroid use, leading to suppression of the hypothalamic-pituitary-adrenal axis and decreased ACTH release, resulting in impaired androgen and cortisol production. Mirtazapine and progestins (eg, medroxyprogesterone acetate and megestrol acetate) have also been reported to induce secondary adrenal insufficiency. Secondary disease typically presents with normal mineralocorticoid concentrations.

CLINICAL PRESENTATION

- Patients commonly complain of weakness, weight loss, GI symptoms, salt craving, headaches, memory impairment, depression, and postural dizziness.
- Signs of adrenal insufficiency include increased skin pigmentation, postural hypotension, fever, decreased body hair, vitiligo, amenorrhea, and cold intolerance.

DIAGNOSIS

- The short cosyntropin stimulation test can be used to assess patients with suspected hypercortisolism. An increase to a cortisol level of 18 mcg/dL or more (500 nmol/L) rules out adrenal insufficiency.
- Patients with Addison disease have an abnormal response to the short cosyntropin stimulation test. Plasma ACTH levels are usually elevated (400–2000 pg/mL or 88–440 pmol/L) in primary insufficiency versus normal to low (5–50 pg/mL or 1.1–11 pmol/L]) in secondary insufficiency. A normal cosyntropin-stimulation test does not rule out secondary adrenal insufficiency.
- Other tests include the insulin hypoglycemia test, the metyrapone test, and the CRH stimulation test.

TREATMENT

- <u>Goals of Treatment</u>: Limit morbidity and mortality, return the patient to a normal functional state, and prevent episodes of acute adrenal insufficiency.

Nonpharmacologic Therapy

- Inform patients of treatment complications, expected outcomes, proper medication administration and adherence, and possible side effects.

Pharmacotherapy

CORTICOSTEROIDS

- **Hydrocortisone, cortisone**, and **prednisone** are the glucocorticoids of choice, administered twice daily at the lowest effective dose while mimicking the normal diurnal adrenal rhythm of cortisol production.
- Recommended starting total daily doses are hydrocortisone 15 to 25 mg daily, which is approximately equivalent to cortisone acetate 25 to 37.5 mg, or prednisone 2.5 mg (Table 18–2). Two thirds of the dose is given in the morning, and one third is given 6 to 8 hours later.
- The patient's symptoms can be monitored every 6 to 8 weeks to assess proper glucocorticoid replacement.

Glucocorticoid	Anti-inflammatory Potency	Equivalent Potency (mg)	Approximate Half-Life (min)	Sodium-Retaining Potency
Cortisone	0.8	25	30	2
Hydrocortisone	1	20	90	2
Prednisone	3.5	5	60	1
Prednisolone	4	5	200	1
Triamcinolone	5	4	300	0
Methylprednisolone	5	4	180	0
Betamethasone	25	0.6	100–300	0
Dexamethasone	30	0.75	100–300	0

TABLE 18–2 Relative Potencies of Glucocorticoids

- In primary adrenal insufficiency, **fludrocortisone acetate** 0.05 to 0.2 mg orally once daily can be used to replace mineralocorticoid loss. If parenteral therapy is needed, 2 to 5 mg of **deoxycorticosterone trimethylacetate** in oil can be administered intramuscularly every 3 to 4 weeks. The major reason for adding the mineralocorticoid is to minimize development of hyperkalemia.
- Because most adrenal crises occur because of glucocorticoid dose reductions or lack of stress-related dose adjustments, patients receiving corticosteroid replacement therapy should add 5 to 10 mg hydrocortisone (or equivalent) to their normal daily regimen shortly before strenuous activities, such as exercise. During times of severe physical stress (eg, febrile illnesses and after accidents), patients should be instructed to double their daily dose until recovery.
- Treatment of secondary adrenal insufficiency is identical to primary disease treatment, with the exception that mineralocorticoid replacement is usually not necessary.

Pharmacotherapy of Acute Adrenal Insufficiency

- Acute adrenal insufficiency (adrenal crisis or addisonian crisis) represents a true endocrine emergency.
- Stressful situations, surgery, infection, and trauma are potential events that increase adrenal requirements, especially in patients with some underlying adrenal or pituitary insufficiency.
- The most common cause of adrenal crisis is HPA-axis suppression brought on by abrupt withdrawal of chronic glucocorticoid use.
- **Hydrocortisone** given parenterally is the corticosteroid of choice because of its combined glucocorticoid and mineralocorticoid activity. The starting dose is 100 mg IV by rapid infusion, followed by a continuous infusion (usually 10 mg/h) or intermittent bolus of 100 to 200 mg every 24 hours. IV administration is continued for 24 to 48 hours. If the patient is stable at that time, oral hydrocortisone can be started at a dose of 50 mg every 6 to 8 hours, followed by tapering to the individual's chronic replacement needs.
- **Fluid replacement** often is required and can be accomplished with IV dextrose 5% in normal saline solution at a rate to support blood pressure.
- If hyperkalemia is present after the hydrocortisone maintenance phase, additional mineralocorticoid supplementation can be achieved with **fludrocortisone acetate** 0.1 mg daily.
- Patients with adrenal insufficiency should carry a card or wear a bracelet or necklace that contains information about their condition. They should also have easy access to injectable hydrocortisone or glucocorticoid suppositories in case of an emergency or during times of physical stress, such as febrile illness or injury.

EVALUATION OF THERAPEUTIC OUTCOMES

- The end point of therapy for adrenal insufficiency is difficult to assess in most patients, but a reduction in excess pigmentation is a good clinical marker. Development of features of Cushing syndrome indicates excessive replacement.

See Chapter 76, Adrenal Gland Disorders, authored by Andrew Y. Hwang, Steven M. Smith, and John G. Gums, for a more detailed discussion of this topic.

- *Diabetes mellitus* (DM) is a group of metabolic disorders characterized by hyperglycemia and abnormalities in carbohydrate, fat, and protein metabolism. It may result in chronic microvascular, macrovascular, and neuropathic complications.

PATHOPHYSIOLOGY

- Type 1 DM (5%–10% of cases) results from autoimmune destruction of pancreatic β-cells, leading to absolute deficiency of insulin. It usually presents in children and adolescents but can occur at any age. The autoimmune process is mediated by macrophages and T lymphocytes with autoantibodies to β-cell antigens (eg, islet cell antibody, insulin antibodies). Amylin (a hormone cosecreted from pancreatic β-cells with insulin) suppresses inappropriate glucagon secretion, slows gastric emptying, and causes central satiety; amylin is also deficient in type 1 DM due to β-cell destruction.
- Type 2 DM (90% of cases) is characterized by multiple defects:
  ✓ *Impaired insulin secretion* is a hallmark finding; β-cell mass and function are both reduced, and β-cell failure is progressive.
  ✓ Normally, the gut incretin hormones glucagon-like peptide-1 (GLP-1) and glucose-dependent insulinotropic peptide (GIP) are released and stimulate insulin secretion when nutrients enter the stomach and intestines. Patients with type 2 DM have a *reduced incretin effect* due to decreased concentrations of or resistance to the effects of these incretin hormones.
  ✓ *Insulin resistance* is manifested by excessive hepatic glucose production, decreased skeletal muscle uptake of glucose, and increased lipolysis and free fatty acid production.
  ✓ *Excess glucagon secretion* occurs because type 2 DM patients fail to suppress glucagon in response to meals because of GLP-1 resistance/deficiency and insulin resistance/deficiency, which directly suppress glucagon.
  ✓ *Sodium-glucose cotransporter-2 (SGLT-2) upregulation in the kidney* increases reabsorption of glucose by proximal renal tubular cells, which may worsen hyperglycemia.
- The *metabolic syndrome* involves multiple metabolic abnormalities and confers a higher risk for developing type 2 DM and subsequent cardiovascular disease (CVD). The current definition includes central obesity (defined as waist circumference with ethnicity-specific values) plus any two of these four factors: (1) raised triglycerides (≥ 150 mg/dL [1.7 mmol/L]); (2) reduced HDL cholesterol (< 40 mg/dL [1.03 mmol/L] in males or < 50 mg/dL [1.29 mmol/L] in females); (3) increased blood pressure (systolic BP ≥ 130 mm Hg, diastolic BP ≥ 85 mm Hg, or treatment of previously-diagnosed hypertension); and (4) raised fasting plasma glucose (≥ 100 mg/dL [5.6 mmol/L] or previous diagnosis of type 2 DM.
- Uncommon causes of diabetes (less than 5% of cases) include gestational diabetes mellitus (GDM), maturity onset diabetes of youth (MODY), endocrine disorders (eg, acromegaly, Cushing syndrome), pancreatic exocrine dysfunction, infections, and medications (eg, glucocorticoids, thiazides, niacin).
- Microvascular complications include retinopathy, neuropathy, and nephropathy. Macrovascular complications include coronary heart disease, stroke, and peripheral vascular disease.

CLINICAL PRESENTATION

TYPE 1 DIABETES MELLITUS

- The most common initial symptoms are polyuria, polydipsia, polyphagia, weight loss, and lethargy accompanied by hyperglycemia.

- Individuals are often thin and are prone to develop diabetic ketoacidosis if insulin is withheld or under conditions of severe stress.
- Between 20% and 40% of patients present with diabetic ketoacidosis after several days of polyuria, polydipsia, polyphagia, and weight loss.

TYPE 2 DIABETES MELLITUS

- Patients are often asymptomatic and may be diagnosed secondary to unrelated blood testing.
- Lethargy, polyuria, nocturia, and polydipsia can be present. Significant weight loss is less common; most patients are overweight or obese.

DIAGNOSIS

- Criteria for diagnosis of DM include any one of the following:
  1. A1C of 6.5% or more (≥0.065; ≥ 48 mmol/mol Hb)
  2. Fasting (no caloric intake for at least 8 hours) plasma glucose of 126 mg/dL or more (≥7.0 mmol/L)
  3. Two-hour plasma glucose of 200 mg/dL or more (≥11.1 mmol/L) during an oral glucose tolerance test (OGTT) using a glucose load containing the equivalent of 75 g anhydrous glucose dissolved in water
  4. Random plasma glucose concentration of 200 mg/dL or more (≥11.1 mmol/L) with classic symptoms of hyperglycemia or hyperglycemic crisis. In the absence of unequivocal hyperglycemia, criteria 1 through 3 should be confirmed by repeat testing.
- Normal fasting plasma glucose (FPG) is less than 100 mg/dL (5.6 mmol/L).
- Impaired fasting glucose (IFG) is FPG 100 to 125 mg/dL (5.6–6.9 mmol/L).
- Impaired glucose tolerance (IGT) is diagnosed when the 2-hour postload sample of OGTT is 140 to 199 mg per dL (7.8–11.0 mmol/L).
- Pregnant women should undergo risk assessment for GDM at first prenatal visit and have glucose testing if there are risk factors for developing diabetes (eg, positive family history, personal history of GDM, marked obesity, or member of a high-risk ethnic group).

TREATMENT

- <u>Goals of Treatment</u>: Ameliorate symptoms, reduce risk of microvascular and macrovascular complications, reduce mortality, and improve quality of life. Desirable plasma glucose and A1C levels are listed in **Table 19–1**.

TABLE 19–1	Glycemic Goals of Therapy for Adults	
Biochemical Index	**ADA**	**ACE and AACE**
A1C	<7%[a] (<0.07; <53 mmol/mol Hb)	≤6.5% (≤0.065; <48 mmol/mol Hb)
Preprandial plasma glucose	80–130 mg/dL (4.4–7.2 mmol/L)	<110 mg/dL (<6.1 mmol/L)
Postprandial plasma glucose	<180 mg/dL[b] (<10 mmol/L)	<140 mg/dL (<7.8 mmol/L)

(AACE, American Association of Clinical Endocrinologists; ACE, American College of Endocrinology; ADA, American Diabetes Association.)

[a]More stringent glycemic goals may be appropriate if accomplished without significant hypoglycemia or adverse effects. Less-stringent goals may also be appropriate in some situations.
[b]Postprandial glucose measurements should be made 1 to 2 hours after the beginning of the meal, generally the time of peak levels in patients with diabetes.

GENERAL APPROACH

- Early treatment to near-normal glycemia reduces risk of microvascular disease complications, but aggressive management of cardiovascular risk factors (ie, smoking cessation, treatment of dyslipidemia, intensive blood pressure [BP] control, and antiplatelet therapy) is needed to reduce macrovascular disease risk.
- Appropriate care requires goal setting for glycemia, BP, and lipid levels; regular monitoring for complications; appropriate food choices; maintaining a healthy weight; engaging in regular physical activity; wise medication selection and use; appropriate self-monitoring of blood glucose (SMBG); and laboratory assessment of appropriate parameters.

NONPHARMACOLOGIC THERAPY

- Medical nutrition therapy is recommended for all patients. For type 1 DM, the focus is on physiologically regulating insulin administration with a balanced diet to achieve and maintain healthy body weight. The meal plan should be moderate in carbohydrates, low in saturated fat (less than 7% of total calories), with all of the essential vitamins and minerals. Weight loss is recommended for all insulin-resistant/overweight or obese patients with type 2 DM.
- Aerobic exercise can improve insulin sensitivity and glycemic control and may reduce cardiovascular risk, contribute to weight control, and improve well-being. Physical activity goals include at least 150 min/week of moderate (50%–70% maximal heart rate) exercise spread over at least 3 days/week with no more than 2 days between activity. Resistance/strength training is recommended at least 2 times/week for patients without proliferative diabetic retinopathy.
- Ongoing diabetes education should emphasize self-care behaviors including healthy eating, being active, monitoring blood glucose (BG) levels, taking medication, problem solving for diabetes control, reducing risk of complications, and healthy coping with stress. Patients must be involved in decision making and have strong knowledge of the disease and associated complications.
- All patients receiving insulin should be instructed on how to recognize and treat hypoglycemia. To minimize overtreatment and avoid rebound hyperglycemia, patients should follow the "rule of 15." If hypoglycemia occurs, the patient should consume 15 g of simple carbohydrate (eg, 8 oz [240 mL] orange juice or milk, 4 glucose tables, or 1 tube of glucose gel and then retest BG 15 minutes later. If BG is < 70 mg/dL (3.9 mmol/L), the patient should repeat the rule of 15 until the BG normalizes.
- Islet cell and whole pancreas transplantation is occasionally used in patients who require immunosuppression for other reasons (eg, kidney transplants). Although many patients are able to stop insulin or require minimal other therapy, at least 80% need to reinitiate some form of insulin therapy within two years after transplantation.

PHARMACOLOGIC THERAPY

TYPE 1 DIABETES MELLITUS

- All patients with type 1 DM require insulin, but the type and manner of delivery differ based on patient preference, lifestyle behaviors, clinician preference, and available resources. Therapy should attempt to match carbohydrate intake with glucose-lowering processes (usually insulin) and physical activity. The goal is to allow the patient to live as normal a life as possible.
- Figure 19–1 depicts the relationship between glucose concentrations and insulin secretion over the course of a day and how various insulin and amylinomimetic regimens may be given. The timing of insulin onset, peak, and duration of effect must match meal patterns and exercise schedules to achieve near-normal blood glucose values throughout the day.

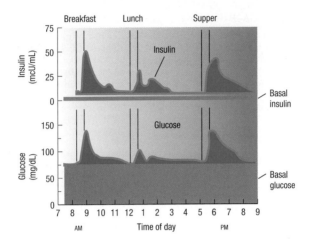

Intensive insulin therapy regimens

	7 AM (meal)	11 AM (meal)	5 PM (meal)	Bedtime
1. 2 doses,[a] R or rapid acting + N	R, L, A, GLU + N		R, L, A, GLU + N	
2. 3 doses, R or rapid acting + N	R, L, A, GLU + N	R, L, A, GLU	R, L, A, GLU + N	
3. 4 doses, R or rapid acting + N	R, L, A, GLU	R, L, A, GLU	R, L, A, GLU	N
4. 4 doses, R or rapid acting + N	R, L, A, GLU + N	R, L, A, GLU	R, L, A, GLU	N
5. 4 doses,[b] R or rapid acting + long acting	R, L, A, GLU	R, L, A, GLU	R, L, A, GLU	G or D[b] (G may be given anytime every 24 hours)
6. CS-II pump	Bolus	← Adjusted basal → Bolus	Bolus	
7. 3 prandial doses pramlintide added to regimens above	P	P	P	

[a]Many clinicians may not consider this intensive insulin therapy.

[b]May be given twice a day in type 1 DM = 5 doses.

(A, Afrezza; A, aspart; CS-II, continuous subcutaneous insulin infusion; D, detemir or degludec; G, glargine; GLU, glulisine; L, lispro; N, NPH; P, pramlintide; R, regular).

FIGURE 19–1. Relationship between insulin and glucose over the course of a day and how various insulin and amylinomimetic regimens could be given.

• The simplest regimen that can approximate physiologic insulin release uses "split-mixed" insulin, consisting of twice-daily premixed doses of an intermediate-acting insulin (eg, **NPH**) and **regular insulin** or a rapid-acting insulin analog (**lispro**, **aspart**, or **glulisine**) given before the morning and evening meals (see **Fig. 19–1**, no. 1). The morning intermediate-acting insulin provides basal insulin during the day and provides "prandial" coverage for the midday meal. The evening intermediate-acting insulin dose provides basal insulin throughout the evening and overnight. Nocturnal hypoglycemia may occur with this regimen; moving the evening NPH dose to bedtime may improve glycemic control and reduce the risk of nocturnal hypoglycemia. Most patients are not sufficiently predictable in their schedule and food intake to allow tight glucose control with this approach, but it may be useful in those who are unable to implement more intense insulin regimens.

- Basal-bolus regimens using multiple daily injections (MDI) attempt to replicate normal insulin physiology with a combination of intermediate (NPH) or long-acting insulin (**detemir**, **glargine**, or **degludec**) as the basal component and a rapid-acting insulin (regular insulin or the analogs lispro, aspart, or glulisine) to provide prandial coverage (see **Fig. 19–1**, nos. 2, 3, 4, and 5). The patient determines the bolus insulin dose based on the preprandial glucose level, anticipated carbohydrate intake from the meal, and anticipated activity in the next 3 to 4 hours. Carbohydrate counting is an effective tool for determining the amount of rapid-acting insulin to be injected for each meal. In type 1 DM, the average daily insulin requirement is 0.5 to 0.6 units/kg, with approximately 50% delivered as basal insulin and the remaining 50% given as bolus insulin divided among meals (eg, 20% before breakfast, 15% before lunch, and 15% before dinner). Requirements may fall to 0.1 to 0.4 units/kg in the honeymoon phase. Higher doses are commonly needed during acute illness or ketosis.

- Continuous subcutaneous insulin infusion (CSII) pump therapy using a basal infusion and rapid-acting insulin analog bolus doses (lispro, aspart, or glulisine) is more likely to achieve excellent glycemic control than MDI (see **Fig. 19–1**, no. 6). CSII can calculate recommended bolus insulin doses based on carbohydrate intake. It can also be paired with continuous glucose monitoring (CGM) to calculate a correction insulin dose and alert the patient to hypo- and hyperglycemia. Patients must still verify that the calculated bolus dose and basal infusion rates are appropriate. The basal insulin infusion rate can be varied throughout the day based on changes in insulin requirements. These features of CSII enable more precise insulin dosing and help patients achieve greater glycemic control. However, it requires greater attention to detail and more frequent SMBG than basal-bolus MDI regimens.

- Erratic gastric emptying can hinder the ability to match insulin with meals. The amylinomimetic **pramlintide** may be appropriate in patients who continue to have erratic postprandial control despite these strategies and proper insulin use (see **Fig. 19–1**, no. 7). When taken prior to each meal, it can modestly improve postprandial glucose control but is not a substitute for bolus insulin and cannot be mixed with insulin. At initiation of therapy, each dose of prandial insulin should be reduced by 30% to 50% to prevent hypoglycemia. Pramlintide should be titrated based on GI adverse effects and postprandial glycemic goals.

TYPE 2 DIABETES MELLITUS

- Consensus treatment algorithms have been published; for example, see the American Diabetes Association (ADA) and the European Association for the Study of Diabetes algorithm (Inzucchi SE et al, *Diabetes Care* 2015;38:140-149).
- Symptomatic patients may initially require insulin or combination oral therapy.
- Patients with A1C 7.5% (0.075, 58 mmol/mol Hb) or less are usually treated with an antihyperglycemic that is unlikely to cause hypoglycemia. Those with A1C above 7.5% but less than 8.5% (0.085, 69 mmol/mol Hb) could be treated initially with a single oral agent or combination therapy. Patients with higher initial A1C values require two agents or insulin.
- Obese patients without contraindications are often started on metformin, titrated to 2000 mg/day. Metformin also works in nonobese patients, but they are more likely to be insulinopenic, necessitating drugs that increase insulin secretion. The durability of metformin response is suboptimal, and patients often require additional therapy over time.

- If the individualized target A1C is not reached with single-drug therapy, adding a second drug to metformin is the next step:
  ✓ An insulin secretagogue (eg, sulfonylurea) is often added second. They are inexpensive but may cause weight gain and hypoglycemia. They also do not produce a durable glycemic response.
  ✓ Dipeptidyl dipeptidase-4 (DPP-4) inhibitors, GLP-1 receptor agonists, and SLGT-2 inhibitors are better choices but they also have therapeutic and safety limitations.
  ✓ Thiazolidinediones (TZDs) produce a more durable glycemic response and are unlikely to cause hypoglycemia, but weight gain, fluid retention, risk of new onset heart failure, and other long-term safe concerns limit their use.
  ✓ Insulin may also be used with metformin.
- If the individualized A1C target is not reached after 3 months of dual-drug therapy, a third drug may be added. Multiple variations are available, and the preferred combination depends on patient- and disease-specific factors.
- If the A1C target is not achieved after about 3 months of triple therapy, further options depend on what the patient is receiving:
  ✓ If on oral therapy, move to injectables;
  ✓ If on a GLP-1 receptor agonist, add basal insulin;
  ✓ If on optimally titrated basal insulin, add a GLP-1 receptor agonist or mealtime insulin; in refractory patients, consider adding a TZD or SLGT-2 inhibitor.
- Nearly all patients ultimately become relatively insulinopenic and require insulin therapy. Higher doses than those used for type 1 DM are required for patients with significant insulin resistance.
  ✓ Patients often transition to insulin by using a bedtime injection of an intermediate- or long-acting basal insulin while continuing oral agents or GLP-1 receptor agonists for daytime control. This strategy is associated with equal efficacy with less weight gain and lower risk of hypoglycemia than starting prandial insulin or split-mix twice-daily insulin. Patients using basal insulin should be monitored for signs/symptoms of hypoglycemia (eg, nocturnal sweating, poor sleep, nightmares, palpitations, tremulousness) as well as SMBG.
  ✓ If there is inadequate control with basal or bedtime insulin, giving a bolus insulin dose prior to the largest meal of the day ("basal plus") may be simpler than implementing MDI. When prandial insulin is added to the evening meal, reducing the bedtime basal insulin dose may be warranted. An alternative to starting prandial insulin is to add a GLP-1 receptor agonist.
  ✓ If a biphasic mixed insulin is used (eg, 70/30 NPH/regular insulin), they should be given twice daily before the first and third meal. If adequate control is not achieved, a third dose of mix insulin may be given with the midday meal.

PHARMACOLOGIC THERAPY: DRUG CLASS INFORMATION

Insulin (Tables 19–2 and 19–3)

- All available insulins are manufactured using recombinant DNA technology and are highly purified. The most commonly used concentration is 100 units/mL (U-100); more concentrated insulins (U-200, U-300, U-500) are reserved for patients requiring larger doses.
- **Regular insulin** given subcutaneously (SC) forms hexamers that undergo conversion to dimers and then monomers before systemic absorption can occur. Thus, it has a relatively slow onset of action when given SC, requiring injection 30 minutes before meals. Regular insulin can also be administered intravenously (IV).
- **Lispro, aspart,** and **glulisine insulins** are analogs that dissociate more rapidly into monomers, resulting in a more rapid onset and peak effect with a shorter duration of action than regular insulin. This permits more convenient SC dosing within 10 minutes of meals (rather than 30 min prior), produces better efficacy in lowering postprandial blood glucose than regular insulin in type 1 DM, and minimizes delayed postmeal hypoglycemia.

TABLE 19–2	Available Insulin and Insulin Analog Preparations	
Generic Name	**Analog[a]**	**Administration Options**
Rapid-acting insulins		
Humalog (insulin lispro)	Yes	Insulin pen 3-mL, 3-mL and 10-mL vial, or 3-mL pen cartridge
NovoLog (insulin aspart)	Yes	Insulin pen 3-mL, 10-mL vial, or 3-mL pen cartridge
Apidra (insulin glulisine)	Yes	Insulin pen 3-mL, 10-mL vial
Short-acting insulins		
Humulin R (regular) U-100	No	10-mL vial, 3-mL vial
Novolin R (regular)	No	10-mL vial
Intermediate-acting insulins		
NPH		
Humulin N	No	3-mL and 10-mL vial, Insulin pen 3-mL
Novolin N	No	10-mL vial
Long-acting insulins		
Lantus (insulin glargine)	Yes	10-mL vial, Insulin pen 3-mL
Levemir (insulin detemir)	Yes	10-mL vial, Insulin pen 3-mL
Tresiba (insulin degludec)	Yes	Insulin pen 3-mL
Premixed insulins		
Premixed insulin analogs		
Humalog Mix 75/25 (75% neutral protamine lispro, 25% lispro)	Yes	10-mL vial, Insulin pen 3-mL
Novolog Mix 70/30 (70% aspart protamine suspension, 30% aspart)	Yes	10-mL vial, Insulin pen 3-mL
Humalog Mix 50/50 (50% neutral protamine lispro/50% lispro)	Yes	10-mL vial, Insulin pen 3-mL
NPH-regular combinations		
Humulin 70/30	No	3-mL and 10-mL vial, Insulin pen 3-mL
Novolin 70/30	No	10-mL vial
Concentrated insulins		
Regular insulin (U-500)	No	20-mL vial, Insulin pen 3-mL
Humalog (U-200 insulin lispro)	Yes	Insulin pen 3-mL
Toujeo (U-300 insulin glargine)	Yes	Insulin pen 1.5-mL
Tresiba (U-200 insulin degludec)	Yes	Insulin pen 3-mL
Inhaled insulin		
Afrezza (Technosphere insulin)	No	4 unit and 8 unit cartridges

[a]All diabetes injectables available in the US are now made by human recombinant DNA technology. An insulin analog is a modified human insulin molecule that imparts particular pharmacokinetic advantages.

- **Neutral protamine Hagedorn (NPH)** is intermediate-acting. Variability in absorption, inconsistent preparation by the patient, and inherent pharmacokinetic differences may contribute to a labile glucose response, nocturnal hypoglycemia, and fasting hyperglycemia.
- **Insulin glargine, degludec,** and **detemir** are long-acting "peakless" insulin analogs that result in less nocturnal hypoglycemia than NPH insulin when given at bedtime. Insulin glargine and degludec are dosed once daily, but detemir at low doses (less than 0.3 units/kg) should be dosed twice daily.
- **Technosphere insulin** (Afrezza) is a dry powder of regular insulin that is inhaled and absorbed through pulmonary tissue. It is rapidly absorbed and reaches maximum

TABLE 19-3	Pharmacokinetics of Select Insulins Administered Subcutaneously				
Type of Insulin	Onset (Hours)	Peak (Hours)	Duration (Hours)	Maximum Duration (Hours)	Appearance
Rapid acting					
Aspart	15–30 minutes	1–2	3–5	5–6	Clear
Lispro	15–30 minutes	1–2	3–4	4–6	Clear
Glulisine	15–30 minutes	1–2	3–4	5–6	Clear
Technosphere[a]	5–10 minutes	0.75–1	~3	~3	Powder
Short-acting					
Regular	0.5–1.0	2–3	4–6	6–8	Clear
Intermediate acting					
NPH	2–4	4–8	8–12	14–18	Cloudy
Long acting					
Detemir	~2 hours	—[b]	14–24	20–24	Clear
Glargine (U-100)	~2–3 hours	—[b]	22–24	24	Clear
Degludec	~2 hours	—[b]	30–36	36	Clear
Glargine (U-300)	~2 hours	—[b]	24–30	30	Clear

[a]Technosphere insulin is inhaled.
[b]Glargine is considered "flat" though there may be a slight peak in effect at 8–12 hours, and with detemir at ~8 hours, but both have exhibited peak effects during comparative testing, and these peak effects may necessitate changing therapy in a minority of type 1 DM patients. Degludec and U-300 insulin glargine appear to have less peak effect compared to U-100 insulin glargine.

blood concentrations in 12 to 15 minutes. Insulin-naïve patients initiating inhaled insulin should start with a 4-unit cartridge before each meal. The most common adverse effects are cough and upper respiratory infections. It is contraindicated in patients with asthma and COPD due to bronchospasm risk.

- Hypoglycemia and weight gain are the most common adverse effects of insulin. Treatment of hypoglycemia is as follows:
  ✓ **Glucose** (10–15 g) given orally for conscious patients is preferred.
  ✓ **Dextrose** IV may be required for unconscious patients.
  ✓ **Glucagon**, 1 g intramuscularly, is preferred in unconscious patients when IV access cannot be established.
- Allergies to human insulin are uncommon. Most injection site reactions dissipate over time; changing to a different type or source of insulin may alleviate mild local reactions. Insulin desensitization protocols are available if allergic reactions persist.
- Lipohypertrophy can occur if patients use the same injection site repeatedly. Insulin should not be injected into these areas because absorption is unpredictable. Lipoatrophy (due to local adipocyte destruction at injection sites) is uncommon.

Biguanides (Table 19–4)

- **Metformin** enhances insulin sensitivity of hepatic and peripheral (muscle) tissues, allowing for increased glucose uptake. It reduces A1C levels by 1.5% to 2% (16–22 mmol/mol Hb), FPG levels by 60 to 80 mg/dL (3.3–4.4 mmol/L), and retains ability to reduce FPG levels when very high (>300 mg/dL or >16.7 mmol/L). Metformin reduces plasma triglycerides and low-density lipoprotein (LDL) cholesterol by 8% to 15% and modestly increases high-density lipoprotein (HDL) cholesterol (2%). Because it does not increase pancreatic insulin release, hypoglycemia is uncommon when used alone.
- Metformin is often the drug of choice in patients with type 2 DM due to its efficacy, low cost, positive pleiotropic effects, and manageable side effect profile. It may cause a modest (2–3 kg) weight loss in overweight and obese patients. Because the

TABLE 19–4 Oral Agents for the Treatment of Type 2 Diabetes Mellitus

Drug Name (Generic Version Available? Y = yes, N = no)	Brand Name	Usual Dose (mg)	Recommended Starting Dosage (mg/day) Nonelderly	Recommended Starting Dosage (mg/day) Elderly	Maximal Dose (mg/day)	Pharmacokinetics/Drug Interactions
Sulfonylureas						
Acetohexamide (Y)	Dymelor		250	125–250	1500	Metabolized in liver; metabolite potency equal to parent compound; renally eliminated First-generation sulfonylureas, which bind to proteins ionically, are more likely to cause drug–drug interactions than second-generation sulfonylureas, which bind nonionically. Drugs that are inducers or inhibitors of CYP450 2C9 should be monitored carefully when used with a sulfonylurea
Chlorpropamide (Y)	Diabinese	250/day	250	100	500	Metabolized in liver; also excreted unchanged renally
Tolazamide (Y)	Tolinase	250/day	100–250	100	1000	Metabolized in liver; metabolite less active than parent compound; renally eliminated
Tolbutamide (Y)	Orinase	500–1000 BID	1000–2000	500–1000	3000	Metabolized in liver to inactive metabolites that are renally excreted
Glipizide (Y)	Glucotrol	5–10/day	5	2.5–5	40	Metabolized in liver to inactive metabolites. ALL: CYP2C9 strong inhibitors
Glipizide (Y)	Glucotrol XL	5–10/day	5	2.5–5	20	Slow-release form; do not cut tablet
Glyburide (Y)	DiaBeta Micronase	5–10/day	5	1.25–2.5	20	Metabolized in liver; elimination 1/2 renal, 1/2 feces. Two active metabolites. Low dose in renal insufficiency
Glyburide, micronized (Y)	Glynase	6/day	3	1.5–3	12	Better absorption from micronized preparation
Glimepiride (Y)	Amaryl	4/day	1–2	0.5–1	8	Metabolized in liver to inactive metabolites. Start lower dose in renal insufficiency

(continued)

TABLE 19–4	Oral Agents for the Treatment of Type 2 Diabetes Mellitus (Continued)					
Drug Name (Generic Version Available? Y = yes, N = no)	Brand Name	Usual Dose (mg)	Recommended Starting Dosage (mg/day)		Maximal Dose (mg/day)	Pharmacokinetics/Drug Interactions
			Nonelderly	Elderly		
Glinides						
Nateglinide (Y)	Starlix	120 with meals	120 with meals	120 with meals	120 mg 3 times a day	Rapidly absorbed and short half-life (1–1.5 hours) Nateglinide is predominantly metabolized by CYP2C9 (70%) and CYP3A4 (30%) to less active metabolites. Glucuronide conjugation then allows rapid renal elimination. No dosage adjustment is needed in moderate to severe renal insufficiency
Repaglinide (Y)	Prandin	2–4 with meals	0.5–1 with meals	0.5–1 with meals	16	Caution with gemfibrozil with trimethoprim—Increased and prolonged hypoglycemic reactions are possible and have been documented Repaglinide is highly protein bound, and is mainly metabolized by oxidative metabolism and glucuronidation. The CYP3A4 and 2C8 system is involved with metabolism Moderate to severe renal insufficiency does not affect repaglinide, but moderate to severe hepatic impairment may
Biguanides						
Metformin (Y)	Glucophage 2 g/day	500 mg twice a day	500 mg twice a day	Assess renal function	2550	Metformin is not metabolized and does not bind to plasma proteins. Metformin is eliminated by renal tubular secretion and glomerular filtration. Half-life of plasma metformin 6 hours, but red blood cells are a second compartment of distribution for metformin, delivering an effective half-life of 17 hours. The main depot of metformin is in the splanchnic tissue, specifically the large intestine Cimetidine competes for renal tubular secretion. May increase metformin levels

Metformin ER (Y)	Glucophage XR	Same as above	500–1000 mg with evening meal	Assess renal function	2550	
Metformin solution	Riomet	Same as above	500 mg daily	Assess renal function	2000	
Thiazolidinediones						
Pioglitazone (Y)	Actos	15–30/day	15	15	45	Pioglitazone is primarily metabolized by CYP2C8, a lesser extent by CYP3A4 (17%), and by hydroxylation/oxidation. The majority of pio-glitazone is eliminated in the feces with 15%–30% appearing in urine as metabolites (M-III and M-IV) are present, which have longer half-lives than parent compound. No dosage adjustment in moderate to severe renal disease, though edema must be monitored. Pioglitazone dose is recommended to be limited to 15 mg daily in combination with gemfibrozil
Rosiglitazone (N)	Avandia	2–4/day	2–4	2	8 mg/day or 4 mg twice a day	Rosiglitazone is metabolized by CYP2C8, and to a lesser extent by CYP2C9, and also by N-demethylation and hydroxylation. Two-thirds is found in urine and one-third in feces. Highly (>99%) bound to albumin. No dosage adjustment in moderate to severe renal disease, though edema must be monitored
α-Glucosidase inhibitors						
Acarbose (Y)	Precose	50 with meals	25 mg 1–3 times a day	25 mg 1–3 times a day	25–100 mg 3 times a day	Acarbose—Metabolites absorbed and eliminated in bile. Slow titration key for tolerability. Miglitol—Eliminated renally after absorption
Miglitol (Y)	Glyset	50 with meals	25 mg 1–3 times a day	25 mg 1–3 times a day	25–100 mg 3 times a day	

(continued)

TABLE 19–4 Oral Agents for the Treatment of Type 2 Diabetes Mellitus (*Continued*)

Drug Name (Generic Version Available? Y = yes, N = no)	Brand Name	Usual Dose (mg)	Recommended Starting Dosage (mg/day)		Maximal Dose (mg/day)	Pharmacokinetics/Drug Interactions
			Nonelderly	Elderly		
Sodium Glucose Cotransporter-2 inhibitors						
Canagliflozin (N)	Invokana	300/day	100–300 mg daily	100 mg daily	300 mg daily	Renal dosing—see text Glucuronidated into two inactive metabolites Systemic exposure to canagliflozin is increased in patients with renal impairment; however, the efficacy is reduced in patients with renal impairment due to the reduced filtered glucose load Canagliflozin—weak P-glycoprotein inhibitor—digoxin levels may need to be monitored. Rifampin—UGT inducer—significantly reduces canagliflozin levels. Use alternative drug
Dapagliflozin (N)	Farxiga	5/day	2.5–5 mg daily	2.5 mg daily	5 mg daily	Renal dosing—see text Dapagliflozin is highly protein bound (>90%) and only 2% is cleared by the kidneys. It is mostly glucuronidated by UGT in the liver to both an inactive (majority) and active (<1%) metabolites. The active metabolite is not produced in dapagliflozin doses below 50 mg
Empagliflozin (N)	Jardiance	25/day	10–25 mg daily	10 mg daily	25 mg daily	Renal dosing—see text Empagliflozin is mostly glucuronidated Rifampin—UGT inducer significantly reduces empagliflozin levels—use alternative drug
Dipeptidyl Peptidase-4 inhibitors						
Sitagliptin (N)	Januvia	100/day	100 mg daily	25–100 mg daily based on renal function	100 mg daily	50 mg daily if estimated creatinine clearance >30 to <50 mL/min (>0.5 to <0.83 mL/s); 25 mg if creatinine clearance <30 mL/min (<0.5 mL/s) Sitagliptin is metabolized approximately 20% by CYP450 3A4 with some CYP450 2C8. Neither an inhibitor nor inducer, but is a p-glycoprotein substrate, but had negligible effects on digoxin and cyclosporine A, increasing the AUC by only 30%

Saxagliptin (N)	Onglyza	5/day	5 mg daily	2.5–5 mg daily based on renal function	5 mg daily	2.5 mg daily if creatinine clearance <50 mL/min (<0.83 mL/s) or if on strong inhibitors of CYP3A4/5 1 active metabolite 5 hydroxy saxagliptin—½ as potent as saxagliptin Metabolism by CYP3A4 and strong inhibitors/inducers will affect levels Saxagliptin is a substrate for P-glycoprotein, but is neither an inhibitor nor inducer. Rifampin, an inducer, can decrease active levels by 50%
Linagliptin (N)	Tradjenta	5/day	5 mg daily	5 mg daily	5 mg daily	Not substantially eliminated by renal, found in feces. Do not use with strong inducer of CYP3A4/P-glycoprotein Excreted unchanged, mostly through bile. Renal excretion less than 5% Linagliptin is a weak to moderate inhibitor of CYP3A4, and a substrate for P-glycoprotein
Alogliptin (N)	Nesina	25 mg/day	25 mg daily	25 mg	25 mg	12.5 mg CrCl <60 mL/min (<1 mL/s), 6.25 mg <30 mL–15 mL/min (<0.5–0.25 mL/s). ~75% eliminated unchanged in urine No significant drug–drug interactions
Bile Acid Sequestrants						
Colesevelam (N)	Welchol	3.75 g/day	6 tablets daily or 3 tablets BID 1.875 g BID or 3.75 g daily	6 tablets daily or 3 tablets BID 1.875 g BID or 3.75 g daily	3.75 g/day	Colesevelam binds bile in the gut Absorption drug–drug interactions: levothyroxine, glyburide, and oral contraceptives Phenytoin, warfarin, digoxin, and fat-soluble vitamins (A, E, D, K) have postmarketing reports of altered absorption. Any fat soluble drug may be affected Medications suspected of an interaction should be moved at least 4 hours prior to dosing the colesevelam

(continued)

TABLE 19–4 Oral Agents for the Treatment of Type 2 Diabetes Mellitus (*Continued*)

Drug Name (Generic Version Available? Y = yes, N = no)	Brand Name	Usual Dose (mg)	Recommended Starting Dosage (mg/day)		Maximal Dose (mg/day)	Pharmacokinetics/Drug Interactions
			Nonelderly	Elderly		
Dopamine Agonist						
Bromocriptine mesylate (N)	Cycloset	3.2–4/day	1.6–4.8 mg daily	1.6–4.8 mg daily	4.8 mg daily	Bromocriptine is a quick release formulation Bioavailability may be increased ~50% if given with a meal. Peak plasma concentration is about 1 hour if taken without food, but with food it is 90–120 minutes Only ~7% reaches the systemic circulation due to gastrointestinal-based metabolism and first-pass metabolism Bromocriptine is extensively metabolized by the CYP3A4 pathway, and the majority (~95%) is excreted in the bile. The half-life is approximately 6 hours. Plasma exposure is increased in females by approximately 18%–30%, but no dosage adjustment is currently recommended Drug–drug interactions: Bromocriptine is extensively metabolized by CYP3A4 and strong inhibitors or inducers may change bromocriptine levels. Because bromocriptine is highly protein bound, it may increase the unbound fraction of other highly protein bound drugs Drug–disease interactions: Antipsychotics and psychotic disorders because they decrease dopamine activity; atypical antipsychotics because they may decrease the effectiveness of bromocriptine; and ergot-based therapy for migraines because bromocriptine may increase migraine and ergot-related nausea and vomiting Sympathomimetic drugs: case reports of hypertension and tachycardia when administered together

durability of response is only fair, many patients require additional therapy within 5 years. Early combination therapy, especially with agents that have low hypoglycemic risk, is recommended if the A1C is > 8.5% (69 mmol/mol Hb). Metformin can be added to any other antihyperglycemic therapy and is often continued when insulin is started; this reduces insulin dose requirements and the risk of hypoglycemia.

- Gastrointestinal side effects (abdominal discomfort, stomach upset, diarrhea) occur in about 30% of patients. These effects are usually mild and can be minimized by slow dose titration and taking it with or immediately after meals. Extended-release metformin may reduce GI side effects. Lactic acidosis occurs rarely; the risk is increased in states that increase lactic acid production or decrease its removal (eg, renal insufficiency, heart failure, shock, septicemia, severe lung or liver disease).
  - ✓ **Metformin immediate-release**: Start at 500 mg orally twice daily with meals and increase by 500 mg weekly as tolerated until reaching glycemic goals or 2500 mg/day. Doses above 2000 mg may be better tolerated given 3 times a day with meals. Metformin 850 mg can be dosed once daily and then increased every 2 weeks to maximum 850 mg three times daily (2550 mg/day).
  - ✓ **Metformin extended-release**: Start with 500 mg orally with the evening meal and increase by 500 mg weekly as tolerated to maximum single evening dose of 2000 mg/day. Administration two or three times daily may reduce GI side effects and improve glycemic control. The 750 mg tablets can be titrated weekly to a maximum dose of 2250 mg/day.
- Dosing in renal insufficiency should be based on estimated glomerular filtration rate (eGFR) rather than serum creatinine: Obtain the eGFR before beginning treatment and at least annually thereafter. Starting treatment in patients with an eGFR between 30 and 45 mL/min/1.73 m^2 is not recommended. If the eGFR falls below 45 mL/min/1.73 m^2 in a patient already taking metformin, assess the benefits and risks of continuing therapy. Metformin is contraindicated in patients with an eGFR <30 mL/min/1.73 m^2.

Glucagon-like Peptide 1 (GLP-1) Receptor Agonists

- GLP-1 receptor agonists enhance insulin secretion and suppress inappropriately high postprandial glucagon secretion, resulting in decreased hepatic glucose production, increased satiety, slowed gastric emptying, and weight loss. Compared to twice-daily exenatide, the once-weekly extended-release product results in greater reductions in A1C (1.6% vs. 0.9%) and FPG (35 mg/dL vs. 12 mg/dL). Liraglutide and dulaglutide reduce A1C by about 0.4% more than twice-daily exenatide. Albiglutide may be slightly less effective than liraglutide.
- Clinical practice guidelines recommend GLP-1 agonists as second-line therapy. It is reasonable to use a GLP-1 agonist instead of basal insulin if the A1C is less than 9% (75 mmol/mol Hb), the patient is overweight/obese, and there is no symptomatic hyperglycemia. The most common adverse effects are nausea, vomiting, and diarrhea.
  - ✓ **Exenatide** (Byetta): Initial dose 5 mcg SC twice daily, titrated to 10 mcg twice daily in 1 month if needed and as tolerated. It should be injected up to 60 minutes before the morning and evening meals.
  - ✓ **Exenatide extended-release** (Bydureon): 2 mg SC once weekly at any time of day, with or without meals.
  - ✓ **Liraglutide** (Victoza): Begin with 0.6 mg SC once daily (independent of meals) for 1 week, then increase to 1.2 mg daily for at least 1 week. If necessary, increase to maximum dose of 1.8 mg daily after at least 1 week.
  - ✓ **Albiglutide** (Tanzeum): Initiate at 30 mg SC once weekly without regard to meals. Dose can be increased to 50 mg once weekly for additional glycemic control.
  - ✓ **Dulaglutide** (Trulicity): Initiate at 0.75 mg SC once weekly at any time of day, with or without food. Dose can be increased to 1.5 mg SC once weekly for additional glycemic control.

Sulfonylureas

- Sulfonylureas enhance insulin secretion by binding to the sulfonylurea receptor SUR1 on pancreatic β-cells. All sulfonylureas are equally effective in lowering blood glucose when administered in equipotent doses. On average, the A1C falls by 1.5% to 2% with FPG reductions of 60 to 70 mg/dL (3.3–3.9 mmol/L). Tachyphylaxis to the insulin secretion effect occurs, leading to poor long-term durability of response in most patients.

- Sulfonylureas are inexpensive and have an extensive track record of safety and effectiveness, but they are generally a second-line option. Diabetologists often avoid them in favor of DPP-4 inhibitors or SLGT-2 inhibitors.

- The most common side effect is hypoglycemia. The lower the FPG upon initiation, the greater the likelihood for hypoglycemia. Those who skip meals, exercise vigorously, or lose a substantial amount of weight are also more prone to hypoglycemia. Weight gain is common (typically 1–2 kg). Patients with sulfa allergy rarely experience crossreactivity with sulfonylureas.

- The usual starting and maximal doses (**Table 19–4**) should be reduced in patients at high risk for hypoglycemia. Dosage can be titrated as soon as every 2 weeks (longer interval with chlorpropamide) to achieve glycemic goals.

Dipeptidyl Peptidase-4 (DPP-4) Inhibitors

- DPP-4 inhibitors prolong the half-life of endogenously produced GLP-1 and GIP, significantly reducing inappropriately elevated postprandial glucagon and improving β-cell response to hyperglycemia.

- DPP4-inhibitors are considered second-line therapy (or later). Monotherapy results in reduced glucose levels without increase in hypoglycemia. They do not alter gastric emptying, cause nausea, have significant effects on satiety, or cause weight gain/loss. In addition, they are given orally once daily, are well tolerated, and do not require dose titration. The average A1C reduction is 0.7% to 1% at maximum doses. Thus, their ability to lower BG is modest and they are expensive.

- The most common side effects include headache, nasopharyngitis, and upper respiratory infection. Urticaria and/or facial edema occur in 1% of patients, and discontinuation is warranted. Rare cases of Stevens–Johnson syndrome have been reported. Saxagliptin causes a dose-related reduction in absolute lymphocyte count; discontinuation should be considered if prolonged infection occurs. The labeling of saxagliptin and alogliptin includes information about increased risk of hospitalizations for heart failure.
  - ✓ **Sitagliptin** (Januvia): Usual dose 100 mg orally once daily. Use 50 mg daily if creatinine clearance (CrCl) is 30 to 50 mL/min and 25 mg daily if CrCl is less than 30 mL/min.
  - ✓ **Saxagliptin** (Onglyza): Usual dose 5 mg orally daily. Reduce to 2.5 mg daily if CrCl is less than 50 mL/min or strong CYP-3A4/5 inhibitors are used concurrently.
  - ✓ **Linagliptin** (Tradjenta): Usual dose 5 mg orally daily; dose adjustment is not required in renal insufficiency.
  - ✓ **Alogliptin** (Nesina): Usual dose 25 mg once daily. Decrease to 12.5 mg daily when CrCl is less than 60 mL/min and 6.25 mg when CrCl is less than 30 mL/min.

Sodium-Glucose Cotransporter-2 (SGLT-2) Inhibitors

- Inhibition of SGLT-2 lowers the renal tubular threshold for glucose reabsorption, and glucosuria occurs at lower plasma glucose concentrations. SGLT-2 inhibitors reduce A1C by 0.5% to 1% and can be used as either monotherapy or add-on therapy. They may also contribute to 1- to 5-kg weight loss and modestly reduce BP. They are unlikely to cause hypoglycemia unless combined with sulfonylureas, meglitinides, or insulin.

- In clinical practice guidelines, SGLT-2 inhibitors are considered second- or third-line therapy. Older adults and patients with stage 4 or 5 chronic kidney disease are not optimal treatment candidates. Concomitant diuretic use may cause orthostatic hypotension and electrolyte abnormalities; loop diuretics may need to be discontinued. Renal impairment decreases the efficacy of SGLT-2 inhibitors.

- The most common adverse effect is genitourinary tract infections, especially yeast infections, which occur more commonly in women and uncircumcised men.
  - ✓ **Canagliflozin** (Invokana): Initial dose is 100 mg orally once daily, taken before the first meal of the day. The dose may be increased to 300 mg once daily in patients with an eGFR 60 mL/min/1.73 m^2 or greater who require additional glycemic control. Limit the dose to 100 mg once daily in patients who have an eGFR between 45 and 60 mL/min/1.73 m^2 and discontinue therapy if the eGFR is less than 45 mL/min/1.73 m^2.
  - ✓ **Dapagliflozin** (Farxiga): Start at 5 mg orally once daily in the morning with or without food. The dose may be increased to 10 mg once daily in patients requiring additional glycemic control. It should not be started or continued if the eGFR is less than 60 mL/min/1.73 m^2.
  - ✓ **Empagliflozin** (Jardiance): Start at 10 mg orally once daily in the morning with or without food. The dose may be increased to 25 mg once daily. Therapy should not be started or continued if the eGFR is less than 45 mL/min/1.73 m^2.

Thiazolidinediones (Glitazones)

- TZDs bind to the peroxisome proliferator activator receptor-γ (PPAR-γ) located primarily on fat and vascular cells, enhancing insulin sensitivity in muscle, liver, and fat tissues indirectly. Insulin must be present in significant quantities, and the drugs are referred to as "insulin sensitizers." At maximal doses, pioglitazone and rosiglitazone reduce A1C by 1% to 1.5% and FPG by 60 to 70 mg/dL (3.3–3.9 mmol/L). Maximum effects may not be seen until 3 to 4 months of therapy.
- Pioglitazone decreases plasma triglycerides by 10% to 20%, whereas rosiglitazone tends to have no effect. Pioglitazone does not cause significant increases in LDL cholesterol, whereas LDL cholesterol may increase by 5% to 15% with rosiglitazone. Both drugs increase HDL, but the magnitude may be greater with pioglitazone.
- Fluid retention may occur, perhaps because of peripheral vasodilation and improved insulin sensitization in the kidney with increased sodium and water retention. This may result in peripheral edema (4%–5% of patients with monotherapy; 15% or more when combined with insulin), heart failure, hemodilution of hemoglobin and hematocrit, and weight gain. Edema is dose related, and if not severe may be managed by dose reduction and use of spironolactone, triamterene, or amiloride. TZDs are contraindicated in patients with New York Heart Association Class III or IV heart failure and should be used with caution in patients with Class I or II heart failure.
- Weight gain of 4 kg is not uncommon; both fluid retention and fat accumulation play roles in this effect. Rarely, rapid gain of a large amount of weight may necessitate discontinuation of therapy. TZDs have also been associated with an increased fracture rate in the upper and lower limbs of postmenopausal women. An increased risk of bladder cancer is controversial.
  - ✓ **Pioglitazone** (Actos): Initially, 15 mg to 30 mg orally once daily. The dose can be increased in 15-mg increments to 45 mg once daily if there is inadequate glycemic control.
  - ✓ **Rosiglitazone** (Avandia): Initiate with 2 to 4 mg orally once daily; the maximum dose is 8 mg/day. A dose of 4 mg twice daily can reduce A1C by 0.2% to 0.3% more than 8 mg taken once daily.

α-Glucosidase Inhibitors

- These agents delay the breakdown of sucrose and complex carbohydrates in the small intestine, prolonging carbohydrate absorption. The net effect is reduction in postprandial glucose (40–50 mg/dL; 2.2–2.8 mmol/L) with relatively unchanged FBG (~10% reduction). Efficacy is modest, with average A1C reduction 0.3% to 1%. Good candidates for these drugs are patients who are near target A1C levels with near-normal FPG levels but high postprandial levels.

- The most common side effects are flatulence, bloating, abdominal discomfort, and diarrhea, which can be minimized by slow dosage titration. If hypoglycemia occurs when used in combination with a hypoglycemic agent (sulfonylurea or insulin), oral or parenteral glucose (dextrose) products or glucagon must be given because the drug will inhibit breakdown and absorption of more complex sugar molecules (eg, sucrose).
  - ✓ **Acarbose** (Precose) and **miglitol** (Glyset): Initiate therapy with very low dose (25 mg orally with one meal a day) and increase very gradually (over several months) to maximum 50 mg three times daily for patients weighing 60 kg or more, or 100 mg three times daily for patients above 60 kg. The drugs should be taken with the first bite of the meal so the drug is present to inhibit enzyme activity.

Short-acting Insulin Secretagogues (Meglitinides or Glinides)

- Glinides stimulate insulin secretion from pancreatic β-cells by binding a site adjacent to the sulfonylurea receptor. They require the presence of glucose to stimulate insulin secretion; as glucose levels decrease to normal, stimulated insulin secretion diminishes. As monotherapy, they reduce postprandial glucose excursions and reduce A1C by 0.8% to 1%.
- These agents have been largely replaced by DPP-4 inhibitors and SGLT-2 inhibitors that offer lower risk of hypoglycemia, single-daily dosing, and similar or better glycemic reductions. Glinides may be useful in patients with renal insufficiency and those with erratic meal schedules.
- Glinides should be administered before each meal (up to 30 minutes prior). If a meal is skipped, the medication should also be skipped.
  - ✓ **Repaglinide** (Prandin): Start with 0.5 to 2 mg orally with maximum 4 mg per meal (up to four meals daily or 16 mg/day).
  - ✓ **Nateglinide** (Starlix): 120 mg orally three times daily before each meal. Initial dose may be lowered to 60 mg per meal in patients who are near goal A1C.

Amylinomimetics

- Pramlintide is a synthetic amylin analog that suppresses inappropriately high postprandial glucagon secretion, increases satiety, and slows gastric emptying. The average A1C reduction is 0.6% in patients with type 2 DM and 0.4% to 0.5% in type 1 DM.
- Clinical practice guidelines favor use of GLP-1 agonists and DPP-4 inhibitors instead of pramlintide to decrease inappropriate glucagon secretion.
- The most common adverse effects are nausea, vomiting, and anorexia. It does not cause hypoglycemia when used alone but is indicated only in patients receiving insulin, so hypoglycemia can occur. If a prandial insulin dose is used, reduce it by 30% to 50% when pramlintide is started to minimize severe hypoglycemic reactions.
- **Pramlintide** (Symlin): In type 1 DM, start with 15 mcg SC prior to each meal, titrating up in 15 mcg increments to maximum 60 mcg prior to each meal if tolerated and warranted. The starting dose for type 2 DM is 60 mcg SC prior to major meals; titrate up to 120 mcg per dose as tolerated and as warranted based on postprandial plasma glucose levels.

Bile Acid Sequestrants

- Colesevelam binds bile acid in the intestinal lumen, decreasing the bile acid pool for reabsorption. Its mechanism in lowering plasma glucose levels is unknown.
- A1C reductions from baseline were ~0.4% when colesevelam 3.8 g/day was added to stable metformin, sulfonylureas, or insulin. FPG was modestly reduced by 5 to 10 mg/dL (0.3–0.6 mmol/L). Colesevelam may also reduce LDL cholesterol by 12% to 16% in patients with type 2 DM. Triglycerides may increase when combined with sulfonylureas or insulin, but not with metformin. Colesevelam is weight neutral and has a low risk of hypoglycemia.

- Good candidates for this alternative medication are patients with type 2 DM who need a small A1C reduction as well as additional LDL-cholesterol lowering.
- The most common side effects are constipation and dyspepsia; it should be taken with a large amount of water. Colesevelam has multiple absorption-related drug–drug interactions.
- **Colesevelam** (Welchol): The dose for type 2 DM is six 625-mg tablets daily (total 3.75 g/day); the dose may be split into three tablets twice daily if desired. A 3.75-gram oral suspension packet dosed once daily or a 1.875-gram oral suspension packet dosed twice daily may also be used. Administer each dose with meals because colesevelam binds to bile acids released during the meal.

Dopamine Agonists

- The mechanisms by which bromocriptine improves glycemic control are unknown but may involve improved hepatic insulin sensitivity and decreased hepatic glucose output. It reduced A1C by 0.3% to 0.6% in clinical trials.
- The role of bromocriptine is unclear; it may be an alternative in combination with other agents.
- Common side effects include nausea, vomiting, constipation, fatigue, headache, dizziness, and asthenia. Somnolence occurs in about 5% of patients. Orthostatic hypotension may also occur.
- **Bromocriptine mesylate** (Cycloset): The initial dose is 0.8 mg orally daily taken with food within 2 hours of waking from sleep. The dose may be increased weekly based on response and side effects to a maximum of 4.8 mg daily. The dose should be skipped if the morning window for administration is missed.

TREATMENT OF COMPLICATIONS

Retinopathy

- Early background retinopathy may reverse with improved glycemic control and optimal BP control. More advanced retinopathy will not fully regress with improved control, and aggressive glucose reduction may acutely worsen retinopathy.
- Laser photocoagulation has markedly improved sight preservation in diabetic patients. Intravitreal antivascular endothelial growth factor (VEGF) therapy is also highly effective for sight preservation. **Bevacizumab** (used off label) and **ranibizumab** are anti-VEGF monoclonal antibodies, and **aflibercept** is a VEGF decoy receptor.

Neuropathy

- Distal symmetrical peripheral neuropathy is the most common complication in patients with type 2 DM. Paresthesias, numbness, or pain are the predominant symptoms. The feet are involved far more often than the hands. Improved glycemic control is the primary treatment and may alleviate some symptoms.
- Pharmacologic therapy is symptomatic and empiric, including low-dose **tricyclic antidepressants, gabapentin, pregabalin, carbamazepine, duloxetine, venlafaxine, topical capsaicin, tramadol**, and **nonsteroidal anti-inflammatory drugs**.
- Gastroparesis can be severe and debilitating. Improved glycemic control, discontinuation of medications that slow gastric motility, and use of **metoclopramide** for only a few weeks at a time or low-dose **erythromycin** may be helpful.
- Diabetic diarrhea is commonly nocturnal and frequently responds to a 10- to 14-day course of an antibiotic such as **doxycycline** or **metronidazole**. **Octreotide** may be useful in unresponsive cases.
- Patients with orthostatic hypotension may require mineralocorticoids or adrenergic agonists.
- Erectile dysfunction is common, and initial therapy should include a trial of an oral phosphodiesterase-5 inhibitor (eg, **sildenafil, vardenafil**, or **tadalafil**).

Nephropathy

- Glucose and BP control are important for preventing and slowing progression of nephropathy.
- Angiotensin-converting enzyme (ACE) inhibitors and angiotensin receptor blockers (ARBs) have shown efficacy in preventing the progression of renal disease in patients with diabetes. Diuretics are frequently necessary due to volume-expanded states and are recommended second-line therapy.

Peripheral Arterial Disease and Foot Ulcers

- Claudication and nonhealing foot ulcers are common in type 2 DM. Smoking cessation, correction of dyslipidemia, good glycemic control, and antiplatelet therapy are important treatment strategies.
- **Cilostazol** (Pletal) may reduce symptoms in select patients. Revascularization is successful with some patients.
- Local debridement and appropriate footwear and foot care are important in the early treatment of foot lesions. Topical treatments and other measures may be beneficial in more advanced lesions.

Coronary Heart Disease

- Multiple risk factor intervention (treatment of dyslipidemia and hypertension, smoking cessation, and antiplatelet therapy) reduces macrovascular events.
- **Aspirin** (75 to 162 mg daily) is recommended in all patients with established CVD. **Clopidogrel** may be used in patients allergic to aspirin. Antiplatelet therapy is recommended for primary prevention if the 10-year risk of CVD is at least 10% or in patients at least 40 years old with an additional risk factor.
- Statin therapy is recommended regardless of baseline lipid levels in patients with overt CVD or without CVD who are over the age of 40 or have CVD risk factors other than diabetes. Patients aged 40 to 75 years with established CVD or an estimated 10-year risk of more than 7.5% should receive high-intensity statin therapy (**atorvastatin** 40 to 80 mg/day; **rosuvastatin** 20–40 mg/day). All others may receive moderate-intensity statin treatment (**atorvastatin** 10–20 mg; **rosuvastatin** 5–10 mg; **simvastatin** 20–40 mg; **pravastatin** 40–80 mg; **lovastatin** 40 mg; **fluvastatin XL** 80 mg). Extremely elevated triglycerides may require additional therapy (eg, fibrates, omega-3 fatty acids, niacin).

Hypertension

- The American Diabetes Association recommends a goal BP less than 140/80 mm Hg in patients with DM. A systolic BP goal of less than 130 mm Hg can be considered in younger patients, patients at high risk of a stroke, or if renal disease is present. **ACE inhibitors** and **ARBs** are recommended for initial therapy. Many patients require multiple agents (three on average), so **diuretics** and **calcium channel blockers** are useful as second and third agents.

EVALUATION OF THERAPEUTIC OUTCOMES

- To follow long-term glycemic control for the previous 3 months, measure A1C at least twice a year in patients meeting treatment goals on a stable therapeutic regimen (see Table 19–1).
- At each visit, ask patients with type 1 DM about the frequency and severity of hypoglycemia. Document any hypoglycemic episodes requiring assistance of another person, medical attention, or hospitalization and take steps to prevent future episodes.
- Screen for complications at the time of diagnosis and thereafter as follows:
  ✓ Obtain yearly dilated eye exams in type 2 DM and an initial exam in the first 5 years in type 1 DM, then yearly.
  ✓ Assess BP at each visit.

✓ Examine the feet at each visit, including palpation of distal pulses and visual inspection for skin integrity, calluses, and deformities.

✓ Screen for pedal sensory loss annually using a 10-g force monofilament.

✓ Screen for nephropathy with urine microalbumin at the time of diagnosis in patients with type 2 DM and 5 years after diagnosis in type 1 DM. At least once a year, assess urinary albumin (urine albumin-to-creatinine ratio) and eGFR in all patients with type 2 DM and in patients with type 1 DM for at least 5 years.

✓ Check fasting lipid panel annually if the patient is on lipid-lowering therapy.

• Administer an annual influenza vaccine and assess for administration of the pneumococcal vaccine and hepatitis B vaccine series along with management of other cardiovascular risk factors (eg, smoking and antiplatelet therapy).

See Chapter 74, Diabetes Mellitus, authored by Curtis L. Triplitt, Thomas Repas, and Carlos Alvarez, for a more detailed discussion of this topic.

Thyroid Disorders

- *Thyroid disorders* involve thyroid hormone production or secretion and result in alterations in metabolic stability.

THYROID HORMONE PHYSIOLOGY

- Thyroid hormones: thyroxine (T_4) and triiodothyronine (T_3) are formed on thyroglobulin, a large glycoprotein synthesized within the thyroid cell. Inorganic iodide enters the thyroid follicular cell and is oxidized by thyroid peroxidase and covalently bound (organified) to tyrosine residues of thyroglobulin.
- Iodinated tyrosine residues monoiodotyrosine (MIT) and diiodotyrosine (DIT) combine (couple) to form iodothyronines in reactions catalyzed by thyroid peroxidase. Thus, two molecules of DIT combine to form T_4, and MIT and DIT join to form T_3.
- Proteolysis within thyroid cells releases thyroid hormone into the bloodstream. T_4 and T_3 are transported by thyroid-binding globulin (TBG), transthyretin, and albumin. Only the unbound (free) thyroid hormone can diffuse into cells, elicit biologic effects, and regulate thyroid-stimulating hormone (TSH) secretion from the pituitary.
- T_4 is secreted solely from the thyroid, but less than 20% of T_3 is produced there; most T_3 is formed from breakdown of T_4 catalyzed by the enzyme 5′-monodeiodinase in peripheral tissues. T_3 is five times more active than T_4. T_4 may also be acted on by 5′-monodeiodinase to form reverse T_3, which has no significant biologic activity.
- Thyroid hormone production is regulated by TSH secreted by the anterior pituitary, which in turn is under negative feedback control by the circulating level of free thyroid hormone and the positive influence of hypothalamic thyrotropin-releasing hormone (TRH). Thyroid hormone production is also regulated by extrathyroidal deiodination of T_4 to T_3, which can be affected by nutrition, nonthyroidal hormones, drugs, and illness.

THYROTOXICOSIS (HYPERTHYROIDISM)

PATHOPHYSIOLOGY

- Thyrotoxicosis results when tissues are exposed to excessive levels of T_4, T_3, or both. Hyperthyroidism, which is one cause of thyrotoxicosis, refers to overproduction of thyroid hormone by the thyroid gland.
- TSH-secreting pituitary tumors occur sporadically and release biologically active hormone that is unresponsive to normal feedback control. The tumors may cosecrete prolactin or growth hormone; therefore, patients may present with amenorrhea, galactorrhea, or signs of acromegaly.
- Resistance to thyroid hormone occurs rarely and can be due to various molecular defects, including mutations in the TRβ gene. Pituitary resistance to thyroid hormone (PRTH) refers to selective resistance of the pituitary thyrotrophs to thyroid hormone.
- Graves' disease is the most common cause of hyperthyroidism, which results from the action of thyroid-stimulating antibodies (TSAb) directed against the thyrotropin receptor on the surface of thyroid cell. These immunoglobulins bind to the receptor and activate the enzyme adenylate cyclase in the same manner as TSH.
- An autonomous thyroid nodule (toxic adenoma) is a thyroid mass whose function is independent of pituitary control. Hyperthyroidism usually occurs with larger nodules (>3 cm in diameter).
- In multinodular goiter, follicles with autonomous function coexist with normal or even nonfunctioning follicles. Thyrotoxicosis occurs when autonomous follicles generate more thyroid hormone than is required.
- Painful subacute (granulomatous or de Quervain) thyroiditis often develops after a viral syndrome, but rarely has a specific virus been identified in thyroid parenchyma.

- Painless (silent, lymphocytic, or postpartum) thyroiditis is a common cause of thyrotoxicosis; its etiology is not fully understood; autoimmunity may underlie most cases.
- Thyrotoxicosis factitia is hyperthyroidism produced by ingestion of exogenous thyroid hormone. This may occur when thyroid hormone is used for inappropriate indications, excessive doses are used for accepted medical indications, there is accidental ingestion, or it is used surreptitiously.
- Amiodarone may induce thyrotoxicosis (2%–3% of patients) or hypothyroidism. It interferes with type I $5'$-deiodinase, leading to reduced conversion of T_4 to T_3, and iodide release from the drug may contribute to iodine excess. Amiodarone also causes a destructive thyroiditis with loss of thyroglobulin and thyroid hormones.

CLINICAL PRESENTATION

- Symptoms of thyrotoxicosis include nervousness, anxiety, palpitations, emotional lability, easy fatigability, heat intolerance, weight loss concurrent with increased appetite, increased frequency of bowel movements, proximal muscle weakness (noted on climbing stairs or arising from a sitting position), and scanty or irregular menses in women.
- Physical signs include warm, smooth, moist skin, and unusually fine hair; separation of the ends of the fingernails from the nail beds (onycholysis); retraction of the eyelids and lagging of the upper lid behind the globe upon downward gaze (lid lag); tachycardia at rest, widened pulse pressure, and systolic ejection murmur; occasional gynecomastia in men; fine tremor of the protruded tongue and outstretched hands; and hyperactive deep tendon reflexes. Thyromegaly is usually present.
- Graves' disease is manifested by hyperthyroidism, diffuse thyroid enlargement, and extrathyroidal findings of exophthalmos, pretibial myxedema, and thyroid acropachy. In severe disease, a thrill may be felt and a systolic bruit may be heard over the gland.
- In subacute thyroiditis, patients have severe pain in the thyroid region, which often extends to the ear. Systemic symptoms include fever, malaise, myalgia, and signs and symptoms of thyrotoxicosis. The thyroid gland is firm and exquisitely tender on physical examination.
- Painless thyroiditis has a triphasic course that mimics painful subacute thyroiditis. Most patients present with mild thyrotoxic symptoms; lid retraction and lid lag are present, but exophthalmos is absent. The thyroid gland may be diffusely enlarged without tenderness.
- Thyroid storm is a life-threatening medical emergency characterized by decompensated thyrotoxicosis, high fever (often >39.4°C [103°F]), tachycardia, tachypnea, dehydration, delirium, coma, nausea, vomiting, and diarrhea. Precipitating factors include infection, trauma, surgery, radioactive iodine (RAI) treatment, and withdrawal from antithyroid drugs.

DIAGNOSIS

- Elevated 24-hour radioactive iodine uptake (RAIU) indicates true hyperthyroidism: the patient's thyroid gland is overproducing T_4, T_3, or both (normal RAIU 10%–30%). A low RAIU indicates that excess thyroid hormone is not a consequence of thyroid gland hyperfunction but is likely caused by thyroiditis or hormone ingestion.
- TSH-induced hyperthyroidism is diagnosed by evidence of peripheral hypermetabolism, diffuse thyroid gland enlargement, elevated free thyroid hormone levels, and elevated serum immunoreactive TSH concentrations. Because the pituitary gland is extremely sensitive to even minimal elevations of free T_4, a "normal" or elevated TSH level in any thyrotoxic patient indicates inappropriate production of TSH.
- TSH-secreting pituitary adenomas are diagnosed by demonstrating lack of TSH response to TRH stimulation, inappropriate TSH levels, elevated TSH α-subunit levels, and radiologic imaging.
- In thyrotoxic Graves' disease, there is an increase in the overall hormone production rate with a disproportionate increase in T_3 relative to T_4 (Table 20–1). Saturation of TBG is increased due to elevated serum levels of T_4 and T_3, which is reflected in elevated T_3

TABLE 20–1	Thyroid Function Tests in Different Thyroid Conditions			
	Total T$_4$	Free T$_4$	Total T$_3$	TSH
Normal	4.5–10.9 mcg/dL	0.8–2.7 ng/dL	60–181 ng/dL	0.5–4.7 milli-international units/L
Hyperthyroid	↑↑	↑↑	↑↑↑	↓↓*
Hypothyroid	↓↓	↓↓	↓	↑↑*
Increased TBG	↑	Normal	↑	Normal

*Primary thyroid disease.

resin uptake. As a result, concentrations of free T$_4$, free T$_3$, and the free T$_4$ and T$_3$ indices are increased to an even greater extent than the measured serum total T$_4$ and T$_3$ concentrations. The TSH level is undetectable due to negative feedback by elevated levels of thyroid hormone at the pituitary. In patients with manifest disease, measurement of serum free T$_4$ (or total T$_4$ and T$_3$ resin uptake), total T$_3$, and TSH will confirm the diagnosis of thyrotoxicosis. If the patient is not pregnant, an increased 24-hour RAIU documents that the thyroid gland is inappropriately using iodine to produce more thyroid hormone when the patient is thyrotoxic.

- For toxic adenomas, because there may be isolated elevation of serum T$_3$ with autonomously functioning nodules, a T$_3$ level must be measured to rule out T$_3$ toxicosis if the T$_4$ level is normal. If autonomous function is suspected, but the TSH is normal, the diagnosis can be confirmed by failure of the autonomous nodule to decrease iodine uptake during exogenous T$_3$ administration sufficient to suppress TSH.
- In multinodular goiters, a thyroid scan shows patchy areas of autonomously functioning thyroid tissue.
- A low RAIU indicates the excess thyroid hormone is not a consequence of thyroid gland hyperfunction. This may be seen in painful subacute thyroiditis, painless thyroiditis, struma ovarii, follicular cancer, and factitious ingestion of exogenous thyroid hormone.
- In subacute thyroiditis, thyroid function tests typically run a triphasic course in this self-limited disease. Initially, serum T$_4$ levels are elevated due to release of preformed thyroid hormone. The 24-hour RAIU during this time is less than 2% because of thyroid inflammation and TSH suppression by the elevated T$_4$ level. As the disease progresses, intrathyroidal hormone stores are depleted, and the patient may become mildly hypothyroid with appropriately elevated TSH level. During the recovery phase, thyroid hormone stores are replenished, and serum TSH elevation gradually returns to normal.
- During the thyrotoxic phase of painless thyroiditis, the 24-hour RAIU is suppressed to less than 2%. Antithyroglobulin and antithyroid peroxidase antibody levels are elevated in more than 50% of patients.
- Thyrotoxicosis factitia should be suspected in a thyrotoxic patient without evidence of increased hormone production, thyroidal inflammation, or ectopic thyroid tissue. The RAIU is low because thyroid gland function is suppressed by exogenous thyroid hormone. Measurement of plasma thyroglobulin reveals presence of very low levels.

TREATMENT

- <u>Goals of Treatment</u>: Eliminate excess thyroid hormone; minimize symptoms and long-term consequences; and provide individualized therapy based on the type and severity of disease, patient age and gender, existence of nonthyroidal conditions, and response to previous therapy.

Nonpharmacologic Therapy

- Surgical removal of the thyroid gland should be considered in patients with a large gland (>80 g), severe ophthalmopathy, or lack of remission on antithyroid drug treatment.

- If thyroidectomy is planned, **methimazole** is usually given until the patient is biochemically euthyroid (usually 6–8 weeks), followed by addition of **iodides** (500 mg/day) for 10 to 14 days before surgery to decrease vascularity of the gland. **Levothyroxine** may be added to maintain the euthyroid state while thionamides are continued.
- **Propranolol** has been used for several weeks preoperatively and 7 to 10 days after surgery to maintain pulse rate less than 90 beats/min. Combined pretreatment with propranolol and 10 to 14 days of **potassium iodide** also has been advocated.

Pharmacologic Therapy

THIOUREAS (THIONAMIDES)

- **Methimazole** and **Propylthiouracil (PTU)** block thyroid hormone synthesis by inhibiting the peroxidase enzyme system of the thyroid, preventing oxidation of trapped iodide and subsequent incorporation into iodotyrosines and ultimately iodothyronine ("organification"); and by inhibiting coupling of MIT and DIT to form T_4 and T_3. PTU (but not methimazole) also inhibits peripheral conversion of T_4 to T_3.
- Usual initial doses include methimazole 30 to 60 mg daily given in two or three divided doses or PTU 300 to 600 mg daily (usually in three or four divided doses). Evidence exists that both drugs can be given as a single daily dose.
- Improvement in symptoms and laboratory abnormalities should occur within 4 to 8 weeks, at which time a tapering regimen to maintenance doses can be started. Make dosage change monthly because the endogenously produced T_4 will reach a new steady-state concentration in this interval. Typical daily maintenance doses are methimazole 5 to 30 mg and PTU 50 to 300 mg. Continue therapy for 12 to 24 months to induce long-term remission.
- Monitor patients every 6 to 12 months after remission. If a relapse occurs, alternate therapy with RAI is preferred to a second course of antithyroid drugs, because subsequent courses are less likely to induce remission.
- Minor adverse reactions include pruritic maculopapular rashes, arthralgias, fever, and benign transient leukopenia (white blood cell count <4000/mm³ or 4×10^9/L). The alternate thiourea may be tried in these situations, but cross-sensitivity occurs in about 50% of patients.
- Major adverse effects include agranulocytosis (with fever, malaise, gingivitis, oropharyngeal infection, and granulocyte count <250/mm³ or 0.25×10^9/L), aplastic anemia, lupus-like syndrome, polymyositis, GI intolerance, hepatotoxicity, and hypoprothrombinemia. If agranulocytosis occurs, it usually develops in the first 3 months of therapy; routine WBC count monitoring is not recommended because of its sudden onset.
- Because of the risk of serious hepatotoxicity, PTU should not be considered first-line therapy in either adults or children. Exceptions to this recommendation include: (1) the first trimester of pregnancy (when the risk of methimazole-induced embryopathy may exceed that of PTU-induced hepatotoxicity), (2) intolerance to methimazole, and (3) thyroid storm.

IODIDES

- **Iodide** acutely blocks thyroid hormone release, inhibits thyroid hormone biosynthesis by interfering with intrathyroidal iodide use, and decreases size and vascularity of the gland.
- Symptom improvement occurs within 2 to 7 days of initiating therapy, and serum T_4 and T_3 concentrations may be reduced for a few weeks.
- Iodides are often used as adjunctive therapy to prepare a patient with Graves' disease for surgery, to acutely inhibit thyroid hormone release and quickly attain the euthyroid state in severely thyrotoxic patients with cardiac decompensation, or to inhibit thyroid hormone release after RAI therapy.
- **Potassium iodide** is available as a saturated solution (**SSKI**, 38 mg iodide per drop) or as **Lugol solution**, containing 6.3 mg of iodide per drop.

- Typical starting dose of SSKI is 3 to 10 drops daily (120–400 mg) in water or juice. When used to prepare a patient for surgery, it should be administered 7 to 14 days preoperatively.
- As an adjunct to RAI, SSKI should not be used before but rather 3 to 7 days after RAI treatment so the RAI can concentrate in the thyroid.
- Adverse effects include hypersensitivity reactions (skin rashes, drug fever, and rhinitis, conjunctivitis), salivary gland swelling, "iodism" (metallic taste, burning mouth and throat, sore teeth and gums, symptoms of a head cold, and sometimes stomach upset and diarrhea), and gynecomastia.

ADRENERGIC BLOCKERS

- β-Blockers are used to ameliorate symptoms such as palpitations, anxiety, tremor, and heat intolerance. They have no effect on peripheral thyrotoxicosis and protein metabolism and do not reduce TSAb or prevent thyroid storm. **Propranolol** and **nadolol** partially block conversion of T_4 to T_3, but this contribution to overall effect is small.
- β-Blockers are usually used as adjunctive therapy with antithyroid drugs, RAI, or iodides when treating Graves' disease or toxic nodules; in preparation for surgery; or in thyroid storm. The only conditions for which β-blockers are primary therapy for thyrotoxicosis are those associated with thyroiditis.
- **Propranolol** doses required to relieve adrenergic symptoms vary, but an initial dose of 20 to 40 mg orally four times daily is effective for most patients (heart rate <90 beats/min). Younger or more severely toxic patients may require 240 to 480 mg/day, perhaps because of increased clearance.
- β-Blockers are contraindicated in decompensated heart failure unless it is caused solely by tachycardia (high output). Other contraindications are sinus bradycardia, concomitant therapy with monoamine oxidase inhibitors or tricyclic antidepressants, and patients with spontaneous hypoglycemia. Side effects include nausea, vomiting, anxiety, insomnia, lightheadedness, bradycardia, and hematologic disturbances.
- Centrally acting sympatholytics (eg, **clonidine**) and calcium channel antagonists (eg, **diltiazem**) may be useful for symptom control when contraindications to β-blockade exist.

RADIOACTIVE IODINE

- **Sodium iodide–131** is an oral liquid that concentrates in the thyroid and initially disrupts hormone synthesis by incorporating into thyroid hormones and thyroglobulin. Over a period of weeks, follicles that have taken up RAI and surrounding follicles develop evidence of cellular necrosis and fibrosis of interstitial tissue.
- RAI is the agent of choice for Graves' disease, toxic autonomous nodules, and toxic multinodular goiters. Pregnancy is an absolute contraindication to use of RAI because radiation would be delivered to the fetal tissue.
- β-Blockers are the primary adjunctive therapy to RAI because they may be given anytime without compromising RAI therapy.
- If iodides are administered, they should be given 3 to 7 days after RAI to prevent interference with uptake of RAI in the thyroid gland.
- Patients with cardiac disease and elderly patients are often treated with thionamides prior to RAI ablation because thyroid hormone levels transiently increase after RAI treatment due to release of preformed thyroid hormone.
- Administering antithyroid drug therapy immediately after RAI may result in a higher rate of posttreatment recurrence or persistent hyperthyroidism.
- Use of lithium as adjunctive therapy to RAI has benefits of increased cure rate, shortened time to cure, and prevention of posttherapy increases in thyroid hormone levels.
- The goal of therapy is to destroy overactive thyroid cells, and a single dose of 4000 to 8000 rad (40–80 Gy) results in a euthyroid state in 60% of patients at 6 months or sooner. A second dose of RAI should be given 6 months after the first RAI treatment if the patient remains hyperthyroid.

TABLE 20–2	Drug Dosages Used in the Management of Thyroid Storm
Drug	**Regimen**
Propylthiouracil	900–1200 mg/day orally in four or six divided doses
Methimazole	90–120 mg/day orally in four or six divided doses
Sodium iodide	Up to 2 g/day IV in single or divided doses
Lugol solution	5–10 drops three times a day in water or juice
Saturated solution of potassium iodide	1–2 drops three times a day in water or juice
Propranolol	40–80 mg every 6 hours
Dexamethasone	5–20 mg/day orally or IV in divided doses
Prednisone	25–100 mg/day orally in divided doses
Methylprednisolone	20–80 mg/day IV in divided doses
Hydrocortisone	100–400 mg/day IV in divided doses

- Hypothyroidism commonly occurs months to years after RAI. The acute, short-term side effects include mild thyroidal tenderness and dysphagia. Long-term follow-up has not revealed an increased risk for development of mutations or congenital defects.

Treatment of Thyroid Storm

- Initiate the following therapeutic measures promptly: (1) suppression of thyroid hormone formation and secretion, (2) antiadrenergic therapy, (3) administration of corticosteroids, and (4) treatment of associated complications or coexisting factors that may have precipitated the storm (Table 20–2).
- **PTU** in large doses may be the preferred thionamide because it blocks peripheral conversion of T_4 to T_3 in addition to interfering with thyroid hormone production. However, β-blockers and corticosteroids serve the same purpose. **Methimazole** has a longer duration of action, which offers a theoretical advantage.
- **Iodides**, which rapidly block the release of preformed thyroid hormone, should be administered after a thionamide is initiated to inhibit iodide utilization by the overactive gland.
- Antiadrenergic therapy with the short-acting agent **esmolol** is preferred because it can be used in patients with pulmonary disease or at risk for cardiac failure and because its effects can be rapidly reversed.
- **Corticosteroids** are generally recommended, but there is no convincing evidence of adrenocortical insufficiency in thyroid storm; their benefits may be attributed to their antipyretic action and stabilization of blood pressure (BP).
- General supportive measures, including **acetaminophen** as an antipyretic (avoid aspirin or other nonsteroidal anti-inflammatory drugs, which may displace bound thyroid hormone), **fluid and electrolyte replacement, sedatives, digoxin, antiarrhythmics, insulin,** and **antibiotics** should be given as indicated.

EVALUATION OF THERAPEUTIC OUTCOMES

- After therapy (surgery, thionamides, or RAI) for hyperthyroidism has been initiated, evaluate patients monthly until they reach a euthyroid condition.
- Assess for clinical signs of continuing thyrotoxicosis or development of hypothyroidism.
- If T_4 replacement is initiated, the goal is to maintain both the free T_4 level and the TSH concentration in the normal range. Once a stable dose of T_4 is identified, monitor the patient every 6 to 12 months.

HYPOTHYROIDISM

PATHOPHYSIOLOGY

- The vast majority of patients have primary hypothyroidism due to thyroid gland failure from chronic autoimmune thyroiditis (Hashimoto disease). Defects in suppressor T lymphocyte function lead to survival of a randomly mutating clone of helper T lymphocytes directed against antigens on the thyroid membrane. The resulting interaction stimulates B lymphocytes to produce thyroid antibodies.
- Iatrogenic hypothyroidism follows exposure to destructive amounts of radiation, after total thyroidectomy, or with excessive thionamide doses used to treat hyperthyroidism. Other causes of primary hypothyroidism include iodine deficiency, enzymatic defects within the thyroid, thyroid hypoplasia, and ingestion of goitrogens.
- Secondary hypothyroidism due to pituitary failure is uncommon. Pituitary insufficiency may be caused by destruction of thyrotrophs by pituitary tumors, surgical therapy, external pituitary radiation, postpartum pituitary necrosis (Sheehan syndrome), trauma, and infiltrative processes of the pituitary (eg, metastatic tumors and tuberculosis).

CLINICAL PRESENTATION

- Symptoms of hypothyroidism include dry skin, cold intolerance, weight gain, constipation, weakness, lethargy, fatigue, muscle cramps, myalgia, stiffness, and loss of ambition or energy. In children, thyroid hormone deficiency may manifest as growth or intellectual retardation.
- Physical signs include coarse skin and hair, cold or dry skin, periorbital puffiness, bradycardia, and slowed or hoarse speech. Objective weakness (with proximal muscles affected more than distal muscles) and slow relaxation of deep tendon reflexes are common. Reversible neurologic syndromes such as carpal tunnel syndrome, polyneuropathy, and cerebellar dysfunction may also occur.
- Most patients with secondary hypothyroidism due to inadequate TSH production have clinical signs of generalized pituitary insufficiency, such as abnormal menses and decreased libido, or evidence of a pituitary adenoma, such as visual field defects, galactorrhea, or acromegaloid features.
- Myxedema coma is a rare consequence of decompensated hypothyroidism manifested by hypothermia, advanced stages of hypothyroid symptoms, and altered sensorium ranging from delirium to coma. Mortality rates of 60% to 70% necessitate immediate and aggressive therapy.

DIAGNOSIS

- A rise in TSH level is the first evidence of primary hypothyroidism. Many patients have a free T_4 level within the normal range (compensated hypothyroidism) and few, if any, symptoms of hypothyroidism. As the disease progresses, the free T_4 drops below normal. The T_3 concentration is often maintained in the normal range despite low T_4. Antithyroid peroxidase antibodies and antithyroglobulin antibodies are usually elevated. The RAIU is not useful in evaluation of hypothyroidism because it can be low, normal, or elevated.
- Pituitary failure (secondary hypothyroidism) should be suspected in patients with decreased T_4 levels and inappropriately normal or low TSH levels.

TREATMENT OF HYPOTHYROIDISM (TABLE 20–3)

- <u>Goals of Treatment</u>: Restore thyroid hormone concentrations in tissue, provide symptomatic relief, prevent neurologic deficits in newborns and children, and reverse the biochemical abnormalities of hypothyroidism.
- **Levothyroxine** (L-thyroxine, T_4) is the drug of choice for thyroid hormone replacement and suppressive therapy because it is chemically stable, relatively inexpensive, active when given orally, free of antigenicity, and has uniform potency. Because T_3 (and not T_4) is the biologically active form, levothyroxine administration results in a pool of thyroid hormone that is readily and consistently converted to T_3.

TABLE 20–3	Thyroid Preparations Used in the Treatment of Hypothyroidism		
Drug/Dosage Form	**Content**	**Relative Dose**	**Comments/Equivalency**
Thyroid USP Armour Thyroid, Nature-Throid, and Westhroid (T_4:T_3 ratio approximately 4.2:1); Armour, 1 grain = 60 mg; Nature-Throid and Westhroid, 1 grain = 65 mg. Doses include 1/4, 1/2, 1, 2, 3, 4, and 5 grain tablets	Desiccated pork thyroid gland	1 grain (equivalent to 74 mcg [~60–100] mcg of T_4)	High T_3:T_4 ratio; inexpensive
Levothyroxine Synthroid, Levothroid, Levoxyl, Levo-T, Unithroid, and other generics 25, 50, 75, 88, 100, 112, 125, 137, 150, 175, 200, 300 mcg tablets; Tirosint 13–150 mcg liquid in gelatin capsule; 200 and 500 mcg per vial injection	Synthetic T_4	100 mcg	Stable; predictable potency; generics may be bioequivalent; when switching from natural thyroid to L-thyroxine, lower dose by one half grain; variable absorption between products; half-life = 7 days, so daily dosing; considered to be drug of choice
Liothyronine Cytomel 5, 25, and 50 mcg tablets	Synthetic T_3	33 mcg (~equivalent to 100 mcg T_4)	Uniform absorption, rapid onset; half-life = 1.5 days, rapid peak and troughs
Liotrix Thyrolar 1/4-, 1/2-, 1-, 2-, and 3-grain tablets	Synthetic T_4:T_3 in 4:1 ratio	Thyrolar 1 = 50 mcg T_4 and 12.5 mcg T_3	Stable; predictable; expensive; risk of T_3 thyrotoxicosis because of high ratio of T_3 relative to T_4

- In patients with long-standing disease and older individuals without known cardiac disease, start therapy with levothyroxine 50 mcg daily and increase after 1 month.
- The recommended initial dose for older patients with known cardiac disease is 25 mcg/day titrated upward in increments of 25 mcg at monthly intervals to prevent stress on the cardiovascular system.
- The average maintenance dose for most adults is ~125 mcg/day, but there is a wide range of replacement doses, necessitating individualized therapy and appropriate TSH monitoring to determine an appropriate dose.
- Although treatment of subclinical hypothyroidism is controversial, patients presenting with marked elevations in TSH (>10 mIU/L) and high titers of thyroid peroxidase antibody or prior treatment with sodium iodide–131 may be most likely to benefit from treatment.
- Levothyroxine is the drug of choice for pregnant women, and the goal is to decrease TSH to the normal reference range for pregnancy.
- Cholestyramine, calcium carbonate, sucralfate, aluminum hydroxide, ferrous sulfate, soybean formula, dietary fiber supplements, and espresso coffee may impair the GI absorption of levothyroxine. Drugs that increase nondeiodinative T_4 clearance include rifampin, carbamazepine, and possibly phenytoin. Selenium deficiency and amiodarone may block conversion of T_4 to T_3.

- **Thyroid USP** (or desiccated thyroid) is usually derived from pig thyroid gland. It may be antigenic in allergic or sensitive patients. Inexpensive generic brands may not be bioequivalent.
- **Liothyronine** (synthetic T_3) has uniform potency but has a higher incidence of cardiac adverse effects, higher cost, and difficulty in monitoring with conventional laboratory tests.
- **Liotrix** (synthetic T_4:T_3 in a 4:1 ratio) is chemically stable, pure, and has a predictable potency but is expensive. It also lacks therapeutic rationale because most T_3 is converted peripherally from T_4.
- Excessive doses of thyroid hormone may lead to heart failure, angina pectoris, and myocardial infarction (MI). Hyperthyroidism leads to reduced bone density and increased risk of fracture.

TREATMENT OF MYXEDEMA COMA

- Immediate and aggressive therapy with IV bolus **levothyroxine**, 300 to 500 mcg, has traditionally been used. Initial treatment with IV **liothyronine** or a combination of both hormones has also been advocated because of impaired conversion of T_4 to T_3.
- Give glucocorticoid therapy with IV **hydrocortisone** 100 mg every 8 hours until coexisting adrenal suppression is ruled out.
- Consciousness, lowered TSH concentrations, and improvement in vital signs are expected within 24 hours.
- Maintenance levothyroxine doses are typically 75 to 100 mcg IV until the patient stabilizes and oral therapy is begun.
- Provide supportive therapy to maintain adequate ventilation, euglycemia, BP, and body temperature. Diagnose and treat underlying disorders such as sepsis and MI.

EVALUATION OF THERAPEUTIC OUTCOMES

- Serum TSH concentration is the most sensitive and specific monitoring parameter for adjustment of levothyroxine dose. Concentrations begin to fall within hours and are usually normalized within 2 to 6 weeks.
- Check both TSH and T_4 concentrations every 6 weeks until a euthyroid state is achieved. An elevated TSH level indicates insufficient replacement. Serum T_4 concentrations can be useful in detecting noncompliance, malabsorption, or changes in levothyroxine product bioequivalence. TSH may also be used to help identify noncompliance.
- In patients with hypothyroidism caused by hypothalamic or pituitary failure, alleviation of the clinical syndrome and restoration of serum T_4 to the normal range are the only criteria available for estimating the appropriate replacement dose of levothyroxine.

See Chapter 75, Thyroid Disorders, authored by Jacqueline Jonklaas and Michael P. Kane, for a more detailed discussion of this topic.

CHAPTER

21

Cirrhosis and Portal Hypertension

CIRRHOSIS

- *Cirrhosis* is a diffuse injury to the liver characterized by fibrosis and a conversion of the normal hepatic architecture into structurally abnormal nodules. The end result is destruction of hepatocytes and their replacement by fibrous tissue.
- The resulting resistance to blood flow results in portal hypertension and the development of varices and ascites. Hepatocyte loss and intrahepatic shunting of blood result in diminished metabolic and synthetic function, which leads to hepatic encephalopathy (HE) and coagulopathy.
- Cirrhosis has many causes (Table 21–1). In the United States, excessive alcohol intake and chronic viral hepatitis (types B and C) are the most common causes.
- Cirrhosis results in elevation of portal blood pressure because of fibrotic changes within the hepatic sinusoids, changes in the levels of vasodilatory and vasoconstrictor mediators, and an increase in blood flow to the splanchnic vasculature. The pathophysiologic abnormalities that cause it result in the commonly encountered problems of ascites, portal hypertension and esophageal varices, HE, and coagulation disorders.
- *Portal hypertension* is noted by elevated pressure gradient between the portal and central venous pressure and is characterized by hypervolemia, increased cardiac index, hypotension, and decreased systemic vascular resistance.
- Ascites is the pathologic accumulation of fluid within the peritoneal cavity. It is one of the earliest and most common presentations of cirrhosis.
- The development of ascites is related to systemic arterial vasodilation mediated by nitric oxide that leads to the activation of the baroreceptors in the kidney and an activation of the renin–angiotensin–aldosterone system, activation of the sympathetic nervous system, and release of antidiuretic hormone in response to the arterial hypotension. These changes cause sodium and water retention.

PORTAL HYPERTENSION AND VARICES

- The most important sequelae of portal hypertension are the development of varices and alternative routes of blood flow resulting in acute variceal bleeding. Portal hypertension is defined by the presence of a gradient of greater than 5 mm Hg (0.7 kPa) between the portal and central venous pressures.
- Progression to bleeding can be predicted by Child-Pugh score, size of varices, and the presence of red wale markings on the varices. First variceal hemorrhage occurs at an annual rate of about 15% and carries a mortality of 7% to 15%.

HEPATIC ENCEPHALOPATHY

- *Hepatic encephalopathy* (HE) is a metabolically induced functional disturbance of the brain that is potentially reversible.
- The symptoms of HE are thought to result from an accumulation of gut-derived nitrogenous substances in the systemic circulation as a consequence of shunting through portosystemic collaterals bypassing the liver. These substances then enter

TABLE 21–1	Etiology of Cirrhosis
Chronic alcohol consumption	
Chronic viral hepatitis (types B and C)	

Metabolic liver disease
    Hemochromatosis
    Wilson's disease
    α_1-antitrypsin deficiency
    Nonalcoholic steatohepatitis ("fatty liver")	

Immunologic disease
    Autoimmune hepatitis
    Primary biliary cirrhosis	

Vascular disease
    Budd–Chiari
    Cardiac failure	

Drugs Isoniazid, methyldopa, amiodarone, amoxicillin-clavulanate, nitrofurantoin, diclofenac, methotrexate, nevirapine, propylthiouracil, valproate	

the central nervous system (CNS) and result in alterations of neurotransmission that affect consciousness and behavior.

- Altered ammonia, glutamate, benzodiazepine receptor agonists, aromatic amino acids, and manganese are potential causes of HE. An established correlation between blood ammonia levels and mental status does not exist.
- Type A HE is induced by acute liver failure, type B results from portal-systemic bypass without intrinsic liver disease, and type C occurs with cirrhosis. HE may be classified as episodic, persistent, or minimal.

COAGULATION DEFECTS

- Complex coagulation derangements can occur in cirrhosis. These derangements include the reduction in the synthesis of procoagulant factors, excessive fibrinolysis, disseminated intravascular coagulation, thrombocytopenia, and platelet dysfunction.
- Naturally occurring anticoagulants, antithrombin, and protein C are decreased; however, two procoagulant factors, factor VIII, and von Willebrand factor, are actually elevated. The net effect of these events could be thrombosis or clinical significant bleeding.

CLINICAL PRESENTATION

- The range of presentation of patients with cirrhosis may be from asymptomatic, with abnormal laboratory or radiographic tests, to decompensated with ascites, spontaneous bacterial peritonitis, HE, or variceal bleeding.
- Some presenting characteristics with cirrhosis are anorexia, weight loss, weakness, fatigue, jaundice, pruritis, gastrointestinal (GI) bleeding, coagulopathy, increased abdominal girth with shifting flank dullness, mental status changes, and vascular spiders. Table 21–2 describes the presenting signs and symptoms of cirrhosis.
- A thorough history including risk factors that predispose patients to cirrhosis should be taken. Quantity and duration of alcohol intake should be determined. Risk factors for hepatitis B and C transmission should be determined.

TABLE 21–2	Clinical Presentation of Cirrhosis

Signs and Symptoms
- Asymptomatic
- Hepatomegaly and splenomegaly
- Pruritus, jaundice, palmar erythema, spider angiomata, and hyperpigmentation
- Gynecomastia and reduced libido
- Ascites, edema, pleural effusion, and respiratory difficulties
- Malaise, anorexia, and weight loss
- Encephalopathy

Laboratory Tests
- Hypoalbuminemia
- Elevated prothrombin time (PT)
- Thrombocytopenia
- Elevated alkaline phosphatase
- Elevated aspartate transaminase (AST), alanine transaminase (ALT), and γ-glutamyl transpeptidase (GGT)

LABORATORY ABNORMALITIES

- There are no laboratory or radiographic tests of hepatic function that can accurately diagnose cirrhosis. Routine liver assessment tests include alkaline phosphatase, bilirubin, aspartate transaminase (AST), alanine aminotransferase (ALT), and γ-glutamyl transpeptidase (GGT). Additional markers of hepatic synthetic activity include albumin and prothrombin time (PT).
- The aminotransferases, AST and ALT, are enzymes that have increased concentrations in plasma after hepatocellular injury. The highest concentrations are seen in acute viral infections and ischemic or toxic liver injury.
- Alkaline phosphatase levels and GGT are elevated in plasma with obstructive disorders that disrupt the flow of bile from hepatocytes to the bile ducts or from the biliary tree to the intestines in conditions such as primary biliary cirrhosis, sclerosing cholangitis, drug-induced cholestasis, bile duct obstruction, autoimmune cholestatic liver disease, and metastatic cancer of the liver.
- Elevations in serum conjugated bilirubin indicate that the liver has lost at least half its excretory capacity. When alkaline phosphatase is elevated and aminotransferase levels are normal, elevated conjugated bilirubin is a sign of cholestatic disease or possible cholestatic drug reactions.
- **Figure 21–1** describes a general algorithm for the interpretation of liver function tests.
- Albumin and coagulation factors are markers of hepatic synthetic activity and are used to estimate hepatocyte functioning in cirrhosis. Thrombocytopenia is a common feature in chronic liver disease
- The Child-Pugh classification system uses a combination of physical and laboratory findings to assess and define the severity of cirrhosis and is a predictor of patient survival, surgical outcome, and risk of variceal bleeding (**Table 21–3**).
- The model for end-stage liver disease (MELD) is a newer scoring system:

$$\text{MELD score} = 0.957 \times \log(\text{serum creatinine mg/dL}) + 0.378 \\ \times \log(\text{bilirubin mg/dL}) + 1.120 \times \log(\text{INR}) + 0.643$$

or using SI units:*

$$\text{MELD score} = 0.957 \times \log_e(\text{creatinine [µmol/L]} \times 0.01131) + 0.378 \\ \times \log_e(\text{bilirubin [µmol/L]} \times 0.05848) + 1.120 \times \log_e(\text{INR}) + 0.643$$

where international normalized ratio (INR) is TK.

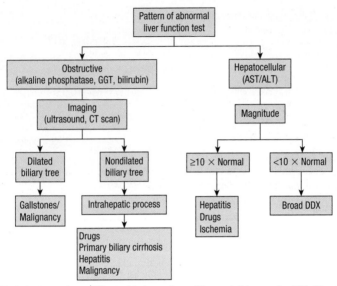

(ALT, alanine transaminase; AST, aspartate transaminase; CT, computed tomography; DDX, differential diagnosis; GGT, γ-glutamyl transpeptidase.)

FIGURE 21–1. Interpretation of liver function tests.

- In MELD, laboratory values less than 1 are rounded up to 1. The formula's score is multiplied by 10 and rounded to the nearest whole number.

TREATMENT

- <u>Goals of Treatment</u>: Treatment goals are resolution of acute complications, such as variceal bleeding, and resolution of hemodynamic instability for an episode of acute variceal hemorrhage. Other goals are prevention of complications, adequate lowering of portal pressure with medical therapy using β-adrenergic blocker therapy, and support of abstinence from alcohol.

TABLE 21–3	Criteria and Scoring for the Child–Pugh Grading of Chronic Liver Disease		
Score	**1**	**2**	**3**
Total bilirubin (mg/dL)	<2 (<34.2 μmol/L)	2–3 (34.2–51.3 μmol/L)	>3 (>51.3 μmol/L)
Albumin (g/dL)	>3.5 (>35 g/L)	2.8–3.5 (28–35 g/L)	<2.8 (<28 g/L)
Ascites	None	Mild	Moderate
Encephalopathy (grade)	None	1 and 2	3 and 4
Prothrombin time (seconds prolonged)	<4	4–6	>6

Grade A, <7 points; grade B, 7–9 points; grade C, 10–15 points.

GENERAL APPROACH TO TREATMENT

- Approaches to treatment include the following:
  - ✓ Identify and eliminate the causes of cirrhosis (eg, alcohol abuse).
  - ✓ Assess the risk for variceal bleeding and begin pharmacologic prophylaxis where indicated, reserving endoscopic therapy for high-risk patients or acute bleeding episodes.
  - ✓ The patient should be evaluated for clinical signs of ascites and managed with pharmacologic treatment (eg, diuretics) and paracentesis. Spontaneous bacterial peritonitis (SBP) should be carefully monitored in patients with ascites who undergo acute deterioration.
  - ✓ HE is a common complication of cirrhosis and requires clinical vigilance and treatment with dietary restriction, elimination of CNS depressants, and therapy to lower ammonia levels.
  - ✓ Frequent monitoring for signs of hepatorenal syndrome, pulmonary insufficiency, and endocrine dysfunction is necessary.

MANAGEMENT OF PORTAL HYPERTENSION AND VARICEAL BLEEDING

- The management of varices involves three strategies: (1) primary prophylaxis to prevent bleeding, (2) treatment of variceal hemorrhage, and (3) secondary prophylaxis to prevent rebleeding in patients who have already bled.

Primary Prophylaxis

- All patients with cirrhosis and portal hypertension should be screened for varices on diagnosis.
- The mainstay of primary prophylaxis is the use of a nonselective β-adrenergic blocking agent such as **propranolol, nadolol, or carvedilol**. These agents reduce portal pressure by reducing portal venous inflow via two mechanisms: decrease in cardiac output and decrease in splanchnic blood flow.
- Therapy for medium, or large varices should be initiated with propranolol, 20 mg twice daily, nadolol, 20 to 40 mg once daily, or carvedilol 6.25 mg daily and titrated every 2 to 3 days to maximal tolerated dose to heart rate of 55 to 60 beats/min. β-adrenergic blocker therapy should be continued indefinitely.
- Patients with contraindications to therapy with nonselective β-adrenergic blockers (ie, those with asthma, insulin-dependent diabetes with episodes of hypoglycemia, and peripheral vascular disease) or intolerance to β-adrenergic blockers should be considered for alternative prophylactic therapy with EVL.

ACUTE VARICEAL HEMORRHAGE

- Figure 21–2 presents an algorithm for the management of variceal hemorrhage. Evidence-based recommendations for selected treatments are presented in Table 21–4.
- Initial treatment goals include (1) adequate blood volume resuscitation, (2) protection of the airway from aspiration of blood, (3) correction of significant coagulopathy and/or thrombocytopenia with fresh frozen plasma and platelets, (4) prophylaxis against SBP and other infections, (5) control of bleeding, (4) prevention of rebleeding, and (5) preservation of liver function.
- Prompt stabilization of blood volume to maintain hemoglobin of 8 g/dL (80 g/L; 4.97 mmol/L) with volume expansion to maintain systolic blood pressure of 90 to 100 mm Hg and heart rate of less than 100 beats/min is recommended. Airway management is critical. Fluid resuscitation involves colloids initially and subsequent blood products. Vigorous resuscitation with saline solution should generally be avoided.
- Combination pharmacologic therapy plus EVL or sclerotherapy (when EVL is not technically feasible) is the most rational approach to treatment of acute variceal bleeding.

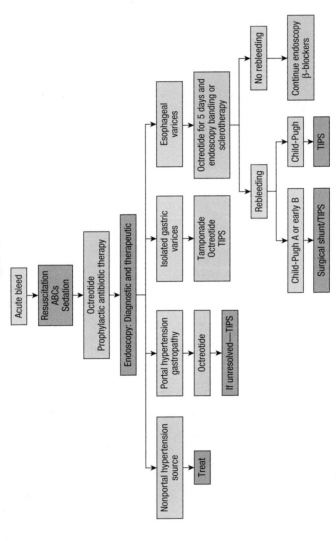

(ABCs, airway, breathing, and circulation; TIPS, transjugular intrahepatic portosystemic shunt.)

FIGURE 21–2. Management of acute variceal hemorrhage.

TABLE 21–4	Evidence-Based Table of Selected Treatment Recommendations: Variceal Bleeding in Portal Hypertension	
Recommendation		**Grade**
Prevention of variceal bleeding		
Nonselective β-blocker therapy should be initiated in:		
Patients with small varices and criteria for increased risk of hemorrhage		IIaC
Patients with medium/large varices without high risk of hemorrhage		IA
Endoscopic variceal ligation (EVL) should be offered to patients who have contraindications or intolerance to nonselective β-blockers		IA
EVL may be recommended for prevention in patients with medium/large varices at high risk of hemorrhage instead of nonselective β-blocker therapy		IA
Treatment of variceal bleeding		
Short-term antibiotic prophylaxis should be instituted on admission		IA
Vasoactive drugs should be started as soon as possible, prior to endoscopy, and maintained for 3–5 days		IA
Endoscopy should be performed within 12 hours to diagnose variceal bleeding and treat bleeding with either sclerotherapy or EVL		IA
Secondary prophylaxis of variceal bleeding		
Nonselective β-blocker therapy plus EVL is the best therapeutic option for prevention of recurrent variceal bleeding		IA

Recommendation grading:
Class I—Conditions for which there is evidence and/or general agreement
Class II—Conditions for which there is conflicting evidence and/or a divergence of opinion
Class IIa—Weight of evidence/opinion is in favor of efficacy
Class IIb—Efficacy less well established
Class III—Conditions for which there is evidence and/or general agreement that treatment is not effective and/or potentially harmful
Level A—Data from multiple randomized trials or meta-analyses
Level B—Data derived from single randomized trial or nonrandomized studies
Level C—Only consensus opinion, case studies, or standard of care

- Vasoactive drug therapy (usually **octreotide**) to stop or slow bleeding is routinely used early in patient management to allow stabilization of the patient. Treatment with octreotide should be initiated early to control bleeding and facilitate endoscopy. Octreotide is administered as an IV bolus of 50 mcg followed by a continuous infusion of 50 mcg/h. It should be continued for 5 days after acute variceal bleeding. Patients should be monitored for hypo- or hyperglycemia.
- **Vasopressin**, alone or in combination with nitroglycerin, is not recommended as first-line therapy for the management of variceal hemorrhage. Vasopressin causes nonselective vasoconstriction and can result in myocardial ischemia or infarction, arrhythmias, mesenteric ischemia, ischemia of the limbs, or cerebrovascular accidents.
- Prophylactic antibiotic therapy should be prescribed for all patients with cirrhosis and acute variceal bleeding. A short course (7 days maximum) of oral **norfloxacin** 400 mg twice daily or IV **ciprofloxacin** when the oral route is not available is recommended.
- EVL is the recommended form of endoscopic therapy for acute variceal bleeding, although endoscopic injection sclerotherapy (injection of 1–4 mL of a sclerosing agent into the lumen of the varices) may be used.
- If standard therapy fails to control bleeding, a salvage procedure such as balloon tamponade (with a Sengstaken-Blakemore tube) or transjugular intrahepatic portosystemic shunt (TIPS) is necessary.

Prevention of Rebleeding

- A nonselective β-adrenergic blocker along with EVL is the best treatment option for prevention of rebleeding.
- **Propranolol** may be given at 20 mg twice daily (or **nadolol**, 20–40 mg once daily) and titrated weekly to achieve a goal of heart rate 55 to 60 beats/min or the maximal tolerated dose. Patients should be monitored for evidence of heart failure, bronchospasm, or glucose intolerance.
- Patients who cannot tolerate or who fail pharmacologic and endoscopic interventions can be considered for tips or surgical shunting to prevent bleeding.

ASCITES

- The therapeutic goals for patients with ascites are to control the ascites, prevent or relieve ascites-related symptoms (dyspnea and abdominal pain and distention), and prevent SBP and hepatorenal syndrome.
- For patients with ascites, a serum–ascites albumin gradient should be determined. If the serum–ascites albumin gradient is greater than or equal to 1.1 g/dL (11 g/L), the patient almost certainly has portal hypertension.
- The treatment of ascites secondary to portal hypertension includes abstinence from alcohol, sodium restriction (to 2 g/day), and diuretics. Fluid loss and weight change depend directly on sodium balance in these patients. A goal of therapy is to increase urinary excretion of sodium to greater than 78 mmol/day.
- Diuretic therapy should be initiated with single morning doses of **spironolactone**, 100 mg, and **furosemide**, 40 mg, titrated every 3 to 5 days (or spironolactone alone), with a goal of 0.5 kg maximum daily weight loss. The dose of each can be increased together, maintaining the 100:40 mg ratio, to a maximum daily dose of 400 mg spironolactone and 160 mg furosemide.
- If tense ascites is present, paracentesis should be performed prior to institution of diuretic therapy and salt restriction.
- Liver transplant should be considered in patients with refractory ascites.

SPONTANEOUS BACTERIAL PERITONITIS

- Antibiotic therapy for prevention of spontaneous bacterial peritonitis (SBP) should be considered in all patients who are at high risk for this complication (those who experience a prior episode of SBP or variceal hemorrhage and those with low-protein ascites).
- Patients with documented or suspected SBP should receive broad-spectrum antibiotic therapy to cover *Escherichia coli, Klebsiella pneumoniae,* and *Streptococcus pneumoniae.*
- **Cefotaxime**, 2 g every 8 hours, or a similar third-generation cephalosporin for 5 days is considered the drug of choice. Oral **ofloxacin**, 400 mg every 12 hours for 8 days, is equivalent to IV cefotaxime.
- Patients who survive an episode of SBP should receive long-term antibiotic prophylaxis with daily norfloxacin 400 mg or double-strength trimethoprim-sulfamethoxazole.

HEPATIC ENCEPHALOPATHY

- The general approach to the management of HE is four pronged and includes the following: care for patients with altered consciousness, identify and treat any other causes besides HE for altered mental status, identify and treat any precipitating factors, and begin empirical HE treatment.
- The grading system for HE is shown in **Table 21–5.**

TABLE 21-5	Grading System for Hepatic Encephalopathy		
Grade	**Level of Consciousness**	**Personality/ Intellect**	**Neurologic Abnormalities**
Unimpaired	Normal	Normal	Normal
Minimal	No clinical evidence of change	No clinical evidence of change/alterations identified on psychometric or neuropsychological testing	No clinical evidence of change
I	Trivial lack of awareness; shortened attention span	Euphoria or anxiety; impairment of addition or subtraction	Altered sleep rhythm
II	Lethargic	Obvious personality changes; inappropriate behavior; apathy	Asterixis; dyspraxia; disoriented for time
III	Somnolent but arousable	Bizarre behavior	Responsive to stimuli; confused; gross disorientation to time and space
IV	Coma/unarousable	None	Does not respond to stimuli

- Treatment approaches include (1) reduction in blood ammonia concentrations by dietary restrictions, with drug therapy aimed at inhibiting ammonia production or enhancing its removal (**lactulose** and antibiotics) and (2) inhibition of γ-aminobutyric acid-benzodiazepine receptors by **flumazenil. Bromocriptine** 30 mg twice daily is indicated for chronic HE treatment in patients who are unresponsive to other therapies.
- To reduce blood ammonia concentrations in patients with episodic HE, protein intake is limited or withheld (while maintaining caloric intake) until the clinical situation improves. Protein intake can be titrated back up based on tolerance to a total of 1.2 to 1.5 g/kg/day.
- To reduce blood ammonia concentrations in episodic HE, lactulose is initiated at 45 mL orally every hour (or 300 mL lactulose syrup with 1 L water given as a retention enema held for 60 minutes) until catharsis begins. The dose is then decreased to 15 to 45 mL orally every 8 to 12 hours and titrated to produce two or three soft stools per day.
- **Rifaximin** 400 to 550 mg twice daily plus lactulose is superior to lactulose alone in patients with a history of recurrent he. Rifaximin should be added on to lactulose therapy in recurrent he following the second recurrence.

EVALUATION OF THERAPEUTIC OUTCOMES

- Table 21-6 summarizes the drug monitoring guidelines patients with cirrhosis and portal hypertension, including monitoring parameters and therapeutic outcomes.

TABLE 21–6	Drug Monitoring Guidelines		
Drug	**Adverse Drug Reaction**	**Monitoring Parameter**	**Comments**
Nonselective β-adrenergic blocker	Heart failure, bronchospasm, glucose intolerance	BP, HR Goal HR: 55–60 beats/min or maximal tolerated dose	Nadolol, propranolol, carvedilol
Octreotide	Bradycardia, hypertension, arrhythmia, abdominal pain	BP, HR, EKG, abdominal pain	
Vasopressin	Myocardial ischemia/infarction, arrhythmia, mesenteric ischemia, ischemia of the limbs, cerebrovascular accident	EKG, distal pulses, symptoms of myocardial, mesenteric, or cerebrovascular ischemia/infarction	
Spironolactone/furosemide	Electrolyte disturbances, dehydration, renal insufficiency, hypotension	Serum electrolytes (especially potassium), SCr, blood urea nitrogen, BP Goal sodium excretion: >78 mmol/day	Spot urine sodium concentration greater than potassium concentration correlates well with daily sodium excretion >78 mmol/day
Lactulose	Electrolyte disturbances	Serum electrolytes Goal number of soft stools per day: 2–3	
Neomycin	Ototoxicity, nephrotoxicity	SCr, annual auditory monitoring	
Metronidazole	Neurotoxicity	Sensory and motor neuropathy	
Rifaximin	Nausea, diarrhea		

(BP, blood pressure; HR, heart rate; beats/min, beats per minute; EKG, electrocardiogram; SCr, serum creatinine; mmol, millimole.)

See Chapter 37, Portal Hypertension and Cirrhosis, authored by Julie M. Sease and Jennifer N. Clements, for a more detailed discussion of this topic.

CHAPTER 22

Constipation

- *Constipation* has been defined as difficult or infrequent passage of stool, at times associated with straining or a feeling of incomplete defecation.

PATHOPHYSIOLOGY

- Constipation may be primary (occurs without an underlying identifiable cause) or secondary (the result of constipating drugs, lifestyle factors, or medical disorders).
- Constipation commonly results from a diet low in fiber, inadequate fluid intake, decreased physical activity, or from use of constipating drugs such as opiates. Constipation may sometimes be psychogenic in origin.
- Diseases or conditions that may cause constipation include the following:
  ✓ Gastrointestinal (GI) disorders: Irritable bowel syndrome (IBS), diverticulitis, upper and lower GI tract diseases, hemorrhoids, anal fissures, ulcerative proctitis, tumors, hernia, volvulus of the bowel, syphilis, tuberculosis, lymphogranuloma venereum, and Hirschsprung disease
  ✓ Metabolic and endocrine disorders: Diabetes mellitus with neuropathy, hypothyroidism, panhypopituitarism, pheochromocytoma, hypercalcemia, and enteric glucagon excess
  ✓ Pregnancy
  ✓ Cardiac disorders (eg, heart failure)
  ✓ Neurogenic constipation: Head trauma, CNS tumors, spinal cord injury, cerebrospinal accidents, and Parkinson disease
  ✓ Psychogenic causes
- Causes of drug-induced constipation are listed in Table 22–1. All opiate derivatives are associated with constipation, but the degree of intestinal inhibitory effects seems to differ among agents. Orally administered opiates appear to have greater inhibitory effect than parenterally administered agents; oral codeine is well known as a potent antimotility agent.

CLINICAL PRESENTATION

- Table 22–2 shows the general clinical presentation of constipation.
- The patient should also be carefully questioned about usual diet and laxative regimens.
- General health status, signs of underlying medical illness (ie, hypothyroidism), and psychological status (eg, depression or other psychological illness) should also be assessed.
- Patients with alarm symptoms, a family history of colon cancer, or those older than 50 years with new symptoms may need further diagnostic evaluation.

TREATMENT

- <u>Goals of Treatment:</u> The major goals of treatment are to (a) relieve symptoms; (b) reestablish normal bowel habits; and (c) improve quality of life by minimizing adverse effects of treatment.

GENERAL APPROACH TO TREATMENT

- General measures believed to be beneficial in managing constipation include dietary modification to increase the amount of fiber consumed daily, exercise, adjustment of bowel habits so that a regular and adequate time is made to respond to the urge to defecate, and increased fluid intake.

TABLE 22–1	Drugs Causing Constipation

Analgesics
    Inhibitors of prostaglandin synthesis
    Opiates	

Anticholinergics
    Antihistamines
    Antiparkinsonian agents (eg, benztropine or trihexyphenidyl)
    Phenothiazines
    Tricyclic antidepressants	

Antacids containing calcium carbonate or aluminum hydroxide	
Barium sulfate	
Calcium channel antagonists	
Clonidine	
Diuretics (non–potassium-sparing)	
Ganglionic blockers	
Iron preparations	
Muscle blockers (D-tubocurarine, succinylcholine)	
Nonsteroidal anti-inflammatory agents	
Polystyrene sodium sulfonate	

- If an underlying disease is recognized as the cause of constipation, attempts should be made to correct it. GI malignancies may be removed through a surgical resection. Endocrine and metabolic derangements are corrected by the appropriate methods.
- If a patient is consuming medications known to cause constipation, consideration should be given to alternative agents. If no reasonable alternatives exist to the medication thought to be responsible for constipation, consideration should be given to lowering the dose. If a patient must remain on constipating medications, more attention must be given to general measures for prevention of constipation.
- The proper management of constipation will require a combination of nonpharmacologic and pharmacologic therapies.

DIETARY MODIFICATION AND BULK-FORMING AGENTS

- The most important aspect of the therapy for constipation is dietary modification to increase the amount of fiber consumed. Gradually increase daily fiber intake to 20 to 25 g, either through dietary changes or through fiber supplements. Fruits, vegetables, and cereals have the highest fiber content.
- A trial of dietary modification with high-fiber content should be continued for at least 1 month. Most patients begin to notice effects on bowel function 3 to 5 days after beginning a high-fiber diet.
- Abdominal distention and flatus may be particularly troublesome in the first few weeks, particularly with high bran consumption.

PHARMACOLOGIC THERAPY

- The laxatives are divided into three classifications: (1) those causing softening of feces in 1 to 3 days (bulk-forming laxatives, **docusates**, and low-dose **polyethylene**

TABLE 22–2	Clinical Presentation of Constipation

Signs and symptoms
- Infrequent bowel movements (<3 per week)
- Stools that are hard, small, or dry
- Difficulty or pain of defecation
- Feeling of abdominal discomfort or bloating, incomplete evacuation, etc.

Alarm signs and symptoms
- Hematochezia
- Melena
- Family history of colon cancer
- Family history of inflammatory bowel disease
- Anemia
- Weight loss
- Anorexia
- Nausea and vomiting
- Severe, persistent constipation that is refractory to treatment
- New-onset or worsening constipation in elderly without evidence of primary cause

Physical examination
- Perform rectal exam for presence of anatomical abnormalities (such as fistulas, fissures, hemorrhoids, rectal prolapse) or abnormalities of perianal descent
- Digital examination of rectum to check for fecal impaction, anal stricture, or rectal mass

Laboratory and other diagnostic tests
- No routine recommendations for lab testing—as indicated by clinical discretion
- In patients with signs and symptoms suggestive of organic disorder, specific testing may be performed (ie, thyroid function tests, electrolytes, glucose, complete blood count) based on clinical presentation
- In patients with alarm signs and symptoms or when structural disease is a possibility, select appropriate diagnostic studies:
  1. Protoscopy
  2. Sigmoidoscopy
  3. Colonoscopy
  4. Barium enema

glycol, and **lactulose**), (2) those resulting in soft or semifluid stool in 6 to 12 hours (**bisacodyl, senna**, and **magnesium sulfate**), and (3) those causing water evacuation in 1 to 6 hours (**saline cathartics, castor oil**, and **polyethylene glycol (PEG)–electrolyte lavage solution**).

- Other agents include the calcium channel activator **lubiprostone**, the guanylate cyclase C agonist **linaclotide**, opioid receptor antagonists (**alvimopan, methylnaltrexone**, and **naloxegol**) and serotonergic agents.
- Dosage recommendations for laxatives and cathartics are provided in Table 22–3.

Recommendations

- A constipation treatment algorithm is presented in Table 22–4.
- The proper management of constipation will require a combination of nonpharmacologic and pharmacologic therapies. Osmotic laxative therapy is considered the preferred first line for the treatment of constipation, in addition to increasing dietary fiber or using fiber supplementation.
- Patients are often encouraged to increase daily fluid intake and physical activity as well dedicate time to respond to the urge to defecate, although efficacy data are conflicting for these measures.

TABLE 22–3	Dosage Recommendations for Laxatives and Cathartics
Agent	**Recommended Dose**
Agents that cause softening of feces in 1–3 days	
Bulk-forming agents/osmotic laxatives	
Methylcellulose	4–6 g/day
Polycarbophil	4–6 g/day
Psyllium	Varies with product
Emollients	
Docusate sodium	50–360 mg/day
Docusate calcium	50–360 mg/day
Docusate potassium	100–300 mg/day
Polyethylene glycol 3350	17 g/dose
Lactulose	15–30 mL orally
Sorbitol	30–50 g/day orally
Agents that result in soft or semifluid stool in 6–12 hours	
Bisacodyl (oral)	5–15 mg orally
Senna	Dose varies with formulation
Magnesium sulfate (low dose)	<10 g orally
Agents that cause watery evacuation in 1–6 hours	
Magnesium citrate	18 g 300 mL water
Magnesium hydroxide	2.4–4.8 g orally
Magnesium sulfate (high dose)	10–30 g orally
Sodium phosphates	Varies with salt used
Bisacodyl	10 mg rectally
Polyethylene glycol-electrolyte preparations	4 L

Emollient Laxatives (Docusates)

- These surfactant agents, **docusates** increase water and electrolyte secretion in the small and large bowel and result in a softening of stools within 1 to 3 days.
- Emollient laxatives are not effective in treating constipation but are used mainly to prevent constipation. They may be helpful in situations where straining at stool should be avoided, such as after recovery from myocardial infarction, with acute perianal disease, or after rectal surgery.
- It is unlikely that these agents are effective in preventing constipation if major causative factors (eg, heavy opiate use, uncorrected pathology, and inadequate dietary fiber) are not concurrently addressed.

TABLE 22–4	Constipation Treatment Algorithm

Diagnosis
1. Treat specific cause
2. No underlying diagnosis, then choose symptomatic therapy
   A. Dietary modification to increase fiber ± supplementation (bulk agents)
   B. Add osmotic laxative (ie, PEG) if no relief; trial 2–4 weeks
   C. Add stimulant laxative (ie, bisacodyl) if no relief or no BM in 2 days
   D. Lubiprostone or linaclotide trial
   E. Opioid-receptor antagonists if opioid-induced constipation

Lactulose and Sorbitol

- **Lactulose** is generally not recommended as a first-line agent for the treatment of constipation because it is costly and may cause flatulence, nausea, and abdominal discomfort or bloating. It may be justified as an alternative for acute constipation and has been found to be particularly useful in elderly patients.
- **Sorbitol**, a monosaccharide, has been recommended as a primary agent in the treatment of functional constipation in cognitively intact patients. It is as effective as lactulose, may cause less nausea, and is much less expensive.

Saline Cathartics

- Saline cathartics are composed of relatively poorly absorbed ions such as magnesium, sulfate, phosphate, and citrate, which produce their effects primarily by osmotic action to retain fluid in the GI tract. These agents may be given orally or rectally.
- A bowel movement may result within a few hours of oral doses and in 1 hour or sooner after rectal administration.
- These agents should be used primarily for acute evacuation of the bowel, which may be necessary before diagnostic examinations, after poisonings, and in conjunction with some anthelmintics to eliminate parasites.
- Agents such as milk of magnesia (an 8% suspension of magnesium hydroxide) may be used occasionally (every few weeks) to treat constipation in otherwise healthy adults.
- Saline cathartics should not be used on a routine basis to treat constipation. With fecal impactions, the enema formulations of these agents may be helpful.

Glycerin

- This agent is usually administered as a suppository and exerts its effect by osmotic action in the rectum. As with most agents given as suppositories, the onset of action is usually less than 30 minutes. Glycerin is considered a safe laxative, although it may occasionally cause rectal irritation. Its use is acceptable on an intermittent basis for constipation, particularly in children.

Polyethylene Glycol–Electrolyte (PEG) Lavage Solution

- Low doses of PEG solution (10–30 g or 17–34 g per 120–240 mL) once or twice daily may be used for treatment of constipation. Daily use in low dose (17 g) may be safe and effective for up to 6 months

Lubiprostone and Linaclotide

- **Lubiprostone** (Amitiza) is approved for chronic idiopathic constipation and constipation-predominant IBS-C in adults and appears safe for long-term treatment (up to 48 weeks). The dose is 24 mg capsule twice daily with food. Lubiprostone may cause headache, diarrhea, and nausea.
- **Linaclotide** (Linzess) is approved for the treatment of constipation and IBS-C. It is approved in a 145-mcg dose and should not be used in patients younger than 18 years of age.

Opioid-Receptor Antagonists

- Alvimopan is an oral GI-specific μ-receptor antagonist for short-term use in hospitalized patients to accelerate recovery of bowel function after large or small bowel resection. It is given 12 mg (capsule) 30 minutes to 5 hours before surgery and then 12 mg twice daily for up to 7 days or until hospital discharge (maximum 15 doses). It is contraindicated in patients receiving therapeutic doses of opioids for more than 7 consecutive days prior to surgery.
- Methylnaltrexone is another μ-receptor antagonist approved for opioid-induced constipation in patients with advanced disease receiving palliative care or when response to laxative therapy has been insufficient.

See Chapter 36, Diarrhea, Constipation, and Irritable Bowel Syndrome, authored by Patricia H. Fabel and Kayce M. Shealy, for a more detailed discussion of this topic.

Diarrhea

23 CHAPTER

- *Diarrhea* is an increased frequency and decreased consistency of fecal discharge as compared with an individual's normal bowel pattern. It is often a symptom of a systemic disease. Acute diarrhea is commonly defined as shorter than 14 days' duration, persistent diarrhea as longer than 14 days' duration, and chronic diarrhea as longer than 30 days' duration. Most cases of acute diarrhea are caused by infections with viruses, bacteria, or protozoa, and are generally self-limited.

PATHOPHYSIOLOGY

- Diarrhea is an imbalance in absorption and secretion of water and electrolytes. It may be associated with a specific disease of the gastrointestinal (GI) tract or with a disease outside the GI tract.
- Four general pathophysiologic mechanisms disrupt water and electrolyte balance, leading to diarrhea; (1) a change in active ion transport by either decreased sodium absorption or increased chloride secretion, (2) a change in intestinal motility, (3) an increase in luminal osmolarity, and (4) an increase in tissue hydrostatic pressure. These mechanisms have been related to four broad clinical diarrheal groups: secretory, osmotic, exudative, and altered intestinal transit.
- Secretory diarrhea occurs when a stimulating substance (eg, vasoactive intestinal peptide [VIP], laxatives, or bacterial toxin) increases secretion or decreases absorption of large amounts of water and electrolytes.
- Inflammatory diseases of the GI tract can cause exudative diarrhea by discharge of mucus, proteins, or blood into the gut. With altered intestinal transit, intestinal motility is altered by reduced contact time in the small intestine, premature emptying of the colon, or bacterial overgrowth.

CLINICAL PRESENTATION

- The clinical presentation of diarrhea is shown in Table 23–1. Most acute diarrhea is self-limiting, subsiding within 72 hours. However, infants, young children, the elderly, and debilitated persons are at risk for morbid and mortal events in prolonged or voluminous diarrhea.
- Many agents, including antibiotics and other drugs, cause diarrhea (Table 23–2). Laxative abuse for weight loss may also result in diarrhea.

TREATMENT

- <u>Goals of Treatment</u>: To manage the diet, prevent excessive water, electrolyte, and acid-base disturbances; provide symptomatic relief; treat curable causes of diarrhea; and manage secondary disorders causing diarrhea. Diarrhea, like a cough, may be a body defense mechanism for ridding itself of harmful substances or pathogens. The correct therapeutic response is not necessarily to stop diarrhea at all costs. If diarrhea is secondary to another illness, controlling the primary condition is necessary.

GENERAL APPROACH TO TREATMENT

- Management of the diet is a first priority for treatment of diarrhea (Figs. 23–1 and 23–2). Most clinicians recommend stopping solid foods for 24 hours and avoiding dairy products.
- Dietary management is a first priority in the treatment of diarrhea. Feeding should continue in children with acute bacterial diarrhea.

| TABLE 23-1 | Clinical Presentation of Diarrhea |

General
- Usually, acute diarrheal episodes subside within 72 hours of onset, whereas chronic diarrhea involves frequent attacks over extended time periods

Signs and symptoms
- Abrupt onset of nausea, vomiting, abdominal pain, headache, fever, chills, and malaise
- Bowel movements are frequent and never bloody, and diarrhea lasts 12–60 hours
- Intermittent periumbilical or lower right quadrant pain with cramps and audible bowel sounds is characteristic of small intestinal disease
- When pain is present in large intestinal diarrhea, it is a gripping, aching sensation with tenesmus (straining, ineffective, and painful stooling). Pain localizes to the hypogastric region, right or left lower quadrant, or sacral region
- In chronic diarrhea, a history of previous bouts, weight loss, anorexia, and chronic weakness are important findings

Physical examination
- Typically demonstrates hyperperistalsis with borborygmi and generalized or local tenderness

Laboratory tests
- Stool analysis studies include examination for microorganisms, blood, mucus, fat, osmolality, pH, electrolyte and mineral concentration, and cultures
- Stool test kits are useful for detecting GI viruses, particularly rotavirus
- Antibody serologic testing shows rising titers over a 3- to 6-day period, but this test is not practical and is nonspecific
- Occasionally, total daily stool volume is also determined
- Direct endoscopic visualization and biopsy of the colon may be undertaken to assess for the presence of conditions such as colitis or cancer
- Radiographic studies are helpful in neoplastic and inflammatory conditions

- If vomiting is present and is uncontrollable with antiemetics, nothing is taken by mouth. As bowel movements decrease, a bland diet is begun.
- Rehydration and maintenance of water and electrolytes are the primary treatment measures until the diarrheal episode ends. If vomiting and dehydration are not severe, enteral feeding is the less costly and preferred method. In the United States, many commercial oral rehydration preparations are available (**Table 23–3**).

PHARMACOLOGIC THERAPY

- Drugs used to treat diarrhea (**Table 23–4**) are grouped into several categories: antimotility, adsorbents, antisecretory compounds, antibiotics, enzymes, and intestinal microflora. Usually, these drugs are not curative but palliative.
- Opiates and opioid derivatives delay the transit of intraluminal content or increase gut capacity, prolonging contact and absorption. The limitations of the opiates are addiction potential (a real concern with long-term use) and worsening of diarrhea in selected infectious diarrheas.
- **Loperamide** is often recommended for managing acute and chronic diarrhea. Diarrhea lasting 48 hours beyond initiating loperamide warrants medical attention.
- **Difenoxin**, a diphenoxylate derivative also chemically related to meperidine, is also combined with atropine and has the same uses, precautions, and side effects.
- Adsorbents (such as **kaolin-pectin**) are used for symptomatic relief (see **Table 23–4**). Adsorbents are nonspecific in their action; they adsorb nutrients, toxins, drugs, and digestive juices. Coadministration with other drugs reduces their bioavailability.
- **Bismuth subsalicylate** is often used for treatment or prevention of diarrhea (traveler's diarrhea) and has antisecretory, anti-inflammatory, and antibacterial effects.

TABLE 23-2	Drugs Causing Diarrhea
Laxatives	
Antacids containing magnesium	
Antineoplastics	
Auranofin (gold salt)	
Antibiotics	
Clindamycin	
Tetracyclines	
Sulfonamides	
Any broad-spectrum antibiotic	
Antihypertensives	
Reserpine	
Guanethidine	
Methyldopa	
Guanabenz	
Guanadrel	
Angiotensin-converting enzyme inhibitors	
Cholinergics	
Bethanechol	
Neostigmine	
Cardiac agents	
Quinidine	
Digitalis	
Digoxin	
Nonsteroidal anti-inflammatory drugs	
Misoprostol	
Colchicine	
Proton pump inhibitors	
H_2-receptor blockers	

Bismuth subsalicylate contains multiple components that might be toxic if given in excess to prevent or treat diarrhea.

- *Lactobacillus* preparation is intended to replace colonic microflora. This supposedly restores intestinal functions and suppresses the growth of pathogenic microorganisms. However, a dairy product diet containing 200 to 400 g of lactose or dextrin is equally effective in recolonization of normal flora.

- Anticholinergic drugs, such as **atropine**, block vagal tone and prolong gut transit time. Their value in controlling diarrhea is questionable and limited by side effects.

- **Octreotide**, a synthetic octapeptide analogue of endogenous somatostatin, is prescribed for the symptomatic treatment of carcinoid tumors and other peptide secreting tumors. The dosage range for managing diarrhea associated with carcinoid tumors is 100 to 600 mcg daily in two to four divided doses, subcutaneously, for 2 weeks. Octreotide is associated with adverse effects such as cholelithiasis, nausea, diarrhea, and abdominal pain.

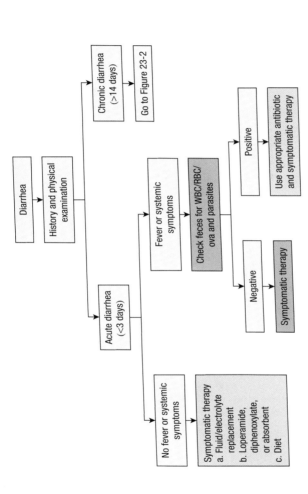

(RBC, red blood cells; WBC, white blood cells.)

FIGURE 23–1. Recommendations for treating acute diarrhea. Follow these steps: (1) Perform a complete history and physical examination. (2) Is the diarrhea acute or chronic? If chronic diarrhea, go to Fig. 23–2. (3) If acute diarrhea, check for fever and/or systemic signs and symptoms (ie, toxic patient). If systemic illness (fever, anorexia, or volume depletion), check for an infectious source. If positive for infectious diarrhea, use the appropriate antibiotic/anthelmintic drug and symptomatic therapy. If negative for infectious cause, use only symptomatic treatment. (4) If no systemic findings, use symptomatic therapy based on severity of volume depletion, oral or parenteral fluid/electrolytes, antidiarrheal agents (see **Table 23–4**), and diet.

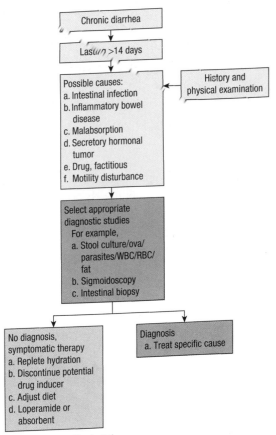

(RBC, red blood cells; WBC, white blood cells.)

FIGURE 23–2. Recommendations for treating chronic diarrhea. Follow these steps: (1) Perform a careful history and physical examination. (2) The possible causes of chronic diarrhea are many. These can be classified into intestinal infections (bacterial or protozoal), inflammatory disease (Crohn disease or ulcerative colitis), malabsorption (lactose intolerance), secretory hormonal tumor (intestinal carcinoid tumor or vasoactive intestinal peptide [VIP]–secreting tumors), drug (antacid), factitious (laxative abuse), or motility disturbance (diabetes mellitus, irritable bowel syndrome, or hyperthyroidism). (3) If the diagnosis is uncertain, appropriate diagnostic studies should be ordered. (4) Once diagnosed, treatment is planned for the underlying cause with symptomatic antidiarrheal therapy. (5) If no specific cause can be identified, symptomatic therapy is prescribed.

EVALUATION OF THERAPEUTIC OUTCOMES

- Therapeutic outcomes are directed to key symptoms, signs, and laboratory studies. The constitutional symptoms usually improve within 24 to 72 hours. Elderly persons with chronic illness as well as infants may require hospitalization for parenteral rehydration and close monitoring. The frequency and character of bowel movements should be checked each day along with the vital signs and improving appetite.

TABLE 23–3	Oral Rehydration Solutions			
	WHO-ORS[a]	Pedialyte[b] (Ross)	CeraLyte (Cera Products)	Enfalyte (Mead Johnson)
Osmolality (mOsm/kg or mmol/kg)	245	250	220	167
Carbohydrates[b] (g/L)	13.5	25	40[c]	30[c]
Calories (cal/L [J/L])	65 (272)	100 (418)	160 (670)	126 (527)
Electrolytes (mEq/L; mmol/L)				
Sodium	75	45	50–90	50
Potassium	20	20	20	25
Chloride	65	35	40–80	45
Citrate	—	30	30	34
Bicarbonate	30	—	—	—
Calcium	—	—	—	—
Magnesium	—	—	—	—
Sulfate	—	—	—	—
Phosphate	—	—	—	—

[a]World Health Organization reduced osmolarity oral rehydration solution.
[b]Carbohydrate is glucose.
[c]Rice syrup solids are carbohydrate source.

TABLE 23–4	Selected Antidiarrheal Preparations	
	Dose Form	Adult Dose
Antimotility		
Diphenoxylate	2.5 mg/tablet 2.5 mg/5 mL	5 mg four times daily; do not exceed 20 mg/day
Loperamide	2 mg/capsule 2 mg/capsule	Initially 4 mg, and then 2 mg after each loose stool; do not exceed 16 mg/day
Paregoric	2 mg/5 mL (morphine)	5–10 mL one to four times daily
Opium tincture	10 mg/mL (morphine)	0.6 mL four times daily
Difenoxin	1 mg/tablet	Two tablets, and then one tablet after each loose stool; up to eight tablets per day
Adsorbents		
Kaolin-pectin mixture	5.7 g kaolin + 130.2 mg pectin/30 mL	30–120 mL after each loose stool
Polycarbophil	500 mg/tablet	Chew 2 tablets four times daily or after each loose stool; do not exceed 12 tablets per day
Attapulgite	750 mg/15 mL 300 mg/7.5 mL 750 mg/tablet 600 mg/tablet 300 mg/tablet	1200–1500 mg after each loose bowel movement or every 2 hours; up to 9000 mg/day

(continued)

TABLE 23–4	Selected Antidiarrheal Preparations (*Continued*)	
	Dose Form	**Adult Dose**
Antisecretory		
Bismuth subsalicylate	1050 mg/30 mL 262 mg/15 mL 524 mg/15 mL 262 mg/tablet	Two tablets or 30 mL every 30 minutes to 1 hour as needed up to eight doses per day
Enzymes (lactase)	1250 neutral lactase units/4 drops 3300 FCC lactase units per tablet	Three to four drops taken with milk or dairy product
Bacterial replacement (*Lactobacillus acidophilus*, *Lactobacillus bulgaricus*)		Two tablets or one granule packet three to four times daily; give with milk, juice, or water
Octreotide	0.05 mg/mL 0.1 mg/mL 0.5 mg/mL	Initial: 50 mcg subcutaneously One to two times per day and titrate dose based on indication up to 600 mcg/day in two to four divided doses

- Monitor body weight, serum osmolality, serum electrolytes, complete blood cell count, urinalysis, and cultures (if appropriate). With an urgent or emergency situation, any change in the volume status of the patient is the most important outcome.
- Toxic patients (those with fever, dehydration, and hematochezia and those who are hypotensive) require hospitalization; they need IV electrolyte solutions and empiric antibiotics while awaiting cultures. With quick management, they usually recover within a few days.

See Chapter 36, Diarrhea, Constipation, and Irritable Bowel Syndrome, authored by Patricia H. Fabel and Kayce M. Shealy, for a more detailed discussion of this topic.

CHAPTER 24 — Gastroesophageal Reflux Disease

- *Gastroesophageal reflux disease* (GERD) is symptoms or complications resulting from refluxed stomach contents into the esophagus, oral cavity (including the larynx), or lungs. Episodic heartburn that is not frequent or painful enough to be bothersome is not included in the definition.

PATHOPHYSIOLOGY

- In some cases, reflux is associated with defective lower esophageal sphincter (LES) pressure or function. Patients may have decreased LES pressure from spontaneous transient LES relaxations, transient increases in intraabdominal pressure, or an atonic LES. Some foods and medications decrease LES pressure (Table 24–1).
- Problems with other normal mucosal defense mechanisms may contribute to development of GERD, including abnormal esophageal anatomy, improper esophageal clearance of gastric fluids, reduced mucosal resistance to acid, delayed or ineffective gastric emptying, inadequate production of epidermal growth factor, and reduced salivary buffering of acid.
- Esophagitis occurs when the esophagus is repeatedly exposed to refluxed gastric contents for prolonged periods. This can progress to erosion of the squamous epithelium of the esophagus (erosive esophagitis).
- Substances that promote esophageal damage upon reflux into the esophagus include gastric acid, pepsin, bile acids, and pancreatic enzymes. Composition and volume of the refluxate and duration of exposure are the primary determinants of the consequences of gastroesophageal reflux.
- An "acid pocket" is thought to be an area of unbuffered acid in the proximal stomach that accumulates after a meal and may contribute to GERD symptoms postprandially. GERD patients are predisposed to upward migration of acid from the acid pocket, which may also be positioned above the diaphragm in patients with hiatal hernia, increasing the risk for acid reflux.
- Reflux and heartburn are common in pregnancy because of hormonal effects on LES tone and increased intraabdominal pressure from an enlarging uterus.
- Obesity is a risk factor for GERD due to increased intra-abdominal pressure. Transient LES relaxations, an incompetent LES, and impaired esophageal motility have also been attributed to obesity.
- Complications from long-term acid reflux include esophagitis, esophageal strictures, Barrett esophagus, and esophageal adenocarcinoma.

CLINICAL PRESENTATION

- *Symptom-based GERD* (with or without esophageal tissue injury) typically presents with heartburn, usually described as a substernal sensation of warmth or burning rising up from the abdomen that may radiate to the neck. It may be waxing and waning in character and aggravated by activities that worsen reflux (eg, recumbent position, bending-over, eating a high-fat meal). Other symptoms are water brash (hypersalivation), belching, and regurgitation. Alarm symptoms that may indicate complications include dysphagia, odynophagia, bleeding, and weight loss. The absence of tissue injury or erosions is termed nonerosive reflux disease (NERD).
- *Tissue injury–based GERD* (with or without esophageal symptoms) may present with esophagitis, esophageal strictures, Barrett esophagus, or esophageal carcinoma. Alarm symptoms may also be present.
- Extraesophageal symptoms may include chronic cough, laryngitis, and asthma.

223

TABLE 24–1	Foods and Medications That May Worsen GERD Symptoms
Foods/Beverages	**Medications**
Decreased lower esophageal sphincter pressure	
Fatty meal	Anticholinergics
Carminatives (peppermint, spearmint)	Barbiturates
Chocolate	Caffeine
Coffee, cola, tea	Dihydropyridine calcium channel blockers
Garlic	Dopamine
Onions	Estrogen
Chili peppers	Nicotine
Alcohol (wine)	Nitrates
	Progesterone
	Tetracycline
	Theophylline
Direct irritants to the esophageal mucosa	
Spicy foods	Aspirin
Orange juice	Bisphosphonates
Tomato juice	Nonsteroidal anti-inflammatory drugs (NSAIDs)
Coffee	Iron
Tobacco	Quinidine
	Potassium chloride

DIAGNOSIS

- Clinical history is sufficient to diagnose GERD in patients with typical symptoms.
- Perform diagnostic tests in patients who do not respond to therapy or who present with alarm symptoms. Endoscopy is preferred for assessing mucosal injury and identifying strictures, Barrett esophagus and other complications.
- Ambulatory pH monitoring, combined impedance–pH monitoring, high-resolution esophageal pressure topography (HREPT), impedance manometry, and an empiric trial of a proton pump inhibitor may be useful in some situations.

TREATMENT

- <u>Goals of Treatment</u>: The goals are to reduce or eliminate symptoms, decrease frequency and duration of gastroesophageal reflux, promote healing of injured mucosa, and prevent development of complications.

GENERAL APPROACH

- Therapy is directed toward decreasing acidity of the refluxate, decreasing the gastric volume available to be refluxed, improving gastric emptying, increasing LES pressure, enhancing esophageal acid clearance, and protecting the esophageal mucosa.
- Treatment is determined by disease severity and includes the following:
  ✓ Lifestyle changes and patient-directed therapy with **antacids** and/or nonprescription acid suppression therapy (**histamine 2–receptor antagonists [H$_2$RAs]** and/or **proton pump inhibitors [PPIs]**)
  ✓ Pharmacologic treatment with prescription-strength acid suppression therapy
  ✓ Antireflux surgery

- The initial intervention depends in part on the patient's condition (symptom frequency, degree of esophagitis, and presence of complications). A step-down approach is most often advocated, starting with a PPI instead of an H$_2$RA, and then stepping down to the lowest dose of acid suppression needed to control symptoms (**Table 24–2**).
- Patient-directed therapy (self-treatment with nonprescription medication) is appropriate for mild, intermittent symptoms. Patients with continuous symptoms for longer than 2 weeks should seek medical attention; such patients are generally started on empiric acid-suppression therapy. Patients not responding satisfactorily or those with alarm symptoms (eg, dysphagia) should undergo endoscopy.

NONPHARMACOLOGIC THERAPY

- Potential lifestyle changes depending on the patient situation:
  - ✓ Elevate head of the bed by placing 6- to 8-in blocks under the headposts. Sleep on a foam wedge.
  - ✓ Weight reduction for overweight or obese patients.
  - ✓ Avoid foods that decrease LES pressure (eg, fats, chocolate)
  - ✓ Include protein-rich meals to augment LES pressure.
  - ✓ Avoid foods with irritant effects on the esophageal mucosa (eg, citrus juices, coffee, pepper)
  - ✓ Eat small meals and avoid eating immediately prior to sleeping (within 3 hours if possible).
  - ✓ Stop smoking.
  - ✓ Avoid alcohol.
  - ✓ Avoid tight-fitting clothes.
  - ✓ For mandatory medications that irritate the esophageal mucosa, take in the upright position with plenty of liquid or food (if appropriate).
- Antireflux surgery (eg, Nissen fundoplication) should be considered when long-term pharmacotherapy is undesirable or when patients have complications. Bariatric surgery, specifically Roux-en-Y gastric bypass surgery, should be considered in obese patients contemplating surgery.
- Radiofrequency ablation is recommended in Barrett esophagus with high grade dysplasia and may be an option in low grade dysplasia.
- A FDA-approved device for magnetic sphincter augmentation can improve lower esophageal resistance and reduce GERD symptoms; many patients can discontinue PPE use. However, there are concerns about long-term safety of this approach.

PHARMACOLOGIC THERAPY

Antacids and Antacid-Alginic Acid Products

- Antacids provide immediate symptomatic relief for mild GERD and are often used concurrently with acid suppression therapies. Patients who require frequent use for chronic symptoms should receive prescription-strength acid suppression therapy instead.
- Some antacid products are combined with alginic acid, which is not a potent acid-neutralizing agent and does not enhance LES pressure, but it does form a viscous solution that floats on the surface of gastric contents. This serves as a protective barrier for the esophagus against reflux of gastric contents and reduces frequency of reflux episodes. The combination product may be superior to antacids alone in relieving GERD symptoms, but efficacy data indicating endoscopic healing are lacking.
- Antacids have a short duration, which necessitates frequent administration throughout the day to provide continuous acid neutralization. Taking antacids after meals can increase duration from approximately 1 hour to 3 hours; however, nighttime acid suppression cannot be maintained with bedtime doses. Antacids may cause constipation or diarrhea depending on the magnesium or aluminum content. These agents have significant drug interactions with tetracycline, ferrous sulfate, isoniazid, sulfonylureas, and quinolone antibiotics.

TABLE 24–2 Therapeutics Approach to GERD in Adults

Recommended Treatment Regimen	Brand Name	Oral Dose	Comments
Intermittent, mild heartburn (individualized lifestyle modifications + patient-directed therapy with antacids and/or nonprescription H₂RAs or nonprescription PPI)			
Individualized lifestyle modifications			Lifestyle modifications should be individualized for each patient
Patient-directed therapy with antacids (≥12 years old)			
Magnesium hydroxide/aluminum hydroxide with simethicone	Maalox	10–20 mL as needed or after meals and at bedtime	If symptoms are unrelieved with lifestyle modifications and nonprescription medications after 2 weeks, patient should seek medical attention; do not exceed 16 teaspoonfuls per 24 hours
Antacid/alginic acid	Gaviscon	2–4 tablets or 10–20 mL after meals and at bedtime	Note: Content of alginic acid varies greatly among products; the higher the alginic acid the better
Calcium carbonate	Tums	500 mg, 2–4 tablets as needed	
Patient-directed therapy with nonprescription H₂RAs (up to twice daily) (≥12 years old)			
Cimetidine	Tagamet HB	200 mg	If symptoms are unrelieved with lifestyle modifications and nonprescription medications after 2 weeks, patient should seek medical attention
Famotidine	Pepcid AC	10–20 mg	
Nizatidine	Axid AR	75 mg	
Ranitidine	Zantac	75–150 mg	
Patient-directed therapy (>18 years old) with nonprescription PPIs (taken once daily)			
Esomeprazole	Nexium 24HR	20 mg	If symptoms are unrelieved with lifestyle modifications and nonprescription medications after 2 weeks, patient should seek medical attention
Lansoprazole	Prevacid 24HR	15 mg	
Omeprazole	Prilosec OTC	20 mg	
Omeprazole/sodium bicarbonate	Zegerid OTC	20 mg/1100 mg	

Symptomatic relief of GERD (individualized lifestyle modifications + prescription-strength H$_2$RAs or prescription-strength PPIs)

Individualized lifestyle modifications			Lifestyle modifications should be individualized for each patient
Prescription-strength H$_2$RAs (for 6–12 weeks)			
Cimetidine (off-label use)	Tagamet	400 mg four times daily or 800 mg twice daily	For typical symptoms, treat empirically with prescription-strength acid suppression therapy
			If symptoms recur, consider maintenance therapy. Note: Most patients will require standard doses for maintenance therapy
Famotidine	Pepcid	20 mg twice daily	
Nizatidine	Axid	150 mg twice daily	
Ranitidine	Zantac	150 mg twice daily	
Prescription-strength PPIs (for 4–8 weeks)			
Dexlansoprazole	Dexilant	30 mg once daily for 4 weeks	For typical symptoms, treat empirically with prescription-strength acid suppression therapy
Esomeprazole	Nexium	20–40 mg once daily	Patients with moderate to severe symptoms should receive a PPI as initial therapy
Lansoprazole	Prevacid	15mg once daily	
Omeprazole	Prilosec	20 mg once daily	If symptoms recur, consider maintenance therapy
Omeprazole/sodium bicarbonate	Zegerid	20 mg once daily	
Pantoprazole (Off-label use)	Protonix	40 mg once daily	
Rabeprazole	Aciphex	20 mg once daily	

Healing of erosive esophagitis or treatment of patients with moderate to severe symptoms or complications (individualized lifestyle modifications + high-dose H$_2$RAs or PPIs or antireflux surgery)

Individualized lifestyle modifications			Lifestyle modifications should be individualized for each patient.

(continued)

TABLE 24–2 Therapeutics Approach to GERD in Adults (*Continued*)

Recommended Treatment

Regimen	Brand Name	Oral Dose	Comments
PPIs (up to twice daily for up to 8 weeks)			
Dexlansoprazole	Dexilant	60 mg daily	For extraesophageal or alarm symptoms, obtain endoscopy with biopsy to evaluate mucosa
Esomeprazole	Nexium	20–40 mg daily	If symptoms are relieved, consider maintenance therapy. PPIs are the most effective maintenance therapy for patients with extraesophageal symptoms, complications, and erosive disease. Start with twice-daily PPI therapy if reflux chest syndrome present
Lansoprazole	Prevacid	30 mg once or twice daily	
Omeprazole	Prilosec	20 mg once or twice daily	
Rabeprazole	Aciphex	20 mg once or twice daily	Patients not responding to pharmacologic therapy, including those with persistent extraesophageal symptoms, should be evaluated via manometry and/or ambulatory reflux monitoring
Pantoprazole	Protonix	40 mg once or twice daily	Twice daily dosing of PPIs is considered off-label use
High-dose H$_2$RAs (for 8–12 weeks)			
Cimetidine	Tagamet	400 mg four times daily or 800 mg twice daily	If high-dose H$_2$RA needed, may consider using PPI to lower cost, increase convenience, and increase tolerability
Famotidine	Pepcid	20–40 mg twice daily	Four times daily H$_2$RA is considered off-label use for nizatidine
Nizatidine	Aciphex	150 mg two-four times daily	
Ranitidine	Zantac	150 mg four times daily	
Interventional therapy			
Antireflux surgery			

(H$_2$RA, histamine$_2$-receptor antagonist; PPI, proton pump inhibitor.)

Proton Pump Inhibitors

- PPIs (**dexlansoprazole**, **esomeprazole**, **lansoprazole**, **omeprazole**, **pantoprazole**, and **rabeprazole**) block gastric acid secretion by inhibiting hydrogen potassium adenosine triphosphatase in gastric parietal cells, resulting in profound and long-lasting antisecretory effects.
- PPIs provide more rapid symptom relief and higher healing rates than H_2RAs in patients with moderate to severe GERD and should be given empirically to patients with troublesome symptoms. Twice-daily use is indicated in patients not responding to standard once-daily therapy.
- Adverse effects include headache, diarrhea, constipation, and abdominal pain. Community-acquired pneumonia has occurred with short-term use. Potential long-term adverse effects include enteric infections, vitamin B_{12} deficiency, hypomagnesemia, and bone fractures. PPIs can decrease the absorption of **ketoconazole** and **itraconazole**, which require an acidic environment for absorption. Inhibition of cytochrome P450 2C19 (CYP2C19) by PPIs (especially omeprazole) may decrease effectiveness of clopidogrel. No drug interactions with lansoprazole, pantoprazole, or rabeprazole have been seen with CYP2C19 substrates such as diazepam, warfarin, and phenytoin.
- PPIs degrade in acidic environments and are therefore formulated in delayed-release capsules or tablets. Dexlansoprazole, esomeprazole, lansoprazole, and omeprazole contain enteric-coated (pH-sensitive) granules in capsules. For patients unable to swallow the capsules, the contents can be mixed in applesauce or orange juice. In patients with nasogastric tubes, the contents can be mixed in 8.4% sodium bicarbonate solution. Esomeprazole granules can be dispersed in water. Esomeprazole, omeprazole, and pantoprazole are also available in a delayed-release oral suspension powder packet, and lansoprazole is available as a delayed-release, orally disintegrating tablet. Patients taking pantoprazole or rabeprazole should be instructed not to crush, chew, or split the delayed-release tablets. Dexlansoprazole is available in a dual delayed-release capsule, with the first release occurring 1 to 2 hours after the dose, and the second release occurring 4 to 5 hours after the dose.
- **Zegerid**® is a combination product containing omeprazole 20 or 40 mg with sodium bicarbonate in immediate-release oral capsules and powder for oral suspension. It should be taken on an empty stomach at least 1 hour before a meal. Zegerid offers an alternative to delayed-release capsules, powder for suspension, or IV formulation in adults with nasogastric tubes.
- **Lansoprazole**, **esomeprazole**, and **pantoprazole** are available in IV formulations for patients who cannot take oral medications, but they are not more effective than oral preparations and are significantly more expensive.
- Patients should take oral PPIs in the morning 30 to 60 minutes before breakfast or their largest meal of the day to maximize efficacy, because these agents inhibit only actively secreting proton pumps. Dexlansoprazole can be taken without regard to meals. If dosed twice daily, the second PPI dose should be taken approximately 10 to 12 hours after the morning dose and prior to a meal or snack.

Histamine 2–Receptor Antagonists

- The H_2RAs **cimetidine**, **ranitidine**, **famotidine**, and **nizatidine** in divided doses are effective for treating mild to moderate GERD. Low-dose nonprescription H_2RAs or standard doses given twice daily may be beneficial for symptomatic relief of mild GERD. Patients not responding to standard doses may be hypersecretors of gastric acid and require higher doses (see **Table 24–2**). However, when standard doses of H_2RAs do not adequately relieve symptoms, it is more cost-effective and effective to switch to a PPI. The efficacy of H_2RAs for GERD treatment is highly variable and frequently lower than desired. Prolonged courses are frequently required.
- The most common adverse effects include headache, fatigue, dizziness, and either constipation or diarrhea. Cimetidine may inhibit the metabolism of theophylline, warfarin, phenytoin, nifedipine, and propranolol, among other drugs.

- Because all H_2RAs are equally efficacious, selection of the specific agent should be based on differences in pharmacokinetics, safety profile, and cost.

Promotility Agents

- Promotility agents may be useful adjuncts to acid-suppression therapy in patients with a known motility defect (eg, LES incompetence, decreased esophageal clearance, delayed gastric emptying). However, these agents are not as effective as acid suppression therapy and have undesirable adverse effects.
- **Metoclopramide**, a dopamine antagonist, increases LES pressure in a dose-related manner and accelerates gastric emptying. However, it does not improve esophageal clearance. Metoclopramide provides symptomatic improvement for some patients, but evidence supporting endoscopic healing is lacking. Common adverse reactions include somnolence, nervousness, fatigue, dizziness, weakness, depression, diarrhea, and rash. In addition, extrapyramidal effects, tardive dyskinesia, and other CNS effects limit its usefulness.
- **Bethanechol** has limited value because of side effects (eg, urinary retention, abdominal discomfort, nausea, flushing).

Mucosal Protectants

- **Sucralfate** is a nonabsorbable aluminum salt of sucrose octasulfate. It has limited value for treatment of GERD but may be useful for management of radiation esophagitis and bile or nonacid reflux GERD.

Combination Therapy

- Combination therapy with an acid-suppressing agent and a promotility agent or mucosal protectant seems logical, but data supporting such therapy are limited. This approach is not recommended unless a patient has GERD with motor dysfunction. Using the omeprazole-sodium bicarbonate immediate-release product in addition to once daily PPI therapy offers an alternative for nocturnal GERD symptoms.

Maintenance Therapy

- Many patients with GERD relapse after medication is withdrawn, so maintenance treatment may be required. Consider long-term therapy to prevent complications and worsening of esophageal function in patients who have symptomatic relapse after discontinuation of therapy or dosage reduction, including patients with Barrett esophagus, strictures, or erosive esophagitis.
- Most patients require standard doses to prevent relapses. PPIs are the drugs of choice for maintenance treatment of moderate to severe esophagitis or symptoms. Usual once-daily doses are omeprazole 20 mg, lansoprazole 30 mg, rabeprazole 20 mg, or esomeprazole 20 mg. Low doses of a PPI or alternate-day regimens may be effective in some patients with milder symptoms. H_2RAs may be effective maintenance therapy in patients with mild disease.
- "On-demand" maintenance therapy, by which patients take their PPI only when they have symptoms, may be effective for patients with endoscopy-negative GERD.

EVALUATION OF THERAPEUTIC OUTCOMES

- Monitor frequency and severity of GERD symptoms, and educate patients on symptoms that suggest presence of complications requiring immediate medical attention, such as dysphagia. Evaluate patients with persistent symptoms for presence of strictures or other complications.
- Monitor patients for adverse drug effects and the presence of extraesophageal symptoms such as laryngitis, asthma, or chest pain. These symptoms require further diagnostic evaluation.

See Chapter 32, Gastroesophageal Reflux Disease, authored by Dianne B. May, Michael Thiman, and Satish Rao, for a more detailed discussion of this topic.

25 Hepatitis, Viral

- *Viral hepatitis* refers to the clinically important hepatotropic viruses responsible for hepatitis A (HAV), hepatitis B (HBV), delta hepatitis, hepatitis C (HCV), and hepatitis E.

HEPATITIS A

- HAV infection usually produces a self-limited disease and acute viral infection, with a low fatality rate, and confers lifelong immunity.
- HAV infection primarily occurs through transmission by the fecal-oral route, person-to-person, or by ingestion of contaminated food or water. The incidence of HAV correlates directly with low socioeconomic status, poor sanitary conditions, and overcrowding. Rates of HAV infection have increased among international travelers, injection drug users, and men who have sex with men.
- The disease exhibits three phases: incubation (averaging 28 days, range 15–50 days), acute hepatitis (generally lasting 2 months), and convalescence. Nearly all individuals will have clinical resolution within 6 months of the infection, and a majority will have done so by 2 months. HAV does not lead to chronic infections.
- The clinical presentation of HAV infection is given in Table 25–1. Children younger than 6 years are typically asymptomatic.
- The diagnosis of acute HAV infection is based on clinical criteria of acute onset of fatigue, abdominal pain, loss of appetite, intermittent nausea and vomiting, jaundice or elevated serum aminotransferase levels, and serologic testing for immunoglobulin (Ig) M anti-HAV.

TREATMENT

- Goals of Treatment: Complete clinical resolution, including reducing complications, normalization of liver function, and reductiong infectivity and transmission. No specific treatment options exist for HAV. Management of HAV infection is primarily supportive. Steroid use is not recommended.

PREVENTION

- The spread of HAV can be best controlled by avoiding exposure. The most important measures to avoid exposure include good handwashing techniques and good personal hygiene practices.
- The current vaccination strategy in the United States includes vaccinating all children at 1 year of age. Groups who should receive HAV vaccine are shown in Table 25–2.
- Three inactivated virus vaccines are currently licensed in the United States: Havrix, Vaqta, and Twinrix. Approved dosing recommendations are shown in Table 25–3. Seroconversion rates of 94% or greater are achieved with the first dose.
- Ig is used when pre- or postexposure prophylaxis against HAV infection is needed in persons for whom vaccination is not an option. It is most effective if given during the incubation phase of infection. A single dose of Ig of 0.02 mL/kg is given intramuscularly for postexposure prophylaxis or short-term (≤5 months) preexposure prophylaxis. For lengthy stays, a single dose of 0.06 mL/kg is used. HAV vaccine may also be given with Ig.
- For people recently exposed to HAV and not previously vaccinated, Ig is indicated for
  ✓ Patients younger than 12 months or older than 40 years, are immunocompromised, have chronic liver disease or have underlying medical conditions, or for whom vaccine is contraindicated.
- Common vaccine side effects include soreness and warmth at the injection site, headache, malaise, and pain.

231

TABLE 25–1	Clinical Presentation of Acute Hepatitis A

Signs and symptoms
- The preicteric phase brings nonspecific influenza-like symptoms consisting of anorexia, nausea, fatigue, and malaise.
- Abrupt onset of anorexia, nausea, vomiting, malaise, fever, headache, and right upper quadrant abdominal pain with acute illness.
- Icteric hepatitis is generally accompanied by dark urine, alcoholic (lightcolored) stools, and worsening of systemic symptoms.
- Pruritus is often a major complaint of icteric patients.

Physical examination
- Icteric sclera, skin, and secretions
- Mild weight loss of 2–5 kg
- Hepatomegaly

Laboratory tests
- Positive-serum Ig M anti–HAV
- Mild elevations of serum bilirubin, γ-globulin, and hepatic transaminase (ALT and AST) values to about twice normal in acute anicteric disease
- Elevations of alkaline phosphatase, γ-glutamyl transferase, and total bilirubin in patients with cholestatic illness

(ALT, alanine transaminase; AST, aspartate transaminase; HAV, hepatitis A virus; Ig, immunoglobulin.)

HEPATITIS B

- HBV is a leading cause of chronic hepatitis, cirrhosis, and hepatocellular carcinoma.
- Transmission of HBV occurs sexually, parenterally, and perinatally. In the United States, transmission occurs predominantly through sexual contact or injection-drug use. International travel is also an important risk factor.
- Patients who continue to have detectable HBsAg for more than 6 months have chronic HBV. Patients with chronic HBV infection may develop complications of decompensated cirrhosis, including hepatic insufficiency and portal hypertension as their compensated cirrhosis progresses to decompensated cirrhosis within a 5-year period. HBV is a risk factor for development of hepatocellular carcinoma.

TABLE 25–2	Recommendations for Hepatitis A Virus Vaccination

All children at 1 year of age.
Children and adolescents between 2 and 18 years who live in states or communities where routine hepatitis A vaccination has been implemented because of high disease incidence.
Persons traveling to or working in countries that have high or intermediate endemicity of infection.[a]
MSM.
Illegal drug users.
Persons with occupational risk for infection (eg, persons who work with HAV-infected primates or with HAV in a research laboratory).
Persons who have clotting factor disorders.
Persons with chronic liver disease.
All previously unvaccinated persons anticipating close personal contact (eg, household contact or regular babysitter) with an international adoptee from a country of high or intermediate endemicity within the first 60 days following the arrival of the adoptee.

(HAV, hepatitis A virus; MSM, men who have sex with men.)
[a]Travelers to Canada, Western Europe, Japan, Australia, or New Zealand are at no greater risk for infection than they are in the United States. All other travelers should be assessed for HAV risk.
From Centers for Disease Control and Prevention

TABLE 25–3	Recommended Dosing of Hepatitis A Vaccines			
Vaccine	Age (Years)	Dose of Hepatitis A Antigen	No. of Doses	Schedule
HAVRIX	1–18	720 ELISA units	2	0, 6–12 months
	≥19	1440 ELISA units	2	0, 6–12 months
VAQTA	1–18	25 units	2	0, 6–18 months
	≥19	50 units	2	0, 6–18 months
TWINRIX[a]	≥18	720 ELISA units	3	0, 1, 6 months
	≥18 (accelerated schedule)	720 ELISA units	4	0, 7 days, 21–30 days, +12 months

(ELISA, enzyme-linked immunosorbent assay.)
[a]Combination hepatitis A and B vaccine, also contains 20 mcg of hepatitis B surface antigen and requires a three-dose schedule.
From Centers for Disease Control and Prevention

- There are phases of chronic HBV infection, with patterns noted in Table 25–4.
- The interpretation of serologic markers for HBV is given in Table 25–5.
- The clinical presentation of chronic HBV is given in Table 25–6.

PREVENTION

- Prophylaxis of HBV can be achieved by vaccination (HBV vaccine) or by passive immunity in postexposure cases with HBV Ig which provides temporary passive immunity.
- The goal of immunization against viral hepatitis is prevention of the short-term viremia that can lead to transmission of infection, clinical disease, and chronic HBV infection.
- Persons who should receive HBV vaccine are listed in Table 25–7.
- Side effects of the vaccines include soreness at the injection site, headache, fatigue, irritability, and fever.

TREATMENT

- Goals of Therapy: The goals of therapy are to suppress HBV replication and prevent disease progression to cirrhosis and HCC. The loss of HBsAg is becoming an increasingly more important goal in therapy.

TABLE 25–4	Patterns of Chronic Hepatitis B Virus Phases			
State	HBeAg Status	ALT Level	HBV DNA IU/mL[a]	Other
Immune tolerant	+	WNL	>20,000	
Immune active	+	High	>2,000	
Immune control	–	WNL	<2,000	Anti-HBe +
Immune escape	–	High	>20,000	Anti-HBe +
Reactivation	±	High	>20,000	Associated with immunosuppressive states or therapies

(ALT, alanine transaminase; DNA, deoxyribonucleic acid; HBeAg, hepatitis B e antigen; HBV, hepatitis B virus; WNL, within normal limits.)
[a]Conversion factor for IU/mL to IU/L is 1000.

TABLE 25–5	Interpretation of Serologic Tests in Hepatitis B Virus	
Tests	**Result**	**Interpretation**
HBsAg	(–)	Susceptible
Anti-HBc	(–)	
Anti-HBs	(–)	
HBsAg	(–)	Immune because of natural infection
Anti-HBc	(+)	
Anti-HBs	(+)	
HBsAg	(–)	Immune because of vaccination (valid only if test performed
Anti-HBc	(c)	1–2 months after third vaccine dose)
Anti-HBs	(+)	
HBsAg	(+)	Acute infection
Anti-HBc	(+)	
IgM anti-HBc	(+)	
Anti-HBs	(–)	
HBsAg	(+)	Chronic infection
Anti-HBc	(+)	
IgM anti-HBc	(–)	
Anti-HBs	(–)	
HBsAg	(–)	Four interpretations possible:
Anti-HBc	(+)	1. Recovery from acute infection
Anti-HBs	(–)	2. Distant immunity and test not sensitive enough to detect low level of HBs in serum
		3. Susceptible with false-positive anti-HBc
		4. May have undetectable level of HBsAg in serum and be chronically infected

(HBc, hepatitis B core; HBs, hepatitis B surface; HBsAg, hepatitis B surface antigen; IgM, immunoglobulin M.)
(From Centers for Disease Control and Prevention. Hepatitis B Serology. http://www.cdc.gov/ncidod/ diseases/hepatitis/b/Bserology.htm)

- Some patients with chronic HBV infection should be treated. Recommendations for treatment consider the patient's age, serum HBV DNA and ALT levels, and histologic evidence and clinical progression of the disease. A suggested treatment algorithm for chronic HBV is shown for patients without (Fig. 25–1) and with cirrhosis (Fig. 25–2).
- All patients with chronic HBV infection should be counseled on preventing disease transmission, avoiding alcohol, and on being immunized against HAV.
- The immune-mediating agents approved as first-line therapy are interferon (IFN)-alfa and pegylated (peg) IFN-alfa. The antiviral agents lamivudine, telbivudine, adefovir, entecavir, and tenofovir are all approved as first-line therapy options for chronic HBV.
- For HBeAg-positive patients, treatment is recommended until HBeAg seroconversion and an undetectable HBV viral load are achieved and for 6 months of additional treatment. In HBeAg-negative patients, treatment should be continued until HBsAg clearance.

HEPATITIS C

- HCV is the most common blood-borne pathogen and is most often acquired through injection drug use. Screening for HCV infection is recommended in groups who are at high risk for infection (Table 25–8). All patients born between 1945 and 1965 should be screened.
- Transmission may occur by sexual contact; hemodialysis; or household, occupational, or perinatal exposure.
- In up to 85% of patients, acute HCV infection leads to chronic infection defined by persistently detectable HCV RNA for 6 months or more.

| TABLE 25–6 | Clinical Presentation of Chronic Hepatitis B[a] |

Signs and symptoms
- Easy fatigability, anxiety, anorexia, and malaise
- Ascites, jaundice, variceal bleeding, and hepatic encephalopathy can manifest with liver decompensation
- Hepatic encephalopathy is associated with hyperexcitability, impaired mentation, confusion, obtundation, and eventually coma
- Vomiting and seizures

Physical examination
- Icteric sclera, skin, and secretions
- Decreased bowel sounds, increased abdominal girth, and detectable fluid wave
- Asterixis
- Spider angiomata

Laboratory tests
- Presence of HBsAg >6 months
- Intermittent elevations of hepatic transaminase (ALT and AST) and HBV DNA >20,000 IU/mL (>20 × 10⁶ IU/L)
- Liver biopsies for pathologic classification as chronic persistent hepatitis, chronic active hepatitis, or cirrhosis

(ALT, alanine transaminase; AST, aspartate transaminase; DNA, deoxyribonucleic acid; HBsAg, hepatitis B surface antigen; HBV, hepatitis B virus.)
[a]Chronic hepatitis B can be present even without all the signs, symptoms, and physical examination findings listed being apparent.

| TABLE 25–7 | Recommendations for Hepatitis B Virus Vaccination |

Infants
Adolescents including all previously unvaccinated children <19 years
All unvaccinated adults aged 19–59 with diabetes mellitus
All unvaccinated adults at risk for infection
All unvaccinated adults seeking vaccination (specific risk factor not required)
Men and women with a history of other STDs and persons with a history of multiple sex partners (>1 partner/6 months)
MSM
Current or recent IDUs
Household contacts and sex partners of persons with chronic hepatitis B infection and healthcare and public safety workers with exposure to blood in the workplace
Clients and staff of institutions for the developmentally disabled
International travelers to regions with high or intermediate levels (HBsAg prevalence ≤2%) of endemic HBV infection
Recipients of clotting factor concentrates
STD clinic patients
HIV patient/HIV-testing patients
Drug abuse treatment and prevention clinic patients
Correctional facilities inmates
Chronic dialysis/ESRD patients including predialysis, peritoneal dialysis, and home dialysis patients
Persons with chronic liver disease

(HBsAg, hepatitis B surface antigen; HBV, hepatitis B virus; HIV, human immunodeficiency virus; ESRD, end-stage renal disease; IDUs, injection drug users; MSM, Men who have sex with men; STDs, sexually transmitted diseases.)

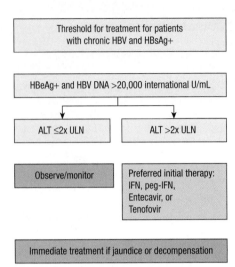

(ALT, alanine transaminases; HBeAg, hepatitis B e antigen; HBsAg, hepatitis B surface antigen; HBV, hepatitis B virus; DNA, deoxyribonucleic acid; IFN, interferon; peg-IFN, pegylated interferon; HBV DNA concentration of >20,000 IU/mL is equivalent to >20 × 10⁶ IU/L.)

FIGURE 25–1. Suggested management algorithm for chronic hepatitis B virus infection based on the recommendations of the American Association for the Study of Liver Diseases. (*Adapted from Lok ASF, McMahon BJ. AASLD practice guidelines: Chronic hepatitis B: Update 2009. Hepatology 2009;50:661-662.*)

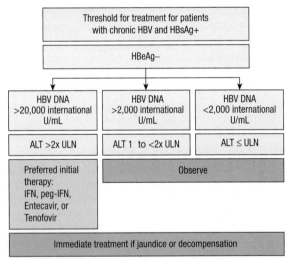

(ALT, alanine transaminases; HBeAg, hepatitis B e antigen; HBsAg, hepatitis B surface antigen; HBV, hepatitis B virus; DNA, deoxyribonucleic acid; IFN, interferon; peg-IFN, pegylated interferon; HBV DNA concentrations of >20,000, >2,000, and ≤2,000 IU/mL are equivalent to >20 × 10⁶, >2 × 10⁶, and ≤2 × 10⁶ IU/L, respectively.)

FIGURE 25–2. Suggested management algorithm based on the recommendations of the American Association for the Study of Liver Diseases for chronic hepatitis B virus–infected patients with cirrhosis. (*Adapted from Lok ASF, McMahon BJ. AASLD practice guidelines: Chronic hepatitis B: Update 2009. Hepatology 2009;50:661-662.*)

TABLE 25-8	Recommendations for Hepatitis C Virus Screening

Anyone born between 1945 and 1965
Current or past use of injection drug use
Coinfection with HIV
Received blood transfusions or organ transplantations before 1992
Received clotting factors before 1987
Patients who have ever been on hemodialysis
Patients with unexplained elevated ALT levels or evidence of liver disease
Healthcare and public safety workers after a needle-stick or mucosal exposure to
    HCV-positive blood
Children born to HCV-positive mothers
Sexual partners of HCV-positive patients

(ALT, alanine transaminase; HCV, hepatitis C virus; HIV, human immunodeficiency virus.)

- Patients with acute HCV are often asymptomatic and undiagnosed. One third of adults will experience some mild and nonspecific symptoms, including persistent fatigue. Additional symptoms include right upper quadrant pain, nausea, or poor appetite.
- HCV cirrhosis poses a 30% risk of developing end-stage liver disease over 10 years as well as a 1% to 2% risk per year of developing hepatocellular carcinoma

TREATMENT

- Goals of Treatment: The goal is to eradicate HCV infection, which prevents the development of chronic HCV infection and sequelae.
- Although treatment for HCV is recommended for all HCV-infected persons, patients with advanced fibrosis, compensated cirrhosis, liver transplant recipients, and patients with severe extrahepatic HCV are recommended for urgent treatment.
- Recommended treatment regimens for HCV infection are given in Table 25–9.

TABLE 25-9	AASLD/IDSA Recommended Treatment Regimens for Treatment-Naïve Patients with Hepatitis C (in order of evidence, then alphabetically)	
HCV Genotype	**No Cirrhosis**	**Compensated Cirrhosis (CTP Class A)**
1a	Elbasvir/Grazoprevir × 12 weeks[a] Ledipasvir/Sofosbuvir × 12 weeks Ombitasvir/Paritaprevir/ritonavir + Dasabuvir and ribavirin × 12 weeks Simeprevir + Sofosbuvir × 12 weeks Sofosbuvir/Velpatasvir × 12 weeks Daclatasvir + Sofosbuvir × 12 weeks	Elbasvir/Grazoprevir × 12 weeks[a] Ledipasvir/Sofosbuvir × 12 weeks Sofosbuvir/Velpatasvir × 12 weeks
1b	Elbasvir/Grazoprevir × 12 weeks Ledipasvir/Sofosbuvir × 12 weeks Ombitasvir/Paritaprevir/ritonavir + Dasabuvir and ribavirin × 12 weeks Simeprevir + Sofosbuvir × 12 weeks Sofosbuvir/Velpatasvir × 12 weeks Daclatasvir plus Sofosbuvir × 12 weeks	Elbasvir/Grazoprevir × 12 weeks Ledipasvir/Sofosbuvir × 12 weeks Ombitasvir/Paritaprevir/ritonavir + Dasabuvir and ribavirin × 12 weeks Sofosbuvir/Velpatasvir × 12 weeks
2	Sofosbuvir/Velpatasvir × 12 weeks	Sofosbuvir/Velpatasvir × 12 weeks
3	Daclatasvir + Sofosbuvir × 12 weeks Sofosbuvir/Velpatasvir × 12 weeks	Sofosbuvir/Velpatasvir × 12 weeks Daclatasvir + Sofosbuvir × 12 weeks

(CTP, Child Turcotte Pugh.)
[a]If no NS5A resistance detected; Pretreatment resistance testing recommended.

- Current guidelines suggest a 12- or 24-week duration of therapy, depending on HCV GT and subtype (1a vs 1b). The need for concomitant ribavirin use varies. Patients who are treatment-experienced, in whom prior peg-IFN and ribavirin therapy failed, and who have cirrhosis may require either a longer treatment duration or the addition of ribavirin.
- Adherence to therapy is a crucial component in response, especially among genotype 1–infected patients.
  ✓ All patients with chronic HCV infection should be vaccinated for HAV and HBV.

PREVENTION

- No HCV vaccine is currently available.

See Chapter 40, Viral Hepatitis, authored by Paulina Deming, for a more detailed discussion of this topic.

26 Inflammatory Bowel Disease

- There are two forms of idopathic *inflammatory bowel disease* (IBD): ulcerative colitis (UC), a mucosal inflammatory condition confined to the rectum and colon, and Crohn's disease, a transmural inflammation of gastrointestinal (GI) mucosa that may occur in any part of the GI tract. The etiologies of both conditions are unknown, but they may have a common pathogenic mechanism.

ETIOLOGY AND PATHOPHYSIOLOGY

- Factors involved in cause of IBD include infectious agents, genetics, the environment, and the immune system. There is thought to be shift toward the presence of more proinflammatory bacteria in the GI tract, often referred to as dysbiosis. Several genetic markers and loci have been identified that occur more frequently in patients with IBD. The inflammatory response with IBD may indicate abnormal regulation of the normal immune response or an autoimmune reaction to self-antigens.
- Th1 cytokine activity is excessive in CD and increased expression of interferon-γ in the intestinal mucosa and production of IL-12 are features of the immune response in CD. In contrast, Th2 cytokine activity is excessive with UC (with excess production of IL-13). Tumor necrosis factor-α (TNF-α) is a pivotal pro-inflammatory cytokine that is increased in the mucosa and intestinal lumen of patients with CD and UC.
- Antineutrophil cytoplasmic antibodies are found in a high percentage of patients with UC and less frequently with CD.
- Smoking appears to be protective for ulcerative colitis but associated with increased frequency of Crohn disease. The use of nonsteroidal anti-inflammatory drugs (NSAIDs) may trigger disease occurrence or lead to disease flares.
- UC and Crohn disease differ in two general respects: anatomical sites and depth of involvement within the bowel wall. There is, however, overlap between the two conditions, with a small fraction of patients showing features of both diseases (**Table 26–1**).

ULCERATIVE COLITIS

- UC is confined to the colon and rectum and affects primarily the mucosa and the submucosa. The primary lesion occurs in the crypts of the mucosa (crypts of Lieberkühn) in the form of a crypt abscess.
- Local complications (involving the colon) occur in the majority of patients with UC. Relatively minor complications include hemorrhoids, anal fissures, and perirectal abscesses.
- A major complication is toxic megacolon, a severe condition that occurs in up to 7.9% of UC patients admitted to hospitals. The patient with toxic megacolon usually has a high fever, tachycardia, distended abdomen, elevated white blood cell count, and a dilated colon.
- The risk of colonic carcinoma is much greater in patients with UC as compared with the general population.
- Patients with UC may have hepatobiliary complications, including fatty liver, pericholangitis, chronic active hepatitis, cirrhosis, sclerosing cholangitis, cholangiocarcinoma, and gallstones.
- Arthritis commonly occurs in patients with IBD and is typically asymptomatic and migratory. Arthritis typically involves one or a few large joints, such as the knees, hips, ankles, wrists, and elbows.
- Ocular complications (iritis, episcleritis, and conjunctivitis) occur in some patients. Skin and mucosal lesions associated with IBD include erythema nodosum, pyoderma gangrenosum, aphthous ulceration, and Sweet syndrome.

TABLE 26–1	Comparison of the Clinical and Pathologic Features of Crohn's Disease and Ulcerative Colitis	
Feature	**Crohn's Disease**	**Ulcerative Colitis**
Clinical		
Malaise, fever	Common	Uncommon
Rectal bleeding	Common	Common
Abdominal tenderness	Common	May be present
Abdominal mass	Common	Absent
Abdominal pain	Common	Unusual
Abdominal wall and internal fistulas	Common	Absent
Distribution	Discontinuous	Continuous
Aphthous or linear ulcers	Common	Rare
Pathologic		
Rectal involvement	Rare	Common
Ileal involvement	Very common	Rare
Strictures	Common	Rare
Fistulas	Common	Rare
Transmural involvement	Common	Rare
Crypt abscesses	Rare	Very common
Granulomas	Common	Rare
Linear clefts	Common	Rare
Cobblestone appearance	Common	Absent

CROHN DISEASE

- Crohn disease is a transmural inflammatory process. The terminal ileum is the most common site of the disorder, but it may occur in any part of the GI tract. Most patients have some colonic involvement. Patients often have normal bowel separating segments of diseased bowel; that is, the disease is often discontinuous.
- Complications of Crohn disease may involve the intestinal tract or organs unrelated to it. Small bowel stricture with subsequent obstruction is a complication that may require surgery. Fistula formation is common and occurs much more frequently than with UC.
- Systemic complications of Crohn disease are common and similar to those found with UC. Arthritis, iritis, skin lesions, and liver disease often accompany Crohn disease.
- Nutritional deficiencies are common with Crohn disease (weight loss, iron deficiency anemia, vitamin B_{12} deficiency, folate deficiency, hypoalbuminemia, hypokalemia, and osteomalacia).

CLINICAL PRESENTATION

ULCERATIVE COLITIS

- There is a wide range of presentation in UC, ranging from mild abdominal cramping with frequent small-volume bowel movements to profuse diarrhea (Table 26–2). Many patients have disease confined to the rectum (proctitis).
- Most patients with UC experience intermittent bouts of illness after varying intervals of no symptoms.

TABLE 26–2	Clinical Presentation of Ulcerative Colitis

Signs and symptoms
- Abdominal cramping
- Frequent bowel movements, often with blood in the stool
- Weight loss
- Fever and tachycardia in severe disease
- Blurred vision, eye pain, and photophobia with ocular involvement
- Arthritis
- Raised, red, tender nodules that vary in size from 1 cm to several centimeters

Physical examination
- Hemorrhoids, anal fissures, or perirectal abscesses may be present
- Iritis, uveitis, episcleritis, and conjunctivitis with ocular involvement
- Dermatologic findings with erythema nodosum, pyoderma gangrenosum, or aphthous ulceration

Laboratory tests
- Decreased hematocrit/hemoglobin
- Increased ESR or CRP
- Leukocytosis and hypoalbuminemia with severe disease
- (+) perinuclear antineutrophil cytoplasmic antibodies

- Mild disease, which afflicts two thirds of patients, has been defined as fewer than four stools daily, with or without blood, with no systemic disturbance and a normal erythrocyte sedimentation rate (ESR).
- Patients with moderate disease have more than four stools per day but with minimal systemic disturbance.
- With severe disease, the patient has more than six stools per day with blood, with evidence of systemic disturbance as shown by fever, tachycardia, anemia, or ESR greater than 30 (8.3 µm/s). And with fulminant disease there is more than 10 bowel movements per day with continuous bleeding, toxicity, abdominal tenderness, requirement for transfusion, and colonic dilation.

CROHN DISEASE

- As with UC, the presentation of Crohn disease is highly variable (Table 26–3). A patient may present with diarrhea and abdominal pain or a perirectal or perianal lesion.

TABLE 26–3	Clinical Presentation of Crohn Disease

Signs and symptoms
- Malaise and fever
- Abdominal pain
- Frequent bowel movements
- Hematochezia
- Fistula
- Weight loss and malnutrition
- Arthritis

Physical examination
- Abdominal mass and tenderness
- Perianal fissure or fistula

Laboratory tests
- Increased white blood cell count, ESR, and CRP
- (+) anti–*Saccharomyces cerevisiae* antibodies

- The course of Crohn disease is characterized by periods of remission and exacerbation. Some patients may be free of symptoms for years, whereas others experience chronic problems despite medical therapy.
- The Crohn Disease Activity Index (CDAI) and the Harvey Bradshaw Index are used to gauge response to therapy and determine remission. Disease activity may be assessed and correlated by evaluation of serum C-reactive protein concentrations.

TREATMENT

- Goals of Treatment: Resolution of acute inflammatory processes, resolution of attendant complications (eg, fistulas or abscesses), alleviation of systemic manifestations (eg, arthritis), maintenance of remission from acute inflammation, or surgical palliation or cure.

NONPHARMACOLOGIC TREATMENT

- Protein–energy malnutrition and suboptimal weight is reported in up to 85% of patients with CD.
- The nutritional needs of the majority of patients can be adequately addressed with enteral supplementation. Parenteral nutrition is generally reserved for patients with severe malnutrition or those who fail enteral therapy or have a contraindication to receiving enteral therapy, such as perforation, protracted vomiting, short bowel syndrome, or severe intestinal stenosis.
- Probiotic formulas have been effective for inducing and maintaining remission in UC, but the data are not conclusive.
- Colectomy may be necessary when the UC patient has disease uncontrolled by maximum medical therapy or when there are complications of the disease such as colonic perforation, toxic megacolon, uncontrolled colonic hemorrhage, or colonic strictures
- The indications for surgery with Crohn disease are not as well established as they are for UC, and surgery is usually reserved for the complications of the disease. There is a high recurrence rate of Crohn disease after surgery.

PHARMACOLOGIC THERAPY

- The major types of drug therapy used in IBD are **aminosalicylates, glucocorticoids,** immunosuppressive agents (**azathioprine, mercaptopurine, cyclosporine,** and **methotrexate**), antimicrobials (**metronidazole** and **ciprofloxacin**), agents to inhibit tumor necrosis factor-α (TNF-α) (anti–TNF-α antibodies), and leukocyte adhesion and migration (**natalizumab and vedolizumab**).
- **Sulfasalazine** combines a sulfonamide (sulfapyridine) antibiotic and mesalamine (5-aminosalicylic acid) in the same molecule. **Mesalamine**-based products are listed in **Table 26–4.**
- Corticosteroids and adrenocorticotropic hormone have been widely used for the treatment of UC and Crohn disease and are used in moderate to severe disease. Prednisone is most commonly used. Immunosuppressive agents such as azathioprine and mercaptopurine (a metabolite of azathioprine) are used in the long-term treatment of IBD. These agents are generally reserved for patients who fail mesalamine therapy or are refractory to or dependent on corticosteroids. Cyclosporine has been of short-term benefit in acute, severe UC when used in a continuous infusion.
- Methotrexate given 15 to 25 mg intramuscularly or subcutaneously once weekly is useful for treatment and maintenance of Crohn's disease and may be steroid sparing.
- Antimicrobial agents, particularly metronidazole and ciprofloxacin, are frequently used in attempts to control Crohn disease, particularly when it involves the perineal area or fistulas. Ciprofloxacin has also been used for treatment of Crohn disease.
- Infliximab is an anti-TNF antibody that is useful in moderate to severe active CD an UC as well as steroid-dependent or fistulizing disease, both as induction and maintenance therapy. Adalimumab is another anti-TNF (fully humanized) antibody that is an option for patients with moderate to severe active Crohn disease or UC previously treated with infliximab who have lost response. Natalizumab and vedolizumab are leukocyte adhesion and migration inhibitors that is used for patients with Crohn disease who are unresponsive to other therapies.

TABLE 26–4	Agents for the Treatment of Inflammatory Bowel Disease		
Drug	**Brand Name**	**Initial Dose (g)**	**Usual Range**
Sulfasalazine	Azulfidine	500 mg–1 g	4–6 g/day
	Azulfidine EN	500 mg–1 g	4–6 g/day
Mesalamine suppository	Rowasa	1 g	1 g daily to three times weekly
Mesalamine enema	Canasa	4 g	4 g daily to three times weekly
Mesalamine (oral)	Asacol HD	1.6 g/day	2.8–4.8 g/day
	Apriso	1.5 g/day	1.5 g/day once daily
	Lialda	1.2–2.4 g/day	1.2–4.8 g/day once daily
	Pentasa	2 g/day	2–4 g/day
	Delzicol	1.2 g/day	2.4–4.8 g/day
Olsalazine	Dipentum	1.5 g/day	1.5–3 g/day
Balsalazide	Colazal	2.25 g/day	2.25–6.75 g/day
Azathioprine	Imuran, Azasan	50–100 mg	1–2.5 mg/kg/day
Cyclosporine	Gengraf	2–4 mg/kg/day IV	2–4 mg/kg/day IV
	Neoral, Sandimmune	2–8 mg/kg/day oral	
Mercaptopurine	Purinethol	50–100 mg	1–2.5 mg/kg/day
Methotrexate	No branded IM injection	15–25 mg IM weekly	15–25 mg IM weekly
Adalimumab	Humira	160 mg SC day 1	80 mg SC 2 (day 15), and then 40 mg every 2 weeks
Certolizumab	Cimzia	400 mg SC	400 mg SC weeks 2 and 4, and then 400 mg SC monthly
Infliximab	Remicade	5 mg/kg IV	5 mg/kg weeks 2 and 6, 5–10 mg/kg every 8 weeks
Natalizumab	Tysabri	300 mg IV	300 mg IV every 4 weeks
Budesonide	Enterocort EC, Uceris	9 mg	6–9 mg daily
Vedolizumab	Entyvio	300 mg IV	300 mg IV weeks 2 and 6 and then every 8 weeks
Golimumab	Simponi	200 mg SC	100 mg SC weeks 2 and 4

(SC, subcutaneous; IM, intramuscular.)

Ulcerative Colitis

MILD TO MODERATE DISEASE

- Most patients with mild to moderate active UC can be managed on an outpatient basis with oral and/or topical mesalamine (Fig. 26–1). When given orally, usually 4 to 6 g/day of sulfasalazine is required to attain control of active inflammation. Sulfasalazine therapy should be instituted at 500 mg/day and increased every few days up to 4 g/day or the maximum tolerated.

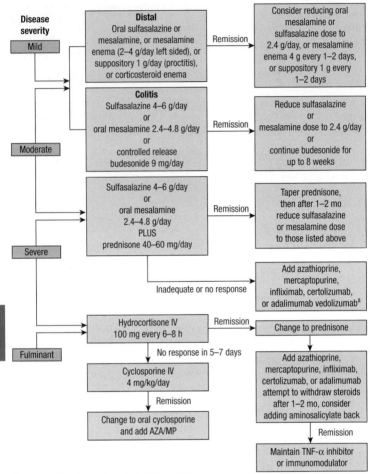

[a]Can be considered as an alternative to TNF-α inhibitors.

FIGURE 26-1. Treatment approaches for ulcerative colitis.

- Oral mesalamine derivatives (such as those listed in Table 26–4) are reasonable alternatives to sulfasalazine for treatment of UC as they are better tolerated.

MODERATE TO SEVERE DISEASE

- Steroids have a place in the treatment of moderate to severe UC or in those who are unresponsive to maximal doses of oral and topical mesalamine. Oral **prednisone** 40 to 60 mg daily is recommended for adult.
- TNF-α inhibitors are an option for patients with moderate to severe disease who are unresponsive to ASAs, corticosteroids, or other immunosuppressive agents.

SEVERE OR INTRACTABLE DISEASE

- Patients with uncontrolled severe colitis or incapacitating symptoms require hospitalization for effective management. Most medication is given by the parenteral route.

- IV hydrocortisone 300 mg daily in three divided doses or methylprednisolone 60 mg once daily is considered a first-line agent. A trial of steroids is warranted in most patients before proceeding to colectomy, unless the condition is grave or rapidly deteriorating.
- Patients who are unresponsive to parenteral corticosteroids after 3 to 7 days can receive cyclosporine or infliximab. A continuous IV infusion of cyclosporine 2 to 4 mg/kg/day is the typical dose range utilized and may delay the need for colectomy.

MAINTENANCE OF REMISSION

- Once remission from active disease has been achieved, the goal of therapy is to maintain the remission.
- Oral agents, including sulfasalazine, mesalamine, and balsalazide, are all effective options for maintenance therapy. The optimal dose to prevent relapse is 2 to 2.4 g/day of mesalamine equivalent, with rates of relapse over 6 to 12 months reported as 40%.
- Steroids do not have a role in the maintenance of remission with UC because they are ineffective. Steroids should be gradually withdrawn after remission is induced (over 2–4 weeks).

Crohn Disease
ACTIVE CROHN DISEASE

- Mesalamine derivatives have not demonstrated significant efficacy in CD. They are often tried as an initial therapy for mild to moderate CD given their favorable adverse effect profile.
- Mesalamine derivatives (e.g., **Pentasa**) that release mesalamine in the small bowel may be more effective than sulfasalazine for ileal involvement.
- Oral **corticosteroids**, such as prednisone 40 to 60 mg/day, are generally considered first-line therapies and are frequently used for the treatment of moderate to severe Crohn disease. Budesonide (Entocort) at a dose of 9 mg daily is a viable first-line option for patients with mild to moderate ileal or right-sided (ascending colonic) disease.
- Metronidazole, given orally as 10 to 20 mg/kg/day in divided doses, may be useful in some patients with CD, particularly for patients with colonic or ileocolonic involvement, those with perineal disease, or those who are unresponsive to sulfasalazine.
- Azathioprine and mercaptopurine are not recommended to induce remission in moderate to severe CD; however, they are effective in maintaining steroid-induced remission and are generally limited to use for patients not achieving adequate response to standard medical therapy or in the setting of steroid dependency. Clinical response to azathioprine and mercaptopurine may be related to whole-blood concentrations of the metabolite 6-thioguanine (TGN). Concentrations of TGN greater than 230 to 260 pmol/8×10^8 erythrocytes have beneficial effects, but monitoring is not routinely performed or may not be available at some sites.
- Patients deficient in thiopurine S-methyltransferase (TPMT) are at greater risk of bone marrow suppression from azathioprine and mercaptopurine. Determination of TPMT or TPMT genotype is recommended to guide dosage.
- Methotrexate, given as a weekly injection of 15–25 mg, has demonstrated some efficacy for induction of remission in Crohn disease, and for corticosteroid sparing effects. The risks are bone marrow suppression, hepatotoxicity, and pulmonary toxicity.
- The TNF-α inhibitors are the most effective and thus the preferred agents in the management of moderate to severe CD. All agents in this class, with the exception of golimumab, which is not approved for use in CD in the United States, have similar rates of efficacy. The use of TNF-α inhibitors in combination with thiopurines has quickly become the preferred approach to treatment of moderate to severe CD.
- The integrin antagonists are options for patients who do not respond to steroids or TNF-α inhibitors.

MAINTENANCE OF REMISSION

- Prevention of recurrence of disease is clearly more difficult with Crohn disease than with ulcerative colitis. Sulfasalazine and oral mesalamine derivatives are effective in preventing acute recurrences in quiescent Crohn disease (**Fig. 26–2**).
- Systemic steroids or budesonide also have no place in the prevention of recurrence of Crohn disease; these agents do not appear to alter the long-term course of the disease. Budesonide can be considered for maintenance therapy for up to 1 year, particularly in patients who have become corticosteroid dependent, for whom switching to budesonide is an option.
- Azathioprine and mercaptopurine are effective in maintaining remission in CD. There is weak evidence to suggest that, methotrexate is effective in maintaining remission in Crohn disease.

SELECTED COMPLICATIONS

Toxic Megacolon

- The treatment required for toxic megacolon includes general supportive measures to maintain vital functions, consideration for early surgical intervention, and antimicrobials.
- Aggressive fluid and electrolyte management are required for dehydration. When the patient has lost significant amounts of blood (through the rectum), blood replacement is also necessary.
- Steroids in high dosages (hydrocortisone 100 mg every 8 hours) should be administered IV to reduce acute inflammation.
- Broad-spectrum antimicrobials that include coverage for gram-negative bacilli and intestinal anaerobes should be used as preemptive therapy in the event that perforation occurs.

Systemic Manifestations

- For arthritis, aspirin or another NSAID may be beneficial, as are corticosteroids. However, NSAID use may exacerbate the underlying IBD and predispose patients to GI bleeding.
- Anemia secondary to blood loss from the GI tract can be treated with oral ferrous sulfate. Vitamin B_{12} or folic acid may also be required.

EVALUATION OF THERAPEUTIC OUTCOMES

- See **Table 26–5** for drug monitoring guidelines.
- Patients receiving sulfasalazine should receive oral **folic acid** supplementation, as sulfasalazine inhibits folic acid absorption.
- The success of therapeutic regimens to treat IBDs can be measured by patient-reported complaints, signs and symptoms, direct physician examination (including endoscopy), history and physical examination, selected laboratory tests, and quality of life measures.
- To create more objective measures, disease-rating scales or indices have been created. The Crohn Disease Activity Index is a commonly used scale, particularly for evaluation of patients during clinical trials. The scale incorporates eight elements: (1) number of stools in the past 7 days, (2) sum of abdominal pain ratings from the past 7 days, (3) rating of general well-being in the past 7 days, (4) use of antidiarrheals, (5) body weight, (6) hematocrit, (7) finding of abdominal mass, and (8) a sum of symptoms present in the past week. Elements of this index provide a guide for those measures that may be useful in assessing the effectiveness of treatment regimens. The Perianal CD Activity Index is used for perianal Crohn disease.
- Standardized assessment tools have also been constructed for UC. Elements in these scales include (1) stool frequency; (2) presence of blood in the stool; (3) mucosal appearance (from endoscopy); and (4) physician's global assessment based on physical examination, endoscopy, and laboratory data.

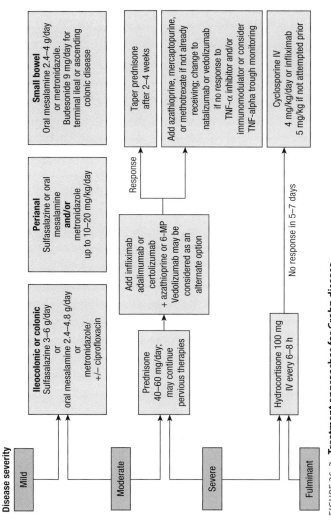

FIGURE 26–2. Treatment approaches for Crohn disease.

TABLE 26–5	Drug Monitoring Guidelines		
Drug(s)	**Adverse Drug Reaction**	**Monitoring Parameters**	**Comments**
Sulfasalazine	Nausea, vomiting, headache Rash, anemia, pneumonitis Hepatotoxicity, nephritis Thrombocytopenia, lymphoma	Folate, complete blood count Liver function tests, Scr, BUN	Increase the dose slowly, over 1–2 weeks
Mesalamine	Nausea, vomiting, headache	GI disturbances	
Corticosteroids	Hyperglycemia, dyslipidemia	Blood pressure, fasting lipid panel	Avoid long-term use if possible or consider budesonide
	Osteoporosis, hypertension, acne	Glucose, vitamin D, bone density	
	Edema, infection, myopathy, psychosis		
Azathioprine/ mercaptopurine	Bone marrow suppression, pancreatitis	Complete blood count	Check TPMT activity
	Liver dysfunction, rash, arthralgia	Scr, BUN, liver function tests, genotype/ phenotype	May monitor TGN
Methotrexate	Bone marrow suppression, pancreatitis	Complete blood count, Scr, BUN	Check baseline pregnancy test
	Pneumonitis, pulmonary fibrosis, hepatitis	Liver function tests	Chest x-ray
Infliximab	Infusion-related reactions (infliximab), infection	Blood pressure/heart rate (infliximab)	Need negative PPD and viral serologies
Adalimumab	Heart failure, optic neuritis, demyelination, injection site reaction, signs of infection	Neurologic exam, mental status	
Certolizumab	Lymphoma	Trough concentrations (infliximab)	
Golimumab		Antidrug antibodies (all agents)	
Natalizumab Vedolizumab	Infusion-related reactions	Brain MRI, mental status, progressive multifocal leukoencephalopathy	Vedolizumab not associated with PML

See Chapter 34, *Inflammatory Bowel Disease*, authored by Brian A. Hemstreet, for a more detailed discussion of this topic.

27 Nausea and Vomiting

- *Nausea* is usually defined as the inclination to vomit or as a feeling in the throat or epigastric region alerting an individual that vomiting is imminent. Vomiting is defined as the ejection or expulsion of gastric contents through the mouth, often requiring a forceful event.

ETIOLOGY AND PATHOPHYSIOLOGY

- Specific etiologies associated with nausea and vomiting are presented in **Table 27–1**.
- **Table 27–2** presents cytotoxic agents categorized by their emetogenic potential. Although some agents may have greater emetogenic potential than others, combinations of agents, high doses, clinical settings, psychological conditions, prior treatment experiences, and unusual stimuli to sight, smell, or taste may alter a patient's response to a drug treatment.
- The three consecutive phases of emesis are nausea, retching, and vomiting. Nausea, the imminent need to vomit, is associated with gastric stasis. Retching is the labored movement of abdominal and thoracic muscles before vomiting. The final phase of emesis is vomiting, the forceful expulsion of gastric contents due to GI retroperistalsis.
- Vomiting is triggered by afferent impulses to the vomiting center, a nucleus of cells in the medulla. Impulses are received from sensory centers, such as the chemoreceptor trigger zone (CTZ), cerebral cortex, and visceral afferents from the pharynx and GI tract. When excited, afferent impulses are integrated by the vomiting center, resulting in efferent impulses to the salivation center, respiratory center, and the pharyngeal, gastrointestinal (GI), and abdominal muscles, leading to vomiting.

CLINICAL PRESENTATION

- The clinical presentation of nausea and vomiting is given in **Table 27–3**. Nausea and vomiting may be classified as either simple or complex.

TREATMENT

- <u>Goal of Treatment</u>: prevent or eliminate nausea and vomiting; ideally accomplished without adverse effects or with clinically acceptable adverse effects.

GENERAL APPROACH TO TREATMENT

- Treatment options for nausea and vomiting include drug and nondrug modalities and depend on associated medical conditions. For patients with simple complaints, perhaps related to food or beverage consumption, avoidance or moderation of dietary intake may be preferable. Patients with symptoms of systemic illness may improve dramatically as their underlying condition improves. Patients in whom these symptoms result from labyrinth changes produced by motion, may benefit quickly by assuming a stable physical position.
- Psychogenic vomiting may benefit from psychological interventions.

PHARMACOLOGIC MANAGEMENT

- Information concerning commonly available antiemetic preparations is compiled in **Table 27–4**. Treatment of simple nausea or vomiting usually requires minimal therapy.
- For most conditions, a single-agent antiemetic is preferred; however, for those patients not responding to such therapy and those receiving highly emetogenic chemotherapy, multiple-agent regimens are usually required.
- The treatment of simple nausea and vomiting usually requires minimal therapy. Both nonprescription and prescription drugs useful in the treatment of simple nausea and vomiting are usually effective in small, infrequently administered doses.

TABLE 27–1	Specific Etiologies of Nausea and Vomiting

GI mechanisms
  Mechanical obstruction
    Gastric outlet obstruction
    Small bowel obstruction
  Functional GI disorders
    Gastroparesis
    Nonulcer dyspepsia
    Chronic intestinal pseudoobstruction
    Irritable bowel syndrome
  Organic GI disorders
    Peptic ulcer disease
    Pancreatitis
    Pyelonephritis
    Cholecystitis
    Cholangitis
    Hepatitis
  Acute gastroenteritis
    Viral
    Bacterial

Cardiovascular diseases
  Acute myocardial infarction
  Congestive heart failure
  Radio-frequency ablation

Neurologic processes
  Increased intracranial pressure
  Migraine headache
  Vestibular disorders

Metabolic disorders
  Diabetes mellitus (diabetic ketoacidosis)
  Addison's disease
  Renal disease (uremia)

Psychiatric causes
  Psychogenic vomiting
  Anxiety disorders
  Anorexia nervosa

Therapy-induced causes
  Cytotoxic chemotherapy
  Radiation therapy
  Theophylline preparations
  Anticonvulsant preparations
  Digitalis preparations
  Opiates
  Antibiotics
  Volatile general anesthetics

Drug withdrawal
  Opiates
  Benzodiazepines

Miscellaneous causes
  Pregnancy
  Noxious odors
  Operative procedures

TABLE 27–2	Emetic Risk of Agents Used in Oncology		
Emetic Risk (If No Prophylactic Medication Is Administered)	**Cytotoxic Agent (in Alphabetical Order)**	**Emetic Risk (If No Prophylactic Medication Is Administered)**	**Cytotoxic Agent (in Alphabetical Order)**
High (>90%)	Combination of either doxorubicin or epirubicin + cyclophosphamide		Etoposide
	Carmustine		Floxuridine
	Cisplatin (>50 mg/m²)		Fluorouracil
	Cyclophosphamide (≥1500 mg/m²)		Gemcitabine
	Dacarbazine		Interferon alfa (<10 million units/m²)
	Ifosfamide (>10 g/m²)		Ixabepilone
	Mechlorethamine		Lapatinib
	Streptozotocin		Methotrexate (<250 mg/m²)
Moderate (30%–90%)	Aldesleukin (>12–15 million units/m²)		Mitomycin
	Amifostine (>300 mg/m²)		Mitoxantrone
	Arsenic trioxide		Paclitaxel
	Azacitidine		Paclitaxel albumin
	Bendamustine		Pemetrexed
	Busulfan		Pentostatin
	Carboplatin		Romidepsin
	Cisplatin (<50 mg/m²)		Sorafenib
	Clofarabine		Sunitinib
	Cytarabine (>200 mg/m²)		Thiotepa
	Cyclophosphamide (<1500 mg/m²)		Topotecan
	Daunorubicin		Trastuzumab
	Dactinomycin	Minimal (<10%)	Alemtuzumab
	Doxorubicin		Asparaginase
	Epirubicin		Bevacizumab
	Idarubicin		Bleomycin
	Ifosfamide		Bortezomib
	Interferon alfa (10 million units/m²)		Cladribine
	Irinotecan		Cytarabine (<200 mg/m²)
	Melphalan		Decitabine
	Methotrexate (>250 mg/m²)		Denileukin diftitox
	Oxaliplatin		Dexrazoxane
	Procarbazine		Fludarabine
	Temozolomide		Ipilimumab
Low (10%–30%)	Cabazitaxel		Nelarabine
	Capecitabine		Ofatumumab
	Cetuximab		Panitumumab
	Cytarabine (≤200 mg/m²)		PEG-asparaginase
	Docetaxel		Rituximab
	Eribulin		Temsirolimus
	Erlotinib		Trastuzumab
			Valrubicin
			Vinblastine
			Vincristine
			Vinorelbine

TABLE 27–3	Clinical Presentation of Nausea and Vomiting

General

Depending on severity of symptoms, patients may present in mild to severe distress

Symptoms

Simple: Self-limiting, resolves spontaneously, and requires only symptomatic therapy

Complex: Not relieved after administration of antiemetics; progressive deterioration of patient secondary to fluid-electrolyte imbalances; usually associated with noxious agents or psychogenic events

Signs

Simple: Patient complaint of queasiness or discomfort

Complex: Weight loss; fever; abdominal pain

Laboratory tests

Simple: None

Complex: Serum electrolyte concentrations; upper/lower GI evaluation

Other information

Fluid input and output

Medication history

Recent history of behavioral or visual changes, headache, pain, or stress

Family history positive for psychogenic vomiting

Drug Class Information

ANTACIDS

- Single or combination nonprescription antacid products, especially those containing **magnesium hydroxide, aluminum hydroxide**, and/or **calcium carbonate**, may provide sufficient relief from simple nausea or vomiting, primarily through gastric acid neutralization. Common antacid dosage regimens for the relief of nausea and vomiting include one or more 15 to 30 mL doses of single- or multiple-agent products.

HISTAMINE$_2$-RECEPTOR ANTAGONISTS

- Histamine$_2$-receptor antagonists (**cimetidine, famotidine, nizatidine**, and **ranitidine**) may be used in low doses to manage simple nausea and vomiting associated with heartburn or gastroesophageal reflux.

ANTIHISTAMINE-ANTICHOLINERGIC DRUGS

- Antiemetic drugs from the antihistaminic-anticholinergic category may be appropriate in the treatment of simple nausea and vomiting, especially associated with motion sickness.
- Adverse reactions that may be apparent with the use of the antihistaminic-anticholinergic agents primarily include drowsiness or confusion, blurred vision, dry mouth, urinary retention, and possibly tachycardia, particularly in elderly patients.

BENZODIAZEPINES

- Benzodiazepines are relatively weak antiemetics and are primarily used to prevent anxiety or anticipatory nausea and vomiting. Both **alprazolam** and **lorazepam** are used as adjuncts to other antiemetics in patients treated with cisplatin-containing regimens.

PHENOTHIAZINES

- **Phenothiazines** are most useful in patients with simple nausea and vomiting. Rectal administration is a reasonable alternative in patients in whom oral or parenteral administration is not feasible.

TABLE 27–4	Common Antiemetic Preparations and Adult Dosage Regimens					
Drug	Adult Dosage Regimen	Dosage Form/ Route	Availability	Adverse Drug Reactions	Monitoring Parameters	Comments
Antacids						
Antacids (various)	15–30 mL every 2–4 hours prn	Liquid/oral	OTC	Magnesium products: diarrhea Aluminum or calcium products: constipation	Assess for symptom relief	Useful with simple nausea/ vomiting
Antihistaminic—anticholinergic agents						
Dimenhydrinate (Dramamine)	50–100 mg every 4–6 hours prn	Tab, chew tab, cap	OTC	Drowsiness, confusion, blurred vision, dry mouth, urinary retention	Assess for episodic relief of motion sickness or nausea/vomiting	Especially problematic in the elderly Increased risk of complications in patients with BPH, narrow angle glaucoma, or asthma
Diphenhydramine (Benadryl)	25–50 mg every 4–6 hours prn 10–50 mg every 2–4 hours prn	Tab, cap, liquid IM, IV	Rx/OTC			
Hydroxyzine (Vistaril, Atarax)	25–100 mg every 4–6 hours prn	IM (unlabeled use)	Rx			
Meclizine (Bonine, Antivert)	12.5–25 mg 1 hour before travel; repeat every 12–24 hours prn	Tab, chew tab	Rx/OTC			
Scopolamine (Transderm Scop)	1.5 mg every 72 hours	Transdermal patch	Rx			

(continued)

TABLE 27-4 Common Antiemetic Preparations and Adult Dosage Regimens (Continued)

Drug	Adult Dosage Regimen	Dosage Form/ Route	Availability	Adverse Drug Reactions	Monitoring Parameters	Comments
Trimethobenzamide (Tigan)	300 mg three to four times daily 200 mg three to four times daily	Cap IM	Rx			
Benzodiazepines						
Alprazolam (Xanax)	0.5–2 mg three times daily prior to chemotherapy	Tab	Rx (C-IV)	Dizziness, sedation, appetite changes, memory impairment	Assess for episodes of ANV	Place in therapy: ANV
Lorazepam (Ativan)	0.5–2 mg on night before and morning of chemotherapy	Tab	Rx (C-IV)			
Butyrophenones						
Haloperidol (Haldol)	1–5 mg every 12 hours prn	Tab, liquid, IM, IV	Rx	Sedation, constipation, hypotension	Observe for additive sedation especially if used with narcotic analgesics	Place in therapy: palliative care
Droperidol (Inapsine)[a]	2.5 mg; additional 1.25 mg may be given	IM, IV	Rx	QT prolongation and/or torsade de pointes	12-Lead electrocardiogram prior to administration, followed by cardiac monitoring for 2–3 hours after administration	Limited use outside of clinical trials

Cannabinoids

Drug	Dosage	Form	Rx/OTC	Adverse Effects	Monitoring	Comments
Dronabinol (Marinol)	5–15 mg/m² every 2–4 hours prn	Cap	Rx (C-III)	Euphoria, somnolence, xerostomia	Assess for symptom relief	May be useful with refractory CINV
Nabilone (Cesamet)	1–2 mg twice daily	Cap	Rx (C-II)	Somnolence, vertigo, xerostomia		

Corticosteroids

Drug	Dosage	Form	Rx/OTC	Adverse Effects	Monitoring	Comments
Dexamethasone	See Tables 27–5 and 27–6	Tab, IV	Rx	Insomnia, GI symptoms, agitation, appetite stimulation	Assess for efficacy as prophylactic agent: episodes of nausea/vomiting and hydration status	Useful as single-agent or combination therapy for prophylaxis of CINV and PONV

Histamine (H2) antagonists

Drug	Dosage	Form	Rx/OTC	Adverse Effects	Monitoring	Comments
Cimetidine (Tagamet HB)	200 mg twice daily prn	Tab	OTC	Headache	Assess for symptom relief	Useful when nausea due to heartburn or GERD
Famotidine (Pepcid AC)	10 mg twice daily prn	Tab	OTC	Constipation, diarrhea		
Nizatidine (Axid AR)	75 mg twice daily prn	Tab	OTC	Diarrhea, headache		
Ranitidine (Zantac 75)	75 mg twice daily prn	Tab	OTC	Constipation, diarrhea		

5-Hydroxytryptamine-3 receptor antagonists

Drug	Dosage	Form	Rx/OTC	Adverse Effects	Monitoring	Comments
	See Tables 27–5 and 27–6	Tab, IV	Rx	Asthenia, constipation, headache	Assess for efficacy as prophylactic agent: episodes of nausea/vomiting and hydration status	Useful as single-agent or combination therapy for prophylaxis of CINV and PONV

(continued)

TABLE 27–4 Common Antiemetic Preparations and Adult Dosage Regimens (*Continued*)

Drug	Adult Dosage Regimen	Dosage Form/ Route	Availability	Adverse Drug Reactions	Monitoring Parameters	Comments
Miscellaneous agents						
Metoclopramide (Reglan)	10 mg four times daily	Tab	Rx	Asthenia, headache, somnolence	Assess for symptom relief	Prokinetic activity useful in diabetic gastroparesis
Olanzapine (Zyprexa)	2.5–5 mg twice daily	Tab	Rx	Sedation	Assess for decrease in episodes of nausea/vomiting	Use with caution in elderly. May be useful in break-through CINV
Phenothiazines						
Chlorpromazine (Thorazine)	10–25 mg every 4–6 hours prn	Tab, liquid	Rx	Constipation, dizziness, tachycardia, tardive dyskinesia	Assess for decrease in episodes of nausea/vomiting	Useful with simple nausea/ vomiting
	25–50 mg every 4–6 hours prn	IM, IV		See above		
Prochlorperazine (Compazine)	5–10 mg three to four times daily prn	Tab, liquid	Rx	Prolonged QT interval, seda- tion, tardive dyskinesia	Assess for decrease in episodes of nausea/vomiting	Useful with simple nausea/ vomiting and for breakthrough CINV
	5–10 mg every 3–4 hours prn	IM				
	2.5–10 mg every 3–4 hours prn	IV	Rx			
	25 mg twice daily prn	Supp	Rx			

Promethazine (Phenergan)	12.5–25 mg every 4–6 hours prn	Tab, liquid, IM, IV, supp	Rx	Drowsiness, sedation	Assess for decreased nausea/vomiting episodes and improvement in hydration status	
Substance P/neurokinin 1 receptor antagonist						
Aprepitant	See Tables 27–5 and 27–6	Cap, IV	Rx	Constipation, diarrhea, headache, hiccups	Assess for efficacy as prophylactic agent: episodes of nausea/vomiting and hydration status	Useful in combination therapy for prophylaxis of CINV and PONV
Fosaprepitant	See Tables 27–5 and 27–6	IV	Rx			
Netupitant/ palonosetron	See Tables 27–5 and 27–6	Cap	Rx	Same as above plus dyspepsia and fatigue		
Rolapitant		Cap	Rx			Long half-life and no drug interactions

(ANV, anticipatory nausea and vomiting; C-II, C-III, and C-IV, controlled substance schedule 2, 3, and 4, respectively; cap, capsule; chew tab, chewable tablet; CINV, chemotherapy-induced nausea and vomiting; GERD, gastroesophageal reflux disease; liquid, oral syrup, concentrate, or suspension; OTC, nonprescription; PONV, postoperative nausea and vomiting; Rx, prescription; supp, rectal suppository; tab, tablet.)

• Problems associated with these drugs are troublesome and potentially dangerous side effects, including extrapyramidal reactions, hypersensitivity reactions with possible liver dysfunction, marrow aplasia, and excessive sedation.

CORTICOSTEROIDS

• **Dexamethasone** is the most commonly used corticosteroid in the management of chemotherapy-induced nausea and vomiting (CINV) and postoperative nausea and vomiting (PONV), either as a single agent or in combination with 5-hydroxytryptamine-3 receptor antagonists (5-HT$_3$-RAs). For CINV, dexamethasone is effective in the prevention of both cisplatin-induced acute emesis and delayed nausea and vomiting with CINV when used alone or in combination.

METOCLOPRAMIDE

• **Metoclopramide** is used for its antiemetic properties in patients with diabetic gastroparesis and with dexamethasone for prophylaxis of delayed nausea and vomiting associated with chemotherapy administration.

CANNABINOIDS

• Oral **nabilone** and oral **dronabinol** are therapeutic options when CINV is refractory to other antiemetics; but are not indicated as first-line agents.

NEUROKININ 1 RECEPTOR ANTAGONISTS

• Substance P is a peptide neurotransmitter with a preferred receptor is NK1 and is believed to be the primary mediator of the delayed phase of CINV and one of two mediators of the acute phase of CINV.

• **Aprepitant** and **fosaprepitant** (injectable form of aprepitant) are NK$_1$ receptor antagonists that are indicated as part of a multiple drug regimen for prophylaxis of nausea and vomiting associated with high-dose cisplatin-based chemotherapy.

• The combination NK1 receptor antagonist/5-HT3-RA products, **netupitant/palonosetron** and the NK1 receptor antagonist, **rolapitant**, are used in patients receiving moderate to highly emetogenic chemotherapy as part of a three-drug combination consisting of an NK1 receptor antagonist, dexamethasone, and a 5-HT3-RA. This combination is now considered the standard of care for CINV

• Numerous potential drug interactions are possible; clinically significant drug interactions with oral contraceptives, warfarin, and oral dexamethasone have been described.

5-HYDROXYTRYPTAMINE-3 RECEPTOR ANTAGONISTS

• 5-HT3-RAs (**dolasetron, granisetron, ondansetron,** and **palonosetron**) are used in the management of CINV, PONV, and radiation-induced nausea and vomiting. The most common side effects associated with these agents are constipation, headache, and asthenia.

CHEMOTHERAPY-INDUCED NAUSEA AND VOMITING

• Nausea and vomiting that occur within 24 hours of chemotherapy administration are defined as acute; nausea and vomiting that starts more than 24 hours after chemotherapy administration are defined as delayed. The emetogenic potential of the chemotherapeutic agent or regimen (see **Table 27–2**) is the primary factor to consider when selecting an antiemetic for **prophylaxis** of CINV.

• Recommendations for antiemetics in patients receiving chemotherapy are presented in Table 27–5.

Prophylaxis of Chemotherapy-Induced Nausea and Vomiting

• Patients receiving chemotherapy that is classified as being of high emetic risk, should receive a combination antiemetic regimen containing three drugs on the day of chemotherapy administration (day 1)—a 5-HT3-RA plus dexamethasone plus an NK1 receptor antagonist.

TABLE 27-5	Dosage Recommendations for CINV for Adult Patients		
Emetogenic Risk	Acute NV Prevention (Day 1)—Prior to Chemotherapy	Delayed NV Prevention (Days 2–4)	
High[b,c]	**Option 1—NK1 + 5-HT3-RA + Steroid**		
	NK1 Antagonist	*5-HT3 receptor antagonist*	*Steroid*
	Aprepitant 125 mg PO × 1	Dolasetron 100 mg PO × 1	Dexamethasone 12 mg PO/IV × 1[a]

Delayed NV Prevention (Days 2–4):

	Day 2	Day 3	Day 4
Aprepitant 125 mg PO × 1	Aprepitant 80 mg PO + Dexamethasone 8 mg IV/PO	Aprepitant 80 mg PO + Dexamethasone 8 mg IV/PO	Dexamethasone 8 mg IV/PO
Fosaprepitant 150 mg IV × 1	Granisetron 2 mg PO × 1 OR 1 mg PO twice daily OR 0.01 mg/kg (Max 1 mg) IV OR 3.1 mg/h transdermal patch applied 24–48 hours prior to chemo	Dexamethasone 8 mg IV/PO	Dexamethasone 8 mg IV/PO twice daily	Dexamethasone 8 mg IV/PO twice daily	Dexamethasone 8 mg IV/PO twice daily

Emetogenic Risk	Acute NV Prevention (Day 1)—Prior to Chemotherapy			Delayed NV Prevention (Days 2–4)		
High[b,c]	**Option 1—NK1 + 5-HT3-RA + Steroid**					
	NK1 Antagonist	*5-HT3 receptor antagonist*	*Steroid*	*Day 2*	*Day 3*	*Day 4*
	Aprepitant 125 mg PO × 1	Dolasetron 100 mg PO × 1	Dexamethasone 12 mg PO/IV × 1[a]	Aprepitant 80 mg PO + Dexamethasone 8 mg IV/PO	Aprepitant 80 mg PO + Dexamethasone 8 mg IV/PO	Dexamethasone 8 mg IV/PO
	Fosaprepitant 150 mg IV × 1	Granisetron 2 mg PO × 1 OR 1 mg PO twice daily OR 0.01 mg/kg (Max 1 mg) IV OR 3.1 mg/h transdermal patch applied 24–48 hours prior to chemo		Dexamethasone 8 mg IV/PO	Dexamethasone 8 mg IV/PO twice daily	Dexamethasone 8 mg IV/PO twice daily	Dexamethasone 8 mg IV/PO twice daily
	Rolapitant 180 mg PO × 1	Ondansetron 16–24 mg PO × 1 OR 8–16 mg IV × 1	Dexamethasone 20 mg PO/IV × 1	Dexamethasone 8 mg IV/PO twice daily	Dexamethasone 8 mg IV/PO twice daily	Dexamethasone 8 mg IV/PO twice daily
		Palonosetron 0.25 mg IV × 1				
	Option 2—NK1/5-HT3-RA + Steroid			*Day 2*	*Day 3*	*Day 4*
	Netupitant 300 mg PO/Palonosetron 0.5 mg PO × 1 + Dexamethasone 12 mg PO/IV × 1			Dexamethasone 8 mg IV/PO	Dexamethasone 8 mg IV/PO	Dexamethasone 8 mg IV/PO
	Option 3—Olanzapine + 5-HT3-RA + Steroid			*Day 2*	*Day 3*	*Day 4*
	Olanzapine 10 mg PO × 1 + Palonosetron 0.25 mg IV + Dexamethasone 20 mg IV × 1			Olanzapine 10 mg PO	Olanzapine 10 mg PO	Olanzapine 10 mg PO

(continued)

TABLE 27-5	Dosage Recommendations for CINV for Adult Patients (Continued)	
Emetogenic Risk	Acute NV Prevention (Day 1)—Prior to Chemotherapy	Delayed NV Prevention (Days 2–4)
Moderate[b,c]	**Options 1–5-HT3-RA (Palonosetron Preferred) + Steroid (Same doses as listed above) ± NK1**	**Options 1–5-HT3-RA Monotherapy, Days 2–3**
		Dolasetron 100 mg PO daily
		Granisetron 1–2 mg PO daily OR 1 mg PO twice daily OR 0.01 mg/kg (Max 1 mg) IV
		Ondansetron 8 mg PO twice daily OR 16 mg PO daily OR 8–16 mg IV daily
		Option 2—Steroid Monotherapy, Days 2–3
		Dexamethasone 8 mg IV/PO daily
		Option 3—NK1 + Steroid, as listed with High-Risk Delayed Regimen
	Option 2—NK1/5-HT3-RA + Steroid at Doses listed above	± Dexamethasone 8 mg IV/PO daily, Days 2–3
	Option 3—Olanzapine + 5-HT3-RA + Steroid at Doses listed above	Olanzapine 10 mg PO daily, Days 2–3
Low[b,c]	Dexamethasone 12 mg IV/PO daily	None
	Metoclopramide 10–40 mg IV/PO, then every 4–6 hours prn	
	Prochlorperazine 10 mg IV/PO, then every 6 hour prn (max 40 mg/day)	
	5-HT3 receptor antagonist	
	Dolasetron 100 mg PO daily	
	Granisetron 1–2 mg PO daily	
	Ondansetron 8–16 mg PO daily	
Minimal	None	None

[a]Use a lower dose of Dexamethasone if Aprepitant or Fosaprepitant is used.
[b]± Use of H2RA or Proton Pump Inhibitor.
[c]± Use of Lorazepam 0.5–2 mg PO/IV/SL every 6 hours prn on Days 1–4.

- The second option includes a two-drug regimen containing the NK1 receptor antagonist/5-HT3 antagonist combination of NEPA, in addition to reduced dose dexamethasone
- Palonosetron is the preferred IV 5-HT3-RA.
- Patients receiving regimens that are classified as being of moderate emetic risk should receive a combination antiemetic regimen containing a $5\text{-}HT_3\text{-}RA$ plus dexamethasone on day 1 then and either a 5-HT3-RA or dexamethasone continued through day 3.
- For prophylaxis of delayed CINV the regimen used in the prevention of acute CINV in each patient will often dictate the regimen to be used for delayed nausea and vomiting. These regimens frequently include continuing dexamethasone or olanzapine for up to 3 days for those receiving HEC. For those who use aprepitant for prevention of acute CINV, aprepitant must be continued for 3 days in addition to dexamethasone. Any of the above regimens, whether it be HEC, MEC, or low risk, may be used in combination with an acid suppressing agent such as an H2RA or a proton pump inhibitor.

POSTOPERATIVE NAUSEA AND VOMITING

- A variety of pharmacologic approaches are available and may be prescribed as single or combination therapy for prophylaxis of PONV. See Table 27–6 for doses of specific agents.

TABLE 27–6	Recommended Prophylactic Doses of Selected Antiemetics for Postoperative Nausea and Vomiting in Adults and Postoperative Vomiting in Children		
Drug	**Adult Dose**	**Pediatric Dose (IV)**	**Timing of Dose[a]**
Aprepitant[b]	40 mg orally	Not labeled for use in pediatrics	Within 3 hours prior to induction
Dexamethasone	4–5 mg IV	150 mcg/kg up to 5 mg	At induction
Dimenhydrinate	1 mg/kg IV	0.5 mg/kg up to 25 mg	Not specified
Dolasetron	12.5 mg IV	350 mcg/kg up to 12.5 mg	At end of surgery
Droperidol[c]	0.625–1.25 mg IV	10–15 mcg/kg up to 1.25 mg	At end of surgery
Granisetron	0.35–3 mg IV	40 mcg/kg up to 0.6 mg	At end of surgery
Haloperidol	0.5–2 mg (IM or IV)	[d]	Not specified
Methylprednisolone	40 mg IV	[d]	At induction
Ondansetron	4 mg IV, 8 mg ODT	50–100 mcg/kg up to 4 mg	At end of surgery
Palonosetron[b]	0.075 mg IV	[d]	At induction
Promethazine[c]	6.25–12.5 mg IV	[d]	At induction
Scopolamine	Transdermal patch	[d]	Prior evening or 4 hours before surgery

[a]Based on recommendations from consensus guidelines.
[b]Labeled for use in PONV but not included in consensus guidelines.
[c]See FDA "black box" warning.
[d]Pediatric dosing not included in consensus guidelines.

- Patients at highest risk of vomiting should receive two or more prophylactic anti-emetics from different pharmacologic classes, while those at moderate risk should receive one or two drugs. Ondansetron is considered the "gold standard" 5-HT3-RA. For prophylaxis of PONV scopolamine patches must be initiated the evening before the surgery or at least 2 hours prior, whereas NK1 antagonists should be given during the induction of anesthesia; all other agents are recommended to be given at the end of the surgery.
- Patients who experience PONV after receiving prophylactic treatment with a combination of 5-HT3-RA plus dexamethasone should be given rescue therapy from a different drug class such as a phenothiazine, metoclopramide, or droperidol. If no prophylaxis was given initially, the recommended treatment is low-dose 5-HT3-RA such as ondansetron 1 mg.

DISORDERS OF BALANCE

- Beneficial therapy for patients with nausea and vomiting associated with disorders of balance can reliably be found among the antihistaminic-anticholinergic agents. Neither the antihistaminic nor the anticholinergic potency appears to correlate well with the ability of these agents to prevent or treat the nausea and vomiting associated with motion sickness.
- Scopolamine (usually administered as a patch) scopolamine is effective for the prevention of motion sickness and is considered first-line for this indication.

ANTIEMETIC USE DURING PREGNANCY

- Initial management of nausea and vomiting of pregnancy (NVP) often involves dietary changes and/or lifestyle modifications.
- Pyridoxine (10–25 mg one to four times daily) is recommended as first-line therapy with or without doxylamine (12.5–20 mg one to four times daily). Patients with persistent NVP or who show signs of dehydration should receive IV fluid replacement with thiamine.
- Patients with persistent NVP or who show signs of dehydration should receive IV fluid replacement with thiamine. Ondansetron, promethazine, and metoclopramide have similar effectiveness for hyperemesis gravidarum, although ondansetron may be better tolerated due to less adverse effects.

ANTIEMETIC USE IN CHILDREN

- For children receiving chemotherapy of high or moderate risk, a corticosteroid (such as dexamethasone) plus 5-HT$_3$-RAs should be administered. The best doses or dosing strategy has not been determined.
- For nausea and vomiting associated with pediatric gastroenteritis, there is greater emphasis on rehydration measures than on pharmacologic intervention.

See Chapter 35, Nausea and Vomiting, authored by Leigh Anne Hylton Gravatt, Krista L. Donohoe, and Cecily V. DiPiro, for a more detailed discussion of this topic.

28 Pancreatitis

- *Acute pancreatitis* (AP) is an inflammatory disorder of the pancreas characterized by upper abdominal pain and pancreatic enzyme elevations.
- *Chronic pancreatitis* (CP) is a progressive disease characterized by long-standing pancreatic inflammation leading to loss of pancreatic exocrine and endocrine function.

ACUTE PANCREATITIS

PATHOPHYSIOLOGY

- Gallstones and alcohol abuse account for most cases in the United States. Diabetes mellitus and autoimmune disorders such as inflammatory bowel disease are also associated with an increase in acute pancreatitis. A cause cannot be identified in some patients (idiopathic pancreatitis).
- Many medications have been implicated (**Table 28–1**), but drug-induced acute pancreatitis is considered to be rare. A causal association is difficult to confirm because ethical and practical considerations prevent rechallenge.
- AP is initiated by premature activation of trypsinogen to trypsin within the pancreas, leading to activation of other digestive enzymes and autodigestion of the gland.
- Activated pancreatic enzymes within the pancreas and surrounding tissues produce damage and necrosis to pancreatic tissue, surrounding fat, vascular endothelium, and adjacent structures. Lipase damages fat cells, producing noxious substances that cause further pancreatic and peripancreatic injury.
- Release of cytokines by acinar cells injures those cells and enhances the inflammatory response. Injured acinar cells liberate chemoattractants that attract neutrophils, macrophages, and other cells to the area of inflammation, causing systemic inflammatory response syndrome (SIRS). Vascular damage and ischemia cause release of kinins, which make capillary walls permeable and promote tissue edema.
- Pancreatic infection may result from increased intestinal permeability and translocation of colonic bacteria.
- Local complications in severe AP include acute fluid collection, pancreatic necrosis, infection, abscess, pseudocyst formation, and pancreatic ascites.
- Systemic complications include respiratory failure and cardiovascular, renal, metabolic, hemorrhagic, and CNS abnormalities.

CLINICAL PRESENTATION

- Clinical presentation depends on severity of the inflammatory process and whether damage is confined to the pancreas or involves local and systemic complications.
- The initial presentation ranges from moderate abdominal discomfort to excruciating pain, shock, and respiratory distress. Abdominal pain occurs in 95% of patients and is usually epigastric, often radiating to the upper quadrants or back. Onset is usually sudden, and intensity is often described as "knife-like" or "boring." Pain usually reaches maximum intensity within 30 minutes and may persist for hours or days. Nausea and vomiting occur in 85% of patients and usually follow onset of pain.
- Signs include marked epigastric tenderness on palpation with rebound tenderness and guarding in severe cases. The abdomen is often distended and tympanic with decreased or absent bowel sounds in severe disease.
- Vital signs may be normal, but hypotension, tachycardia, and low-grade fever are often observed, especially with widespread pancreatic inflammation and necrosis. Dyspnea and tachypnea are signs of acute respiratory complications.
- Jaundice and altered mental status may be present; other signs of alcoholic liver disease may be present in patients with alcoholic pancreatitis.

TABLE 28–1	Medications Associated with Acute Pancreatitis		
Well-Supported Association	**Probable Association**	**Possible Association**	
5-Aminosalicylic acid	Acetaminophen	Aldesleukin	Indinavir
Asparaginase	Atorvastatin	Amiodarone	Indomethacin
Azathioprine	Hydrochlorothiazide	Atorvastatin	Infliximab
Bortezomib	Ifosfamide	Asparaginase	Ketoprofen
Carbamazepine	Interferon α_{2b}	Calcium	Ketorolac
Cimetidine	Maprotiline	Ceftriaxone	Lipid emulsion
Corticosteroids	Methyldopa	Capecitabine	Liraglutide
Cisplatin	Oxaliplatin	Carboplatin	Lisinopril
Cytarabine	Simvastatin	Celecoxib	Mefenamic acid
Didanosine		Clozapine	Metformin
Enalapril		Cholestyramine	Metolazone
Erythromycin		Ciprofloxacin	Metronidazole
Estrogens		Clarithromycin	Nitrofurantoin
Furosemide		Clonidine	Omeprazole
Hydrochlorothiazide		Cyclosporine	Ondansetron
Mercaptopurine		Danazol	Paclitaxel
Mesalamine		Diazoxide	Pravastatin
Octreotide		Etanercept	Propofol
Olsalazine		Ethacrynic acid	Propoxyphene
Opiates		Exenatide	Rifampin
Pentamidine		Famciclovir	Sertraline
Pentavalent antimonials		Glyburide	Sitagliptin
Sulfasalazine		Gold therapy	Sorafenib
Sulfamethoxazole and trimethoprim		Granisetron	Sulindac
Sulindac		Ibuprofen	Zalcitabine
Tamoxifen		Imatinib	
Tetracyclines			
Valproic acid/salts			

DIAGNOSIS

- Diagnosis of AP requires two of the following: (1) upper abdominal pain, (2) serum lipase or amylase at least three times the upper limit of normal, and (3) characteristic findings on imaging studies.
- Transabdominal ultrasound should be performed in all patients to detect dilated biliary ducts and gallstones. Contrast-enhanced computed tomography (CECT) is used if the diagnosis cannot be made from clinical and laboratory findings. Magnetic resonance cholangiopancreatography (MRCP) is useful for detecting retained common bile duct stones.

- AP may be associated with leukocytosis, hyperglycemia, and hypoalbuminemia. Hepatic transaminases, alkaline phosphatase, and bilirubin are usually elevated in gallstone pancreatitis and in patients with intrinsic liver disease. Marked hypocalcemia indicates severe necrosis and is a poor prognostic sign.
- Serum amylase usually rises 4 to 8 hours after symptom onset, peaks at 24 hours, and returns to normal over the next 8 to 14 days. Concentrations greater than three times the upper limit of normal are highly suggestive of AP.
- Serum lipase is specific to the pancreas, and concentrations are elevated and parallel the serum amylase elevations. Increases persist longer than serum amylase elevations and can be detected after the amylase has returned to normal.
- Hematocrit may be normal, but hemoconcentration results from multiple factors (eg, vomiting). Hematocrit greater than 47% predicts severe AP, and hematocrit less than 44% predicts mild disease.
- C-reactive protein levels greater than 150 mg/dL at 48 to 72 hours predict severe AP.
- Thrombocytopenia and increased international normalized ratio (INR) occur in some patients with severe AP and associated liver disease.

TREATMENT (FIG. 28–1)

- <u>Goals of Treatment</u>: Relieve abdominal pain and nausea; replace fluids; correct electrolyte, glucose, and lipid abnormalities; minimize systemic complications; and manage pancreatic necrosis and infection.

Nonpharmacologic Therapy

- **Nutritional support** is important because AP creates a catabolic state that promotes nutritional depletion. Patients with mild AP can begin oral feeding when pain is decreasing and inflammatory markers are improving. Nutritional support should begin when it is anticipated that oral nutrition will be withheld for longer than 1 week. Enteral feeding via nasogastric or nasojejunal tube is preferred over parenteral nutrition (PN) in severe AP, if it can be tolerated. If enteral feeding is not possible or is inadequate, PN should be implemented before protein and calorie depletion become advanced.

Pharmacologic Therapy

- Patients with AP often require IV antiemetics for nausea.
- Patients requiring ICU admission should be treated with antisecretory agents if they are at risk of stress-related mucosal bleeding.
- Vasodilation from the inflammatory response, vomiting, and nasogastric suction contribute to hypovolemia and fluid and electrolyte abnormalities, necessitating replacement. Patients should receive aggressive fluid replacement to reduce the risks of persistent SIRS and organ failure. Different guidelines recommend goal-directed IV fluid with either lactated Ringer's at an initial rate of 5 to 10 mL/kg/hour or crystalloids at a rate of 250 to 500 mL/hour.
- Parenteral opioid analgesics are used to control abdominal pain. Parenteral **morphine** is often used, and patient-controlled analgesia should be considered in patients who require frequent opioid dosing (eg, every 2–3 hours).
- Prophylactic antibiotics are not recommended in patients with acute pancreatitis without signs or symptoms of infection, including those with necrosis. However, empiric antimicrobial therapy may be considered in patients with necrosis who deteriorate or fail to improve within 7 to 10 days.
- Selective digestive tract decontamination using minimally-absorbed antibiotics (eg, polymyxin E, tobramycin, amphotericin B) to eradicate intestinal flora may reduce the risk of pancreatic infection, but more studies are needed before this approach can be recommended.
- Patients with known or suspected infected AP should receive broad-spectrum antibiotics that cover the range of enteric aerobic gram-negative bacilli and anaerobic organisms. **Imipenem–cilastatin** (500 mg IV every 8 hours) has been widely used but has been replaced on many formularies by newer carbapenems (eg, **meropenem**). A fluoroquinolone (eg, **ciprofloxacin** or **levofloxacin**) combined with **metronidazole** should be considered for penicillin-allergic patients.

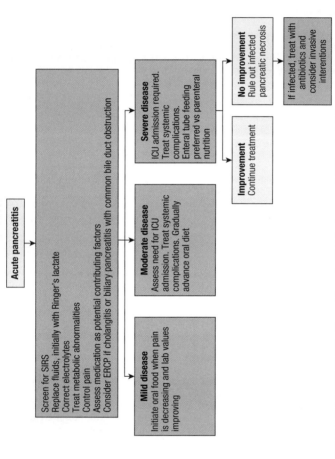

Acute pancreatitis

Screen for SIRS
Replace fluids, initially with Ringer's lactate
Correct electrolytes
Treat metabolic abnormalities
Control pain
Assess medication as potential contributing factors
Consider ERCP if cholangitis or biliary pancreatitis with common bile duct obstruction

Mild disease
Initiate oral food when pain is decreasing and lab values improving

Moderate disease
Assess need for ICU admission. Treat systemic complications. Gradually advance oral diet

Severe disease
ICU admission required. Treat systemic complications. Enteral tube feeding preferred vs parenteral nutrition

Improvement
Continue treatment

No improvement
Rule out infected pancreatic necrosis

If infected, treat with antibiotics and consider invasive interventions

(ERCP, endoscopic retrograde cholangiopancreatography; ICU, intensive care unit; SIRS, systemic inflammatory response syndrome.)

FIGURE 28–1. Algorithm of guidelines for evaluation and treatment of acute pancreatitis.

- There are insufficient data to support routine use of somatostatin or octreotide for treatment of AP. Parenteral histamine2-receptor antagonists and proton pump inhibitors do not improve the overall outcome of patients with AP.

EVALUATION OF THERAPEUTIC OUTCOMES

- In patients with mild AP, assess pain control, fluid and electrolyte status, and nutrition periodically depending on the degree of abdominal pain and fluid loss.
- Transfer patients with severe AP to an intensive care unit for close monitoring of vital signs, fluid and electrolyte status, white blood cell count, blood glucose, lactate dehydrogenase, aspartate aminotransferase, serum albumin, hematocrit, blood urea nitrogen, serum creatinine, and INR. Continuous hemodynamic and arterial blood gas monitoring is essential. Serum lipase, amylase, and bilirubin require less frequent monitoring. Monitor for signs of infection, relief of abdominal pain, and adequate nutritional status. Severity of disease and patient response should be assessed using an evidence-based method.

CHRONIC PANCREATITIS

PATHOPHYSIOLOGY

- CP results from long-standing pancreatic inflammation and leads to irreversible destruction of pancreatic tissue with fibrin deposition and loss of exocrine and endocrine function.
- Chronic ethanol consumption accounts for about two thirds of cases in Western society. Most of the remaining cases are idiopathic, and a small percentage are due to rare causes such as autoimmune, hereditary, and tropical pancreatitis.
- The exact pathogenesis is unknown. Activation of pancreatic stellate cells by toxins, oxidative stress, and/or inflammatory mediators appears to be the cause of fibrin deposition.
- Abdominal pain may be caused by abnormal pain processing in the central nervous system and sensitization of visceral nerves. This may explain the hyperalgesia that CP patients often experience with the need for various methods of pain management. Impaired inhibition of somatic and visceral pain pathways may also cause pain in areas distant to the pancreas.

CLINICAL PRESENTATION

- The main features of CP are abdominal pain, malabsorption with steatorrhea, weight loss, and diabetes. Jaundice occurs in ~10% of patients.
- Patients typically report deep, penetrating epigastric or abdominal pain that may radiate to the back. Pain often occurs with meals and at night and may be associated with nausea and vomiting.
- Steatorrhea and azotorrhea occur in most patients. Steatorrhea is often associated with diarrhea and bloating. Weight loss may occur.
- Pancreatic diabetes is a late manifestation commonly associated with pancreatic calcification.

DIAGNOSIS

- Diagnosis is based primarily on clinical presentation and either imaging or pancreatic function studies. Noninvasive imaging includes abdominal ultrasound, computed tomography (CT), and magnetic resonance cholangiopancreatography (MRCP). Invasive imaging includes endoscopic ultrasonography (EUS) and ERCP.
- Serum amylase and lipase are usually normal or only slightly elevated but may be increased in acute exacerbations.
- Total bilirubin, alkaline phosphatase, and hepatic transaminases may be elevated with ductal obstruction. Serum albumin and calcium may be low with malnutrition.

- Pancreatic function tests include
  ✓ Serum trypsinogen (<20 ng/mL is abnormal)
  ✓ Fecal elastase (<200 mcg/g of stool is abnormal)
  ✓ Fecal fat estimation (>7 g/day is abnormal; stool must be collected for 72 hours)
  ✓ Secretin stimulation (evaluates duodenal bicarbonate secretion)
  ✓ ^{13}C-mixed triglyceride breath test (not available in the U.S.)

TREATMENT

- <u>Goals of Treatment</u>: Major goals for uncomplicated CP are to relieve abdominal pain, treat complications of malabsorption and glucose intolerance, and improve quality of life. Secondary goals are to delay development of complications and treat associated disorders such as depression and malnutrition.

Nonpharmacologic Therapy

- Lifestyle modifications should include abstinence from alcohol and smoking cessation.
- Advise patients with steatorrhea to eat smaller, more frequent meals and reduce dietary fat intake.
- Reduction in dietary fat may be needed if symptoms are uncontrolled with enzyme supplementation. Consumption of a low-fat purified amino acid elemental diet may reduce pain. Supplementation with medium-chain triglycerides should be considered for patients with steatorrhea who are unable to gain weight.. Enteral nutrition via a feeding tube is recommended for patients who cannot consume adequate calories, have continued weight loss, experience complications, or require surgery.
- Invasive procedures and surgery are used primarily to treat uncontrolled pain and the complications of chronic pancreatitis.

Pharmacologic Therapy

- Pain management should begin with weak opioid analgesics (eg, tramadol, codeine) scheduled around the clock (rather than as needed) to maximize efficacy. Administration of short-acting analgesics prior to meals may decrease postprandial pain. Severe pain requires more potent opioids. Unless contraindicated, oral opioids should be used before parenteral, transdermal, or other dosage forms.
  ✓ **Tramadol** 50 to 100 mg every 4 to 6 hours, not to exceed 400 mg/day
  ✓ **Codeine** 30 to 60 mg every 6 hours
  ✓ **Hydrocodone** 5 to 10 mg every 4 to 6 hours
  ✓ **Morphine sulfate (extended-release)** 30 to 60 mg every 8 to 12 hours
  ✓ **Oxycodone** 5 to 10 mg every 6 hours
  ✓ **Methadone** 2.5 to 10 mg every 8 to 12 hours
  ✓ **Hydromorphone** 0.5 to 1 mg every 4 to 6 hours
  ✓ **Fentanyl patch** 25 to 100 mcg/hour every 72 hours
- Adjuvant agents should be added if patients have inadequate relief from opioids alone. **Pregabalin** (75 mg twice daily initially; maximum 300 mg twice daily) has the best evidence. Selective serotonin reuptake inhibitors (eg, **paroxetine**), serotonin/norepinephrine reuptake inhibitors (eg, **duloxetine**), and tricyclic antidepressants can be considered in difficult-to-manage patients.
- Adding pancreatic enzyme supplements for pain control (eg, 4–8 tablets/capsules of a preferred product with each meal plus a histamine$_2$-receptor antagonist or proton pump inhibitor) may be considered in select patients, but no clinical trial data support this approach for pain management.
- Pancreatic enzyme supplementation and reduction in dietary fat intake are the primary treatments for malabsorption due to CP (Fig. 28–2). This combination enhances nutritional status and reduces steatorrhea. The enzyme dose required to

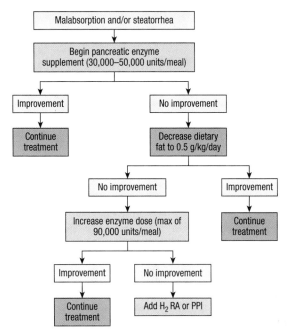

(H$_2$RA, histamine$_2$-receptor antagonist; PPI, proton pump inhibitor.)

FIGURE 28–2. Algorithm for the treatment of malabsorption and steatorrhea in chronic pancreatitis.

minimize malabsorption is 30,000 to 50,000 units of lipase administered with each meal. The dose may be increased to a maximum of 90,000 units per meal. Products containing enteric-coated microspheres or mini-microspheres may be more effective than other dosage forms (Table 28–2).

- Adverse effects from pancreatic enzyme supplements are generally benign, but high doses can lead to nausea, diarrhea, and intestinal upset. A more serious but uncommon adverse effect is fibrosing colonopathy. Deficiencies in fat-soluble vitamins have been reported, and appropriate monitoring (especially of vitamin D) is warranted.
- Addition of a histamine$_2$-receptor antagonist or proton pump inhibitor may increase the effectiveness of pancreatic enzyme therapy by increasing gastric and duodenal pH.
- Exogenous insulin is the primary means for treating diabetes mellitus associated with CP. Metformin may be initiated in early CP and has the added benefit of reducing the risk of pancreatic cancer.

EVALUATION OF THERAPEUTIC OUTCOMES

- Assess the severity and frequency of abdominal pain periodically to determine efficacy of the analgesic regimen. Patients receiving opioids should be prescribed laxatives on an as-needed or scheduled basis and be monitored for constipation.
- For patients receiving pancreatic enzymes for malabsorption, monitor body weight and stool frequency and consistency periodically.
- Monitor blood glucose carefully in diabetic patients.

TABLE 28-2	Commercially Available Pancreatic Enzyme (Pancrelipase) Preparations

	Enzyme Content Per Unit Dose (USP Units)		
Product	**Lipase**	**Amylase**	**Protease**
Tablets			
Viokace™ 10,440 lipase units	10,440	39,150	39,150
Viokace™ 20,880 lipase units	20,880	78,300	78,300
Enteric-coated beads			
Zenpep® 3,000 lipase units	3,000	16,000	10,000
Zenpep® 5,000 lipase units	5,000	27,000	17,000
Zenpep® 10,000 lipase units	10,000	55,000	34,000
Zenpep® 15,000 lipase units	15,000	82,000	51,000
Zenpep® 20,000 lipase units	20,000	109,000	68,000
Zenpep® 25,000 lipase units	25,000	136,000	85,000
Zenpep® 40,000 lipase units	40,000	218,000	136,000
Enteric-coated microspheres with bicarbonate buffer			
Pertzye™ 8,000 lipase units	8,000	30,250	28,750
Pertzye™ 16,000 lipase units	16,000	60,500	57,500
Enteric-coated minimicrospheres			
Creon® 3,000 lipase units	3,000	15,000	9,500
Creon® 6,000 lipase units	6,000	30,000	19,000
Creon® 12,000 lipase units	12,000	60,000	38,000
Creon® 24,000 lipase units	24,000	120,000	76,000
Creon® 36,000 lipase units	36,000	180,000	114,000
Enteric-coated minitablets/microtablets			
Pancreaze® 4,200 lipase units	4,200	17,500	10,000
Pancreaze® 10,500 lipase units	10,500	43,750	25,000
Pancreaze® 16,800 lipase units	16,800	70,000	40,000
Pancreaze® 21,000 lipase units	21,000	61,000	37,000
Ultresa™ 13,800 lipase units	13,800	27,600	27,600
Ultresa™ 20,700 lipase units	20,700	41,400	41,400
Ultresa™ 23,000 lipase units	23,000	46,000	46,000

(USP, United States Pharmacopeia.)

See Chapter 39, Pancreatitis, authored by Scott Bolesta and Patricia A. Montgomery, for a more detailed discussion of this topic.

CHAPTER 29

Peptic Ulcer Disease

- *Peptic ulcer disease* (PUD) refers to ulcerative disorders of the upper gastrointestinal (GI) tract that require acid and pepsin for their formation. The three common etiologies include: (1) *Helicobacter pylori* infection, (2) nonsteroidal anti-inflammatory drug (NSAID) use, and (3) stress-related mucosal damage (SRMD).

PATHOPHYSIOLOGY

- Benign gastric ulcers, erosions, and gastritis can occur anywhere in the stomach, although the antrum and lesser curvature represent the most common locations. Most duodenal ulcers occur in the first part of the duodenum (duodenal bulb).
- Pathophysiology is determined by the balance between aggressive factors (gastric acid and pepsin) and protective factors (mucosal defense and repair). Gastric acid, *H. pylori* infection, and NSAID use are independent factors that contribute to disruption of mucosal integrity. Increased acid secretion may be involved in duodenal ulcers, but patients with gastric ulcer usually have normal or reduced acid secretion (hypochlorhydria).
- Mucus and bicarbonate secretion, intrinsic epithelial cell defense, and mucosal blood flow normally protect the gastroduodenal mucosa from noxious endogenous and exogenous substances. Endogenous prostaglandins (PGs) facilitate mucosal integrity and repair. Disruptions in normal mucosal defense and healing mechanisms allow acid and pepsin to reach the gastric epithelium.
- HP infection causes gastric mucosal inflammation in all infected individuals, but only a minority develop an ulcer or gastric cancer. Bacterial enzymes (urease, lipases, and proteases), bacterial adherence, and *H. pylori* virulence factors produce gastric mucosal injury. HP induces gastric inflammation by altering the host inflammatory response and damaging epithelial cells.
- Nonselective NSAIDs (including aspirin) cause gastric mucosal damage by two mechanisms: (1) a direct or topical irritation of the gastric epithelium, and (2) systemic inhibition of endogenous mucosal PG synthesis. COX-2 selective inhibitors have a lower risk of ulcers and related GI complications than nonselective NSAIDs. Addition of aspirin to a selective COX-2 inhibitor reduces its ulcer-sparing benefit and increases ulcer risk.
- Use of corticosteroids alone does not increase risk of ulcer or complications, but ulcer risk is doubled in corticosteroid users taking NSAIDs concurrently.
- Cigarette smoking has been linked to PUD, impaired ulcer healing, and ulcer recurrence. Risk is proportional to amount smoked per day.
- Psychological stress has not been shown to cause PUD, but ulcer patients may be adversely affected by stressful life events.
- Carbonated beverages, coffee, tea, beer, milk, and spices may cause dyspepsia but do not appear to increase PUD risk. Ethanol ingestion in high concentrations is associated with acute gastric mucosal damage and upper GI bleeding but is not clearly the cause of ulcers.

CLINICAL PRESENTATION

- Abdominal pain is the most frequent PUD symptom. Pain is often epigastric and described as burning but can present as vague discomfort, abdominal fullness, or cramping. Nocturnal pain may awaken patients from sleep, especially between 12 AM and 3 AM.
- Pain from duodenal ulcers often occurs 1 to 3 hours after meals and is usually relieved by food, whereas food may precipitate or accentuate ulcer pain in gastric ulcers. Antacids provide rapid pain relief in most ulcer patients.

271

- Heartburn, belching, and bloating often accompany pain. Nausea, vomiting, and anorexia are more common in gastric than duodenal ulcers and may be signs of an ulcer-related complication.
- Severity of symptoms varies among patients and may be seasonal, occurring more frequently in spring or fall.
- Presence or absence of epigastric pain does not define an ulcer. Ulcer healing does not necessarily render the patient asymptomatic. Conversely, absence of pain does not preclude an ulcer diagnosis, especially in the elderly who may present with a "silent" ulcer complication.
- Ulcer complications include upper GI bleeding, perforation into the peritoneal cavity, penetration into an adjacent structure (eg, pancreas, biliary tract, or liver), and gastric outlet obstruction. Bleeding may be occult or present as melena or hematemesis. Perforation is associated with sudden, sharp, severe pain, beginning first in the epigastrium but quickly spreading over the entire abdomen. Symptoms of gastric outlet obstruction typically occur over several months and include early satiety, bloating, anorexia, nausea, vomiting, and weight loss.

DIAGNOSIS

- Physical examination may reveal epigastric tenderness between the umbilicus and the xiphoid process that less commonly radiates to the back.
- Routine blood tests are not helpful in establishing a diagnosis of PUD. Hematocrit, hemoglobin, and stool guaiac tests are used to detect bleeding.
- Diagnosis of PUD depends on visualizing the ulcer crater either by upper GI radiography or endoscopy. Endoscopy is preferred because it provides a more accurate diagnosis and permits direct visualization of the ulcer.
- Diagnosis of *H. pylori* infection can be made using endoscopic or nonendoscopic (urea breath test [UBT], serologic antibody detection, and fecal antigen) tests. Testing for HP is only recommended if eradication therapy is planned. If endoscopy is not planned, serologic antibody testing is reasonable to determine HP status. The UBT and fecal antigen tests are the preferred nonendoscopic methods to verify HP eradication but must be delayed at least 4 weeks after completion of treatment to avoid confusing bacterial suppression with eradication.

TREATMENT

- <u>Goals of Treatment</u>: Overall goals are to relieve ulcer pain, heal the ulcer, prevent ulcer recurrence, and reduce ulcer-related complications. In *H. pylori*-positive patients with an active ulcer, previously documented ulcer, or history of an ulcer-related complication, goals are to eradicate *H. pylori*, heal the ulcer, and cure the disease with a cost-effective drug regimen. The primary goal for a patient with an NSAID-induced ulcer is to heal the ulcer as rapidly as possible.

NONPHARMACOLOGIC TREATMENT

- Patients with PUD should eliminate or reduce psychological stress, cigarette smoking, and use of NSAIDs (including aspirin). If possible, alternative agents such as **acetaminophen** or a nonacetylated salicylate (eg, **salsalate**) should be used for pain relief.
- Although there is no need for a special diet, patients should avoid foods and beverages that cause dyspepsia or exacerbate ulcer symptoms (eg, spicy foods, caffeine, and alcohol).
- Elective surgery is rarely performed because of highly effective medical management. Emergency surgery may be required for bleeding, perforation, or obstruction.

PHARMACOLOGIC TREATMENT

- **Figure 29–1** depicts an algorithm for evaluation and management of a patient with dyspeptic or ulcer-like symptoms.

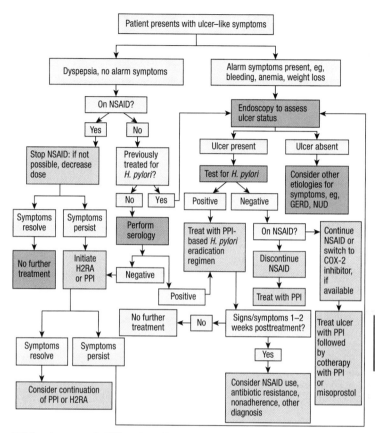

(COX-2, cyclooxygenase-2; GERD, gastroesophageal reflux disease; *H. pylori, Helicobacter pylori*; H2RA, histamine₂-receptor antagonist; NSAID, nonsteroidal anti-inflammatory drug; NUD, nonulcer dyspepsia; PPI, proton pump inhibitor.)

FIGURE 29–1. Guidelines for the evaluation and management of a patient who presents with dyspeptic or ulcer-like symptoms.

- Indications for treatment of HP include gastric or duodenal ulcer, mucosa-associated lymphoid tissue (MALT) lymphoma, postendoscopic resection of gastric cancer, and uninvestigated dyspepsia. Treatment should be effective, well tolerated, convenient, and cost-effective.
- First-line therapy to eradicate HP infection is usually initiated with a proton pump inhibitor (PPI)–based, three-drug regimen for 14 days. If a second treatment course is required, the salvage regimen should contain different antibiotics or a four-drug regimen with a bismuth salt, metronidazole, tetracycline, and a PPI (Table 29–1).
- Bismuth-based quadruple therapy is recommended as an alternative for patients allergic to penicillin. All medications except the PPI should be taken with meals and at bedtime.
- In sequential therapy, the antibiotics are administered in a sequence rather than all together. The rationale is to treat initially with antibiotics that rarely promote resistance (eg, amoxicillin) to reduce bacterial load and preexisting resistant organisms and then to follow with different antibiotics (eg, clarithromycin and metronidazole)

TABLE 29–1	Drug Regimens Used to Eradicate *Helicobacter pylori*		
Drug #1	Drug #2	Drug #3	Drug #4
PPI-based triple therapy[a]			
PPI once or twice daily[b]	Clarithromycin 500 mg twice daily	Amoxicillin 1 g twice daily or metronidazole 500 mg twice daily	
Bismuth-based quadruple therapy[a]			
PPI or H2RA once or twice daily[b,c]	Bismuth subsalicylate[d] 525 mg four times daily	Metronidazole 250–500 mg four times daily	Tetracycline 500 mg four times daily
Non-bismuth quadruple or "concomitant" therapy[e]			
PPI once or twice daily on days 1 through 10[b]	Clarithromycin 250–500 mg twice daily on days 1–10	Amoxicillin 1 g twice daily on days 1 through 10	Metronidazole 250–500 mg twice daily on days 1 through 10
Sequential therapy[e]			
PPI once or twice daily on days 1 through 10[b]	Amoxicillin 1 g twice daily on days 1 through 5	Metronidazole 250–500 mg twice daily on days 6 through 10	Clarithromycin 250–500 mg twice daily on days 6 through 10
Hybrid therapy[e]			
PPI once or twice daily on days 1 through 14[b]	Amoxicillin 1 g twice daily on days 1 through 14	Metronidazole 250–500 mg twice daily on days 7 through 14	Clarithromycin 250–500 mg twice daily on days 7 through 14
Second-line (salvage) therapy for persistent infections			
PPI or H2RA once or twice daily[b,c]	Bismuth subsalicylate[d] 525 mg four times daily	Metronidazole 250–500 mg four times daily	Tetracycline 500 mg four times daily
PPI once or twice daily[b,f]	Amoxicillin 1 g twice daily	Levofloxacin 250 mg twice daily	

(H2RA, H_2-receptor antagonist; PPI, proton pump inhibitor.)
[a]Although treatment is minimally effective if used for 7 days, 10–14 days is recommended. The antisecretory drug may be continued beyond antimicrobial treatment for patients with a history of a complicated ulcer (eg, bleeding), or in heavy smokers.
[b]Standard PPI peptic ulcer healing dosages given once or twice daily.
[c]Standard H2RA peptic ulcer healing dosages may be used in place of a PPI.
[d]Bismuth subcitrate potassium (biskalcitrate) 140 mg, as the bismuth salt, is contained in a prepackaged capsule (Pylera), along with metronidazole 125 mg and tetracycline 125 mg; three capsules are taken with each meal and at bedtime; a standard PPI dosage is added to the regimen and taken twice daily. All medications are taken for 10 days.
[e]Requires validation as first-line therapy in the United States.
[f]Requires validation as rescue therapy in the United States.

to kill any remaining organisms. The potential advantages of superior eradication rates requires validation in the United States before this regimen can be recommended as first-line *H. pylori* eradication therapy.

• *Nonbismuth quadruple therapy* (also called "concomitant" therapy) contains a PPI, amoxicillin, clarithromycin, and metronidazole taken together at standard doses for 10 days. *Hybrid therapy* involves 7 days of dual therapy (PPI and amoxicillin) followed by 7 days of quadruple therapy (PPI, amoxicillin, clarithromycin, and metronidazole). Both non-bismuth quadruple therapy and hybrid therapy have demonstrated higher eradication rates than traditional triple-therapy, although similar eradication rates are likely in areas of low antimicrobial resistance.

- If initial treatment fails to eradicate HP, second-line (salvage) treatment should: (1) use antibiotics that were not included in the initial regimen, (2) use antibiotics that are not associated with resistance, (3) use a drug that has a topical effect (eg, bismuth), and (4) extend the treatment duration to 14 days. A 14-day course of the PPI-based bismuth-containing quadruple regimen is the most commonly used second-line therapy after failure of a PPI–amoxicillin–clarithromycin regimen. Levofloxacin-based triple therapy with amoxicillin and a PPI may be an alternative second-line eradication regimen and may be better tolerated than PPI-based bismuth-containing quadruple therapy.

- Patients with NSAID-induced ulcers should be tested to determine *H. pylori* status. If *H. pylori* positive, start treatment with a PPI-based three-drug regimen. If *H. pylori* negative, discontinue the NSAID and treat with a standard four-week regimen of a PPI, histamine$_2$-receptor antagonist (H2RA), or sucralfate (Table 29–2). PPIs are preferred because they provide more rapid symptom relief and ulcer healing. If the NSAID must be continued despite ulceration, initiate treatment with a PPI (if *H. pylori* negative) or a PPI-based three-drug regimen (if *H. pylori* positive). PPI treatment should be continued for 8 to 12 weeks if the NSAID must be continued. Cotherapy with a PPI or misoprostol or switching to a selective cyclooxygenase-2 (COX-2) inhibitor is recommended for patients at risk of developing an ulcer-related complication.

TABLE 29–2	Drug Dosing Table		
Drug	**Brand Name**	**Initial Dose**	**Usual Range**
Proton pump inhibitors			
Omeprazole	Prilosec, various	40 mg daily	20–40 mg/day
Omeprazole + sodium bicarbonate	Zegerid	40 mg daily	20–40 mg/day
Lansoprazole	Prevacid, various	30 mg daily	15–30 mg/day
Rabeprazole	Aciphex	20 mg daily	20–40 mg/day
Pantoprazole	Protonix, various	40 mg daily	40–80 mg/day
Esomeprazole	Nexium	40 mg daily	20–40 mg/day
Dexlansoprazole	Dexilant	30–60 mg daily	30–60 mg/day
H$_2$-receptor antagonists			
Cimetidine	Tagamet, various	300 mg four times daily, 400 mg twice daily, or 800 mg at bedtime	800–1600 mg/day in divided doses
Famotidine	Pepcid, various	20 mg twice daily, or 40 mg at bedtime	20–40 mg/day
Nizatidine	Axid, various	150 mg twice daily, or 300 mg at bedtime	150–300 mg/day
Ranitidine	Zantac, various	150 mg twice daily, or 300 mg at bedtime	150–300 mg/day
Mucosal protectants			
Sucralfate	Carafate, various	1 g four times daily, or 2 g twice daily	2–4 g/day
Misoprostol	Cytotec	100–200 mcg four times daily	400–800 mcg/day

- Limit maintenance therapy with a PPI or H2RA to high-risk patients with ulcer complications, patients who fail HP eradication, and those with *H. pylori*-negative ulcers.
- Patients with ulcers refractory to treatment should undergo upper endoscopy to confirm a nonhealing ulcer, exclude malignancy, and assess *H. pylori* status. *H. pylori*-positive patients should receive eradication therapy. In *H. pylori*-negative patients, higher PPI doses (eg, omeprazole 40 mg/day) heal the majority of ulcers. Continuous PPI treatment is often necessary to maintain healing. Patients with refractory gastric ulcer may require surgery because of the possibility of malignancy.

EVALUATION OF THERAPEUTIC OUTCOMES

- Monitor patients for symptomatic relief of ulcer pain, potential adverse drug effects, and drug interactions.
- Ulcer pain typically resolves in a few days when NSAIDs are discontinued and within 7 days upon initiation of antiulcer therapy. Patients with uncomplicated PUD are usually symptom free after treatment with any of the recommended antiulcer regimens.
- Persistent or recurrent symptoms within 14 days after the end of treatment suggests failure of ulcer healing or *H. pylori* eradication or presence of an alternative diagnosis such as gastroesophageal reflux disease.
- Most patients with uncomplicated HP-positive ulcers do not require confirmation of ulcer healing or HP eradication.
- Monitor patients taking NSAIDs closely for signs and symptoms of bleeding, obstruction, penetration, and perforation.
- Follow-up endoscopy is justified in patients with frequent symptomatic recurrence, refractory disease, complications, or suspected hypersecretory states.

See Chapter 33, Peptic Ulcer Disease and Related Disorders, authored by Bryan L. Love and Phillip L. Mohorn, for a more detailed discussion of this topic.

CHAPTER 30 — Contraception

- *Contraception* is the prevention of pregnancy by inhibiting sperm from reaching a mature ovum or by preventing a fertilized ovum from implanting in the endometrium.

THE MENSTRUAL CYCLE

- The median length of the menstrual cycle is 28 days (range 21–40 days). The first day of menses is day 1, which marks the beginning of the follicular phase. Ovulation usually occurs on day 14. After ovulation, the luteal phase starts and lasts until the beginning of the next cycle.
- The hypothalamus secretes gonadotropin-releasing hormone, which stimulates the anterior pituitary to secrete gonadotropins, follicle-stimulating hormone (FSH), and luteinizing hormone (LH).
- In the follicular phase, FSH levels increase and cause recruitment of a small group of follicles for continued growth. Between days 5 and 7, one of these becomes the dominant follicle, which later ruptures to release the oocyte. The dominant follicle develops increasing amounts of estradiol and inhibin, providing a negative feedback on the secretion of gonadotropin-releasing hormone and FSH.
- The dominant follicle continues to grow and synthesizes estradiol, progesterone, and androgen. Estradiol stops the menstrual flow from the previous cycle, thickens the endometrial lining, and produces thin, watery cervical mucus. FSH regulates aromatase enzymes that induce conversion of androgens to estrogens in the follicle.
- The pituitary releases a midcycle LH surge that stimulates the final stages of follicular maturation and ovulation. Ovulation occurs 24 to 36 hours after the estradiol peak and 10 to 16 hours after the LH peak.
- The LH surge is the most clinically useful predictor of approaching ovulation. Conception is most successful when intercourse takes place from 2 days before ovulation to the day of ovulation.
- After ovulation, the remaining luteinized follicles become the corpus luteum, which synthesizes androgen, estrogen, and progesterone (Fig. 30–1).
- If pregnancy occurs, human chorionic gonadotropin prevents regression of the corpus luteum and stimulates continued production of estrogen and progesterone. If pregnancy does not occur, the corpus luteum degenerates, progesterone declines, and menstruation occurs.

TREATMENT

- <u>Goal of Treatment</u>: the prevention of pregnancy following sexual intercourse.

NONPHARMACOLOGIC THERAPY

- A comparison of methods of nonhormonal contraception is shown in Table 30–1.
- The abstinence (rhythm) method is associated with relatively high pregnancy rates.

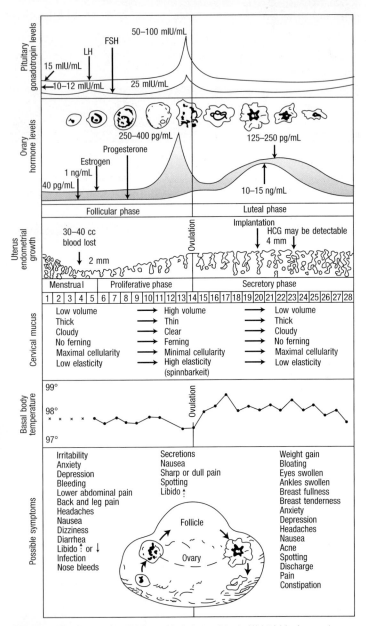

(FSH, follicle-stimulating hormone; HCG, human chorionic gonadotropin; LH, luteinizing hormone.)
LH: 15 mIU/mL = 15 IU/L; 50 to 100 mIU/mL = 50 to 100 IU/L.
FSH: 10 to 12 mIU/mL = 10 to 12 IU/L; 25 mIU/mL = 25 IU/L.
Estrogen: 40 pg/mL = ~150 pmol/L; 250 to 400 pg/mL = ~920 to 1470 pmol/L; 125 to 250 pg/mL = ~460 to 920 pmol/L.
Progesterone: 1 ng/mL = 3 nmol/L; 10 to 15 ng/mL = ~30 to 50 nmol/L.
Temperatures: 99°F = 37.2°C; 98°F = 36.7°C; 97°F = 36.1°C.

FIGURE 30–1. Menstrual cycle events, idealized 28-day cycle. (*Hatcher RA, Trussell J, Nelson AL, et al. Contraceptive Technology. 21st ed. Ardent New York: Median, Inc.; 2015.*)

TABLE 30-1 Comparison of Methods of Nonhormonal Contraception

Method	Absolute Contraindications	Advantages	Disadvantages	Perfect Use	Typical Use
Condoms, male	Allergy to latex or rubber	Inexpensive STD protection, including HIV (latex only)	High user failure rate Poor acceptance Possibility of breakage Efficacy decreased by oil-based lubricants Possible allergic reactions to latex in either partner	2	18
Condoms, female	Allergy to polyurethane History of TSS	Can be inserted just before intercourse or ahead of time STD protection, including HIV	High user failure rate Dislike ring hanging outside vagina Cumbersome	5	21
Diaphragm with spermicide	Allergy to latex, rubber, or spermicide Recurrent UTIs History of TSS Abnormal gynecologic anatomy	Low cost Decreased incidence of cervical neoplasia Some protection against STDs	High user failure rate Decreased efficacy with increased frequency of intercourse Increased incidence of vaginal yeast UTIs, TSS Efficacy decreased by oil-based lubricants Cervical irritation	6	12
Cervical cap (FemCap)	Allergy to spermicide History of TSS Abnormal gynecologic anatomy Abnormal Papanicolaou smear	Low cost Latex-free Some protection against STDs FemCap reusable for up to 2 years	High user failure rate Decreased efficacy with parity Cannot be used during menses	9	16[b]

(continued)

279

TABLE 30–1 Comparison of Methods of Nonhormonal Contraception (*Continued*)

Method	Absolute Contraindications	Advantages	Disadvantages	Percent of Women with Pregnancy[a]	
				Perfect Use	Typical Use
Spermicides alone	Allergy to spermicide	Inexpensive	High user failure rate Must be reapplied before each act of intercourse May enhance HIV transmission No protection against STDs	18	28
Sponge (Today)	Allergy to spermicide Recurrent UTIs History of TSS Abnormal gynecologic anatomy	Inexpensive	High user failure rate Decreased efficacy with parity Cannot be used during menses No protection against STDs	9[c]	12[d]

(HIV, human immunodeficiency virus; STD, sexually transmitted disease; TSS, toxic shock syndrome; UTI, urinary tract infection.)
[a]Failure rates in the United States during first year of use.
[b]Failure rate with FemCap reported to be 24% per package insert.
[c]Failure rate with Today sponge reported to be 20% in parous women.
[d]Failure rate with Today sponge reported to be 32% in parous women.

Barrier Techniques

- Diaphragms are effective because they are barriers and because of the spermicide placed in the diaphragm before insertion. It should be inserted up to 6 hours before intercourse and must be left in place for at least 6 hours after. It should not be left in place for more than 24 hours because of the risk of toxic shock syndrome (TSS).
- The cervical cap can be inserted 6 hours prior to intercourse, and should not remain in place for longer than 48 hours to reduce the risk of TSS. With use of diaphragms or cervical caps, a condom should also be used to protect against sexually transmitted diseases (STDs) including human immunodeficiency virus (HIV).
- Most condoms made in the United States are latex, which is impermeable to viruses, but ~5% are made from lamb intestine, which is not impermeable to viruses. Mineral oil–based vaginal drug formulations (eg, Cleocin vaginal cream, Premarin vaginal cream,) can decrease the barrier strength of latex. Condoms with spermicides are not recommended, as they provide no additional protection against pregnancy or STDs and may increase vulnerability to HIV.
- The female condom (Reality) covers the labia, as well as the cervix. However, the pregnancy rate is higher than with male condoms.

PHARMACOLOGIC THERAPY

- Table 30–2 compares unintended pregnancy rates and continuation rates for pharmacologic contraceptive methods.

Spermicides and Spermicide Implanted Barrier Techniques

- Most spermicides contain nonoxynol-9, a surfactant that destroys sperm cell walls and blocks entry into the cervical os. They offer no protection against STDs, and when used more than twice daily, nonoxynol-9 may increase the transmission of HIV.
- The **vaginal contraceptive sponge (Today)** contains nonoxynol-9 and provides protection for 24 hours. After intercourse, the sponge must be left in place for at least 6 hours before removal. It should not be left in place for more than 24 to 30 hours to reduce the risk of TSS. It is available without a prescription.

Hormonal Contraception

COMPOSITION AND FORMULATIONS

- Hormonal contraceptives contain either a combination of synthetic estrogen and synthetic progestin or a progestin alone.

TABLE 30–2	Pregnancy and Continuation Rates for Various Pharmacologic Contraceptive Methods		
Method	**Pregnancy Typical Use (%)**	**Pregnancy Ideal Use (%)**	**Continuation After 1 Year (%)**
Combined oral contraceptive	9	<1	71
Combined hormonal transdermal contraceptive patch	9	<1	–
Combined hormonal vaginal contraceptive ring	9	<1	–
Depot medroxyprogesterone acetate	6	<1	70
Copper IUD	<1	<1	78
Levonorgestrel IUD	<1	<1	80
Progestin-only implant	<1	<1	88

- Progestins thicken cervical mucus, delay sperm transport, and induce endometrial atrophy. They also block the LH surge and thus inhibit ovulation. Estrogens suppress FSH release (which may contribute to blocking the LH surge) and also stabilize the endometrial lining and provide cycle control.

COMPONENTS

- Table 30–3 lists available oral contraceptives (OCs) by brand name and hormonal composition. **Mestranol** must be converted to **ethinyl estradiol (EE)** in the liver to be active. It is ~50% less potent than EE.
- Progestins vary in their progestational activity and differ with respect to inherent estrogenic, antiestrogenic, and androgenic effects. Their estrogenic and antiestrogenic properties occur because progestins are metabolized to estrogenic substances. Androgenic activity depends on the presence of sex hormone (testosterone) binding globulin and the androgen-to-progesterone activity ratio. If sex hormone binding globulin decreases, free testosterone levels increase, and androgenic side effects are more prominent.

CONSIDERATIONS WITH USE OF COMBINED HORMONAL CONTRACEPTIVES (CHC)

- Obtain a medical history and blood pressure measurement, and discuss the risks, benefits, and adverse effects with the patient before prescribing a CHC.
- Noncontraceptive benefits of OCs include decreased menstrual cramps and ovulatory pain; decreased menstrual blood loss; improved menstrual regularity; decreased iron deficiency anemia; reduced risk of ovarian and endometrial cancer; and reduced risk of ovarian cysts, ectopic pregnancy, pelvic inflammatory disease, endometriosis, uterine fibroids, and benign breast disease.
- Serious symptoms that may be associated with CHCs and monitoring of hormonal contraception are shown in Tables 30–4 and 30–5, respectively.
- An important concern about CHCs is their lack of protection against STDs. Encourage use of condoms to prevent STDs.
- Table 30–6 shows graded eligibility criteria for contraceptive use.

Women over 35 Years of Age

- Use of CHCs containing less than 50 mcg estrogen may be considered in healthy nonsmoking women older than 35 years.
- CHCs are not recommended for women older than 35 years with migraine, uncontrolled hypertension, smoking, or diabetes with vascular disease.
- Studies have not demonstrated an increased risk of cardiovascular disease with low-dose CHCs in healthy, nonobese women.

Women Who Smoke

- Women older than 35 years who smoke and take OCs have an increased risk of myocardial infarction; therefore, clinicians should prescribe CHCs with caution, if at all, in this group. Smoking 15 or more cigarettes per day by women over 35 years is a contraindication to the use of CHCs, and the risks generally outweigh the benefits even in those who smoke fewer than 15 cigarettes per day. Progestin-only methods should be considered in this group.

Hypertension

- CHCs, regardless of estrogen dose, can cause small increases in blood pressure (6–8 mm Hg). In women with hypertension, OCs have been associated with an increased risk of myocardial infarction (MI) and stroke. Use of low-dose CHCs is acceptable in women younger than 35 years with well-controlled and monitored hypertension.
- Systolic blood pressure greater than or equal to 160 mm Hg or diastolic blood pressure greater than or equal to 100 mm Hg is a contraindication to use of CHCs. Women with a systolic blood pressure of 140 to 159 or a diastolic blood pressure of 90 to 99 mm Hg should also avoid CHC, as the risks generally outweigh the benefits.

TABLE 30-3 Composition of Commonly Prescribed Oral Contraceptives[a]

Product	Estrogen	Micrograms[b]	Progestin	Milligrams[b]	Spotting and Breakthrough Bleeding
50 mcg estrogen					
Ogestrel 0.5/50	Ethinyl estradiol	50	Norgestrel	0.5	4.5
Zovia 1/50	Ethinyl estradiol	50	Ethynodiol diacetate	1	13.9
Sub-50 mcg estrogen monophasic					
Aubra, Aviane, Falmina, Lessina, Lutera, Orsythia, Sronyx, levonorgestrel/EE	Ethinyl estradiol	20	Levonorgestrel	0.1	26.5
Brevicon, Modicon, Necon 0.5/35, Nortrel 0.5/35 Wera	Ethinyl estradiol	35	Norethindrone	0.5	24.6
Zovia 1/35, Kelnor 1/35	Ethinyl estradiol	35	Ethynodiol diacetate	1	37.4
Apri, Desogen, desogestrel/EE, Emoquette, Ortho-Cept, Reclipsen, Enskyce	Ethinyl estradiol	30	Desogestrel	0.15	13.1
Levora, ChatealPortia, Altavera, Kurvelo, Marlissa	Ethinyl estradiol	30	Levonorgestrel	0.15	14
Gildess Fe 1/20, Junel Fe 1/20, Junel Fe 1.5/30, Loestrin 1/20; Fe 1/20, Microgestin 1/20; Fe 1/20, Trina Fe 1/20	Ethinyl estradiol	20	Norethindrone 1 mg	1	26.5
Gildess Fe 1.5/30, Junel 1.5/30, Junel Fe 1.5/30, Loestrin Fe 1.5/30, Microgestin 1.5/30, Microgestin Fe 1.5/30, Larin (Fe) 1.5/30	Ethinyl estradiol	30	Norethindrone acetate	1.5	25.2
Cryselle, Elinest, Lo-Ovral, Low-Ogestrel	Ethinyl estradiol	30	Norgestrel	0.3	9.6
Necon 1/35, Norinyl 1+35, Nortrel 1/35, Ortho-Novum 1/35, Alyacen 1/35, Cyclafem 1/35, Dasetta 1/35, Pirmella 1/35	Ethinyl estradiol	35	Norethindrone	1	14.7
Estarylla, Norgestimate/ethinyl estradiolOrtho-Cyclen, Mononessa, Mono-Linyah, Previfem, Sprintec	Ethinyl estradiol	35	Norgestimate	0.25	14.3
Balziva, Femcon Fe chewable, Zenchent, Briellyn, Gildagia, Philith, Wymzya chewable, Vyfemla	Ethinyl estradiol	35	Norethindrone	0.4	11

(continued)

TABLE 30-3 Composition of Commonly Prescribed Oral Contraceptives[a] (*Continued*)

Product	Estrogen	Micrograms[b]	Progestin	Milligrams[b]	Spotting and Breakthrough Bleeding
Yasmin, Ocella, Safyral, Syeda, Zarah, drospirenone/EE	Ethinyl estradiol	30	Drospirenone	3	14.5
Generess Fe chewable, Layolis Fe, norethindrone/EE	Ethinyl estradiol	25	Norethindrone	0.8	14.5
Sub-50 mcg estrogen monophasic extended cycle					
Lo Loestrin-24 FE[c]	Ethinyl estradiol	10	Norethindrone	1	50[e]
Larin (Fe) 1/20, Minastrin 24 Fe chewable	Ethinyl estradiol	20	Norethindrone	1	50[e]
Amethia Lo, Camrese Lo, levonorgestrel/EE, LoSeasonique	Ethinyl estradiol	20/10	Levonorgestrel	0.1	50[e]
Amethyst	Ethinyl estradiol	20	Levonorgestrel	0.09	52[e]
Introvale, levonorgestrel/EE, Jolessa, Quasense[d]	Ethinyl estradiol	30	Levonorgestrel	0.15	58.5[e]
Amethia, Ashlyna, Daysee, Seasonique	Ethinyl estradiol	30/10	Levonorgestrel	0.15	50[e]
Quartette	Ethinyl estradiol	20/25/30/10	Levonorgestrel	0.15	50[e]
Beyaz, Gianvi, Loryna, Nikki; Vestura, Yazc	Ethinyl estradiol	20	Drospirenone	3	52.5[e]
Sub-50 mcg estrogen multiphasic					
Caziant, Cyclessa, Velivet	Ethinyl estradiol	25 (7) 25 (7) 25 (7)	Desogestrel	0.1 (7) 0.125 (7) 0.15 (7)	11.1
Tilia Fe, Tri-Legest Fe	Ethinyl estradiol Ethinyl estradiol Ethinyl estradiol	20 (5) 30 (7) 35 (9)	Norethindrone acetate Norethindrone acetate Norethindrone acetate	1 (5) 1 (7) 1 (9)	21.7
Kariva, Mircette, Azurette, Viorele	Ethinyl estradiol Ethinyl estradiol	20 (21) 10 (5)	Desogestrel Desogestrel	0.15 (21)	19.7
Necon 10/11	Ethinyl estradiol Ethinyl estradiol	35 (10) 35 (11)	Norethindrone Norethindrone	0.5 (10) 1 (11)	17.6

	Estrogen	Dose (days)	Progestin	Dose (days)	%
Ortho-Novum 7/7/7, Nortrel 7/7/7, Necon 7/7/7, Cyclafem 7/7/7, Alyacen 7/7/7, Dasetta 7/7/7, Pirmella 7/7/7	Ethinyl estradiol Ethinyl estradiol Ethinyl estradiol	35 (7) 35 (7) 35 (7)	Norethindrone Norethindrone Norethindrone	0.5 (7) 0.75 (7) 1 (7)	14.5
Ortho Tri-Cyclen, Trinessa, Tri-Previfem, Tri-Sprintec, Tri-Estarylla, Tri-Linyah, Norgestimate/EE	Ethinyl estradiol Ethinyl estradiol Ethinyl estradiol	35 (7) 35 (7) 35 (7)	Norgestimate Norgestimate Norgestimate	0.18 (7) 0.215 (7) 0.25 (7)	17.7
Ortho Tri-Cyclen Lo, Norgestimate/EE	Ethinyl estradiol Ethinyl estradiol Ethinyl estradiol	25 (7) 25 (7) 25 (7)	Norgestimate Norgestimate Norgestimate	0.18 (7) 0.215 (7) 0.25 (7)	11.5
Aranelle, Leena, Tri-Norinyl	Ethinyl estradiol Ethinyl estradiol Ethinyl estradiol	35 (7) 35 (9) 35 (5)	Norethindrone Norethindrone Norethindrone	0.5 (7) 1 (9) 0.5 (5)	25.5
Enpresse, Trivora, Levonest Myzilra	Ethinyl estradiol Ethinyl estradiol Ethinyl estradiol	30 (6) 40 (5) 30 (10)	Levonorgestrel Levonorgestrel Levonorgestrel	0.05 (6) 0.075 (5) 0.125 (10)	
Natazia	Estradiol valerate	3 (2) 2 (22) 1 (2)	Dienogest	0 (2) 2 (5) 3 (17) 0 (4)	
Progestin only					
Camilla, Errin, Heather, Jencycla,Jolivette, Lyza, Ortho Micronor, Nor-QD, Nora-BE, norethindrone	Ethinyl estradiol	–	Norethindrone	0.35	42.3

a28-day regimen (21-day active pills, then 7-day pill-free interval) unless otherwise noted.
bNumber in parentheses refers to the number of days the dose is received in multiphasic oral contraceptives.
c28-day regimen (24-day active pills, then 4-day pill-free interval).
d91-day regimen (84-day active pills, then 7-day pill-free interval).
ePercent reporting after 6 to 12 months of use.

TABLE 30–4	Symptoms of a Serious or Potentially Serious Nature in Individuals Taking Combined Hormonal Contraception
Symptom	**Possible Cause**
SERIOUS: Stop immediately	
Loss of vision, proptosis, diplopia, papilledema	Retinal artery thrombosis
Unilateral numbness, weakness, or tingling	Hemorrhagic or thrombotic stroke
Severe pains in chest, left arm, or neck	MI
Hemoptysis	PE
Severe pains, tenderness or swelling, warmth or palpable cord in legs	Thrombophlebitis or thrombosis
Slurring of speech	Hemorrhagic or thrombotic stroke
Hepatic mass or tenderness	Liver neoplasm
POTENTIALLY SERIOUS: May continue with caution while being evaluated	
Absence of menses	Pregnancy
Spotting or breakthrough bleeding	Cervical endometrial or vaginal cancer
Breast mass, pain or swelling	Breast cancer
Right upper-quadrant pain	Cholecystitis, cholelithiasis or liver neoplasm
Mid-epigastric pain	Thrombosis of abdominal artery or vein, MI or PE
Migraine headache	Vascular spasm which may precede thrombosis
Severe nonvascular headache	Hypertension, vascular spasm
Galactorrhea	Pituitary adenoma
Jaundice, pruritus	Cholestatic jaundice
Depression, sleepiness	B6 deficiency
Uterine size increase	Leiomyomata, adenomyosis, pregnancy

(MI, myocardial infarction; PE, pulmonary embolism.)

Diabetes

• Except for some levonorgestrel-containing products, formulations containing low doses of progestins do not significantly alter insulin, glucose, or glucagon release after a glucose load in healthy women or in those with a history of gestational diabetes. Women younger than 35 years with diabetes but no vascular disease who do not smoke can safely use CHCs. Diabetic women with vascular disease or diabetics of more than 20 years' duration should not use CHCs.

Dyslipidemia

• Generally, synthetic progestins decrease high-density lipoprotein (HDL) and increase low-density lipoprotein (LDL). Estrogens decrease LDL but increase HDL and may moderately increase triglycerides. Most low-dose CHCs (with the possible exception of levonorgestrel pills, which may reduce HDL levels in some patients) have no significant impact on HDL, LDL, triglycerides, or total cholesterol.
• The mechanism for the increased cardiovascular disease in CHC users is believed to be thromboembolic and thrombotic changes, not atherosclerosis.
• Women with controlled dyslipidemias can use low-dose CHCs, with monitoring of fasting lipid profiles. Women with uncontrolled dyslipidemia (LDL >160 mg/dL [4.14 mmol/L], HDL <35 mg/dL [0.91 mmol/L], triglycerides >250 mg/dL [2.83 mmol/L]) and additional risk factors (eg, coronary artery disease, diabetes, hypertension, smoking, or a positive family history) should use an alternative method of contraception.

TABLE 30–5 Monitoring Patients Taking Hormonal Contraceptives

Drug (or Drug Class)	Adverse Drug Reactions	Monitoring Parameter	Comments
Combined hormonal contraception	Nausea/vomiting	Patient symptoms	Typically improves after two to three cycles; consider changing to lower estrogenic
	Breast tenderness	Patient symptoms	
	Weight gain	Weight	
	Acne, oily skin	Visual inspection	Consider changing to lower androgenic
	Depression, fatigue	Depression screening	Data are limited and conflicting
	Breakthrough bleeding/spotting	Menstrual symptoms	Consider changing to higher estrogenic
	Application site reaction (transdermal)	Visual inspection	
	Vaginal irritation (vaginal ring)	Patient symptoms	
Depot medroxypro-gesterone acetate	Menstrual irregularities	Menstrual symptoms	Typically improves after 6 months
	Weight gain	Weight	
	Acne	Visual inspection	
	Hirsutism	Visual inspection	
	Depression	Depression screening	Data are limited and conflicting
	Decreased bone density	BMD	Do not routinely screen with DXA
Levonorgestrel IUD	Menstrual irregularities	Menstrual symptoms	Typically spotting, amenorrhea
	Insertion-related complications	Cramping, pain	Prophylactic NSAIDs or local anesthetic may reduce occurrence
		Cramping, pain, spotting, dyspareunia, missing strings	IUD strings should be checked regularly by women to ensure IUD properly placed
	Expulsion	Lower abdominal pain, unusual vaginal discharge, fever	Overall risk of developing is rare, but counseling on STD prevention is important
	Pelvic inflammatory disease		
Copper IUD	See levonorgestrel IUD above	See levonorgestrel IUD above	Menstrual irregularities; typically heavier menses with copper IUD
Progestin-only implant	Menstrual irregularities	Menstrual symptoms	Typically well-tolerated and resolve without treatment, infection is rare
	Insertion-site reactions	Pain, bruising, skin irritation, erythema, pus, fever	

(BMD, bone mineral density; DXA, dual energy x-ray absorptiometry; IUD, intrauterine device; STD, sexually transmitted disease.)

TABLE 30-6	U.S. Medical Eligibility Criteria for Contraceptive Use: Classifications for Combined Hormonal Contraceptives

Category 4: Unacceptable health risk (method not to be used)
- Breastfeeding or nonbreastfeeding <21 days postpartum
- Current breast cancer
- Severe (decompensated) cirrhosis
- History/risk of or current deep venous thrombosis/pulmonary embolism (not on anticoagulant therapy); thrombogenic mutations
- Major surgery with prolonged immobilization
- Migraines with aura, any age
- Systolic blood pressure ≥160 mm Hg or diastolic ≥100 mm Hg
- Hypertension with vascular disease
- Current and history of ischemic heart disease
- Benign hepatocellular adenoma or malignant liver tumor
- Moderately or severely impaired cardiac function; normal or mildly impaired cardiac function <6 months
- Smoking ≥15 cigarettes per day and age ≥35
- Complicated solid organ transplantation
- History of cerebrovascular accident
- SLE; positive or unknown antiphospholipid antibodies
- Complicated valvular heart disease

Category 3: Theoretical or proven risks usually outweigh the advantages
- Breastfeeding 21–30 days postpartum with or without risk factors for VTE
- Nonbreastfeeding 21–42 days postpartum with other risk factors for VTE
- Past breast cancer and no evidence of disease for 5 years
- History of DVT/PE (not on anticoagulant therapy or established on anticoagulant therapy for at least 3 months), but lower risk for recurrent DVT/PE
- Current gallbladder disease, symptomatic and medically treated
- Migraines without aura, age ≥35 (*category 4 with continued use*)
- History of bariatric surgery; malabsorptive procedures
- History of cholestasis, past COC-related
- Hypertension; systolic blood pressure 140–159 mm Hg or diastolic 90–99 mm Hg
- Normal or mildly impaired cardiac function ≥6 months
- Postpartum 21–42 days with other risk factors for VTE
- Smoking <15 cigarettes per day and age ≥35
- Use of ritonavir-boosted protease inhibitors
- Use of certain anticonvulsants (phenytoin, carbamazepine, barbiturates, primidone, topiramate, oxcarbazepine, and lamotrigine)
- Use of rifampicin or rifabutin therapy
- Diabetes with vascular disease or >20 years duration (*possibly category 4 depending upon severity*)
- Multiple risk factors for arterial cardiovascular disease (older age, smoking, diabetes, and hypertension) (*possibly category 4 depending on category and severity*)

Category 2: Advantages generally outweigh theoretical or proven risks
- Age ≥40 (in the absence of other comorbid conditions that increase CVD risk)
- Sickle-cell disease
- Undiagnosed breast mass
- Cervical cancer and awaiting treatment; cervical intraepithelial neoplasia
- Family history (first-degree relatives) of DVT/PE
- Major surgery without prolonged immobilization
- Diabetes mellitus (type 1 or type 2), nonvascular disease
- Gallbladder disease; symptomatic and treated by cholecystectomy or asymptomatic
- Migraines without aura, age <35 (*category 3 with continued use*)
- History of pregnancy-related cholestasis
- History of high blood pressure during pregnancy

TABLE 30–6	U.S. Medical Eligibility Criteria for Contraceptive Use: Classifications for Combined Hormonal Contraceptives (*Continued*)

- Benign liver tumors; focal nodular hyperplasia
- Obesity
- Breastfeeding 30 days or more postpartum
- Postpartum 21–42 days without other risk factors
- Nonbreastfeeding 21–42 days postpartum without risk factors for VTE
- Rheumatoid arthritis on or off immunosuppressive therapy
- Smoking and <35 years old
- Uncomplicated sold organ transplantation
- Superficial thrombophlebitis
- Stable SLE without antiphospholipid antibodies
- Unexplained vaginal bleeding before evaluation
- Uncomplicated valvular heart disease
- Use of nonnucleoside reverse transcriptase inhibitors
- Hyperlipidemia (*possibly category 3 based upon type, severity, and other risk factors*)
- Inflammatory bowel disease (*possibly category 3 for those with increased risk of VTE*)

Category 1: No restriction (method can be used)
- Thalassemia, iron deficiency anemia
- Mild compensated cirrhosis
- Benign ovarian tumors
- Benign breast disease or family history of cancer
- Family history of cancer
- Schistosomiasis
- Viral hepatitis (carrier/chronic)
- Minor surgery without immobilization
- Depression
- Gestational diabetes mellitus
- Endometrial cancer/hyperplasia, endometriosis
- Epilepsy
- Gestational trophoblastic disease
- Nonmigrainous headaches (category 2 for continued use)
- History of bariatric surgery; restrictive procedures
- History of pelvic surgery
- HIV infected or high risk
- Malaria
- Ovarian cancer
- Past ectopic pregnancy
- PID
- Postabortion
- More than 42 days postpartum
- Severe dysmenorrhea
- Sexually transmitted infections
- Varicose veins
- Thyroid disorders
- Tuberculosis
- Uterine fibroids
- Use of nucleoside reverse transcriptase inhibitors
- Use of broad-spectrum antibiotics, antifungals, and antiparasitics

(CHC, combined hormonal contraception; HIV, human immunodeficiency virus; VTE, venous thromboembolism; PE, pulmonary embolism; CVD, cardiovascular disease; PID, pelvic inflammatory disease.)

Thromboembolism

- Estrogens have a dose-related effect in the development of venous thromboembolism (VTE) and pulmonary embolism, especially in women with underlying hypercoagulable states or who have acquired conditions (eg, obesity, pregnancy, immobility, trauma, surgery, and certain malignancies) that predispose them to coagulation abnormalities.
- OCs containing the newer progestins (eg, **drospirenone, desogestrel, norgestimate**) carry a slightly increased risk of thrombosis compared to other progestins.
- The transdermal patch and vaginal ring provide continuous higher exposure to estrogen and have an increased thromboembolic risk.
- The risk of VTE in women using OCs is three times the risk in nonusers. However, this risk is less than the risk of thromboembolic events during pregnancy.
- For women at increased risk of thromboembolism (older than 35 years, obesity, smoking, personal or family history of venous thrombosis, prolonged immobilization), consider low-dose oral estrogen contraceptives containing older progestins or progestin-only methods.

Migraine Headache

- Women with migraines may experience a decreased or increased frequency of migraines when using CHCs. CHCs may be considered for healthy, nonsmoking women with migraines without aura. Women of any age who have migraine with aura and women over 35 years with any type of migraine should not use CHCs. Women who develop migraines (with or without aura) while receiving CHCs should immediately discontinue their use and consider a progestin-only option.

Breast Cancer

- There is a small increase in the relative risk of having breast cancer while combined OCs are taken and for up to 10 years following discontinuation. Cancers diagnosed in women who used combined OCs were less advanced than cancers diagnosed in women who had not used OCs.
- The choice to use CHCs should not be influenced by the presence of benign breast disease or a family history of breast cancer with either BRCA1 or BRCA2 mutation, but women with a current or past history of breast cancer should not use CHCs.

Systemic Lupus Erythematosus

- OCs with less than 50 mcg EE do not increase the risk of flare among women with stable systemic lupus erythematosus (SLE) and without antiphospholipid/anticardiolipin antibodies. CHCs should be avoided in women with SLE and antiphospholipid antibodies or vascular complications. Progestin-only contraceptives can be used in these women.

Obesity

- OCs have lower efficacy in obese women, and low-dose OCs may be especially problematic. Obese women are at increased risk for VTE. The transdermal contraceptive patches should not be used as a first choice in women weighing greater than 90 kg (198 lb), and progestin-only contraception may be better for obese women over 35 years.

GENERAL CONSIDERATIONS FOR ORAL CONTRACEPTIVES

- With perfect use, OC efficacy is more than 99%, but with typical use, up to 8% of women may experience unintended pregnancy.
- Monophasic OCs contain a constant amount of estrogen and progestin for 21 days, followed by 7 days of placebo. Biphasic and triphasic pills contain variable amounts of estrogen and progestin for 21 days and are followed by a 7-day placebo phase.
- Extended-cycle pills and continuous combination regimens may offer some side effect and convenience benefits. One particular extended-cycle OC increases the number of hormone-containing pills from 21 to 84 days, followed by a 7-day placebo phase, resulting in four menstrual cycles per year.

- The progestin-only "minipills" tend to be less effective than combination OCs, and they are associated with irregular and unpredictable menstrual bleeding. They must be taken every day of the menstrual cycle at approximately the same time of day to maintain contraceptive efficacy. They are associated with more ectopic pregnancies than other hormonal contraceptives.
- In the first-day start method, women take the first pill on the first day of the next menstrual cycle. In the Sunday start method, the first pill is taken on the first Sunday after starting the menstrual cycle. Women should use a second contraceptive method for 7 to 30 days after OC initiation.
- The World Health Organization's Selected Practice Recommendations for Contraceptive Use can be used for guidance when instructing women what to do if a pill is missed.

CHOICE OF AN ORAL CONTRACEPTIVE

- In women without coexisting medical conditions, an OC containing 35 mcg or less of EE and less than 0.5 mg of norethindrone is recommended.
- Adolescents, underweight women (<50 kg [110 lb]), women older than 35 years, and those who are perimenopausal may have fewer side effects with OCs containing 20 to 25 mcg of EE. However, these low-estrogen OCs are associated with more breakthrough bleeding and an increased risk of contraceptive failure if doses are missed.

MANAGING SIDE EFFECTS

- Many symptoms occurring in the first cycle of OC use (eg, breakthrough bleeding, nausea, and bloating) improve by the third cycle of use. Table 30–5 shows side effect monitoring of women taking hormonal contraceptives.
- Table 30–4 shows symptoms of a serious or potentially serious nature associated with CHC.
- Instruct women to immediately discontinue CHCs if they experience warning signs referred to by the mnemonic ACHES (abdominal pain, chest pain, headaches, eye problems, and severe leg pain).

DRUG INTERACTIONS

- Tell women to use an alternative method of contraception if there is a possibility of a drug interaction compromising OC efficacy.
- **Rifampin** reduces the efficacy of OCs. Advise women to use an additional non-hormonal contraceptive agent during and for at least 7 to 28 days after the course of rifampin therapy.
- Tell women about the small risk of interaction with other antibiotics, and that additional nonhormonal contraceptives can be considered if desired. If there is breakthrough bleeding in women taking concomitant antibiotics and OCs, an alternate method of contraception should be used during the time of concomitant use.
- **Phenobarbital, carbamazepine**, and **phenytoin** potentially reduce the efficacy of OCs, and many anticonvulsants are known teratogens. Intrauterine devices (IUDs), **injectable medroxyprogesterone**, or nonhormonal options may be considered for women taking these drugs.
- Combined OCs may decrease the efficacy of **lamotrigine** and increase the risk of seizures.
- Certain **antiretroviral therapies** may decrease the efficacy of OCs.

DISCONTINUATION OF THE ORAL CONTRACEPTIVE, RETURN OF FERTILITY

- In several large cohort and case-control studies, infants conceived in the first month after an OC was discontinued had no greater chance of miscarriage or a birth defect than those born in the general population. There is no evidence that use of OCs, transdermal patches, or vaginal rings decreases subsequent fertility.

EMERGENCY CONTRACEPTION (EC)

- Progestin-only and progesterone receptor modulator products are approved by the FDA and recommended as first-line EC options. They will not disrupt the fertilized egg if implantation has already occurred. Use of higher doses of CHCs is another option for EC (Yuzpe method), but this option is not widely used and may cause more side effects.
- The progestin-only formulation containing one 1.5 mg tablet of **levonorgestrel (Next Choice One Dose; Plan B One Step**) is approved for EC in the United States. The levonorgestrel-containing formulation is the regimen of choice. These one-dose options are to be given within 72 hours (3 days) of unprotected intercourse, but the sooner it is taken, the greater the efficacy. There is some evidence that it may be effective for up to 5 days after unprotected intercourse, but in this situation **ulipristal (Ella)** or a copper IUD may be a better option.
- Levonorgestrel-containing EC products are now available without a prescription in the United States.
- Ulipristal is a selective progesterone receptor modulator available by prescription as a single dose of 30 mg taken within 120 hours (5 days) of unprotected intercourse. It is considered noninferior to levonorgestrel containing ECs.
- Nausea and vomiting occur significantly less often with progestin-only and progesterone receptor modulator EC compared to the **Yuzpe method**.
- Backup nonhormonal contraceptive methods should be used after EC for at least 7 days.

TRANSDERMAL CONTRACEPTIVES

- A combination contraceptive is available as a transdermal patch (**Ortho Evra**), which may have improved adherence compared with OCs. It is as effective as CHCs in women weighing less than 90 kg (198 lb), so the patch is not recommended as a first-line option in women weighting more than 90 kg. The patch should be applied to the abdomen, buttocks, upper torso, or upper arm at the beginning of the menstrual cycle and replaced every week for 3 weeks. The fourth week is patch-free.
- Women using the patch are exposed to ~60% more estrogen than if they were taking an OC containing 35 mcg of EE, possibly leading to increased thromboembolic risk, and the approved labeling for the patch includes a warning in this regard.

VAGINAL RINGS

- **NuvaRing** releases ~15 mcg/day of EE and 120 mcg/day of etonogestrel over a 3-week period. On first use, the ring should be inserted on or prior to the fifth day of the cycle, remain in place for 3 weeks, and then be removed. One week should lapse before the new ring is inserted on the same day of the week as it was for the last cycle. A second form of contraception should be used for the first 7 days of ring use or if the ring has been expelled for more than 3 hours.

LONG-ACTING INJECTABLE AND IMPLANTABLE CONTRACEPTIVES

- Women who particularly benefit from progestin-only methods, including minipills, are those who are breast-feeding, intolerant of estrogens, and those with concomitant medical conditions in which estrogen is not recommended. Injectable and implantable contraceptives are also beneficial for women with adherence issues. Contraceptive failure rates with long-acting progestin contraception are lower than with CHC.

Injectable Progestins

- **Depot medroxyprogesterone acetate (DMPA)** 150 mg is administered by deep intramuscular injection in the gluteal or deltoid muscle within 5 days of onset of menstrual bleeding, and the dose should be repeated every 12 weeks. Another formulation contains 104 mg of DMPA (Depo-SubQ Provera 104), which is injected subcutaneously into the thigh or abdomen. Exclude pregnancy in women more than 1 week late for repeat injection of the intramuscular formulation or 2 weeks late for repeat injection of the subcutaneous formulation. Return of fertility may be delayed after discontinuation.

- DMPA can be given immediately postpartum in women who are not breastfeeding, but in women who are breast-feeding, delay administration until 6 weeks postpartum. The median time to conception from the first omitted dose is 10 months.
- The most frequent adverse effect of DMPA is menstrual irregularity, which decreases after the first year. Breast tenderness, weight gain, and depression occur less frequently.
- DMPA is associated with a reduction in bone mineral density (BMD), but there are no clear data that demonstrate the effects of DMPA on fracture risk. Loss of BMD seems to be greater with increasing duration of use, and effects on BMD may not be completely reversible upon discontinuation. DMPA should not be continued beyond 2 years unless other contraceptive methods are inadequate.

Subdermal Progestin Implants

- **Nexplanon**, an etonogestrel implant which is radiopaque, is a 4 cm implant, containing 68 mg of etonogestrel that is placed under the skin of the upper arm. It releases 60 mcg daily for the first month, decreasing gradually to 30 mcg/day at the end of the 3 years of recommended use. Efficacy exceeds 99%, but it may be less in women more than 130% of their ideal body weight.
- The major adverse effect is irregular menstrual bleeding. Other side effects are headache, vaginitis, weight gain, acne, and breast and abdominal pain. It does not appear to decrease BMD. Fertility returns within 30 days of removal.

INTRAUTERINE DEVICES

- The contraceptive activity occurs before implantation. Endometrial suppression is caused by progestin-releasing IUDs. Efficacy rates are greater than 99%.
- The risk of pelvic inflammatory disease among users is low.
- **ParaGard** (copper) can be left in place for 10 years. Disadvantages of ParaGard are increased menstrual blood flow and dysmenorrhea.
- **Mirena, Liletta**, and **Skyla** release levonorgestrel. They must be replaced after 5 years (Mirena) and 3 years (Skyla and Liletta). They cause a reduction in menstrual blood loss.

EVALUATION OF THERAPEUTIC OUTCOMES

- Monitor blood pressure annually in all CHC users.
- Monitor glucose levels closely when CHCs are started or stopped in women with a history of glucose intolerance or diabetes mellitus.
- For all contraceptive users do annual cytologic screening (more often if they are at risk for STDs), pelvic and breast examination, and well woman consultation. Also, regularly evaluate for problems that may relate to the CHCs (eg, breakthrough bleeding, amenorrhea, weight gain, and acne). These screenings do not have to occur before prescribing hormonal contraceptives.
- Annually monitor women using Nexplanon for menstrual cycle disturbances, weight gain, local inflammation or infection at the implant site, acne, breast tenderness, headaches, and hair loss.
- Evaluate women using DMPA every 3 months for weight gain, menstrual cycle disturbances, and fractures.
- Monitor women with IUDs at 1 to 3 month intervals for proper positioning of the IUD, changes in menstrual bleeding patterns, upper genital tract infection, and protection against STDs.
- Clinicians should monitor and when indicated screen for HIV and STDs. Counsel all women about healthy sexual practices, including the use of condoms to prevent transmission of STDs when necessary.

See Chapter 79, Contraception, authored by Sarah P. Shrader and Kelly R. Ragucci, for a more detailed discussion of this topic.

31 Menopausal, Perimenopausal, and Postmenopausal Hormone Therapy

- *Perimenopause* begins with the onset of menstrual irregularity and ends 12 months after the last menstrual period which marks the beginning of menopause. *Menopause* is the permanent cessation of menses caused by the loss of ovarian follicular activity. Women spend about 40% of their lives in postmenopause.

PHYSIOLOGY

- The hypothalamic-pituitary-ovarian axis controls reproductive physiology. Follicle-stimulating hormone (FSH) and luteinizing hormone (LH), produced by the pituitary in response to gonadotropin-releasing hormone from the hypothalamus, regulate ovarian function. Gonadotropins are also influenced by negative feedback from the sex steroids estradiol (produced by the dominant follicle) and progesterone (produced by the corpus luteum). Other sex steroids are androgens, primarily testosterone and androstenedione, secreted by the ovarian stroma.
- As women age, circulating FSH progressively rises, and ovarian inhibin-B and anti-Mullerian hormone declines. In menopause, there is a 10- to 15-fold increase in circulating FSH, a 4- to 5-fold increase in LH, and a greater than 90% decrease in circulating estradiol concentrations.

CLINICAL PRESENTATION

- Symptoms of perimenopause and menopause include vasomotor symptoms (hot flushes and night sweats), sleep disturbances, depression, anxiety, poor concentration and memory, vaginal dryness and dyspareunia, headache, sexual dysfunction, and arthralgia.
- Signs include urogenital atrophy in menopause and dysfunctional uterine bleeding in perimenopause. Other potential causes of dysfunctional uterine bleeding should be ruled out.
- Additionally, loss of estrogen production results in metabolic changes; increase in central abdominal fat; and effects on lipids, vascular function, and bone metabolism.

DIAGNOSIS

- Menopause is determined retrospectively after 12 consecutive months of amenorrhea. FSH on day 2 or 3 of the menstrual cycle greater than 10 to 12 IU/L indicates diminished ovarian reserve.
- The diagnosis of menopause should include a comprehensive medical history and physical examination, complete blood count, and measurement of serum FSH. When ovarian function has ceased, serum FSH concentrations exceed 40 IU/L. Altered thyroid function and pregnancy must be excluded.

TREATMENT

- <u>Goals of Treatment</u>: The goals are to relieve symptoms, improve quality of life, and minimize medication adverse effects.
- Mild vasomotor and/or vaginal symptoms can often be alleviated by lowering the room temperature; decreasing intake of caffeine, spicy foods, and hot beverages; smoking cessation; exercise; and a healthy diet.
- Mild vaginal dryness can sometimes be relieved by nonestrogenic vaginal creams, but significant vaginal dryness often requires local or systemic estrogen therapy.
- Figure 31–1 outlines the pharmacologic treatment of women with menopausal symptoms. Food and Drug Administration (FDA)-approved indications and contraindications for menopausal hormone therapy (MHT) are shown in Table 31–1.

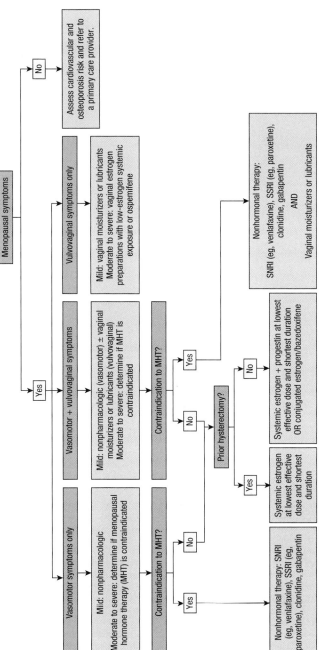

FIGURE 31-1. Algorithm for pharmacologic management of menopause symptoms.

TABLE 31–1	FDA-Labeled Indications and Contraindications for Menopausal Hormone Therapy with Estrogen and Progestins
Indications	
For systemic use	Treatment of moderate to severe vasomotor symptoms (ie, moderate to severe hot flushes)
For intravaginal use (low systemic exposure)	Treatment of moderate to severe symptoms of vulvar and vaginal atrophy (ie, moderate to severe vaginal dryness, dyspareunia, and atrophic vaginitis)
Contraindications	
Absolute contraindications	Undiagnosed abnormal genital bleeding Known, suspected, or history of cancer of the breast Known or suspected estrogen- or progesterone-dependent neoplasia Active deep vein thrombosis, pulmonary embolism, or a history of these conditions Active or recent (eg, within the past year) arterial thromboembolic disease (eg, stroke, myocardial infarction) Liver dysfunction or disease
Relative contraindications	Elevated blood pressure Hypertriglyceridemia Impaired liver function and past history of cholestatic jaundice Hypothyroidism Fluid retention Severe hypocalcemia Ovarian cancer Exacerbation of endometriosis Exacerbation of asthma, diabetes mellitus, migraine, systemic lupus erythematosus, epilepsy, porphyria, and hepatic hemangioma

- Perimenopausal women should not use estrogen-containing contraceptives if they smoke or have a history of estrogen-dependent cancer, heart disease, high blood pressure, diabetes, or thromboembolism.
- Approved indications for MHT are moderate to severe vasomotor symptoms, moderate to severe vulvovaginal atrophy, and prevention of postmenopausal osteoporosis.
- As new data are continuously published, the most current guidelines and consensus statements should always be consulted (eg, United States Preventive Services Task Force, American Association of Clinical Endocrinologists, North American Menopause Society).

MENOPAUSAL HORMONE THERAPY

- Evidence-based guidelines for hormone therapy for menopausal symptoms are shown in Table 31–2.
- When urogenital symptoms, such as vaginal dryness and dyspareunia, are the only menopausal complaint, **intravaginal estrogen cream, tablet, or ring** should be considered before oral therapy. Intravaginal estrogen minimizes systemic absorption and is more effective for vaginal symptoms than oral therapy. **Ospemifene**, a selective estrogen receptor modulator (SERM), is another option. Intravaginal estrogen reduces the risk of recurrent urinary tract infections and may improve urge incontinence and overactive bladder.
- Menopausal hormone therapy is the most effective treatment for moderate to severe vasomotor symptoms, and impaired sleep quality. **Estrogen-only** therapy may decrease heart disease and all cause mortality in 50- to 59-year-old women with a history of hysterectomy.

TABLE 31–2	Evidence-Based Hormone Therapy Guidelines for Menopausal Symptom Management
Recommendation	**Recommendation Grade[a]**
In the absence of contraindications, estrogen-based postmenopausal hormone therapy should be used for treatment of moderate to severe vasomotor symptoms	A1
Systemic or vaginal estrogen therapy should be used for treatment of urogenital symptoms and vaginal atrophy	A1
Postmenopausal women taking estrogen-based therapy should be followed up every year, taking into account findings from new clinical trials	A1
Postmenopausal women taking estrogen-based therapy should be informed about potential risks	A1
Safety and tolerability may vary substantially with the type and regimen of hormone therapy	B2
Breast cancer risk increases after use of continuous combined hormone therapy for longer than 5 years	A1
Breast cancer risk does not increase after long-term estrogen-only therapy (6.8 years) in postmenopausal women with hysterectomy	A1
Hormone therapy should not be used for primary or secondary prevention of coronary heart disease	A1
Oral hormone therapy increases risk of venous thromboembolism	A1
Non-oral hormone therapy may be safer for postmenopausal women at risk for venous thromboembolism who choose to take hormone therapy	B2
Oral hormone therapy increases risk of ischemic stroke	A1
Although hormone therapy decreases risk of osteoporotic fractures, it cannot be recommended as a first-line therapy for the treatment of osteoporosis	A1
Potential harm (cardiovascular disease, breast cancer, and thromboembolism) from long-term hormone therapy (use greater than 5 years) outweighs potential benefits	A1
Young women with primary ovarian insufficiency have severe menopausal symptoms and increased risk for osteoporosis and cardiovascular disease. Decisions on whether and how these young women must be treated should not be based on studies of hormone therapy in women older than 50 years	B3

Quality of evidence: 1, evidence from more than one properly randomized controlled trial; 2, evidence from more than one well-designed clinical trial with randomization from cohort or case-controlled analytic studies or multiple time series, or dramatic results from uncontrolled experiments; 3, evidence from opinions of respected authorities based on clinical experience, descriptive studies, or reports of expert communities.
[a]*Strength of recommendations:* A, good evidence to support recommendation; B, moderate evidence to support recommendation; C, poor evidence to support recommendation.

- Menopausal hormone therapy is effective and appropriate for prevention of osteoporosis-related fractures in recently menopausal women at risk.
- In women with an intact uterus, MHT consists of an **estrogen plus a progestogen** or **estrogen agonist/antagonist** (eg, **bazedoxifine**; see Fig. 31–1). In women who have undergone hysterectomy, estrogen therapy is given unopposed by a progestogen. Concomitant progestogen therapy is unnecessary when low-dose vaginal estrogen is used.
- The **continuous combined oral estrogen–progestogen** arm of the Women's Health Initiative (WHI) study was terminated after a mean of 5.2-year follow-up because of the occurrence of a prespecified level of invasive breast cancer. This study also found increased coronary disease events, stroke, and pulmonary embolism. Beneficial effects included decreases in hip, spine, and wrist fracture and colorectal cancer.
- The oral estrogen-alone arm of the WHI was stopped after a mean of 6.8-year follow-up. Estrogen-only therapy caused no increase in coronary heart disease risk or in breast cancer risk, but the risk of stroke and venous thromboembolism was increased.
- Women with vasomotor symptoms taking MHT have better mental health and fewer depressive symptoms compared with those taking placebo, but hormone therapy may worsen quality of life in women without vasomotor symptoms.

Estrogens

- Estrogen products and doses for MHT are shown in Table 31–3. The oral and transdermal routes are used most frequently and are considered equally effective.
- **Conjugated equine estrogens** are composed of **estrone sulfate** (50%–60%) and other estrogens such as **equilin** and **17α-dihydroequilin**.
- **Estradiol** is the predominant and most active form of endogenous estrogens. Given orally, it is metabolized by the intestinal mucosa and liver, and resultant estrone concentrations are three to six times those of estradiol.
- **Ethinyl estradiol** is a semisynthetic estrogen that has similar activity following oral or parenteral administration.
- **Nonoral estrogens**, including transdermal, intranasal, and vaginal products, avoid first-pass metabolism and result in a more physiologic estradiol:estrone ratio (ie, estradiol concentrations greater than estrone concentrations). Transdermal estrogen is also less likely to increase sex hormone–binding globulin, triglycerides, blood pressure, or C-reactive protein levels. Transdermal dosage forms may also have a lower risk for deep vein thrombosis, stroke, and myocardial infarction.
- Variability in absorption is common with the **percutaneous preparations** (gels, creams, and emulsions).
- **Estradiol pellets** (unavailable in the United States) contain pure **crystalline 17β-estradiol** and are placed subcutaneously (abdomen or buttock). They are difficult to remove.
- **Vaginal creams**, **tablets**, and **rings** are used for treatment of urogenital atrophy. Most tablets and rings provide local estrogen, but Femring is designed to achieve systemic estrogen concentrations and is indicated for moderate to severe vasomotor symptoms.
- New evidence indicates that lower doses of estrogens are effective in controlling postmenopausal symptoms and reducing bone loss. **Low-dose estrogen regimens** include 0.3 to 0.45 mg conjugated estrogens, 0.5 mg micronized 17β-estradiol, and 0.014 to 0.0375 mg transdermal 17β-estradiol patch. Topical gels, creams and sprays are also available in low doses. Lower doses typically have fewer adverse effects, and may have better benefit to risk profiles than standard doses. The lowest effective dose should be used.
- Further study is needed to clarify the efficacy of **phytoestrogens** and their effects on the breast, bone, and endometrium.

Progestogens

- In women who have not undergone hysterectomy, a **progestogen** should be added because estrogen monotherapy is associated with endometrial hyperplasia and cancer.
- The most commonly used oral progestogens are **medroxyprogesterone acetate**, **micronized progesterone**, and **norethindrone** (also known as **norethisterone**) **acetate**.

TABLE 31–3 FDA-Approved Estrogen Products for Menopausal Hormone Therapy

Systemic Estrogen Products (for the treatment of moderate and severe vasomotor symptoms ± urogenital symptoms)

Oral estrogens[b]

Drug	Brand Name[a]	Initial Dose/Low Dose	Usual Dose Range	Comments
Conjugated equine estrogens	Premarin	0.3 or 0.45 mg once daily	0.3–1.25 mg once daily	Dosage form available as 0.3, 0.45, 0.625, 0.9, 1.25 mg
Synthetic conjugated estrogens	Cenestin, Enjuvia	0.3 mg once daily	0.3–1.25 mg once daily	Dosage form available as 0.3, 0.45, 0.625, 0.9, 1.25 mg
Esterified estrogens (75%–85% estrone + 6%–15% equilin)	Menest	0.3 mg once daily	0.3–2.5 mg once daily	Administer 3 weeks on and 1 week off
				Dosage form available as 0.3, 0.625, 1.25, 2.5 mg
Estropipate (piperazine estrone sulfate)	Ogen, Ortho-Est, Generics	0.75 once daily	0.75–6 mg once daily	Dosage form available as 0.75, 1, 5, 3, 6 mg
Estradiol acetate	Femtrace	0.45 mg once daily	0.45–1.8 mg once daily	Dosage form available as 0.45, 0.9, 1.8 mg
Micronized 17β-estradiol	Estrace Generics	1 mg once daily	1 or 2 mg once daily	Administer 3 weeks on and 1 week off
				Dosage form available as 1, 2 mg

(continued)

TABLE 31–3 FDA-Approved Estrogen Products for Menopausal Hormone Therapy (Continued)

Transdermal estrogens patches

17β-estradiol	Alora	0.025 mg/day (patch applied twice weekly)c	0.025–0.1 mg/day (patch applied twice weekly)c	Dosage form available as 0.025, 0.05, 0.075, 0.1 mg/day
	Climara	0.025 mg/day (patch applied twice weekly)c	0.025–0.1 mg/day (patch applied twice weekly)c	Dosage form available as 0.025, 0.0375, 0.05, 0.06, 0.075, 0.1 mg/day
	Menostar	0.014 mg/day (patch applied once weekly)c,d	0.014 mg/day (patch applied once weekly)c,d	Dosage form available as 0.014 mg/day
	Estraderm	—	0.05 or 0.1 mg/day (patch applied twice weekly)c	Dosage form available as 0.05, 0.1 mg/day
	Minivelle, Vivelle, Vivelle Dot	0.025 mg/day (patch applied twice weekly)c	0.025–0.1 mg/day, 0.05 is standard dose (patch applied twice weekly)c	Dosage form available as 0.025, 0.0375, 0.05 (standard dose), 0.075, 0.1 mg/day

Other topical forms of estrogen

17β-estradiol topical emulsion	Estrasorb 0.25% emulsion	—	Two pouches once daily (which delivers 0.05 mg of estradiol per day)	Apply to legs
17β-estradiol topical gel	EstroGel 0.06% metered-dose pump	—	1.25 g/day once daily (contains 0.75 mg estradiol)	Apply from wrist to shoulder
	Elestrin 0.06% metered-dose pump		1–2 unit doses once daily (1 unit dose: 0.87 g, which contains 0.52 mg estradiol)	Apply to upper arm
	Divigel 0.1% (topical once daily)	0.25 g once daily	0.25–1 g (provides 0.25–1 mg of estradiol)	Apply to upper thigh. Dosage form available as 0.25, 0.5, 1 g

	[a]		
17β-estradiol transdermal spray	Evamist	1 spray once daily	2–3 sprays once daily (1.53 mg of estradiol per spray)	Apply to inner surface of forearm
Implanted estrogens[e]			
Implanted 17β-estradiol	Estradiol pellets	25 mg implanted subcutaneously every 6 months	50–100 mg implanted subcutaneously every 6 months
Vaginal estrogens			
Estradiol acetate vaginal ring	Femring	12.4 mg every 3 months	12.4, 24.8 mg ring (delivers 0.05 or 0.1 mg estradiol/day)
Intravaginal estrogen products (for the treatment of urogenital symptoms only/low systemic exposure)			
Conjugated equine estrogens (CEE) vaginal cream	Premarin		0.5–2 g/day (contains 0.625 mg CEE per g)
17β-estradiol vaginal cream	Estrace		1 g/day (contains 0.1 mg estradiol per g)
17β-estradiol vaginal ring	Estring	2 mg replaced every 90 days	2 mg ring (delivers 0.0075 mg/day) replaced every 90 days
Estradiol hemihydrate vaginal tablet	Vagifem	10 mcg twice weekly	10 or 25 mcg twice weekly

[a] United States brand names.

[b] Orally administered estrogens stimulate synthesis of hepatic proteins and increase circulating concentrations of sex hormone-binding globulin, which in turn may compromise the bioavailability of androgens and estrogens. Women with elevated triglyceride concentrations or significant liver function abnormalities are candidates for non-oral estrogen therapy.

[c] Do not apply estrogen patches on or near breasts. Avoid waistline as patch may rub off with tight-fitting clothing.

[d] FDA-approved for prevention of postmenopausal osteoporosis only.

[e] Not available in the United States.

TABLE 31-4	Progestogen Dosing for Endometrial Protection (Cyclic Administration)	
Progestogen	**Brand Name**	**Dosage**
Dydrogesterone[a]	Duphaston	10–20 mg/day for 12–14 days per calendar month (oral dosage form available as 10 mg tablets)
Medroxyprogesterone acetate	Provera	5–10 mg/day for 12–14 days per calendar month (oral dosage form available as 2.5, 5, 10 mg tablets)
Micronized progesterone	Prometrium	200 mg/day for 12–14 days per calendar month (oral dosage form available as 100 and 200 mg tablets)
Norethindrone acetate	Aygestin[b]	5 mg/day for 12–14 days per calendar month (oral dosage form available as 2.5, 5 mg tablets)

[a]Not available in the United States.
[b]Not approved for postmenopausal hormone therapy in the United States.

- Several progestogen regimens to prevent endometrial hyperplasia are shown in Table 31–4. **Combination estrogen–progestogen** regimens are shown in Table 31–5. Methods of administration include the following:
  - ✓ **Continuous-cyclic estrogen-progestogen (sequential)** results in scheduled vaginal withdrawal bleeding in approximately 90% of women. The progestogen is administered 12 to 14 days of the 28-day cycle.
  - ✓ **Continuous-combined estrogen-progestogen** causes endometrial atrophy but prevents monthly bleeding. It may initially cause unpredictable spotting or bleeding.
  - ✓ **Continuous long-cycle estrogen-progestogen (cyclic withdrawal).** Estrogen is given daily, and progestogen is given six times yearly (every other month) for 12 to 14 days, resulting in six periods per year.
  - ✓ **Intermittent-combined estrogen-progestogen (continuous pulsed)** lowers the incidence of uterine bleeding. It consists of 3 days of estrogen therapy alone, followed by 3 days of combined estrogen and progestogen, which is then repeated without interruption. It causes fewer side effects than regimens with higher progestogen doses.

ALTERNATIVE DRUG TREATMENTS

- For women with contraindications to or who cannot tolerate estrogens and/or progestogens, other treatment options for hot flushes can be considered (Table 31–6). Some clinicians consider **selective serotonin reuptake inhibitors** (eg, **paroxetine**) or serotonin-norepinephrine reuptake inhibitors (eg, venlafaxine) to be first-line agents. **Clonidine** can be effective, but side effects are often problematic (eg, sedation, dry mouth, hypotension).

Androgens

- **Testosterone** use in women, although controversial, is becoming more common, even in the absence of androgen deficiency. Testosterone, with or without estrogen, may improve the quality of the sexual experience in postmenopausal women.
- Absolute contraindications to androgen therapy include pregnancy or lactation and known or suspected androgen-dependent neoplasia.
- Excessive dosage may cause virilization, fluid retention, and adverse lipoprotein lipid effects, which are more likely with oral administration. Evidence on the efficacy and safety of testosterone in women in lacking, and its use is currently not recommended.

TABLE 31-5	Common Combination Menopausal Hormone Therapy Regimens	
Regimen	**Brand name**	**Dosage**
Oral regimens		
Conjugated equine estrogen (CEE) + medroxyprogesterone acetate (MPA)	Prempro (continuous)	0.625 mg/2.5 MPA, 0.625 mg/ 5 mg daily Low dose: 0.3 mg/1.5 mg, 0.45 mg/1.5 mg daily
	Premphase (continuous sequential)	0.625 mg CEE daily only in the first 2 weeks of a 4-week cycle then 0.625 mg daily CEE + 5 mg MPA daily in the last 2 weeks of a 4-week cycle
Conjugated equine estrogen (CEE) + bazedoxifene	Duavee (continuous)	0.45 mg/20 mg daily
Ethinyl estradiol (EE) + norethindrone acetate (NETA)	Generic, Femhrt (continuous)	5 mcg EE/1 mg NETA daily Low dose (Femhrt only): 2.5 mcg EE/0.5 mg NETA daily
Estradiol (E) + drospirenone (DRSP)	Angeliq (continuous)	1 mg E/5 mg DRSP daily Low dose: 0.5 mg E/0.25 mg DRSP daily
Estradiol (E) + norgestimate	Prefest (estrogen/intermittent progestogen)	1 mg E daily for first 3 days then 1 mg E/0.09 mg norgestimate daily for next 3 days; this pattern is repeated continuously
Estradiol (E) + norethindrone acetate (NETA)	Activella (continuous) Mimvey (continuous)	1 mg E/0.5 mg NETA daily Low-dose: 0.5 mg E/0.1 mg NETA daily 1 mg E/0.5 mg NETA daily
Transdermal regimens		
Estradiol + norethindrone acetate patch	CombiPatch (continuous) CombiPatch (continuous sequential)	Continuous: 0.05/0.14 mg, 0.05/0.25 mg (apply 1 patch twice weekly) Continuous sequential: 0.05 mg of an estradiol only patch (apply 1 patch twice weekly) in the first 2 weeks of a 4-week cycle then either dose of the CombiPatch (apply 1 patch twice weekly) in the last 2 weeks of a 4-week cycle
Estradiol (E) + levonorgestrel patch	Climara Pro (continuous)	0.045 mg E/0.015 mg/day (apply 1 patch once weekly)

(CEE, conjugated equine estrogen; DRSP, drospirenone; E, estradiol; EE, ethinyl estradiol; NETA, norethindrone acetate; MPA, medroxyprogesterone acetate.)

Selective Estrogen Receptor Modulators (SERMs)

- SERMs are nonsteroidal compounds that act as estrogen agonists in some tissues such as bone and as estrogen antagonists in other tissues such as breast through high-affinity binding to the estrogen receptor.
- **Tamoxifen** is an antagonist in breast tissue and an agonist on the bone and endometrium (see Chapter 60).

TABLE 31–6 Alternatives to Estrogen for Treatment of Hot Flushes[a]

Drug	Brand Name[b]	Initial Dose	Usual Dose Range	Comments
Tibolone[c]	Livial (not available in the United States)	2.5 mg	2.5 mg/day	Tibolone is not recommended during the perimenopause period because it may cause irregular bleeding
Venlafaxine	Effexor, Effexor XR	37.5 mg	37.5–150 mg/day	Adverse effects include nausea, headache, somnolence, dizziness, insomnia, nervousness, xerostomia, anorexia, constipation, diaphoresis, weakness, and hypertension
Desvenlafaxine	Pristiq	100–150 mg	100–150 mg/day	Adverse effects include nausea, headache, somnolence, dizziness, insomnia, xerostomia, anorexia, constipation, diaphoresis, and weakness
Paroxetine, paroxetine CR[d]	Brisdelle,[e] Paxil, Paxil CR, Pexeva	17.5 mg/day (paroxetine),[e] 10 mg/day (paroxetine), or 12.5 mg/day (paroxetine CR)	7.5 mg/day;[e] 10–20 mg/day or 12.5–25 mg/day	Adverse effects include nausea, somnolence, insomnia, headache, dizziness, xerostomia, constipation, diarrhea, weakness, and diaphoresis
Megestrol acetate	Megace	20 mg/day	20–40 mg/day	Progesterone may be linked to breast cancer etiology; also, there is concern regarding the safety of progestational agents in women with preexisting breast cancer

Clonidine	Catapres and generic tablets (oral) Catapres-TTS (transdermal) Kapvay tablets (extended release; oral)	0.1 mg/day	0.1 mg/day	Adverse effects include drowsiness, dizziness, hypotension, and dry mouth, especially with higher doses
Gabapentin	Gralise, Neurontin	300 mg at bedtime	900 mg/day (divided in three daily doses), doses up to 2,400 mg/day (divided in three daily doses) have been studied	Adverse effects include somnolence and dizziness; these symptoms often can be obviated with a gradual increase in dosing

(CR, controlled release.)

aTreatment of postmenopausal hot flushes is an off-label indication in the United States for all medications listed except for one formulation of paroxetine (paroxetine mesylate).

bUnited States brand names.

cNot available in the United States.

dOther selective serotonin reuptake inhibitors (eg, citalopram, escitalopram, fluoxetine, and sertraline) have also been studied and may be used for the treatment of hot flushes.

eThe brand Brisdelle contains 7.5 mg of paroxetine and is FDA-approved to treat moderate to severe vasomotor symptoms of menopause. This specific product is not FDA-approved for treating psychiatric conditions.

- **Raloxifene** is approved for prevention and treatment of postmenopausal osteoporosis and reduction in risk of invasive breast cancer in postmenopausal women with osteoporosis. The dose is 60 mg once daily.
- The third-generation SERM, **bazedoxifene**, is used in conjunction with conjugated estrogen, and is FDA-approved for moderate to severe vasomotor symptoms and prevention of osteoporosis.
- **Ospemifene** is recently approved for moderate to severe dyspareunia from menopausal vulvar and vaginal atrophy. It has a boxed warning for increased risk of endometrial cancer in women with a uterus who use ospemifene (an estrogen agonist in the endometrium) without a progestogen to reduce endometrial hyperplasia. It also has a boxed warning about the possible risk of stroke and venous thromboembolism. It also increases hot flushes.

Tibolone

- **Tibolone** (unavailable in the United States) has combined estrogenic, progestogenic, and androgenic activity. Tibolone improves mood, libido, menopausal symptoms, and vaginal atrophy. It protects against bone loss and reduces the risk of vertebral fractures. It reduces total cholesterol, triglyceride, lipoprotein (a), but may decrease high-density lipoprotein concentrations. It decreases the risk of breast and colon cancer in women ages 60 to 85 years.
- Adverse effects include weight gain and bloating. It may increase the risk of stroke in elderly women. It is associated with breast cancer recurrence, and it may increase endometrial cancer risk.

RISKS OF HORMONE THERAPY

- Adverse effects of **estrogen** include nausea, headache, breast tenderness, and heavy bleeding. More serious adverse effects include increased risk for stroke, venous thromboembolism, and gall bladder disease. Transdermal estrogen is less likely than oral estrogen to cause breast tenderness, gallbladder disease, and deep vein thrombosis.
- Adverse effects of progestogens include irritability, headache, mood swings, fluid retention, and sleep disturbance.
- The WHI trial showed an overall increase in the risk of coronary heart disease in healthy postmenopausal women ages 50 to 79 years taking **estrogen–progestogen therapy** compared with those taking placebo. The estrogen-alone arm of the WHI showed no effect (either increase or decrease) in the risk of coronary heart disease. A more recent analysis from the WHI, which included only adherent participants, found that the risk of coronary heart disease with estrogen plus progestogen is increased in the first 2 years of treatment, even in women aged 50 to 59 years at study entry. However, the risk of coronary heart disease in women who initiated therapy within 10 years of menopause appears to decrease after 6 years of treatment. Menopausal hormone therapy should not be initiated or continued solely for prevention of cardiovascular disease.
- Risk of venous thromboembolism and stroke increases with oral MHT containing estrogen, but the absolute risk is low in women below 60 years of age. Transdermal MHT and low-dose oral estrogen therapy appear to have a lower risk of venous thromboembolism and stroke compared to standard-dose oral estrogen regimens. The norpregnane progestogens also appear to be thrombogenic. Menopausal hormone therapy should be avoided in women at high risk for thromboembolic events (eg, those with Factor V Leiden mutation, obesity, or history of previous thromboembolic events).
- Menopausal hormone therapy is contraindicated in women with a personal history of breast cancer. The risk of MHT-related breast cancer appears to be associated with the addition of progestogen to estrogen and increased after 5 or more years of continuous combined use. However, use of estrogen alone appears to decrease rather than increase breast cancer risk.
- The WHI trial suggests that combined oral MHT does not increase endometrial cancer risk compared with placebo, but estrogen alone given to women with an intact uterus significantly increases uterine cancer risk.

- The WHI trial suggested that oral combined MHT does not increase the risk of ovarian cancer. An observational study concurred, but noted an increase in risk for ovarian cancer in postmenopausal women taking estrogen-only therapy for more than 10 years.
- The WHI study found that postmenopausal women 65 years or older taking **estrogen plus progestogen** therapy had twice the rate of dementia, including Alzheimer disease than those taking placebo. Combined therapy did not prevent mild cognitive impairment. The estrogen-alone arm showed similar findings.

EVALUATION OF THERAPEUTIC OUTCOMES

- Management of patients taking hormone therapy is summarized in **Table 31–7**.

TABLE 31–7 Management of Patients Taking Hormone Therapy Regimens

Initiation of hormone therapy

Hormone therapy should be used only as long as vasomotor symptom control is necessary (usually 2–3 years)

6-week follow-up visit

- To discuss patient concerns about hormone therapy
- To evaluate the patient for symptom relief, adverse effects, and patterns of withdrawal bleeding (if continuous sequential hormone therapy is given)

Drug	Adverse drug reaction	Monitoring parameter	Suggested change
Estrogen		Persistence of hot flushes	Increase estrogen dose
Estrogen	Breast tenderness		Reduce estrogen dose; switch to a transdermal regimen
Progestogen	Bloating Premenstrual-like symptoms		Switch to another progestogen

Annual follow-up visit

Annual monitoring: medical history, physical examination (including pelvic examination), blood pressure measurement, and routine endometrial cancer surveillance (as indicated). Additional follow-up is determined based on the patient's initial response to therapy and the need for any modification of the regimen

Breast examinations: annual mammograms (scheduled based on patient's age and risk factors)

Osteoporosis prevention: BMD should be measured in women 65 years and older and in women younger than 65 years with risk factors for osteoporosis. Repeat testing should be performed as clinically indicated.

In women taking sequential hormone therapy	Transvaginal ultrasound, and where indicated an endometrial biopsy should be performed if vaginal bleeding occurs at any time other than the expected time of withdrawal bleeding or when heavier or more prolonged withdrawal bleeding occurs (if endometrial pathology cannot be excluded by endovaginal ultrasonography, further evaluation may be required, such as hysteroscopy)
In women taking continuous combined hormone therapy	Endometrial evaluation should be considered when irregular bleeding persists for more than 6 months after initiating therapy

(BMD, bone mineral density.)

CONCLUSIONS

- Menopausal hormone therapy should be considered for healthy women with moderate to severe vasomotor symptoms who are within 10 years of menopause or age younger than 60 years and who do not have contraindications. The duration of estrogen-progestogen therapy is limited by the risk of breast cancer at 3 to 5 years of use; estrogen-only therapy allows for more flexibility up to 7 years of use.
- Long-term use of MHT or initiation in older women is associated with greater risks.
- All types and routes of administration of estrogen are equally effective for vasomotor symptoms and vulvovaginal atrophy. A dose-dependent relationship between estrogen administration and suppression of hot flushes is established.
- Starting with low doses of estrogen often minimizes adverse effects.
- Avoid oral estrogen in favor of transdermal administration in women with hypertriglyceridemia, liver disease, and gallbladder disease. Transdermal estradiol is also less likely than oral estrogen to cause nausea and headache.

See Chapter 82, Hormone Therapy in Women, authored by Sophia N. Kalantaridou, Laura M. Borgelt, Devra K. Dang, and Karim Anton Calis, for a more detailed discussion of this topic.

32

Pregnancy and Lactation: Therapeutic Considerations

- Resources on the use of drugs in pregnancy and lactation include the Food and Drug Administration (FDA) categorization system (A, B, C, D, and X), the primary literature, tertiary compendia, textbooks, and computerized databases (eg, www.motherisk.org and www.toxnet.nlm.nih.gov).

PHYSIOLOGIC AND PHARMACOKINETIC FACTORS

- The duration of pregnancy is approximately 280 days (measured from the first day of the last menstrual period to birth). Pregnancy is divided into three periods of three calendar months (ie, trimesters).
- Drug absorption during pregnancy may be altered by delayed gastric emptying and vomiting. An increased gastric pH may affect absorption of weak acids and bases. Hepatic perfusion increases. Higher estrogen and progesterone levels may alter liver enzyme activity and increase elimination of some drugs but cause accumulation of others.
- Maternal plasma volume, cardiac output, and glomerular filtration increase by 30% to 50% or higher during pregnancy, possibly lowering the plasma concentration of renally cleared drugs. Body fat increases; thus, volume of distribution of fat-soluble drugs may increase. Plasma albumin concentrations decrease; thus volume of distribution of highly protein bound drugs may increase. However, there may be little change in serum concentration, as these unbound drugs are more rapidly cleared by the liver and kidneys.
- The placenta is the organ of exchange between the mother and fetus for drugs. Drugs with molecular weights less than 500 Da transfer readily, drugs with molecular weights from 600 to 1000 Da cross more slowly, and drugs with molecular weights greater than 1000 Da (eg, insulin and heparin) do not cross in significant amounts.
- Lipophilic drugs (eg, opiates and antibiotics) cross more easily than do water-soluble drugs. Certain protein-bound drugs may achieve higher plasma concentrations in the fetus than in the mother.

DRUG SELECTION DURING PREGNANCY

- The incidence of congenital malformation is approximately 3% to 6%, and it is estimated that less than 1% of all birth defects are caused by medication exposure.
- Adverse effects on the fetus depend on drug dosage, route of administration, and stage of pregnancy when the exposure occurred.
- Fetal exposure to a teratogen in the first 2 weeks after conception may have an "all or nothing" effect (ie, could destroy the embryo or have no ill effect). Exposure during organogenesis (18–60 days postconception) may cause structural anomalies (eg, **methotrexate, cyclophosphamide, diethylstilbestrol, lithium, retinoids, thalidomide,** some **antiepileptic drugs [AEDs]**, and **coumarin derivatives).**
- Exposure after this point may result in growth retardation, central nervous system (CNS) or other abnormalities, or death. **Nonsteroidal anti-inflammatory drugs (NSAIDs)** and **tetracycline derivatives** are more likely to exhibit effects in the second or third trimester.
- Principles for drug use during pregnancy include (1) selecting drugs that have been used safely for a long time; (2) prescribing doses at the lower end of the dosing range; (3) eliminating nonessential medication and discouraging self-medication; and (4) avoiding medications known to be harmful.

PRECONCEPTION PLANNING

- **Folic acid** supplementation between 0.4 and 0.9 mg daily is recommended throughout the reproductive years to reduce the risk for neural tube (NTD) defects in offspring. Women of child-bearing potential who take AED medications should take prenatal vitamins with folic acid 0.4 to 5 mg/day. Higher folate doses should be used in women who have previously delivered a child with a NTD and those taking valproic acid.
- Reduction in the use of alcohol, tobacco, and other substances prior to pregnancy improves outcomes. For smoking cessation, behavioral interventions are preferred. Use of **nicotine replacement therapy** during pregnancy is controversial.

PREGNANCY-INFLUENCED ISSUES

GASTROINTESTINAL TRACT

- Constipation commonly occurs during pregnancy. Institute education, physical exercise, and increased intake of dietary fiber and fluid. If additional therapy is warranted, give **supplemental fiber** and/or a stool softener. **Polyethylene glycol**, **lactulose**, and **sorbitol**, can be used intermittently. **Senna** and **bisacodyl** can also be used occasionally. Magnesium and sodium salts can cause electrolyte imbalance. Avoid **castor oil** and **mineral oil**.
- Therapy for gastroesophageal reflux disease includes lifestyle and dietary modifications, for example, small, frequent meals; alcohol, tobacco, and caffeine avoidance; food avoidance before bedtime; and elevation of the head of the bed. If necessary, initiate **aluminum**, **calcium**, or **magnesium antacids**; **sucralfate**; **cimetidine**, or **ranitidine**. Proton pump inhibitors are options if response to histamine 2 (H_2)–receptor blockers is inadequate. Avoid **sodium bicarbonate** and **magnesium trisilicate**.
- Therapy for hemorrhoids includes high intake of dietary fiber, adequate oral fluid intake, and use of sitz baths. If response is inadequate, laxatives and stool softeners can be used. Topical anesthetics, skin protectants, and astringents may help irritation and pain. Topical hydrocortisone may reduce inflammation and pruritus.
- Nonpharmacologic treatments for nausea and vomiting include eating small, frequent meals; avoiding fatty and spicy foods; and acupressure. Pharmacotherapy may include ginger, antihistamines (eg, **doxylamine**), and **pyridoxine**. The American College of Obstetricians and Gynecologists considers pyridoxine alone or in combination with doxylamine to be first line treatment. Metoclopramide and phenothiazines are considered safe, but may cause sedation and extrapyramidal effects. **Ondansetron** may cause oral clefts.
- **Corticosteroids** have been effective for hyperemesis gravidarum (ie, severe nausea and vomiting causing weight loss >5% of prepregnancy weight, dehydration, and ketonuria), but the risk of oral clefts is increased. They should not be used during the first trimester.

GESTATIONAL DIABETES MELLITUS

- First-line therapy for all women with gestational diabetes mellitus (GDM) includes exercise, dietary modification, and caloric restrictions for obese women. Daily self-monitoring of blood glucose is required. If lifestyle interventions fail to achieve glycemic control, drug therapy is indicated. Glycemic control is pre-prandial capillary glucose concentrations at or below 95 mg/dL (5.3 mmol/L) along with one of the following: a 1-hour postprandial glucose at or below 140 mg/dL (7.8 mmol/L), or a 2-hour postprandial glucose of 120 mg/dL (6.7 mmol/L) or below. **Human insulin** is the drug of choice for diabetes management during pregnancy, because it does not cross the placenta. **Glyburide** and **metformin** are alternatives, but long-term safety data are limited. The American College of Obstetricians and Gynecologists (ACOG) support either insulin, glyburide, or metformin for first-line therapy.

HYPERTENSION

- Hypertensive disorders of pregnancy include (1) preeclampsia-eclampsia, (2) chronic hypertension (HTN; preexisting HTN or developing before 20 weeks' gestation), (3) chronic hypertension with superimposed preeclampsia, and (4) gestational HTN (ie, HTN without proteinuria developing after 20 weeks' gestation). Eclampsia, a medical emergency, is preeclampsia with seizures. HTN in pregnancy is either systolic blood pressure above 140 mm Hg or diastolic blood pressure above 90 mm Hg based on two or more measurements at least 4 hours apart.
- For women at risk for preeclampsia, low-dose **aspirin** (60–81 mg/day) beginning late in the first trimester reduces the risk for preeclampsia by 17%. Aspirin also reduces the risk of preterm birth by 8% and fetal and neonatal death by 14%. **Calcium**, 1 to 2 g/day, decreases the relative risk of HTN by 35% and preeclampsia by 55%. ACOG states that these recommendations do not apply to populations with adequate calcium intake, such as the United States.
- Antihypertensive drug therapy is discussed later under Chronic Illnesses in Pregnancy below.
- **Magnesium sulfate** decreases the risk of progression of preeclampsia to eclampsia by almost 60%, and it also treats eclamptic seizures. Avoid **diazepam** and **phenytoin**.

THYROID ABNORMALITIES

- Gestational transient thyrotoxicosis usually resolves by 20 weeks' gestation. Antithyroid medication is usually not needed.
- Pregnant women with overt hyperthyroidism should be treated with **methimazole** or **propylthiouracil**, and those with overt hypothyroidism should receive thyroid replacement therapy (ie, **levothyroxine**).

VENOUS THROMBOEMBOLISM (VTE)

- For treatment of acute thromboembolism during pregnancy, **low-molecular-weight heparin (LMWH)** is preferred over **unfractionated heparin** or **warfarin**. Continue treatment throughout pregnancy and for 6 weeks after delivery. Duration of therapy should not be less than 3 months. Avoid fondaparinux, lepirudin, and bivalirudin unless a severe allergy to heparin exists. Dabigatran, rivaroxaban, and apixaban are not recommended. Avoid **warfarin** because it may cause fetal bleeding, nasal hypoplasia, stippled epiphyses, or CNS anomalies.
- For women at intermediate or high risk for recurrent VTE, provide antepartum prophylaxis with LMWH plus 6-week postpartum prophylaxis with LMWH or warfarin. For women with prosthetic heart valves, thrombophilias, and those at very high risk for VTE, consult current guidelines.

ACUTE CARE ISSUES IN PREGNANCY

HEADACHE

- For tension and migraine headaches during pregnancy, first-line therapies are nonpharmacologic, including relaxation, stress management, and biofeedback.
- For tension headache, **acetaminophen** or **ibuprofen** can be used if necessary. All NSAIDs and aspirin are contraindicated in the third trimester because of the potential for closure of the ductus arteriosus. Aspirin may also cause maternal and fetal bleeding, and decreased uterine contractility. **Opioids** are rarely used.
- For migraine headache, acetaminophen and ibuprofen can be used. Opioids have been used, but they can contribute to nausea, and long-term use can cause neonatal withdrawal. For nonresponsive migraines, **sumatriptan** can be used. **Ergotamine** and **dihydroergotamine** are contraindicated. For migraine-associated nausea, **promethazine**, **prochlorperazine**, and **metoclopramide** can be used.
- For pregnant women with severe headaches (usually migraine) not responsive to other treatments, propranolol, at the lowest effective dose, can be used as preventive treatment. Alternatives include amitriptyline or nortriptyline, 10 to 25 mg daily by mouth.

URINARY TRACT INFECTION

- The principal infecting organism is *Escherichia coli*, but *Proteus mirabilis*, *Klebsiella pneumoniae*, and group B *Streptococcus* cause some infections. Untreated bacteriuria may result in pyelonephritis, preterm labor, hypertension, anemia, transient renal failure, and low birth weight.
- Treatment of asymptomatic bacteriuria is necessary to reduce the risk of pyelonephritis and premature delivery. Treatment of asymptomatic bacteriuria and cystitis for 7 to 14 days is common.
- The most commonly used antibiotics for asymptomatic bacteriuria and cystitis are the β-lactams (penicillins and cephalosporins) and nitrofurantoin. *E. coli* resistance to ampicillin and amoxicillin is problematic. **Nitrofurantoin** is not active against *Proteus* and should not be used after week 37 in patients with glucose-6-phosphate dehydrogenase deficiency due to concern for hemolytic anemia in the newborn. **Sulfa-containing drugs** may increase the risk for kernicterus in the newborn and should be avoided during the last weeks of gestation. **Folate antagonists**, such as **trimethoprim**, are relatively contraindicated during the first trimester because of their association with cardiovascular malformations. Regionally, increased rates of *E. coli* resistance to trimethoprim-sulfa limit its use. **Fluoroquinolones** and **tetracyclines** are contraindicated.
- Inpatient therapy for pyelonephritis has included parenteral administration of second- or third-generation cephalosporins, ampicillin plus gentamicin, or ampicillin-sulbactam. Switching to oral antibiotics can occur after the woman is afebrile for 48 hours, but avoid nitrofurantoin. The total duration of antibiotic therapy for pyelonephritis is 10 to 14 days.

SEXUALLY TRANSMITTED DISEASES

- Pharmacotherapy for selected sexually transmitted infections is shown in **Table 32–1**.
- Complications of *Chlamydia trachomatis* include pelvic inflammatory disease, ectopic pregnancy, and infertility. *Chlamydia* infection can be transmitted at birth to the neonate and cause conjunctivitis and a subacute, afebrile pneumonia.
- **Benzathine Penicillin G** is the drug of choice for all stages of syphilis except neurosyphilis, which is treated with **Aqueous Penicillin G**. Penicillin is effective for preventing transmission to the fetus and treating the already infected fetus.
- *Neisseria gonorrhoeae* is a risk factor for pelvic inflammatory disease and preterm delivery. Symptoms in the neonate (eg, rhinitis, vaginitis, urethritis, ophthalmia neonatorum, and sepsis) usually start within 2 to 5 days of birth. Blindness can occur. Oral cephalosporins have been removed as a preferred treatment option for Gonorrhea because of antimicrobial resistance. Coinfection with Chlamydia is common, so usually treatment of Gonorrhea includes treatment for Chlamydia.
- The overriding concern with genital herpes is transmission of the virus to the neonate during birth. Maternal use of **acyclovir** during the first trimester is not associated with an increased risk of birth defects. **Valacyclovir** is an alternative.
- Bacterial vaginosis is caused by anaerobic bacteria, mycoplasmas, and *Gardnerella vaginalis*. It is a risk factor for premature rupture of membranes, preterm labor, preterm birth, intraamniotic infection, and postpartum endometritis.
- Trichomoniasis is associated with an increased risk of premature rupture of membranes, premature delivery, and low birth weight. Treatment may prevent respiratory or genital infection in the neonate.

CHRONIC ILLNESSES IN PREGNANCY

- **Table 32–2** shows treatment of some chronic illnesses in pregnancy.

ALLERGIC RHINITIS AND ASTHMA

- Diagnosis and staging of asthma during pregnancy is the same as in nonpregnant women, but more frequent follow-up is necessary. The risks of medication use to the fetus are lower than the risks of untreated asthma.

TABLE 32–1	Management of Sexually Transmitted Infections in Pregnancy		
STI	Drug Name (Brand Name)	Usual Dose	Monitoring	Comments
Bacterial vaginosis	*Recommended:* Metronidazole (Flagyl) **OR** Metronidazole 0.75% gel *Alternatives*: Clindamycin (Cleocin)	• 500 mg by mouth two times daily × 7 days • 5 g intravaginally once daily × 5 days	Follow-up testing not required if symptoms resolve	No link between intravaginal clindamycin and newborn complications Oral or vaginal preparations can be used
Chlamydia	*Recommended:* Azithromycin (Zithromax) *Alternatives*: Amoxicillin (Amoxil) Erythromycin base Erythromycin ethylsuccinate	1 g by mouth × 1 dose	Test-of-cure at 3–4 weeks after therapy completion; retest all after 3 months	Gonorrheal coinfection common; both are treated concurrently Chlamydia is asymptomatic in men and women Women below age 25 years and those at high risk should be retested in the third trimester
Genital herpes	*Recommended:* Acyclovir (Zovirax) **OR** Valacyclovir	400 mg by mouth three times a day 500 mg by mouth twice a day	Routine serologic testing for HSV-2 is not recommended	Start treatment at 36 weeks of gestation
Gonorrhea	*Recommended:* Ceftriaxone (Rocephin) *PLUS* Azithromycin (Zithromax)	250 mg IM × 1 dose 1 g by mouth × 1 dose	Because of high reinfection rate, repeat testing for gonorrhea 3 months after treatment	Chlamydial coinfection common; both are treated concurrently Consult with infectious disease specialist if cephalosporin allergy

(continued)

TABLE 32-1 Management of Sexually Transmitted Infections in Pregnancy (*Continued*)

STI	Drug Name (Brand Name)	Usual Dose	Monitoring	Comments
Syphilis[b]				
Primary, secondary, early latent	*Recommended:* Benzathine penicillin G (Bicillin L-A)	2.4 million units IM × 1 dose; a second dose can be given 1 week after initial dose	Nontreponemal serologic evaluation[c] at 6 and 12 months	For treatment failure or reinfection, use same drug and dose but increase to 3 weekly doses unless neurosyphilis is present
Tertiary, late latent	*Recommended:* Benzathine penicillin G (Bicillin L-A)	2.4 million units IM × 3 doses at 1-week intervals	Nontreponemal serologic evaluation[c] at 6, 12, and 24 months. CSF examination may be required	Use this regimen for late latent or latent syphilis of unknown duration
Neurosyphilis	*Recommended:* Aqueous penicillin G (Pfizerpen) *Alternative:* Procaine penicillin (Wycillin, Pfizerpen-AS) PLUS Probenecid	3–4 million units IV every 4 hours or 18–24 million units IV continuously × 10–14 days 2.4 million units IM daily × 10–14 days 500 mg by mouth four times daily × 10–14 days	If initial elevation of leukocytes in CSF, repeat CSF examination every 6 months until normalization	Consider repeat treatment if CSF leukocytes or protein do not normalize after 2 years Use alternative regimen only if compliance can be ensured
Trichomoniasis	*Recommended:* Metronidazole	2 g by mouth × 1 dose	Rescreen HIV patients at 3 months after treatment	While tinidazole is an alternative for nonpregnant women, avoid during pregnancy

(CSF, cerebrospinal fluid; IM, intramuscular; STI, sexually transmitted infection.)
[a]Refer to reference 50 for specific dosing recommendations.
[b]Pregnant women with history of penicillin allergy should undergo penicillin desensitization as no proven alternatives exist.
[c]Nontreponemal evaluation consists of VDRL (Venereal Disease Research Laboratory) and RPR (rapid plasma regain).

TABLE 32–2	Treatment of Chronic Illnesses in Pregnancy	
Chronic Illness	**Treatment**	**Comments**
Allergic rhinitis	Intranasal corticosteroids Intranasal cromolyn First generation antihistamines (chlorpheniramine, diphenhydramine, hydroxyzine)	Budesonide and beclomethasone most widely studied intranasal corticosteroids Second generation antihistamines do not appear to increase fetal risk, but are less extensively studied than first generation products Use of external nasal dilator, short-term topical oxymetazoline, or ICS may be preferable to oral decongestants
Asthma		Budesonide is the preferred ICS, but any may be used Alternatives are cromolyn (less effective), leukotriene receptor antagonists (less experience in pregnancy), and theophylline (more potential toxicity) Systemic corticosteroids recommended to gain control in patients with most severe disease
Step 1 (intermittent)	SABA (albuterol)	
Step 2 and above (persistent)	SABA (albuterol) Step-appropriate ICS LABA	
Epilepsy	Probably Safest AEDs • Carbamazepine • Lamotrigine • Levetiracetam • Phenytoin Lower risk than VPA • Gabapentin • Oxcarbazepine • Zonisamide Significant risk greater than other AEDs • Phenobarbital • Topiramate • VPA	Polytherapy carries higher risk of major malformations than monotherapy Rates of major malformation with probably safest AEDs clusters around 2%–5% Phenytoin, lamotrigine, and carbamazepine may cause cleft palate Phenobarbital is associated with cardiac malformations Risk for most AED-associated malformations is dose-related Emerging evidence suggests risk of structural teratogenesis with levetiracetam is low

(continued)

TABLE 32–2	Treatment of Chronic Illnesses in Pregnancy (Continued)	
Chronic Illness	**Treatment**	**Comments**
HIV	Currently receiving ART: Continue current regimen if viral load is suppressed ART-naïve, no evidence of resistance: • Dual NRTI backbone **PLUS** • Ritonavir-boosted PI **OR** • NNRTI **OR** • Integrase inhibitor	In women currently receiving ART, antiretroviral drug resistance testing should be performed to guide ART If efavirenz is part of current ART, continue use since NTDs usually occur through weeks 5–6 of gestation and pregnancy often is not recognized during that time period If ART-naïve, any regimen containing efavirenz should be initiated after first 8 weeks of pregnancy
Hypertension, chronic	Initial treatment: Labetalol Nifedipine Methyldopa	ACE inhibitors, ARBs, renin inhibitors, mineralocorticoid receptor antagonists are not recommended Atenolol has been associated with fetal growth restriction Thiazide diuretics theoretically lower the increase in plasma volume during pregnancy, but are considered second-line
Thyroid disorders	Hypothyroid Levothyroxine Hyperthyroid • PTU • Methimazole	For hypothyroidism, attain a TSH of 0.1–2.5, 0.2–3, and 0.3–3 milli-international units/L (mIU/L) in the first, second, and third trimester, respectively Use PTU in first trimester followed by switch to methimazole in second and third trimester to balance the risk of PTU-induced hepatotoxicity and methimazole embryopathy

(ACE, angiotensin converting enzyme, AED, antiepileptic drug; ARB, angiotensin receptor blocker; ART, antiretroviral therapy; ICS, inhaled corticosteroid; LABA, long-acting beta agonist; NNRTI, non-nucleoside reverse transcriptase inhibitor; NRTI, nucleoside reverse transcriptase inhibitor; NTD, neural tube defects; PI, protease inhibitor; PTU, propylthiouracil; SABA, short-acting beta agonist; TSH, thyroid stimulating hormone; VPA, valproic acid.)
^aList is not all-inclusive.

- Treatment of asthma follows a stepwise approach. As step 1, all pregnant patients with asthma should have access to a short-acting inhaled β_2-agonist (**albuterol** is the preferred agent). For persistent asthma (step 2 or higher), low, medium, or high doses of controller corticosteroids are foundational. Budesonide is preferred, but corticosteroids used before pregnancy can be continued. Long-acting β_2-agonists are safe. **Cromolyn, leukotriene receptor antagonists,** and **theophylline** are considered alternative agents, but they are not preferred. For patients with the most severe disease, systemic corticosteroids are recommended.
- First-line medications for allergic rhinitis during pregnancy include intranasal **corticosteroids, nasal cromolyn,** and first-generation antihistamines (eg, **chlorpheniramine, diphenhydramine,** and **hydroxyzine**). **Intranasal corticosteroids** are the most effective treatment and have a low risk for systemic effect. **Beclomethasone** and **budesonide** have been used most. **Loratadine** and **cetirizine** do not appear to increase fetal risk, but they have not been extensively studied.
- Use of an external nasal dilator, short-term **topical oxymetazoline**, or **inhaled corticosteroids** may be preferred over oral decongestants, especially during early pregnancy.

DIABETES MELLITUS

- Glycemic control can change dramatically during pregnancy, and frequent adjustments may be needed. Self-monitored blood glucose should occur before and after meals, and sometimes between 2 and 4 am. Patients with type 1 diabetes may continue human insulin. Evidence supports insulin detemir as the first-line long-acting insulin analogue. Glyburide and metformin are considered first-line for GDM, so they may be potential treatment alternatives for type 2 diabetes during pregnancy.

EPILEPSY

- Major malformations are two to three times more likely in children born to women taking AEDs than to those who do not, but the risks of untreated epilepsy to the fetus are considered to be greater than those associated with the AEDs.
- Major malformations with valproic acid therapy are dose related and range from 6% to 9%. When possible, avoid **valproic acid** during pregnancy to minimize the risk of neural tube defects, facial clefts, and cognitive teratogenicity. **Phenobarbital** should also be avoided. If either is used during pregnancy, the lowest effective dose should be used.
- Drug therapy should be optimized prior to conception, and AED monotherapy is recommended when possible.
- If drug withdrawal is planned, it should be fully completed prior to conception.
- All women taking AEDs should take **folic acid**, 4 to 5 mg daily, starting before pregnancy and continuing through at least the first trimester and preferably through the entire pregnancy.

HUMAN IMMUNODEFICIENCY VIRUS INFECTION (HIV)

- In women newly diagnosed with HIV, or who have not previously received antiretroviral therapy (ART), ART should be initiated as soon as pregnancy is determined, since risk of perinatal transmission is lower with earlier viral suppression. ART therapy is selected from those recommended for nonpregnant adults (with consideration given to the teratogenic profiles of each drug). Women already taking ART therapy should continue their regimen provided that viral suppression below the level of detection is documented.
- For ART-naïve women, use of a three-drug combination regimen is recommended. The clinical guidelines provided at https://aidsinfo.nih.gov are the most current.
- Pregnant women with HIV RNA levels above 1000 copies/mL (1000×10^3/L) approaching delivery should have cesarean section at 38 weeks gestation to reduce the risk of perinatal HIV transmission. Cesarean section is not recommended if HIV RNA levels are at or below that level. If maternal viral load is greater than that

level or unknown, IV zidovudine should be initiated with a 1-hour load (2 mg/kg) followed by a continuous infusion (1 mg/kg/h) for 2 hours (cesarean) or until vaginal delivery. Women with a viral load at or below 1000 copies/mL (1000 × 10^3/L) near delivery do not require zidovudine IV, but should continue their ART.

HYPERTENSION

- Hypertension occurring before 20 weeks of gestation, the use of antihypertensive medications before pregnancy, or the persistence of hypertension beyond 12 weeks postpartum defines chronic hypertension in pregnancy. It is classified as mild/nonsevere (systolic blood pressure [sBP] 140–159 mm Hg or diastolic blood pressure [dBP] 90–109 mm Hg), or severe (sBP 160 mm Hg or higher or dBP 110 mm Hg or higher). Chronic HTN can cause maternal complications, fetal growth restriction, and hospital admission.
- Treatment of nonsevere HTN reduces risks of severe HTN by 50% but does not substantially affect fetal outcomes. According to ACOG, drug therapy is recommended for pregnant women with persistent chronic HTN with a blood pressure of 160/105 mm Hg and above. When antihypertensive therapy is used, maintenance of sBP between 120 and 160 mm Hg and dBP between 80 and 105 mm Hg is recommended. If there is no evidence of end organ damage, and sBP is below 160 mm Hg and dBP is below 105 mm Hg, drug therapy is not suggested.
- Severe HTN in pregnancy requires treatment, and lowering of BP should occur over a period of hours to prevent compromise of uteroplacental blood flow. Recommended agents are parenteral **labetalol** and **hydralazine**, but hydralazine is associated with more maternal and fetal adverse effects. Oral **nifedipine** may also be used. Limited evidence supports the use of **magnesium sulfate**, except when it is being used concomitantly for preeclampsia. **Nitroprusside, diazoxide**, and **nitroglycerin** should be reserved for refractory HTN in an appropriately monitored environment.

DEPRESSION

- In general, monotherapy is preferred over polytherapy even if higher doses are required. If antidepressants are used, the lowest possible dose should be used for the shortest possible time to minimize adverse fetal and maternal pregnancy outcomes.
- Pregnant women who stopped taking antidepressants are more likely to relapse than women who completed treatment.
- The **selective serotonin reuptake inhibitors (SSRIs)** are not considered major teratogens with the exception of paroxetine. Initiation of paroxetine, for women who intend to become pregnant, or are in their first trimester of pregnancy, should be considered only after other treatment options have been evaluated because of the risk for cardiovascular malformations in the fetus. The **serotonin/norepinephrine reuptake inhibitors (SNRIs)** are less well defined. Use of SSRIs and SNRIs in the latter part of pregnancy is associated with persistent pulmonary HTN of the newborn and prenatal antidepressant exposure syndrome (ie, cardiac, respiratory, neurologic, gastrointestinal [GI], and metabolic complications from drug toxicity or withdrawal of drug therapy). Tricyclic antidepressants are not considered major teratogens but have been associated with neonatal withdrawal syndrome when used late in pregnancy.

THYROID DISORDERS

- For hypothyroidism in pregnancy, initiate levothyroxine 0.1 mg/day. Women receiving thyroid replacement therapy before pregnancy may require increased dosage during pregnancy. Monitor thyroid-stimulating hormone (TSH) levels every 4 to 6 weeks during pregnancy to allow for dose titration according to TSH levels.
- Hyperthyroidism therapy includes the thioamides (eg, methimazole, propylthiouracil [PTU]). The goal of therapy is to attain free thyroxine concentrations near the upper limit of normal.

LABOR AND DELIVERY

PRETERM LABOR

- Preterm labor is labor that occurs between 20 and 37 weeks of gestation when changes in cervical dilations and/or effacement happen along with regular uterine contractions or when the initial presentation includes regular contractions and cervical dilation of at least 2 cm.

Tocolytic Therapy

- The goals of tocolytic therapy are to postpone delivery long enough to allow for maximum effect of antenatal steroids, for transportation of the mother to a facility equipped to deal with high-risk deliveries, or to prolong pregnancy when there are underlying self-limited conditions that can cause labor. Tocolytics can be started when there are regular uterine contractions with cervical change. They are not generally used beyond 34 weeks of gestation. Do not use them in cases of previability, intrauterine fetal demise, a lethal fetal anomaly, intrauterine infection, fetal distress, severe preeclampsia, vaginal bleeding, or maternal hemodynamic instability.
- There are four classes of tocolytics in the United States: **β-agonists**, **magnesium sulfate**, **prostaglandin inhibitors** (i.e., **NSAIDs**), and **calcium channel blockers**. Prolongation of pregnancy with tocolytics is not associated with significant reduction in rates of respiratory distress syndrome, neonatal death, or birth before 37 weeks of gestation. Prostaglandin inhibitors and calcium channel blockers may be preferable, based on delaying delivery and improving neonatal outcomes.
- β-Agonists (**terbutaline** and **ritodrine** [unavailable in the United States] have a higher risk for maternal side effects. A common dose of terbutaline is 250 mcg subcutaneously which may be repeated in 15 to 30 minutes for inadequate response, with a maximum of 500 mcg given in a 4-hour period. An FDA black box warning cautions against oral dosing or prolonged parenteral use (beyond 48–72 hours) because of maternal cardiotoxicity and death.
- A Cochrane review does not support the effectiveness of **magnesium sulfate** for tocolysis. However, it can be used IV during preterm labor to decrease the occurrence of moderate to severe cerebral palsy.
- **Nifedipine** is associated with fewer side effects than magnesium or β-agonist therapy and decreases risk of delivery within 7 days compared to β-agonist. Nifedipine loading doses range between 10 and 40 mg, with subsequent dosing of 10 to 20 mg every 4 to 6 hours, with dose adjustment based on patterns of preterm contractions. Five to 10 mg nifedipine may be administered sublingually every 15 to 20 minutes for three doses. Once stabilized, 10 to 20 mg may be administered orally every 4 to 6 hours for preterm contractions. It can cause hypotension and a change in uteroplacental blood flow.
- **Indomethacin**, 50 to 100 mg orally or rectally, followed by 25 to 50 mg orally every 6 hours for 48 hours has been used. Premature constriction of the ductus arteriosus has been reported.

Antenatal Glucocorticoids

- A Cochrane review shows the benefit of antenatal **corticosteroids** for fetal lung maturation to prevent respiratory distress syndrome, intraventricular hemorrhage, and death in infants delivered prematurely.
- Current recommendations are **betamethasone**, 12 mg IM every 24 hours for two doses, or **dexamethasone**, 6 mg IM every 12 hours for four doses, to pregnant women between 24 and 34 weeks' gestation who are at risk for preterm delivery within the next 7 days. Benefits from antenatal glucocorticoid administration are believed to begin within 24 hours.

GROUP B *STREPTOCOCCUS* INFECTION

- Prenatal screening (vaginal/rectal cultures) for group B *Streptococcus* colonization of all pregnant women at 35 to 37 weeks' gestation is recommended. If cultures are positive, or if the woman had a previous infant with invasive group B *Streptococcus* disease, or if the woman had group B *Streptococcus* bacteriuria, antibiotics are given.

- The currently recommended regimen for group B *Streptococcus* disease is **penicillin G**, 5 million units IV, followed by 2.5 million units IV every 4 hours until delivery. Alternatives include **ampicillin**, 2 g IV, followed by 1 g IV every 4 hours; **cefazolin**, 2 g IV, followed by 1 g every 8 hours; **clindamycin**, 900 mg IV every 8 hours; or **erythromycin**, 500 mg IV every 6 hours. In penicillin-allergic women in whom sensitivity testing shows resistance to clindamycin and erythromycin, **vancomycin**, 1 g IV every 12 hours until delivery, can be used.

CERVICAL RIPENING AND LABOR INDUCTION

- Prostaglandin E_2 analogues (eg, **dinoprostone [Prepidil Gel** and **Cervidil Vaginal Insert]**) are commonly used for cervical ripening. Fetal heart rate monitoring is required when Cervidil Vaginal Insert is used and for 15 minutes after its removal. **Misoprostol**, a prostaglandin E_1 analogue, is effective and inexpensive, but it has been associated with uterine rupture.
- **Oxytocin** is the most commonly used agent for labor induction after cervical ripening.

LABOR ANALGESIA

- The IV or IM administration of narcotics is commonly used for pain associated with labor. Compared with epidural analgesia, parenteral **opioids** are associated with lower rates of oxytocin augmentation, shorter stages of labor, and fewer instrumental deliveries.
- Epidural analgesia involves administering an opioid and/or an anesthetic (eg, **fentanyl** and/or **bupivacaine**) through a catheter into the epidural space to provide pain relief. Epidural analgesia is associated with longer stages of labor, more instrumental deliveries, and maternal fever compared with parenteral narcotic analgesia. Patient-controlled epidural analgesia results in a lower total dose of local anesthetic. Complications of epidural analgesia include hypotension, itching, and urinary retention.
- Other options for labor analgesia include spinal analgesia, combined spinal-epidural analgesia, and nerve blocks.

LACTATION ISSUES

DRUG USE DURING LACTATION

- Medications enter breast milk via passive diffusion of nonionized and non-protein-bound medication. Drugs with high molecular weights, lower lipid solubility, and higher protein binding are less likely to cross into breast milk, or they transfer more slowly or in smaller amounts. The higher the maternal serum concentration of drug, the higher the concentration will be in breast milk. Drugs with longer half-lives are more likely to maintain higher levels in breast milk. The timing and frequency of feedings and the amount of milk ingested by the infant are also important.
- Strategies for reducing infant risk from drugs transferred into breast milk include selecting medications for the mother that would be considered safe for use in the infant and choosing medications with shorter half-lives, higher protein binding, lower bioavailability, and lower lipid solubility.

RELACTATION

- For relactation use **metoclopramide**, 10 mg three times daily for 7 to 14 days only if nondrug therapy is ineffective.

See Chapter 78, Pregnancy and Lactation: Therapeutic Considerations, authored by Kristina E. Ward, for a more detailed discussion of this topic.

CHAPTER 33

Anemias

- *Anemia* is a group of diseases characterized by a decrease in either hemoglobin (Hb) or the volume of red blood cells (RBCs), resulting in decreased oxygen-carrying capacity of blood. The World Health Organization defines anemia as Hb less than 13 g/dL (<130 g/L; <8.07 mmol/L) in men or less than 12 g/dL (<120 g/L; <7.45 mmol/L) in women.

PATHOPHYSIOLOGY

- The functional classification of anemias is found in Fig. 33–1. The most common anemias are included in this chapter.
- Morphologic classifications are based on cell size. Macrocytic cells are larger than normal and are associated with deficiencies of vitamin B_{12} or folic acid. Microcytic cells are smaller than normal and are associated with iron deficiency, whereas normocytic anemia may be associated with recent blood loss or chronic disease.
- Iron-deficiency anemia (IDA) can be caused by inadequate dietary intake, inadequate gastrointestinal (GI) absorption, increased iron demand (eg, pregnancy), blood loss, and chronic diseases.
- Vitamin B_{12}– and folic acid–deficiency anemias can be caused by inadequate dietary intake, decreased absorption, and inadequate utilization. Deficiency of intrinsic factor causes decreased absorption of vitamin B_{12} (ie, pernicious anemia). Folic acid–deficiency anemia can be caused by hyperutilization due to pregnancy, hemolytic anemia, myelofibrosis, malignancy, chronic inflammatory disorders, long-term dialysis, or growth spurt. Drugs can cause anemia by reducing absorption of folate (eg, **phenytoin**) or through folate antagonism (eg, **methotrexate**).
- Anemia of inflammation (AI) is a newer term used to describe both anemia of chronic disease and anemia of critical illness. AI is an anemia that traditionally has been associated with infectious or inflammatory processes, tissue injury, and conditions associated with release of proinflammatory cytokines. See Table 33–1 for diseases associated with AI. For information on anemia of chronic kidney disease, see Chapter 74.
- Age-related reductions in bone marrow reserve can render elderly patients more susceptible to anemia caused by multiple minor and often unrecognized diseases (eg, nutritional deficiencies) that negatively affect erythropoiesis.
- Pediatric anemias are often due to a primary hematologic abnormality. The risk of IDA is increased by rapid growth spurts and dietary deficiency.

CLINICAL PRESENTATION

- Signs and symptoms depend on rate of development and age and cardiovascular status of the patient. Acute-onset anemia is characterized by cardiorespiratory symptoms such as palpitations, angina, orthostatic light-headedness, and breathlessness. Chronic anemia is characterized by weakness, fatigue, headache, orthopnea, dyspnea on exertion, vertigo, faintness, cold sensitivity, pallor, and loss of skin tone.
- IDA is characterized by glossal pain, smooth tongue, reduced salivary flow, pica (compulsive eating of nonfood items), and pagophagia (compulsive eating of ice).

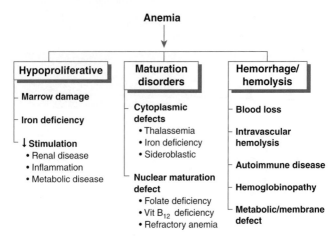

FIGURE 33–1. Functional classification of anemia. Each of the major categories of anemia (hypoproliferative, maturation disorders, and hemorrhage/hemolysis) can be further subclassified according to the functional defect in the several components of normal erythropoiesis.

- Neurologic effects (eg, numbness and ataxia) of vitamin B_{12} deficiency may occur in absence of hematologic changes. Psychiatric findings, including irritability, depression, and memory impairment, may also occur with vitamin B_{12} deficiency. Anemia with folate deficiency is not associated with neurologic symptoms.

DIAGNOSIS

- Rapid diagnosis is essential because anemia is often a sign of underlying pathology.
- Initial evaluation of anemia involves a complete blood cell count (CBC), reticulocyte index, and examination of the stool for occult blood. **Figure 33–2** shows a broad, general algorithm for the diagnosis of anemia based on laboratory data.
- The earliest and most sensitive laboratory change for IDA is decreased serum ferritin (storage iron), which should be interpreted in conjunction with decreased transferrin saturation and increased total iron-binding capacity (TIBC). Hb, hematocrit (Hct), and RBC indices usually remain normal until later stages of IDA.
- In macrocytic anemias, mean corpuscular volume is usually elevated to greater than 100 fL. Vitamin B_{12} and folate concentrations can be measured to differentiate between the two deficiency anemias. A vitamin B_{12} value less than 200 pg/mL (<148 pmol/L), together with appropriate peripheral smear and clinical symptoms, is diagnostic of vitamin B_{12}–deficiency anemia. A decreased RBC folate concentration (<150 ng/mL [<340 nmol/L]) appears to be a better indicator of folate-deficiency anemia than a decreased serum folate concentration (<3 ng/mL [<7 nmol/L]).
- The diagnosis of AI is usually one of exclusion, with consideration of coexisting iron and folate deficiencies. Serum iron is usually decreased, but, unlike IDA, serum ferritin is normal or increased, and TIBC is decreased. The bone marrow reveals an abundance of iron; the peripheral smear reveals normocytic anemia.
- Elderly patients with symptoms of anemia should undergo a CBC with peripheral smear and reticulocyte count and other laboratory studies as needed to determine the etiology of anemia.
- The diagnosis of anemia in pediatric populations requires use of age- and sex-adjusted norms for laboratory values.

TABLE 33–1	Diseases Causing Anemia of Inflammation

Common causes
  Chronic infections
    Tuberculosis
    Other chronic lung infections (eg, lung abscess, bronchiectasis)
    Human immunodeficiency virus
    Subacute bacterial endocarditis
    Osteomyelitis
    Chronic urinary tract infections
  Chronic inflammation
    Rheumatoid arthritis
    Systemic lupus erythematosus
    Inflammatory bowel disease
    Inflammatory osteoarthritis
    Gout
    Other (collagen vascular) diseases
    Chronic inflammatory liver diseases
  Malignancies
    Carcinoma
    Lymphoma
    Leukemia
    Multiple myeloma

Less common causes
  Alcoholic liver disease
  Congestive heart failure
  Thrombophlebitis
  Chronic obstructive pulmonary disease
  Ischemic heart disease

TREATMENT

- Goals of Treatment: The goals are to alleviate signs and symptoms, correct the underlying etiology (eg, restore substrates needed for RBC production), replace body stores, and prevent long-term complications.

IRON-DEFICIENCY ANEMIA

- **Oral iron** therapy with soluble ferrous iron salts, which are not enteric coated and not slow or sustained release, is recommended at a daily dosage of 150 to 200 mg elemental iron in two or three divided doses (see Table 33–2).
- Iron is best absorbed from meat, fish, and poultry. Administer iron at least 1 hour before meals because food interferes with absorption, but administration with food may be needed to improve tolerability.
- Consider **parenteral iron** for patients with iron malabsorption, intolerance of oral iron therapy, or nonadherence. The following formula can be used to estimate the total dose of parenteral iron needed to correct anemia:

Dose of iron (mg) = whole blood hemoglobin deficit (g/dL) × body weight (lb) or
Dose of iron (mg) = whole blood hemoglobin deficit (g/L) × body weight (kg) × 0.22

- An additional quantity of iron to replenish stores should be added (about 600 mg for women and 1000 mg for men).

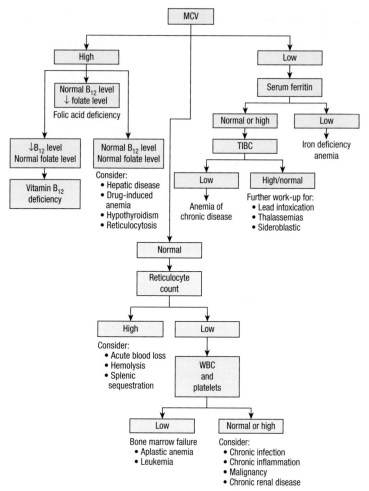

(↓, decreased; MCV, mean corpuscular volume; TIBC, total iron-binding capacity; WBC, white blood cells.)

FIGURE 33–2. General algorithm for diagnosis of anemias.

- **Iron dextran, sodium ferric gluconate, iron sucrose, ferumoxytol,** and **ferric carboxymaltose** are available parenteral iron preparations with similar efficacy but different molecular size, pharmacokinetics, bioavailability, and adverse effect profiles (see Table 74–3).

VITAMIN B₁₂–DEFICIENCY ANEMIA

- Oral vitamin B_{12} supplementation is as effective as parenteral, even in patients with pernicious anemia, because the alternate vitamin B_{12} absorption pathway is independent of intrinsic factor. Initiate oral **cobalamin** at 1 to 2 mg daily for 1 to 2 weeks, followed by 1 mg daily.

TABLE 33–2	Oral Iron Products	
Iron Salt	Percent Elemental Iron	Common: Formulations and Elemental Iron Provided
Ferrous sulfate	20	60–65 mg/324–325 mg tablet 60 mg/5 mL syrup 44 mg/ 5 mL elixir 15 mg/1 mL
Ferrous sulfate (exsiccated)	30	65 mg/200 mg tablet 50 mg/160 mg tablet
Ferrous gluconate	12	38 mg/325 mg tablet 28–29 mg/240–246 mg tablet
Ferrous fumarate	33	66 mg/200 mg tablet 106 mg/324–325 mg tablet

- Parenteral therapy acts more rapidly than oral therapy and is recommended if neurologic symptoms are present. A popular regimen is IM **cyanocobalamin**, 1000 mcg daily for 1 week, then weekly for 1 month, and then monthly. Initiate daily oral cobalamin administration after symptoms resolve.

FOLATE-DEFICIENCY ANEMIA

- Oral **folate**, 1 mg daily for 4 months, is usually sufficient for treatment of folic acid–deficiency anemia, unless the etiology cannot be corrected. If malabsorption is present, a dose of 1 to 5 mg daily may be necessary.

ANEMIA OF INFLAMMATION

- Treatment of anemia of inflammation (AI) is less specific than that of other anemias and should focus on correcting reversible causes. Reserve iron therapy for an established IDA; iron is not effective when inflammation is present. RBC transfusions are effective but should be limited to episodes of inadequate oxygen transport and Hb of 7 to 8 g/dL (70–80 g/L; 4.34–4.97 mmol/L).
- **Erythropoiesis-stimulating agents (ESAs)** can be considered, but response can be impaired in patients with AI (off-label use). The initial dosage for **epoetin alfa** is 50 to 100 units/kg three times weekly and **darbepoetin alfa** 0.45 mcg/kg once weekly. ESA use may result in iron deficiency. Many practitioners routinely supplement ESA therapy with oral iron therapy.
- Potential toxicities of exogenous ESA administration include increases in blood pressure, nausea, headache, fever, bone pain, and fatigue. Hb must be monitored during ESA therapy. An increase in Hb greater than 12 g/dL (>120 g/L; >7.45 mmol/L) with treatment or a rise of greater than 1 g/dL (>10 g/L; >0.62 mmol/L) every 2 weeks has been associated with increased mortality and cardiovascular events.
- In patients with anemia of critical illness, parenteral iron is often used but is associated with a theoretical risk of infection. Routine use of ESAs or RBC transfusions is not supported by clinical studies.

ANEMIA IN PEDIATRIC POPULATIONS

- Infants aged 9 to 12 months: administer iron sulfate 3 to 6 mg/kg/day (elemental iron) divided once or twice daily between meals for 4 weeks. Continue for two additional months in responders to replace storage iron pools. The dose and schedule of vitamin B_{12} should be titrated according to clinical and laboratory response. The daily dose of folate is 1 mg.

EVALUATION OF THERAPEUTIC OUTCOMES

- IDA: Positive response to oral iron therapy characterized by modest reticulocytosis in a few days with an increase in Hb seen at 2 weeks. Reevaluate the patient if reticulocytosis does not occur. Hb should return to normal after 2 months; continue iron therapy until iron stores are replenished and serum ferritin normalized (up to 12 months).
- Megaloblastic anemia: Signs and symptoms usually improve within a few days after starting vitamin B_{12} or folate therapy. Neurologic symptoms can take longer to improve or can be irreversible, but should not progress during therapy. Reticulocytosis should occur within 3 to 5 days. Hb begins to rise a week after starting vitamin B_{12} therapy and should normalize in 1 to 2 months. Hct should rise within 2 weeks after starting folate therapy and should normalize within 2 months.
- ESAs: Reticulocytosis should occur within a few days. Monitor iron, TIBC, transferrin saturation, and ferritin levels at baseline and periodically during therapy. The optimal form and schedule of iron supplementation are unknown. Discontinue ESAs if a clinical response does not occur after 8 weeks.
- Pediatrics: Monitor Hb, Hct, and RBC indices 4 to 8 weeks after initiation of iron therapy. Monitor Hb or Hct weekly in premature infants.

See Chapter 100, Anemias, authored by Kristen Cook for a more detailed discussion of this topic.

CHAPTER 34

Sickle Cell Disease

- *Sickle cell syndromes*, which can be divided into sickle cell trait (SCT) and sickle cell disease (SCD), are hereditary conditions characterized by the presence of sickle hemoglobin (HbS) in red blood cells (RBCs).
- SCT is the heterozygous inheritance of one normal β-globin gene producing hemoglobin A (HbA) and one sickle gene producing HbS (HbAS) gene. Individuals with SCT are asymptomatic.
- SCD can be of homozygous or compounded heterozygous inheritance. Homozygous HbS (HbSS) has historically been referred to as sickle cell anemia (SCA).

PATHOPHYSIOLOGY

- Clinical manifestations of SCD are due to impaired circulation, RBC destruction, and stasis of blood flow and ongoing inflammatory responses. These changes result from disturbances in RBC polymerization and to membrane damage. In addition to sickling, other factors contributing to the clinical manifestations include functional asplenia (and increased risk of bacterial infection), deficient opsonization, and coagulation abnormalities.
- Polymerization allows deoxygenated hemoglobin to exist as a semisolid gel that protrudes into the cell membrane, distorting RBCs into sickle shapes. Sickle-shaped RBCs increase blood viscosity and encourage sludging in the capillaries and small vessels, leading to local tissue hypoxia that accentuates the pathologic process.
- Repeated cycles of sickling, upon deoxygenation, and unsickling, upon oxygenation, damage the RBC membrane and cause irreversible sickling. Rigid, sickled RBCs are easily trapped, resulting in shortened circulatory survival and chronic hemolysis.

CLINICAL PRESENTATION

- SCD involves multiple organ systems. Clinical manifestations depend on the genotype (Table 34–1).
- Cardinal features of SCD are hemolytic anemia and vasoocclusion. Symptoms are delayed until 4 to 6 months of age when HbS replaces fetal hemoglobin (HbF). Common findings include pain with fever, pneumonia, splenomegaly, and, in infants, pain and swelling of the hands and feet (eg, hand-and-foot syndrome or dactylitis).
- Usual clinical signs and symptoms of SCD include chronic anemia; fever; pallor; arthralgia; scleral icterus; abdominal pain; weakness; anorexia; fatigue; enlarged liver, spleen, and heart; and hematuria.
- Acute complications of SCD include fever and infection (eg, sepsis caused by encapsulated pathogens such as *Streptococcus pneumoniae*), stroke, acute chest syndrome, and priapism. Acute chest syndrome is characterized by pulmonary infiltration, respiratory symptoms, and equivocal response to antibiotic therapy.
- Acute episodes of pain can be precipitated by infection, dehydration, stresses, and sudden temperature changes. The most common type is vasoocclusive pain, which is manifested by pain over the involved areas without change in Hb. Aplastic crisis is characterized by acute decrease in Hb with decreased reticulocyte count manifested as fatigue, dyspnea, pallor, and tachycardia. Acute splenic sequestration is the sudden massive enlargement of the spleen due to sequestration of sickled RBCs. The trapping of sickled RBCs by the spleen leads to hypotension and shock, and can cause sudden death in young children. Repeated infarctions lead to autosplenectomy; therefore, incidence declines as adolescence approaches.

SECTION 7 | Hematologic Disorders

TABLE 34-1	Clinical Features of Sickle Cell Trait and Common Types of Sickle Cell Disease
Type	**Clinical Features**
Sickle cell trait (SCT)	Rare painless hematuria; normal Hb level; heavy exercise under extreme conditions can provoke gross hematuria and complications (normal Hb)
Sickle cell anemia (SCA- HbSS)	Pain episodes, microvascular disruption of organs (spleen, liver, bone marrow, kidney, brain, and lung), gallstones, priapism, leg ulcers; anemia (Hb 6–9 g/dL [60–90 g/L; 3.72–5.59 mmol/L])
Sickle cell hemoglobin C (HbSC)	Painless hematuria and rare aseptic necrosis of bone; pain episodes are less common and occur later in life; other complications are ocular disease and pregnancy-related problems; mild anemia (Hb 9–14 g/dL [90–140 g/L; 5.59–8.69 mmol/L])
Sickle cell β⁺-thalassemia (HbSβ⁺-thal)	Rare pain; milder severity than HbSS because production of some HbA; Hb 9–12 g/dL (90–120 g/L; 5.59–7.45 mmol/L) with microcytosis
Sickle cell β⁰-thalassemia (HbSβ⁰-thal)	No HbA production; severity similar to SCA; Hb 7–9 g/dL (70–90 g/L; 4.34–5.59 mmol/L) with microcytosis

(Hb, hemoglobin; HbA, hemoglobin A.)

- Chronic complications involve many organs and include pulmonary hypertension, bone and joint destruction, ocular problems, cholelithiasis, cardiovascular abnormalities, depression, and hematuria and other renal complications. Children experience delayed growth and sexual maturation.
- Patients with SCT are usually asymptomatic, except for rare painless hematuria.

DIAGNOSIS

- SCD is usually identified by routine neonatal screening programs using isoelectric focusing, high-performance liquid chromatography, or electrophoresis.
- Laboratory findings include low hemoglobin; increased reticulocyte, platelet, and white blood cell counts; and sickled red cell forms on the peripheral smear.

TREATMENT

- <u>Goals of Treatment</u>: The goals are to reduce hospitalizations, complications, and mortality.

GENERAL PRINCIPLES

- Patients with SCD require lifelong multidisciplinary care that combines general symptomatic supportive care, preventative medical therapies and specific disease modifying therapies.
- Routine immunizations plus influenza, meningococcal, and pneumococcal vaccinations are recommended.
- Prophylactic **penicillin** is recommended until at least 5 years of age. An effective regimen is penicillin V potassium, 125 mg orally twice daily until 3 years of age and then 250 mg orally twice daily until age 5 years.

FETAL HEMOGLOBIN INDUCERS

- HbF directly effects polymer formation. Increases in HbF correlate with decreased RBC sickling and adhesion. Patients with low HbF levels have more frequent pain and higher mortality. HbF levels of 20% or greater reduce the risk of acute sickle cell complications.

- **Hydroxyurea**, a chemotherapeutic agent, stimulates HbF production and increases the number of HbF-containing reticulocytes and intracellular HbF. It is indicated for patients with frequent painful episodes, severe symptomatic anemia, acute chest syndrome, or other severe vasoocclusive complications. The starting dose is 15 mg/kg as a single daily dose (Fig. 34–1).
- Chronic RBC transfusions are indicated for primary and secondary stroke prevention in children. Transfusions are usually given every 3 to 4 weeks or as needed to maintain desired HbS levels. The optimal duration of primary prophylactic transfusion therapy in children is unknown. Risks include alloimmunization, hyperviscosity, viral transmission (requiring hepatitis A and B vaccination), volume and iron overload, and transfusion reactions.
- Allogeneic hematopoietic stem cell transplantation is the only curative therapy for SCD. The best candidates are younger than 16 years, have severe complications, and have human leukocyte antigen–matched donors. Risks must be carefully considered and include mortality, graft rejection, and secondary malignancies.

TREATMENT OF COMPLICATIONS

- Educate patients to recognize conditions that require urgent evaluation. Balanced fluid status and oxygen saturation of at least 92% are important to avoid exacerbation during acute illness.
- RBC transfusions are indicated for acute exacerbation of baseline anemia (eg, aplastic crisis, hepatic or splenic sequestration, or severe hemolysis), severe vasoocclusive episodes, and procedures requiring general anesthesia. Transfusions can be useful in patients with complicated obstetric problems, refractory leg ulcers, or refractory and protracted painful episodes and for primary or secondary stroke prevention.
- Promptly evaluate fever of 38.5°C (101.3°F) or higher. Empiric antibiotic therapy should provide coverage against encapsulated organisms (eg, **ceftriaxone** for outpatients and **cefotaxime** for inpatients; **clindamycin** for cephalosporin-allergic patients).
- Initiate incentive spirometry; appropriate fluid therapy; broad-spectrum antibiotics, including a **macrolide** or **quinolone**; and, for hypoxia or acute distress, oxygen therapy in acute chest syndrome. Other potential therapies include steroids and nitric oxide.
- Priapism has been treated with analgesics, antianxiety agents, and vasoconstrictors to force blood out of the corpus cavernosum (eg, **phenylephrine** and **epinephrine**), and vasodilators to relax smooth muscle (eg, **terbutaline** and **hydralazine**).
- Treatment of aplastic crisis is primarily supportive. Blood transfusions may be indicated for severe or symptomatic anemia.
- Treatment options for splenic sequestration include observation alone, especially for adults because they tend to have milder episodes; chronic transfusion in children younger than 2 years of age to delay splenectomy; and splenectomy after a life-threatening crisis, after repetitive episodes, or for chronic hypersplenism.
- Hydration and analgesics are mainstays of treatment for vasoocclusive (painful) crisis. Administer fluids IV or orally at 1 to 1.5 times the maintenance requirement; monitor closely to avoid volume overload. Consider an infectious etiology and initiate empiric therapy if indicated.
- Tailor analgesic therapy to the individual because of the variable frequency and severity of pain. Pain scales should be used to quantify the degree of pain.
- Use **nonsteroidal anti-inflammatory drugs (NSAIDs)** or **acetaminophen** for mild to moderate pain. Consider adding an opioid if mild to moderate pain persists. (e.g., **codeine** or **hydrocodone**).
- Treat severe pain aggressively with an opioid, such as **morphine**, **hydromorphone**, **fentanyl**, or **methadone**. **Meperidine** should be avoided because accumulation of the normeperidine metabolite can cause neurotoxicity, especially in patients with impaired renal function.

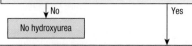

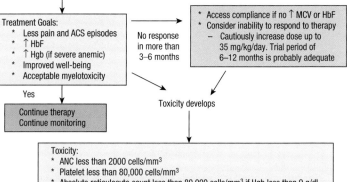

HbSS or Sβ⁰–thalassemia with
* 3 or more severe vasoocclusive pain episodes and/or ACS per year or
* Severe symptomatic anemia

Baseline laboratory: CBC, reticulocyte, HbF, chemistries (include creatinine, bilirubin, ALT), pregnancy test (if menstruating)
Baseline physical examination and history

* Pregnancy test negative
* Use contraception for sexually active men and women
* Compliance with daily dosing, frequent laboratory monitoring, and medical appointments

No → No hydroxyurea

Yes

Hydroxyurea: 15 mg/kg/day for adults and 20 mg/kg/day for children. May increase by 5 mg/kg/day every 8 weeks up to 35 mg/kg/day
Monitoring:
* CBC: every 4 wks until maximum tolerated dose achieved for 8–12 wks, then every 8 wks
* HbF every 3 months × 2 then every 6 months
* Bilirubin, ALT, and creatinine every 12–24 wks
* Pregnancy test PRN (if positive, stop therapy and provide teratogen risk counseling)
* History and PE: every 4 wks until maximum dose achieved for 8–12 wks, then every 8 wks

Treatment Goals:
* Less pain and ACS episodes
* ↑ HbF
* ↑ Hgb (if severe anemic)
* Improved well-being
* Acceptable myelotoxicity

No response in more than 3–6 months

* Access compliance if no ↑ MCV or HbF
* Consider inability to respond to therapy
  – Cautiously increase dose up to 35 mg/kg/day. Trial period of 6–12 months is probably adequate

Yes

Continue therapy
Continue monitoring

Toxicity develops

Toxicity:
* ANC less than 2000 cells/mm³
* Platelet less than 80,000 cells/mm³
* Absolute reticulocyte count less than 80,000 cells/mm³ if Hgb less than 9 g/dL
* Hgb less than 5 g/dL or more than 20% below baseline
* Increased serum creatinine 50% above baseline
* Increased ALT 100% above baseline

Stop hydroxyurea for at least 1 wk and until toxicity resolves

* Resume hydroxyurea at 2.5–5 mg/kg/day less than previous dose
* May resume previous dose if no toxicity recurs after 12 wks of the lower dose
  – If toxicity recurs on higher dose, stop hydroxyurea again until resolves, then resume at the lowest tolerated dose

(ACS, acute chest syndrome; ALT, alanine aminotransferase; ANC, absolute neutrophil count; CBC, complete blood cell count; Hb, hemoglobin; HbF, fetal hemoglobin; HbSS, homozygous sickle cell hemoglobin; HbSSβ⁰, sickle cell β⁰-thalassemia; MCV, mean corpuscular volume; PE, physical examination; PRN, as needed; RBC, red blood cell.)

FIGURE 34–1. Hydroxyurea use in sickle cell disease. (Data from McCavit TL. Sickle cell disease. Pediatr Rev 2012;33:195–204, quiz 5–6; Wong TE, Brandow AM, Lim W, Lottenberg R. Update on the use of hydroxyurea therapy in sickle cell disease. Blood 2014;124:3850–3857; National Institutes of Health, National Heart Lung and Blood Institute. Evidence-Based Management of Sickle Cell Disease: Expert Panel Report. http://www.nhlbi.nih.gov/health-pro/guidelines/sickle-cell-disease-guidelines/. Last accessed, October 15, 2015.)

- Treat severe pain with an IV opioid titrated to pain relief and then administered on a scheduled basis with as-needed dosing for breakthrough pain. Patient-controlled analgesia is commonly utilized.
- Suspicion of addiction commonly leads to suboptimal pain control. Factors that minimize dependence include aggressive pain control, frequent monitoring, and tapering medication according to response.
- Treatment of chronic pain in SCD requires a multidisciplinary approach. Guidelines for chronic pain management are available.

EVALUATION OF THERAPEUTIC OUTCOMES

- Evaluate patients on a regular basis to establish baseline symptoms, monitor changes, and provide age-appropriate education.
- Evaluate CBC and reticulocyte counts every 3 to 6 months up to 2 years of age, then every 6 to 12 months. Screen HbF level annually until 2 years of age. Evaluate renal, hepatobiliary, and pulmonary function annually. Screen patients for retinopathy.
- Assess efficacy of hydroxyurea by monitoring the number, severity, and duration of sickle cell crises.

See Chapter 102, Sickle Cell Disease, authored by C. Y. Jennifer Chan and Melissa Frei-Jones, for a more detailed discussion of this topic.

CHAPTER

35

Antimicrobial Regimen Selection

- A systematic approach to the selection and evaluation of an antimicrobial regimen is shown in Table 35–1. An "empiric" antimicrobial regimen is begun before the offending organism is identified and sometimes before the documentation of the presence of infection, whereas a "definitive" regimen is instituted when the causative organism is known.

CONFIRMING THE PRESENCE OF INFECTION

FEVER

- *Fever* is defined as a controlled elevation of body temperature above the expected 37°C (98.6°F) (measured orally) and is a manifestation of many disease states other than infection.
- Many drugs have been identified as causes of fever. Drug-induced fever is defined as persistent fever in the absence of infection or other underlying condition. The fever must coincide temporally with the administration of the offending agent and disappear promptly upon its withdrawal, after which the temperature remains normal.

SIGNS AND SYMPTOMS

- Most infections result in elevated white blood cell (WBC) counts (leukocytosis) because of the mobilization of granulocytes and/or lymphocytes to destroy invading microbes. Normal values for WBC counts are between 4000 and 10,000 cells/mm^3.
- Bacterial infections are associated with elevated granulocyte counts (neutrophils and basophils), often with increased numbers of immature forms (band neutrophils) seen in peripheral blood smears (left-shift). With infection, peripheral leukocyte counts may be high, but they are rarely higher than 30,000 to 10,000 cells/mm^3 (4×10^9 and 10×10^9/L). Low neutrophil counts (neutropenia) after the onset of infection indicate an abnormal response and are generally associated with a poor prognosis for bacterial infection.
- Relative lymphocytosis, even with normal or slightly elevated total WBC counts, is generally associated with tuberculosis and viral or fungal infections. Many types of infections, however, may be accompanied by a completely normal WBC count and differential.
- Pain and inflammation may accompany infection and are sometimes manifested by swelling, erythema, tenderness, and purulent drainage. Unfortunately, these signs may be apparent only if the infection is superficial or in a bone or joint.
- The manifestations of inflammation with deep-seated infections such as meningitis, pneumonia, endocarditis, and urinary tract infection must be ascertained by examining tissues or fluids. For example, the presence of polymorphonuclear leukocytes (neutrophils) in spinal fluid, lung secretions (sputum), and urine is highly suggestive of bacterial infection.

IDENTIFICATION OF THE PATHOGEN

- Infected body materials must be sampled, if at all possible or practical, before the institution of antimicrobial therapy. A Gram stain of the material may reveal bacteria, or an acid-fast stain may detect mycobacteria or actinomycetes. A delay

TABLE 35–1	Systematic Approach for Selection of Antimicrobials

Confirm the presence of infection
    Careful history and physical examination
    Signs and symptoms
    Predisposing factors	

Identification of the pathogen (see Chapter e25 in 10th edition of PAPA)
    Collection of infected material
    Stains
    Serologies
    Culture and sensitivity	

Selection of presumptive therapy considering every infected site
    Host factors
    Drug factors	

Monitor therapeutic response
    Clinical assessment
    Laboratory tests
    Assessment of therapeutic failure	

in obtaining infected fluids or tissues until after therapy is started may result in false-negative culture results or alterations in the cellular and chemical composition of infected fluids.

- Blood cultures should be performed in the acutely ill, febrile patient. Less accessible fluids or tissues are obtained when needed to assess localized signs or symptoms (eg, spinal fluid in meningitis and joint fluid in arthritis). Abscesses and cellulitic areas should also be aspirated.
- Caution must be used in the evaluation of positive culture results from normally sterile sites (eg, blood, cerebrospinal fluid [CSF], and joint fluid). The recovery of bacteria normally found on the skin in large quantities (eg, coagulase-negative staphylococci and diphtheroids) from one of these sites may be a result of contamination of the specimen rather than a true infection.

SELECTION OF PRESUMPTIVE THERAPY

- A variety of factors must be considered to select rational antimicrobial therapy, including the severity and acuity of the disease, host factors, factors related to the drugs used, and the necessity for use of multiple agents.
- The drugs of choice for the treatment of most pathogens are compiled from a variety of sources and are intended as guidelines rather than specific rules for antimicrobial use (see Table 35–2).
- Important considerations when selecting empiric antimicrobial therapy include: (1) prior knowledge of colonization or infections, (2) previous antimicrobial use, (3) the site of infection and the organisms most likely pathogens, and (4) local antibiogram and resistance patterns for important pathogens.

HOST FACTORS

- When a patient for initial or empiric therapy is evaluated, the following factors should be considered:
  ✓ Allergy or history of adverse drug reactions.
  ✓ Age of patient.
  ✓ Pregnancy.
  ✓ Metabolic or genetic variation.
  ✓ *Renal and hepatic function*: Patients with diminished renal and/or hepatic function will accumulate certain drugs unless the dosage is adjusted.

TABLE 35–2 Drugs of Choice, First Choice, *Alternative(s)*

GRAM-POSITIVE COCCI

Enterococcus faecalis (generally not as resistant to antibiotics as *Enterococcus faecium*)
- Serious infection (endocarditis, meningitis, pyelonephritis with bacteremia)
  - Ampicillin (or penicillin G) + (gentamicin or streptomycin)
  - *Vancomycin + (gentamicin or streptomycin), daptomycin, linezolid, tedizolid, telavancin, tigecycline[a]*
- Urinary tract infection
  - Ampicillin, amoxicillin
  - *Fosfomycin or nitrofurantoin*

E. faecium (generally more resistant to antibiotics than *E. faecalis*)
- Recommend consultation with infectious disease specialist
  - *Linezolid, quinupristin/dalfopristin, daptomycin, tigecycline[a]*

Staphylococcus aureus/Staphylococcus epidermidis
- Methicillin (oxacillin)-sensitive
  - Nafcillin or oxacillin
  - *FGC,[b,c] trimethoprim–sulfamethoxazole, clindamycin, BL/BLI[d]*
- Hospital-acquired methicillin (oxacillin)–resistant
  - Vancomycin ± (gentamicin or rifampin)
  - *Ceftaroline, daptomycin, linezolid, telavancin, tigecycline,[a] trimethoprim–sulfamethoxazole, quinupristin–dalfopristin*
- Community-acquired methicillin (oxacillin)–resistant
  - Clindamycin, trimethoprim.sulfamethoxazole, doxycycline[a]
  - *Ceftaroline, dalbavancin, daptomycin, linezolid, oritivancin, tedizolid, telavancin, tigecycline,[a] or vancomycin*

Streptococcus (groups A, B, C, G, and *Streptococcus bovis*)
- Penicillin G or V or ampicillin
- *FGC,[b,c] erythromycin, azithromycin, clarithromycin*

Streptococcus pneumoniae
- Penicillin-sensitive (minimal inhibitory concentration [MIC] <0.1 mcg/mL [mg/L])
  - Penicillin G or V or ampicillin
  - *FGC,[b,c] doxycycline,[a] azithromycin, clarithromycin, erythromycin*
- Penicillin intermediate (MIC 0.1–1 mcg/mL [mg/L])
  - High-dose penicillin (12 million units/day for adults) or ceftriaxone[c] or cefotaxime[c]
  - *Levofloxacin,[a] moxifloxacin,[a] gemifloxacin,[a] or vancomycin*
- Penicillin-resistant (MIC ≥1.0 mcg/mL [mg/L])
  - Recommend consultation with infectious disease specialist.
    – Vancomycin ± rifampin
    – *Per sensitivities: ceftaroline, cefotaxime, ceftriaxone,[c] levofloxacin,[a] moxifloxacin,[a] or gemifloxacin[a]*

Streptococcus, viridans group
- Penicillin G ± gentamicin[e]
- *Cefotaxime,[c] ceftriaxone,[c] erythromycin, azithromycin, clarithromycin, or vancomycin ± gentamicin*

GRAM-NEGATIVE COCCI

Moraxella (Branhamella) catarrhalis
- Amoxicillin–clavulanate, ampicillin–sulbactam
- *Trimethoprim–sulfamethoxazole, erythromycin, azithromycin, clarithromycin, doxycycline,[a] SGC,[c,f] cefotaxime,[c] ceftriaxone,[c] or TGCPO[c,g]*

Neisseria gonorrhoeae (also give concomitant treatment for *Chlamydia trachomatis*)
- Disseminated gonococcal infection
  - Ceftriaxone[c] or cefotaxime[c]
  - *Oral follow up: cefpodoxime,[c] ciprofloxacin,[a] or levofloxacin[a]*

(continued)

TABLE 35–2 Drugs of Choice, First Choice, *Alternative(s)* (*Continued*)

- Uncomplicated infection
  - Ceftriaxone,[c] cefotaxime,[c] or cefpodoxime[c]
  - Ciprofloxacin[a] or levofloxacin[a]

Neisseria meningitides
- Penicillin G
- Cefotaxime[c] or ceftriaxone[c]

GRAM-POSITIVE BACILLI

Clostridium perfringens
- Penicillin G ± clindamycin
- Metronidazole,[a] clindamycin, doxycycline,[a] cefazolin,[c] carbapenem[h,i]

Clostridium difficile
- Oral metronidazole[a]
- Oral vancomycin or fidaxomicin

GRAM-NEGATIVE BACILLI

Acinetobacter spp.
- Doripenem, imipenem, or meropenem ± aminoglycoside[j] (amikacin usually most effective)
- Ampicillin–sulbactam, polymyxins,[i] or tigecycline[a]

Bacteroides fragilis (and others)
- Metronidazole[a]
- BL/BLI,[d] clindamycin, cefoxitin,[c] cefotetan,[c] ceftolozaneazobactam, ceftazidime-avibactam, or carbapenem[h,i]

Enterobacter spp.
- Carbapenem[h] or cefepime ± aminoglycoside[j]
- Ceftolozane-tazobactam, ceftazidime-avibactam, ciprofloxacin,[a] levofloxacin,[a] piperacillin–tazobactam, ticarcillin–clavulanate

Escherichia coli
- Meningitis
  - Cefotaxime,[c] ceftriaxone,[c] meropenem
- Systemic infection
  - Cefotaxime[c] or ceftriaxone[c]
  - BL/BLI,[d] fluoroquinolone,[a,k] carbapenem[h,i]
- Urinary tract infection
  - Most oral agents: check sensitivities
  - Ampicillin, amoxicillin–clavulanate, doxycycline,[a] or cephalexin[c]
  - Aminoglycoside,[j] FGC,[b,c] nitrofurantoin, fluoroquinolone[a,k]

Gardnerella vaginalis
- Metronidazole[a]
- Clindamycin

Haemophilus influenzae
- Meningitis
  - Cefotaxime[c] or ceftriaxone[c]
  - Meropenem[i]
- Other infections
  - BL/BLI,[d] or if β-lactamase-negative, ampicillin or amoxicillin
  - Trimethoprim–sulfamethoxazole, cefuroxime,[c] azithromycin, clarithromycin, or fluoroquinolone[a,k]

Klebsiella pneumoniae
- BL/BLI,[d] cefotaxime,[c] ceftriaxone,[c] cefepime[c]
- Carbapenem,[h,i] ceftolozane-tazobactam, ceftazidimeavibactam, fluoroquinolone[a,k]

(continued)

TABLE 35–2	Drugs of Choice, First Choice, *Alternative(s)* (*Continued*)

Legionella spp.
- Azithromycin, erythromycin ± rifampin, or fluoroquinolone[a,k]
- Trimethoprim–sulfamethoxazole, clarithromycin, or doxycycline[a]

Pasteurella multocida
- Penicillin G, ampicillin, amoxicillin
- Doxycycline,[a] BL/BLI,[d] trimethoprim–sulfamethoxazole or ceftriaxone[c]

Proteus mirabilis
- Ampicillin
- Trimethoprim–sulfamethoxazole

Proteus (indole-positive) (including *Providencia rettgeri, Morganella morganii,* and *Proteus vulgaris*)
- Cefotaxime,[c] ceftriaxone,[c] or fluoroquinolone[a,k]
- BL/BLI,[d] aztreonam,[i] aminoglycosides,[j] carbapenem,[h,i] ceftolozane-tazobactam, ceftazidime-avibactam

Providencia stuartii
- Amikacin, cefotaxime,[c] ceftriaxone,[c] fluoroquinolone[a,k]
- Trimethoprim–sulfamethoxazole, aztreonam,[i] carbapenem[h,i]

Pseudomonas aeruginosa
- Urinary tract infection only
  - Aminoglycoside[j]
  - Ciprofloxacin,[a] levofloxacin[a]
- Systemic infection
  - Cefepime,[c] ceftazidime,[c] doripenem,[i] imipenem,[i] meropenem,[i] piperacillin–tazobactam, or ticarcillin–clavulanate + aminoglycoside[j]
  - Aztreonam,[i] ceftolozane-tazobactam, ceftazidime-avibactam, ciprofloxacin,[a] levofloxacin,[a] polymyxin[i]

Salmonella typhi
- Ciprofloxacin,[a] levofloxacin,[c] ceftriaxone,[c] cefotaxime[c]
- Trimethoprim–sulfamethoxazole

Serratia marcescens
- Ceftriaxone,[c] cefotaxime,[c] cefepime,[c] ciprofloxacin,[a] levofloxacin[a]
- Aztreonam,[i] carbapenem,[h,i] piperacillin–tazobactam, ticarcillin–clavulanate

Stenotrophomonas (Xanthomonas) maltophilia (generally very resistant to all antimicrobials)
- Trimethoprim–sulfamethoxazole.
- Check sensitivities to ceftazidime,[c] doxycycline,[a] minocycline,[a] and ticarcillin–clavulanate

MISCELLANEOUS MICROORGANISMS

Chlamydia pneumoniae
- Doxycycline[a]
- Azithromycin, clarithromycin, erythromycin, or fluoroquinolone[a,k]

C. trachomatis
- Azithromycin or doxycycline[a]
- Levofloxacin,[a] erythromycin

Mycoplasma pneumoniae
- Azithromycin, clarithromycin, erythromycin, fluoroquinolone[a,k]
- Doxycycline[a]

SPIROCHETES

Treponema pallidum
- Neurosyphilis
  - Penicillin G
  - Ceftriaxone[c]

(*continued*)

TABLE 35-2	Drugs of Choice, First Choice, *Alternative(s)* *(Continued)*

- *Primary or secondary*
  - Benzathine, penicillin G
  - *Ceftriaxone[c] or doxycycline[a]*

Borrelia burgdorferi (choice depends on stage of disease)
- Ceftriaxone[c] or cefuroxime axetil,[c] doxycycline,[a] amoxicillin
- High-dose penicillin, cefotaxime[c]

[a]Not for use in pregnant patients or children.
[b]First-generation cephalosporins—IV: cefazolin; orally: cephalexin, cephradine, or cefadroxil.
[c]Some penicillin-allergic patients may react to cephalosporins.
[d]β-Lactam/β-lactamase inhibitor combination—IV: ampicillin–sulbactam, piperacillin–tazobactam, and ticarcillin–clavulanate; orally: amoxicillin–clavulanate.
[e]Gentamicin should be added if tolerance or moderately susceptible (MIC >0.1 mcg/mL [mg/L]) organisms are encountered; streptomycin is used but can be more toxic.
[f]Second-generation cephalosporins—IV: cefuroxime; orally: cefaclor, cefditoren, cefprozil, cefuroxime axetil, and loracarbef.
[g]Third-generation cephalosporins—orally: cefdinir, cefixime, cefetamet, cefpodoxime proxetil, and ceftibuten.
[h]Carbapenem: doripenem, ertapenem, imipenem/cilastatin, and meropenem.
[i]Reserve for serious infection.
[j]Aminoglycosides: gentamicin, tobramycin, and amikacin; use per sensitivities.
[k]Fluoroquinolones IV/orally: ciprofloxacin, levofloxacin, and moxifloxacin.
[l]Generally reserved for patients with hypersensitivity reactions to penicillin.

✓ *Concomitant drug therapy*: Any concomitant therapy the patient is receiving may influence the selection of drug therapy, the dose, and monitoring. A list of selected drug interactions involving antimicrobials is provided in Table 35–3.
✓ *Concomitant disease states.*

DRUG FACTORS

- Integration of both pharmacokinetic and pharmacodynamic properties of an agent is important when choosing antimicrobial therapy to ensure efficacy and prevent resistance. Antibiotics may demonstrate concentration-dependent (aminoglycosides and fluoroquinolones) or time-dependent (β-lactams) bactericidal effects.
- The importance of tissue penetration varies with the site of infection. The central nervous system (CNS) is one body site where the importance of antimicrobial penetration is relatively well defined, and correlations with clinical outcomes are established. Drugs that do not reach significant concentrations in CSF should either be avoided or instilled directly when treating meningitis.
- Apart from the bloodstream, other body fluids in which drug concentration data are clinically relevant are urine, synovial fluid, and peritoneal fluid.
- Pharmacokinetic parameters such as area under the concentration-time curve (AUC) and maximal plasma concentration can be predictive of treatment outcome when specific ratios of AUC or maximal plasma concentration to the minimum inhibitory concentration (MIC) are achieved. For some agents, the ratio of AUC to MIC, peak-to-MIC ratio, or the time that the drug concentration is above the MIC may predict efficacy.
- The most important pharmacodynamic relationship for antimicrobials that display time-dependent bactericidal effects (such as penicillins and cephalosporins) is the duration that drug concentrations exceed the MIC.

COMBINATION ANTIMICROBIAL THERAPY

- Combinations of antimicrobials are generally used to broaden the spectrum of coverage for empiric therapy, achieve synergistic activity against the infecting organism, and prevent the emergence of resistance.

TABLE 35-3 Major Drug Interactions with Antimicrobials

Antimicrobial	Other Agent(s)	Mechanism of Action/Effect	Clinical Management
Aminoglycosides	Neuromuscular blocking agents	Additive adverse effects	Avoid
	Nephrotoxins (N) or ototoxins (O) (eg, amphotericin B [N], cisplatin [N/O], cyclosporine [N], furosemide [O], NSAIDs [N], radiocontrast [N], vancomycin [N])	Additive adverse effects	Monitor aminoglycoside SDC and renal function
Amphotericin B	Nephrotoxins (eg, aminoglycosides, cidofovir, cyclosporine, foscarnet, pentamidine)	Additive adverse effects	Monitor renal function
Azoles	See Chapter 98 in 10th edition of PAPA		
Chloramphenicol	Phenytoin, tolbutamide, ethanol	Decreased metabolism of other agents	Monitor phenytoin SDC, blood glucose
Foscarnet	Pentamidine IV	Increased risk of severe nephrotoxicity/hypocalcemia	Monitor renal function/serum calcium
Isoniazid	Carbamazepine, phenytoin	Decreased metabolism of other agents (nausea, vomiting, nystagmus, ataxia)	Monitor drug SDC
Macrolides/azalides	Digoxin	Decreased digoxin bioavailability and metabolism	Monitor digoxin SDC; avoid if possible
	Theophylline	Decreased metabolism of theophylline	Monitor theophylline SDC
Metronidazole	Ethanol (drugs containing ethanol)	Disulfiram-like reaction	Avoid
Penicillins and cephalosporins	Probenecid, aspirin	Blocked excretion of β-lactams	Use if prolonged high concentration of β-lactam desirable
Ciprofloxacin/norfloxacin	Theophylline	Decreased metabolism of theophylline	Monitor theophylline

(continued)

TABLE 35–3	Major Drug Interactions with Antimicrobials (*Continued*)		
Antimicrobial	Other Agent(s)	Mechanism of Action/Effect	Clinical Management
Quinolones	Classes Ia and III antiarrhythmics	Increased Q-T interval	Avoid
	Multivalent cations (antacids, iron, sucralfate, zinc, vitamins, dairy, citric acid), didanosine	Decreased absorption of quinolone	Separate by 2 hours
Rifampin	Azoles, cyclosporine, methadone propranolol, PIs, oral contraceptives, tacrolimus, warfarin	Increased metabolism of other agent	Avoid if possible
Sulfonamides	Sulfonylureas, phenytoin, warfarin	Decreased metabolism of other agent	Monitor blood glucose, SDC, PT
Tetracyclines	Antacids, iron, calcium, sucralfate	Decreased absorption of tetracycline	Separate by 2 hours
	Digoxin	Decreased digoxin bioavailability	Monitor digoxin SDC; avoid if possible

(PI, protease inhibitor; PT, prothrombin time; SDC, serum drug concentrations.)

Azalides: azithromycin; azoles: fluconazole, itraconazole, ketoconazole, and voriconazole; macrolides: erythromycin and clarithromycin; protease inhibitors: amprenavir, indinavir, lopinavir/ritonavir, nelfinavir, ritonavir, and saquinavir; quinolones: ciprofloxacin, gemifloxacin, levofloxacin, and moxifloxacin.

- Increasing the coverage of antimicrobial therapy is generally necessary in mixed infections in which multiple organisms are likely to be present, such as intra-abdominal and female pelvic infections in which a variety of aerobic and anaerobic bacteria may produce disease. Another clinical situation in which increased spectrum of activity is desirable is with nosocomial infection.

Synergism

- The achievement of synergistic antimicrobial activity is advantageous for infections caused by gram-negative bacilli in immunosuppressed patients.
- Traditionally, combinations of aminoglycosides and β-lactams have been used because these drugs together generally act synergistically against a wide variety of bacteria. However, the data supporting superior efficacy of synergistic over nonsynergistic combinations are weak.
- Synergistic combinations may produce better results in infections caused by *Pseudomonas aeruginosa*, as well as in certain infections caused by *Enterococcus* spp.
- The use of combinations to prevent the emergence of resistance is widely applied but not often realized. The only circumstance in which this has been clearly effective is in the treatment of tuberculosis.

Disadvantages of Combination Therapy

- Although there are potentially beneficial effects from combining drugs, there are also potential disadvantages, including increased cost, greater risk of drug toxicity, and superinfection with even more resistant bacteria.
- Some combinations of antimicrobials are potentially antagonistic. For example, agents that are capable of inducing β-lactamase production in bacteria (eg, cefoxitin) may antagonize the effects of enzyme-labile drugs such as penicillins or imipenem.

MONITORING THERAPEUTIC RESPONSE

- After antimicrobial therapy has been instituted, the patient must be monitored carefully for a therapeutic response. Culture and sensitivity reports from specimens collected must be reviewed.
- Use of agents with the narrowest spectrum of activity against identified pathogens is recommended.
- Patient monitoring should include a variety of parameters, including WBC count, temperature, signs and symptoms of infection, appetite, radiologic studies as appropriate, and determination of antimicrobial concentrations in body fluids.
- As the patient improves, the route of antibiotic administration should be reevaluated. Switching to oral therapy is an accepted practice for many infections. Criteria favoring the switch to oral therapy include the following:

  ✓ Overall clinical improvement
  ✓ Lack of fever for 8 to 24 hours
  ✓ Decreased WBC
  ✓ A functioning gastrointestinal (GI) tract

FAILURE OF ANTIMICROBIAL THERAPY

- A variety of factors may be responsible for the apparent lack of response to therapy. It is possible that the disease is not infectious or nonbacterial in origin, or there is an undetected pathogen. Other factors include those directly related to drug selection, the host, or the pathogen. Laboratory error in identification and/or susceptibility testing errors are rare.

Failures Caused by Drug Selection

- Factors directly related to the drug selection include an inappropriate selection of drug, dosage, or route of administration. Malabsorption of a drug product due to GI disease (eg, short-bowel syndrome) or a drug interaction (eg, complexation of fluoroquinolones with multivalent cations resulting in reduced absorption) may lead to potentially subtherapeutic serum concentrations.

- Accelerated drug elimination is also a possible reason for failure and may occur in patients with cystic fibrosis or during pregnancy, when more rapid clearance or larger volumes of distribution may result in low serum concentrations, particularly for aminoglycosides.
- A common cause of failure of therapy is poor penetration into the site of infection. This is especially true for the so-called privileged sites, such as the CNS, the eye, and the prostate gland.

Failures Caused by Host Factors

- Patients who are immunosuppressed (eg, granulocytopenia from chemotherapy and acquired immunodeficiency syndrome) may respond poorly to therapy because their own defenses are inadequate to eradicate the infection despite seemingly adequate drug regimens.
- Other host factors are related to the necessity for surgical drainage of abscesses or removal of foreign bodies and/or necrotic tissue. If these situations are not corrected, they result in persistent infection and, occasionally, bacteremia, despite adequate antimicrobial therapy.

Failures Caused by Microorganisms

- Factors related to the pathogen include the development of drug resistance during therapy. Primary resistance refers to the intrinsic resistance of the pathogens producing the infection. However, acquisition of resistance during treatment has become a major problem as well.
- The increase in resistance among pathogenic organisms is believed to be due, in large part, to continued overuse of antimicrobials in the community, as well as in hospitals, and the increasing prevalence of immunosuppressed patients receiving long-term suppressive antimicrobials for the prevention of infections.

See Chapter 105, Antimicrobial Regimen Selection, authored by Grace C. Lee and David S. Burgess, for a more detailed discussion of this topic.

- Central Nervous System (CNS) infections include a wide variety of clinical conditions and etiologies: meningitis, meningoencephalitis, encephalitis, brain and meningeal abscesses, and shunt infections. The focus of this chapter is meningitis.

PATHOPHYSIOLOGY

- Central nervous system infections are the result of hematogenous spread from a primary infection site, seeding from a parameningeal focus, reactivation from a latent site, trauma, or congenital defects in the CNS.
- Passive and active exposure to cigarette smoke and the presence of a cochlear implant that includes a positioner, both increase the risk of bacterial meningitis.
- CNS infections may be caused by a variety of bacteria, fungi, viruses, and parasites. The most common causes of bacterial meningitis are *Streptococcus pneumoniae*, group B *Streptococcus*, *Neisseria meningitidis*, *Haemophilus influenzae*, and *Listeria monocytogenes*.
- The critical first step in the acquisition of acute bacterial meningitis is nasopharyngeal colonization of the host by the bacterial pathogen. The bacteria first attach themselves to nasopharyngeal epithelial cells and are then phagocytized into the host's bloodstream.
- A common characteristic of most CNS bacterial pathogens (eg, *H. influenzae, Escherichia coli*, and *N. meningitidis*) is the presence of an extensive polysaccharide capsule that is resistant to neutrophil phagocytosis and complement opsonization.
- The neurologic sequelae of meningitis occur due to the activation of host inflammatory pathways. Bacterial cell death causes the release of cell wall components such as lipopolysaccharide, lipid A (endotoxin), lipoteichoic acid, teichoic acid, and peptidoglycan, depending on whether the pathogen is gram-positive or gram-negative. These cell wall components cause capillary endothelial cells and CNS macrophages to release cytokines (interleukin-1, tumor necrosis factor, and other inflammatory mediators). Proteolytic products and toxic oxygen radicals cause an alteration of the blood–brain barrier, whereas platelet-activating factor activates coagulation, and arachidonic acid metabolites stimulate vasodilation. These events lead to cerebral edema, elevated intracranial pressure, cerebrospinal fluid (CSF) pleocytosis, decreased cerebral blood flow, cerebral ischemia, and death.

CLINICAL PRESENTATION

- Meningitis causes CSF fluid changes, and these changes can be used as diagnostic markers of infection (Table 36–1).
- Clinical presentation varies with age; generally, the younger the patient, the more atypical and the less pronounced is the clinical picture.
- Patients may receive antibiotics before a diagnosis of meningitis is made, delaying presentation to the hospital. Prior antibiotic therapy may cause the Gram stain and CSF culture to be negative, but the antibiotic therapy rarely affects CSF protein or glucose.
- Classic signs and symptoms include fever, nuchal rigidity, altered mental status, chills, vomiting, photophobia, and severe headache. Kernig and Brudzinski signs may be present but are poorly sensitive and frequently absent in children.
- Clinical signs and symptoms in young children may include bulging fontanelle, apneas, purpuric rash, and convulsions, in addition to those just mentioned.
- Purpuric and petechial skin lesions typically indicate meningococcal involvement, although the lesions may be present with *H. influenzae* meningitis. Rashes rarely occur with pneumococcal meningitis.

TABLE 36–1	Mean Values of the Components of Normal and Abnormal Cerebrospinal Fluid				
Type	Normal	Bacterial	Viral	Fungal	Tuberculosis
WBC (cells/mm³ or 10⁶/L)	<5 (<30 in newborns)	1000–5000	5–500	100–400	25–500
Differentialª	Monocytes	Neutrophils	Lymphocytes	Lymphocytes	Variable
Protein (mg/dL)	<50 (<500 mg/L)	Elevated	Mild elevation	Elevated	Elevated
Glucose (mg/dL)	45–80 (2.5–4.4 mmol/L)	Low	Normal	Low	Low
CSF/blood glucose ratio	50%–60%	Decreased	Normal	Decreased	Decreased

ªInitial cerebrospinal fluid (CSF), while blood cell (WBC) count may reveal a predominance of polymorphonuclear neutrophils (PMNs).

- *Bacterial Meningitis Score is a validated clinical decision tool aimed to identify children older than 2 months with CSF pleocytosis who are at low risk of acute bacterial meningitis. This tool incorporates clinical features such as positive CSF Gram stain, presence of seizure, serum absolute neutrophil count of 10,000 cells/mm³ or more ($\geq 10 \times 10^9$/L), CSF protein ≥ 80 mg/dL (≥ 800 mg/L), and CSF neutrophil count ≥ 1000 cells/mm³ ($\geq 1 \times 10^9$/L). Treatment is recommended when one or more criteria are present. An elevated CSF protein of 50 mg/dL or more and a CSF glucose concentration less than 50% of the* simultaneously obtained peripheral value suggest bacterial meningitis (see Table 36–1).
- Gram stain and culture of the CSF are the most important laboratory tests performed for bacterial meningitis. When performed before antibiotic therapy is initiated, Gram stain is both rapid and sensitive and can confirm the diagnosis of bacterial meningitis in 75% to 90% of cases.
- Polymerase chain reaction (PCR) techniques can be used to diagnose meningitis caused by *N. meningitidis, S. pneumoniae*, and *H. influenzae* type b (Hib). Latex fixation, latex coagglutination, and enzyme immunoassay tests provide for the rapid identification of several bacterial causes of meningitis, including *S. pneumoniae, N. meningitidis*, and Hib. The rapid antigen tests should be used in situations in which the Gram stain is negative.
- Diagnosis of tuberculosis meningitis employs acid-fast staining, culture, and PCR of the CSF.

TREATMENT

- Goals of Treatment: Eradication of infection with amelioration of signs and symptoms preventing morbidity and mortality, initiating appropriate antimicrobials, providing supportive care, and preventing disease through timely introduction of vaccination and chemoprophylaxis.
- The administration of fluids, electrolytes, antipyretics, analgesia, and other supportive measures are particularly important for patients presenting with acute bacterial meningitis.

PHARMACOLOGIC TREATMENT

- Empiric antimicrobial therapy should be instituted as soon as possible to eradicate the causative organism (see Table 36–2). Antimicrobial therapy should last at least 48 to 72 hours or until the diagnosis of bacterial meningitis can be ruled out. Continued therapy should be based on the assessment of clinical improvement, cultures, and susceptibility testing results. Once a pathogen is identified, antibiotic therapy should be tailored to the specific pathogen. The first dose of antibiotic should not be withheld even when lumbar puncture is delayed or neuroimaging is being performed.

TABLE 36–2	Bacterial Meningitis: Most Likely Etiologies and Empirical Therapy by Age Group	
Age	Most Likely Organisms	Empirical Therapy[a]
<1 month	S. agalactiae Gram-negative enterics[b] L. monocytogenes	Ampicillin + cefotaxime or ampicillin + aminoglycoside
1–23 months	S. pneumoniae N. meningitidis H. influenzae S. agalactiae	Vancomycin[c] + 3rd generation cephalosporin (cefotaxime or ceftriaxone)
2–50 years	N. meningitidis S. pneumoniae	Vancomycin[c] + 3rd generation cephalosporin (cefotaxime or ceftriaxone)
>50 years	S. pneumoniae N. meningitidis Gram-negative enterics[b] L. monocytogenes	Vancomycin[c] + ampicillin + 3rd generation cephalosporin (cefotaxime or ceftriaxone

[a]All recommendations are A-III.
[b]E. coli, Klebsiella spp, Enterobacter spp common.
[c]Vancomycin use should be based on local incidence of penicillin-resistant S. pneumoniae and until cefotaxime or ceftriaxone minimum inhibitory concentration results are available.
Strength of recommendation: (A) Good evidence to support a recommendation for use; should always be offered. (B) Moderate evidence to support a recommendation for use; should generally be offered.
Quality of evidence: (I) Evidence from 1 or more properly randomized, controlled trial. (II) Evidence from 1 or more well-designed clinical trial, without randomization; from cohort or case-controlled analytic studies (preferably from 1 or more center) or from multiple time-series. (III) Evidence from opinions of respected authorities, based on clinical experience, descriptive studies, or reports of expert committees.

- With increased meningeal inflammation, there will be greater antibiotic penetration (see Table 36–3). Problems of CSF penetration were traditionally overcome by direct instillation of antibiotics intrathecally, intracisternally, or intraventricularly. Advantages of direct instillation, however, must be weighed against the risks of invasive CNS procedures. Intrathecal administration of antibiotics is unlikely to produce therapeutic concentrations in the ventricles possibly owing to the unidirectional flow of CSF.
- Table 36–4 for antimicrobial agents of first choice and alternatives for treatment of meningitis caused by gram-positive and gram-negative microorganisms.

Dexamethasone as an Adjunctive Treatment for Meningitis

- In addition to antibiotics, **dexamethasone** is a commonly used therapy for the treatment of pediatric meningitis.
- Current recommendations call for the use of adjunctive dexamethasone in infants and children with H. influenzae meningitis. The recommended IV dose is 0.15 mg/kg every 6 hours for 2 to 4 days, initiated 10 to 20 minutes prior to or concomitant with, but not after, the first dose of antimicrobials. Clinical outcome is unlikely to improve if dexamethasone is given after the first dose of antimicrobial and should therefore be avoided. If adjunctive dexamethasone is used, careful monitoring of signs and symptoms of gastrointestinal (GI) bleeding and hyperglycemia should be employed.

Neisseria meningitidis (Meningococcus)

- The presence of petechiae may be the primary clue that the underlying pathogen is N. meningitidis. Approximately 60% of adults and up to 90% of pediatric patients with meningococcal meningitis have purpuric lesions, petechiae, or both. N. meningitidis meningitis is the leading cause of bacterial meningitis in children and young adults in the United States and around the world. Most cases occur in the winter or spring, at a time when viral meningitis is relatively uncommon.

TABLE 36-3 Penetration of Antimicrobial Agents into the CSF[a]

Therapeutic Levels in CSF With or Without Inflammation

Acyclovir	Levofloxacin
Chloramphenicol	Linezolid
Ciprofloxacin	Metronidazole
Fluconazole	Moxifloxacin
Flucytosine	Pyrazinamide
Foscarnet	Rifampin
Fosfomycin	Sulfonamides
Ganciclovir	Trimethoprim
Isoniazid	Voriconazole

Therapeutic Levels in CSF With Inflammation of Meninges

Ampicillin ± sulbactam	Imipenem
Aztreonam	Meropenem
Cefepime	Nafcillin
Cefotaxime	Ofloxacin
Ceftazidime	Penicillin G
Ceftriaxone	Piperacillin/tazobactam[b]
Cefuroxime	Pyrimethamine
Colistin	Quinupristin/dalfopristin
Daptomycin	Ticarcillin ± clavulanic acid[b]
Ethambutol	Vancomycin

Nontherapeutic Levels in CSF With or Without Inflammation

Aminoglycosides	Cephalosporins (second generation)d
Amphotericin B	Doxycycline[e]
β-Lactamase inhibitors[c]	Itraconazole[f]
Cephalosporins (first generation)	

[a]Using recommended CNS dosing and compared to MIC of target pathogens.
[b]May not achieve therapeutic levels against organisms with higher MIC, as in *P. aeruginosa*. Tazobactam does not penetrate BBB.
[c]Includes clavulanic acid, sulbactam, and tazobactam.
[d]Cefuroxime is an exception.
[e]Documented effectiveness for *B. burgdorferi*.
[f]Achieves therapeutic concentrations for *Cryptococcus neoformans* therapy.

- Approximately 10 to 14 days after the onset of the disease and despite successful treatment, the patient develops a characteristic immunologic reaction of fever, arthritis (usually involving large joints), and pericarditis. The synovial fluid is characterized by a large number of polymorphonuclear cells, elevated protein concentrations, normal glucose concentrations, and sterile cultures.
- Deafness unilaterally, or more commonly bilaterally, may develop early or late in the disease course.

TREATMENT AND PREVENTION

- Third-generation cephalosporins (ie, cefotaxime and ceftriaxone) are the recommended empiric treatment for meningococcal meningitis
- Close contacts of patients contracting *N. meningitidis* meningitis are at an increased risk of developing meningitis. Prophylaxis of contacts should be started only after consultation with the local health department.
- In general, rifampin, ceftriaxone, ciprofloxacin, or azithromycin is given for prophylaxis. For regions with reported ciprofloxacin resistance, one dose of azithromycin 500 mg is recommended for prophylaxis.

Streptococcus pneumoniae (Pneumococcus or Diplococcus)

- *S. pneumoniae* is the leading cause of meningitis in patients 2 months of age or older in the United States.
- Neurologic complications, such as coma and seizures, are common.
- The treatment of choice until susceptibility of the organism is known is the combination of **vancomycin** plus **ceftriaxone.** Penicillin may be used for drug-susceptible isolates with minimum inhibitory concentrations of 0.06 mcg/mL or less, but for intermediate isolates ceftriaxone is used, and for highly drug-resistant isolates a combination of ceftriaxone and vancomycin should be used. A high percent of *S. pneumoniae* is either intermediately or highly resistant to penicillin. Ceftriaxone and cefotaxime have served as alternatives to penicillin in the treatment of penicillin-resistant pneumococci. Therapeutic approaches to cephalosporin resistant pneumococcus include the addition of vancomycin and rifampin. Meropenem is recommended as an alternative to a third-generation cephalosporin in penicillin nonsusceptible isolates. IV linezolid and daptomycin have emerged as therapeutic options for treating multidrug-resistant gram-positive infections.
- The Centers for Disease Control and Prevention (CDC) recommends use of 23-valent pneumococcal vaccine (PPV 23) for persons over 65 years of age; persons 2 to 64 years of age who have a chronic illness, who live in high-risk environments, and who lack a functioning spleen; and immunocompromised persons over 2 years, including those with human immunodeficiency virus (HIV) infection. All healthy infants younger than 2 years of age should be immunized with the 13-valent pneumococcal conjugate vaccine (PCV13) at 2, 4, 6, and 12 to 15 months. PCV13 should be used in series with PPV23 for all adults who are 65 years of age or older.

Haemophilus influenzae

- In the past, *H. influenzae* was the most common cause of meningitis in children 6 months to 3 years of age, but this has declined dramatically since the introduction of effective vaccines.
- Because approximately 20% of *H. influenzae* are ampicillin resistant, many clinicians use a third-generation cephalosporin (**cefotaxime** or **ceftriaxone**) for initial antimicrobial therapy. Cefepime and fluoroquinolones are suitable alternatives regardless of β-lactamase activity.
- Prophylaxis of close contacts should be started only after consultation with the local health department and the CDC.
- Vaccination with Hib conjugate vaccines is usually begun in children at 2 months. The vaccine should be considered in patients older than 5 years with sickle cell disease, asplenia, or immunocompromising diseases.

Listeria monocytogenes

- *L. monocytogenes* is a gram-positive, diphtheroid-like organism and is responsible for 10% of all reported cases of meningitis in those older than 65 years.
- The combination of **penicillin G** or **ampicillin** with an aminoglycoside results in a bactericidal effect. Patients should be treated a minimum of 3 weeks. Combination therapy is given for the first 7 to 10 days with the remainder completed with penicillin G or ampicillin alone.
- **Trimethoprim–sulfamethoxazole** and **meropenem** may be an effective alternative because adequate CSF penetration is achieved with these agents.

Gram-Negative Bacillary Meningitis

- Elderly debilitated patients are at an increased risk of gram-negative meningitis but typically lack the classic signs and symptoms of the disease.

TABLE 36–4 Antimicrobial Agents of First Choice and Alternative Choice in the Treatment of Meningitis Caused by Gram-Positive and Gram-Negative Microorganisms

Organism	Antibiotics of First Choice	Alternative Antibiotics	Recommended Duration of Therapy
Gram-Positive Organisms			
Streptococcus pneumoniae[a]			10–14 days
Penicillin susceptible MIC ≤ 0.06 mcg/mL (mg/L)	Penicillin G or Ampicillin (A-III)	Cefotaxime (A-III), Ceftriaxone (A-III), Cefepime (B-II), or Meropenem (B-II)	
Penicillin resistant MIC > 0.06 mcg/mL (mg/L)	Vancomycin[b,c] + Cefotaxime or Ceftriaxone (A-III)	Moxifloxacin (B-II)	
Ceftriaxone resistant MIC > 0.5 mcg/mL (mg/L)	Vancomycin[b,c] + Cefotaxime or Ceftriaxone (A-III)	Moxifloxacin (B-II)	
Staphylococcus aureus			14–21 days
Methicillin susceptible	Nafcillin or Oxacillin (A-III)	Vancomycin (A-III) or Meropenem (B-III)	
Methicillin resistant	Vancomycin[b,c] (A-III)	TMP-SMX or Linezolid (B-III)	
Group B *Streptococcus*	Penicillin G or Ampicillin (A-III) ± Gentamicin[b,c]	Ceftriaxone or Cefotaxime (B-III)	14–21 days
S. epidermidis	Vancomycin[b,c] (A-III)	Linezolid (B-III)	14–21 days[d]
L. monocytogenes	Penicillin G or Ampicillin ± Gentamicin[b,c,e] (A-III)	Trimethoprim-sulfamethoxazole (A-III), Meropenem (B-III)	≥21 days
Gram-Negative Organisms			
Neisseria meningitis			7–10 days
Penicillin susceptible	Penicillin G or Ampicillin (A-III)	Cefotaxime or Ceftriaxone (A-II)	
Penicillin resistant	Cefotaxime or Ceftriaxone (A-II)	Meropenem or Moxifloxacin (A-III)	

Haemophilus influenzae		7–10 days
β-lactamase negative	Ampicillin (A-III)	
β-lactamase positive	Cefotaxime or Ceftriaxone (A-I)	
	Cefotaxime (A-III), Ceftriaxone (A-III), Cefepime (A-III) or Moxifloxacin (A-II)	
	Cefepime (A-I) or Moxifloxacin (A-III)	
Enterobacteriaceae[f]	Cefotaxime or Ceftriaxone (A-II)	21 days
	Cefepime (A-III), Moxifloxacin (A-III), Meropenem (A-III) or Aztreonam (A-III)	
Pseudomonas aeruginosa	Cefepime or Ceftazidime (A-II) ± Tobramycin[b,c] (A-III)	21 days
	Ciprofloxacin (A-III), Meropenem (A-III), Piperacillin plus Tobramycin[a,b] (A-III), Colistin sulfomethate[g] (B-III), Aztreonam (A-III)	

[a]European Guidelines recommend considering the addition of rifampin to vancomycin therapy.
[b]Direct CNS administration maybe considered if failed conventional treatment.
[c]Monitor serum drug levels.
[d]Based on clinical experience; no clear recommendations.
[e]European guidelines recommend adding gentamicin for the first 7 days of treatment.
[f]Includes *E. coli* and *Klebsiella* spp.
[g]Should be reserved for multidrug-resistant pseudomonal or *Actinetobacter* infections for which all other therapeutic options have been exhausted.

- Optimal antibiotic therapies for gram-negative bacillary meningitis have not been fully defined. Meningitis caused by *Pseudomonas aeruginosa* is initially treated with an extended-spectrum β-lactam such as **ceftazidime** or **cefepime**, or alternatively aztreonam, ciprofloxacin, or meropenem. The addition of an aminoglycoside—usually tobramycin—to one of the above agents should also be considered (see Table 36–4).
- If the pseudomonad is suspected to be antibiotic resistant or becomes resistant during therapy, an intraventricular aminoglycoside (preservative-free) should be considered along with IV aminoglycoside.
- Gram-negative organisms, other than *P. aeruginosa*, that cause meningitis can be treated with a third- or fourth-generation cephalosporin such as **cefotaxime, ceftriaxone, ceftazidime**, or **cefepime**.
- Therapy for gram-negative meningitis is continued for a minimum of 21 days. CSF cultures may remain positive for several days or more on a regimen that will eventually be curative.

See Chapter 106, Central Nervous System Infections, authored by Ramy H. Elshaboury, Aileen S. Ahiskali, Jessica S. Holt, and John C. Rotschafer, for a more detailed discussion of this topic.

CHAPTER 37

Endocarditis

- *Endocarditis* is an inflammation of the endocardium, the membrane lining the chambers of the heart and covering the cusps of the heart valves. *Infective endocarditis* (IE) refers to infection of the heart valves by microorganisms, primarily bacteria.
- Endocarditis is often referred to as either acute or subacute depending on the clinical presentation. Acute bacterial endocarditis is a fulminating infection associated with high fevers, systemic toxicity, and death within days to weeks if untreated. Subacute infectious endocarditis is a more indolent infection, usually occurring in a setting of prior valvular heart disease.

ETIOLOGY

- Most patients with IE have risk factors, such as preexisting cardiac valve abnormalities. Many types of structural heart disease resulting in turbulence of blood flow will increase the risk for IE. Some of the most important risk factors include the following:
  ✓ Highest risk: presence of a prosthetic valve or previous endocarditis
  ✓ Congenital heart disease, chronic intravenous access, diabetes mellitus, healthcare-related exposure, acquired valvular dysfunction (eg, rheumatic heart disease), hypertrophic cardiomyopathy, mitral valve prolapse with regurgitation, and intravenous (IV) drug abuse.
- Three groups of organisms cause most cases of IE: streptococci, staphylococci, and enterococci (**Table 37–1**).

CLINICAL PRESENTATION

- The clinical presentation of patients with IE is highly variable and nonspecific (**Table 37–2**). Fever is the most common finding. The mitral and aortic valves are most often affected.
- Important clinical signs, especially prevalent in subacute illness, may include the following peripheral manifestations ("stigmata") of endocarditis: Osler nodes, Janeway lesions, splinter hemorrhages, petechiae, clubbing of the fingers, Roth's spots, and emboli.
- Without appropriate antimicrobial therapy and surgery, IE is usually fatal. With proper management, recovery can be expected in most patients.
- Factors associated with increased mortality include the following: congestive heart failure, culture-negative endocarditis, endocarditis caused by resistant organisms such as fungi and gram-negative bacteria, left-sided endocarditis caused by *Staphylococcus aureus*, prosthetic valve endocarditis (PVE).
- Ninety percent to 90% to 95% of patients with IE have a positive blood culture. Anemia, leukocytosis, and thrombocytopenia may be present. The erythrocyte sedimentation rate (ESR) and C-reactive protein (CRP) may be elevated in approximately 60% of patients.
- Transesophageal echocardiography is important in identifying and localizing valvular lesions in patients suspected of having IE. It is more sensitive for detecting vegetations (85%–90%), compared with transthoracic echocardiography (58%–75%).
- The Modified Duke criteria, encompassing major findings of persistent bacteremia and echocardiographic findings and other minor findings, are used to categorize patients as "definite IE" or "possible IE."

TREATMENT

- <u>Goals of Treatment</u>: relieve the signs and symptoms of disease. Decrease morbidity and mortality associated with infection. Eradicate the causative organism with minimal drug exposure. Provide cost-effective antimicrobial therapy. Prevent IE in high-risk patients with appropriate prophylactic antimicrobials.

TABLE 37–1	Etiologic Organisms in Infective Endocarditis[a]
Agent	**Percentage of Cases**
Staphylococci	30–70
Coagulase positive	20–68
Coagulase negative	3–26
Streptococci	9–38
Viridans streptococci	10–28
Other streptococci	3–14
Enterococci	5–18
Gram-negative aerobic bacilli	1.5–13
Fungi	1–9
Miscellaneous bacteria	<5
Mixed infections	1–2
"Culture negative"	<5–17

[a]Values encompass community-acquired, healthcare-associated, native valve, and prosthetic valve infective endocarditis.

- The most important approach to treatment of IE is isolation of the infecting pathogen and determination of antimicrobial susceptibilities, followed by high-dose, bactericidal antibiotics for an extended period.
- Treatment usually is started in the hospital, but in select patients, it may be completed in the outpatient setting as long as defervescence has occurred and followup blood cultures show no growth.

TABLE 37–2	Clinical Presentation of Infective Endocarditis

General

The clinical presentation of infective endocarditis is highly variable and nonspecific

Symptoms

The patient may complain of fever, chills, weakness, dyspnea, night sweats, weight loss, and/or malaise

Signs

Fever is common, as is a heart murmur (sometimes new or changing). The patient may have embolic phenomenon, splenomegaly, or skin manifestations (eg, Osler's nodes, Janeway's lesions)

Laboratory tests

The patient's white blood cell count may be normal or only slightly elevated

Nonspecific findings include anemia (normocytic, normochromic), thrombocytopenia, an elevated erythrocyte sedimentation rate or C-reactive protein, and altered urinary analysis (proteinuria/microscopic hematuria)

The hallmark laboratory finding is continuous bacteremia; three sets of blood cultures should be collected over 24 hours

Other diagnostic tests

An electrocardiogram, chest radiograph, and echocardiogram are commonly performed. Echocardiography to determine the presence of valvular vegetations plays a key role in the diagnosis of infective endocarditis; it should be performed in all suspected cases

- Large doses of parenteral antimicrobials usually are necessary to achieve bactericidal concentrations within vegetations. An extended duration of therapy is required, even for susceptible pathogens, because microorganisms are enclosed within valvular vegetations and fibrin deposits.
- Drug dosing for treatment of IE is given in Table 37–3.

NONPHARMACOLOGIC THERAPY

- Surgery is an important adjunct to management of endocarditis in certain patients. In most cases, valvectomy and valve replacement are performed to remove infected tissues and restore hemodynamic function. Indications for surgery include heart failure, persistent bacteremia, persistent vegetation, an increase in vegetation size, or recurrent emboli despite prolonged antibiotic treatment, valve dysfunction, paravalvular extension (eg, abscess), or endocarditis caused by resistant organisms.

STREPTOCOCCAL ENDOCARDITIS

- Streptococci are a common cause of IE, with most isolates being viridans group streptococci.
- Most viridans group streptococci are highly sensitive to penicillin G with minimum inhibitory concentrations (MICs) of 0.12 mcg/mL [mg/L] or less. The MIC should be determined for all viridans streptococci and the results used to guide therapy. Approximately 10% to 20% are moderately susceptible (MIC 0.12–0.5 mcg/mL [mg/L]).
- Recommended therapy in the uncomplicated case caused by fully susceptible strains in native valves is 4 weeks of either high-dose **penicillin G** or **ceftriaxone**, or 2 weeks of combined penicillin G or ceftriaxone therapy plus **gentamicin** (Table 37–4).
- The following conditions should all be present to consider a 2-week treatment regimen:
  - ✓ The isolate is penicillin sensitive (MIC ≤0.1 mcg/mL [mg/L]).
  - ✓ There are no cardiovascular risk factors such as heart failure, aortic insufficiency, or conduction abnormalities.
  - ✓ No evidence of thromboembolic disease
  - ✓ Native valve infection
  - ✓ No vegetation greater than 5 mm diameter on echocardiogram
  - ✓ Low risk of nephrotoxicity
  - ✓ Not at risk for *Clostridium difficile* infection
  - ✓ Clinical response is evident within 7 days.
- Vancomycin is effective and is the drug of choice for the patient with a history of immediate-type hypersensitivity reaction to penicillin. When vancomycin is used, the addition of gentamicin is not recommended.
- For patients with complicated infection (eg, extracardiac foci) or when the organism is relatively resistant (MIC = 0.12–0.5 mcg/mL[mg/L]), combination therapy with an aminoglycoside and penicillin (higher dose) or ceftriaxone for the first 2 weeks is recommended followed by penicillin or ceftriaxone alone for an additional 2 weeks.
- In patients with endocarditis of prosthetic valves or other prosthetic material caused by viridans streptococci and *Streptococcus bovis*, treatment courses are extended to 6 weeks (Table 37–5).

STAPHYLOCOCCAL ENDOCARDITIS

- *S. aureus* has become more prevalent as a cause of endocarditis because of increased IV drug abuse, frequent use of peripheral and central venous catheters, and valve replacement surgery. Coagulase-negative staphylococci (usually *Staphylococcus epidermidis*) are prominent causes of PVE.
- The recommended therapy for patients with left-sided IE caused by methicillin-sensitive *S. aureus* (MSSA) is 6 weeks of **nafcillin** or **oxacillin**, often combined with a short course of gentamicin (see Table 37–4).
- If a patient has a mild, delayed allergy to penicillin, **first-generation cephalosporins** are effective alternatives but should be avoided in patients with an immediate-type hypersensitivity reaction.

TABLE 37-3 Drug Dosing Table for Treatment of Infective Endocarditis[a]

Drug	Brand Name	Recommended Dose	Pediatric (Ped) Dose[b]	Additional Information
Ampicillin	NA	2 g IV every 4 hours	50 mg/kg every 4 hours or 75 mg/kg every 6 hours	24-hour total dose may be administered as a continuous infusion: 12 g IV every 24 hours
Ampicillin–sulbactam	Unasyn®	2 g IV every 4 hours	50 mg/kg every 4 hours or 75 mg/kg every 6 hours	
Aqueous crystalline penicillin G sodium	NA			24-hour total dose may be administered as a continuous infusion: 12–18 million units IV every 24 hours (Ped: 200,000 units/kg IV/24 hours)
• MIC <0.12 mcg/mL (mg/L) (native valve only)		3 million units IV every 4 hours or every 6 hours	50,000 units/kg IV every 6 hours	
• All other indications		4 million units IV every 4 hours or 6 million units IV every 6 hours	50,000 units/kg IV every 4 hours or 75,000 units/kg IV every 6 hours	24 million units IV every 24 hours (Ped: 300,000 units/kg IV every 24 hours)
Cefazolin	Ancef®	2 g IV every 8 hours	33 mg/kg IV every 8 hours	
Cefepime	Maxipime®	2 g IV every 8 hours	50 mg/kg IV every 8 hours	
Ceftriaxone sodium	Rocephin®	2 g IV or IM every 24 hours 2 g IV or IM every 12 hours (E. faecalis only)	100 mg/kg IV or IM every 24 hours	
Ciprofloxacin	Cipro®	400 mg IV every 12 hours or 500 mg po every 12 hours	20–30 mg/kg IV or po every 12 hours	Avoid use if possible in patients <18 years of age
Daptomycin	Cubicin®	≥8 mg/kg IV every 24 hours	6 mg/kg IV every 24 hours	Doses as high as 10–12 mg/kg IV every 24 hours have been used in adults with enterococcus resistant to penicillin, aminoglycosides and vancomycin; doses should be calculated using actual body weight

Doxycline	Vibramycin®	100 mg IV or po every 12 hours	1–2 mg/kg IV or orally every 12 hours	
Gentamicin sulfate	NA	3 mg/kg IV or IM every 24 hours or 1 mg/kg IV or IM every 8 hours^c	1 mg/kg IV or IM every 8 hours	Once-daily dosing is only recommended for treatment of streptococcal infections.
Linezolid	Zyvox®	600 mg IV or po every 12 hours	10 mg/kg IV every 8 hours	
Nafcillin or oxacillin	NA	2 g IV every 4 hours	50 mg/kg IV every 6 hours	
Rifampin	Rifadin®	300 mg IV or po every 8 hours	5–7 mg/kg IV or orally every 8 hours	
Streptomycin	NA	7.5 mg/kg IV or IM every 12 hours		
Vancomycin	Vancocin®	15–20 mg/kg IV every 8 hours or every 12 hours	15 mg/kg IV every 6 hours	A loading dose of 25–30 mg/kg may be administered in adults; doses should be calculated using actual body weight; single doses should not exceed 2 g

aAll doses assume normal renal function.
bShould not exceed adult dosage.
cActual body weight should be used when the full aminoglycoside dose is administered once daily; when administered in three divided doses, use ideal body weight or adjusted body weight when actual body weight is >120% ideal body weight.

TABLE 37–4 Treatment Options for Native Valve Endocarditis by Causative Organism

Agent	Duration	Strength of Recommendation	Comments
Highly penicillin-susceptible (MIC ≤ 0.12 mcg/mL [mg/L]) viridans group streptococci and S. gallolyticus			
Aqueous crystalline penicillin G sodium[a]	4 weeks	IIaB	2-week regimens are not intended for the following patients:
Ceftriaxone	4 weeks	IIaB	• Most patients >65 years of age
Aqueous crystalline penicillin G sodium[a] plus gentamicin	2 weeks	IIaB	• Children • Impairment of the eighth cranial nerve function • Renal function with a creatinine clearance <20 mL/min (<0.33 mL/s)
Ceftriaxone plus gentamicin	2 weeks	IIaB	• Known cardiac or extracardiac abscess • Infection with Abiotrophia, Granulicatella, or Gemella species
Vancomycin	4 weeks	IIaB	Recommended only for patients unable to tolerate penicillin or ceftriaxone
Viridans group streptococci and S. gallolyticus relatively resistant to penicillin (MIC >0.12 to ≤0.5 mcg/mL [mg/L])			
Aqueous crystalline penicillin G sodium[a] plus gentamicin	4 weeks 2 weeks	IIaB	
Ceftriaxone plus gentamicin	4 weeks 2 weeks	IIbC	
Vancomycin	4 weeks	IIaB	Recommended only for patients unable to tolerate penicillin or ceftriaxone
Oxacillin-susceptible staphylococci[b]			
Nafcillin or oxacillin	6 weeks	1C	
Cefazolin	6 weeks	1B	For use in patients with nonanaphylactoid-type penicillin allergies; patients with an unclear history of immediate-type hypersensitivity to penicillin should be considered for skin testing

Vancomycin	6 weeks	1B	For use in patients with anaphylactoid-type hypersensitivity to penicillin and/or cephalosporins
Daptomycin	6 weeks	IIaB	For use in patients with immediate-type hypersensitivity reactions to penicillin
Oxacillin-resistant staphylococci			
Vancomycin	6 weeks	1C	
Daptomycin	6 weeks	IIbB	

[a]May use ampicillin in the event of a penicillin shortage.
[b]Regimens indicate treatment for left-sided endocarditis or complicated right-sided endocarditis; uncomplicated right-sided endocarditis may be treated for shorter durations and is described in the text.

TABLE 37–5	Treatment Options for Prosthetic Valve Endocarditis (PVE) by Causative Organism		
Agent	Duration	Strength of Recommendation	Comments
Highly penicillin-susceptible (MIC ≤ 0.12 mcg/mL [mg/L]) viridans group streptococci and S. gallyoticus			
Aqueous crystalline penicillin G sodium[a] with or without gentamicin	6 weeks 2 weeks	IIaB	Combination therapy with gentamicin has not demonstrated superior cure rates compared with monotherapy with a penicillin or cephalosporin and should be avoided in patients with CrCl <30 mL/min (<0.50 mL/s)
Ceftriaxone with or without gentamicin	6 weeks 2 weeks	IIaB	
Vancomycin	6 weeks	IIaB	Recommended only for patients unable to tolerate penicillin or ceftriaxone
Relatively resistant or fully resistant (MIC > 0.12 mcg/mL [mg/L]) viridans group streptococci and S. gallolyticus			
Aqueous crystalline penicillin G sodium[a] plus gentamicin	6 weeks	IIaB	
Ceftriaxone plus gentamicin	6 weeks	IIaB	
Vancomycin[b]	6 weeks	IIaB	Recommended only for patients unable to tolerate penicillin or ceftriaxone
Oxacillin-susceptible staphylococci			
Nafcillin or oxacillin plus rifampin plus gentamicin	≥6 weeks ≥6 weeks 2 weeks	1B	Cefazolin may be substituted for nafcillin or oxacillin in patients with nonimmediate-type hypersensitivity
Vancomycin plus rifampin plus gentamicin	≥6 weeks ≥6 weeks 2 weeks	1B	Recommended only for patients with anaphylactoid-type hypersensitivity to penicillin and/or cephalosporins
Oxacillin-resistant staphylococci			
Vancomycin plus rifampin plus gentamicin	≥6 weeks ≥6 weeks 2 weeks	1B	

[a]May use ampicillin in the event of a penicillin shortage.
[b]The ESC 2015 guidelines recommend gentamicin (3 mg/kg/day) be administered with vancomycin for the initial 2 weeks of therapy in patients with relatively resistant strains to penicillin.

- In a patient with a positive penicillin skin test or a history of immediate hypersensitivity to penicillin, **vancomycin** is an option. Vancomycin, however, kills *S. aureus* slowly and is generally regarded as inferior to penicillinase-resistant penicillins for MSSA. Penicillin-allergic patients who fail on vancomycin therapy should be considered for penicillin desensitization. **Daptomycin** (at a dose of 6 mg/kg/day) is a recommended alternative.

- **Vancomycin** is the drug of choice for methicillin-resistant staphylococci because most methicillin-resistant *S. aureus* (MRSA) and most coagulase-negative staphylococci are susceptible. Reports of *S. aureus* strains resistant to vancomycin are emerging.

Treatment of *Staphylococcus* Endocarditis in IV Drug Abusers

- IE in IV drug abusers is most frequently (60%–70%) caused by *S. aureus*, although other organisms may be more common in certain geographic locations.
- A 2-week course of **nafcillin, oxacillin, or daptomycin** without an aminoglycoside is recommended.
- Selection of a 2-week duration of treatment may be appropriate as long as the following criteria are fulfilled: the pathogen is identified as MSSA, there is good response to treatment, there is absence of metastatic sites of infection or empyema, cardiac and extracardiac complications, associated prosthetic valve or left sided valve infection, and severe immunosuppression. Also, vegetation size is less than 20 mm.

Treatment of Staphylococcal Prosthetic Valve Endocarditis

- PVE that occurs within 2 months of cardiac surgery is usually caused by staphylococci implanted at the time of surgery. Methicillin-resistant organisms are common. Vancomycin is the cornerstone of therapy.
- Because of the high morbidity and mortality associated with PVE and refractoriness to therapy, combinations of antimicrobials are usually recommended.
- For methicillin-resistant staphylococci (both MRSA and coagulase-negative staphylococci), **vancomycin** is used with rifampin for 6 weeks or more (see Table 37–5). An **aminoglycoside** is added for the first 2 weeks if the organism is susceptible.
- For methicillin-susceptible staphylococci, a **penicillinase-resistant penicillin** is used in place of vancomycin. If an organism is identified other than staphylococci, the treatment regimen should be guided by susceptibilities and should be at least 6 weeks in duration.

ENTEROCOCCAL ENDOCARDITIS

- Enterococci are the third leading cause of endocarditis and are noteworthy for the following reasons: (1) no single antibiotic is bactericidal; (2) MICs to penicillin are relatively high (1–25 mcg/mL[mg/L]); (3) they are intrinsically resistant to all cephalosporins and relatively resistant to aminoglycosides (ie, "low-level" aminoglycoside resistance); (4) combinations of a cell wall–active agent, such as a penicillin or vancomycin, plus an aminoglycoside are necessary for killing; and (5) resistance to all available drugs is increasing.
- Enterococcal endocarditis ordinarily requires 4 to 6 weeks of high-dose **penicillin G** or **ampicillin**, plus **gentamicin** for cure (Table 37–6). Ampicillin plus ceftriaxone is as effective as ampicillin plus gentamicin and should be considered as a treatment option. A 6-week course is recommended for patients with symptoms lasting longer than 3 months and those with PVE.
- In addition to isolates with high-level aminoglycoside resistance, β-lactamase-producing enterococci (especially *Enterococcus faecium*) are increasingly reported. If these organisms are discovered, use of vancomycin or ampicillin–sulbactam in combination with gentamicin should be considered.

EVALUATION OF THERAPEUTIC OUTCOMES

- The evaluation of patients treated for IE includes assessment of signs and symptoms, blood cultures, microbiologic tests (eg, MIC, minimum bactericidal concentration [MBC], or serum bactericidal titers), serum drug concentrations, and other tests to evaluate organ function.
- Persistence of fever beyond 1 week may indicate ineffective antimicrobial therapy, emboli, infections of intravascular catheters, or drug reactions. In some patients, low-grade fever may persist even with appropriate antimicrobial therapy.

TABLE 37-6 Treatment Options for Native or Prosthetic Valve Endocarditis Caused by Enterococci

Agent	Duration[a]	Strength of Recommendation	Comments
Ampicillin-, penicillin-, and vancomycin-susceptible strains			
Ampicillin plus gentamicin	4–6 weeks	IIaB	Native valve plus symptoms present for <3 months: use 4-week regimen
Aqueous crystalline penicillin G sodium plus gentamicin	4–6 weeks	IIAB	Prosthetic valve or native valve plus symptoms present for >3 months: use 6-week regimen
Ampicillin plus ceftriaxone	6 weeks	IIaB	Recommended regimen if creatinine clearance is <50 mL/min (<0.83 mL/s; at baseline or due to therapy with a gentamicin-containing regimen)
Vancomycin plus gentamicin	6 weeks	IIaB	Recommended only for patients unable to tolerate penicillin or ampicillin
Gentamicin-resistant strains			
If susceptible, use streptomycin in place of gentamicin in the regimens listed above as long as creatinine clearance is >50 mL/min (>0.83 mL/s), cranial nerve VIII function is intact and there is laboratory capability for rapid streptomycin serum concentrations.			
Penicillin-resistant strains			
Ampicillin–sulbactam plus gentamicin (β-lactamase–producing strain)	6 weeks	IIbC	
Vancomycin plus gentamicin (intrinsic penicillin resistance[b])	6 weeks	IIbC	May also use in patients with β-lactamase–producing strains who have known intolerance to ampicillin–sulbactam
***Enterococcus faecium* strains resistant to penicillin, aminoglycosides, and vancomycin[c]**			
Linezolid	>6 weeks	IIbC	Antimicrobial cure rates may be <50%; bacteriologic cure may only be achieved with cardiac valve replacement
Daptomycin	>6 weeks	IIbC	

[a]All patients with prosthetic valves should be treated for at least 6 weeks.
[b]Infectious disease consult highly recommended.
[c]Patients should be managed by a multidisciplinary team that includes specialists in cardiology, cardiovascular surgery, infectious diseases, and clinical pharmacy.

- With effective therapy, blood cultures should be negative within a few days, although microbiologic response to vancomycin may be unusually slower. After the initiation of therapy, blood cultures should be rechecked until they are negative. During the remainder of the therapy, frequent blood culturing is not necessary.
- If bacteria continue to be isolated from blood beyond the first few days of therapy, it may indicate that the antimicrobials are inactive against the pathogen or that the doses are not producing adequate concentrations at the site of infection.
- For all isolates from blood cultures, MICs (not MBCs) should be determined.

PREVENTION OF ENDOCARDITIS

- Antimicrobial prophylaxis is used to prevent IE in patients believed to be at high risk.
- The use of antimicrobials for this purpose requires consideration of the types of patients who are at risk; the procedures causing bacteremia; the organisms that are likely to cause endocarditis; and the pharmacokinetics, spectrum, cost, and ease of administration of available agents. The objective of prophylaxis is to diminish the likelihood of IE in high-risk individuals who are undergoing procedures that cause transient bacteremia.
- The literature lacks adequate evidence to prove the effectiveness or ineffectiveness of antibiotic prophylaxis, and the common practice of using antimicrobial therapy in this setting remains controversial.

TABLE 37–7 Prophylaxis of Infective Endocarditis

Highest Risk Cardiac Conditions	Presence of a prosthetic heart valve Prior diagnosis of infective endocarditis Cardiac transplantation with subsequent valvulopathy Congenital heart disease (CHD)[a]	
Types of Procedures	Any that require perforation of the oral mucosa or manipulation of the periapical region of the teeth of gingival tissue	
Antimicrobial Options	**Adult Doses[b]**	**Pediatric Doses[b] (mg/kg)**
Oral amoxicillin	2 g	50
IM or IV ampicillin[c]	2 g	50
IM or IV cefazolin or ceftriaxone[c,d,e]	1 g	50
Oral cephalexin[d,e,f]	2 g	50
Oral clindamycin[e]	600 mg	20
Oral azithromycin or clarithromycin[e]	500 mg	15
IV or IM clindamycin[c,e]	600 mg	20

[a]Includes only the following: unrepaired cyanotic CHD, prophlyaxis within the first 6 months of implanting prosthetic material to repair a congenital heart defect, and repaired CHD with residual defects at or adjacent to prosthetic material.
[b]All one-time doses administered 30–60 minutes prior to initiation of the procedure.
[c]For patients unable to tolerate oral medication.
[d]Should be avoided in patients with immediate-type hypersensitivity reaction to penicillin or ampicillin (eg, anaphylaxis, urticaria, or angioedema).
[e]Option for patients with nonimmediate hypersensitivity reaction to penicillin or ampicillin.
[f]May substitute with an alternative first- or second-generation cephalosporin at an equivalent dose.

- Prophylaxis for dental procedures should be recommended only for patients with underlying cardiac conditions associated with the highest risk; for those with high-risk underlying cardiac conditions, prophylaxis is recommended for all dental procedures involving manipulation of gingival tissue or the periapical region of teeth or perforation of the oral mucosa; prophylaxis is not recommended based solely on an increased lifetime risk of acquisition of infective endocarditis; and administration of antibiotics solely to prevent endocarditis is not recommended for patients who undergo a genitourinary or GI tract procedure.
- Antibiotic regimens for a dental procedure are given in Table 37–7.

See Chapter 111, Infective Endocarditis, authored by Angie Veverka, Brian L. Odle, and Jeffrey A. Kyle for a more detailed discussion of this topic.

SPECIFIC FUNGAL INFECTIONS

HISTOPLASMOSIS

- *Histoplasmosis* is caused by inhalation of dust-borne microconidia of the dimorphic fungus *Histoplasma capsulatum*. In the United States, most disease is localized along the Ohio and Mississippi river valleys.

Clinical Presentation and Diagnosis

- In the vast majority of patients, low-inoculum exposure to *H. capsulatum* results in mild or asymptomatic pulmonary histoplasmosis. The course of disease is generally benign, and symptoms usually abate within a few weeks of onset. Patients exposed to a higher inoculum during a primary infection or reinfection may experience an acute, self-limited illness with flu-like pulmonary symptoms, including fever, chills, headache, myalgia, and nonproductive cough.

- Chronic pulmonary histoplasmosis generally presents as an opportunistic infection imposed on a preexisting structural abnormality, such as lesions resulting from emphysema. Patients demonstrate chronic pulmonary symptoms and apical lung lesions that progress with inflammation, calcified granulomas, and fibrosis. Progression of disease over a period of years, seen in 25% to 30% of patients, is associated with cavitation, bronchopleural fistulas, extension to the other lung, pulmonary insufficiency, and often death.

- In patients exposed to a large inoculum and in immunocompromised hosts, progressive illness, disseminated histoplasmosis, occurs. The clinical severity of the diverse forms of disseminated histoplasmosis (Table 38–1) generally parallels the degree of macrophage parasitization observed.

- Acute (infantile) disseminated histoplasmosis is seen in infants and young children and (rarely) in adults with Hodgkin disease or other lymphoproliferative disorders. It is characterized by unrelenting fever; anemia; leukopenia or thrombocytopenia; enlargement of the liver, spleen, and visceral lymph nodes; and GI symptoms, particularly nausea, vomiting, and diarrhea. Untreated disease is uniformly fatal in 1 to 2 months

- Most adults with disseminated histoplasmosis demonstrate a mild, chronic form of the disease. Untreated patients are often ill for 10 to 20 years, with long asymptomatic periods interrupted by relapses characterized by weight loss, weakness, and fatigue.

- Adult patients with acquired immunodeficiency syndrome (AIDS) demonstrate an acute form of disseminated disease that resembles the syndrome seen in infants and children. Progressive disseminated histoplasmosis can occur as the direct result of initial infection or because of reactivation of dormant foci.

- In most patients, serologic evidence remains the primary method in the diagnosis of histoplasmosis. Results obtained from complement fixation, immunodiffusion, and latex antigen agglutination antibody tests are used alone or in combination. Detection of Histoplasma antigen by enzyme immunoassay (EIA) in the urine, blood, or bronchoalveolar lavage fluid of infected patients provides rapid diagnostic information and is particularly useful in patients who are severely ill.

Treatment

- Recommended therapy for the treatment of histoplasmosis is summarized in Table 38–1.

- Asymptomatic or mildly ill patients and patients with sarcoid-like disease generally do not benefit from antifungal therapy. Therapy may be helpful in symptomatic patients whose conditions have not improved during the first month of infection.

TABLE 38–1	Clinical Manifestations and Therapy of Histoplasmosis	
Type of Disease and Common Clinical Manifestations	**Approximate Frequency (%)[a]**	**Therapy/Comments**
Nonimmunosuppressed host		
Acute pulmonary histoplasmosis		
Asymptomatic or mild to moderate disease	50–99	*Asymptomatic, mild, or symptoms <4 weeks:* No therapy generally required. Itraconazole (200 mg three times daily for 3 days and then 200 mg once or twice daily for 6–12 weeks) is recommended for patients who continue to have symptoms for 11 months *Symptoms >4 weeks:* Itraconazole 200 mg once daily × 6–12 weeks[b]
Self-limited disease	1–50	*Self-limited disease:* Amphotericin B[c] 0.3–0.5 mg/kg/day × 2–4 weeks (total dose 500 mg) or ketoconazole 400 mg orally daily × 3–6 months can be beneficial in patients with severe hypoxia following inhalation of large inocula; antifungal therapy generally not useful for arthritis or pericarditis; NSAIDs or corticosteroids can be useful in some cases
Mediastinal granulomas	1–50	Most lesions resolve spontaneously; surgery or antifungal therapy with amphotericin B 40–50 mg/day × 2–3 weeks or itraconazole 400 mg/day orally × 6–12 months can be beneficial in some severe cases; mild to moderate disease can be treated with itraconazole for 6–12 months
Moderately severe to severe diffuse pulmonary disease		Lipid amphotericin B 3–5 mg/kg/day followed by itraconazole 200 mg twice daily for 3 days then twice daily for a total of 12 weeks of therapy; alternatively, in patients at low risk for nephrotoxicity, amphotericin B deoxycholate 0.7–1 mg/kg/day can be utilized; methylprednisolone (0.5–1 mg/kg daily IV) during the first 1–2 weeks of antifungal therapy is recommended for patients who develop respiratory complications, including hypoxemia or significant respiratory distress
Inflammatory/fibrotic disease	0.02	*Fibrosing mediastinitis:* The benefit of antifungal therapy (itraconazole 200 mg twice daily × 3 months) is controversial but should be considered, especially in patients with elevated ESR or CF titers ≤1:32; surgery can be of benefit if disease is detected early; late disease cannot respond to therapy *Sarcoid-like:* NSAIDs or corticosteroids[d] can be of benefit for some patients *Pericarditis:* Severe disease: corticosteroids 1 mg/kg/day or pericardial drainage procedure

(continued)

| TABLE 38–1 | Clinical Manifestations and Therapy of Histoplasmosis (*Continued*) |

Type of Disease and Common Clinical Manifestations	Approximate Frequency (%)[a]	Therapy/Comments
Chronic cavitary pulmonary histoplasmosis	0.05	Antifungal therapy generally recommended for all patients to halt further lung destruction and reduce mortality *Mild–moderate disease:* Itraconazole 200 mg three times daily for 3 days and then one or two times daily for at least 1 year; some clinicians recommend therapy for 18–24 months due to the high rate of relapse; itraconazole plasma concentrations should be obtained after the patient has been receiving this agent for at least 2 weeks *Severe disease:* Amphotericin B 0.7 mg/kg/day for a minimum total dose of 25–35 mg/kg is effective in 59%–100% of cases and should be used in patients who require hospitalization or are unable to take itraconazole because of drug interactions, allergies, failure to absorb drug, or failure to improve clinically after a minimum of 12 weeks of itraconazole therapy
Histoplasma endocarditis		Amphotericin B (lipid formulations may be preferred, due to their lower rate of renal toxicity) plus a valve replacement is recommended; if the valve cannot be replaced, lifelong suppression with itraconazole is recommended
CNS histoplasmosis		Amphotericin B should be used as initial therapy (lipid formulations at 5 mg/kg/day, for a total dosage of 175 mg/kg may be preferred, due to their lower rate of renal toxicity) for 4–6 weeks, followed by an oral azole (fluconazole or itraconazole 200 mg two or three times daily) for at least a year; some patients may require lifelong therapy; response to therapy should be monitored by repeat lumbar punctures to assess *Histoplasma* antigen levels, WBC, and CF antibody titers; blood levels of itraconazole should be obtained to ensure adequate drug exposure
Immunosuppressed host		
Disseminated histoplasmosis	0.02–0.05	*Disseminated histoplasmosis:* Untreated mortality 83%–93%; relapse 5%–23% in non-AIDS patients; therapy is recommended for all patients
Acute (Infantile)		*Nonimmunosuppressed patients:* Ketoconazole 400 mg/day orally × 6–12 months or amphotericin B 35 mg/kg IV over 3–4 months
Subacute		*Immunosuppressed patients (non-AIDS) or endocarditis or CNS disease:* Amphotericin B >35 mg/kg over 3 months followed by fluconazole or itraconazole 200 mg orally twice daily × 12 months

(*continued*)

TABLE 38-1	Clinical Manifestations and Therapy of Histoplasmosis (*Continued*)	
Type of Disease and Common Clinical Manifestations	**Approximate Frequency (%)[a]**	**Therapy/Comments**
Progressive histoplasmosis (immunocompetent patients and immunosuppressed patients without AIDS)		*Moderately severe to severe:* Liposomal amphotericin B (3 mg/kg daily), amphotericin B lipid complex (ABLC, 5 mg/kg daily), or deoxycholate amphotericin B (0.7–1 mg/kg daily) for 1–2 weeks, followed by itraconazole (200 mg twice daily for at least 12 months) *Mild to moderate:* Itraconazole (200 mg twice daily for at least 12 months)
Progressive disease of AIDS	25–50[e]	Amphotericin B 15–30 mg/kg (1–2 g over 4–10 weeks)[f] or itraconazole 200 mg three times daily for 3 days then twice daily for 12 weeks, followed by lifelong suppressive therapy with itraconazole 200–400 mg orally daily; although patients receiving secondary prophylaxis (chronic maintenance therapy) might be at low risk for recurrence of systemic mycosis when their $CD4^+$ T-lymphocyte counts increase to >100 cells/μL (>0.1 × 10^9/L) in response to HAART, the number of patients who have been evaluated is insufficient to warrant a recommendation to discontinue prophylaxis

(AIDS, acquired immunodeficiency syndrome; CF, complement fixation; ESR, erythrocyte sedimentation rate; HAART, highly active antiretroviral therapy; NSAIDs, nonsteroidal anti-inflammatory drugs; PO, orally.)

[a]As a percentage of all patients presenting with histoplasmosis.

[b]Itraconazole plasma concentrations should be measured during the second week of therapy to ensure that detectable concentrations have been achieved. If the concentration is below 1 mcg/mL (mg/L; 1.4 μmol/L), the dose may be insufficient or drug interactions can be impairing absorption or accelerating metabolism, requiring a change in dosage. If plasma concentrations are greater than 10 mcg/mL (mg/L; 14 μmol/L), the dosage can be reduced.

[c]Deoxycholate amphotericin B.

[d]Effectiveness of corticosteroids is controversial.

[e]As a percentage of AIDS patients presenting with histoplasmosis as the initial manifestation of their disease.

[f]Liposomal amphotericin B (AmBisome) may be more appropriate for disseminated disease.

- Patients with mild, self-limited disease, chronic disseminated disease, or chronic pulmonary histoplasmosis who have no underlying immunosuppression usually can be treated with either oral itraconazole or IV amphotericin B.
- In AIDS patients, intensive 12-week primary antifungal therapy (induction and consolidation therapy) is followed by lifelong suppressive (maintenance) therapy with itraconazole. Amphotericin B dosages of 50 mg/day (up to 1 mg/kg per day) should be administered IV to a cumulative dose of 15 to 35 mg/kg (1–2 g) in patients who require hospitalization.
- Response to therapy should be measured by resolution of radiologic, serologic, and microbiologic parameters and improvement in signs and symptoms of infection.
- Once the initial course of therapy for histoplasmosis is completed, lifelong suppressive therapy with oral azoles or amphotericin B (1–1.5 mg/kg weekly or biweekly) is recommended, because of the frequent recurrence of infection.
- Relapse rates in AIDS patients not receiving preventive maintenance are 50% to 90%.

BLASTOMYCOSIS

- North American *blastomycosis* is a systemic fungal infection caused by *Blastomyces dermatitidis*.

Clinical Presentation and Diagnosis

- Acute pulmonary blastomycosis is generally an asymptomatic or self-limited disease characterized by fever, shaking chills, and a productive, purulent cough, with or without hemoptysis in immunocompetent individuals.
- Sporadic pulmonary blastomycosis may present as a more chronic or subacute disease, with low-grade fever, night sweats, weight loss, and a productive cough resembling that of TB rather than bacterial pneumonia. Chronic pulmonary blastomycosis is characterized by fever, malaise, weight loss, night sweats, chest pain, and productive cough.
- The simplest and most successful method of diagnosing blastomycosis is by direct microscopic visualization of the large, multinucleated yeast with single, broad-based buds in sputum or other respiratory specimens, following digestion of cells and debris with 10% potassium hydroxide. Histopathologic examination of tissue biopsies and culture of secretions should be used to identify *B. dermatitidis*.

Treatment

- In the immunocompetent host, acute pulmonary blastomycosis can be mild and self-limited and may not require treatment. However, consideration should be given to treating all infected individuals to prevent extrapulmonary dissemination. All individuals with moderate to severe pneumonia, disseminated infection, or those who are immunocompromised require antifungal therapy (**Table 38–2**).
- Some authors recommend azole therapy for the treatment of self-limited pulmonary disease, with the hope of preventing late extrapulmonary disease.
- **Itraconazole**, 200 to 400 mg/day, demonstrated 90% efficacy as a first-line agent in the treatment of non-life-threatening, non-CNS blastomycosis and 95% success rate for compliant patients who completed at least 2 months of therapy.
- All patients with disseminated blastomycosis and those with extrapulmonary disease require therapy.

COCCIDIOIDOMYCOSIS

- *Coccidioidomycosis* is caused by infection with *Coccidioides immitis*. The endemic regions encompass the semiarid areas of the southwestern United States from California to Texas, known as the Lower Sonoran Zone. It encompasses a spectrum of illnesses ranging from primary uncomplicated respiratory tract infection that resolves spontaneously to progressive pulmonary or disseminated infection.

Clinical Presentation and Diagnosis

- Approximately 60% of those infected are asymptomatic or have nonspecific symptoms that are often indistinguishable from those of ordinary upper respiratory infections, including fever, cough, headache, sore throat, myalgias, and fatigue. A fine, diffuse rash may appear during the first few days of illness. Chronic, persistent pneumonia or persistent pulmonary coccidioidomycosis (primary disease lasting >6 weeks) is complicated by hemoptysis, pulmonary scarring, and the formation of cavities or bronchopleural fistulas.
- Disseminated infection occurs in less than 1% of infected patients. Dissemination may occur to the skin, lymph nodes, bone, meninges, spleen, liver, kidney, and adrenal gland. CNS infection occurs in ~16% of patients with disseminated infection.
- The diagnoses of coccidioidomycosis generally utilize identification or recovery of *Coccidioides* spp. from clinical specimens and detection of specific anticoccidioidal antibodies in serum or other body fluids.

Treatment

- Therapy of coccidioidomycosis is difficult, and the results are unpredictable. Only 5% of infected persons require therapy.

TABLE 38–2	Therapy of Blastomycosis
Type of Disease	**Preferred Treatment**
Pulmonary[a]	
Moderately severe to severe disease	Lipid formulation of amphotericin B 3–5 mg/kg IV daily or amphotericin B[b] 0.7–1 mg/kg IV daily (total dose 1.5–2.5 g) × 1–2 weeks or until improvement is noted, followed by itraconazole[c,d] 200 mg orally three times daily for 3 days, then 200 mg twice daily, over a total of 6–12 months
Mild to moderate disease	Itraconazole[c,d] 200 mg orally three times daily for 3 days, then 200 mg twice daily, for a total of 6 months[c]
CNS disease	*Induction:* Lipid formulation of amphotericin B 5 mg/kg IV daily × 4–6 weeks, followed by an oral azole as consolidation therapy *Consolidation:* Fluconazole[d] 800 mg orally daily, or itraconazole[d] 200 mg two or three times orally daily, or voriconazole[d] 200–400 mg orally twice daily, for ≥12 months and until resolution of CSF abnormalities
Disseminated or extrapulmonary disease	
Moderately severe to severe disease	Lipid formulation of amphotericin B 3–5 mg/kg IV daily or amphotericin B[b] 0.7–1 mg/kg IV daily × 1–2 weeks or until improvement is noted, followed by itraconazole[c,d] 200 mg orally three times daily for 3 days, then 200 mg twice daily × 6–12 months. Treat osteoarticular disease with 12 months of antifungal therapy Most clinicians prefer to step-down to itraconazole[d] therapy once the patient's condition improves
Mild to moderate	Itraconazole[c,d] 200 mg orally three times daily for 3 days, then 200 mg once or twice daily × ≥12 months. Treat osteoarticular disease with 12 months of antifungal therapy
Immunocompromised host (including patients with AIDS, transplants, or receiving chronic glucocorticoid therapy)	
Acute disease	Lipid formulation of amphotericin B 3–5 mg/kg IV daily or amphotericin B[b] 0.7–1 mg/kg IV daily × 1–2 weeks or until improvement is noted, then give suppressive therapy for a total of at least 12 months of therapy
Suppressive therapy	Itraconazole[c,d] 200 mg orally three times daily for 3 days, then 200 mg twice daily for a total of at least 12 months of therapy; lifelong suppressive therapy with oral itraconazole[d] 200 mg daily may be required for immunosuppressed patients in whom immunosuppression cannot be reversed, and in patients who experience relapse despite appropriate therapy

(AIDS, acquired immunodeficiency syndrome.)
[a]In the immunocompetent host, acute pulmonary blastomycosis can be mild and self-limited and may not require treatment.
[b]Desoxycholate amphotericin B.
[c]Serum levels of itraconazole should be determined after the patient has received itraconazole for ≥2 weeks, to ensure adequate drug exposure.
[d]Azoles should not be used during pregnancy.

- Azole antifungals, primarily fluconazole and itraconazole, have replaced amphotericin B as initial therapy for most chronic pulmonary or disseminated infections. Specific antifungals (and their usual dosages) for the treatment of coccidioidomycosis include amphotericin B IV (0.5–1.5 mg/kg/day), **ketoconazole** (400 mg orally daily), IV or oral **fluconazole** (usually 400–800 mg daily, although dosages as high as 1200 mg/day have been used without complications), and itraconazole (200–300 mg orally twice daily as either capsules or solution). If itraconazole is used, measurement of serum concentrations may be helpful to ascertain whether oral bioavailability is adequate.
- Amphotericin B is generally preferred as initial therapy in patients with rapidly progressive disease, whereas azoles are generally preferred in patients with subacute or chronic presentations. Lipid formulations of amphotericin B have not been extensively studied for coccidioidomycosis but can offer a means of giving more drugs with less toxicity. Treatments for primary respiratory diseases (mainly symptomatic patients) are 3- to 6-month courses of therapy.
- Patients with disease outside the lungs should be treated with 400 mg/day of an oral azole. For meningeal disease, fluconazole 400 mg/day orally should be used; however, some clinicians initiate therapy with 800 or 1000 mg/day, and itraconazole doses of 400 to 600 mg/day are comparable.

CRYPTOCOCCOSIS

- *Cryptococcosis* is a noncontagious, systemic mycotic infection caused by the ubiquitous encapsulated soil yeast *Cryptococcus neoformans*.

Clinical Presentation and Diagnosis

- Primary cryptococcosis in humans almost always occurs in the lungs. Symptomatic infections are usually manifested by cough, rales, and shortness of breath that generally resolve spontaneously.
- Disease may remain localized in the lungs or disseminate to other tissues, particularly the CNS, although the skin can also be affected.
- In the non-AIDS patient, the symptoms of cryptococcal meningitis are nonspecific. Headache, fever, nausea, vomiting, mental status changes, and neck stiffness are generally observed. In AIDS patients, fever and headache are common, but meningismus and photophobia are much less common than in non-AIDS patients.
- Examination of cerebrospinal fluid (CSF) in patients with cryptococcal meningitis generally reveals an elevated opening pressure, CSF pleocytosis (usually lymphocytes), leukocytosis, a decreased CSF glucose, an elevated CSF protein, and a positive cryptococcal antigen.
- Antigens to *C. neoformans* can be detected by latex agglutination. *C. neoformans* can be detected in ~60% of patients by India ink smear of CSF and cultured in more than 96% of patients.

Treatment

- Treatment of cryptococcosis is detailed in Table 38–3. For asymptomatic, immunocompetent persons with isolated pulmonary disease and no evidence of CNS disease, careful observation may be warranted. With symptomatic infection, **fluconazole** for 6 to 12 months is warranted.
- The use of intrathecal **amphotericin B** is not recommended for the treatment of cryptococcal meningitis except in very ill patients or in those with recurrent or progressive disease despite aggressive IV amphotericin B therapy. The dosage of amphotericin B employed is usually 0.5 mg administered via the lumbar, cisternal, or intraventricular (via an Ommaya reservoir) route two or three times weekly.
- **Amphotericin B** with **flucytosine** is the initial treatment of choice for acute therapy of cryptococcal meningitis in AIDS patients. Many clinicians will initiate therapy with amphotericin B, 0.7 to 1 mg/kg/day IV (with flucytosine, 100 mg/kg/day). After 2 weeks, consolidation therapy with **fluconazole** 400 mg/day orally can be administered for 8 weeks or until CSF cultures are negative.

369

TABLE 38–3 Therapy of Cryptococcosis[a,b]

Type of Disease and Common Clinical Manifestations	Therapy/Comments
Nonimmunocompromised patients (non–HIV-infected, nontransplant)	
Meningoencephalitis *without* neurological complications, in patients in whom CSF yeast cultures are negative after 2 weeks of therapy	*Induction:* Amphotericin B[c] IV 0.7–1 mg/kg/day *plus* flucytosine 100 mg/kg/day orally in four divided doses × ≥4 weeks A lipid formulation of amphotericin B may be substituted for amphotericin B in the second 2 weeks
Follow all regimens with suppressive therapy	*Consolidation:* Fluconazole 400–800 mg orally daily × 8 weeks *Maintenance:* Fluconazole 200 mg orally daily × 6–12 months
Meningoencephalitis *with* neurological complications	*Induction:* Same as for patients without neurologic complications, but consider extending the induction therapy for a total of 6 weeks. A lipid formulation of amphotericin B may be given for the last 4 weeks of the prolonged induction period *Consolidation:* Fluconazole 400 mg orally daily × 8 weeks
Mild-to-moderate pulmonary disease (Nonmeningeal disease)	Fluconazole 400 mg orally daily × 6–12 months
Severe pulmonary cryptococcosis	*Same as CNS disease × 12 months*
Cryptococcemia (nonmeningeal, nonpulmonary disease)	*Same as CNS disease × 12 months*
Immunocompromised patients	
Severe pulmonary cryptococcosis	*Same as CNS disease × 12 months*
HIV-infected patients	
Primary therapy; induction and consolidation[g]	*Preferred regimen:* *Induction:* Amphotericin B[d] IV 0.7–1 mg/kg IV daily *plus* flucytosine 100 mg/kg/day orally in four divided doses for ≥2 weeks
Follow all regimens with suppressive therapy	*Consolidation:* Fluconazole 400 mg [6 mg/kg] orally daily × ≥8 weeks Liposomal amphotericin B 3–4 mg/kg IV daily, or amphotericin B lipid complex (ABLC) 5 mg/kg IV daily, for ≥2 weeks can be substituted for amphotericin B[d] in patients with or at risk for renal dysfunction *Alternative regimens, in order of preference:* Amphotericin B[d] IV 0.7–1 mg/kg IV daily × 4–6 weeks *or* liposomal amphotericin B 3–4 mg/kg IV daily[f] × 4–6 weeks *or* ABLC 5 mg/kg IV daily × 4–6 weeks *or* Amphotericin B[d] IV 0.7 mg/kg IV daily, *plus* fluconazole 800 mg (12 mg/kg) orally daily × 2 weeks, followed by fluconazole 800 mg (12 mg/kg) orally daily × ≥8weeks *or* Fluconazole ≥800 mg (1200 mg/day is preferred) orally daily *plus* flucytosine 100 mg/kg/day orally in four divided doses × 6 weeks

(continued)

TABLE 38–3 Therapy of Cryptococcosis[a,b] *(Continued)*

Type of Disease and Common Clinical Manifestations	Therapy/Comments
	or Fluconazole 800–1200 mg/day orally daily × 10–12 weeks (a dosage ≥1200 mg/day is preferred when fluconazole is used alone)[e] *or* Itraconazole 200 mg orally twice daily × 10–12 weeks (use of itraconazole, which produces minimal concentrations of active drug in the CSF is discouraged)[i]
Suppressive/maintenance therapy[h]	Preferred: Fluconazole 200 mg orally daily × ≥1 year *or* Itraconazole[i] 200 mg orally twice daily × ≥1 year *or* Amphotericin B[j] IV 1 mg/kg weekly × ≥1 year
Organ transplant recipients	
Mild-moderate non-CNS disease or mild-to-moderate symptoms without diffuse pulmonary infiltrates	Fluconazole 400 mg (6 mg/kg) orally daily × 6–12 months
CNS disease, moderately severe or severe CNS disease or disseminated disease without CNS disease, or severe pulmonary disease without evidence of extrapulmonary or disseminated disease	*Induction:* Liposomal amphotericin B 3–4 mg/kg IV daily,[f] or ABLC 5 mg/kg IV daily *plus* flucytosine 100 mg/kg/day orally in four divided doses × ≥2 weeks If induction therapy does not include flucytosine, consider a lipid formulation of amphotericin B for ≥4–6 weeks of induction therapy. Consider the use of a lipid formulation of amphotericin B lipid formulation (6 mg/kg IV daily) in patients with a high-fungal burden disease or relapse of disease *Consolidation:* Fluconazole 400–800 mg (6–12 mg/kg) per day orally for 8 weeks *Maintenance:* Fluconazole 200–400 mg per day orally for 6–12 months

(HIV, human immunodeficiency virus; IT, intrathecal.)

[a]When more than one therapy is listed, they are listed in order of preference.
[b]See the text for definitions of induction, consolidation, suppressive/maintenance therapy, and prophylactic therapy.
[c]Deoxycholate amphotericin B.
[d]In patients with significant renal disease, lipid formulations of amphotericin B can be substituted for deoxycholate amphotericin B during the induction.
[e]Or until cerebrospinal fluid (CSF) cultures are negative.
[f]Liposomal amphotericin B has been given safely up to 6 mg/kg daily; could be considered in treatment failure or in patients with a high fungal burden.
[g]Initiate HAART therapy 2–10 weeks after commencement of initial antifungal treatment.
[h]Consider discontinuing suppressive therapy during HAART in patients with a CD4 cell count ≥100 cells/μL (≥0.1 × 10⁹/L) and an undetectable or very low HIV RNA level sustained for ≥3months (with a minimum of 12 months of antifungal therapy). Consider reinstitution of maintenance therapy if the CD4 cell count decreases to <100 cells/μL (<0.1 × 10⁹/L).
[i]Drug level monitoring is strongly advised.
[j]Use is discouraged except in azole intolerant patients, since it is less effective than azole therapy, and is associated with a risk of IV catheter-related infections.

- Relapse of *C. neoformans* meningitis occurs in ~50% of AIDS patients after completion of primary therapy. HIV-infected patients requiring chronic suppressive therapy of cryptococcal meningitis can receive **Fluconazole** (200 mg daily) for chronic suppressive therapy.

CANDIDA INFECTIONS

- Eight species of *Candida* are regarded as clinically important pathogens in human disease: *C. albicans*, *C. tropicalis*, *C. parapsilosis*, *C. krusei*, *C. stellatoidea*, *C. guilliermondii*, *C. lusitaniae*, and *C. glabrata*.

Hematogenous candidiasis

- Dissemination of *C. albicans* can result in infection in single or multiple organs, particularly the kidney, brain, myocardium, skin, eye, bone, and joints
- *Candida* is generally acquired via the gastrointestinal (GI) tract, although organisms may also enter the bloodstream via indwelling IV catheters. Immunosuppressed patients, including those with lymphoreticular or hematologic malignancies, diabetes, immunodeficiency diseases, or those receiving immunosuppressive therapy with high-dose corticosteroids, immunosuppressants, antineoplastic agents, or broad-spectrum antimicrobial agents are at high risk for invasive fungal infections. Major risk factors include the use of central venous catheters, total parenteral nutrition, receipt of multiple antibiotics, extensive surgery and burns, renal failure and hemodialysis, mechanical ventilation, and prior fungal colonization.
- Treatment of candidiasis is presented in Table 38–4.

ASPERGILLUS INFECTIONS

- Aspergillus fumigatus is the most commonly observed pathogen, followed by Aspergillus flavus.
- Invasive aspergillosis commonly affects immunocompromised patients and patients with acute myeloid leukemia (AML) and those who undergo allogeneic HSCT who have prolonged durations (more than 10 days) of neutropenia. Aspergillosis is generally acquired by inhalation of airborne conidia that are small enough (2.5–3 mm) to reach the alveoli or the paranasal sinuses.
- Superficial or locally invasive infections of the ear, skin, or appendages can often be managed with topical antifungal therapy.

Allergic Bronchopulmonary Aspergillosis

- Allergic manifestations of *Aspergillus* range in severity from mild asthma to allergic bronchopulmonary aspergillosis characterized by severe asthma with wheezing, fever, malaise, weight loss, chest pain, and a cough productive of blood-streaked sputum.
- Therapy is aimed at minimizing the quantity of antigenic material released in the tracheobronchial tree.
- Antifungal therapy is generally not indicated in the management of allergic manifestations of aspergillosis, although some patients have demonstrated a decrease in their glucocorticoid dose following therapy with itraconazole.

Aspergilloma

- In the nonimmunocompromised host, *Aspergillus* infections of the sinuses most commonly occur as saprophytic colonization (aspergillomas, or "fungus balls") of previously abnormal sinus tissue. Treatment consists of removal of the aspergilloma. Therapy with glucocorticoids and surgery is generally successful.
- Although IV amphotericin B is generally not useful in eradicating aspergillomas, intracavitary instillation of amphotericin B has been employed successfully in a limited number of patients. Hemoptysis generally ceases when the aspergilloma is eradicated.

TABLE 38–4	Antifungal Therapy of Invasive Candidiasis

Type of Disease and Common Clinical Manifestations	Therapy/Comments
Prophylaxis of candidemia	
Nonneutropenic patients[a]	Not recommended except for severely ill/high-risk patients in whom fluconazole IV/oral 400 mg daily should be used (see the text)
Neutropenic patients[a]	The optimal duration of therapy is unclear but at a minimum should include the period at risk for neutropenia: Fluconazole IV/oral 400 mg daily *or* itraconazole solution 2.5 mg/kg every 12 hours orally *or* micafungin 50 mg (1 mg/kg in patients under 50 kg) IV daily
Solid-organ transplantation, liver transplantation	*Patients with two or more key risk factors[b]:* Amphotericin B IV 10–20 mg daily *or* liposomal amphotericin B (AmBisome) 1 mg/kg/day *or* fluconazole 400 mg orally daily
Empirical (preemptive) antifungal therapy	
Suspected disseminated candidiasis in febrile nonneutropenic patients	None recommended; data are lacking defining subsets of patients who are appropriate for therapy (see the text)
Initial antifungal therapy (documented Candidemia with unknown Candida species)	
Febrile neutropenic patients with prolonged fever despite 4–6 days of empirical antibacterial therapy	*Treatment duration:* Until resolution of neutropenia An echinocandin[d] is a reasonable alternative; voriconazole can be used in selected situations (see the text)
Less critically ill patients with no recent azole exposure	An echinocandin[d] or fluconazole (loading dose of 800 mg [12 mg/kg], then 400 mg [6 mg/kg] daily)
Additional mold coverage is desired	Voriconazole
Antifungal therapy of documented Candidemia and acute hematogenously disseminated Candidiasis, unknown species	
Nonimmunocompromised host[c]	*Treatment duration:* 2 weeks after the last positive blood culture and resolution of signs and symptoms of infection *Remove existing central venous catheters when feasible plus fluconazole (loading dose of 800 mg [12 mg/kg], then 400 mg [6 mg/kg] daily) or an echinocandin[d]*
Patients with recent azole exposure, moderately severe or severe illness, or who are at high risk of infection due to *C. glabrata* or *C. krusei*	An echinocandin[d] Transition from an echinocandin to fluconazole is recommended for patients who are clinically stable and have isolates (eg, *C. albicans*) likely to be susceptible to fluconazole
Patients who are less critically ill and who have had no recent azole exposure	Fluconazole

(continued)

TABLE 38–4 Antifungal Therapy of Invasive Candidiasis (*Continued*)

Type of Disease and Common Clinical Manifestations	Therapy/Comments
Antifungal therapy of specific pathogens	

C. albicans, C. tropicalis, and *C. parapsilosis*	Fluconazole IV/oral 6 mg/kg/day *or* an echinocandin[d] or amphotericin B IV 0.7 mg/kg/day *plus* fluconazole IV/orally 800 mg/day; amphotericin B deoxycholate 0.5–1 mg/kg daily or a lipid formulation of amphotericin B (3–5 mg/kg daily) are alternatives in patients who are intolerant to other antifungals; transition from amphotericin B deoxycholate or a lipid formulation of amphotericin B to fluconazole is recommended in patients who are clinically stable and whose isolates are likely to be susceptible to fluconazole (eg, *C. albicans*); voriconazole (400 mg [6 mg/kg] twice daily × two doses then 200 mg [3 mg/kg] twice daily thereafter) is efficacious, but offers little advantage over fluconazole; it may be utilized as step-down oral therapy for selected cases of candidiasis due to *C. krusei* or voriconazole-susceptible *C. glabrata*
	Patients intolerant or refractory to other therapy[e]*:*
	  Amphotericin B lipid complex IV 5 mg/kg/day
	  Liposomal amphotericin B IV 3–5 mg/kg/day
	  Amphotericin B colloid dispersion IV 2–6 mg/kg/day

C. krusei	Amphotericin B IV ≤1 mg/kg/day *or* an echinocandin[d]
C. lusitaniae	Fluconazole IV/orally 6 mg/kg/day
C. glabrata	An echinocandin[d] (transition to fluconazole or voriconazole therapy is not recommended without confirmation of isolate susceptibility)
Neutropenic host[f]	*Treatment duration:* Until resolution of neutropenia *Remove existing central venous catheters when feasible, plus:* Amphotericin B IV 0.7–1 mg/kg/day (total dosages 0.5–1 g) *or patients failing therapy with traditional amphotericin B:* Lipid formulation of amphotericin B IV 3–5 mg/kg/day
Chronic disseminated candidiasis (hepatosplenic candidiasis)	*Treatment duration:* Until calcification or resolution of lesions *Stable patients:* Fluconazole IV/orally 6 mg/kg/day *Acutely ill or refractory patients:* Amphotericin B IV 0.6–0.7 mg/kg/day

(*continued*)

TABLE 38–4	Antifungal Therapy of Invasive Candidiasis (*Continued*)
Type of Disease and Common Clinical Manifestations	**Therapy/Comments**
Urinary candidiasis	*Asymptomatic disease:* Generally no therapy is required *Symptomatic or high-risk patients*[g]: Removal of urinary tract instruments, stents, and Foley catheters, +7–14 days therapy with fluconazole 200 mg orally daily *or* amphotericin B IV 0.3–1 mg/kg/day

(PO, orally.)

[a]Patients at significant risk for invasive candidiasis include those receiving standard chemotherapy for acute myelogenous leukemia, allogeneic bone marrow transplants, or high-risk autologous bone marrow transplants. However, among these populations, chemotherapy or bone marrow transplant protocols do not all produce equivalent risk, and local experience should be used to determine the relevance of prophylaxis.

[b]Risk factors include retransplantation, creatinine of more than 2 mg/dL (177 μmol/L), choledocho-jejunostomy, intraoperative use of 40 units or more of blood products, and fungal colonization detected within the first 3 days after transplantation.

[c]Therapy is generally the same for acquired immunodeficiency syndrome (AIDS)/non-AIDS patients except where indicated and should continued for 2 weeks after the last positive blood culture and resolution of signs and symptoms of infection. All patients should receive an ophthalmologic examination. Amphotericin B can be switched to fluconazole (IV or oral) for the completion of therapy. Susceptibility testing of the infecting isolate is a useful adjunct to species identification during selection of a therapeutic approach because it can be used to identify isolates that are unlikely to respond to fluconazole or amphotericin B. However, this is not currently available at most institutions.

[d]Echinocandin = caspofungin 70 mg loading dose, then 50 mg IV daily maintenance dose, or micafungin 100 mg daily, or anidulafungin 200 mg loading dose, then 100 mg daily maintenance dose.

[e]Often defined as failure of ≥500 mg amphotericin B, initial renal insufficiency (creatinine ≥2.5 mg/dL [≥221 μmol/L] or creatinine clearance <25 mL/min [< 0.42 mL/s]), a significant increase in creatinine (to 2.5 mg/dL [221 μmol/L] for adults or 1.5 mg/dL [133 μmol/L] for children), or severe acute administration-related toxicity.

[f]Patients who are neutropenic at the time of developing candidemia should receive a recombinant cytokine (granulocyte colony-stimulating factor or granulocyte–monocyte colony-stimulating factor) that accelerates recovery from neutropenia.

[g]Patients at high risk for dissemination include neutropenic patients, low-birth-weight infants, patients with renal allografts, and patients who will undergo urologic manipulation.

Invasive Aspergillosis

- Patients often present with classic signs and symptoms of acute pulmonary embolus: pleuritic chest pain, fever, hemoptysis, a friction rub, and a wedge-shaped infiltrate on chest radiographs.
- Demonstration of *Aspergillus* by repeated culture and microscopic examination of tissue provides the most firm diagnosis.
- In the immunocompromised host, aspergillosis is characterized by vascular invasion leading to thrombosis, infarction, and necrosis of tissue.

Treatment

- Voriconazole is the drug of choice for primary therapy of most patients with aspergillosis as it provided improved survival and fewer side effects.
- In patients who cannot tolerate voriconazole, amphotericin B can be used. Full doses (1–1.5 mg/kg/day) are generally recommended, with response measured by defervescence and radiographic clearing. The lipid-based formulations may be preferred as initial therapy in patients with marginal renal function or in patients receiving other nephrotoxic drugs. The optimal duration of treatment is unknown.

- **Caspofungin** is indicated for treatment of invasive aspergillosis in patients who are refractory to or intolerant of other therapies such as amphotericin B.
- The use of prophylactic antifungal therapy to prevent primary infection or reactivation of aspergillosis during subsequent courses of chemotherapy is controversial.

See Chapter 121 Invasive Fungal Infections, authored by Peggy L. Carver, for a more detailed discussion of this topic.

39 Gastrointestinal Infections

- *Gastrointestinal* (GI) infections are among the more common causes of morbidity and mortality around the world. Most are caused by viruses, and some are caused by bacteria or other organisms. In underdeveloped and developing countries, acute gastroenteritis involving diarrhea is the leading cause of mortality in infants and children younger than 5 years of age. In the United States, there are 179 million episodes of acute gastroenteritis each year, causing over 600,000 hospitalizations and over 5000 deaths.
- Public health measures such as clean water supply and sanitation facilities, as well as quality control of commercial products are important for the control of most enteric infections. Sanitary food handling and preparation practices significantly decrease the incidence of enteric infections.

REHYDRATION, ANTIMOTILITY, AND PROBIOTIC THERAPY

- Treatment of dehydration includes rehydration, replacement of ongoing losses, and continuation of normal feeding. Fluid replacement is the cornerstone of therapy for diarrhea regardless of etiology.
- Initial assessment of fluid loss is essential for rehydration. Weight loss is the most reliable means of determining the extent of water loss. Clinical signs such as changes in skin turgor, sunken eyes, dry mucous membranes, decreased tearing, decreased urine output, altered mentation, and changes in vital signs can be helpful in determining approximate deficits (Table 39–1).
- The necessary components of oral rehydration solution (ORS) include glucose, sodium, potassium chloride, and water (Table 39–2). ORS should be given in small frequent volumes (5 mL every 2–3 min) in a teaspoon or oral syringe.
- Severely dehydrated patients should be resuscitated initially with lactated Ringer solution or normal intravenous (IV) saline. Guidelines for rehydration therapy based on the degree of dehydration and replacement of ongoing losses are outlined in Table 39–1.
- Early refeeding as tolerated is recommended. Age-appropriate diet may be resumed as soon as dehydration is corrected. Early initiation of feeding shortens the course of diarrhea. Initially, easily digested foods, such as bananas, applesauce, and cereal may be added as tolerated. Foods high in fiber, sodium, and sugar should be avoided.
- Antimotility drugs such as **diphenoxylate** and **loperamide** offer symptomatic relief in patients with watery diarrhea by reducing the number of stools. Antimotility drugs are not recommended in patients with many toxin-mediated dysenteric diarrheas (ie, enterohemorrhagic *Escherichia coli* [EHEC], pseudomembranous colitis, and shigellosis).
- Individual studies have not shown significant benefit from probiotics and meta-analyses have shown conflicting results. Probiotics should not be recommended for prophylaxis or treatment of initial antibiotic-associated diarrhea.

BACTERIAL INFECTIONS

- Antibiotic therapy is recommended in severe cases of diarrhea, moderate-to-severe cases of traveler's diarrhea, most cases of febrile dysenteric diarrhea, and culture-proven bacterial diarrhea. Antibiotics are not essential in the treatment of most mild diarrheas, and empirical therapy for acute GI infections may result in unnecessary antibiotic courses. Antibiotic choices for bacterial infections are given in Table 39–3.

TABLE 39–1	Clinical Assessment of Degree of Dehydration in Children Based on Percentage of Body Weight Loss[a]		
Variable	Minimal or No Dehydration (<3% Loss of Body Weight)	Mild to Moderate (3%–9% Loss of Body Weight)	Severe (≥10% Loss of Body Weight)
Blood pressure	Normal	Normal	Normal to reduced
Quality of pulses	Normal	Normal or slightly decreased	Weak, thready, or not palpable
Heart rate	Normal	Normal to increased	Increased (bradycardia in severe cases)
Breathing	Normal	Normal to fast	Deep
Mental status	Normal	Normal to listless	Apathetic, lethargic, or comatose
Eyes	Normal	Sunken orbits/ decreased tears	Deeply sunken orbits/absent tears
Mouth and tongue	Moist	Dry	Parched
Thirst	Normal	Eager to drink	Drinks poorly; too lethargic to drink
Skin fold	Normal	Recoil in <2 seconds	Recoil in >2 seconds
Extremities	Warm, normal capillary refill	Cool, prolonged capillary refill	Cold, mottled, cyanotic, prolonged capillary refill
Urine output	Normal to decreased	Decreased	Minimal
Hydration therapy	None	ORS 50–100 mL/kg over 3–4 hours	Lactated Ringer's solution or normal saline 20 mL/kg over 15–30 minutes IV until mental status or perfusion improves. Followed by 5% dextrose/ 0.45% sodium chloride IV at higher maintenance rates or ORS 100 mL/kg over 4 hours.
Replacement of ongoing losses	For each diarrheal stool or emesis <10 kg body weight: 60–120 mL ORS >10 kg body weight: 120–240 mL ORS	Same as minimal dehydration	If unable to tolerate ORS, administer through nasogastric tube or administer 5% dextrose/0.45% sodium chloride with 20 mEq/L (20 mmol/L) potassium chloride IV

(ORS, oral rehydration solution.)
[a]Percentages vary among authors for each dehydration category; hemodynamic and perfusion status is most important; when unsure of category, therapy for more severe category is recommended.

TABLE 39–2	Comparison of Common Solutions Used in Oral Rehydration and Maintenance				
Product	Na (mEq/L)[b]	K (mEq/L)[b]	Base (mEq/L)	Carbohydrate (mmol/L)	Osmolarity (mOsm/L)
WHO/UNICEF (2002)	75	20	30	75	245
Pedialyte	45	20	30	140	250
Infalyte	50	25	30	70	200
Oralyte	60	20	0	90	260
Rehydralyte	75	20	30	140	250
Cola[a]	2	0	13	700	750
Apple juice[a]	5	32	0	690	730s
Chicken broth[a]	250	8	0	0	500
Sports beverage[a]	20	3	3	255	330

[a]These solutions should be avoided in dehydration.
[b]Concentration of monovalent ions expressed in mEq/L is numerically equivalent to mmol/L concentration.

TABLE 39–3	Recommendations for Antibiotic Therapy	
Pathogen	Children	Adults
Watery diarrhea		
Enterotoxigenic Escherichia coli	Azithromycin 10 mg/kg/day given orally once daily × 3 days; ceftriaxone 50 mg/kg/day given IV once daily × 3 days	Ciprofloxacin 750 mg orally once daily × 1–3 days. Alternatives: rifaximin 200 mg orally three times daily × 3 days; azithromycin 1000 mg orally × 1 day or 500 mg orally daily × 3 days
Vibrio cholerae O1	Erythromycin 30 mg/kg/day divided every 8 hours orally × 3 days; azithromycin 10 mg/kg/day given orally once daily × 3 days	Doxycycline 300 mg orally × 1 day Alternatives: tetracycline 500 mg orally four times daily × 3 days; erythromycin 250 mg orally every 8 hours × 3 days; azithromycin 500 mg orally once daily × 3 days
Dysenteric diarrhea		
Campylobacter species[a]	Azithromycin 10 mg/kg/day given orally once daily × 3–5 days; erythromycin 30 mg/kg/day divided into two to four doses orally × 3–5 days	Azithromycin 500 mg orally once daily × 3 days; erythromycin 500 mg orally every 6 hours × 3 days
Salmonella Nontyphoidal[a]	Ceftriaxone 100 mg/kg/day divided IV every 12 hours × 7–10 days; azithromycin 20 mg/kg/day orally once daily × 7 days	Ciprofloxacin 750 mg orally once daily × 7–10 days; levofloxacin 500 mg orally once daily × 7–10 days Alternatives: azithromycin 500 mg orally once daily × 7 days For immunocompromised patients, duration should be increased to 14 days for both fluoroquinolones and azithromycin

(continued)

TABLE 39–3	Recommendations for Antibiotic Therapy (*Continued*)	
Pathogen	**Children**	**Adults**
Shigella species[a]	Azithromycin 10 mg/kg/day given orally once daily × 3 days; ceftriaxone 50 mg/kg/day given IV once daily × 3 days	Ciprofloxacin 750 mg orally once daily × 3 days; levofloxacin 500 mg orally once daily × 3 days Alternatives: azithromycin 500 mg orally once daily × 3 days
Yersinia species[a]	Treat as shigellosis	Treat as shigellosis
Clostridium difficile-associated diarrhea		
Clostridium difficile	Metronidazole 7.5 mg/kg (maximum: 500 mg) orally or IV every 8 hours × 10–14 days; vancomycin 10 mg/kg (maximum: 125 mg) orally every 6 hours × 10–14 days	Mild to moderate disease: metronidazole 500 mg orally or IV every 8 hours daily × 10–14 days Severe disease: vancomycin 125 mg orally every 6 hours × 10–14 days Alternatives: fidaxomicin 200 mg orally every 12 hours × 10–14 days
Traveler's diarrhea		
Prophylaxis[a]		Norfloxacin 400 mg or ciprofloxacin 750 mg orally daily; rifaximin 200 mg one to three times daily up to 2 weeks
Treatment		Ciprofloxacin 750 mg orally × 1 day or 500 mg orally every 12 hours × 3 days; levofloxacin 1000 mg orally × 1 day or 500 mg orally daily × 3 days; rifaximin 200 mg three times daily × 3 days; azithromycin 1000 mg orally × 1 day or 500 mg orally daily × 3 days

[a]For high-risk patients only. See the preceding text for the high-risk patients in each infection.

- Common pathogens responsible for watery diarrhea in the United States are norovirus and ETEC, while those most commonly associated with dysentery diarrhea are Campylobacter spp., EHEC, Salmonella spp., and Shigella sppc *E. coli*. ETEC is also the most common cause of traveler's diarrhea and a common cause of food- and water-associated outbreaks Cholera is caused by toxigenic *Vibrio cholera*.

TRAVELER'S DIARRHEA

- Traveler's diarrhea describes the clinical syndrome caused by contaminated food or water that is manifested by malaise, anorexia, and abdominal cramps followed by the sudden onset of diarrhea that incapacitates many travelers.
- The most common pathogens are bacterial in nature and include enterotoxigenic *Escherichia coli* (ETEC) (20%–72%), Shigella (3%–25%), Campylobacter (3%–17%), and Salmonella (3%–7%). Viruses (up to 30%) are also potential causes, as are parasites.
- Although the efficacy of prophylactic antibiotics has been documented, their use is not recommended for most travelers due to the potential side effects of antibiotics. Prophylactic antibiotics are recommended only in high-risk individuals or in situations in which short-term illness could ruin the purpose of the trip, such as a military mission. A fluoroquinolone is the drug of choice when traveling to most areas of the world. Azithromycin can be considered when traveling to South and Southeast Asia.

Bismuth subsalicylate 524 mg (2 tablets or 2 tablespoonfuls) orally four times daily for up to 3 weeks is a commonly recommended prophylactic regimen.

- The goals of treatment of traveler's diarrhea are to avoid dehydration, reduce the severity and duration of symptoms, and prevent interruption to planned activities.
- Fluid and electrolyte replacement should be initiated at the onset of diarrhea.
- Antibiotics used for treatment are found in Table 39–3.
- For symptom relief, **loperamide** (preferred because of its quicker onset and longer duration of relief relative to bismuth) may be taken (4 mg orally initially and then 2 mg with each subsequent loose stool to a maximum of 16 mg/day in patients without bloody diarrhea and fever). Loperamide should be discontinued if symptoms persist for more than 48 hours. Other symptomatic therapy in mild diarrhea includes bismuth subsalicylate 524 mg every 30 minutes for up to eight doses. There is insufficient evidence to warrant the recommendation of probiotics.

Clostridium difficile

- *Clostridium difficile* is the most commonly recognized cause of infectious diarrhea in healthcare settings with high rates of disease in long-term care facilities and in the elderly. CDI is associated with use of broad-spectrum antimicrobials and accounts for approximately 20% to 30% of all cases of antibiotic-associated diarrhea. The antibiotics most commonly associated with CDI include clindamycin, ampicillin, cephalosporins, and fluoroquinolones.
- Those at high risk for *C. difficile* infection (CDI) include the elderly or debilitated, patients undergoing surgery or nasogastric intubation, those with cancer, and those receiving antibiotics, proton pump inhibitors (PPIs), or frequent laxatives.
- The spectrum of disease ranges from mild diarrhea to life-threatening toxic megacolon and pseudomembranous enterocolitis. Fulminant disease is characterized by severe abdominal pain, perfuse diarrhea, high fever, marked leukocytosis, and classic pseudomembrane formation evident with sigmoidoscopic examination.
- Diagnosis is established by detection of toxin A or B in the stool, stool culture for *C. difficile*, or endoscopy.
- Once determination of disease severity has been made, treatment should be initiated with an antibiotic effective against *C. difficile*. Metronidazole, vancomycin, and fidaxomicin are the most commonly prescribed agents. Initial therapy should also include discontinuation of the offending agent. The patient should be supported with fluid and electrolyte replacement.
- **Metronidazole,** 250 mg orally four times daily or 500 mg three times daily for 10 to 14 days, is the drug of choice for mild to moderate CDI. In patients with severe disease, contraindication or intolerance to metronidazole, and inadequate response to metronidazole, oral vancomycin, or fidaxomicin is recommended. In patients with severe or complicated CDI, practice guidelines suggest combination therapy with IV metronidazole and vancomycin.
- Relapse can occur in 25% of patients within 30 days. Management of a first relapse is identical to the primary episode. The optimal management of multiple relapses is not clear. Fecal transplantation is sometimes used.
- A prolonged tapered and pulse-dosing of oral vancomycin has been suggested for second episodes of relapse. Other regimens that have shown efficacy include stepped therapy with vancomycin followed by rifaximin. Alternative treatments effective against CDI include intravenous immunoglobulin (IVIG) and fecal microbiota transplantation (FMT)

VIRAL INFECTIONS

- Viruses are now recognized as the leading cause of diarrhea in the world.
- In infants and children rotavirus, a double-stranded, wheel-shaped RNA virus is the most common cause of diarrhea worldwide and 1 million people die annually from the infection.

TABLE 39–4	Characteristics of Agents Responsible for Acute Viral Gastroenteritis				
Virus	Peak Age of Onset	Time of Year	Duration	Mode of Transmission	Common Symptoms
Rotavirus	6 months to 2 years	October to April	3–7 days	Fecal–oral, water, food	Nausea, vomiting, diarrhea, fever, abdominal pain, lactose intolerance
Norovirus	All age groups	Peak in winter	2–3 days	Fecal–oral, food, water, environment	Nausea, vomiting, diarrhea, abdominal cramps, myalgia
Astrovirus	<7 years	Winter	1–4 days	Fecal–oral, water, shellfish	Diarrhea, headache, malaise, nausea
Enteric adenovirus	<2 years	Year-round	7–9 days	Fecal–oral	Diarrhea, respiratory symptoms, vomiting, fever
Pestivirus	<2 years	NR	3 days	NR	Mild
Coronavirus-like particles	<2 years	Fall and early winter	7 days	NR	Respiratory disease
Enterovirus	NR	NR	NR	NR	Mild diarrhea, secondary organ damage

(NR, not reported.)

- In the United States, routine rotavirus vaccination is recommended for all infants beginning at age 2 months. There are two vaccines, RotaTeq (RV5) and Rotarix (RV1) available for reducing rotaviral gastroenteritis.
- Characteristics of agents responsible for viral gastroenteritis are found in **Table 39–4**.

See Chapter 113, Gastrointestinal Infections and Enterotoxigenic Poisonings, authored by Andrew Roecker, Brittany Bates, and Steven Martin for a more detailed discussion of this topic.

- Table 40–1 presents the case definition for adult, adolescent, and children, respectively, for *human immunodeficiency virus* (HIV) infection.

ETIOLOGY AND PATHOGENESIS

- Infection with HIV occurs through three primary modes: sexual, parenteral, and perinatal. Sexual intercourse, primarily anal and vaginal intercourse, is the most common vehicle for transmission. The highest risk appears to be from receptive anorectal intercourse at about 1.4 transmissions per 100 sexual acts. Condom use reduces the risk of transmission by approximately 80%. Individuals with genital ulcers or sexually transmitted diseases are at great risk for contracting HIV.
- The risk of HIV transmission from sharing needles is approximately 0.67 per 100 episodes.
- Healthcare workers have a small risk of occupationally acquiring HIV, mostly through accidental injury, most often percutaneous needlestick injury.
- Perinatal infection, or vertical transmission, is the most common cause of pediatric HIV infection. The risk of mother-to-child transmission is ~25% in the absence of antiretroviral therapy. Breast-feeding can also transmit HIV.

CLINICAL PRESENTATION AND DIAGNOSIS

- Clinical presentations of primary HIV infection vary, but patients often have a viral syndrome or mononucleosis-like illness with fever, pharyngitis, and adenopathy (Table 40–2). Symptoms may last for 2 weeks.
- Most children born with HIV are asymptomatic. On physical examination, they often present with unexplained physical signs such as lymphadenopathy, hepatomegaly, splenomegaly, failure to thrive, weight loss or unexplained low birth weight, and fever of unknown origin. Laboratory findings include anemia, hypergammaglobulinemia, altered mononuclear cell function, and altered T-cell subset ratios. The normal range for CD4 cell counts in children is much different than for adults.
- Clinical presentations of the opportunistic infections are presented in Infectious Complications of HIV below.
- The probability of progression to AIDS is related to RNA viral load; viral load is a major prognostic factor for disease progression, CD4 count decline, and death.
- The presence of HIV infection is screened with an enzyme-linked immunosorbent assay (ELISA), which detects antibodies against HIV-1. Positive screening tests are confirmed with another enzyme immunoassay to specify if the antibodies are to HIV-1 versus HIV-2. Rare false-positive results can occur particularly in those with autoimmune disorders. False-negative results also occur and may be attributed to the "window-period" before adequate production of antibodies or antigen.
- Once diagnosed, HIV disease is monitored primarily by two surrogate biomarkers, viral load and CD4 cell count. The viral load test quantifies viremia by measuring the amount of viral RNA. There are several methods used for determining the amount of HIV RNA: reverse transcriptase–coupled polymerase chain reaction, branched DNA, transcription-mediated amplification, and nucleic acid sequence–based assay.
- The number of CD4 lymphocytes in the blood is a surrogate marker of disease progression. The normal adult CD4 lymphocyte count ranges between 500 and 1600 cells/mm^3 (500 and 1600 $\times$ 10^6/L), or 40% to 70% of all lymphocytes.

TABLE 40–1	Surveillance Case Definition for HIV Infection Stage Based on CD4+ T-lymphocyte Counts, United States, 2014

	Age on date of CD4+ T-lymphocyte test					
	<1 year		**1–5 years**		**≥6 years**	
Stage	Cells/μL (×10⁶/L)	%	Cells/μL (×10⁶/L)	%	Cells/μL (×10⁶/L)	%
1	≥1500	≥34	≥1000	≥30	≥500	≥26
2	750–1499	26–33	500–999	22–29	200–499	14–25
3 (AIDS)	<750	<26	<500	<22	<200	<14

AIDS indicator conditions

Bacterial infections, multiple or recurrent (specific to children <6 years)

Candidiasis of bronchi, trachea, or lungs	Lymphoma, Burkitt
Candidiasis, esophageal	Lymphoma, immunoblastic
Cervical cancer, invasive (specific to adults, adolescents, children >6 years)	Lymphoma, primary, or brain
Coccidioidomycosis, disseminated or extrapulmonary	*Mycobacterium avium* complex or *Mycobacterium kansasii*, disseminated or extrapulmonary
Cryptococcosis, extrapulmonary	*Mycobacterium tuberculosis*, any site (pulmonary or extrapulmonary)
Cryptosporidiosis, chronic intestinal (duration >1 month)	*Mycobacterium*, other species or unidentified species, disseminated or extrapulmonary
Cytomegalovirus disease (other than liver, spleen, or nodes), onset at age > 1 month	*Pneumocystis jirovecii* pneumonia (PCP)
Cytomegalovirus retinitis (with loss of vision)	Pneumonia, recurrent (specific to adults, adolescents, children >6 years)
Encephalopathy, HIV-related	Progressive multifocal leukoencephalopathy
Herpes simplex: chronic ulcer(s) (duration >1 month); or bronchitis, pneumonitis, or esophagitis, onset at age > 1 month	*Salmonella* septicemia, recurrent Toxoplasmosis of brain, onset at age >1 month Wasting syndrome due to HIV
Histoplasmosis, disseminated or extrapulmonary Isosporiasis, chronic intestinal (duration >1 month) Kaposi's sarcoma	

TABLE 40–2	Clinical Presentation of Primary Human Immunodeficiency Virus Infection in Adults

Signs and symptoms

Most common: Fever, headache, sore throat, fatigue, GI upset (diarrhea, nausea, vomiting) weight loss, myalgia, morbilliform or maculopapular rash usually involving the trunk, lymphadenopathy, night sweats

Less common: Aseptic meningitis, oral ulcers, leukopenia

Other

High viral load (may exceed 1,000,000 copies per milliliter or 10⁹/L)

Persistent decrease in CD4 lymphocytes

TREATMENT

- Goal of Treatment: The central goal of antiretroviral therapy is to decrease morbidity and mortality, improve quality of life, restore and preserve immune function, and prevent further transmission through maximum suppression of HIV replication (HIV RNA level that is less than the lower limit of quantitation (ie, undetectable; usually <50 copies/mL [<50 × 10^3/L]).).

GENERAL APPROACH

- Regular, periodic measurement of plasma HIV RNA levels and CD4 cell counts is necessary to determine the risk of disease progression in an HIV-infected individual and to determine when to initiate or modify antiretroviral treatment regimens.
- The use of potent combination antiretroviral therapy to suppress HIV replication to below the levels of detection of sensitive plasma HIV RNA assays limits the potential for selection of antiretroviral-resistant HIV variants, the major factor limiting the ability of antiretroviral drugs to inhibit virus replication and delay disease progression. Maximum achievable suppression of HIV replication should be the goal of therapy.
- The most effective means to accomplish durable suppression of HIV replication is the simultaneous initiation of combinations of effective anti-HIV drugs with which the patient has not been previously treated and that are not cross-resistant with antiretroviral agents with which the patient has been treated previously. Each of the antiretroviral drugs used in combination therapy regimens should always be used according to optimum schedules and dosages. Combinations of three active antiretroviral agents from two pharmacologic classes profoundly inhibit HIV replication to undetectable plasma levels, prevent and reverse immune deficiency, and substantially decrease morbidity and mortality.
- Women should receive optimal antiretroviral therapy regardless of pregnancy status.
- The same principles of antiretroviral therapy apply to both HIV-infected children and adults, although the treatment of HIV-infected children involves unique pharmacologic, virologic, and immunologic considerations.
- Persons with acute primary HIV infections should be treated with combination antiretroviral therapy to suppress virus replication to levels below the limit of detection of sensitive plasma HIV RNA assays.
- HIV-infected persons, even those with viral loads below detectable limits, should be considered infectious and should be counseled to avoid sexual and drug-use behaviors that are associated with transmission or acquisition of HIV and other infectious pathogens.
- An excellent source for information on treatment guidelines can be found at *http://aidsinfo.nih.gov/*.
- Untreated HIV is harmful even at high CD4 counts and immediate ART confers individual- and population-level benefit compared with delayed ART. Major policymakers now recommend immediate ART regardless of CD4 count. Treatment of HIV infection in antiretroviral-naïve persons is shown in **Table 40–3**.

PHARMACOLOGIC THERAPY

Antiretroviral Agents

- Inhibiting viral replication with a combination of potent antiretroviral therapy has been the most clinically successful strategy in the treatment of HIV infection. There have been four primary groups of drugs used: entry inhibitors, reverse transcriptase inhibitors, integrase strand transfer inhibitors (InSTIs), and HIV protease inhibitors (PIs) (**Table 40–4**).
- Reverse transcriptase inhibitors are of two types: those that are derivatives of purine- and pyrimidine-based nucleosides and nucleotides (NRTIs) and those that are not nucleoside- or nucleotide-based (NNRTIs).

TABLE 40–3	Treatment of Human Immunodeficiency Virus Infection: Antiretroviral Regimens Recommended in Antiretroviral-Naïve Persons	
	Preferred Regimens	**Selected Limitations**
HIV PI based	Darunavir + ritonavir + tenofovir disoproxil fumarate + emtricitabine (AI)	Rash (darunavir has sulfonamide moiety); GI; food requirement; CYP3A4 drug interactions
InSTI based	Raltegravir + tenofovir disoproxil fumarate + emtricitabine (AI)	Twice daily (not once daily); interactions with polyvalent antacids; creatine kinase increases
	Elvitegravir + cobicistat + tenofovir disoproxil fumarate + emtricitabine (coformulated) (AI)	Only if CLcr ≥70 mL/min (≥1.17 mL/s); food requirement; interactions with polyvalent antacids; CYP3A4 drug interactions; cobicistat inhibits creatinine secretion increasing Scr—distinguish vs renal dysfunction
	Elvitegravir + cobicistat + tenofovir alafenamide fumarate + emtricitabine (coformulated) (AI)	Only if CLcr ≥30 mL/min (≥0.5 mL/s); same as above
	Dolutegravir + abacavir + lamivudine (coformulated) (AI)	Only if HLA-B5701 negative; interactions with polyvalent antacids; dolutegravir inhibits creatinine secretion increasing Scr—distinguish vs renal dysfunction
	Dolutegravir + tenofovir disoproxil fumarate + emtricitabine (AI)	Same as above without HLA-B5701 negative requirement
Selected alternative regimens (some potential disadvantages vs preferred regimens)		
NNRTI based	Efavirenz + tenofovir disoproxil fumarate + emtricitabine (coformulated) (BI)	CNS side effects with efavirenz; CYP450 drug interactions; empty stomach dosing; teratogenic in non human primates—avoid in women planning to conceive
	Rilpivirine + tenofovir disoproxil fumarate + emtricitabine (coformulated) (BI)	Not recommended when HIV-RNA >100,000 copies/mL (>100,000 × 10^3/L) or CD4 <200 cells/μL (<200 × 10^6/L); no proton-pump inhibitors (rilpivirine); food requirement; antacid interactions
HIV PI based	Atazanavir + ritonavir (or cobicistat) + tenofovir disoproxil fumarate + emtricitabine (BI)	GI; food requirement; CYP3A4 drug interactions; hyperbilirubinemia leading to drug discontinuation especially in those with Gilbert's; only for CLcr ≥ 70 mL/min (≥1.17 mL/s) as cobicistat inhibits creatinine secretion increasing Scr—distinguish vs renal dysfunction
	Darunavir + ritonavir (or cobicistat) + abacavir + lamivudine (BII for ritonavir and BIII for cobicistat)	Only if HLA-B5701 negative; see issues above
	Darunavir + cobicistat + tenofovir disoproxil fumarate + emtricitabine (BII)	Only for CLcr ≥70 mL/min (≥1.17 mL/s) as cobicistat inhibits creatinine secretion increasing Scr—distinguish vs renal dysfunction; see issues above

(continued)

TABLE 40–3	Treatment of Human Immunodeficiency Virus Infection: Antiretroviral Regimens Recommended in Antiretroviral-Naïve Persons (*Continued*)
Preferred Regimens	**Selected Limitations**

Selected regimens or components that should not be used at any time

Regimen or Component	Comment
Any all NRTI regimen (AIBII)	Inferior virologic efficacy
Didanosine + tenofovir (AII)	Inferior virologic efficacy, CD4 declines
Didanosine + Stavudine (AII)	Toxicity including subcutaneous fat loss, peripheral neuropathy, and lactic acidosis
2 NNRTI combinations (AI)	Higher adverse events, drug interactins
Emtricitabine + lamivudine or zidovudine + stavudine (AIIAIII)	Analogs of same nucleobase, No additive benefit (or antagonistic)
Unboosted PIs (ie, darunavir, saquinavir, tipranavir) (AII)	Inadequate bioavailability
Etravirine + selected boosted PIs (AII)	Possible induction of PI metabolism, doses not established
Nevirapine in ARV naïve with higher CD4 counts (>250 for women, >400 for men) (BI)	High incidence of symptomatic hepatotoxicity

Evidence-based rating definition.
Rating strength of recommendation:
A: Strong recommendation.
B: Moderate recommendation.
C: Optional recommendation.
Rating Quality of Evidence Supporting the Recommendation:
I: Evidence from at least one correctly randomized, controlled trial with clinical outcomes and/or validated laboratory endpoints.
II: Evidence from at least one well-designed clinical trial without randomization or observational cohorts with long-term clinical outcomes.
III: Expert opinion.
Lamivudine and emtricitabine are considered interchangeable.

- Current recommendations for initial treatment of HIV infection advocate a minimum of three active antiretroviral agents: **tenofovir disoproxil fumarate** plus **emtricitabine** with either a ritonavir-enhanced PI (**darunavir** or **atazanavir**), the NNRTI **efavirenz**, or the InSTI, **raltegravir**. Multiple alternative regimens are also safe and effective, but have one or two disadvantages compared with the preferred regimens such as lack of long-term follow-up, weaker virologic responses with high viral loads, lower tolerability, or greater risk of long-term toxicities such as subcutaneous fat loss.
- Significant drug interactions can occur with many antiretroviral agents. The latest information on drug interactions of antiretroviral drugs should be consulted.
  ✓ **Ritonavir** is a potent inhibitor of cytochrome P450 enzyme 3A and is used to reduce clearance of other PIs. **Rifampin** may substantially reduce the concentrations of PIs and is contraindicated with the use of most PIs. Saint John's wort is a potent inducer of metabolism and is contraindicated with PIs, NNRTIs, and **maraviroc**.

TREATMENT DURING PREGNANCY

- In general, pregnant women should be treated like nonpregnant adults with some exceptions. Efavirenz should be avoided when possible in pregnant women during the first trimester or in women trying to conceive because of potential teratogenicity. Drugs that cross the placental barrier should be avoided, such as **abacavir**, emtricitabine, **lamivudine**, tenofovir, or **zidovudine**.

387

TABLE 40–4 Pharmacologic Characteristics of Selected Antiretroviral Compounds

Drug	F (%)	$t_{1/2}$ (h)[a]	Adult Dose[b] (Doses/Day)	Plasma C_{max}/C_{min} (μM)	Distinguishing Adverse Effect(s)
Integrase inhibitors (InSTI)					
Dolutegravir	?	14	50 mg (1)	8.3/2.5	Insomnia, headache, rash (can be severe)
Elvitegravir (coformulated with cobicistat)	?	13	150 mg (1)	3.8/1	Diarrhea, nausea
Raltegravir	?	9	400 mg (2)	1.74/0.22	Rash (can be severe), creatine phosphokinase increases
Nucleoside (nucleotide) reverse transcriptase inhibitors (NtRTIs)					
Abacavir	83	1.5/20	300 mg (2) or 600 mg (1)	5.2/0.03	Hypersensitivity (HLA-B5701 test to predict)
Didanosine	42	1.4/24	200 mg (2) or 400 mg (1)	2.8/0.03	Peripheral neuropathy, pancreatitis
				5.6[c]	
Emtricitabine	93	10/39	200 mg (1)	7.3/0.04	Rarely pigmentation on soles and palms in nonwhites
Lamivudine	86	5/22	150 mg (2) or 300 mg (1)	6.3/1.6	Headache
				10.5/0.5	
Stavudine	86	1.4/7	40 mg (2)	2.4/0.04	Lipoatrophy, peripheral neuropathy
Tenofovir alafenamide	?	35/150 (tenofovir component)	10 mg (1) (when combined with cobicistat)	0.07/0.03	Increased lipids
Tenofovir disoproxil fumarate	25	17/150 (tenofovir component)	300 mg (1)	1.04/0.4	Renal dysfunction (proximal tubulopathy), bone de-mineralization
Zidovudine	85	2/7	200 mg (3) or 300 mg (2)	0.2	Anemia, neutropenia, myopathy
				3[c]	

Nonnucleoside reverse transcriptase inhibitors (NNRTIs)

Delavirdine	85	5.8	400 mg (3) or 600 mg (2)	35/14	Rash, elevated liver function tests
Efavirenz	43	48	600 mg (1)	12.9/5.6	CNS disturbances and potential teratogenicity
Etravirine	?	41	200 mg (2)	1.69/0.86	Rash, nausea
Nevirapine	93	25	200 mg (2)[d]	22/14	Potentially serious rash and hepatotoxicity
Rilpivirine	?	50	25 mg (1)	0.7/0.3	Possibly depression
Protease inhibitors (PIs)					
Fosamprenavir[e]		8	1400 mg (1)[ef] 400 mg (1)	14.3/2.9	Rash
Atazanavir	68	7	or 300 mg (1)[f]	3.3/0.23 6.2/0.9	Unconjugated hyperbilirubinemia
Darunavir	82	15	800 mg (1)[f] or 600 mg (2)[f]	11.9/6.5	Hepatitis, rash
Indinavir	60	1.5	800 mg (3) or 400–800 mg (2)[f]	13/0.25	Nephrolithiasis
Lopinavir[g]	?	5.5	800 mg (1) or 400 mg (2)	13.6/7.5	Hyperlipidemia/GI intolerance

(continued)

TABLE 40–4 Pharmacologic Characteristics of Selected Antiretroviral Compounds (Continued)

Drug	F (%)	$t_{1/2}$ (h)[a]	Adult Dose[b] (doses/day)	Plasma C_{max}/C_{min} (µM)	Distinguishing Adverse Effect(s)
Nelfinavir	?	2.6	750 mg (3) or 1250 mg (2)	5.3/1.76 7/1.2	Diarrhea
Ritonavir	60	3–5	600 mg (2)[d] or "Boosting doses"	16/5	GI intolerance
Saquinavir	4	3	1000 mg (2)[f]	3.9/0.55	QT prolongation
Tipranavir	?	6	500 mg (2)[f]	77.6/35.6	Hepatotoxicity, intracranial hemorrhage
Entry inhibitors—fusion inhibitor					
Enfuvirtide	84	3.8	90 mg (2)	1.1/0.73	Injection-site reactions
Coreceptor inhibitor					
Maraviroc	33	15	300 mg (2)	1.2/0.066	Hepatitis, allergic reaction

C_{max}, maximum plasma concentration; C_{min}, minimum plasma concentration; F, bioavailability; $t_{1/2}$, elimination half-life.
[a]NtRTIs: Plasma NtRTI $t_{1/2}$/intracellular (peripheral blood mononuclear cells) NtRTI-triphosphate $t_{1/2}$; plasma $t_{1/2}$ only for other classes.
[b]Dose adjustment may be required for weight, renal or hepatic disease, and drug interactions.
[c]C_{min} concentration typically below the limit of quantification.
[d]Initial dose escalation recommended to minimize side effects.
[e]Fosamprenavir is a tablet phosphate prodrug of amprenavir. Amprenavir is no longer available.
[f]Must be boosted with low doses of ritonavir (100–200 mg).
[g]Available as coformulation 4:1 lopinavir to ritonavir.

- Intravenous (IV) zidovudine is recommended intrapartum depending on the mother's viral load, based on early studies demonstrating clear prophylactic effectiveness as well as extensive familiarity with the side effect profile. Infants also receive zidovudine (± several doses of **nevirapine**) prophylaxis for 6 weeks after birth.

POSTEXPOSURE PROPHYLAXIS

- Postexposure prophylaxis with a triple-drug regimen consisting of two NRTIs and a boosted PI is recommended for percutaneous blood exposure involving significant risk (ie, large-bore needle or large volume of blood or blood from patients with advanced AIDS).
- Two NRTIs may be offered to healthcare workers with lower risk of exposure such as that involving either the mucous membrane or skin. Treatment is not necessary if the source of exposure is urine or saliva.
- The optimal duration of treatment is unknown, but at least 4 weeks of therapy is advocated. Ideally, treatment should be initiated within 1 to 2 hours of exposure, but treatment is recommended for up to 72 hours postexposure.

EVALUATION OF THERAPEUTIC OUTCOMES

- Following the initiation of therapy, patients are usually monitored at 3-month intervals with immunologic (ie, CD4 count), virologic (HIV RNA), and clinical assessments.
- There are two general indications to change therapy: significant toxicity and treatment failure.
- Specific criteria to indicate treatment failure have not been established through controlled clinical trials. As a general guide, the following events should prompt consideration for changing therapy:
  ✓ Less than a 1 $\log_{10}$ reduction in HIV RNA 1 to 4 weeks after the initiation of therapy, or a failure to achieve less than 200 copies/mL ($<200 \times 10^3$/L) by 24 weeks or less than 50 copies/mL ($<50 \times 10^3$/L) by 48 weeks
  ✓ After HIV RNA suppression, repeated detection of HIV-RNA
  ✓ Clinical disease progression, usually the development of a new opportunistic infection

THERAPEUTIC FAILURE

- The most important measure of therapeutic failure is suboptimal suppression of viral replication.
- Therapeutic failure may be the result of nonadherence to medication, development of drug resistance, intolerance to one or more medications, adverse drug–drug interactions, or pharmacokinetic–pharmacodynamic variability.
- Patients should be treated with at least two (preferably three) fully active antiretroviral drugs based on medication history, resistance tests, and new mechanistic drug classes (eg, maraviroc and raltegravir). The goal of therapy is to suppress HIV-RNA to less than 50 copies/mL ($<50 \times 10^3$/L). In cases when less than 50 copies/mL ($<50 \times 10^3$/L) cannot be attained, maintenance on the regimen is preferred over drug discontinuation so as to prevent rapid immunological and clinical decline.

INFECTIOUS COMPLICATIONS OF HUMAN IMMUNODEFICIENCY VIRUS

- The development of certain opportunistic infections is directly or indirectly related to the level of CD4 lymphocytes. The principle in the management of opportunistic infections (OIs) is treating HIV infection to enable CD4 cells to recover and be maintained above safe levels. Other important principles are:
  ✓ Preventing exposure to opportunistic pathogens
  ✓ Using vaccinations to prevent first episodes of disease
  ✓ Initiating primary chemoprophylaxis at certain CD4 thresholds to prevent first episodes of disease
  ✓ Treating emergent OIs
  ✓ Initiating secondary chemoprophylaxis to prevent disease recurrence
  ✓ Discontinuing prophylaxis with sustained immune recovery
- The spectrum of infectious diseases observed in HIV-infected individuals and recommended first-line therapies are shown in **Table 40–5.**

TABLE 40–5	Selected Therapies for Common Opportunistic Pathogens in HIV-Infected Individuals	
Clinical Disease	Preferred Initial Therapies for Acute Infection in Adults (Strength of Recommendation in Parentheses)	Common Drug- or Dose-Limiting Adverse Reactions
Fungi		
Candidiasis, oral	Fluconazole 100 mg orally for 7–14 days (AI)	Elevated liver function tests, hepatotoxicity, nausea, and vomiting
	or	
	Nystatin 500,000 units oral swish (~5 mL) four times daily for 7–14 days (BII)	Taste, patient acceptance
Candidiasis, esophageal	Fluconazole 100–400 mg orally or IV daily for 14–21 days (AI)	Same as above
	or	
	Itraconazole 200 mg/day orally for 14–21 days (AI)	Elevated liver function tests, hepatotoxicity, nausea, and vomiting
Pneumocystis jiroveci pneumonia	Trimethoprim–sulfamethoxazole IV or orally 15–20 mg/kg/day as trimethoprim component in three to four divided doses for 21 days[a] (AI) moderate or severe therapy should be started IV	Skin rash, fever, leucopenia Thrombocytopenia
	or	
	Pentamidine IV 4 mg/kg/day for 21 days[a] (AI)	Azotemia, hypoglycemia, hyperglycemia, arrhythmias
	Mild episodes	
	Atovaquone suspension 750 mg (5 mL) orally twice daily with meals for 21 days[a] (BI)	Rash, elevated liver enzymes, diarrhea
Cryptococcal meningitis	Liposomal amphotericin B 3–4 mg/kg/day IV for a minimum of 2 weeks with flucytosine 100 mg/kg/day orally in four divided doses (AI) *followed by*	Nephrotoxicity, hypokalemia, anemia, fever, chills Bone marrow suppression
	Fluconazole 400 mg/day, orally for 8 weeks or until CSF cultures are negative (AI)[a]	Same as above
Histoplasmosis	Liposomal amphotericin B 3 mg/kg/day IV for 2 weeks (AI) *followed by*	Same as above
	Itraconazole 200 mg orally thrice daily for 3 days then twice daily, for 12 months (AII)[a]	
Coccidioidomycosis	Liposomal amphotericin B 4–6 mg/kg/day IV until clinical improvement (usually after 500–1000 mg) then switch to azole (AIII)[a]	Same as above
	or	
	Fluconazole 400–800 mg once daily (meningeal disease) (AII)[a]	Same as above
Protozoa		
Toxoplasmic encephalitis	Pyrimethamine 200 mg orally once, then 50–75 mg/day	Bone marrow suppression
	plus	
	Sulfadiazine 1–1.5 g orally four times daily	Rash, drug fever
	and	
	Leucovorin 10–25 mg orally daily for 6 weeks (AI)[a]	

Isosporiasis	Trimethoprim and sulfamethoxazole: 160 mg trimethoprim and 800 mg sulfamethoxazole orally or IV four times daily for 10 days (AII)[a]	Same as above
Bacteria		
Mycobacterium avium complex	Clarithromycin 500 mg orally twice daily, *plus* ethambutol 15 mg/kg/day orally (AI) for at least 12 months	GI intolerance, optic neuritis, peripheral neuritis, elevated liver tests
Salmonella enterocolitis or bacteremia	Ciprofloxacin 500–750 mg orally (or 400 mg IV) twice daily for 14 days (longer duration for bacteremia or advanced HIV) (AIII)	GI intolerance, headache, dizziness
Campylobacter enterocolitis (mild to moderate)	Ciprofloxacin 500–750 mg orally (or 400 mg IV) twice daily for 7–10 days (or longer with bacteremia) (BII)	Same as above
Shigella enterocolitis	Ciprofloxacin 500–750 mg orally (or 400 mg IV) twice daily for 7–10 days (or 14 days for bacteremia) (AIII)	Same as above
Viruses		
Mucocutaneous herpes simplex	Acyclovir 5 mg/kg IV every 8 hours until lesions regress, then acyclovir 400 mg orally three times daily until complete healing (famciclovir or valacyclovir is alternative) (AIII)	GI intolerance, crystalluria
Primary varicella-zoster	Acyclovir 10–15 mg/kg every 8 hours IV for 7–10 days (severe cases), then switch to oral valacyclovir 1 g three times daily after defervescence (famciclovir or acyclovir is alternative) (AIII)	Obstructive nephropathy, CNS symptoms
Cytomegalovirus (retinitis)	Intravitreal ganciclovir (2 mg) one to four doses over 7–10 days (for sight threatening lesions) *plus* valganciclovir 900 mg twice daily for 14–21 days then once daily until immune recovery from ART (AIII)[a]	Neutropenia, thrombocytopenia
Cytomegalovirus esophagitis or colitis	Ganciclovir 5 mg/kg IV every 12 hours for 21–42 days may switch to valganciclovir 900 mg orally every 12 hours when oral therapy can be tolerated (BI)	Same as above

(continued)

393

TABLE 40-5 Selected Therapies for Common Opportunistic Pathogens in HIV-Infected Individuals (*Continued*)

Therapies for prophylaxis of select first-episode opportunistic diseases in adults and adolescents

Pathogen	Indication	First Choice (Strength of Recommendation in Parentheses)
I. Standard of care		
Pneumocystis jirovecii	CD4+ count <200/mm³ (<200 × 10⁶/L) *or* oropharyngeal candidiasis	Trimethoprim–sulfamethoxazole, one double-strength tablet orally once daily (AI) *or* one single-strength tablet orally once daily (AI)
Histoplasma capsulatum	CD4+ count <150/mm³, (<150 × 10⁶/L) endemic geographic area and high risk for exposures	Intraconazole 200 mg orally once daily (BI)
Mycobacterium tuberculosis	(Active TB should be ruled out):	
Isoniazid-sensitive	+ test for latent TB infection with no prior TB treatment history (AI) *or* − test for latent TB infection, but close contact with case of active tuberculosis (AII)	Isoniazid 300 mg orally plus pyridoxine, 25 mg orally once daily for 9 months (AII) *or* Isoniazid 900 mg orally twice weekly by directly observed therapy (BII) plus pyridoxine 25 mg orally daily for 9 months (BII)
For exposure to drug-resistant TB	Consult public health authorities	
Toxoplasma gondii	Immunoglobulin G antibody to *Toxoplasma* and CD4+ count <100/mm³ (<100 × 10⁶/L)	Trimethoprim–sulfamethoxazole one double-strength tablet orally once daily (AII)
Mycobacterium avium complex	CD4+ count <50/mm³ (<50 × 10⁶/L)	Azithromycin 1200 mg orally once weekly (AI) *or* 600 mg orally twice weekly (BIII) or clarithromycin 500 mg orally twice daily (AI)

Varicella zoster virus (VZV)	Preexposure: CD4 ≥200/mm³ (≥200 × 10⁶/L), no history of varicella vaccination or infection, or, if available, negative antibody to VZV. Varicella vaccination; two doses, 3 months apart (CIII) Postexposure: Significant exposure to chicken pox or shingles for patients who have no history of vaccination or either condition or, if available, negative antibody to VZV. Varicella-zoster immune globulin, 125 IU per 10 kg (maximum of 625 IU) IM, as soon as possible and within 10 days after exposure (AIII)
Streptococcus pneumoniae	Any individual regardless of CD4 count. 13-valent polysaccharide vaccine, 0.5 mL intramuscularly once (AI) followed by 23-valent polysaccharide vaccine 0.5 mL 8 weeks later (CIII) Re-vaccinate with 23-valent polysaccharide vaccine every 5 years
Hepatitis B virus	All susceptible patients. HBV vaccine IM (Engerix-B 20 mcg/mL or Recombivax HB 10 mcg/mL), 0, 1, and 6 months (AII) Anti-HBs should be obtained 1 month after the vaccine series completion (BIII)
Influenza virus	All patients (annually, before influenza season). Inactivated trivalent influenza virus vaccine (annual): 0.5 mL intramuscularly (AIII) (live-attenuated vaccine is contraindicated in all HIV-infected patients)
Hepatitis A virus	All susceptible (anti-hepatitis A virus–negative) patients at increased risk for hepatitis A infection (eg, chronic liver disease, injection drug users, men who have sex with men). Hepatitis A vaccine: two doses (AII) antibody response should be assessed 1 month after vaccination; with revaccination as needed when CD4 >200 cells/μL (>200 × 10⁶/L)(BIII)
Human papillomavirus (HPV) infection	13 to 26-year-old males and females. HPV quadrivalent vaccine months 0, 1–2, and 6 (BIII)

(ART, antiretroviral therapy; CSF, cerebrospinal fluid; HIV, human immunodeficiency virus.)
Maintenance therapy is recommended.
See Table 40–3 for levels of evidence-based recommendations.

Pneumocystis carinii (Pneumocystis jiroveci)

- *Pneumocystis jiroveci* pneumonia is the most common life-threatening opportunistic infection in patients with AIDS. The taxonomy of the organism is unclear, having been classified as both protozoan and fungal.

CLINICAL PRESENTATION

- Characteristic symptoms include fever and dyspnea; clinical signs are tachypnea, with or without rales or rhonchi, and a nonproductive or mildly productive cough. Chest radiographs may show florid or subtle infiltrates or may occasionally be normal, although infiltrates are usually interstitial and bilateral. Arterial blood gases may show minimal hypoxia (partial pressure of oxygen [PaO_2] 80 to 95 mm Hg [10.6–12.6 kPa]) but in more advanced disease may be markedly abnormal.
- The onset of *P. carinii* pneumonia (PCP) is often insidious, occurring over a period of weeks. Clinical signs are tachypnea with or without rales or rhonchi and a non-productive or mildly productive cough occurring over a period of weeks, although more fulminant presentations can occur.

TREATMENT

- Treatment with **trimethoprim–sulfamethoxazole** or parenteral pentamidine is associated with a 60% to 100% response rate. Trimethoprim–sulfamethoxazole is the regimen of choice for treatment and subsequent prophylaxis of PCP in patients with and without HIV.
- Trimethoprim–sulfamethoxazole is given in doses of 15 to 20 mg/kg/day (based on the trimethoprim component) as three or four divided doses for the treatment of PCP. Treatment duration is typically 21 days but must be based on clinical response.
- Trimethoprim–sulfamethoxazole is usually initiated by the IV route, although oral therapy (as oral absorption is high) may suffice in mildly ill and reliable patients or to complete a course of therapy after a response has been achieved with IV administration.
- The more common adverse reactions seen with trimethoprim–sulfamethoxazole are rash (including Stevens–Johnson syndrome), fever, leukopenia, elevated serum trans-aminases, and thrombocytopenia. The incidence of these adverse reactions is higher in HIV-infected individuals than in those not infected with HIV.
- For pentamidine, side effects include hypotension, tachycardia, nausea, vomiting, severe hypoglycemia or hyperglycemia, pancreatitis, irreversible diabetes mellitus, elevated transaminases, nephrotoxicity, leukopenia, and cardiac arrhythmias.
- The early addition of adjunctive glucocorticoid therapy to anti-PCP regimens has been shown to decrease the risk of respiratory failure and improve survival in patients with AIDS and moderate to severe PCP (PaO_2 ≤70 mm Hg [≤9.3 kPa]or [alveolar–arterial] gradient greater than or equal to 35 mm Hg [≥4.7 kPa]).

PROPHYLAXIS

- Currently, PCP prophylaxis is recommended for all HIV-infected individuals who have already had previous PCP. Prophylaxis is also recommended for all HIV-infected persons who have a CD4 lymphocyte count less than 200 cells/mm³ (ie, their CD4 cells are <14% of total lymphocytes) or a history of oropharyngeal candidiasis.
- Trimethoprim–sulfamethoxazole is the preferred therapy for both primary and secondary prophylaxis of PCP in adults and adolescents. The recommended dose in adults and adolescents is one double-strength tablet daily.

See Chapter 126, Human Immunodeficiency Virus Infection, authored by Peter L. Anderson, Thomas N. Kakuda, and Courtney V. Fletcher, for a more detailed discussion of this topic.

CHAPTER 41

Influenza

- *Influenza* is a viral illness associated with high mortality and high hospitalization rates. The highest rates of severe illness, hospitalization, and death occur among those older than age 65 years, young children (younger than 2 years old), and those who have underlying medical conditions, including pregnancy and cardiopulmonary disorders.
- The route of influenza transmission is person-to-person via inhalation of respiratory droplets, which can occur when an infected person coughs or sneezes. The incubation period for influenza ranges between 1 and 7 days, with an average incubation of 2 days. Adults are considered infectious from the day before their symptoms begin through 7 days after the onset of illness, whereas children can be infectious for longer than 10 days after the onset of illness. Viral shedding can persist for weeks to months in severely immunocompromised people.

CLINICAL PRESENTATION

- The presentation of influenza is similar to a number of other respiratory illnesses.
- The clinical course and outcome are affected by age, immunocompetence, viral characteristics, smoking, comorbidities, pregnancy, and the degree of preexisting immunity.
- Complications of influenza may include exacerbation of underlying comorbidities, primary viral pneumonia, secondary bacterial pneumonia or other respiratory illnesses (eg, sinusitis, bronchitis, and otitis), encephalopathy, transverse myelitis, myositis, myocarditis, pericarditis, and Reye syndrome.

SIGNS AND SYMPTOMS

- Classic signs and symptoms of influenza include rapid onset of fever, myalgia, headache, malaise, nonproductive cough, sore throat, and rhinitis.
- Nausea, vomiting, and otitis media are also commonly reported in children.
- Signs and symptoms typically resolve in 3 to 7 days, although cough and malaise may persist for more than 2 weeks.

LABORATORY TESTS

- The gold standard for diagnosis of influenza are reverse-transcription polymerase chain reaction (RT-PCR) or viral culture.
- Rapid influenza diagnostic tests [(RIDTs), also known as point-of-care (POC) tests], direct (DFA) or indirect (IFA) fluorescence antibody tests, and the RT-PCR assay may be used for rapid detection of virus.
- Chest radiograph should be obtained if pneumonia is suspected.

PREVENTION

- The best means to decrease the morbidity and mortality associated with influenza is to prevent infection through vaccination. Appropriate infection control measures, such as hand hygiene, basic respiratory etiquette (cover your cough and throw tissues away), and contact avoidance, are also important in preventing the spread of influenza.
- Annual vaccination is recommended for all persons age 6 months or older and caregivers (eg, parents, teachers, babysitters, nannies) of children less than 6 months of age.
- Vaccination is also recommended for those who live with and/or care for people who are at high risk, including household contacts and healthcare workers.

- The Advisory Committee on Immunization Practices (ACIP) has made the following recommendations regarding the vaccinations of persons with reports of egg allergy: (a) Vaccination with any age appropriate IIV or RIV3 vaccine, for persons with a history of egg allergy that involves only hives. (b) Persons with severe allergic reactions (i.e., symptoms other than hives), such as angioedema, respiratory distress, lightheadedness, or recurrent emesis or required epinephrine after an egg exposure may be immunized with any licensed IIV or RIV3 that is appropriate for age and health status. Vaccine should be administered in an inpatient or outpatient medical setting (including but not necessarily limited to hospitals, clinics, health departments, and physician offices), under the supervision of a health care provider who is able to recognize and manage severe allergic conditions. (c) Severe allergic reaction to influenza vaccine is a contraindication to receiving future vaccinations. (d) Vaccine providers should consider observing all patients for 15 minutes after vaccination to decrease the risk for injury should a patient experiences syncope.

✓ The ideal time for vaccination is October or November to allow for the development and maintenance of immunity during the peak of the influenza season.

✓ The two vaccines currently available for prevention of influenza are the inactivated vaccine IIV and the LAIV. The specific strains included in the vaccine each year change based on antigenic drift.

✓ IIV is FDA approved for use in people over 6 months of age, regardless of their immune status. Of note, several commercial products are available and are approved for different age groups (Table 41–1).

✓ Adults older than 65 years benefit from influenza vaccination, including prevention of complications and decreased risk of influenza-related hospitalization and death. However, people in this population may not generate a strong antibody response to the vaccine and may remain susceptible to infection.

✓ The most frequent adverse effect associated with IIV is soreness at the injection site that lasts for less than 48 hours. IIV may cause fever and malaise in those who have not previously been exposed to the viral antigens in the vaccine. Allergic-type reactions (hives and systemic anaphylaxis) rarely occur after influenza vaccination and are likely a result of a reaction to residual egg protein in the vaccine.

✓ Vaccination should be avoided in persons who are not at high risk for influenza complications and who have experienced Guillain–Barré syndrome within 6 weeks of receiving a previous influenza vaccine.

✓ LAIV is made with live, attenuated viruses and is approved for intranasal administration in healthy people between 2 and 49 years of age (Table 41–2). Advantages of LAIV include its ease of administration, intranasal rather than intramuscular administration, and the potential induction of broad mucosal and systemic immune response.

✓ LAIV is only approved for children over the age of 2 years in part because of data showing an increase in asthma or reactive airway disease in those younger than 5 years.

✓ The adverse effects typically associated with LAIV administration include runny nose, congestion, sore throat, and headache.

✓ LAIV should not be given to immunosuppressed patients or given by healthcare workers who are severely immunocompromised.

POSTEXPOSURE PROPHYLAXIS

- Antiviral drugs available for prophylaxis of influenza should be considered adjuncts but are not replacements for annual vaccination.
- **Amantadine** and **rimantadine** are currently not recommended for prophylaxis or treatment in the United States because of the rapid emergence of resistance.
- The neuraminidase inhibitors **oseltamivir** and **zanamivir** are effective prophylactic agents against influenza in terms of preventing laboratory-confirmed influenza when used for seasonal prophylaxis and preventing influenza illness among persons exposed to a household contact who were diagnosed with influenza. Table 41–3 gives dosing recommendations. Peramivir is not approved for chemoprophylaxis.

TABLE 41-1 Approved Influenza Vaccines for Different Age Groups—United States, 2016-2017 Season

Vaccine	Trade Name	Manufacturer	Dose/Presentation	Thimerosal Mercury Content (mcg Hg/0.5 mL Dose)	Age Group	Number of Doses
Inactivated						
IIV3	Fluvirin	Seqirus Vaccines	0.5-mL prefilled syringe	≤1	≥4 years	1 or 2[a]
			5-mL multi-dose vial	25	≥4 years	1 or 2[a]
IIV3	Afluria	Seqirus	0.5-mL prefilled syringe	0	≥9 years	1
			5-mL multi-dose vial	24.5	≥9 years via needle/ syringe or 18–64 years via jet injector	1
ccIIV4	Quadrivalent	Seqirus Vaccines	0.5-mL prefilled syringe	0	≥4 years	1
RIV3	Flublok	Protein Sciences	0.5-mL single-dose vial	0	≥18 years	1
IIV3 High Dose	Fluzone HD	Sanofi Pasteur	0.5-mL prefilled syringe	0	≥65 years	1
aIIV3	Fluad	Seqirus	0.5 mL single-dose prefilled syringe	0	≥65 years	1
IIV4	Quadrivalent	ID Biomedical Corporation	5-mL multi-dose vial	<25	≥3 years	1
IIV4	Fluarix Quadrivalent	GlaxoSmithKline	0.5-mL prefilled syringe	0	≥3 years	1
IIV4	Fluzone Quadrivalent	Sanofi Pasteur	0.25-mL prefilled syringe	0	≥6–35 months	1 or 2[a]
			0.5-mL prefilled syringe	0	≥36 months	1 or 2[a]
			0.5-mL single-dose vial	0	≥36 months	1 or 2[a]
			5-mL multi-dose vial	25	≥6 months	1 or 2[a]

(continued)

Vaccine	Trade Name	Manufacturer	Dose/Presentation	Thimerosal Mercury Content (mcg Hg/0.5 mL Dose)	Age Group	Number of Doses
IIV4 intradermal	Fluzone Intradermal Quadrivalent	Sanofi Pasteur	0.1-mL prefilled micro-injection system	0	18–64 years	1[b]
LAIV	FluMist Quadrivalent[c]	MedImmune	0.2-mL sprayer	0	2–49 years	1 or 2[d]

(LAIV, live-attenuated influenza vaccine; IIV3, trivalent influenza vaccine; IIV4, quadrivalent influenza vaccine; ccIIV3, cell culture-based trivalent influenza vaccine; RIV3, recombinant trivalent influenza vaccine; aIIV3, adjuvanted inactivated influenza vaccine, trivalent, standard dose.)

[a]Two doses administered at least 1 month apart are recommended for children aged 6 months to less than 9 years who are receiving influenza vaccine for the first time or received one dose in first year of vaccination during the previous influenza season.

[b]Given intradermally. A 0.1-mL dose contains 9 mcg of each vaccine antigen (27 mcg total).

[c]ACIP recommends that FLumist (LAIV4) not be used during the 2016-2017 season.

[d]Two doses administered 4 weeks apart are recommended for children aged 2 to less than 9 years who are receiving influenza vaccine for the first time.

TABLE 41–1 Approved Influenza Vaccines for Different Age Groups—United States, 2016-2017 Season (Continued)

TABLE 41-2	Comparison of Inactivated Influenza Vaccine (IIV) and Live-Attenuated Influenza Vaccine (LAIV)	
Characteristic	**IIV (IIV3/IIV4)**	**LAIV**
Age groups approved for use	>6 months	2–49 years
Immune status requirements	Immunocompetent or immunocompromised	Immunocompetent
Viral properties	Inactivated (killed) influenza A (H3N2), A (H1N1), and B viruses	Live-attenuated influenza A (H3N2), A (H1N1), and B viruses
Route of administration	Intramuscular/Intradermal	Intranasal
Immune system response	High serum IgG antibody response	Lower IgG response and high serum IgA mucosal response

- In those patients who did not receive the influenza vaccination and are receiving an antiviral drug for prevention of disease during the influenza season, the medication should optimally be taken for the entire duration of influenza activity in the community.
- Prophylaxis should be considered during influenza season for the following groups of patients:
  ✓ Persons at high risk of serious illness and/or complications who cannot be vaccinated.
  ✓ Persons at high risk of serious illness and/or complications who are vaccinated after influenza activity has begun in their community because the development of sufficient antibody titers after vaccination takes ~2 weeks.
  ✓ Persons with severe immune deficiency or who may have an inadequate response to vaccination (e.g., advanced human immunodeficiency virus [HIV] disease, persons receiving immunosuppressive medications), after exposure to an infectious person. Long-term care facility residents, regardless of vaccination status, when an outbreak has occurred in the institution.
- LAIV should not be administered until 48 hours after influenza antiviral therapy has stopped, and influenza antiviral drugs should not be administered for 2 weeks after the administration of LAIV because the antiviral drugs inhibit influenza virus replication.
- Pregnant women, regardless of trimester, should receive annual influenza vaccination with IIV but not with LAIV.
- The adamantanes and neuraminidase inhibitors are not recommended during pregnancy because of concerns regarding the effects of the drugs on the fetus.
- Immunocompromised hosts should receive annual influenza vaccination with IIV but not LAIV.

TREATMENT

- Goals of Therapy: The four primary goals of therapy of influenza are as follows: (1) control symptoms, (2) prevent complications, (3) decrease work and/or school absenteeism, and (4) prevent the spread of infection.
- Antiviral drugs are most effective if started within 48 hours of the onset of illness. Adjunct agents, such as acetaminophen for fever or an antihistamine for rhinitis, may be used concomitantly with the antiviral drugs.
- Patients suffering from influenza should get adequate sleep and maintain a low level of activity. They should stay home from work and/or school in order to rest and prevent the spread of infection. Appropriate fluid intake should be maintained. Cough/throat lozenges, warm tea, or soup may help with symptom control (cough and sore throat).

TABLE 41–3 Recommended Daily Dosage of Influenza Antiviral Medications for Treatment and Prophylaxis—United States

Drug	Adult Treatment	Adult Prophylaxis[a]	Pediatric Treatment[b]	Pediatric Prophylaxis[c]
Oseltamivir	75-mg capsule twice daily for 5 days	75-mg capsule daily	<1 year: 3 mg/kg/dose twice daily 9–11 months[d]: 3.5 mg/kg/dose twice daily ≥1 year ≤15 kg: 30 mg twice daily 16–23 kg: 45 mg twice daily 23–40 kg: 60 mg twice daily >40 kg: 75 mg twice daily Duration: All for 5 days	3–8 months, 3 mg/kg/dose daily Not recommended if <3 months 9–11 months, 3.5 mg/kg/dose daily ≥1 year ≤15 kg: 30 mg daily 16–23 kg: 45 mg daily 23–40 kg: 60 mg daily >40 kg: 75 mg daily Duration: All for 10 days
Zanamivir	2 inhalations twice daily × 5 days	2 inhalations daily	2 inhalations twice daily × 5 days for ≥7 years old	2 inhalations daily for ≥5 years old for 10 days
Peramivir[e]	600 mg via intravenous infusion for 15–30 minutes once	None	None	None
Rimantadine[f]	200 mg/day in one to two doses × 7 days	200 mg/day in one to two doses	1–9 years old or <40 kg: 6.6 mg/kg/day divided twice daily (maximum 150 mg/day) ≥10 years old: 200 mg/day in one to two doses Treat 5–7 days	1–9 years old: 5 mg/kg daily (maximum 150 mg/day) ≥10 years old: 200 mg/day in one to two doses

Amantadine[f]	200 mg/day in one to two doses until 24–48 hours after symptom resolution	Same as treatment doses	>12 years old: same as adult; 1–9 years old: 5 mg/kg/day in one to two doses; maximum 150 mg/day; ≥10–12 years old: 100 mg orally twice daily	Same as treatment doses

[a] If influenza vaccine is administered, prophylaxis can generally be stopped 14 days after vaccination for noninstitutionalized persons. When prophylaxis is being administered following an exposure, prophylaxis should be continued for 10 days after the last exposure. In persons at high risk for complications from influenza for whom vaccination is contraindicated or expected to be ineffective, chemoprophylaxis should be continued for the duration that influenza viruses are circulating in the community during influenza season.

[b] Oseltamivir dosing for preterm infants—<38 weeks, 1 mg/kg/dose every 12 h; 38–40 weeks, 1.5mg/kg/dose every 12; >40 weeks, 3mg/kg/dose every 12 hours.

[c] Alternate dosing by IDSA/PIDS (2011) is: 3–8 months—3 mg/kg/dose daily; 9–23 months—3.5 mg/kg/dose daily.

[d] Unlabeled dosing.

[e] Only approved for use in adults ≥18 years. Adjust dose if CrCl <50 mL/min (<0.83 mL/s).

[f] *Note:* Although amantadine and rimantadine have been used historically for the treatment and prophylaxis of influenza A viruses, due to high resistance, the CDC no longer recommends the use of these agents for the treatment and/or prophylaxis of influenza.

PHARMACOLOGIC THERAPY

- The neuraminidase inhibitors are the only antiviral drugs available for treatment and prophylaxis of influenza and are oseltamivir and zanamivir. IV peramivir is another NA inhibitor under investigation for treatment of influenza. The adamantanes (amantadine and rimantadine) are no longer recommended due to high resistance among influenza viruses.
- Oseltamivir, zanamivir, and **peramivir** have activity against both influenza A and influenza B viruses. When administered within 48 hours of the onset of illness, oseltamivir and zanamivir may reduce the duration of illness by ~1 day versus placebo. Benefits are highly dependent on the timing of initiation of treatment, ideally being within 12 hours of illness onset.
- Oseltamivir is approved for treatment in those older than 14 days; zanamivir is approved for treatment in those older than 7 years, and peramivir for those 18 years and older. The recommended dosages vary by agent and age (see Table 41–3), and the recommended duration of treatment for both agents is 5 days for oseltamivir and zanamivir and one does for one day for peramivir.
- Neuropsychiatric complications consisting of delirium, seizures, hallucinations, and self-injury in pediatric patients have been reported following treatment with oseltamivir and peramivir.
- Oseltamivir and zanamivir have been used in pregnancy, but solid clinical safety data are lacking. Both the adamantanes and the neuraminidase inhibitors are excreted in breast milk and should be avoided by mothers who are breast-feeding their infants. More studies are needed in these populations who are at high risk for serious disease and complications from influenza.

EVALUATION OF THERAPEUTIC OUTCOMES

- Patients should be monitored daily for resolution of signs and symptoms associated with influenza, such as fever, myalgia, headache, malaise, nonproductive cough, sore throat, and rhinitis. These signs and symptoms will typically resolve within ~1 week. If the patient continues to exhibit signs and symptoms of illness beyond 10 days or a worsening of symptoms after 7 days, a physician visit is warranted, as this may be an indication of a secondary bacterial infection.

See Chapter 109, Influenza, authored by Jessica C. Njoku for a more detailed discussion of this topic.

CHAPTER 42

Intra-Abdominal Infections

- Intra-abdominal infections are those contained within the peritoneum or retroperitoneal space. Two general types of intra-abdominal infections are discussed throughout this chapter: peritonitis and abscess.
- Peritonitis is defined as the acute, inflammatory response of peritoneal lining to microorganisms, chemicals, irradiation, or foreign body injury. It may be classified as either primary or secondary. With primary peritonitis, an intra-abdominal focus of disease may not be evident. In secondary peritonitis, a focal disease process is evident within the abdomen.
- An abscess is a purulent collection of fluid separated from surrounding tissue by a wall consisting of inflammatory cells and adjacent organs. It usually contains necrotic debris, bacteria, and inflammatory cells.

PATHOPHYSIOLOGY

- Table 42–1 summarizes many of the potential causes of bacterial peritonitis. Appendicitis is the most frequent cause of abscess. Intra-abdominal infection results from entry of bacteria into the peritoneal or retroperitoneal spaces or from bacterial collections within intra-abdominal organs. When peritonitis results from peritoneal dialysis, skin surface flora are introduced via the peritoneal catheter.
- In primary peritonitis, bacteria may enter the abdomen via the bloodstream or the lymphatic system, by transmigration through the bowel wall, through an indwelling peritoneal dialysis catheter, or via the fallopian tubes in female patients.
- In secondary peritonitis, bacteria most often enter the peritoneum or retroperitoneum as a result of disruption of the integrity of the gastrointestinal (GI) tract caused by diseases or traumatic injuries.
- When bacteria become dispersed throughout the peritoneum, the inflammatory process involves the majority of the peritoneal lining. Fluid and protein shift into the abdomen (called "third spacing") may decrease circulating blood volume and cause shock.
- Peritonitis often results in death because of the effects on major organ systems. Fluid shifts and endotoxins may cause hypotension and shock.
- An abscess begins by the combined action of inflammatory cells (eg, neutrophils), bacteria, fibrin, and other inflammatory components. Within the abscess, oxygen tension is low, and anaerobic bacteria thrive.

MICROBIOLOGY

- Primary bacterial peritonitis is often caused by a single organism. In children, the pathogen is usually group A *Streptococcus, Escherichia coli, Streptococcus pneumoniae,* or *Bacteroides* species. When peritonitis occurs in association with cirrhotic ascites, *E. coli* is isolated most frequently.
- Peritonitis in patients undergoing peritoneal dialysis is most often caused by common skin organisms: coagulase negative staphylococci, *Staphylococcus aureus,* streptococci, and enterococci. Gram-negative bacteria associated with peritoneal dialysis infections include *E. coli, Klebsiella,* and *Pseudomonas.*
- Secondary intra-abdominal infections are often polymicrobial. The mean number of isolates of microorganisms from infected intra-abdominal sites has ranged from 2.9 to 3.7, including an average of 1.3 to 1.6 aerobes and 1.7 to 2.1 anaerobes. The frequencies with which specific bacteria were isolated in intra-abdominal infections are given in Table 42–2.
- The combination of aerobic and anaerobic organisms appears to greatly the severity of infection. In intra-abdominal infections, facultative bacteria may provide an environment conducive to the growth of anaerobic bacteria.

TABLE 42–1	Causes of Bacterial Peritonitis
Primary (spontaneous) bacterial peritonitis	
Peritoneal dialysis	
Cirrhosis with ascites	
Nephrotic syndrome	
Secondary bacterial peritonitis	
Miscellaneous causes	
Diverticulitis	
Appendicitis	
Inflammatory bowel diseases	
Salpingitis	
Biliary tract infections	
Necrotizing pancreatitis	
Neoplasms	
Intestinal obstruction	
Perforation	
Mechanical GI problems	
Any cause of small bowel obstruction (adhesions, hernia)	
Vascular causes	
Mesenteric arterial or venous occlusion (atrial fibrillation)	
Mesenteric ischemia without occlusion	
Trauma	
Blunt abdominal trauma with rupture of intestine	
Penetrating abdominal trauma	
Iatrogenic intestinal perforation (endoscopy)	
Intraoperative events	
Solid organ transplant in the abdomen	
Peritoneal contamination during abdominal operation	
Leakage from GI anastomosis	

(GI, gastrointestinal.)

- Aerobic enteric bacteria and anaerobic bacteria are both pathogens in intra-abdominal infection. Aerobic bacteria, particularly *E. coli*, appear responsible for the early mortality from peritonitis, whereas anaerobic bacteria are major pathogens in abscesses, with *Bacteroides fragilis* predominating.
- The role of *Enterococcus* as a pathogen is not clear. Enterococcal infection occurs more commonly in postoperative peritonitis, in the presence of specific risk factors indicating failure of the host defenses, or with the use of broad-spectrum antibiotics.

CLINICAL PRESENTATION

- Intra-abdominal infections have a wide spectrum of clinical features often depending on the specific disease process, the location and the magnitude of bacterial contamination, and concurrent host factors. Patients with primary and secondary peritonitis present quite differently (**Table 42–3**).
- If peritonitis continues untreated, the patient may experience hypovolemic shock from fluid loss into the peritoneum, bowel wall, and lumen. This may be accompanied by generalized sepsis. Intra-abdominal abscess may pose a diagnostic challenge, as the symptoms are neither specific nor dramatic.
- The overall outcome from intra-abdominal infection depends on five key factors: inoculum size, virulence of the organisms, the presence of adjuvants within the peritoneal cavity that facilitate infection, the adequacy of host defenses, and the adequacy of initial treatment.

TABLE 42–2	Pathogens Isolated from Patients with Intra-Abdominal Infection		
	Secondary Peritonitis (%)	Community-Acquired Infection (%)	Nosocomial Infection (%)
Gram-negative bacteria			
Escherichia coli	32–61	29	22.5
Enterobacter	8–26	5.2	8.0
Klebsiella	6–26	2.8	4.5
Proteus	4–23	1.7	2.4
Pseudomonas	5–13	5	13
Gram-positive bacteria			
Enterococcus	18–24	10.6	18
Streptococcus	6–55	13.7	10
Staphylococcus	6–16	3.1	4.8
Anaerobic bacteria			
Bacteroides	25–80	13.7	10.3
Clostridium	5–18	3.5	3.4
Fungi	2–5	3	4

TREATMENT

- The goals of treatment are the correction of intra-abdominal disease processes or injuries that have caused infection and the drainage of collections of purulent material (eg, abscess). A secondary objective is to achieve resolution of infection without major organ system complications or adverse treatment effects.
- The three major modalities for the treatment of intra-abdominal infection are prompt surgical drainage of the infected site, hemodynamic resuscitation and support of vital functions, and early administration of appropriate antimicrobial therapy to treat infection not removed by surgery.
- Antimicrobials are an important adjunct to drainage procedures in the treatment of intra-abdominal infections; however, the use of antimicrobial agents without surgical intervention is usually inadequate. For most cases of primary peritonitis, drainage procedures may not be required, and antimicrobial agents become the mainstay of therapy.
- In the early phase of serious intra-abdominal infections, attention should be given to the maintenance of organ system functions. With generalized peritonitis, large volumes of IV fluids are required to restore vascular volume, to improve cardiovascular function, and to maintain adequate tissue perfusion and oxygenation.

NONPHARMACOLOGIC TREATMENT

- Secondary peritonitis is treated surgically; this is called "source control," which refers to the physical measures undertaken to eradicate the focus of infection. Abdominal laparotomy may be used to correct the cause of peritonitis.
- Aggressive fluid repletion and management are required for the purposes of achieving or maintaining proper intravascular volume to ensure adequate cardiac output, tissue perfusion, and correction of acidosis.
- The Surviving Sepsis Campaign: International Guidelines for Management of Severe Sepsis and Septic Shock recommend treatment goals during the first 6 hours or resuscitation: (a) central venous pressure (CVP) 8 to 12 mm Hg, (b) mean arterial pressure (MAP) more than or equal to 65 mm Hg, and (c) maintain urine output more than or equal to 0.5 mL/kg/h.

TABLE 42–3	Clinical Presentation of Peritonitis

Primary Peritonitis

General
The patient may not be in acute distress, particularly with peritoneal dialysis

Signs and symptoms
The patient may complain of loss of appetite, bloating, nausea, vomiting (sometimes with diarrhea), and abdominal tenderness
Temperature may be only mildly elevated or not elevated in patients undergoing peritoneal dialysis
Bowel sounds are hypoactive
The cirrhotic patient may have worsening encephalopathy
Cloudy dialysate fluid with peritoneal dialysis

Laboratory tests
The patient's WBC count may be only mildly elevated
Ascitic fluid usually contains greater than 250 leukocytes/mm³ (0.25 × 10⁹/L), and bacteria may be evident on Gram stain of a centrifuged specimen
In 60%–80% of patients with cirrhotic ascites, the Gram stain is negative

Other diagnostic tests
Culture of peritoneal dialysate or ascitic fluid should be positive, particularly if collected prior to initiation of antibiotics
Procalcitonin in conjunction with clinical findings is a sensitive test for bacterial peritonitis

Secondary Peritonitis

Signs and symptoms
Generalized abdominal pain
Tachypnea
Tachycardia
Nausea and vomiting
Temperature is normal initially then increases to 37.8–38.9°C (100–102°F) within the first few hours and may continue to rise for the next several hours
Hypotension, hypoperfusion, and shock if volume is not restored
Decreased urine output due to vascular volume depletion

Physical examination
Voluntary abdominal guarding changing to involuntary guarding and a "board-like abdomen"
Abdominal tenderness and distension
Faint bowel sounds that cease over time

Laboratory tests
Leukocytosis (15,000–20,000 WBC/mm³ [15 × 10⁹ to 20 × 10⁹/L]), with neutrophils predominating and an elevated percentage of immature neutrophils (bands)
Elevated hematocrit and blood urea nitrogen because of dehydration
Patient progresses from early alkalosis because of hyperventilation and vomiting to metabolic acidosis

Other diagnostic tests
Abdominal radiographs may be useful because free air in the abdomen (indicating intestinal perforation) or distension of the small or large bowel is often evident

(WBC, white blood cell.)

- In the initial hour of treatment, a large volume of IV solution (lactated Ringer solution) may need to be administered to restore intravascular volume. This may be followed by up to 1 L/h until fluid balance is restored in a few hours.
- In patients with significant blood loss (hematocrit ≤25%), blood should be given. This is generally in the form of packed red blood cells.
- Enteral or parenteral nutrition facilitates improved immune function and wound healing to ensure recovery.

PHARMACOLOGIC THERAPY

- The goals of antimicrobial therapy are to control bacteremia and to establish the metastatic foci of infection, to reduce suppurative complications after bacterial contamination, and to prevent local spread of existing infection.
- An empiric antimicrobial regimen should be started as soon as the presence of intra-abdominal infection is suspected on the basis of likely pathogens.

Recommendations

- Table 42–4 presents recommended and alternative regimens for community-acquired complicated intra-abdominal infections. Guidelines for initial antimicrobial treatment of specific intra-abdominal infections are presented in Table 42–5.
- Evidence-based treatment principles for complicated intra-abdominal infections are given in Table 42–6.
- The selection of a specific agent or combination should be based on culture and susceptibility data for peritonitis that occurs from chronic peritoneal dialysis. If microbiologic data are unavailable, empiric therapy should be initiated.
- For established intra-abdominal infections, most patients are adequately treated with 4 to 7 days of antimicrobial therapy.
- Intraperitoneal administration of antibiotics is preferred over IV therapy in the treatment of peritonitis that occurs in patients undergoing continuous ambulatory peritoneal dialysis. Initial antibiotic regimens should be effective against both gram-positive and gram-negative organisms.

TABLE 42–4	Recommended Agents for the Treatment of Community-Acquired Complicated Intra-Abdominal Infections in Adults
Agents Recommended for Mild-to-Moderate Infections	**Agents Recommended for High Risk or High Severity Infections**
Single agent	
Cefoxitin[a]	Piperacillin–tazobactam
Moxifloxacin[b]	Imipenem–cilastatin,[c] meropenem,[c]
Ertapenem[c]	doripenem[c]
Combination regimens	
Cefazolin,[a] cefuroxime,[a] ceftriaxone, cefotaxime each in combination with metronidazole	Cefepime or ceftazidime each in combination with metronidazole
Ciprofloxacin[b] or levofloxacin[b] each in combination with metronidazole	Ciprofloxacin[b] or levofloxacin[b] each in combination with metronidazole

[a]Empiric first- and second-generation cephalosporin use should be avoided unless local antibiograms show >80% to 90% susceptibility of *E. coli* to these agents.
[b]Use of quinolones may be associated with treatment failure due to increasing resistance of enteric pathogens including *E. coli*. Empiric quinolone use should be avoided unless local antibiograms show >80% to 90% susceptibility of *E. coli* to quinolones.
[c]Carbapenems should be reserved for settings where there is a high risk of resistance to other agents.

TABLE 42–5 Guidelines for Empiric Antimicrobial Agents for Intra-Abdominal Infections

	Primary Agents	Alternatives
Primary (spontaneous) bacterial peritonitis		
Cirrhosis	Ceftriaxone, cefotaxime	1. Piperacillin–tazobactam, carbapenems
		2. Aztreonam combined with an agent active against *Streptococcus* spp. (eg, vancomycin) or quinolones with significant *Streptococcus* spp. activity (levofloxacin, moxifloxacin)
Peritoneal dialysis	Initial empiric regimens should be active against both Gram-positive (including *S. aureus*) and Gram-negative pathogens: Gram-positive agent (first-generation cephalosporin or vancomycin) plus a Gram-negative agent (third-generation cephalosporin or aminoglycoside)	1. Cefepime or carbapenems may be used alone
		2. Aztreonam or an aminoglycoside may be used in place of ceftazidime or cefepime as long as combined with a Gram-positive agent
		3. Quinolones may be used in place of Gram-negative agents if local susceptibilities allow
	1. *Staphylococcus* spp: oxacillin/nafcillin or first-generation cephalosporin	1. Vancomycin should be used if concern for methicillin-resistant *Staphylococcus* spp.
		2. Add rifampin for 5–7 days with vancomycin for methicillin-resistant *S. aureus*
	2. *Streptococcus* or *Enterococcus*: ampicillin	1. An aminoglycoside may be added for *Enterococcus* spp.
		2. Linezolid or daptomycin should ideally be used to treat vancomycin-resistant *Enterococcus* spp. not susceptible to ampicillin
	3. Aerobic Gram-negative bacilli: ceftazidime or cefepime	1. The regimen should be based on in vitro sensitivity tests
	4. *Pseudomonas aeruginosa*: two agents with differing mechanisms of action, such as an oral quinolone plus ceftazidime, cefepime, tobramycin, or piperacillin	
Secondary bacterial peritonitis		
Perforated peptic ulcer	First-generation cephalosporins	1. Ceftriaxone, cefotaxime, or antianaerobic cephalosporins[a]
Other	Third- or fourth-generation cephalosporin with metronidazole, piperacillin–tazobactam or carbapenem	1. Ciprofloxacin[b] or levofloxacin[b] each with metronidazole or moxifloxacin[b] alone
		2. Aztreonam with vancomycin and metronidazole
		3. Antianaerobic cephalosporins[a]

Abscess		
General	Third- or fourth-generation cephalosporin with metronidazole, or piperacillin–tazobactam	1. Imipenem–cilastatin, meropenem, doripenem, or ertapenem 2. Ciprofloxacin[b] or levofloxacin[b] each with metronidazole or moxifloxacin alone
Liver	As above	Use metronidazole if amoebic liver abscess is suspected
Spleen	Ceftriaxone or cefotaxime	Moxifloxacin[b] or levofloxacin[b]
Other intra-abdominal infections		
Appendicitis	Same management as for community-acquired complicated intra-abdominal infections	
Community-acquired acute cholecystitis	Ceftriaxone or cefotaxime	Severe infection, piperacillin/tazobactam, antipseuodomonal carbapenem, aztreonam with metronidazole
Cholangitis	Ceftriaxone or cefotaxime each with or without metronidazole	Vancomycin with aztreonam with or without metronidazole
Acute contamination from abdominal trauma	Antianaerobic cephalosporins[a] or metronidazole with either ceftriaxone or cefotaxime	1. Piperacillin/tazobactam or a carbapenem 2. Ciprofloxacin[b] or levofloxacin[b] each with metronidazole or moxifloxacin alone

[a]Cefoxitin or ceftizoxime; these agents should be avoided empirically unless local antibiograms show >80% to 90% susceptibility of E. coli to these agents.

[b]Use of quinolones may be associated with treatment failure due to increasing resistance of enteric pathogens including E. coli. Empiric quinolone use should be avoided unless local antibiograms show >80% to 90% susceptibility of E. coli to quinolones.

TABLE 42–6 Evidence-Based Recommendations for Treatment of Complicated Intra-Abdominal Infections

	Grade of Recommendation[a]
Elements of appropriate intervention	
An appropriate source control procedure to drain infected foci, control ongoing peritoneal contamination by diversion or resection, and restore anatomic and physiological function to the extent feasible is recommended for nearly all patients with intra-abdominal infection	B-2
Community-acquired infections of mild-to-moderate severity in adults	
Antibiotics used for empiric treatment of community-acquired intra-abdominal infections should be active against enteric Gram-negative aerobic and facultative bacilli and enteric Gram-positive streptococci	A-1
For patients with mild-to-moderate community-acquired infections regimens with substantial anti-pseudomonal activity are not required	A-1
Empiric coverage of *Enterococcus* is not necessary in patients with mild-to-moderate severity community-acquired intra-abdominal infection	A-1
The use of agents listed as appropriate for higher-severity community-acquired infection and healthcare-associated infection is not recommended for patients with mild-to-moderate community-acquired infection, because such regimens may carry a greater risk of toxicity and facilitate acquisition of more resistant organisms	B-2
High-risk or high-severity community-acquired infections in adults[b]	
The empiric use of antimicrobial regimens with broad-spectrum activity against Gram-negative organisms including *Pseudomonas* spp., such as meropenem, imipenem–cilastatin, doripenem, piperacillin–tazobactam, ciprofloxacin or levofloxacin in combination with met-ronidazole, or ceftazidime or cefepime in combination with metronidazole, is recommended for patients with high-severity community-acquired intra-abdominal infection	A-1
Aztreonam plus metronidazole is an alternative, but addition of an agent effective against Gram-positive cocci is recommended	B-3
Healthcare-associated infections in adults	
Empiric antibiotic therapy for healthcare-associated intra-abdominal infection should be driven by local microbiologic results	A-2
To achieve empiric coverage of likely pathogens, multidrug regimens that include agents with expanded spectra of activity against Gram-negative aerobic and facultative bacilli may be needed. These agents include meropenem, imipenem–cilastatin, doripenem, piperacillin–tazobactam, or ceftazidime or cefepime in combination with metronidazole. Aminoglycosides or colistin may be required	B-3

Antimicrobial agents not recommended

Ampicillin–sulbactam is not recommended for use because of high rates of resistance to this agent among community-acquired *E. coli* B-2

Quinolone-resistant *E. coli* have become common in some communities, and quinolones should not be used unless hospital surveys indicate 90% susceptibility of *E. coli* to quinolones A-2

Cefotetan and clindamycin are not recommended for use because of increasing prevalence of resistance to these agents among *Bacteroides fragilis* B-2

Because of the availability of less toxic agents demonstrated to be at least equally effective, aminoglycosides are not recommended for routine use in adults with community-acquired intra-abdominal infection B-2

Oral completion therapy

For adults recovering from intra-abdominal infection, completion of the antimicrobial course with oral forms of moxifloxacin, ciprofloxacin plus metronidazole, levofloxacin plus metronidazole, an oral cephalosporin with metronidazole, or amoxicillin–clavulanic acid is acceptable in patients able to tolerate an oral diet and in patients in whom susceptibility studies do not demonstrate resistance B-2

Duration of therapy

Antimicrobial therapy of established infection should be limited to 4 days, unless it is difficult to achieve adequate source control. Longer durations of therapy have not been associated with improved outcome[c] A-1

For acute stomach and proximal jejunum perforations, in the absence of acid-reducing therapy or malignancy and when source control is achieved within 24 hours, prophylactic anti-infective therapy directed at aerobic Gram-positive cocci for 24 hours is adequate B-2

Bowel injuries attributable to penetrating, blunt, or iatrogenic trauma that are repaired within 12 hours and any other intraoperative contamination of the operative field by enteric contents should be treated with antibiotics for ≤24 hours A-1

Acute appendicitis without evidence of perforation, abscess, or local peritonitis requires only prophylactic administration of narrow spectrum regimens active against aerobic and facultative and obligate anaerobes; treatment should be discontinued within 24 hours A-1

The administration of prophylactic antibiotics to patients with severe necrotizing pancreatitis prior to the diagnosis of infection is not recommended A-1

Anaerobic coverage

Coverage for obligate anaerobic bacilli should be provided for distal small bowel, appendiceal, and colon-derived infection and for more proximal GI perforations in the presence of obstruction or paralytic ileus A-1

Antifungal therapy

Antifungal therapy for patients with severe community-acquired or healthcare-associated infection is recommended if *Candida* is grown from intra-abdominal cultures B-2

(continued)

TABLE 42–6 Evidence-Based Recommendations for Treatment of Complicated Intra-Abdominal Infections (*Continued*)

	Grade of Recommendation[a]
Anti-MRSA therapy	
Empiric antimicrobial coverage directed against MRSA should be provided to patients with healthcare-associated intra-abdominal infection who are known to be colonized with the organism or who are at risk of having an infection due to this organism because of prior treatment failure and significant antibiotic exposure	B-2
Vancomycin is recommended for treatment of suspected or proven intra-abdominal infection due to MRSA	A-3
Antienterococcal therapy	
Antimicrobial therapy for enterococci should be given when enterococci are recovered from patients with healthcare-associated infection	B-III
Empiric antienterococcal therapy is recommended for patients with high-risk community-acquired infections and healthcare-associated intra-abdominal infections, particularly those with postoperative infection, those who have previously received cephalosporins or other antimicrobial agents selecting for *Enterococcus* species, immunocompromised patients, and those with valvular heart disease or prosthetic intravascular materials	B-II
Initial empiric antienterococcal therapy should be directed against *Enterococcus faecalis*. Antibiotics that can potentially be used against this organism, on the basis of susceptibility testing of the individual isolate, include ampicillin, piperacillin/tazobactam, and vancomycin	B-III
Empiric therapy directed against vancomycin-resistant *Enterococcus faecium* is not recommended unless the patient is at very high risk for an infection due to this organism, such as a liver transplant recipient with an intra-abdominal infection originating in the hepatobiliary tree or a patient known to be colonized with vancomycin-resistant *E. faecium*	B-III

(MRSA, methicillin-resistant *Staphylococcus aureus*.)

[a]Strength of recommendations: A, B, C = good, moderate, and poor evidence to support recommendation, respectively. Quality of evidence: 1 = Evidence from ≥1 properly randomized, controlled trial. 2 = Evidence from ≥1 well-designed clinical trial without randomization, from cohort or case-controlled analytic studies; from multiple time series, or from dramatic results from uncontrolled experiments. 3 = Evidence from opinions of respected authorities, based on clinical experience, descriptive studies, or reports of expert communities.

[b]Criteria for high risk or high severity community-acquired infection: APACHE II score ≥15, delay in initial intervention >24 hours), advanced age, comorbidity and degree of organ dysfunction, low albumin level, poor nutritional status, degree of peritoneal involvement or diffuse peritonitis, inability to achieve adequate debridement or control of drainage, and presence of malignancy.

[c]After IDSA/SIS guideline publication a randomized controlled trial was published and demonstrated that 4 days of therapy after source control is adequate.[47]

- Suitable antibiotics for initial empiric treatment of continuous ambulatory peritoneal dialysis–associated peritonitis are **cefazolin** (loading dose [LD] 500 mg/L; maintenance dose [MD] 125 mg/L) or **vancomycin** (LD 1000 mg/L; MD 25 mg/L) in cases of high prevalence of methicillin-resistant *Staphylococcus aureus* (MRSA) or β-lactam allergy may be utilized for Gram-positive coverage. One of these Gram-positive agents should be combined with a Gram-negative agent such as **ceftazidime** (LD 500 mg/L; MD 125 mg/L) or **cefepime** (LD 500 mg/L; MD 125 mg/L) or an aminoglycoside (**gentamicin** or **tobramycin** LD 8 mg/L; MD 4 mg/L).
- Antimicrobial therapy should be continued for at least 1 week after the dialysate fluid is clear and for a total of at least 14 days.

EVALUATION OF THERAPEUTIC OUTCOMES

- The patient should be continually reassessed to determine the success or failure of therapies.
- Once antimicrobials are initiated and other important therapies described earlier in the Treatment section are used, most patients should show improvement within 2 to 3 days. Usually, temperature will return to near normal, vital signs should stabilize, and the patient should not appear in distress, with the exception of recognized discomfort and pain from incisions, drains, and nasogastric tube.
- At 24 to 48 hours, aerobic bacterial culture results should return. If a suspected pathogen is not sensitive to the antimicrobial agents being given, the regimen should be changed if the patient has not shown sufficient improvement.
- If the isolated pathogen is susceptible to one antimicrobial, and the patient is progressing well, concurrent antimicrobial therapy may often be deescalated.
- With present anaerobic culturing techniques and the slow growth of these organisms, anaerobes are often not identified until 4 to 7 days after culture, and sensitivity information is difficult to obtain. For this reason, there are usually few data with which to alter the antianaerobic component of the antimicrobial regimen.
- Superinfection in patients being treated for intra-abdominal infection is often due to *Candida*; however, enterococci or opportunistic gram-negative bacilli such as *Pseudomonas* or *Serratia* may be involved.
- Treatment regimens for intra-abdominal infection can be judged successful if the patient recovers from the infection without recurrent peritonitis or intra-abdominal abscess and without the need for additional antimicrobials. A regimen can be considered unsuccessful if a significant adverse drug reaction occurs, if reoperation is necessary, or if patient improvement is delayed beyond 1 or 2 weeks.

See Chapter 114, Intra-Abdominal Infections, authored by Alan E. Gross, Keith M. Olsen, and Joseph T. DiPiro, for a more detailed discussion of this topic.

Respiratory Tract Infections, Lower

BRONCHITIS

ACUTE BRONCHITIS

- Acute bronchitis is characterized by inflammation of the epithelium of the large airways resulting from infection or exposure to irritating environmental triggers (eg, air pollution and cigarette smoke). The disease entity is frequently classified as either acute or chronic. Acute bronchitis occurs in all ages, whereas chronic bronchitis primarily affects adults.
- Acute bronchitis most commonly occurs during the winter months. Cold, damp climates and/or the presence of high concentrations of irritating substances such as air pollution or cigarette smoke may precipitate attacks.
- Respiratory viruses are the predominant infectious agents associated with acute bronchitis. The most common infecting agents include influenza A and B, respiratory syncytial virus (RSV), and parainfluenza virus, whereas the common cold viruses (rhinovirus and coronavirus) and adenovirus are encountered less frequently. Common bacterial pathogens are those associated with community-acquired pneumonia (CAP), including *Mycoplasma pneumoniae*, *Streptococcus pneumonia*, *Haemophilus influenzae*, and *Moraxella catarrhalis*.
- Infection of the trachea and bronchi causes hyperemic and edematous mucous membranes and an increase in bronchial secretions. Destruction of respiratory epithelium can range from mild to extensive and may affect bronchial mucociliary function. In addition, the increase in bronchial secretions, which can become thick and tenacious, further impairs mucociliary activity. Recurrent acute respiratory infections may be associated with increased airway hyperreactivity and possibly the pathogenesis of chronic obstructive lung disease.

Clinical Presentation

- Acute bronchitis usually begins as an upper respiratory infection. Cough is the hallmark of acute bronchitis. It occurs early and will persist despite the resolution of nasal or nasopharyngeal complaints. Frequently, the cough is initially nonproductive but progresses, yielding mucopurulent sputum.
- Bacterial cultures of expectorated sputum are generally of limited utility because of the inability to avoid normal nasopharyngeal flora by the sampling technique. Similarly, viral cultures are unnecessary. For the vast majority of affected patients, an etiologic diagnosis is unnecessary and will not change the prescribing of routine supportive care for the management of these patients.

Treatment

- **Goals of Therapy:** The goal is to provide comfort to the patient and, in the unusually severe case, to treat associated dehydration and respiratory compromise.
- The treatment of acute bronchitis is symptomatic and supportive in nature. Reassurance and antipyretics alone are often sufficient. Bed rest and mild analgesic-antipyretic therapy are often helpful in relieving the associated lethargy, malaise, and fever. Patients should be encouraged to drink fluids to prevent dehydration and possibly decrease the viscosity of respiratory secretions.
- **Aspirin** or **acetaminophen** (650 mg in adults or 10–15 mg/kg per dose in children with a maximum daily adult dose of <4 g and 60 mg/kg for children) or **ibuprofen** (200–800 mg in adults or 10 mg/kg per dose in children with a maximum daily dose of 3.2 g for adults and 40 mg/kg for children) is administered every 4 to 6 hours.
- In children, aspirin should be avoided and acetaminophen used as the preferred agent because of the possible association between aspirin use and the development of Reye syndrome.

- Mist therapy and/or the use of a vaporizer may further promote the thinning and loosening of respiratory secretions. In otherwise healthy patients, no meaningful benefits have been described with the use of oral or aerosolized β_2-receptor agonists and/or oral or aerosolized corticosteroids.
- Persistent, mild cough, which may be bothersome, may be treated with **dextromethorphan**; more severe coughs may require intermittent **codeine** or other similar agents.
- Routine use of antibiotics in the treatment of acute bronchitis is strongly discouraged; however, in patients who exhibit persistent fever or respiratory symptomatology for more than 5 to 7 days, the possibility of a concurrent bacterial infection should be suspected.
- When possible, antibiotic therapy is directed toward anticipated respiratory pathogen(s) (ie, *Streptococcus pneumoniae* and *H. influenzae*).
- *M. pneumoniae*, if suspected by history or if confirmed by culture, serology, or PCR may be treated with **azithromycin.** Also, a fluoroquinolone with activity against these pathogens (**levofloxacin**) may be used in adults.
- See Chapter 41 for recommendations to treat influenza.

CHRONIC BRONCHITIS

- Chronic bronchitis is a result of several contributing factors, including cigarette smoking; exposure to occupational dusts, fumes, and environmental pollution; host factors [eg, genetic factors]; and bacterial or viral infections.
- Chronic bronchitis is defined clinically as the presence of a chronic cough productive of sputum lasting more than three consecutive months of the year for two consecutive years without an underlying etiology of bronchiectasis or tuberculosis.

Clinical Presentation

- The hallmark of chronic bronchitis is a cough that may range from a mild to severe, incessant coughing productive of purulent sputum. Expectoration of the largest quantity of sputum usually occurs upon arising in the morning, although many patients expectorate sputum throughout the day. The expectorated sputum is usually tenacious and can vary in color from white to yellow-green. The diagnosis of chronic bronchitis is based primarily on clinical assessment and history.
- The most common bacterial isolates (expressed in percentages of total cultures) identified from sputum culture in patients experiencing an acute exacerbation of chronic bronchitis are given in **Table 43–1.**
- With the exception of pulmonary findings, the physical examination of patients with mild to moderate chronic bronchitis is usually unremarkable (**Table 43–2**).

Treatment

- **Goals of Therapy**: The goal is to reduce the severity of symptoms, to ameliorate acute exacerbations, and to achieve prolonged infection-free intervals.

TABLE 43–1	Common Bacterial Pathogens Isolated from Sputum of Patients with Acute Exacerbation of Chronic Bronchitis
Pathogen	**Percent of Cultures**
H. influenzae[a,b]	45
M. catarrhalis[a]	30
S. pneumoniae[c]	20
E. coli, Enterobacter species, *Klebsiella* species, *P. aeruginosa*	5

[a]Often β-lactamase positive.
[b]Vast majority are nontypable strains.
[c]More than 25% of strains may have intermediate or high resistance to penicillin.

TABLE 43–2	Clinical Presentation of Chronic Bronchitis

Signs and symptoms
  Excessive sputum expectoration
  Cough
  Cyanosis (advanced disease)

Physical examination
  Chest auscultation usually reveals inspiratory and expiratory rales, rhonchi, and mild wheezing with an expiratory phase that is frequently prolonged
  Hyperresonance on percussion with obliteration of the area of cardiac dullness
  Normal vesicular breathing sounds are diminished
  Clubbing of digits (advanced disease)
  Obesity

Chest radiograph
  Increase in anteroposterior diameter of the thoracic cage (barrel chest)
  Depressed diaphragm with limited mobility

Laboratory tests
  Erythrocytosis (advanced disease), that is, increased hematocrit

Pulmonary function tests
  Decreased vital capacity
  Prolonged expiratory flow

- A complete occupational/environmental history for the determination of exposure to noxious and irritating gases, as well as cigarette smoking must be assessed. Exposure to bronchial irritants should be reduced.
- Attempts must be made to reduce the patient's exposure to known bronchial irritants (eg, smoking and workplace pollution).
- Pulmonary rehabilitation programs individualized for patients with chronic respiratory impairment can improve quality of life by optimizing each patient's physical and social performance and autonomy.
- Chest physiotherapy (pulmonary toilet) can be instituted. Humidification of inspired air may promote the hydration (liquefaction) of tenacious secretions, allowing for more effective sputum production. The use of mucolytic aerosols (eg, N-acetylcysteine and deoxyribonuclease) is of questionable therapeutic value. Mucolytic was associated with a small reduction in acute exacerbations and did not cause any harm, improve quality of life, or slow the decline of lung function.
- For patients with moderate to severe chronic obstructive pulmonary disease (COPD), combination therapy with a long-acting β_2-agonist and inhaled corticosteroid led to decreased exacerbations and rescue medication use while it also improved quality of life, lung function, and symptom scores compared with long-acting β_2–agonist monotherapy.

PHARMACOLOGIC THERAPY

- For patients who consistently demonstrate clinical limitation in airflow, a therapeutic challenge of a short-acting β_2-receptor agonist bronchodilator (eg, as albuterol aerosol) should be considered. Regular use of a long-acting β_2-receptor agonist aerosol (eg, salmeterol and formoterol) in responsive patients are more effective and probably more convenient than short-acting β_2-receptor agonists. Chronic inhalation of the salmeterol/fluticasone combination has been associated with improved pulmonary function and quality of life.
- Long-term inhalation of **ipratropium** (or **tiotropium**) decreases the frequency of cough, severity of cough, and volume of expectorated sputum.
- Inhaled long-acting muscarinic antagonists (LAMAs) alone or more frequently when administered in combination with a long-acting β_2-receptor agonist improves lung function and provides benefits in symptom control and reductions in the number of acute exacerbations.

- The role of roflumilast in chronic lung disease is evolving but many guidelines suggest its greatest use is in the more severely affected patients.
- Use of antimicrobials for treatment of chronic bronchitis has been controversial but is becoming more accepted. The goal is to select the most effective antibiotic drug for the patient based on their history of previous exacerbations and response to drug therapy (Fig. 43–1).
- The Anthonisen criteria can be used to determine if antibiotic therapy is indicated. The patient will most likely benefit from antibiotic therapy if two or three of the following are present: (1) increase of shortness of breath, (2) increase in sputum volume, or (3) production of purulent sputum.

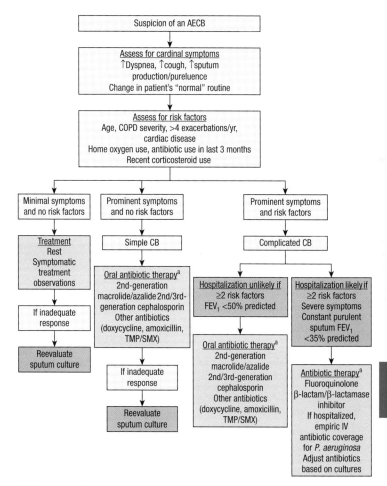

(AECB, acute exacerbation of chronic bronchitis; COPD, chronic obstructive pulmonary disease; CB, chronic bronchitis; TMP/SMX, trimethoprim/sulfamethoxazole.) ªSee Table 43–3 for commonly used antibiotics and doses.

FIGURE 43–1. Clinical algorithm for the diagnosis and treatment of chronic bronchitic patients with an acute exacerbation incorporating the principles of the clinical classification system.

TABLE 43–3	Oral Antibiotics Commonly Used for the Treatment of Acute Respiratory Exacerbations in Chronic Bronchitis		
Antibiotic	**Brand Name**	**Usual Adult Dose (mg)**	**Dose Schedule (Doses/Day)**
Preferred drugs			
Ampicillin	–	250–500	4–3
Amoxicillin	–	500–875	3–2
Amoxicillin/clavulanate	Augmentin®	500–875	3–2
Ciprofloxacin	Cipro®	500–750	2
Levofloxacin	Levaquin®	500–750	1
Moxifloxacin	Avelox®	400	1
Doxycycline	Monodox®	100	2
Minocycline	Minocin®	100	2
Tetracycline HCl	–	500	4
Trimethoprim/sulfamethoxazole[a]	Bactrim DS™/Septra DS®	1 DS	2
Supplemental drugs			
Azithromycin	Zithromax®	250–500	1
Erythromycin	Ery-Tab®/Erythrocin®	500	4
Clarithromycin	Biaxin®	250–500	2
Cephalexin	Keflex®	500	4

[a]DS, double-strength tablet (160-mg trimethoprim/800-mg sulfamethoxazole).

- Selection of antibiotics should consider that up to 30% to 40% of *H. influenzae* and 95% to 100% of *M. catarrhalis* are β-lactamase producers; up to 40% of *S. pneumoniae* demonstrate penicillin resistance, with 20% being highly resistant.
- Antibiotics commonly used in the treatment of these patients and their respective adult starting doses are outlined in Table 43–3. Duration of symptom-free periods may be enhanced by antibiotic regimens using the upper limit of the recommended daily dose for 5 to 7 days.

BRONCHIOLITIS

- Bronchiolitis is an acute viral infection of the lower respiratory tract of infants that affects ~50% of children during the first year of life and 100% by 2 years.
- Respiratory syncytial virus is the most common cause of bronchiolitis, accounting for up to 75% of all cases. Other detectable viruses include parainfluenza, adenovirus, and influenza. Bacteria serve as secondary pathogens in a small minority of cases.

Clinical Presentation

- The most common clinical signs of bronchiolitis are found in Table 43–4. A prodrome suggesting an upper respiratory tract infection, usually lasting from 1 to 4 days, precedes the onset of clinical symptoms. As a result of limited oral intake due to coughing combined with fever, vomiting, and diarrhea, infants are frequently dehydrated.
- The diagnosis of bronchiolitis is based primarily on history and clinical findings. Identification of *respiratory syncytial virus* (RSV) by PCR should be available routinely from most clinical laboratories, but its relevance to the clinical management of bronchiolitis remains obscure and routine testing is not recommended.

TABLE 43–4	Clinical Presentation of Bronchiolitis

Signs and symptoms
Prodrome with irritability, restlessness, and mild fever
Cough and coryza
Vomiting, diarrhea, noisy breathing, and increased respiratory rate as symptoms progress
Labored breathing with retractions of the chest wall, nasal flaring, and grunting

Physical examination
Tachycardia and respiratory rate of 40–80/min in hospitalized infants
Wheezing and inspiratory rales
Mild conjunctivitis in one third of patients
Otitis media in 5%–10% of patients

Laboratory tests
Peripheral white blood cell count normal or slightly elevated
Abnormal arterial blood gases (hypoxemia and, rarely, hypercarbia)

Treatment

- Bronchiolitis is a self-limiting illness and usually requires no therapy (other than reassurance, antipyretics, and adequate fluid intake) unless the infant is hypoxic or dehydrated. Otherwise healthy infants can be treated for fever, provided generous amounts of oral fluids, and observed closely for evidence of respiratory deterioration.
- In severely affected children, the mainstays of therapy for bronchiolitis are oxygen therapy and intravenous (IV) fluids.
- Aerosolized β-adrenergic therapy appears to offer little benefit for the majority of patients but may be useful in the child with a predisposition toward bronchospasm.
- Because bacteria do not represent primary pathogens in the etiology of bronchiolitis, antibiotics should not be routinely administered. However, many clinicians frequently administer antibiotics initially while awaiting culture results because the clinical and radiographic findings in bronchiolitis are often suggestive of a possible bacterial pneumonia.
- **Ribavirin** may be considered for bronchiolitis caused by respiratory syncytial virus in a subset of patients (severely ill patients, especially those with chronic lung disease, congenital heart disease, prematurity, and immunodeficiency—especially severe combined immunodeficiency and human immunodeficiency virus [HIV] infection). Use of the drug requires special equipment (small-particle aerosol generator) and specifically trained personnel for administration via oxygen hood or mist tent.

PNEUMONIA

- Pneumonia remains one of the most common causes of severe sepsis and infectious cause of death in children and adults in the United States, with a mortality rate of 30% to 40%. Table 43–5 presents the classification of pneumonia and risk factors.

PATHOPHYSIOLOGY

- Microorganisms gain access to the lower respiratory tract by three routes: they may be inhaled as aerosolized particles, they may enter the lung via the bloodstream from an extrapulmonary site of infection, or aspiration of oropharyngeal contents may occur.
- Lung infections with viruses suppress the bacterial clearing activity of the lung by impairing alveolar macrophage function and mucociliary clearance, thus setting the stage for secondary bacterial pneumonia.
- The most prominent pathogen causing community-acquired pneumonia in otherwise healthy adults is *S. pneumoniae* (up to 35% of all cases). Other common bacterial causes are *H. influenza*, the "atypical" pathogens including *M. pneumoniae*, *Legionella* species, *Chlamydophila pneumoniae*, and a variety of viruses.

TABLE 43–5	Pneumonia Classifications and Risk Factors	
Type of Pneumonia	**Definition**	**Risk Factors**
Community acquired (CAP)	Pneumonia developing in patients with no contact to a medical facility	• Age >65 years • Diabetes mellitus • Asplenia • Chronic cardiovascular, pulmonary, renal and/or liver disease • Smoking and/or alcohol abuse
Hospital acquired (HAP)	Pneumonia developing >48 hours after hospital admission	• Witnessed aspiration • COPD, ARDS, or coma • Administration of antacids, H_2-antagonists, or proton pump inhibitor • Supine position • Enteral nutrition, nasogastric tube • Reintubation, tracheostomy, or patient transport • Head trauma, ICP monitoring • Age >60 years • MDR risk (eg. MRSA, MDR *Pseudomonas*) if IV antibiotic use within 90 days
Ventilator associated (VAP)	Pneumonia developing >48 hours after intubation and mechanical ventilation	• Same as hospital acquired • MDR risk with septic shock, ARDS, acute renal replacement therapy, or 5+ days of hospitalization

ARDS, adult respiratory distress syndrome; CAP, community-acquired pneumonia; COPD, chronic obstructive pulmonary disease; HAP, hospital-acquired pneumonia; ICP, intracranial pressure; MDR, multidrug resistant; MRSA, methicillin-resistant S. aureus VAP, ventilator-associated pneumonia.

• Gram-negative aerobic bacilli and *Staphylococcus aureus* and multidrug resistant pathogens are also the leading causative agents in hospital-acquired pneumonia.
• Anaerobic bacteria are the most common etiologic agents in pneumonia that follows the gross aspiration of gastric or oropharyngeal contents.
• In the pediatric age group, most pneumonias are due to viruses, especially respiratory syncytial virus, parainfluenza, and adenovirus. *S. pneumoniae* is the major bacterial pathogen, followed by group *A Streptococcus, S. aureus,* and *H. influenzae* type b.

CLINICAL PRESENTATION

Gram-Positive and Gram-Negative Bacterial Pneumonia

• The clinical presentation of pneumonia is found in Table 43–6.
• The chest radiograph and sputum examination and culture are the most useful diagnostic tests for gram-positive and gram-negative bacterial pneumonia. Typically, the chest radiograph reveals a dense lobar or segmental infiltrate.

Anaerobic Pneumonia

• Anaerobic pneumonitis is most likely to occur in individuals predisposed to aspiration by impaired consciousness or dysphagia as the source for the anaerobic bacteria is generally the oral cavity/gingival crevice. The most common organisms identified are *Bacteroides melaninogenicus,* Fusobacteria, and anaerobic streptococci; polymicrobial infections with anaerobes and aerobes, such as *S. aureus, S. pneumoniae,* and

TABLE 43-6	Clinical Presentation of Pneumonia

Signs and symptoms
Abrupt onset of fever, chills, dyspnea, and productive cough
Rust-colored sputum or hemoptysis
Pleuritic chest pain

Physical examination
Tachypnea and tachycardia
Dullness to percussion
Increased tactile fremitus, whisper pectoriloquy, and egophony
Chest wall retractions and grunting respirations
Diminished breath sounds over affected area
Inspiratory crackles during lung expansion

Chest radiograph
Dense lobar or segmental infiltrate

Laboratory tests
Leukocytosis with predominance of polymorphonuclear cells
Low oxygen saturation on arterial blood gas or pulse oximetry

gram-negative bacilli, are common. The course of anaerobic pneumonia is typically indolent with cough, low-grade fever, and weight loss, although an acute presentation may occur.

Mycoplasma Pneumoniae

- *M. pneumoniae* pneumonia presents with a gradual onset of fever, headache, and malaise, with the appearance 3 to 5 days after the onset of illness of a persistent, hacking cough that initially is nonproductive. Sore throat, ear pain, and rhinorrhea are often present. Lung findings are generally limited to rales and rhonchi; findings of consolidation are rarely present.
- Nonpulmonary manifestations are extremely common and include nausea, vomiting, diarrhea, myalgias, arthralgias, polyarticular arthritis, skin rashes, myocarditis and pericarditis, hemolytic anemia, meningoencephalitis, cranial neuropathies, and Guillain–Barré syndrome. Systemic symptoms generally clear in 1 to 2 weeks, whereas respiratory symptoms may persist up to 4 weeks.
- Radiographic findings include patchy or interstitial infiltrates, which are most commonly seen in the lower lobes.

Viral Pneumonia

- The clinical pictures produced by respiratory viruses are sufficiently variable and overlap to such a degree that an etiologic diagnosis cannot confidently be made on clinical grounds alone. Serologic tests for virus-specific antibodies are often used in the diagnosis of viral infections. The diagnostic fourfold rise in titer between acute and convalescent phase sera may require 2 to 3 weeks to develop; however, same-day diagnosis of viral infections is now possible through the use of indirect immunofluorescence tests on exfoliated cells from the respiratory tract.
- Radiographic findings are nonspecific and include bronchial wall thickening and perihilar and diffuse interstitial infiltrates.

Hospital-Acquired Pneumonia

- The strongest predisposing factor for hospital-acquired pneumonia (HAP) is mechanical ventilation. Factors predisposing patients to HAP include severe illness, long duration of hospitalization, supine positioning, witnessed aspiration, coma, acute respiratory distress syndrome, patient transport, and prior antibiotic exposure.

TABLE 43–7   Evidence-Based Empirical Antimicrobial Therapy for Pneumonia in Adults[a]

Clinical Setting	Usual Pathogens	Empirical Therapy
Outpatient/community acquired		
Previously healthy	S. pneumoniae, M. pneumoniae, H. influenzae, C. pneumoniae, M. catarrhalis	Macrolide,[b] or tetracycline[c]
Comorbidities (diabetes, heart/lung/liver/renal disease, and alcoholism)	Viral	Oseltamivir or zanamivir if <48° from onset of symptoms
	MDR S. pneumoniae	Fluoroquinolone[d] or β-lactam + macrolide[b]
Elderly	S. pneumoniae, gram-negative bacilli	Piperacillin/tazobactam or cephalosporin[e] or carbapenem[f]
Regions with >25% rate of macrolide-resistant S. pneumoniae		Fluoroquinolone[d] or β-lactam + macrolide[b]/tetracycline
Inpatient/community acquired		
Non-ICU	S. pneumoniae, H. influenzae, M. pneumoniae, C. pneumoniae, Legionella sp.	Fluoroquinolone[d] or β-lactam + macrolide[b]/tetracycline
ICU	S. pneumoniae, S. aureus, Legionella sp., gram-negative bacilli, H. influenzae	β-Lactam + macrolide[b]/fluoroquinolone[d]
	If P. aeruginosa suspected	Piperacillin/tazobactam or meropenem or cefepime + fluoroquinolone[d]/AMG/azithromycin; or β-lactam + AMG + azithromycin/respiratory fluoroquinolone[d]
	If MRSA suspected	Above + vancomycin or linezolid
	Viral	Oseltamivir or zanamivir ± antibiotics for 2° infection
Hospital acquired or ventilator associated		
No risk factors for MDR pathogens (single agent Pseudomonal coverage)	S. pneumoniae, H. influenzae, MSSA, enteric gram-negative bacilli	Piperacillin/tazobactam, cefepime, levofloxacin, imipenem or meropenem
Risk factors for MDR pathogen (dual agent Pseudomonal coverage)	P. aeruginosa, K. pneumoniae (ESBL), Acinetobacter sp.	Antipseudomonal cephalosporin[e] or antipseudomonal carbapenem or β-lactam/β-lactamase + antipseudomonal fluoroquinolone[d] or AMG[g]
	If MRSA or Legionella sp. suspected	Above + vancomycin or linezolid

| Aspiration | S. aureus, enteric gram-negative bacilli | Penicillin or clindamycin or piperacillin/tazobactam + AMG[g] |
| | Anaerobes | Clindamycin, β-lactam/β-lactamase, or carbapenem |

Atypical pneumonia

Legionella pneumophila		Fluoroquinolone,[d] doxycycline, or azithromycin
Mycoplasma pneumonia		Fluoroquinolone,[d] doxycycline, or azithromycin
Chlamydophila pneumonia		Fluoroquinolone,[d] doxycycline, or azithromycin
SARS		Fluoroquinolone[d] or macrolides[b]
Avian influenza		Oseltamivir
H1N1 influenza		Oseltamivir

(MRSA, methicillin-resistant *Staphylococcus aureus*; AMG, aminoglycoside; SARS, severe acute respiratory syndrome; ESBL, extended-spectrum β-lactamases; MDR, multidrug resistant; MSSA, methicillin-sensitive *Staphylococcus aureus*.)

[a] See the section Selection of Antimicrobial Agents.
[b] Macrolide/azalide: erythromycin, clarithromycin, and azithromycin.
[c] Tetracycline: tetracycline, HCl, and doxycycline.
[d] Fluoroquinolone: ciprofloxacin, levofloxacin, and moxifloxacin.
[e] Antipseudomonal cephalosporin: cefepime and ceftazidime.
[f] Antipseudomonal carbapenem: imipenem and meropenem.
[g] Aminoglycoside: amikacin, gentamicin, and tobramycin.

TABLE 43-8	Empirical Antimicrobial Therapy for Pneumonia in Pediatric Patients[a]	
Clinical Setting	**Usual Pathogen(s)**	**Empirical Therapy**
Outpatient/community acquired		
<1 month	Group B *Streptococcus*, *H. influenzae* (nontypable), *E. coli*, *S. aureus*, *Listeria* CMV, RSV, adenovirus	Ampicillin/sulbactam, cephalosporin,[b] carbapenem[c] Ribavirin for RSV[d]
1–3 months	*C. pneumoniae*, possibly *Ureaplasma*, CMV, *Pneumocystis carinii* (afebrile pneumonia syndrome) *S. pneumoniae*, *S. aureus*	Macrolide/azalide,[e] trimethoprim–sulfamethoxazole Semisynthetic penicillin[f] or cephalosporin[g]
Preschool-aged children	Viral (rhinovirus, RSV, influenza A and B, parainfluenzae, adenovirus, human meta-pneumovirus, coronavirus)	Antimicrobial therapy not routinely required
Previously healthy, fully immunized infants and preschool children with suspected mild–moderate bacterial CAP	*S. pneumoniae* *M. pneumoniae*, other atypical	Amoxicillin, cephalosporin[b,g] Macrolide/azalide or fluoroquinolone
Previously healthy, fully immunized school-aged children and adolescents with mild–moderate CAP	*S. pneumoniae* *M. pneumoniae*, other atypical	Amoxicillin, cephalosporin,[b,g] or fluoroquinolone Macrolide/azalide, fluoroquinolone, or tetracycline
Moderate–severe CAP during influenza virus outbreak	Influenza A and B, other viruses	Oseltamivir or zanamivir
Inpatient/community acquired		
Fully immunized infants and school-aged children	*S. pneumoniae* CA-MRSA *M. pneumoniae*, *C. pneumoniae*	Ampicillin, penicillin G, cephalosporin[b] β-Lactam + vancomycin/clindamycin β-Lactam + macrolide/fluoroquinolone/doxycycline
Not fully immunized infants and children; regions with invasive penicillin-resistant pneumococcal strains; patients with life-threatening infections	*S. pneumoniae*, PCN resistant MRSA *M. pneumoniae*, other atypical pathogens	Cephalosporin[b] Add vancomycin/clindamycin Macrolide/azalide[e] + β-lactam/doxycycline/fluoroquinolone

(CMV, cytomegalovirus; RSV, respiratory syncytial virus; CAP, community-acquired pneumonia; MRSA, methicillin resistant *Staphylococcus aureus*.)
[a]See the section Selection of Antimicrobial Agents.
[b]Third-generation cephalosporin: ceftriaxone and cefotaxime. Note that cephalosporins are not active against *Listeria*.
[c]Carbapenem: imipenem–cilastatin and meropenem.
[d]See text for details regarding possible ribavirin treatment for RSV infection.
[e]Macrolide/azalide: erythromycin and clarithromycin/azithromycin.
[f]Semisynthetic penicillin: nafcillin, and oxacillin.
[g]Second-generation cephalosporin: cefuroxime and cefprozil.

TABLE 43–9 Antibiotic Doses for Treatment of Bacterial Pneumonia

Antibiotic class	Antibiotic	Brand name	Daily Antibiotic Dose[a]	
			Pediatric	Adult (Total Dose/Day)
Penicillin	Ampicillin ± sulbactam	Unasyn®	150–200 mg/kg/day	6–12 g
	Amoxicillin ± clavulanate[b]	Augmentin®	45–100 mg/kg/day	0.75–1 g
	Piperacillin/tazobactam	Zosyn®	200–300 mg/kg/day	12–18 g
	Penicillin		100,000–250,000 units/kg/day	12–18 million units
Extended-spectrum cephalosporins	Ceftriaxone	Rocephin®	50–75 mg/kg/day	1–2 g
	Cefotaxime	Claforan®	150 mg/kg/day	2–12 g
	Ceftazidime	Fortaz®/Tazicef®	90–150 mg/kg/day	4–6 g
	Cefepime	Maxipime®	100–150 mg/kg/day	2–6 g
Macrolide/azalide	Clarithromycin	Biaxin®	15 mg/kg/day	0.5–1 g
	Erythromycin	Ery-Tab®	30–50 mg/kg/day	1–2 g
	Azithromycin	Zithromax®	10 mg/kg × 1 day (× 2 days if parenteral), and then 5 mg/kg days 2–5	500 mg × 1 day (× 2 days if parenteral), and then 250 mg days 2–5
Fluoroquinolones[c]	Moxifloxacin	Avelox®	–	400 mg
	Gemifloxacin	Factive®	–	320 mg
	Levofloxacin	Levaquin®	8–20 mg/kg/day	750 mg
	Ciprofloxacin	Cipro®	30 mg/kg/day	1.2 g
Tetracycline[d]	Doxycycline	Monodox®/Doxy 100™	2–5 mg/kg/day	100–200 mg
	Tetracycline HCl		25–50 mg/kg/day	1–2 g
Aminoglycosides	Gentamicin		7.5–10 mg/kg/day	7.5 mg/kg
	Tobramycin		7.5–10 mg/kg/day	7.5 mg/kg
Carbapenems	Imipenem	Primaxin®	60–100 mg/kg/day	2–4 g
	Meropenem	Merrem®	30–60 mg/kg/day	1–3 g

(continued)

TABLE 43-9 Antibiotic Doses for Treatment of Bacterial Pneumonia (*Continued*)

Antibiotic class	Antibiotic	Brand name	Daily Antibiotic Dose[a]	
			Pediatric	Adult (Total Dose/Day)
Other	Vancomycin		45–60 mg/kg/day	2–3 g
	Linezolid	Zyvox®	20–30 mg/kg/day	1.2 g
	Clindamycin	Cleocin®	30–40 mg/kg/day	1.8 g

[a]Doses can be increased for more severe disease and may require modification for patients with organ dysfunction.

[b]Higher-dose amoxicillin and amoxicillin/clavulanate (eg, 90 mg/kg/day) are used for penicillin-resistant *S. pneumoniae*.

[c]Fluoroquinolones have been avoided for pediatric patients because of the potential for cartilage damage; however, they have been used for MDR bacterial infection safely and effectively in infants and children (see text).

[d]Tetracyclines are rarely used in pediatric patients, particularly in those younger than 8 years because of tetracycline-induced permanent tooth discoloration.

- The diagnosis of nosocomial pneumonia is usually established by the presence of a new infiltrate on chest radiograph, fever, worsening respiratory status, and the appearance of thick, neutrophil-laden respiratory secretions.

TREATMENT

- Eradication of the offending organism and complete clinical cure are the primary objectives. Associated morbidity should be minimized (eg, renal, pulmonary, or hepatic dysfunction).
- The first priority on assessing the patient with pneumonia is to evaluate the adequacy of respiratory function and to determine whether there are signs of systemic illness, specifically dehydration, or sepsis with resulting circulatory collapse.
- The supportive care of the patient with pneumonia includes the use of humidified oxygen for hypoxemia, fluid resuscitation, administration of bronchodilators (albuterol) when bronchospasm is present, and chest physiotherapy with postural drainage if there is evidence of retained secretions.
- Important therapeutic adjuncts include adequate hydration (by IV route if necessary), optimal nutritional support, and fever control.
- The treatment of bacterial pneumonia initially involves the empiric use of a relatively broad-spectrum antibiotic (or antibiotics) effective against probable pathogens after appropriate cultures and specimens for laboratory evaluation have been obtained. Therapy should be narrowed to cover specific pathogens once the results of cultures are known.
- Appropriate empiric choices for the treatment of bacterial pneumonias relative to a patient's underlying disease are shown in **Table 43–7** for adults and **Table 43–8** for children. Dosages for antibiotics to treat pneumonia are provided in **Table 43–9**.
- Antibiotic concentrations in respiratory secretions in excess of the pathogen minimum inhibitory concentration (MIC) are necessary for successful treatment of pulmonary infections.
- The benefit of antibiotic aerosols or direct endotracheal instillation has not been consistently demonstrated.

EVALUATION OF THERAPEUTIC OUTCOMES

- With community-acquired pneumonia, time for resolution of cough, sputum production, and presence of constitutional symptoms (eg, malaise, nausea or vomiting, and lethargy) should be assessed. Progress should be noted in the first 2 days, with complete resolution in 5 to 7 days.
- With nosocomial pneumonia, the above parameters should be assessed along with white blood cell counts, chest radiograph, and blood gas determinations.

See Chapter 107, Lower Respiratory Tract Infections, authored by Martha G. Blackford, Mark L. Glover, and Michael D. Reed for a more detailed discussion of this topic.

OTITIS MEDIA

- *Otitis media* is an inflammation of the middle ear that is most common in infants and children. There are three subtypes of otitis media: acute otitis media, otitis media with effusion, and chronic otitis media. The three are differentiated by (a) acute signs of infection, (b) evidence of middle ear inflammation, and (c) presence of fluid in the middle ear.
- There are more than 709 million cases of otitis media worldwide each year; half of these cases occur in children under 5 years of age.

PATHOPHYSIOLOGY

- Bacteria have been found in more than 90% of cases of otitis media. Common bacterial pathogens include *Streptococcus pneumoniae*, nontypeable *Haemophilus influenzae*, and *Moraxella catarrhalis*.
- Acute otitis media usually follows a viral upper respiratory tract infection that impairs the mucociliary apparatus and causes Eustachian tube dysfunction in the middle ear.
- Up to 40% of *S. pneumonia* isolates in the United States are penicillin nonsusceptible, and up to half of these have high-level penicillin resistance. Approximately 30% to 40% of *H. influenzae* and greater than 90% of *M. catarrhalis* isolates from the upper respiratory tract produce β-lactamases.

CLINICAL PRESENTATION

- Irritability and tugging on the ear are often the first clues that a child has acute otitis media.
- Children should be diagnosed with acute otitis media if they have middle ear effusion and either (1) moderate to severe bulging of the tympanic membrane or new onset otorrhea not due to acute otitis externa or (2) mild bulging of the tympanic membrane and onset of ear pain within the last 48 hours or intense erythema of the tympanic membrane.
- Nonverbal children with ear pain might hold, rub, or tug their ear. Very young children might cry, be irritable, and have difficulty sleeping. Signs and symptoms include: bulging of the tympanic membrane, otorrhea, otalgia (considered to be moderate or severe if pain lasts at least 48 hours), and fever (considered to be severe if temperature is 39°C [102.2°F] or higher).

TREATMENT

- Goals of Treatment: The goals are pain management, prudent antibiotic use, and secondary disease prevention. Acute otitis media should first be differentiated from otitis media with effusion or chronic otitis media.
- Primary prevention of acute otitis media with vaccines should be considered. The seven-valent pneumococcal conjugate vaccine reduced the occurrence of acute otitis media by 6% to 7% during infancy.
- Pain of otitis media should be addressed with oral analgesics. **Acetaminophen** or a nonsteroidal antiinflammatory agent, such as **ibuprofen**, should be offered early to relieve pain of acute otitis media.
- Children 6 months to 12 years of age, with moderate to severe ear pain or temperature of 39°C (102.2°F) or higher should receive antibiotics. Children 6 to 23 months of age, with nonsevere bilateral acute otitis media should also receive antibiotics. Children 6 to 23 months, with nonsevere unilateral acute otitis media, and children

24 months to 12 years of age, with nonsevere acute otitis media, may receive initial antibiotics or initial observation.

- The central principle is to administer antibiotics quickly when the diagnosis is certain, but to withhold antibiotics, at least initially, when the diagnosis is uncertain.
- High-dose **amoxicillin** (80–90 mg/kg/day) is recommended for most patients. Children who have received amoxicillin in the last 30 days, have concurrent purulent conjunctivitis, or have a history of recurrent infection unresponsive to amoxicillin should receive high-dose **amoxicillin-clavulanate** (90 mg/kg/day of amoxicillin, with 6.4 mg/kg/day of clavulanate, in two divided doses) instead of amoxicillin.
- Treatment recommendations for acute otitis media are found in **Table 44–1**.
- If treatment failure occurs with amoxicillin, an agent should be chosen with activity against β-lactamase-producing *H. influenzae* and *M. catarrhalis*, as well as drug-resistant *S. pneumoniae*, such as high-dose amoxicillin–clavulanate (recommended) or cefuroxime, cefdinir, cefpodoxime, or intramuscular or intravenous ceftriaxone.
- In children at least 6 years old who have mild to moderate acute otitis media, a 5- to 7-day course of antibiotics may be used. Some experts have speculated that patients can be treated for as little as 3 to 5 days but short-course treatment is not recommended in children younger than 2 years of age.

TABLE 44–1	Antibiotics and Doses for Acute Otitis Media		
Antibiotic	**Brand Name**	**Dose**	**Comments[a]**
Initial diagnosis			
Amoxicillin	Amoxil®	80–90 mg/kg/day orally divided twice daily	First-line
Amoxicillin-clavulanate	Augmentin®	90 mg/kg/day orally of amoxicillin plus 6.4 mg/kg/day orally of clavulanate, divided twice daily	First-line if certain criteria are present[b]
Cefdinir, cefuroxime, cefpodoxime	Omnicef®, Ceftin®, Vantin®	cefdinir (14 mg/kg/day orally in 1–2 doses) cefuroxime (30 mg/kg/day orally in 2 divided doses) cefpodoxime (10 mg/kg/day orally in 2 divided doses)	Second-line or nonsevere penicillin allergy
Ceftriaxone (1–3 days)	Rocephin®	50 mg/kg/day IM or IV for 3 days	Second-line or nonsevere penicillin allergy
Failure at 48–72 hours			
Amoxicillin-clavulanate[b]	Augmentin®	90 mg/kg/day orally of amoxicillin plus 6.4 mg/kg/day orally of clavulanate, divided twice daily	First-line
Ceftriaxone (1–3 days)	Rocephin®	50 mg/kg/day IM or IV for 3 days	First-line or nonsevere penicillin allergy
Clindamycin	Cleocin®	30–40 mg/kg/day orally in 3 divided doses plus third-generation cephalosporin	Second-line or nonsevere penicillin allergy

(IM, intramuscular; IV, intravenous; po, orally.)
[a]If a patient has received amoxicillin in the last 30 days, has concurrent purulent conjunctivitis, or has a history of recurrent infection unresponsive to amoxicillin.
[b]Amoxicillin-clavulanate 90:6.4 or 14:1 ratio is available in the United States; 7:1 ratio is available in Canada (use amoxicillin 45 mg/kg for one dose, amoxicillin 45 mg/kg with clavulanate 6.4 mg/kg for second dose).

- Surgical insertion of tympanostomy tubes (T tubes) is an effective method for the prevention of recurrent otitis media. Patients with acute otitis media should be reassessed after 48 to 72 hours, with most children being asymptomatic at 7 days.

PHARYNGITIS

- *Pharyngitis* is an acute infection of the oropharynx or nasopharynx that results in 1% to 2% of all outpatient visits. Although viral causes are most common, group A β-hemolytic *Streptococcus* (GABHS), or *Streptococcus pyogenes*, is the primary bacterial cause.
- Viruses (eg, rhinovirus, coronavirus, and adenovirus) cause most of the cases of acute pharyngitis. A bacterial etiology for acute pharyngitis is far less likely. Of all of the bacterial causes, GABHS is the most common (10%–30% of cases in pediatric patients and 5%–15% in adults).
- Nonsuppurative complications of GABHS pharyngitis include acute rheumatic fever, acute glomerulonephritis, reactive arthritis, peritonsillar abscess, retropharyngeal abscess cervical lymphadenitis, mastoiditis, otitis media, rhinosinusitis, and necrotizing fasciitis.

CLINICAL PRESENTATION

- The most common symptom of pharyngitis is sore throat. The clinical presentation of group A streptococcal pharyngitis is presented in **Table 44–2**.

TREATMENT

- <u>Goals of Treatment</u>: The goal is to improve clinical signs and symptoms, minimize adverse drug reactions, prevent transmission to close contacts, and prevent acute rheumatic fever and suppurative complications such as peritonsillar abscess, cervical lymphadenitis, and mastoiditis.
- Antimicrobial therapy should be limited to those who have clinical and epidemiologic features of GABHS pharyngitis, preferably with a positive laboratory test.
- Because pain is often the primary reason for visiting a physician, emphasis on analgesics such as **acetaminophen** and nonsteroidal anti-inflammatory drugs (NSAIDs) to aid in pain relief is strongly recommended.

TABLE 44–2	CLINICAL PRESENTATION: Group A Streptococcal Pharyngitis

General
- A sore throat of sudden onset that is mostly self-limited
- Fever and constitutional symptoms resolving in about 3–5 days
- Clinical signs and symptoms are similar for viral causes and nonstreptococcal bacterial causes

Signs and symptoms of GABHS pharyngitis
- Sore throat
- Pain on swallowing
- Fever
- Headache, nausea, vomiting, and abdominal pain (especially in children)
- Erythema/inflammation of the tonsils and pharynx with or without patchy exudates
- Enlarged, tender lymph nodes
- Red swollen uvula, petechiae on the soft palate, and a scarlatiniform rash

Signs suggestive of viral origin for pharyngitis
- Conjunctivitis
- Coryza
- Cough

Laboratory tests
- Throat swab and culture
- Rapid antigen-detection test (RADT)

- Penicillin and amoxicillin are the treatments of choice. Antimicrobial treatment should be limited to those who have clinical and epidemiologic features of GABHS pharyngitis with a positive laboratory test (**Table 44–3**). **Table 44–4** presents antibiotics and doses for eradication of GABHS in chronic carriers. The duration of therapy for GABHS pharyngitis is 10 days, except for benzathine penicillin and azithromycin, to maximize bacterial eradication.
- Most cases of pharyngitis are self-limited; however, antimicrobial therapy will hasten resolution when given early to proven cases of GABHS. Symptoms generally resolve by 3 or 4 days even without therapy. Follow-up testing is generally not necessary for index cases or in asymptomatic contacts of the index patient.

TABLE 44–3	Antibiotics and Doses for Group A β-Hemolytic Streptococcal Pharyngitis			
Antibiotic	**Brand Name**	**Dose**	**Duration**	**Rating**
Preferred antibiotics				
Penicillin V	Pen-V®	Children: 250 mg twice daily or three times daily orally. Adult: 250 mg four times daily or 500 mg twice daily orally	10 days	IB
Penicillin G benzathine	Bicillin L-A®	< 27 kg: 0.6 million units; 27 kg or greater: 1.2 million units intramuscularly	One dose	IB
Amoxicillin[a]	Amoxil®	50 mg/kg once daily (maximum 1000 mg); 25 mg/kg (maximum 500 mg) twice daily	10 days	IB
Penicillin allergy				
Cephalexin	Keflex®	20 mg/kg/dose orally twice daily (maximum 500 mg/dose)	10 days	IB
Cefadroxil	Duricef®	30 mg/kg orally once daily (maximum 1 g)	10 days	IB
Clindamycin	Cleocin®	7 mg/kg/dose orally thrice daily (maximum 300 mg/dose)	10 days	IIaB
Azithromycin[b]	Zithromax®	12 mg/kg orally once daily (maximum 500 mg) for one day, then 6 mg/kg orally once daily (maximum 250 mg) for four days	5 days	IIaB
Clarithromycin[b]	Biaxin®	15 mg/kg orally per day divided in two doses (maximum 250 mg twice daily)	10 days	IIaB

These guidelines provide a systematic weighting of the strength of the recommendation (Class I, conditions for which there is evidence and/or general agreement that a given procedure or treatment is beneficial, useful, and effective; Class II, conditions for which there is conflicting evidence and/or a divergence of opinion about the usefulness/efficacy of a procedure or treatment; Class IIa, weight of evidence/opinion is in favor of usefulness/efficacy; Class IIb, usefulness/efficacy is less well established by evidence/opinion; Class III, conditions for which there is evidence and/or general agreement that a procedure/treatment is not useful/effective and in some cases may be harmful) and quality of evidence (A, data derived from multiple randomized clinical trials or meta-analyses; B, data derived from a single randomized trial or nonrandomized studies; C, only consensus opinion of experts, cases studies, or standard of care).
[a]Standard formulation, not extended release.
[b]Resistance of group A β-hemolytic *Streptococcus* (GABHS) to these agents may vary and local susceptibilities should be considered with these agents.

TABLE 44–4	Antibiotics and Doses for Eradication of Group A β-Hemolytic Streptococcal Pharyngitis in Chronic Carriers	
Antibiotic	**Brand Name**	**Dose**
Clindamycin	Cleocin®	20–30 mg/kg/day orally in three divided doses (maximum 300 mg/dose)
Amoxicillin-clavulanate	Augmentin®	40 mg/kg/day orally in three divided doses (maximum 2000 mg/day of amoxicillin)
Penicillin V and rifampin	Pen-V®, Rifadin®	Penicillin V: 50 mg/kg/day orally in four doses for 10 days (maximum 2000 mg/day); *and* rifampin: 20 mg/kg/day orally in one dose for the last 4 days of treatment (maximum 600 mg/day)
Penicillin G benzathine and rifampin	Bicillin L-A®, Rifadin®	Penicillin G benzathine: < 27 kg—0.6 million units; 27 kg or greater—1.2 million units intramuscularly; *and* rifampin: 20 mg/kg/day orally in two doses during last 4 days of treatment with penicillin (maximum 600 mg/day)

ACUTE BACTERIAL RHINOSINUSITIS

- *Sinusitis* is an inflammation and/or infection of the paranasal sinus mucosa. The term *rhinosinusitis* is now preferred, because sinusitis typically also involves the nasal mucosa. The majority of these infections are viral in origin. It is important to differentiate between viral and bacterial sinusitis to aid in optimizing treatment decisions.
- Acute bacterial sinusitis is most often caused by the same bacteria implicated in acute otitis media: *S. pneumoniae* and *H. influenzae*. These organisms are responsible for ~50% to 70% of bacterial causes of acute sinusitis in both adults and children.

CLINICAL PRESENTATION

- The typical clinical presentation of bacterial rhinosinusitis is presented in Table 44–5.

TABLE 44–5	CLINICAL PRESENTATION: Acute Bacterial Rhinosinusitis

General

There are three clinical presentations that are most consistent with acute bacterial versus viral rhinosinusitis:
- Onset with *persistent* signs or symptoms compatible with acute rhinosinusitis, lasting for ≥ 10 days without any evidence of clinical improvement
- Onset with *severe* signs or symptoms of high fever (≥39°C [102.2°F]) and purulent nasal discharge or facial pain lasting for at least 3–4 consecutive days at the beginning of illness
- Onset with *worsening* signs or symptoms characterized by new-onset fever, headache, or increase in nasal discharge following a typical viral URI that lasted 5–6 days and were initially improving ("double sickening")

Signs and Symptoms
- Purulent anterior nasal discharge, purulent or discolored posterior nasal discharge, nasal congestion or obstruction, facial congestion or fullness, facial pain or pressure, fever, headache, ear pain/pressure/fullness, halitosis, dental pain, cough, and fatigue

TREATMENT

- <u>Goals of Treatment</u>: reduce signs and symptoms, achieving and maintaining patency of the ostia, limiting antimicrobial treatment to those who may benefit, eradicating bacterial infection with appropriate antimicrobial therapy, minimizing the duration of illness, preventing complications, and preventing progression from acute disease to chronic disease.
- Nasal decongestant sprays such as **phenylephrine** and **oxymetazoline** that reduce inflammation by vasoconstriction are often used in nonbacterial rhinosinusitis. Use should be limited to the recommended duration of the product (no more than 3 days) to prevent development of tolerance and/or rebound congestion. Oral decongestants may also aid in nasal or sinus patency. Irrigation of the nasal cavity with saline and steam inhalation may be used to increase mucosal moisture, and mucolytics (eg, guaifenesin) may be used to decrease the viscosity of nasal secretions. Antihistamines and oral decongestants should not be used for acute bacterial sinusitis in view of their anticholinergic effects that can dry mucosa and disturb clearance of mucosal secretions.
- Antimicrobial therapy is superior to placebo in reducing or eliminating symptoms, although the benefit is small.
- **Amoxicillin-clavulanate** is first-line treatment for acute bacterial rhinosinusitis. The approach to treating acute bacterial rhinosinusitis in children and adults is given in **Tables 44–6 and 44–7**.

TABLE 44–6	Antibiotics and Doses for Acute Bacterial Rhinosinusitis in Children		
Antibiotic	**Brand Name**	**Dose**	**Comments**
Initial empirical therapy			
Amoxicillin-clavulanate	Augmentin®	45 mg/kg/day orally twice daily	First-line
Amoxicillin-clavulanate	Augmentin®	90 mg/kg/day orally twice daily	Second-line
β-Lactam allergy			
Clindamycin plus cefixime or cefpodoxime	Cleocin®, Suprax®, Vantin®	Clindamycin (30–40 mg/kg/day orally three times daily) plus cefixime (8 mg/kg/day orally twice daily) or cefpodoxime (10 mg/kg/day orally twice daily)	Non–type 1 allergy
Levofloxacin	Levaquin®	10–20 mg/kg/day orally every 12–24 hours	Type 1 allergy
Risk for antibiotic resistance or failed initial therapy			
Amoxicillin-clavulanate	Augmentin®	90 mg/kg/day orally twice daily	
Clindamycin plus cefixime or cefpodoxime	Cleocin®, Suprax®, Vantin®	Clindamycin (30–40 mg/kg/day orally three times daily) plus cefixime (8 mg/kg/day orally twice daily) or cefpodoxime (10 mg/kg/day orally twice daily)	
Levofloxacin	Levaquin®	10–20 mg/kg/day orally every 12–24 hours	
Severe infection requiring hospitalization			
Ampicillin-sulbactam	Unasyn®	200–400 mg/kg/day IV every 6 hours	
Ceftriaxone	Rocephin®	50 mg/kg/day IV every 12 hours	
Cefotaxime	Claforan®	100–200 mg/kg/day IV every 6 hours	
Levofloxacin	Levaquin®	10–20 mg/kg/day IV every 12–24 hours	

TABLE 44-7	Antibiotics and Doses for Acute Bacterial Rhinosinusitis in Adults		
Antibiotic	**Brand Name**	**Dose**	**Comments**
Initial empirical therapy			
Amoxicillin-clavulanate	Augmentin®	500 mg/125 mg orally three times daily, or 875 mg/125 mg orally twice daily	First-line
Amoxicillin-clavulanate	Augmentin®	2000 mg/125 mg orally twice daily	Second-line
Doxycycline		100 mg orally twice daily or 200 mg orally once daily	Second-line
β-Lactam allergy			
Doxycycline		100 mg orally twice daily or 200 mg orally once daily	
Levofloxacin	Levaquin®	500 mg orally once daily	
Moxifloxacin	Avelox®	400 mg orally once daily	
Risk for antibiotic resistance or failed initial therapy			
Amoxicillin-clavulanate	Augmentin®	2000 mg/125 mg orally twice daily	
Levofloxacin	Levaquin®	500 mg orally once daily	
Moxifloxacin	Avelox®	400 mg orally once daily	
Severe infection requiring hospitalization			
Ampicillin-sulbactam	Unasyn®	1.5–3 g IV every 6 hours	
Levofloxacin	Levaquin®	500 mg orally once daily	
Moxifloxacin	Avelox®	400 mg orally once daily	
Ceftriaxone	Rocephin®	1–2 g IV every 12–24 hours	
Cefotaxime	Claforan®	2 g IV every 4–6 hours	

- High-dose amoxicillin-clavulanate is preferred in the following situations: (a) geographic regions with high endemic rates (10% or greater) of invasive penicillin-nonsusceptible *S. pneumoniae,* (b) severe infection, (c) attendance at daycare, (d) age less than 2 or greater than 65 years, (e) recent hospitalization, (f) antibiotic use within the last month, and (g) immunocompromised persons
- The duration of antimicrobial therapy for the treatment of acute bacterial rhinosinusitis is not well established. Most trials have used 10- to 14-day antibiotic courses for uncomplicated rhinosinusitis. For adults, the recommended duration is 5 to 7 days.

See Chapter 108, Upper Respiratory Tract Infections, authored by Christopher Frei and Bradi Frei, for a more detailed discussion of this topic.

CHAPTER 45

Sepsis and Septic Shock

- The definitions of terms related to *sepsis* are given in **Table 45–1**. Physiologically similar systemic inflammatory response syndrome can be seen even in the absence of identifiable infection.

ETIOLOGY AND PATHOPHYSIOLOGY

- The sites of infections that most frequently lead to sepsis are the respiratory tract (39%–50%), urinary tract (5%–37%), and intra-abdominal space (8%–16%). Sepsis may be caused by gram-negative (50%–62% of sepsis) or gram-positive bacteria (37%–47%), as well as by fungi (5%) or other microorganisms.
- *Escherichia coli, Klebsiella species,* and *Pseudomonas aeruginosa* are the most commonly isolated gram-negative pathogens in sepsis. Other common gram-negative pathogens are *Serratia* spp., *Enterobacter* spp., and *Proteus* spp. *P. aeruginosa* is the most frequent cause of sepsis fatality. Common gram-positive pathogens are *Staphylococcus aureus, Streptococcus pneumoniae,* coagulase-negative staphylococci, and *Enterococcus* species.
- *Candida* species (particularly *Candida albicans*) are common fungal etiologic agents of bloodstream infections. The 30-day mortality rate for sepsis due to candidemia was 54%.
- The pathophysiologic focus of gram-negative sepsis has been on the lipopolysaccharide (endotoxin) component of the gram-negative cell wall. Lipid A is a part of the endotoxin molecule from the gram-negative bacterial cell wall that is highly immunoreactive and is responsible for most of the toxic effects.
- Sepsis involves a complex interaction of proinflammatory (eg, tumor necrosis factor-α [TNF-α]; interleukin [IL]-1, IL-6) and anti-inflammatory mediators (eg, IL-1 receptor antagonist, IL-4, and IL-10). IL-8, platelet-activating factor, leukotrienes, and thromboxane A_2 are also important.
- TNF-α is considered the primary mediator of sepsis. Concentrations are elevated early in the inflammatory response during sepsis, and there is a correlation with the severity of sepsis. TNF-α release leads to activation of other cytokines associated with cellular damage, and it stimulates release of arachidonic acid metabolites that contribute to endothelial cell damage.
- A primary mechanism of injury with sepsis is through endothelial cells. With inflammation, endothelial cells allow circulating cells (eg, granulocytes) and plasma constituents to enter inflamed tissues, which may result in organ damage.
- A key endogenous substance involved in inflammation of sepsis is activated protein C, which enhances fibrinolysis and inhibits inflammation. Levels of protein C are reduced in patients with sepsis.
- Shock is the most ominous complication associated with gram-negative sepsis and causes death in about one half of patients. Another complication is disseminated intravascular coagulation (DIC), which occurs in up to 50% of patients with septic shock. DIC is the inappropriate activation of the clotting cascade that causes formation of microthrombi, resulting in consumption of coagulation factors, organ dysfunction, and bleeding. Acute respiratory distress syndrome (ARDS) is another common complication of sepsis.
- The hallmark of the hemodynamic effect of sepsis is the hyperdynamic state characterized by high cardiac output and an abnormally low systemic vascular resistance.

CLINICAL PRESENTATION

- The signs and symptoms of early sepsis are variable and include fever, chills, and a change in mental status. Hypothermia may occur instead of fever. The patient may be hypoxic. Signs and symptoms of early and late sepsis are found in **Table 45–2**.

TABLE 45–1	Definitions Related to Sepsis
Condition	**Definition**
Bacteremia (fungemia)	Presence of viable bacteria (fungi) in the bloodstream
Infection	Inflammatory response to invasion of normally sterile host tissue by the microorganisms
SIRS	Systemic inflammatory response to a variety of clinical insults, which can be infectious or noninfectious. The response is manifested by two or more of the following conditions: temperature >38°C (>100.4°F) or <36°C (<96.8°F); HR >90 beats/min; RR >20 breaths/min or $PaCO_2$ <32 mm Hg (<4.3 kPa); WBC >12,000 cells/mm³ (>12 × 10⁹/L), <4,000 cells/mm³ (<4 × 10⁹/L), or >10% (>0.10) immature (band) forms
Sepsis	SIRS secondary to suspected or documented infection Additional criteria include general variables (altered mental status, positive fluid balance of >20 mL/kg over 24 hours, hyperglycemia >120 mg/dL [>6.7 mmol/L]); inflammatory variables (plasma C-reactive protein/procalcitonin >2 SD above normal value); hemodynamic variables (arterial hypotension <90mm Hg (<12.0 kPa) or MAP <70 mm Hg (<9.3 kPa), elevated mixed venous oxygen saturation of >70% (>0.70); CI >3.5 L/min (>0.058 L/s); organ-dysfunction variables (arterial hypoxemia; acute oliguria of <0.5ml/kg/hr or 45 ml/hr for at least 2 hr, creatinine increase >0.5 mg/dL (>0.44 µmol/L), coagulation abnormalities, paralytic ileus, platelets <100,000 /mm³ (<100 × 10⁹/L), bilirubin >4 mg/dL (>68 µmol/L); tissue-perfusion variable (hyperlactatemia >1 mmol/L, decreased capillary refill)
Severe sepsis	Sepsis associated with one or more organ dysfunctions, hypoperfusion, or hypotension. Hypoperfusion and perfusion abnormalities may include but not limited to arterial hypoxemia (PaO_2/FiO_2<300) lactic acidosis, oliguria, increase in creatinine, coagulation abnormalities (INR>1.5), and elevated bilirubin
Septic shock	Sepsis with persistent hypotension despite fluid resuscitation (intravenous fluid of 30 mL/kg) or hyperlactatemia >1 mmol/L

(CI, cardiac index; HR, heart rate; INR, international normalized ratio; RR, respiratory rate; SD, standard deviation; SIRS, systemic inflammatory response syndrome; T, temperature; WBC, white blood cell (count).)

Adapted from Levy MM, Fink MP, Marshall JC, et al. 2001 SCCM/ESICM/ACCP/ATS/SIS International Sepsis Definitions Conference. Crit Care Med 2003;31:1250-1256.

- Progression of uncontrolled sepsis leads to evidence of organ dysfunction, which may include oliguria, hemodynamic instability with hypotension or shock, lactic acidosis, hyperglycemia or hypoglycemia, possibly leukopenia, DIC, thrombocytopenia, ARDS, GI (gastrointestinal) hemorrhage, or coma.

TREATMENT

- The primary goals for treatment of sepsis are as follows: timely diagnosis and identification of the pathogen, rapid elimination of the source of infection, early initiation of aggressive antimicrobial therapy, interruption of the pathogenic sequence leading to septic shock, and avoidance of organ failure.
- Evidence-based treatment recommendations for sepsis and septic shock from the *Surviving Sepsis* campaign are presented in **Table 45–3.**

TABLE 45–2	Signs and Symptoms Associated with Sepsis
Early Sepsis	**Late Sepsis**
Fever or hypothermia	Lactic acidosis
Rigors, chills	Oliguria
Tachycardia	Leukopenia
Tachypnea	DIC
Nausea, vomiting	Myocardial depression
Hyperglycemia	Pulmonary edema
Myalgia	Hypotension (shock)
Lethargy, malaise	Hypoglycemia
Proteinuria	Azotemia
Hypoxia	Thrombocytopenia
Leukocytosis	ARDS
Hyperbilirubinemia	GI hemorrhage
Delirium	Coma

(ARDS, acute respiratory distress syndrome; DIC, disseminated intravascular coagulation.)

TABLE 45–3	Evidence-Based Treatment Recommendations for Sepsis and Septic Shock	
Recommendations		**Recommendation Grades[a]**
Initial resuscitation (first 6 hours)		
Quantitative resuscitation of patients with sepsis-induced tissue hypoperfusion, CVP 8–12 mm Hg (1.1–1.6 kPa), MAP ≥65 mm Hg (≥8.6 kPa), urine output > 0.5 mL/kg/h, SCVO$_2$ ≥70% (≥0.70)		1C
Antibiotic therapy		
IV broad-spectrum antibiotic within 1 hour of diagnosis of septic shock and severe sepsis against likely bacterial/fungal pathogens		1B
Reassess antibiotic therapy daily with microbiology and clinical data to narrow coverage (de-escalation)		1B
Combination empirical therapy for neutropenic patients with severe sepsis and patients with difficult-to-treat, multidrug-resistant bacterial pathogens such as *Acinetobacter* and *Pseudomonas* spp. for no more than 3–5 days and then de-escalate		2B
Fluid therapy		
Crystalloids as the initial fluid of choice		1B
Minimum of 30 mL/kg of crystalloids for initial fluid challenge, but more rapid and greater amount may be needed		1C
Albumin when patients require substantial amounts of crystalloids		2C
Vasopressors		
Initiate vasopressor therapy to maintain MAP ≥65 mm Hg (≥8.6 kPa)		1C
Norepinephrine as the first choice vasopressor		1B
Epinephrine when an additional agent is needed to maintain adequate blood pressure		2B

(*continued*)

TABLE 45–3	Evidence-Based Treatment Recommendations for Sepsis and Septic Shock (*Continued*)
Recommendations	**Recommendation Grades**[a]
Dopamine as an alternative vasopressor to norepinephrine in selective patients with low risk of tachyarrhythmia and bradycardia	2C
Inotropic therapy	
Use dobutamine up to 20 mcg/kg/min or added to vasopressor when cardiac output remains low or ongoing signs of hypoperfusion despite adequate MAP	1C
Glucose control	
Use insulin dosing protocol in ICU patients when 2 consecutive blood glucose levels are >180 mg/dL (>10 mmol/L), targeting an upper blood glucose <180 mg/dL (≤10 mmol/L)	1A
Steroids	
IV hydrocortisone 200 mg per day for septic shock only when hypotension remains poorly responsive to adequate fluid resuscitation and vasopressors	2C
Hydrocortisone should be tapered when vasopressors are no longer required	2D
Deep vein thrombosis prophylaxis	
Use daily low-molecular-weight heparin and intermittent pneumatic compression device whenever possible	1B
If creatinine clearance is <30 mL/min (<0.5 mL/s), use unfractionated heparin or dalteparin	1A, 1A
If heparin is contraindicated, use mechanical prophylactic treatment	2C
Stress ulcer prophylaxis	
Stress ulcer prophylaxis should be given to patients who have bleeding risk factors	1B
Proton pump inhibitors are preferred over H2 receptor blockers	2C

(CVP, central venous pressure; MAP, mean arterial pressure.)

[a]Grades of Recommendation, Assessment, Development, and Evaluation (GRADE) system: a structured system for rating quality of evidence and grading strength of recommendation in clinical practice. Quality of evidence: high (grade A), moderate (grade B), low (grade C), or very low (grade D). Strength of recommendation: strong (grade 1) or weak (grade 2).

Adapted from Dellinger RP, Levy MM, Rhodes A, et al. Surviving sepsis campaign: International guidelines for management of severe sepsis and septic shock: 2012. Crit Care Med 2013;41:580-637.

ANTIMICROBIAL THERAPY

- The Surviving Sepsis Campaign guidelines recommended starting IV administration of one or more antibiotics within 1 hour of recognition of septic shock and severe sepsis without septic shock. The regimen selected should be based on the suspected site of infection, likely pathogens and the local antibiotic susceptibility patterns, whether the organism was acquired from the community or a hospital, the patient's immune status, recent exposure to antibiotics within past 3 months, and the antibiotic susceptibility and resistance profile for the institution.
- The antibiotics that may be used for empiric treatment of sepsis are listed in **Table 45–4.**
- If *P. aeruginosa* is suspected, or with sepsis from hospital-acquired infections, an antipseudomonal cephalosporin (**ceftazidime** or **cefepime**), antipseudomonal fluoroquinolone (**ciprofloxacin** or **levofloxacin**), or an aminoglycoside should be included in the regimen.

TABLE 45–4 Empiric Antimicrobial Regimens in Sepsis

| Infection (site or type) | Antimicrobial Regimen | |
	Community-acquired	Hospital-acquired
Urinary tract	Ceftriaxone or ciprofloxacin/levofloxacin	Ciprofloxacin/levofloxacin or ceftriaxone or ceftazidime
Respiratory tract	Levofloxacin[a]/moxifloxacin or ceftriaxone + clarithromycin/azithromycin	Piperacillin/tazobactam or ceftazidime or cefipime + levofloxacin/ciprofloxacin or aminoglycoside carbapenem[b]
Intraabdominal	Ertapenem or ciprofloxacin/levofloxacin + metronidazole	Piperacillin/tazobactam or carbapenem[b]
Skin/soft tissue	Vancomycin or linezolid or daptomycin	Vancomycin + piperacillin/tazobactam
Catheter-related		Vancomycin
Unknown		Piperacillin/tazobactam or ceftazidime/cefipime or imipenem/meropenem } ± vancomycin

[a]750 mg orally once daily.
[b]Imipenem, meropenem, and doripenem.

- Empiric combination therapy should not be administered for longer than 3 to 5 days. The antimicrobial regimen should be reassessed daily based on the microbiological and clinical data.
- When *S. aureus* is likely to be methicillin-resistant, linezolid may be preferred to vancomycin because of the poor penetration of vancomycin into the lungs, as well as the worldwide emergence of glycopeptide intermediately resistant *S. aureus*.
- The average duration of antimicrobial therapy in the normal host with sepsis is 7 to 10 days, and fungal infections can require 10 to 14 days.
- Treatment of invasive candidiasis involves echinocandins, triazoles, or a formulation of amphotericin B. The choice depends on the clinical status of the patient, the fungal species and its susceptibility, relative drug toxicity, presence of organ dysfunction that would affect drug clearance, and the patient's prior exposure to antifungal agents. In general, suspected systemic mycotic infection leading to sepsis in nonneutropenic patients should be treated empirically with parenteral fluconazole or an echinocandin.

HEMODYNAMIC SUPPORT

- The Surviving Sepsis Guidelines recommend a MAP of at least 65 mm Hg (8.6 kPa) in patients with septic shock.
- Rapid fluid resuscitation is the best initial therapeutic intervention for treatment of hypotension in sepsis. The goal is to maximize cardiac output by increasing the left ventricular preload, which will ultimately restore tissue perfusion.
- Fluid administration should be titrated to clinical end points such as heart rate, urine output, blood pressure (BP), and mental status. Isotonic crystalloids, such as 0.9% sodium chloride or lactated Ringer solution, are commonly used for fluid resuscitation.
- Iso-oncotic colloid solutions (plasma and plasma protein fractions), such as 5% albumin and 6% hetastarch, offer the advantage of more rapid restoration of intravascular volume with less volume infused, however, synthetic colloids cause dose-related renal impairment and increased bleeding Crystalloid solutions are generally recommended for fluid resuscitation because of the absence of any clear benefit with colloids solutions in addition to the lower cost of crystalloids.

441

TABLE 45–5	Receptor Activity of Cardiovascular Agents Commonly Used in Septic Shock				
Agent	α_1	α_2	β_1	β_2	Dopaminergic
Dopamine	++/+++	?	++++	++	++++
Dobutamine	+	+	++++	++	0
Norepinephrine	+++	+++	+++	+/++	0
Phenylephrine	++/+++	+	?	0	0
Epinephrine	++++	++++	++++	+++	0

(α_1, α_1-adrenergic receptor; α_2, α_2-adrenergic receptor; β_1, β_1-adrenergic receptor; β_2, β_2-adrenergic receptor; 0, no activity; ++++, maximal activity; ?, unknown activity.)

INOTROPE AND VASOACTIVE DRUG SUPPORT

- When fluid resuscitation is insufficient to maintain tissue perfusion, the use of inotropes and vasoactive drugs is necessary. Selection and dosage are based on the pharmacologic properties of various catecholamines and how they influence hemo-dynamic parameters (Table 45–5).

Suggested Protocol for the Use of Inotropes and Vasoactive Agents

- For the septic patients with clinical signs of shock and significant hypotension unresponsive to aggressive fluid therapy, norepinephrine is the preferred agent for increasing MAP. In comparison to dopamine, it is less arrhythmogenic and studies have shown benefits in mortality. Epinephrine is an alternative to norepinephrine for refractory hypotension. Dopamine and epinephrine are more likely to induce or exacerbate tachycardia than norepinephrine. Phenylephrine is only recommended as a salvage therapy only if tachycardia or arrhythmia makes norepinephrine and epinephrine intolerable. In a septic patient with low CI after adequate fluid therapy and adequate MAP, dobutamine is the first-line agent for its strong inotropic effect, increasing cardiac output with minimal effect on SVR.

Initial Resuscitation

- Initial resuscitation of a patient in severe sepsis or sepsis induced tissue hypoperfusion should begin within 6 hours of recognition of the syndrome. The goals during the first 6 hours included central venous pressure (CVP) of 8 to 12 mm Hg (1.1–1.6 kPa), MAP more than or equal to 65 mm Hg (≥8.6 kPa), urine output more than or equal to 0.5 mL/kg/h, and a central venous or mixed venous oxygen saturation (Scvo2) more than or equal to 70% (≥0.70).

Adjunctive Therapy

- Recommended blood glucose levels to initiate an insulin protocol are more than 180 mg/dL (>10 mmol/L) with an upper target blood glucose level than 180 mg/dL (10 mmol/L) for the majority of critically ill patients to improve the outcome while reducing the risk of hypoglycemia.
- Cortisol levels vary widely in patients with septic shock, and some studies have suggested increased mortality associated with both low and high serum cortisol levels. IV hydrocortisone should be used only if hemodynamic stability is not achieved after adequate fluid resuscitation and vasopressor therapy, regardless of the state of adrenal insufficiency, negating the ACTH stimulation test.

See Chapter 119, Severe Sepsis and Septic Shock, authored by S. Lena Kang-Birken, for a more detailed discussion of this topic.

46 Sexually Transmitted Diseases

- The spectrum of sexually transmitted diseases (STDs) includes the classic venereal diseases—gonorrhea, syphilis, chancroid, lymphogranuloma venereum, and granuloma inguinale—as well as a variety of other pathogens known to be spread by sexual contact (Table 46–1). Common clinical syndromes associated with STDs are listed in Table 46–2. The most current information on epidemiology, diagnosis, and treatment of STDs provided by the Centers for Disease Control and Prevention (CDC) can be found at *www.cdc.gov*.

GONORRHEA

- *Neisseria gonorrhoeae* is a gram-negative diplococcus estimated to cause over 300,000 new infections per year in the United States. Humans are the only known host of this intracellular parasite.

CLINICAL PRESENTATION

- Infected individuals may be symptomatic or asymptomatic, have complicated or uncomplicated infections, and have infections involving several anatomical sites.
- The most common clinical features of gonococcal infections are presented in Table 46–3. Approximately 15% of women with gonorrhea develop pelvic inflammatory disease. Left untreated, pelvic inflammatory disease can be an indirect cause of infertility and ectopic pregnancies.
- In 0.5% to 3% of patients with gonorrhea, the gonococci invade the bloodstream and produce disseminated disease. The usual clinical manifestations of disseminated gonococcal infection are tender necrotic skin lesions, tenosynovitis, and monoarticular arthritis.
- Diagnosis of gonococcal infections can be made by gram-stained smears, culture (the most reliable method), or newer methods based on the detection of cellular components of the gonococcus (eg, enzymes, antigens, DNA, or lipopolysaccharide) in clinical specimens.
- Although culture of infected fluids is not the most sensitive of diagnostic tests for gonorrhea, it is still the diagnostic test of choice because of the high specificity.
- Alternative methods of diagnosis include enzyme immunoassay, DNA probes, and nucleic acid amplification techniques.

TREATMENT

- Parenteral **ceftriaxone**-based regimens are the only treatments recommended for gonorrhea (Table 46–4). A 400 mg oral dose of **cefixime** may be substituted if ceftriaxone is unavailable, however, a test of cure is recommended 2 weeks later.
- Coexisting chlamydial infection, which is documented in up to 50% of women and 20% of men with gonorrhea, constitutes the major cause of postgonococcal urethritis, cervicitis, and salpingitis in patients treated for gonorrhea. As a result, concomitant treatment with azithromycin is currently preferred to doxycycline and is recommended in all patients treated for gonorrhea.
- Pregnant women infected with *N. gonorrhoeae* should be treated with ceftriaxone. For presumed *Chlamydia trachomatis* infection, azithromycin is the preferred treatment.
- Treatment of gonorrhea during pregnancy is essential to prevent ophthalmia neonatorum. The CDC recommends that erythromycin (0.5%) ophthalmic ointment be instilled in each conjunctival sac immediately postpartum to prevent ophthalmia neonatorum.

TABLE 46-1	Sexually Transmitted Diseases
Disease	**Associated Pathogens**
Bacterial	
Gonorrhea	*Neisseria gonorrhoeae*
Syphilis	*Treponema pallidum*
Chancroid	*Haemophilus ducreyi*
Granuloma inguinale	*Calymmatobacterium granulomatis*
Enteric disease	*Salmonella* spp., *Shigella* spp., *Campylobacter fetus*
Campylobacter infection	*Campylobacter jejuni*
Bacterial vaginosis	*Gardnerella vaginalis, Mycoplasma hominis, Bacteroides* spp., *Mobiluncus* spp.
Group B streptococcal infections	Group B *Streptococcus*
Chlamydial	
Nongonococcal urethritis	*Chlamydia trachomatis*
Lymphogranuloma venereum	*C. trachomatis*, type L
Viral	
Acquired immunodeficiency syndrome	Human immunodeficiency virus
Herpes genitalis	Herpes simplex virus, types I and II
Viral hepatitis	Hepatitis A, B, C, and D viruses
Condylomata acuminata	Human papillomavirus
Molluscum contagiosum	Poxvirus
Cytomegalovirus infection	Cytomegalovirus
Mycoplasmal	
Nongonococcal urethritis	*Mycoplasma genitalium*
Protozoal	
Trichomoniasis	*Trichomonas vaginalis*
Amebiasis	*Entamoeba histolytica*
Giardiasis	*Giardia lamblia*
Fungal	
Vaginal candidiasis	*Candida albicans*
Parasitic	
Scabies	*Sarcoptes scabiei*
Pediculosis pubis	*Phthirus pubis*
Enterobiasis	*Enterobius vermicularis*

SYPHILIS

- The causative organism of syphilis is *Treponema pallidum*, a spirochete.
- Syphilis is usually acquired by sexual contact with infected mucous membranes or cutaneous lesions, although on rare occasions it can be acquired by nonsexual personal contact, accidental inoculation, or blood transfusion.

TABLE 46–2	Selected Syndromes Associated with Common Sexually Transmitted Pathogens	
Syndrome	Commonly Implicated Pathogens	Common Clinical Manifestations[a]
Urethritis	*Chlamydia trachomatis*, herpes simplex virus, *Neisseria gonorrhoeae*, *Trichomonas vaginalis*, *Ureaplasma Mycoplasma genitalium*	Urethral discharge, dysuria
Epididymitis	*C. trachomatis*, *N. gonorrhoeae*	Scrotal pain, inguinal pain, flank pain, urethral discharge
Cervicitis/vulvovaginitis	*C. trachomatis*, *Gardnerella vaginalis*, herpes simplex virus, human papillomavirus, *N. gonorrhoeae*, *T. vaginalis*	Abnormal vaginal discharge, vulvar itching/irritation, dysuria, dyspareunia
Genital ulcers (painful)	*Haemophilus ducreyi*, herpes simplex virus	Usually multiple vesicular/pustular (herpes) or papular/pustular (*H. ducreyi*) lesions that can coalesce; painful, tender lymphadenopathy[b]
Genital ulcers (painless)	*Treponema pallidum*	Usually single papular lesion
Genital/anal warts	Human papillomavirus	Multiple lesions ranging in size from small papular warts to large exophytic condylomas
Pharyngitis	*C. trachomatis* (?), herpes simplex virus, *N. gonorrhoeae*	Symptoms of acute pharyngitis, cervical lymphadenopathy, fever[c]
Proctitis	*C. trachomatis*, herpes simplex virus, *N. gonorrhoeae*, *T. pallidum*	Constipation, anorectal discomfort, tenesmus, mucopurulent rectal discharge
Salpingitis	*C. trachomatis*, *N. gonorrhoeae*	Lower abdominal pain, purulent cervical or vaginal discharge, adnexal swelling, fever[d]

[a]For some syndromes, clinical manifestations can be minimal or absent.
[b]Recurrent herpes infection can manifest as a single lesion.
[c]Most cases of pharyngeal gonococcal infection are asymptomatic.
[d]Salpingitis increases the risk of subsequent ectopic pregnancy and infertility.

CLINICAL PRESENTATION

• The clinical presentation of syphilis is varied, with progression through multiple stages possible in untreated or inadequately treated patients (Table 46–5).

Primary Syphilis

• Primary syphilis is characterized by the appearance of a chancre on cutaneous or mucocutaneous tissue. Chancres persist only for 1 to 8 weeks before spontaneously disappearing.

Secondary Syphilis

• The secondary stage of syphilis is characterized by a variety of mucocutaneous eruptions, resulting from widespread hematogenous and lymphatic spread of *T. pallidum*.
• Signs and symptoms of secondary syphilis disappear in 4 to 10 weeks; however, in untreated patients, lesions may recur at any time within 4 years.

445

TABLE 46–3	Presentation of Gonorrhea Infections	
	Males	**Females**
General	Incubation period 1–14 days	Incubation period 1–14 days
	Symptom onset in 2–8 days	Symptom onset in 10 days
Site of infection	Most common: urethra	Most common: endocervical canal
	Others: rectum (usually caused by rectal intercourse in MSM), oropharynx, eye	Others: urethra, rectum (usually caused by perineal contamination), oropharynx, eye
Symptoms	Commonly symptomatic, may be asymptomatic	Can be asymptomatic or minimally symptomatic
	Urethral infection: dysuria and urinary frequency	Endocervical infection: usually asymptomatic or mildly symptomatic
	Anorectal infection: asymptomatic to severe rectal pain	Urethral infection: dysuria, urinary frequency
	Pharyngeal infection: asymptomatic to mild pharyngitis	Anorectal and pharyngeal infection; symptoms same as for men
Signs	Purulent urethral or rectal discharge can be scant to profuse Anorectal: pruritus, mucopurulent discharge, bleeding	Abnormal vaginal discharge or uterine bleeding; purulent urethral or rectal discharge can be scant to profuse
Complications	Rare (epididymitis, prostatitis, inguinal lymphadenopathy, urethral stricture)	Pelvic inflammatory disease and associated complications (ie, ectopic pregnancy, infertility)
	Disseminated gonorrhea	Disseminated gonorrhea (three times more common than in men)

(MSM, men who have sex with men.)

Latent Syphilis

- Persons with a positive serologic test for syphilis but with no other evidence of disease have latent syphilis.
- Most untreated patients with latent syphilis have no further sequelae; however, ~25% to 30% progress to either neurosyphilis or late syphilis with clinical manifestations other than neurosyphilis.

Tertiary Syphilis and Neurosyphilis

- Forty percent of patients with primary or secondary syphilis exhibit CNS infection.

DIAGNOSIS

- Because *T. pallidum* is difficult to culture in vitro, diagnosis is based primarily on dark-field or direct fluorescent antibody microscopic examination of serous material from a suspected syphilitic lesion or on results from serologic testing.
- Serologic tests are the mainstay in the diagnosis of syphilis and are categorized as nontreponemal or treponemal. Common nontreponemal tests include the Venereal Disease Research Laboratory (VDRL) slide test, rapid plasma reagin (RPR) card test, unheated serum reagin (USR) test, and the toluidine red unheated serum test (TRUST).

TABLE 46–4 Treatment of Gonorrhea

Type of Infection	Recommended Regimens[a]	Alternative Regimens[a]
Uncomplicated infections of the cervix, urethra, and rectum in adults	Ceftriaxone 250 mg IM once *plus* Azithromycin 1 g orally once	Cefixime 400 mg orally once *plus* Azithromycin 1 g orally once, or doxycycline 100 mg orally twice daily for 7 days[b,c] or Gemifloxacin 320 mg orally once or gentamicin 240 mg IM[e] *plus* Azithromycin 2 g orally once
Uncomplicated infections of the pharynx	Ceftriaxone 250 mg IM once *plus* Azithromycin 1 g orally once	Consult with infectious disease expert
Disseminated gonococcal infection in adults (>45 kg)	Ceftriaxone 1–2 g IM or IV every 12–24 hour[e] *plus* Azithromycin 1 g orally once	Cefotaxime 1 g IV every 8 hours[e] or ceftizoxime 1 g IV every 8 hours[e] *plus* Azithromycin 1 g orally once
Uncomplicated infections of the cervix, urethra, pharynx, and rectum in children (<45 kg)	Ceftriaxone 25–50 mg/kg IV or IM once (not to exceed 125 mg)	
Disseminated gonococcal infection in children (<45 kg)	Ceftriaxone 50 mg/kg IV or IM once daily (not to exceed 1 g)	
Gonococcal conjunctivitis in adults	Ceftriaxone 1 g IM once[f]	
Ophthalmia neonatorum	Ceftriaxone 25–50 mg/kg IV or IM once (not to exceed 125 mg)	

(continued)

TABLE 46–4 Treatment of Gonorrhea (*Continued*)

Type of Infection	Recommended Regimens[a]	Alternative Regimens[a]
Disseminated gonococcal infection in neonates	Ceftriaxone 25–50 mg/kg/day IV or IM once daily or cefotaxime 25 mg/kg IV or IM twice daily for 7 days, or 10–14 days if meningitis is suspected[h]	
Infants born to mothers with gonococcal infection (prophylaxis)	Erythromycin (0.5%) ophthalmic ointment in a single application[g] Ceftriaxone 25–50 mg/kg IM or IV once (not to exceed 125 mg)	

(CDC, Centers for Disease Control and Prevention; C. *trachomatis*, *Chlamydia trachomatis*; NAAT, Nucleic Acid Amplification Test; N. *gonorrhoeae*, *Neisseria gonorrhoeae*.)

[a]Recommendations are those of the CDC.

[b]Tetracyclines are contraindicated during pregnancy. Pregnant women should be treated with recommended cephalosporin-based combination therapy. In severe cephalosporin allergy, consultation with an infectious diseases expert is recommended.

[c]Patients who are treatment failures with alternative regimens should be treated with ceftriaxone 250 mg IM once plus azithromycin 1 g PO once in consultation with an infectious disease expert.

[d]For patients with severe cephalosporin allergy.

[e]Parenteral treatment duration should be determined in consultation with an infectious diseases expert. Parenteral therapy for meningitis should be continued for at least 10–14 days and at least 4 weeks in endocarditis.

[f]A single lavage of the infected eye with normal saline should be considered; empiric therapy for C. *trachomatis* is recommended.

[g]Efficacy in preventing chlamydial ophthalmia is unclear.

[h]Caution should be taken when administering ceftriaxone to hyperbilirubinemic neonates.

TABLE 46–5	Presentation of Syphilis Infections
General	
Primary	Incubation period 10–90 days (mean, 21 days)
Secondary	Develops 2–8 weeks after initial infection in untreated or inadequately treated individuals
Latent	Develops 4–10 weeks after secondary stage in untreated or inadequately treated individuals
Tertiary	Develops in approximately 30% of untreated or inadequately treated individuals 10–30 years after initial infection
Site of infection	
Primary	External genitalia, perianal region, mouth, and throat
Secondary	Multisystem involvement secondary to hematogenous and lymphatic spread
Latent tertiary	Potentially multisystem involvement (dormant)
	CNS, heart, eyes, bones, and joints
Signs and symptoms	
Primary	Single, painless, indurated lesion (chancre) that erodes, ulcerates, and eventually heals (typical); regional lymphadenopathy is common; multiple, painful, purulent lesions possible but uncommon
Secondary	Pruritic or nonpruritic rash, mucocutaneous lesions, flulike symptoms, lymphadenopathy
Latent	Asymptomatic
Tertiary	Cardiovascular syphilis (aortitis or aortic insufficiency), neurosyphilis (meningitis, general paresis, dementia, tabes dorsalis, eighth cranial nerve deafness, blindness), gummatous lesions involving any organ or tissue

(CNS, central nervous system.)

- Treponemal tests are more sensitive than nontreponemal tests and are used to confirm the diagnosis (ie, the fluorescent treponemal antibody absorption).

TREATMENT

- Treatment recommendations from the CDC for syphilis are presented in **Table 46–6**. Parenteral **penicillin G** is the treatment of choice for all stages of syphilis. Benzathine penicillin G is the only penicillin effective for single-dose therapy.
- Patients with abnormal cerebrospinal fluid findings should be treated as having neurosyphilis.
- For pregnant patients, penicillin is the treatment of choice at the dosage recommended for that particular stage of syphilis. To ensure treatment success and prevent transmission to the fetus, some experts advocate an additional intramuscular dose of benzathine penicillin G, 2.4 million units, 1 week after completion of the recommended regimen.
- Most patients treated for primary and secondary syphilis experience the Jarisch–Herxheimer reaction after treatment, characterized by flu-like symptoms such as transient headache, fever, chills, malaise, arthralgia, myalgia, tachypnea, peripheral vasodilation, and aggravation of syphilitic lesions. The Jarisch–Herxheimer reaction should not be confused with penicillin allergy. Most reactions can be managed symptomatically with analgesics, antipyretics, and rest.

TABLE 46–6 Drug Therapy and Follow-Up of Syphilis

Stage/Type of Syphilis	Recommended Regimens[a,b]	Follow-up Serology
Primary, secondary, or early latent syphilis (<1 year's duration)	Adults: Benzathine penicillin G 2.4 million units IM in a single dose Children: Benzathine penicillin G 50,000 units/kg IM in a single dose, up to 2.4 million units	Quantitative nontreponemal tests at 6 and 12 months for primary and secondary syphilis; at 6, 12, and 24 months for early latent syphilis[c]
Late latent syphilis (>1 year's duration) or latent syphilis of unknown duration or tertiary syphilis or retreatment	Adults: Benzathine penicillin G 2.4 million units IM once a week for 3 successive weeks (7.2 million units total) Children: Benzathine penicillin G 50,000 units/kg IM once a week for 3 successive weeks, up to 7.2 million units total	Quantitative nontreponemal tests at 6, 12, and 24 months[d,e]
Neurosyphilis	Aqueous crystalline penicillin G 18–24 million units IV (3–4 million units every 4 hours or by continuous infusion) for 10–14 days[f] or Aqueous procaine penicillin G 2.4 million units IM daily plus probenecid 500 mg orally four times daily, both for 10–14 days[f]	CSF examination every 6 months until the cell count is normal; if it has not decreased at 6 months or is not normal by 2 years, retreatment should be considered
Congenital syphilis (infants with proven or highly probable disease)	Aqueous crystalline penicillin G 50,000 units/kg/dose IV every 12 hours during the first 7 days of life and every 8 hours thereafter for a total of 10 days or Procaine penicillin G 50,000 units/kg IM daily for 10 days	Serologic follow-up only recommended if antimicrobials other than penicillin are used

Penicillin-allergic patients[g]

Primary, secondary, or early latent syphilis	Doxycycline 100 mg orally two times daily for 14 days[g,h]	Same as for non–penicillin-allergic patients
	or	
	Tetracycline 500 mg orally four times daily for 14 days[h]	
	or	
	Ceftriaxone 1–2 g IM or IV daily for 10–14 days	
Late latent syphilis (>1 year's duration) or syphilis of unknown duration	Doxycycline 100 mg orally twice a day for 28 days[h,i]	Same as for non–penicillin-allergic patients
	or	
	Tetracycline 500 mg orally four times daily for 28 days[h,i]	

(CDC, Centers for Disease Control and Prevention; CSF, cerebrospinal fluid; HIV, human immunodeficiency virus.)

[a]Recommendations are those of the CDC.

[b]The CDC recommends that all patients diagnosed with syphilis be tested for HIV infection.

[c]More frequent follow-up (ie, 3, 6, 9, 12, and 24 months) recommended for HIV-infected patients.

[d]More frequent follow-up (ie, 6, 12, 18, and 24 months) recommended for HIV-infected patients.

[e]No specific recommendations exist for tertiary syphilis because of the lack of available data.

[f]Some experts administer benzathine penicillin G 2.4 million units IM once per week for up to 3 weeks after completion of the neurosyphilis regimens to provide a total duration of therapy comparable to that used for late syphilis in the absence of neurosyphilis.

[g]For nonpregnant patients; pregnant patients should be treated with penicillin after desensitization.

[h]Pregnant patients allergic to penicillin should be desensitized and treated with penicillin.

[i]Limited data suggest that ceftriaxone may be effective, although the optimal dosage and treatment duration are unclear.

- CDC recommendations for serologic follow-up of patients treated for syphilis are given in Table 46–6.
- For women treated during pregnancy, monthly, quantitative, nontreponemal tests are recommended in those at high risk of reinfection.

CHLAMYDIA

- Infections caused by *C. trachomatis* are believed to be the most common STD in the United States. *C. trachomatis* is an obligate intracellular parasite that has some similarities to viruses and bacteria.

CLINICAL PRESENTATION

- In comparison with gonorrhea, chlamydial genital infections are more frequently asymptomatic, and when present, symptoms tend to be less noticeable. Table 46–7 summarizes the usual clinical presentation of chlamydial infections.
- Similar to gonorrhea, chlamydia may be transmitted to an infant during contact with infected cervicovaginal secretions. Nearly two thirds of infants acquire chlamydial infection after endocervical exposure, with the primary morbidity associated with seeding of the infant's eyes, nasopharynx, rectum, or vagina.
- Culture of endocervical or urethral epithelial cell scrapings is the most specific method (close to 100%) for detection of chlamydia, but sensitivity is as low as 70%. Between 3 and 7 days are required for results.
- Tests that allow rapid identification of chlamydial antigens and nucleic acid provide more rapid results, are technically less demanding, are less costly, and in some situations have greater sensitivity than culture. Commonly used nonculture tests for detection of *C. trachomatis* are the enzyme immunosorbent assay (EIA), DNA hybridization probe, and nucleic acid amplification tests (NAATs).

TABLE 46–7	Presentation of *Chlamydia* Infections	
	Males	**Females**
General	Incubation period: 35 days Symptom onset: 7–21 days	Incubation period: 7–35 days Usual symptom onset: 7–21 days
Site of infection	Most common: urethra Others: rectum (receptive anal intercourse), oropharynx, eye	Most common: endocervical canal Others: urethra, rectum (usually caused by perineal contamination), oropharynx, eye
Symptoms	More than 50% of urethral and rectal infections are asymptomatic Urethral infection: mild dysuria, discharge Pharyngeal infection: asymptomatic to mild pharyngitis	More than 66% of cervical infections are asymptomatic Urethral infection: usually subclinical; dysuria and frequency uncommon Rectal and pharyngeal infection: symptoms same as for men
Signs	Scant to profuse, mucoid to purulent urethral or rectal discharge Rectal infection: pain, discharge, bleeding	Abnormal vaginal discharge or uterine bleeding, purulent urethral or rectal discharge can be scant to profuse
Complications	Epididymitis, Reiter's syndrome (rare)	Pelvic inflammatory disease and associated complications (ie, ectopic pregnancy, infertility) Reiter's syndrome (rare)

TABLE 46-8	Treatment of *Chlamydial* Infections	
Infection	**Recommended Regimens**[a]	**Alternative Regimen**
Uncomplicated urethral, endocervical, or rectal infection in adults	Azithromycin 1 g orally once, or doxycycline 100 mg orally twice daily for 7 days	Erythromycin base 500 mg orally four times daily for 7 days, or erythromycin ethylsuccinate 800 mg orally four times daily for 7 days, or levofloxacin 500 mg orally once daily for 7 days, or ofloxacin 300 mg orally twice daily for 7 days
Urogenital infections during pregnancy	Azithromycin 1 g orally as a single dose or amoxicillin 500 mg orally three times daily for 7 days	Amoxicillin 500 mg orally three times daily for 7 days, or erythromycin base 500 mg orally four times daily for 7 days, or erythromycin base 250 mg orally four times daily for 14 days, or erythromycin ethylsuccinate 800 mg orally four times daily for 7 days, or erythromycin ethylsuccinate 400 mg orally four times daily for 14 days
Conjunctivitis of the newborn or pneumonia in infants	Erythromycin base or ethylsuccinate 50 mg/kg/day orally in four divided doses for 14 days[b,c]	Azithromycin suspension 20 mg/kg/day orally once daily for 3 days[c]

(CDC, Centers for Disease Control and Prevention; IHPS, infantile hypertrophic pyloric stenosis.)
[a]Recommendations are those of the CDC.
[b]Topical therapy alone is inadequate for ophthalmia neonatorum and is unnecessary when systemic therapy is administered. Effectiveness of erythromycin treatment is approximately 80%; therefore, a second course of therapy may be required.
[c]An association between oral erythromycin and azithromycin and IHPS has been reported in infants aged <6 weeks. Infants treated with either of these antimicrobials should be followed for signs and symptoms of IHPS.

TREATMENT

- Recommended regimens for treatment of chlamydial infections are given in Table 46-8. Single-dose **azithromycin** and 7-day **doxycycline** are the agents of choice.
- Treatment of chlamydial infections with the recommended regimens is highly effective; therefore, posttreatment cultures are not routinely recommended.
- Infants with pneumonitis should receive follow-up testing because erythromycin is only 80% effective.

GENITAL HERPES

- The term *herpes* is used to describe two distinct but antigenically related serotypes of herpes simplex virus (HSV). HSV type 1 (HSV-1) is most commonly associated with oropharyngeal disease; type 2 (HSV-2) is most closely associated with genital disease.

CLINICAL PRESENTATION

- A summary of the clinical presentation of genital herpes is provided in Table 46-9.
- Tissue culture is the most specific (100%) and sensitive method (80%–90%) of confirming the diagnosis of first-episode genital herpes; however, culture is relatively insensitive in detecting HSV in ulcers in the latter stages of healing and in recurrent infections.

TABLE 46–9	Presentation of Genital Herpes Infections
General	Incubation period 2–14 days (mean, 4 days) Can be caused by either HSV-1 or HSV-2
Classification of infection	
First-episode primary	Initial genital infection in individuals lacking antibody to either HSV-1 or HSV-2
First-episode nonprimary	Initial genital infection in individuals with clinical or serologic evidence of prior HSV (usually HSV-1) infection
Recurrent	Appearance of genital lesions at some time following healing of first-episode infection
Signs and symptoms	
First-episode infections	Most primary infections are asymptomatic or minimally symptomatic Multiple painful pustular or ulcerative lesions on external genitalia developing over a period of 7–10 days; lesions heal in 2–4 weeks (mean, 21 days) Flulike symptoms (eg, fever, headache, malaise) during first few days after appearance of lesions Others—local itching, pain, or discomfort; vaginal or urethral discharge, tender inguinal adenopathy, paresthesias, urinary retention Severity of symptoms greater in females than in males Symptoms are less severe (eg, fewer lesions, more rapid lesion healing, fewer or milder systemic symptoms) with nonprimary infections Symptoms more severe and prolonged in the immunocompromised On average viral shedding lasts approximately 11–12 days for primary infections and 7 days for nonprimary infections
Recurrent	Prodrome seen in approximately 50% of patients prior to appearance of recurrent lesions; mild burning, itching, or tingling are typical prodromal symptoms Compared to primary infections, recurrent infections associated with (1) fewer lesions that are more localized, (2) shorter duration of active infection (lesions heal within 7 days), and (3) milder symptoms Severity of symptoms greater in females than in males Symptoms more severe and prolonged in the immunocompromised On average viral shedding lasts approximately 4 days Asymptomatic viral shedding is more frequent during the first year after infection with HSV
Therapeutic implications of HSV-1 versus HSV-2 genital infection	Primary infections caused by HSV-1 and HSV-2 virtually indistinguishable Recurrent infections and subclinical viral shedding are less frequent with HSV-1 Recurrent infections with HSV-2 tend to be more severe
Complications	Secondary infection of lesions; extragenital infection because of autoinoculation; disseminated infection (primarily in immunocompromised patients); meningitis or encephalitis; neonatal transmission

(HSV-1, herpes simplex virus type 1; HSV-2, herpes simplex virus type 2.)

TREATMENT

- <u>Goals of Treatment</u>: to relieve symptoms and to shorten the clinical course, prevent complications and recurrences, and to decrease disease transmission.
- Palliative and supportive measures are the cornerstone of therapy for patients with genital herpes. Pain and discomfort usually respond to warm saline baths or the use of analgesics, antipyretics, or antipruritics.
- Specific treatment recommendations are given in Table 46–10.
- Oral **acyclovir, valacyclovir**, and **famciclovir** are the treatments of choice for outpatients with first-episode genital herpes. Treatment does not prevent latency or alter the subsequent frequency and severity of recurrences.
- Suppressive oral antiviral therapy reduces the frequency and the severity of recurrences in 70% to 80% of patients experiencing frequent recurrences.
- Acyclovir, valacyclovir, and famciclovir have been used to prevent reactivation of infection in patients seropositive for HSV who undergo transplantation procedures or induction chemotherapy for acute leukemia.
- The safety of **acyclovir, famciclovir, and valacyclovir** therapy during pregnancy is not established, although there is no evidence of teratogenic effects of acyclovir in humans.

TRICHOMONIASIS

- Trichomoniasis is caused by *Trichomonas vaginalis*, a flagellated, motile protozoan that is responsible for 3 million to 5 million cases per year in the United States.
- Coinfection with other STDs (eg, gonorrhea) is common in patients diagnosed with trichomoniasis.

CLINICAL PRESENTATION

- The typical presentation of trichomoniasis in men and women is presented in Table 46–11.
- *T. vaginalis* produces nonspecific symptoms also consistent with bacterial vaginosis; thus, laboratory diagnosis is required.
- The simplest and most reliable means of diagnosis is a wet-mount examination of the vaginal discharge. Trichomoniasis is confirmed if characteristic pear-shaped, flagellating organisms are observed. Newer diagnostic tests such as monoclonal antibody or DNA probe techniques, as well as polymerase chain reaction tests, are highly sensitive and specific.

TREATMENT

- **Metronidazole** and **tinidazole** are the only antimicrobial agents available in the United States that are consistently effective in *T. vaginalis* infections.
- Treatment recommendations for *Trichomonas* infections are given in Table 46–12.
- GI complaints (eg, anorexia, nausea, vomiting, and diarrhea) are the most common adverse effects with the single 2 g dose of metronidazole or tinidazole, occurring in 5% to 10% of treated patients. Some patients complain of a bitter, metallic taste in the mouth.
- Patients intolerant of the single 2 g dose because of GI adverse effects usually tolerate the multidose regimen.
- To achieve maximal cure rates and prevent relapse with the single 2 g dose of metronidazole, simultaneous treatment of infected sexual partners is necessary.
- Patients who fail to respond to an initial course usually respond to a second course of metronidazole or tinidazole therapy.
- Patients taking metronidazole should be instructed to avoid alcohol ingestion during therapy and for 1 or 2 days after completion of therapy because of a possible disulfiram-like effect.
- At present no satisfactory treatment is available for pregnant women with *Trichomonas* infections. Metronidazole and tinidazole are contraindicated during the first trimester of pregnancy.

TABLE 46–10 Treatment of Genital Herpes

Type of Infection	Recommended Regimens[a,b]	Alternative Regimen
First clinical episode of genital herpes[c]	Acyclovir 400 mg orally three times daily for 7–10 days,[d] or Acyclovir 200 mg orally five times daily for 7–10 days,[d] or Famciclovir 250 mg orally three times daily for 7–10 days,[d] or Valacyclovir 1 g orally twice daily for 7–10 days[d]	Acyclovir 5–10 mg/kg IV every 8 hours for 2–7 days or until clinical improvement occurs, followed by oral therapy to complete at least 10 days of total therapy[e]
Recurrent infection		
Episodic therapy	Acyclovir 400 mg orally three times daily for 5 days,[f] or Acyclovir 800 mg orally twice daily for 5 days,[f] or Acyclovir 800 mg orally three times daily for 2 days,[f] or Famciclovir 125 mg orally twice daily for 5 days,[f] or Famciclovir 1 g orally twice daily for 1 day,[f] or Famciclovir 500 mg orally once, followed by 250 mg orally twice daily for 2 days,[f] or Valacyclovir 500 mg orally twice daily for 3 days,[f] or Valacyclovir 1 g orally once daily for 5 days[f]	
Suppressive therapy	Acyclovir 400 mg orally twice daily, or Famciclovir 250 mg orally twice daily[h], or Valacyclovir 500 mg or 1,000 mg orally once daily[i]	

(CDC, Centers for Disease Control and Prevention; HIV, human immunodeficiency virus; IV, intravenous.)
[a]Recommendations are those of the CDC.
[b]HIV-infected patients can require more aggressive therapy.
[c]Primary or nonprimary first episode.
[d]Treatment duration can be extended if healing is incomplete after 10 days.
[e]Only for patients with severe symptoms or complications that necessitate hospitalization. HSV encephalitis requires 21 days of IV therapy.
[f]Requires initiation of therapy within 24 hours of lesion onset or during the prodrome that precedes some outbreaks.
[g]Consider discontinuation of treatment after one year to assess frequency of recurrence.
[h]Famcicolvir appears less effective for suppression of viral shedding.
[i]Valacyclovir 500 mg appears less effective than other valacyclovir and acyclovir regimens in patients with 10 or more recurrences per year.

TABLE 46–11	Presentation of Trichomonas Infections	
	Males	**Females**
General	Incubation period 3–28 days Organism can be detectable within 48 hours after exposure to infected partner	Incubation period 3–28 days
Site of infection	Most common: urethra Others: rectum (usually caused by rectal intercourse in MSM), oropharynx, eye	Most common: endocervical canal Others: urethra, rectum (usually caused by perineal contamination), oropharynx, eye
Symptoms	Can be asymptomatic (more common in males than females) or minimally symptomatic Urethral discharge (clear to mucopurulent) Dysuria, pruritus	Can be asymptomatic or minimally symptomatic Scant to copious, typically malodorous vaginal discharge (50%-75%) and pruritus (worse during menses) Dysuria, dyspareunia
Signs	Urethral discharge	Vaginal discharge Vaginal pH 4.5–6 Inflammation/erythema of vulva, vagina, and/or cervix Urethritis
Complications	Epididymitis and chronic prostatitis (uncommon) Male infertility (decreased sperm motility and viability)	Pelvic inflammatory disease and associated complications (ie, ectopic pregnancy, infertility) Premature labor, premature rupture of membranes, and low–birth-weight infants (risk of neonatal infections is low) Cervical neoplasia

(MSM, men who have sex with men.)

- Follow-up is considered unnecessary in patients who become asymptomatic after treatment with metronidazole.
- When patients remain symptomatic, it is important to determine if reinfection has occurred. In these cases, a repeat course of therapy, as well as identification and treatment or retreatment of infected sexual partners, is recommended.

OTHER SEXUALLY TRANSMITTED DISEASES

- Several STDs other than those previously discussed occur with varying frequency in the United States and throughout the world. Although an in-depth discussion of these diseases is beyond the scope of this chapter, recommended treatment regimens are given in **Table 46–13**.

TABLE 46–12	Treatment of Trichomoniasis	
Type	**Recommended Regimen[a]**	**Alternative Regimen**
Symptomatic and asymptomatic infections	Metronidazole 2 g orally in a single dose *or* Tinidazole 2 g orally in a single dose[b]	Metronidazole 500 mg orally two times daily for 7 days[c,d]
Persistent or recurrent infections	Metronidazole 500 mg orally two times daily for 7 days[c]	Metronidazole 2 g orally for 7 days[e] *or*
Treatment in pregnancy	Metronidazole 2 g orally in a single dose[e]	Tinidazole 2 g orally for 7 days[e]

(CDC, Centers for Disease Control and Prevention; HIV, human immunodeficiency virus.)
[a]Recommendations are those of the CDC.
[b]Randomized controlled trials comparing single 2 g doses of metronidazole and tinidazole suggest that tinidazole is equivalent to, or superior to, metronidazole in achieving parasitologic cure and resolution of symptoms.
[c]Metronidazole labeling approved by the FDA does not include this regimen. Dosage regimens for treatment of trichomoniasis included in the product labeling are the single 2 g dose; 250 mg three times daily for 7 days; and 375 mg twice daily for 7 days. The 250 mg and 375 mg dosage regimens are currently not included in the CDC recommendations.
[d]Recommended treatment regimen for women with HIV coinfection.
[e]For treatment failures with metronidazole 2 g as a single dose and metronidazole 500 mg orally two times daily for 7 days.
[f]Symptomatic pregnant women can be treated with this regimen at any stage of pregnancy.

TABLE 46–13	Treatment Regimens for Miscellaneous Sexually Transmitted Diseases	
Infection	**Recommended Regimen[a]**	**Alternative Regimen**
Chancroid (*Haemophilus ducreyi*)	Azithromycin 1 g orally in a single dose, *or* Ceftriaxone 250 mg IM in a single dose, *or* Ciprofloxacin 500 mg orally twice daily for 3 days[b] *or* Erythromycin base 500 mg orally four times daily for 7 days	
Lymphogranuloma venereum	Doxycycline 100 mg orally twice daily for 21 days[c]	Erythromycin base 500 mg orally four times daily for 21 days[d]
HPV infection		
External genital/perianal warts	*Provider-Administered Therapies:* Cryotherapy (eg, liquid nitrogen or cryoprobe); repeat weekly as necessary, *or* Podophyllin resin 10%-25% in compound tincture of benzoin applied to lesions; repeat weekly as necessary,[e,f] *or* TCA 80%-90% *or* BCA 80%-90% applied to warts; repeat weekly as necessary, *or* Surgical removal (tangential scissor excision, tangential shave excision, curettage, or electrosurgery)	Intralesional interferon *or* Photodynamic therapy *or* Topical cidofovir

(continued)

TABLE 46–13	Treatment Regimens for Miscellaneous Sexually Transmitted Diseases (*Continued*)	
Infection	Recommended Regimen[a]	Alternative Regimen
	Patient-Applied Therapies:	
	Podofilox 0.5% solution or gel applied twice daily for 3 days, followed by 4 days of no therapy; cycle is repeated as necessary for up to four cycles,[f] *or*	
	Imiquimod 3.75% or 5% cream applied at bedtime three times weekly for up to 16 weeks,[f] *or*	
	Sinecatechins 15% ointment applied three times daily for up to 16 weeks	
Vaginal and anal warts	Cryotherapy with liquid nitrogen, or TCA or BCA 80%-90% as for external HPV warts; repeat weekly as necessary[g]	
	Surgical removal (not for vaginal or urethral meatus warts)	
Urethral meatus warts	Cryotherapy with liquid nitrogen, or podophyllin resin 10%-25% in compound tincture of benzoin applied at weekly intervals[f,h]	
Prevention	Gardasil® (HPV quadrivalent [types 6, 11, 16, and 18]) recombinant vaccine 0.5 mL IM on day 1; a second and third dose are administered 2 and 6 months following the first dose[i,j,k]	
	Cervarix® (HPV bivalent [types 16 and 18]) recombinant vaccine 0.5 mL IM on day 1; a second and third dose are administered 1 and 6 months following the first dose[i,l]	
	Gardasil9®(HPV 9-valent [types 6, 11, 16, 18, 31, 33, 45, 52, 58]) recombinant vaccine 0.5 mL IM on day 1; a second and third dose are administered 1 and 6 months following the first dose[i]	

(BCA, bichloracetic acid; HPV, human papillomavirus; TCA, trichloroacetic acid.)
[a]Recommendations are those of the Centers for Disease Control and Prevention (CDC).
[b]Ciprofloxacin is contraindicated for pregnant and lactating women and for persons aged <18 years.
[c]Azithromycin 1 g PO once weekly for 3 weeks can be effective.
[d]Pregnant patients should be treated with erythromycin.
[e]Some experts recommended washing podophyllin off after 1–4 hours to minimize local irritation.
[f]Safety during pregnancy is not established.
[g]Surgical removal of anal warts is also a recommended treatment.
[h]Some specialists recommend the use of podofilox and imiquimod for treating distal meatal warts.
[i]CDC recommendations: vaccination is recommended in girls 11–12 years of age, and in females aged 13–26 years who either were not previously vaccinated, or who did not complete the vaccination series.
[j]FDA approved labeling for Gardasil®: indicated in girls and women 9 through 26 years of age for the prevention of cervical, vulvar, vaginal, and anal cancer caused by HPV types 16 and 18, genital warts (condyloma acuminata) caused by HPV types 6 and 11, and precancerous or dysplastic lesions caused by HPV types 6, 11, 16, and 18.
[k]Vaccination is recommended in males aged 9–26 years to prevent genital warts and anal cancer.
[l]FDA approved labeling for Cervarix®: indicated in females 9 through 25 years of age for the prevention of cervical cancer, cervical intraepithelial neoplasia grade 2 or worse, adenocarcinoma in situ, and cervical intraepithelial neoplasia grade 1 caused by HPV types 16 and 18.

See Chapter 117, Sexually Transmitted Diseases, authored by Leroy C. Knodel, Bryson Duhon, and Jacqueline Argamany for a more detailed discussion of this topic.

Skin and Soft-Tissue Infections

- Bacterial infections of the skin can be classified as primary or secondary (Table 47–1). Primary bacterial infections are usually caused by a single bacterial species and involve areas of generally healthy skin (eg, impetigo and erysipelas). Secondary infections, however, develop in areas of previously damaged skin and are frequently polymicrobic.
- The conditions that may predispose a patient to the development of skin and soft-tissue infections (SSTIs) include (1) a high concentration of bacteria; (2) excessive moisture of the skin; (3) inadequate blood supply; (4) availability of bacterial nutrients; and (5) damage to the corneal layer, allowing for bacterial penetration.
- The majority of SSTIs are caused by gram-positive organisms and, less commonly, gram-negative bacteria present on the skin surface. *Staphylococcus aureus* and *Streptococcus pyogenes* account for the majority of SSTIs. Community-associated methicillin-resistant *S. aureus* (CA-MRSA) has emerged and is often isolated in otherwise healthy patients.

ERYSIPELAS

- *Erysipelas* (Saint Anthony's fire) is an infection of the superficial layers of the skin and cutaneous lymphatics. The infection is almost always caused by β-hemolytic streptococci, with *S. pyogenes* (group A *streptococci*) responsible for most infections.
- The lower extremities are the most common sites for erysipelas. Patients often experience flu-like symptoms (fever and malaise) prior to the appearance of the lesions. The infected area is painful, often a burning pain. Erysipelas lesions are bright red and edematous with lymphatic streaking and clearly demarcated raised margins. Leukocytosis is common, and C-reactive protein is generally elevated.
- Mild to moderate cases of erysipelas in adults are treated with intramuscular **procaine penicillin G** or **penicillin VK**. For more serious infections, aqueous penicillin G, 2 million to 8 million units daily, should be administered intravenously (IV). Penicillin-allergic patients can be treated with clindamycin or erythromycin.
- Evidence-based recommendations for treatment of SSTIs are found in Table 47–2, and recommended drugs and dosing regimens for outpatient treatment of mild to moderate SSTIs are found in Tables 47–3 and 47–4.

IMPETIGO

- *Impetigo* is a superficial skin infection that is seen most commonly in children. It is highly communicable and spreads through close contact. Most cases are caused by *S. pyogenes*, but *S. aureus* either alone or in combination with *S. pyogenes* has emerged as a principal cause of impetigo.

CLINICAL PRESENTATION

- Exposed skin, especially the face, is the most common site for impetigo.
- Pruritus is common, and scratching of the lesions may further spread infection through excoriation of the skin. Other systemic signs of infection are minimal.
- Weakness, fever, and diarrhea are sometimes seen with bullous impetigo.
- Nonbullous impetigo manifests initially as small, fluid-filled vesicles. These lesions rapidly develop into pus-filled blisters that readily rupture. Purulent discharge from the lesions dries to form golden yellow crusts that are characteristic of impetigo.
- In the bullous form of impetigo, the lesions begin as vesicles and turn into bullae containing clear yellow fluid. Bullae soon rupture, forming thin, light brown crusts.
- Regional lymph nodes may be enlarged.

TABLE 47–1	Bacterial Classification of Important Skin and Soft-Tissue Infections
Primary infections	
Erysipelas	Group A streptococci (*Streptococcus pyogenes*)
Impetigo	*Staphylococcus aureus* (including methicillin-resistant strains), group A streptococci
Lymphangitis	Group A streptococci; occasionally *S. aureus*
Cellulitis	Group A streptococci, *S. aureus* (potentially including methicillin-resistant strains); occasionally other gram-positive cocci, gram-negative bacilli, and/or anaerobes
Necrotizing fasciitis	
Type I	Anaerobes (*Bacteroides* spp., *Peptostreptococcus* spp.) and facultative bacteria (streptococci, Enterobacteriaceae)
Type II	Group A streptococci
Type III	*Clostridium perfringens*
Secondary infections	
Diabetic foot infections	*S. aureus*, streptococci, Enterobacteriaceae, *Bacteroides* spp., *Peptostreptococcus* spp., *Pseudomonas aeruginosa*
Pressure sores	*S. aureus* including methicillin-resistant strains, streptococci, Enterobacteriaceae, *Bacteroides* spp., *Peptostreptococcus* spp., *P. aeruginosa*
Bite wounds	
Animal	*Pasteurella* spp., *S. aureus*, streptococci, *Bacteroides* spp.
Human	*Eikenella corrodens*, *S. aureus*, streptococci, *Corynebacterium* spp., *Bacteroides* spp., *Peptostreptococcus* spp.
Burn wounds	*P. aeruginosa*, Enterobacteriaceae, *S. aureus*, streptococci

TREATMENT

- Topical mupirocin ointment or retapamulin ointment for 5 days are recommended as first-line treatment of mild cases of impetigo not involving multiple lesions or the face.
- Penicillinase-resistant penicillins (eg, **dicloxacillin**) are the systemic agents of choice because of the increased isolation of *S. aureus*. First-generation cephalosporins (eg, cephalexin) are also effective (see Table 47–3). **Penicillin** may be used for impetigo caused by *S. pyogenes*. It may be administered as either a single intramuscular dose of benzathine penicillin G (300,000–600,000 units in children, 1.2 million units in adults) or as oral penicillin VK given for 7. Penicillin-allergic patients can be treated with oral **clindamycin, doxycycline, or trimethoprim-sulfamethoxazole**. Recommended doses for antimicrobials are found in Table 47–4.

CELLULITIS

- Cellulitis is an acute, spreading infectious process that initially affects the epidermis and dermis and may subsequently spread within the superficial fascia. This process is characterized by inflammation but with little or no necrosis or suppuration of soft tissue.

461

TABLE 47–2 Evidence-Based Recommendations for Treatment of Skin and Soft-Tissue Infections

Recommendations	Recommendation Grade[a]
Folliculitis, furuncles, carbuncles	
Gram stain and culture of pus from carbuncles and abscesses are recommended, but treatment without cultures is reasonable in most patients	Strong, moderate
Carbuncles, abscesses and large furuncles of mild severity should be treated with incision and drainage	Strong, high
Administration of antibiotics with activity against *Staphylococcus aureus* as an adjunct to incision and drainage should be based on presence or absence of systemic signs of infection	Strong, low
Antibiotics with activity against MRSA are recommended for patients with carbuncles or abscesses of higher severity who have failed initial antibiotic therapy, have severe systemic signs of infection, or are immunocompromised	Strong, low
Erysipelas	
Most infections are caused by *Streptococcus pyogenes*. Penicillin (oral or IV depending on clinical severity) is the drug of choice	A-I
If *S. aureus* is suspected, a penicillinase-resistant penicillin or first-generation cephalosporin should be used	A-I
Impetigo	
Gram stain and culture of pus or exudates should be obtained to help identify causative pathogens	Strong, moderate
Bullous and nonbullous impetigo should be treated with either mupirocin or retapamulin for 5 days	Strong, high
Impetigo should be treated with oral antibiotics active against *S. aureus* unless cultures show streptococci alone. Dicloxacillin or cephalexin is recommended for 7 days. Doxycycline, clindamycin, or sulfamethoxazole-trimethoprim should be used when MRSA is suspected or confirmed	Strong, moderate
Cellulitis	
Cultures of blood or cutaneous aspirates, biopsies or swabs are not routinely recommended	Strong, moderate
Blood cultures are recommended, and cultures of cutaneous aspirates, biopsies, or swabs should be considered, in patients receiving chemotherapy for malignancies, neutropenia, severe cell-mediated immunodeficiency, immersion injuries, or animal bites	Strong, moderate (blood) Weak, moderate (other cultures)
Typical cases of mild nonpurulent cellulitis should be treated with antibiotics active against streptococci	Strong, moderate
Systemic antibiotics are recommended for moderate nonpurulent cellulitis with systemic signs of infection. Use of antibiotics active against methicillin-susceptible *S. aureus* could be considered	Weak, low

Patients with severe nonpurulent cellulitis associated with penetrating trauma, MRSA infection in another location, MRSA nasal colonization, injection drug use, or systemic signs of infection should be treated with vancomycin or other antibiotics active against both MRSA and streptococci	Strong, moderate
Broad-spectrum antibiotic therapy with vancomycin plus either piperacillin–tazobactam, imipenem, or meropenem may be considered for empiric treatment of severe nonpurulent cellulitis in severely immunocompromised patients	Weak, moderate (need for broad-spectrum therapy) Strong, moderate (recommended broad-spectrum antibiotic regimen if used)
A treatment duration of 5 days is recommended for cellulitis, but may be extended if lack of clinical response within that time	Strong, high
Elevation of the affected area and treatment of predisposing factors are recommended for cellulitis	Strong, moderate
Systemic corticosteroids for 7 days can be considered for adjunctive treatment of cellulitis in nondiabetic patients	Weak, moderate
Patients with mild nonpurulent cellulitis who do not have systemic signs of infection, altered mental status, or hemodynamic instability should be treated as outpatients	Strong, moderate
Hospitalization is recommended for patients with moderate to severe nonpurulent cellulitis who have failed outpatient therapy, have poor adherence to therapy, are immunocompromised, or in whom there is a concern for deeper or necrotizing infection	Strong, moderate
Empiric antibiotics for outpatients with purulent cellulitis should provide activity against community-associated MRSA; coverage of β-hemolytic streptococci is likely not required. Mild–moderate infections can generally be treated with oral agents (dicloxacillin, cephalexin, clindamycin) unless resistance is high in the community	A-II
Recommended antibiotics for empiric coverage of MRSA in outpatients include orally administered trimethoprim–sulfamethoxazole, doxycycline, minocycline, clindamycin, and linezolid	A-II for all listed options
If coverage of both β-hemolytic streptococci and community-associated MRSA is desired, empiric antibiotic regimens for outpatient therapy include orally administered clindamycin alone; linezolid alone; or trimethoprim–sulfamethoxazole, doxycycline, or minocycline in combination with amoxicillin	A-II for all listed options
Hospitalized patients with complicated or purulent cellulitis should receive IV antibiotics with activity against MRSA pending culture data. Antibiotic options include vancomycin, linezolid, daptomycin, telavancin, and clindamycin	A-I for all except clindamycin; clindamycin A-III
In the treatment of S. aureus infections, trough serum vancomycin concentrations should always be maintained >10 mg/L (>7 μmol/L) to avoid development of resistance	B-III

(continued)

TABLE 47–2 Evidence-Based Recommendations for Treatment of Skin and Soft-Tissue Infections (*Continued*)

Recommendations	Recommendation Grade[a]
Necrotizing fasciitis	
Patients with severe nonpurulent cellulitis characterized by aggressive infection and associated with signs of systemic toxicity, necrotizing fasciitis, or gas gangrene should have prompt surgical consultation	Strong, low
Early and aggressive surgical debridement of all necrotic tissue is essential	A-III
Necrotizing fasciitis should be empirically treated with broad-spectrum antibiotics such as vancomycin or linezolid plus piperacillin–tazobactam or a carbapenem, or vancomycin or linezolid plus ceftriaxone and metronidazole	Strong, low
Necrotizing fasciitis caused by *S. pyogenes* should be treated with the combination of clindamycin and penicillin	Strong, low
In the treatment of necrotizing fasciitis caused by methicillin-resistant *S. aureus* infections, trough serum vancomycin concentrations of 15–20 mg/L (10–14 μmol/L) are recommended	B-II
Clostridial gas gangrene (myonecrosis) should be treated with clindamycin and penicillin	B-III
Diabetic foot infections	
Clinically uninfected wounds should not be treated with antibiotics	A-III
Empiric antibiotic regimens should be selected based on severity of infection and likely pathogens	A-III
Antibiotic therapy should target only aerobic gram-positive cocci in patients with mild to moderate infection who have not received antibiotics within the previous month	C-III
Broad-spectrum empiric antibiotic therapy should be initiated in most patients with severe infections, until culture and susceptibility data are available	A-III
Empiric antibiotics directed against *Pseudomonas aeruginosa* are usually unnecessary except in patients with specific risk factors for infection with this pathogen: patient has been soaking feet, patient has failed previous antibiotic therapy with nonpseudomonal agents, or clinically severe infection	A-III
Empiric antibiotics directed against MRSA should be considered in patients with specific risk factors, including: prior history of infection or colonization with MRSA, high local prevalence of MRSA (eg, ≥50% for mild infections, ≥30% for severe infection), or clinically severe infection	C-III
Oral agents with high bioavailability may be used in the treatment of most mild, and many moderate, infections	A-II
Parenteral therapy is initially preferred for all severe, and some moderate, infections. After initial response, step-down therapy to oral agents can be considered	C-III
Definitive therapy should be based on results of appropriately collected cultures and sensitivities, as well as clinical response to empiric antimicrobial agents	A-III

Appropriate wound care, in addition to appropriate antimicrobial therapy, is often necessary for healing of infected wounds	A-III
Antibiotic therapy should only be continued until resolution of signs/symptoms of infection, but not necessarily until the wound is fully healed. The duration of therapy should initially be 1–2 weeks for mild infections and 2–3 weeks for moderate to severe infection	C-III

Animal bites

Preemptive early antibiotics should be administered for 3–5 days in patients with any of the following: immunocompromised; asplenic; advanced liver disease; preexisting or resultant edema of the bitten area; moderate to severe bite-related injuries, especially to the hands or face; or bite injuries that have penetrated the periosteum or joint capsule	Strong, low
Amoxicillin–clavulanic acid or other antibiotics active against both aerobic and anaerobic bacteria should be used for treatment of infected animal bites	Strong, moderate
Serious infections requiring IV antimicrobial therapy can be treated with a β-lactam/β-lactamase inhibitor combination or second-generation cephalosporin with activity against anaerobes (eg, cefoxitin)	B-II
Penicillinase-resistant penicillins, first-generation cephalosporins, macrolides, clindamycin should not be used for treatment of infected wounds because of their poor activity against *Pasteurella multocida*	D-III

Human bites

Antimicrobial therapy should provide coverage against *Eikenella corrodens*, *S. aureus*, and β-lactamase–producing anaerobes	B-III

aCited evidence-based guidelines utilize different systems for grading the strengths of recommendation and quality of the associated evidence. Qualitative (descriptive) recommendations are from reference 16; letter- and roman numeral-based recommendations are from the other cited guidelines. Readers are advised to consult the original documents for full explanations of the grading systems and definitions used in individual guidelines.

Strength of recommendation: A, good evidence for use; B, moderate evidence for use; C, poor evidence for use, optional; D, moderate evidence to support not using; E, good evidence to support not using. *Quality of evidence:* I, evidence from ≥1 properly randomized controlled trials; II, evidence from ≥1 well-designed clinical trials without randomization, case–control analytic studies, multiple time series, or dramatic results from uncontrolled experiments; III, evidence from expert opinion, clinical experience, descriptive studies, or reports of expert committees.

Qualitative (descriptive) recommendations: *Strong, high:* strong recommendation, high-quality evidence from well-performed randomized controlled trials (RCTs) or exceptionally strong evidence from unbiased observational studies; *Strong, moderate:* strong recommendation, moderate quality evidence from RCTs with important limitations or exceptionally strong evidence from unbiased observational studies; *Strong, low:* strong recommendation, low-quality evidence for at least 1 critical outcome from observational studies, RCTs with serious flaws, or indirect evidence; *Weak, moderate:* weak recommendation, moderate quality evidence from RCTs with important limitations or exceptionally strong evidence from unbiased observational studies; *Weak, low:* weak recommendation, low-quality evidence for at least one critical outcome from observational studies, RCTs with serious flaws, or indirect evidence.

TABLE 47–3	Recommended Oral Drugs for Outpatient Treatment of Mild–Moderate Skin and Soft-Tissue Infections	
Infection	**Adults**	**Children**
Folliculitis	None; warm saline compresses usually sufficient	
Furuncles and carbuncles	Trimethoprim–sulfamethoxazole[a,b] Doxycycline[a,b] Minocycline[a,b]	Trimethoprim–sulfamethoxazole[a,b] Clindamycin[a,b]
Erysipelas	Procaine penicillin G Penicillin VK Clindamycin[a] Erythromycin[a]	Penicillin VK Clindamycin[a] Erythromycin[a]
Impetigo	Mupirocin ointment[a] Retapamulin ointment[a] Dicloxacillin Cephalexin Trimethoprim–sulfamethoxazole[a,b] Clindamycin[a,b] Doxycycline[a,b]	Mupirocin ointment[a] Retapamulin ointment[a] Dicloxacillin Cephalexin Trimethoprim–sulfamethoxazole[a,b] Clindamycin[a,b]
Lymphangitis	Initial IV therapy, followed by penicillin VK Clindamycin[a]	Initial IV therapy, followed by penicillin VK Clindamycin[a]
Diabetic foot infections	Dicloxacillin Clindamycin Cephalexin Amoxicillin–clavulanate Levofloxacin ± metronidazole or clindamycin[a,c] Ciprofloxacin ± metronidazole or clindamycin[a,c] Moxifloxacin	
Bite wounds (animal or human)	Amoxicillin–clavulanate Doxycycline[a] Moxifloxacin[a] Trimethoprim–sulfamethoxazole + metronidazole or clindamycin[a] Levofloxacin or ciprofloxacin + metronidazole or clindamycin[a] Cefuroxime axetil + metronidazole or clindamycin Dicloxacillin + penicillin VK	Amoxicillin–clavulanate Trimethoprim–sulfamethoxazole + metronidazole or clindamycin[a] Cefuroxime axetil + metronidazole or clindamycin Dicloxacillin + penicillin VK

[a]May be used in patients with penicillin allergy.
[b]Recommended if CA-MRSA is suspected.
[c]Fluoroquinolone alone may be suitable for mild infections, while addition of drugs with antianaerobic activity may be recommended for more severe infections.

TABLE 47–4 Drug Dosing Table[a]

Drug	Brand Name	Initial Dose	Usual Range	Special Population Dose	Other
Oral agents					
Amoxicillin–clavulanate	Augmentin®	875/125 mg orally two times daily	875/125 mg orally two times daily	Pediatric: 40 mg/kg (of the amoxicillin component) orally in two divided doses	
Cefaclor	Ceclor®	500 mg orally every 8 hours	500 mg orally every 8 hours	Pediatric: 20–40 mg/kg/day (not to exceed 1 g) orally in three divided doses	
Cefadroxil	Duricef®	500 mg orally every 12 hours	250–500 mg orally every 12 hours	Pediatric: 30 mg/kg orally in two divided doses	
Cefuroxime axetil	Ceftin®	500 mg orally every 12 hours	250–500 mg orally every 12 hours	Pediatric: 20–30 mg/kg orally in two divided doses	
Cephalexin	Keflex®	250–500 mg orally every 6 hours	250–500 mg orally every 6 hours	Pediatric: 25–50 mg/kg orally in four divided doses	
Ciprofloxacin	Cipro®	500 mg orally every 12 hours	500–750 mg orally every 12 hours		
Clindamycin	Cleocin®	300–600 mg orally every 6–8 hours	300–600 mg orally every 6–8 hours	Pediatric: 10–30 mg/kg/day orally in three to four divided doses[4]	May be used for oral treatment of MRSA infection
Dicloxacillin	Dynapen®	250–500 mg orally every 6 hours	250–500 mg orally every 6 hours	Pediatric: 25–50 mg/kg orally in four divided doses	
Doxycycline	Vibramycin®	100–200 mg orally every 12 hours	100–200 mg orally every 12 hours		May be used for oral treatment of MRSA infection
Erythromycin	E-Mycin® Erythrocin®	250–500 mg orally every 6 hours	250–500 mg orally every 6 hours	Pediatric: 30–50 mg/kg orally in four divided doses[a]	
Levofloxacin	Levaquin®	500–750 mg orally once daily	500–750 mg orally once daily		

(continued)

TABLE 47–4	Drug Dosing Table[a] (Continued)			
Drug	Brand Name	Initial Dose	Usual Range	Special Population Dose	Other
Linezolid	Zyvox®	600 mg orally every 12 hours	600 mg orally every 12 hours	Pediatric: 20–30 mg/kg/day orally in two to three divided doses	For oral treatment of MRSA infection
Metronidazole	Flagyl®	250–500 mg orally every 8 hours	250–500 mg orally every 8 hours	Pediatric: 30 mg/kg orally in three to four divided doses	
Moxifloxacin	Avelox®	400 mg orally once daily	400 mg orally once daily		
Mupirocin ointment	Bactroban®	Apply to affected areas every 8 hours	Apply to affected areas every 8 hours	Pediatric: apply to affected areas every 8 hours	
Penicillin VK	Veetids® Pen-V®	250–500 mg orally every 6 hours	250–500 mg orally every 6 hours	Pediatric: 25,000–90,000 units/kg orally in four divided doses	
Retapamulin ointment	Altabax®	Apply to affected area every 12 hours	Apply to affected area every 12 hours	Pediatric: apply to affected area every 12 hours	
Tedizolid	Sivextro®	200 mg orally once daily	200 mg orally once daily		For oral treatment of MRSA infection
Trimethoprim–sulfamethoxazole	Bactrim® Septra® Cotrimoxazole®	160/800 mg orally every 12 hours	160/800 mg orally every 12 hours	Pediatric: 4–6 mg/kg (of the trimethoprim component) orally every 12 hours	Up to double the usual dose may be considered for oral treatment of MRSA infection
Parenteral agents					
Ampicillin	Omnipen® Polycillin® Principen®	2 g IV every 6 hours	1–2 g IV every 4–6 hours	Pediatric: 200–300 mg/kg/day IV in four to six divided doses	
Aztreonam	Azactam®	1 g IV every 6 hours	1 g IV every 6 hours	Pediatric: 100–150 mg/kg/day IV in four divided doses	

Cefazolin	Ancef® Kefzol®	1 g IV every 8 hours	1 g IV every 6–8 hours	Pediatric: 75 mg/kg/dayIV in three divided doses
Cefepime	Maxipime®	2 g IV every 12 hours	1–2 g IV every 12 hours	Pediatric: 100 mg/kg/day IV in two divided doses
Cefotaxime	Claforan®	2 g IV every 6 hours	1–2 g IV every 6 hours	150–200 mg/kg/day in three to four divided doses
Cefoxitin	Mefoxin®	1–2 g IV every 6 hours	1–2 g IV every 6 hours	Pediatric: 30–40 mg/kg/day IV in four divided doses
Ceftazidime	Fortaz®	2 g IV every 8 hours	1–2 g IV every 8 hours	Pediatric: 150 mg/kg/day IV in three divided doses
Ceftaroline	Teflaro®	600 mg IV every 12 hours	600 mg IV every 12 hours	For MRSA infection
Ceftriaxone	Rocephin®	1 g IV once daily	1 g IV once daily	
Cefuroxime	Zinacef®	1.5 g IV every 8 hours	0.75–1.5 g IV every 8 hours	Pediatric: 150 mg/kg/day IV in three divided doses
Ciprofloxacin	Cipro®	400 mg IV every 8–12 hours	400 mg IV every 8–12 hours	
Clindamycin	Cleocin®	300–600 mg IV every 6–8 hours	300–600 mg IV every 6–8 hours; 600–900 mg IV every 6–8 hours for necrotizing fasciitis	Pediatric: 30–50 mg/kg/day IV in three to four divided doses
Dalbavancin	Dalvance®	1000 mg IV once on Day 1 of therapy	500 mg IV once on Day 8 of therapy	For MRSA infection
Daptomycin	Cubicin®	4 mg/kg IV once daily	4 mg/kg IV once daily	For MRSA infection
Doripenem	Doribax®	500 mg IV every 8 hours	500 mg IV every 8 hours	
Ertapenem	Invanz®	1 g IV once daily	1 g IV once daily	Pediatric: 30 mg/kg/day IV in one to two divided doses

(continued)

TABLE 47–4	Drug Dosing Table[a] (Continued)			
Drug	Brand Name	Initial Dose	Usual Range	Special Population Dose	Other
Gentamicin	Garamycin®	Traditional: 2 mg/kg loading dose, followed by 1.5 mg/kg IV every 8 hours. Alternative: 5–7 mg/kg IV once daily	Traditional dosing: guided by measured serum concentrations	Pediatric: 5–7 mg/kg/day IV in three divided doses; doses guided by serum concentrations	
Imipenem–cilastatin	Primaxin®	500 mg IV every 6 hours	250–500 mg IV every 6–8 hours	Pediatric: 40–80 mg/kg/day IV in four divided doses	
Levofloxacin	Levaquin®	750 mg IV once daily	500–750 mg IV once daily		
Linezolid	Zyvox®	600 mg IV every 12 hours	600 mg IV every 12 hours	Pediatric: 20–30 mg/kg/day IV in two to three divided doses	For MRSA infection
Meropenem	Merrem®	1 g IV every 8 hours	1 g IV every 8 hours	Pediatric: 60 mg/kg/day IV in three divided doses	
Metronidazole	Flagyl®	500 mg IV every 8 hours	500 mg IV every 8 hours	Pediatric: 30–50 mg/kg/day IV in three divided doses	
Moxifloxacin	Avelox®	400 mg IV once daily	400 mg IV once daily		
Nafcillin	Nafcil®	2 g IV every 6 hours	1–2 g IV every 4–6 hour	Pediatric: 100–200 mg/kg/day IV in four to six equally divided doses	
Oritavancin	Orbactiv®	1200 mg IV once	(no additional doses)		For MRSA infection
Penicillin G	Pfizerpen® Bicillin® Wycillin®	1–2 million units IV every 4–6 hours	1–2 million units IV every 4–6 hours	Pediatric: 100,000–200,000 units/kg/day IV in four divided doses[a]	

Drug	Trade name	Dose		Pediatric	Comments
Piperacillin–tazobactam	Zosyn®	4.5 g IV every 6 hours	3.375–4.5 g IV every 6 hours	Pediatric: 250–350 mg/kg/day IV in three to four divided doses	
Procaine penicillin G	Bicillin C-R®	600,000 units IM every 12 hours	600,000–1.2 million units IM every 12 hours	Pediatric: 25,000–50,000 units/kg (maximum 1.2 million units) IM once daily	
Tedizolid	Sivextro®	200 mg IV once daily	200 mg IV once daily		For MRSA infection
Telavancin	Vibativ®	10 mg/kg IV once daily	10 mg/kg IV once daily		For MRSA infection
Tigecycline	Tigacil®	100 mg IV once, and then 50 mg IV every 12 hours	100 mg IV once, and then 50 mg IV every 12 hours		
Tobramycin	Nebcin®	Traditional: 2 mg/kg loading dose, followed by 1.5 mg/kg IV every 8 hours. Alternative: 5–7 mg/kg IV once daily	Traditional dosing: guided by measured serum concentrations	Pediatric: 5–7 mg/kg/day IV in three divided doses; doses guided by serum concentrations	
Vancomycin	Vancocin®	30–40 mg/kg/day IV in two divided doses	Dosing guided by serum concentrations to achieve trough of 15–20 mg/L	Pediatric: 40–60 mg/kg/day IV in three to four divided doses; doses guided by serum concentrations	For MRSA infection

(IM, intramuscularly; MRSA, methicillin-resistant *S. aureus*.)
[a]Dosing guidelines in patients with normal renal function.

- Cellulitis is most often caused by *S. pyogenes* or *S. aureus* (see Table 47–1).
- *S. aureus* is the most common pathogen isolated from injection drug users; the incidence of MRSA is also rising. Anaerobic bacteria, especially oropharyngeal anaerobes, are also found commonly, particularly in polymicrobic infections.

CLINICAL PRESENTATION

- Cellulitis is characterized by erythema and edema of the skin. The lesion, which may be extensive, is painful and nonelevated and has poorly defined margins. Tender lymphadenopathy associated with lymphatic involvement is common. Malaise, fever, and chills are also commonly present. There is usually a history of an antecedent wound from minor trauma, an ulcer, or surgery.
- A Gram stain of a smear obtained by injection and aspiration of 0.5 mL of saline (using a small-gauge needle) into the advancing edge of the erythematous lesion may help in making the microbiologic diagnosis but often yields negative results. Blood cultures are useful, as bacteremia may be present in 30% of cases.

TREATMENT

- <u>Goal of Treatment</u>: The goal for acute bacterial cellulitis is rapid eradication of the infection and prevention of further complications. Antimicrobial therapy of bacterial cellulitis is directed toward the type of bacteria either documented to be present or suspected. Local care of cellulitis includes elevation and immobilization of the involved area to decrease local swelling. Incision and drainage is the primary therapy for infections such as small abscesses and furuncles, and in otherwise uncomplicated patients with mild infections. Systemic antibiotic therapy is often unnecessary in such cases.
- Antibiotic therapy is recommended along with incision and drainage in patients with more complicated abscesses associated with the following: severe or extensive disease involving multiple sites of infection; rapidly progressive infection in the presence of associated cellulitis; signs and symptoms of systemic illness; complicating factors such as extremes of age, comorbidities, or immunosuppression; abscesses in areas that are difficult to drain, such as hands, face, and genitalia; or lack of response to previous drainage alone.
- Oral agents recommended for moderate purulent cellulitis include trimethoprim-sulfamethoxazole and doxycycline (**Figure 47–1**). Oral linezolid is also recommended in such cases but is significantly more expensive and apparently no more efficacious than other treatment options.
- Patients with severe purulent cellulitis should be hospitalized for empiric treatment with parenteral antibiotics having activity against MRSA. Vancomycin, daptomycin, linezolid, televancin, and ceftaroline are all acceptable treatment options with comparable efficacy in adults (see Figure 47–1).
- Empiric therapy of nonpurulent cellulitis is directed primarily against Group A β-hemolytic streptococci. Recommended empiric therapy of mild nonpurulent cellulitis (i.e., no focus of purulence or systemic signs of infection) consists of an orally administered β-lactam such as penicillin VK, cephalexin, or dicloxacillin.

DIABETIC FOOT INFECTIONS

- Three key factors are involved in the causation of diabetic foot problems: neuropathy, ischemia, and immunologic defects. Any of these disorders can occur in isolation; however, they frequently occur together.
- There are three major types of diabetic foot infections: deep abscesses, cellulitis of the dorsum, and mal perforans ulcers of the sole of the foot. Osteomyelitis may occur in 30% to 40% of infections.
- Mild cases of diabetic foot infections (DFI) are often monomicrobial. However, more severe infections are typically polymicrobic; up to 60% of hospitalized patients have polymicrobial infections. Staphylococci and streptococci are the most common pathogens, although gram-negative bacilli and anaerobes occur in 50% of cases.

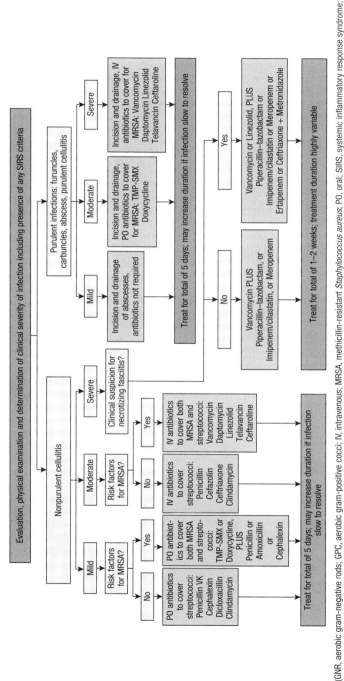

(GNR, aerobic gram-negative rods; GPC, aerobic gram-positive cocci; IV, intravenous; MRSA, methicillin-resistant *Staphylococcus aureus*; PO, oral; SIRS, systemic inflammatory response syndrome; TMP-SMX, trimethoprim–sulfamethoxazole.)

FIGURE 47–1. **Recommended treatment algorithm for initial empiric management of selected purulent and nonpurulent skin and soft tissue infections.**

- Patients with peripheral neuropathy often do not experience pain but seek medical attention for swelling or erythema. Lesions vary in size and clinical features. A foul-smelling odor suggests anaerobic organisms. Temperature may be mildly elevated or normal.

TREATMENT

- Goal of Treatment: (a) Successfully treat infected wounds by using effective nondrug and antibiotic therapy; (b) prevent additional infectious complications; (c) preserve as much normal limb function as possible; (d) avoid unnecessary use of antimicrobials that contribute to increased resistance; and (e) minimize toxicities and cost while increasing patient quality of life.
- Up to 90% of infections can be treated successfully with a comprehensive treatment approach that includes both wound care and antimicrobial therapy.
- Diabetic glycemic control should be maximized to ensure optimal healing.
- The patient should initially be restricted to bed rest, leg elevation, and control of edema, if present.
- Suggested antibiotic regimens for empiric treatment of diabetic foot infections are found in Table 47–5. Treatment algorithms for initial management of mild to moderate DFI and severe DFI are shown in Figs. 47–2 and 47–3.

INFECTED PRESSURE ULCERS

- A pressure sore is also called a "decubitus ulcer" or "bed sore." A classification system for pressure sores is presented in Table 47–6. Many factors are thought to predispose patients to the formation of pressure ulcers: paralysis, paresis, immobilization, malnutrition, anemia, infection, and advanced age. Factors thought to be most critical to their formation are pressure, shearing forces, friction, and moisture; however, there is still debate as to the exact pathophysiology of pressure sore formation. The areas of highest pressure are generated over the bony prominences.
- Most pressure sores are colonized by bacteria; however, bacteria frequently infect healthy tissue. A large variety of aerobic gram-positive and gram-negative bacteria, as well as anaerobes, is frequently isolated.

CLINICAL PRESENTATION

- Most pressure sores are in the pelvic region and lower extremities. The most common sites are the sacral and coccygeal areas, ischial tuberosities, and greater trochanter.
- Clinical infection is recognized by the presence of redness, heat, and pain. Purulent discharge, foul odor, and systemic signs (fever and leukocytosis) may be present.
- Pressure sores vary greatly in their severity, ranging from an abrasion to large lesions that can penetrate into the deep fascia involving both bone and muscle.

PREVENTION AND TREATMENT

- Goal of Treatment: The primary goal for pressure sores is prevention. Once a pressure sore has developed, the goals of therapy are prevention of complications (i.e., infections), preventing sores from growing larger, and preventing the development of sores in other locations. The goal of therapy is to clean and decontaminate the ulcer in order to permit formation of healthy granulation tissue that promotes wound healing or prepares the wound for an operative procedure. The main factors to be considered for successful wound care are (1) relief of pressure; (2) debridement of necrotic tissue; (3) wound cleansing; (4) dressing selection; and (5) prevention, diagnosis, and treatment of infection.
- Prevention is the single most important aspect in the management of pressure sores. Friction and shearing forces can be minimized by proper positioning. Skin care and prevention of soilage are important, with the intent being to keep the surface relatively free from moisture. Relief of pressure (even for 5 minutes once every 2 hours) is probably the single most important factor in preventing pressure sore formation.

TABLE 47–5 Suggested Antibiotic Regimens for Empiric Treatment of Diabetic Foot Infections

Severity of Infection	Probable Pathogens	Drug(s)[a]	Duration of Therapy
Mild	*Staphylococcus aureus* (MSSA) *Streptococcus* spp. *S. aureus* (MRSA) • Patients with history of MRSA infection or colonization in past year • Prevalence of MRSA ≥50% in local geographic area • Recent hospitalization	Amoxicillin–clavulanate Cephalexin Dicloxacillin Clindamycin Levofloxacin Moxifloxacin[b]	1–2 weeks; may increase up to 4 weeks if infection slow to resolve
Moderate to severe (initially oral or IV antibiotics for moderately severe infections, IV antibiotics for severe infections)	MSSA *Streptococcus* spp. Enterobacteriaceae Obligate anaerobes	Ampicillin/Sulbactam Cefoxitin Ceftriaxone Imipenem/cilastatin Ertapenem Levofloxacin Moxifloxacin Tigecycline Levofloxacin or ciprofloxacin + clindamycin	Moderately severe infection: 1–3 weeks; severe infection: 2–4 weeks
	MRSA • Patients with history of MRSA infection or colonization in past year • Prevalence of MRSA ≥30% in local geographic area • Recent hospitalization • Infection severe enough that not empirically covering MRSA poses unacceptable risk of treatment failure	Add to one of the above regimens: • Vancomycin • Linezolid • Daptomycin	

(continued)

TABLE 47-5 Suggested Antibiotic Regimens for Empiric Treatment of Diabetic Foot Infections (*Continued*)

Severity of Infection	Probable Pathogens	Drug(s)[a]	Duration of Therapy
	Pseudomonas aeruginosa • Patient has been soaking feet • Patient has previously failed therapy with nonpseudomonal antibiotic regimen • Severe infection	Piperacillin/tazobactam	
	Mixed infections potentially including all of the above	Cefepime, ceftazidime, or aztreonam + metronidazole or clindamycin + vancomycin[c] *Or* piperacillin–tazobactam or imipenem–cilastatin or meropenem[b] + vancomycin[c]	

(MRSA, methicillin-resistant *S. aureus*; MSSA, methicillin-susceptible *S. aureus*.)
[a]Agents not shown in any particular order of preference.
[b]Not specifically recommended in IDSA guidelines but may be appropriate treatment option.
[c]Linezolid or daptomycin may be used in place of vancomycin.

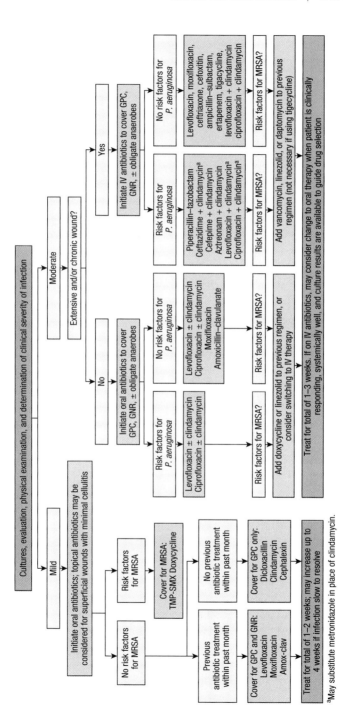

FIGURE 47–2. **Recommended treatment algorithm for initial empiric management of mild to moderate diabetic foot infections.**

(GNR, aerobic gram-negative rods; GPC, aerobic gram-positive cocci; MRSA, methicillin-resistant *Staphylococcus aureus*; TMP-SMX, trimethoprim–sulfamethoxazole.)

[a]May substitute metronidazole in place of clindamycin.

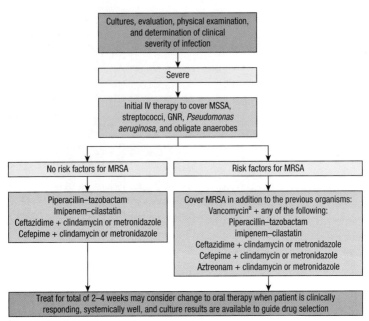

Cultures, evaluation, physical examination, and determination of clinical severity of infection

↓

Severe

↓

Initial IV therapy to cover MSSA, streptococci, GNR, *Pseudomonas aeruginosa*, and obligate anaerobes

No risk factors for MRSA | Risk factors for MRSA

Piperacillin–tazobactam
Imipenem–cilastatin
Ceftazidime + clindamycin or metronidazole
Cefepime + clindamycin or metronidazole

Cover MRSA in addition to the previous organisms:
Vancomycin[a] + any of the following:
Piperacillin–tazobactam
imipenem–cilastatin
Ceftazidime + clindamycin or metronidazole
Cefepime + clindamycin or metronidazole
Aztreonam + clindamycin or metronidazole

Treat for total of 2–4 weeks may consider change to oral therapy when patient is clinically responding, systemically well, and culture results are available to guide drug selection

[a]May substitute linezolid or daptomycin for vancomycin.

(GNR, aerobic gram-negative rods; MRSA, methicillin-resistant *Staphylococcus aureus*; MSSA, methicillin-susceptible *S. aureus*.)

FIGURE 47–3. Recommended treatment algorithm for initial empiric management of severe diabetic foot infections.

- Medical management is generally indicated for lesions that are of moderate size and of relatively shallow depth (stage 1 or 2 lesions) and are not located over a bony prominence.
- Debridement can be accomplished by surgical, mechanical (wet-to-dry dressing changes), or chemical means. Other effective therapies are hydrotherapy, wound irrigation, and dextranomers. Pressure sores should be cleaned with normal saline.
- A short, 2-week trial of topical antibiotic (**silver sulfadiazine** or **triple antibiotic**) is recommended for a clean ulcer that is not healing or is producing a moderate amount of exudate despite appropriate care.

INFECTED BITE WOUNDS

- Patients at risk of acquiring an infection after a bite have had a puncture wound, have not sought medical attention within 8 hours of injury, or are older than 50 years.
- An infected dog or cat bite is usually characterized by erythema, and clear or purulent discharge at the wound site. If *Pasteurella multocida* is present, a rapidly progressing cellulitis is observed within 24 to 48 hours of initial injury.
- Most infections from dog and cat bites are polymicrobial. Pasteurella is the most frequent isolate.
- Wounds should be thoroughly irrigated with a sterile saline solution. Proper irrigation will reduce the bacterial count in the wound.
- The role of antimicrobials for noninfected dog-bite wounds remains controversial. A 3- to 5-day antibiotic prophylaxis regimen is recommended in patients with the following factors associated with increased risk for infection: immunocompromised;

TABLE 47–6	Pressure Sore Classification
Suspected deep-tissue injury	Area of discolored intact skin or blood-filled blister due to damage of underlying soft tissue from pressure and/or shear. Area may be preceded by tissue that is painful, firm, mushy, boggy, warmer or cooler as compared with adjacent tissue
Stage 1	Pressure sore is generally reversible, is limited to the epidermis, and resembles an abrasion. Intact skin with nonblanchable redness of a localized area, usually over a bony prominence. The area may be painful, firm, soft, warmer or cooler as compared with adjacent tissue
Stage 2	A stage 2 sore also may be reversible; partial thickness loss of dermis presenting as a shallow open ulcer with a red pink wound bed. May also present as an intact or open/ruptured serum-filled blister, or as a shiny or dry shallow ulcer
Stage 3[a]	Full thickness tissue loss. Subcutaneous fat may be visible, but bone, tendon, or muscles are not exposed. May include under-mining and tunneling. Depth of the ulcer varies by anatomical location; may range from shallow to extremely deep over areas of significant adiposity
Stage 4[a]	Full thickness tissue loss with exposed bone, tendon, or muscle; can extend into muscle and/or supporting structures (eg, fascia, tendon, or joint capsule) making osteomyelitis possible. Often includes undermining and tunneling; depth of the ulcer varies by anatomical location
Unstageable[a]	Full thickness tissue loss in which the base of the ulcer is covered by slough (yellow, tan, gray, green, or brown) and/or eschar (tan, brown, or black) in the wound bed. True depth, and therefore stage, cannot be determined

[a]Stage 3, stage 4, and unstageable lesions are unlikely to resolve on their own and often require surgical intervention.

asplenic; advanced liver disease; preexisting or resultant edema of the affected area; moderate to severe bite-related injuries, especially to the hands or face; or bite injuries that have penetrated the periosteum or joint capsule.

- Empiric antibiotics for the treatment of established infection of dog and cat bite wounds should be directed at a variety of aerobic and anaerobic flora. **Amoxicillin–clavulanic** acid is commonly recommended for oral outpatient therapy. Alternative oral agents include **moxifloxacin** or **doxycycline** alone, or **trimethoprim–sulfamethoxazole, levofloxacin, ciprofloxacin**, or a second- or third-generation cephalosporin in combination with metronidazole or clindamycin to provide activity against oropharyngeal anaerobes.
- Treatment options for patients requiring IV therapy include β-lactam–β-lactamase inhibitors (**ampicillin–sulbactam** and **piperacillin–tazobactam**), second-generation cephalosporins with antianaerobic activity (**cefoxitin**), and **ertapenem**. Therapy should generally be continued from 7 to 14 days.
- If the immunization history of a patient with anything other than a clean minor wound is not known, tetanus/diphtheria toxoids should be administered. Both tetanus/diphtheria toxoids and tetanus immunoglobulin should be administered to patients who have never been immunized.
- If a patient has been exposed to rabies, the treatment objectives consist of thorough irrigation of the wound, tetanus prophylaxis, antibiotic prophylaxis (if indicated), and immunization. Postexposure prophylaxis immunization consists of both passive antibody administration and vaccine administration.

HUMAN BITES

- Infections caused by these injuries are most often caused by the normal oral flora, which includes both aerobic and anaerobic microorganisms. Human bite wounds are notable for potential involvement of *Eikenella corrodens* in approximately 30% of infections.

- Management of bite wounds consists of aggressive irrigation and topical wound dressing, surgical debridement, and immobilization of the affected area. Primary closure for human bites is not generally recommended. Tetanus toxoid and antitoxin may be indicated.

- All patients with human bite injuries should receive prophylactic antibiotic therapy ("early preemptive therapy") for 3 to 5 days due to high infection risk.

- **Amoxicillin–clavulanic** acid (500 mg every 8 hours) is commonly recommended. Alternatives for penicillin-allergic patients include fluoroquinolones or **trimethoprim–sulfamethoxazole** in combination with **clindamycin** or **metronidazole**.

- Patients with serious injuries or clenched-fist injuries should be started on IV antibiotics. Treatment options for patients requiring IV therapy include β-lactam–β-lactamase inhibitor combinations (**ampicillin–sulbactam, piperacillin–tazobactam**), second-generation cephalosporins with antianaerobic activity (eg, **cefoxitin**), and ertapenem.

See Chapter 110, Skin and Soft-Tissue Infections, authored by Douglas N. Fish for a more detailed discussion of this topic.

48 Surgical Prophylaxis

- Antibiotics administered prior to the contamination of previously sterile tissues or fluids are considered prophylactic. The goal of prophylactic antibiotics is to prevent an infection from developing.
- Presumptive antibiotic therapy is administered when an infection is suspected but not yet proven. Therapeutic antibiotics are required for established infection.
- *Surgical-site infections* (SSIs) are classified as either incisional (eg, cellulitis of the incision site) or involving an organ or space (eg, with meningitis). Incisional SSIs may be superficial (skin or subcutaneous tissue) or deep (fascial and muscle layers). Both types, by definition, occur by postoperative day 30. This period extends to 1 year in the case of deep infection, associated with prosthesis implantation.

RISK FACTORS FOR SURGICAL WOUND INFECTION

- The traditional classification system developed by the National Research Council (NRC) stratifying surgical procedures by infection risk is reproduced in **Table 48–1**. The NRC wound classification for a specific procedure is determined intraoperatively and is the primary determinant of whether antibiotic prophylaxis is warranted.
- The Study on the Efficacy of Nosocomial Infection Control (SENIC) analyzed more than 100,000 surgery cases and identified abdominal operations, operations lasting more than 2 hours, contaminated or dirty procedures, and more than three underlying medical diagnoses as factors associated with an increased incidence of SSI. When the NRC classification described in Table 48–1 was stratified by the number of SENIC risk factors present, the infection rates varied by as much as a factor of 15 within the same operative category.
- The SENIC risk assessment technique has been modified to include the American Society of Anesthesiologists preoperative assessment score (**Table 48–2**). An American Society of Anesthesiologists score greater than or equal to three was associated with increased SSI risk.

BACTERIOLOGY

- Bacteria involved in SSI are acquired either from the patient's normal flora (endogenous) or from contamination during the surgical procedure (exogenous).
- Loss of protective flora via antibiotics can upset the balance and allow pathogenic bacteria to proliferate and increase infectious risk.
- Normal flora can become pathogenic when translocated to a normally sterile tissue site or fluid during surgical procedures.
- The five most common pathogens encountered in surgical wounds are *Staphylococcus aureus*, coagulase-negative staphylococci, Enterococci, *Escherichia coli*, and *Pseudomonas aeruginosa*.
- Impaired host defenses, vascular occlusive states, traumatized tissues, and the presence of a foreign body greatly decrease the number of bacteria required to cause an SSI.

ANTIBIOTIC ISSUES

SCHEDULING ANTIBIOTIC ADMINISTRATION

- The following principles must be considered when providing antimicrobial surgical prophylaxis:
  - ✓ Antimicrobials should be delivered to the surgical site prior to the initial incision. They should be administered with anesthesia, just prior to initial incision. Antibiotics should not be prescribed to be given "on-call to the OR [operating room]."

TABLE 48–1	National Research Council Wound Classification, Risk of Surgical Site Infection, and Indication for Antibiotics			
	SSI Rate (%)			
Classification	**Preoperative Antibiotics**	**No Preoperative Antibiotics**	**Criteria**	**Antibiotics**
Clean	5.1	0.8	No acute inflammation or transection of GI, oropharyngeal, genitourinary, biliary, or respiratory tracts; elective case, no technique break	Not indicated unless high-risk procedure[a]
Clean–contaminated	10.1	1.3	Controlled opening of aforementioned tracts with minimal spillage/minor technique break; clean procedures performed emergently or with major technique breaks	Prophylactic antibiotics indicated
Contaminated	21.9	10.2	Acute, nonpurulent inflammation present; major spillage/technique break during clean–contaminated procedure	Prophylactic antibiotics indicated
Dirty	N/A	N/A	Obvious preexisting infection present (abscess, pus, or necrotic tissue present)	Therapeutic antibiotics required

(N/A, not applicable; SSI, surgical site infection.)
[a]High-risk procedures include implantation of prosthetic materials and other procedures where surgical site infection is associated with high morbidity (see the text).

    ✓ Bactericidal antibiotic tissue concentrations should be maintained throughout the surgical procedure.
- Strategies to ensure appropriate antimicrobial prophylaxis use are described in Table 48–3.

ANTIMICROBIAL SELECTION

- The choice of the prophylactic antimicrobial depends on the type of surgical procedure, most likely pathogenic organisms, safety and efficacy of the antimicrobial, and current literature evidence supporting its use and cost.
- Typically, gram-positive coverage is included in the choice of surgical prophylaxis because organisms such as *S. aureus* and *S. epidermidis* are common skin flora.

TABLE 48–2	Surgical Site Infection Incidence (%) Stratified by NRC Wound Classification and SENIC Risk Factors[a]			
Number of SENIC Risk Factors	**Clean**	**Clean–Contaminated**	**Contaminated**	**Dirty**
0	1.1	0.6	N/A	N/A
1	3.9	2.8	4.5	6.7
2	8.4	8.4	8.3	10.9
3	15.8	17.7	11.0	18.8
4	N/A	N/A	23.9	27.4

(N/A, not applicable; NRC, National Research Council; SENIC, Study on the Efficacy of Nosocomial Infection Control.)

[a]Study on the Efficacy of Nosocomial Infection Control (SENIC) risk factors include abdominal operation, operations lasting >2 hours, contaminated or dirty procedures by National Research Council (NRC) classification, and more than three underlying medical diagnoses.

Used with permission from Wilson AP, Hodgson B, Liu M, et al. Reduction in wound infection rates by wound surveillance with postdischarge follow-up and feedback. Br J Surg 2006;93:630-638. Copyright © 2006 Wiley & Sons.

- Parenteral antibiotic administration is favored because of its reliability in achieving suitable tissue concentrations.
- First-generation cephalosporins (particularly cefazolin) are the preferred choice, particularly for clean surgical procedures. Antianaerobic cephalosporins (eg, cefoxitin or cefotetan) are appropriate choices when broad-spectrum anaerobic and gram-negative coverage is desired.
- Vancomycin may be considered for prophylactic therapy in surgical procedures involving implantation of a prosthetic device in which the rate of methicillin-resistant *S. aureus* (MRSA) is high. If the risk of MRSA is low and a β-lactam hypersensitivity exists, clindamycin can be used instead of cefazolin in order to limit vancomycin use.

TABLE 48–3	Strategies for Implementing an Institutional Program to Ensure Appropriate Use of Antimicrobial Prophylaxis in Surgery

1. Educate

Develop an educational program that enforces the importance and rationale of timely antimicrobial prophylaxis

Make this educational program available to all healthcare practitioners involved in the patient's care

2. Standardize the ordering process

Establish a protocol (eg, a preprinted order sheet) that standardizes antibiotic choice according to current published evidence, formulary availability, institutional resistance patterns, and cost

3. Standardize the delivery and administration process

Use system that ensures antibiotics are prepared and delivered to the holding area in a timely fashion

Standardize the administration time to <1 hour preoperatively

Designate responsibility and accountability for antibiotic administration

Provide visible reminders to prescribe/administer prophylactic antibiotics (eg, checklists)

Develop a system to remind surgeons/nurses to readminister antibiotics intraoperatively during long procedures

4. Provide feedback

Follow up with regular reports of compliance and infection rates

RECOMMENDATIONS FOR SPECIFIC TYPES OF SURGERIES

- Specific recommendations are summarized in **Table 48–4**.

GASTRODUODENAL SURGERY

- The risk of infection rises with conditions that increase gastric pH and subsequent bacterial overgrowth, such as obstruction, hemorrhage, malignancy, and acid-suppression therapy (clean-contaminated).
- A single dose of intravenous (IV) **cefazolin** will provide adequate prophylaxis for most cases. Oral **ciprofloxacin** may be used for patients with β-lactam hypersensitivity.
- Postoperative therapeutic antibiotics may be indicated if perforation is detected during surgery, depending on whether an established infection is present.

BILIARY TRACT SURGERY

- Antibiotic prophylaxis has been proven beneficial for surgery involving the biliary tract.
- Most frequently encountered organisms include *E. coli, Klebsiella,* and Enterococci. Single-dose prophylaxis with **cefazolin** is currently recommended. **Ciprofloxacin** and **levofloxacin** are alternatives for patients with β-lactam hypersensitivity.
- For low-risk patients undergoing elective laparoscopic cholecystectomy, antibiotic prophylaxis is of no benefit and is not recommended.
- Some surgeons use presumptive antibiotics for cases of acute cholecystitis or cholangitis and defer surgery until the patient is afebrile, in an attempt to decrease infection rates further, but this practice is controversial.
- Detection of an active infection during surgery (gangrenous gallbladder or suppurative cholangitis) is an indication for therapeutic postoperative antibiotics.

COLORECTAL SURGERY

- Anaerobes and gram-negative aerobes predominate in SSIs (see Table 48–4), although gram-positive aerobes are also important. Therefore, the risk of an SSI in the absence of an adequate prophylactic regimen is substantial.
- Reducing bacteria load with a thorough bowel preparation regimen (4 L of polyethylene glycol solution or 90 mL of sodium phosphate solution administered orally the day before surgery) is controversial, even though it is used by most surgeons.
- The combination of 1 g of **neomycin** and 1 g of **erythromycin base** given orally 19, 18, and 9 hours preoperatively is the most commonly used oral regimen in the United States.
- Whether perioperative parenteral antibiotics, in addition to the standard preoperative oral antibiotic regimen, will lower SSI rates further is controversial. Patients who cannot take oral medications should receive parenteral antibiotics.
- Postoperative antibiotics are unnecessary in the absence of any untoward events or findings during surgery.

APPENDECTOMY

- A cephalosporin with antianaerobic activity such as **cefoxitin** or **cefotetan** is currently recommended as a first-line agent. Cefotetan may be superior for longer operations because of its longer duration of action.
- Single-dose therapy with cefotetan is adequate. Intraoperative dosing of cefoxitin may be required if the procedure extends beyond 3 hours.

UROLOGIC PROCEDURES

- As long as the urine is sterile preoperatively, the risk of SSI after urologic procedures is low, and the benefit of prophylactic antibiotics in this setting is controversial. *E. coli* is the most frequently encountered organism.
- Antibiotic prophylaxis is warranted for all patients undergoing transurethral resection of the prostate or bladder tumors, shock wave lithotripsy, percutaneous renal surgery, or ureteroscopy.

TABLE 48–4 Most Likely Pathogens and Specific Recommendations for Surgical Prophylaxis

Type of Operation	Likely Pathogens	Recommended Prophylaxis Regimen[a]	Comments	Grade of Recommendation[b]
GI surgery				
Gastroduodenal	Enteric gram-negative bacilli, gram-positive cocci, oral anaerobes	Cefazolin 1 g × 1	High-risk patients only (obstruction, hemorrhage, malignancy, acid suppression therapy, morbid obesity)	IA
Cholecystectomy	Enteric gram-negative bacilli, anaerobes	Cefazolin 1 g × 1 for high-risk patients Laparoscopic: none	High-risk patients only (open biliary tract procedures, acute cholecystitis, common duct stones, previous biliary surgery, jaundice, age >60 years, obesity, diabetes mellitus)	IA
Transjugular intrahepatic portosystemic shunt (TIPS)	Enteric gram-negative bacilli, anaerobes	Ceftriaxone 1 g × 1	Longer-acting cephalosporins preferred	IA
Appendectomy	Enteric gram-negative bacilli, anaerobes	Cefoxitin or cefotetan 1 g × 1 or cefazolin 1 g × 1 plus metronidazole 1 g × 1	Second intraoperative dose of cefoxitin may be required if procedure lasts longer than 3 hours	IA
Colorectal	Enteric gram-negative bacilli, anaerobes	Orally: neomycin 1 g + erythromycin base 1 g at 1, 2, and 11 PM 1 day preoperatively plus mechanical bowel preparation IV: cefoxitin or cefotetan 1 g × 1	Role of mechanical bowel preparation is controversial. It is widely used despite evidence suggesting it may have no effect on SSI or other clinical outcomes	IA
GI endoscopy	Variable, depending on procedure, but typically enteric gram-negative bacilli, gram-positive cocci, oral anaerobes	Orally: amoxicillin 2 g × 1 IV: ampicillin 2 g × 1 or cefazolin 1 g × 1	Recommended only for high-risk patients undergoing high-risk procedures (see the text)	IA

(continued)

TABLE 48–4 Most Likely Pathogens and Specific Recommendations for Surgical Prophylaxis (*Continued*)

Type of Operation	Likely Pathogens	Recommended Prophylaxis Regimen[a]	Comments	Grade of Recommendation[b]
Urologic surgery				
Prostate resection, shock-wave lithotripsy, ureteroscopy	*Escherichia coli*	Ciprofloxacin 500 mg orally or Trimethoprim–sulfamethoxazole 1 DS tablet	All patients with positive preoperative urine cultures should receive a course of antibiotic treatment	IA–IB
Removal of external urinary catheters, cystography, urodynamic studies, simple cystourethroscopy	*E. coli*	Ciprofloxacin 500 mg orally or Trimethoprim–sulfamethoxazole 1 DS tablet	Should be considered only in patients with risk factors (see the text)	IB
Gynecological surgery				
Cesarean section	Enteric gram-negative bacilli, anaerobes, group B streptococci, enterococci	Cefazolin 2 g × 1	Most guidelines recommend administration before incision. Administration after cord clamping may be as effective based on conflicting studies.	IA
Hysterectomy	Enteric gram-negative bacilli, anaerobes, group B streptococci, enterococci	Vaginal: cefazolin 1 g × 1 Abdominal: cefotetan 1 g × 1 or cefazolin 1 g × 1	Metronidazole 1 g IV × 1 is recommended alternative for penicillin allergy	IA
Head and neck surgery				
Maxillofacial surgery	*Staphylococcus aureus*, streptococci oral anaerobes	Cefazolin 2 g or clindamycin 600 mg	Repeat intraoperative dose for operations longer than 4 hours	IA
Head and neck cancer resection	*S. aureus*, streptococci oral anaerobes	Clindamycin 600 mg at induction and every 8 hours × 2 more doses	Add gentamicin for clean-contaminated procedures	IA

Surgery	Organisms	Recommendation	
Cardiothoracic surgery			
Cardiac surgery	S. aureus, S. epidermidis, Corynebacterium	Cefazolin 1 g every 8 hours × 48 hours Intranasal mupirocin twice daily for 5 days preoperatively for patients colonized with S. aureus	Patients >80 kg (>176 lb) should receive 2 g of cefazolin instead; in areas with high prevalence of S. aureus resistance, vancomycin should be considered	IA
Thoracic surgery	S. aureus, S. epidermidis, Corynebacterium, enteric gram-negative bacilli	Cefuroxime 750 mg IV every 8 hours × 48 hours	First-generation cephalosporins are deemed inadequate, and shorter durations of prophylaxis have not been adequately studied	IA
Vascular surgery			
Abdominal aorta and lower extremity vascular surgery	S. aureus, S. epidermidis, enteric gram-negative bacilli	Cefazolin 1 g at induction and every 8 hours × 2 more doses	Although complications from infections may be infrequent, graft infections are associated with significant morbidity	IB
Orthopedic surgery			
Joint replacement	S. aureus, S. epidermidis	Cefazolin 1 g × 1 preoperatively, then every 8 hours × 2 more doses Intranasal mupirocin twice daily for 5 days preoperatively for patients colonized with S. aureus	Vancomycin reserved for penicillin-allergic patients or where institutional prevalence of methicillin-resistant S. aureus warrants use	IA
Hip fracture repair	S. aureus, S. epidermidis	Cefazolin 1 g × 1 preoperatively, then every 8 hours for 48 hours	Compound fractures are treated as if infection is presumed	IA
Open/compound fractures	S. aureus, S. epidermidis, gram-negative bacilli, polymicrobial	Cefazolin 1 g × 1 preoperatively, then every 8 hours for a course of presumed infection	Gram-negative coverage (ie, gentamicin) often indicated for severe open fractures	IA

(continued)

TABLE 48–4 Most Likely Pathogens and Specific Recommendations for Surgical Prophylaxis (Continued)

Type of Operation	Likely Pathogens	Recommended Prophylaxis Regimen[a]	Comments	Grade of Recommendation[b]
Neurosurgery				
CSF shunt procedures	S. aureus, S. epidermidis	Cefazolin 1 g every 8 hours × 3 doses or ceftriaxone 2 g × 1	No agents have been shown to be better than cefazolin in randomized comparative trials	IA
Spinal surgery	S. aureus, S. epidermidis	Cefazolin 1 g × 1	Limited number of clinical trials comparing different treatment regimens	IB
CSF shunt procedures	S. aureus, S. epidermidis	Cefazolin 1 g every 8 hours × 3 doses or ceftriaxone 2 g × 1	No agents have been shown to be better than cefazolin in randomized comparative trials	IA
Craniotomy	S. aureus, S. epidermidis	Cefazolin 1 g × 1 or cefotaxime 1 g × 1	Vancomycin 1 g IV × 1 can be substituted for patients with penicillin allergy	IA

(CSF, cerebrospinal fluid; DS, double strength.)

[a]One-time doses are optimally infused at induction of anesthesia except as noted. Repeat doses may be required for long procedures. See the text for references.

[b]Strength of recommendations:

Category IA: Strongly recommended and supported by well-designed experimental, clinical, or epidemiologic studies.

Category IB: Strongly recommended and supported by some experimental, clinical, or epidemiologic studies and strong theoretical rationale.

Category II: Suggested and supported by suggestive clinical or epidemiologic studies or theoretical rationale.

- Specific recommendations are listed in Table 48–4.
- Urologic procedures requiring an abdominal approach such as a nephrectomy or cystectomy require prophylaxis appropriate for a clean-contaminated abdominal procedure.

CESAREAN SECTION

- Antibiotics are efficacious to prevent SSIs for women undergoing cesarean section regardless of underlying risk factors.
- **Cefazolin**, 2 g IV, remains the drug of choice. Providing a broader spectrum by using cefoxitin against anaerobes or piperacillin for better coverage against *Pseudomonas* or enterococci, for example, does not lower postoperative infection rates any further in comparative studies.
- The timing of antibiotic administration is controversial, as some advocate administration just after the umbilical cord is clamped, avoiding exposure of the infant to the drug, whereas others advocate administration before the initial incision.

HYSTERECTOMY

- Vaginal hysterectomies are associated with a high rate of postoperative infection when performed without the benefit of prophylactic antibiotics.
- A single preoperative dose of **cefazolin** or **cefoxitin** is recommended for vaginal hysterectomy. For patients with β-lactam hypersensitivity, a single preoperative dose of **metronidazole** or **doxycycline** is effective.
- Abdominal hysterectomy SSI rates are correspondingly lower than vaginal hysterectomy rates. However, prophylactic antibiotics are still recommended regardless of underlying risk factors.
- Both cefazolin and antianaerobic cephalosporins (eg, **cefoxitin** and **cefotetan**) have been studied extensively for abdominal hysterectomy. First-, second-, or third-generation cephalosporins can be used for prophylaxis.

HEAD AND NECK SURGERY

- Use of prophylactic antibiotics during head and neck surgery depends on the procedure type. Clean procedures, such as parotidectomy or a simple tooth extraction, are associated with low rates of SSI. Head and neck procedures involving an incision through a mucosal layer carry a high risk of SSI.
- Specific recommendations for prophylaxis are listed in Table 48–4.
- Although typical doses of **cefazolin** are ineffective for anaerobic infections, the recommended 2 g dose produces concentrations high enough to be inhibitory to these organisms. A 24-hour duration has been used in most studies, but single-dose therapy may also be effective.

CARDIAC SURGERY

- Although most cardiac surgeries are technically clean procedures, prophylactic antibiotics have been shown to lower rates of SSI.
- The usual pathogens are skin flora (see Table 48–4) and, rarely, gram-negative enteric organisms.
- Risk factors for developing an SSI after cardiac surgery include obesity, renal insufficiency, connective tissue disease, reexploration for bleeding, and poorly timed administration of antibiotics.
- **Cefazolin** has been extensively studied and is currently considered the drug of choice. Patients weighing more than 80 kg should receive 2 g cefazolin rather than 1 g. Doses should be administered no earlier than 60 minutes before the first incision and no later than the beginning of induction of anesthesia.
- Extending antibiotic administration beyond 48 hours does not lower SSI rates.
- **Vancomycin** use may be justified in hospitals with a high incidence of SSI with MRSA or when sternal wounds are to be explored for possible mediastinitis.

489

NONCARDIAC VASCULAR SURGERY

• Prophylactic antibiotics are beneficial, especially in procedures involving the abdominal aorta and the lower extremities.
• Twenty-four hours of prophylaxis with IV **cefazolin** is adequate. For patients with β-lactam allergy, 24 hours of oral **ciprofloxacin** is effective.

ORTHOPEDIC SURGERY

• Prophylactic antibiotics are beneficial in cases involving implantation of prosthetic material (pins, plates, and artificial joints).
• The most likely pathogens mirror those of other clean procedures and include staphylococci and, infrequently, gram-negative aerobes.
• **Cefazolin** is the best-studied antibiotic and is thus the drug of choice. For hip fracture repairs and joint replacements, it should be administered for 24 hours. **Vancomycin** is not recommended unless a patient has a history of β-lactam hypersensitivity or the propensity for MRSA infection at the institution necessitates its use.

NEUROSURGERY

• The use of prophylactic antibiotics in neurosurgery is controversial.
• Single doses of **cefazolin** or, where required, **vancomycin** appears to lower SSI risk after craniotomy.

See Chapter 123, Antimicrobial Prophylaxis in Surgery, authored by Salmaan Kanji, for a more detailed discussion of this topic.

- *Tuberculosis* (TB) is a communicable infectious disease caused by *Mycobacterium tuberculosis*. It can produce silent, latent infection, as well as progressive, active disease. Globally, 2 billion people are infected and roughly 1.5 million people die from TB each year.
- *M. tuberculosis* is transmitted from person to person by coughing or other activities that cause the organism to be aerosolized. Close contacts of TB patients are most likely to become infected.
- Human immunodeficiency virus (HIV) is the most important risk factor for progressing to active TB, especially among people 25 to 44 years of age. An HIV-infected individual with TB infection is over 100-fold more likely to develop active disease than an HIV-seronegative patient.
- Approximately 90% of patients who experience primary disease have no further clinical manifestations other than a positive skin test either alone or in combination with radiographic evidence of stable granulomas. Tissue necrosis and calcification of the originally infected site and regional lymph nodes may occur, resulting in the formation of a radiodense area referred to as a *Ghon complex.*
- All clinical specimens suspected of containing mycobacteria should be cultured.
- Approximately 5% of patients (usually children, the elderly, or the immunocompromised) experience progressive primary disease at the site of the primary infection (usually the lower lobes) and frequently by dissemination, leading to meningitis and often to involvement of the upper lobes of the lung as well.
- Approximately 10% of patients develop reactivation disease, which arises subsequent to the hematogenous spread of the organism. In the United States, most cases of TB are believed to result from reactivation.
- Occasionally, a massive inoculum of organisms may be introduced into the bloodstream, causing widely disseminated disease and granuloma formation known as *miliary TB.*

CLINICAL PRESENTATION AND DIAGNOSIS

- The classic presentation of pulmonary TB is weight loss, fatigue, a productive cough, fever, and night sweats (Table 49–1). The onset of TB may be gradual. Physical examination is nonspecific but suggestive of progressive pulmonary disease.
- Clinical features associated with extrapulmonary TB vary depending on the organ system(s) involved but typically consist of slowly progressive decline of organ function with low-grade fever and other constitutional symptoms.
- Patients with HIV may have atypical presentation. HIV-positive patients are less likely to have positive skin tests, cavitary lesions, or fever. They have a higher incidence of extrapulmonary TB and are more likely to present with progressive primary disease.
- TB in the elderly is easily confused with other respiratory diseases. It is far less likely to present with positive skin tests, fevers, night sweats, sputum production, or hemoptysis. TB in children may present as typical bacterial pneumonia and is called **progressive primary TB**.
- The most widely used screening method for tuberculous infection is the tuberculin skin test, which uses purified protein derivative (PPD). Populations most likely to benefit from skin testing are listed in Table 49–2.
- The Mantoux method of PPD administration consists of the intracutaneous injection of PPD containing five tuberculin units. The test is read 48 to 72 hours after injection by measuring the diameter of the zone of induration.
- Some patients may exhibit a positive test 1 week after an initial negative test; this is referred to as a *booster effect.*

TABLE 49–1	Clinical Presentation Tuberculosis

Signs and Symptoms
- Patients typically present with cough weight loss, fatigue, fever, and night sweats.
- Frank hemoptysis usually occurs late in the course of disease but may present earlier.

Physical Examination
- Dullness to chest percussion, rales, and increased vocal fremitus are observed frequently on auscultation but a normal lung examination is very common compared to the degree of radiological lung involvement.
- Patient is usually thin with evidence or recent weight loss.

Laboratory Tests
- Moderate elevations in the white blood cell (WBC) count with a lymphocyte predominance.
- High platelet count (thrombocytosis) and mild to moderate anemia are common.

Diagnostic Considerations
- Positive-sputum smear
- Fiber-optic bronchoscopy (if sputum tests are inconclusive and suspicion is high)

Chest Radiograph
- Patchy or nodular infiltrates in the apical areas of the upper lobes or the superior segment of the lower lobes.
- Cavitation that may show air–fluid levels as the infection progresses.

TABLE 49–2	Criteria for Tuberculin Positivity by Risk Group	
Reaction 5 mm of Induration	**Reaction ≥10 mm of Induration**	**Reaction ≥15 mm of Induration**
HIV-positive persons	Recent immigrants (ie, within the last 5 years) from high-prevalence countries	Persons with no risk factors for TB
Recent contacts of TB case patients	Injection-drug users	
Fibrotic changes on chest radiograph consistent with prior TB	Residents and employees[a] of the following high-risk congregate settings: prisons and jails, nursing homes and other long-term care facilities for the elderly, hospitals and other healthcare facilities, residential facilities for patients with AIDS, homeless shelters	
Patients with organ transplants and other immunosuppressed patients (receiving the equivalent of ≥15 mg/day of prednisone for 1 month or more)[b]	Mycobacteriology laboratory personnel Persons with the following clinical conditions that place them at high risk: silicosis, diabetes mellitus, chronic renal failure, some hematologic disorders (eg, leukemias and lymphomas), other specific malignancies (eg, carcinoma of the head or neck and lung), weight loss of ≥10% of ideal body weight, gastrectomy, jejunoileal bypass Children younger than 4 years or infants, children, and adolescents exposed to adults at high risk	

(AIDS, acquired immunodeficiency syndrome; HIV, human immunodeficiency virus; TB, tuberculosis.)
[a]For persons who are otherwise at low risk and who are tested at the start of employment, a reaction of ≥15 mm induration is considered positive.
[b]Risk of TB for patients treated with corticosteroids increases with higher dose and longer duration.
Adapted from Screening for tuberculosis and tuberculosis infection in high-risk populations: Recommendations of the Advisory Council for the Elimination of Tuberculosis. MMWR Recomm Rep 1995;44(RR-11):19-34.

- Confirmatory diagnosis of a clinical suspicion of TB must be made via chest radiograph and microbiologic examination of sputum or other infected material to rule out active disease.
- When active TB is suspected, attempts should be made to isolate *M. tuberculosis* from the infected site. Daily sputum collection over three consecutive days is recommended.
- Tests to measure release of interferon-γ in the patient's blood in response to TB antigens may provide quick and specific results for identifying *M. tuberculosis*.

TREATMENT

- <u>Goals of Treatment</u>: (1) Rapid identification of a new TB case. (2) Initiation of specific anti-TB treatment. (3) Eradicating *M. tuberculosis* infection. (4) Achievement of a noninfectious state in the patient, thus ending isolation. (5) Preventing the development of resistance. (6) Adherence to the treatment regimen by the patient. (7) Cure of the patient as quickly as possible (generally at least 6 months of treatment).
- Drug treatment is the cornerstone of TB management. A minimum of two drugs, and generally three or four drugs, must be used simultaneously. Directly observed therapy (DOT) by a healthcare worker is a cost effective way to ensure completion of treatment and is considered the standard of care.
- Drug treatment is continued for at least 6 months, and 18–24 months for cases of multidrug-resistant TB (MDR-TB).
- Debilitated patients may require therapy for other medical conditions, including substance abuse and HIV infection, and some may need nutritional support.
- Surgery may be needed to remove destroyed lung tissue, space-occupying lesions, and some extrapulmonary lesions.

PHARMACOLOGIC TREATMENT

Latent Infection

- As described in **Table 49–3**, chemoprophylaxis should be initiated in patients to reduce the risk of progression to active disease.
- **Isoniazid**, 300 mg (5–10 mg/kg of body weight) daily in adults, is the preferred treatment for latent TB in the United States, generally given for 9 months.
- **Rifampin**, 600 mg daily for 4 months, can be used when isoniazid resistance is suspected or when the patient cannot tolerate isoniazid. Rifabutin, 300 mg daily, may be substituted for rifampin for patients at high risk of drug interactions.
- The CDC recommends the 12-week isoniazid/**rifapentine** regimen as an equal alternative to 9 months of daily isoniazid for treating latent tuberculosis infection (LTBI) in otherwise healthy patients aged 12 years or older who have a predictive factor for greater likelihood of TB developing, which included recent exposure to contagious TB, conversion from negative to positive on an indirect test for infection (ie, interferon-gamma release assays [IGRA] or tuberculin skin test), and radiographic findings of healed pulmonary TB.
- Pregnant women, alcoholics, and patients with poor diets who are treated with isoniazid should receive pyridoxine, 10 to 50 mg daily, to reduce the incidence of central nervous system (CNS) effects or peripheral neuropathies.

Treating Active Disease

- See **Figure 49–1** for treatment algorithm for TB.
- **Table 49–4** lists options for treatment of culture-positive pulmonary TB caused by drug-susceptible organisms. Doses of antituberculosis drugs are given in **Table 49–5**. Other sources should be consulted for treatment recommendations when TB is concurrent with HIV infection. The standard TB treatment regimen is isoniazid, rifampin, pyrazinamide, and ethambutol for 2 months, followed by isoniazid and rifampin for 4 months. Ethambutol can be stopped if susceptibility to isoniazid, rifampin, and pyrazinamide is shown.

TABLE 49-3	Recommended Drug Regimens for Treatment of LTBI in Adults		Rating^a (Evidence)^b	
Drug	**Interval and Duration**	**Comments**	**HIV−**	**HIV+**
Isoniazid	Daily for 9 months^b,c	In HIV-infected patients, isoniazid may be administered concurrently with NRTIs, protease inhibitors, or NNRTIs	A (II)	A (II)
	Twice weekly for 9 months^b,c	DOT must be used with twice-weekly dosing	B (II)	B (II)
Isoniazid	Daily for 6 months^c	Not indicated for HIV-infected persons, those with fibrotic lesions on chest radiographs, or children	B (I)	C (I)
	Twice weekly for 6 months^c	DOT must be used with twice-weekly dosing	B (II)	C (I)
Rifampin	Daily for 4 months	For persons who are contacts of patients with isoniazid-resistant, rifampin-susceptible TB who cannot tolerate pyrazinamide	B (II)	B (III)
Isoniazid and rifapentine	Once weekly for 3 months	DOT must be used with once-weekly dosing. Not recommended for the following: children <2 years old, HIV/AIDS patients taking anti-retroviral treatment, isoniazid- or rifampin-resistant strains, pregnant women or women expecting to become pregnant within the 12-week regimen	B (II)	B (II)

(AIDS, acquired immunodeficiency syndrome; DOT, directly observed therapy; HIV, human immunodeficiency virus; LTBI, latent tuberculosis infection; NNRTIs, non-nucleoside reverse transcriptase inhibitors; NRTIs, nucleoside reverse transcriptase inhibitors.)
^aStrength of recommendation: A, preferred; B, acceptable alternative; C, offer when A and B cannot be given.
^bQuality of evidence: I, randomized clinical trial data; II, data from clinical trials that are not randomized or were conducted in other populations; III, expert opinion.
^cRecommended regimen for children younger than 18 years of age.
Adapted from Targeted tuberculin testing and treatment of latent tuberculosis infection. MMWR Recomm Rep 2000;49(RR06):31. A Joint Statement of the American Thoracic Society (ATS) and the Centers for Disease Control and Prevention (CDC).

- Appropriate samples should be sent for culture and susceptibility testing prior to initiating therapy for all patients with active TB. The data should guide the initial drug selection for the new patient. If susceptibility data are not available, the drug resistance pattern in the area where the patient likely acquired TB should be used.
- If the patient is being evaluated for the retreatment of TB, it is imperative to know what drugs were used previously and for how long.
- The standard TB treatment regimen is isoniazid, rifampin, pyrazinamide, and ethambutol for 2 months, followed by isoniazid and rifampin for 4 months, a total of 6 months of treatment.
- Patients who are slow to respond, those who remain culture positive at 2 months of treatment, those with cavitary lesions on chest radiograph, and HIV-positive patients should be treated for 9 months and for at least 6 months from the time they convert to smear and culture negativity.

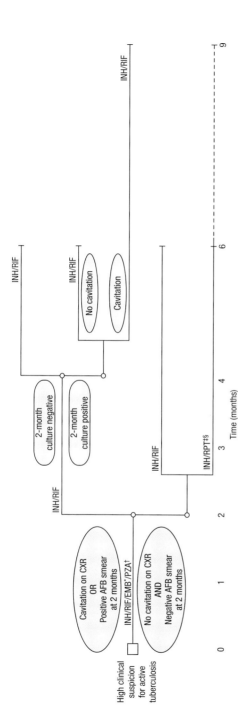

FIGURE 49–1. Treatment algorithm for tuberculosis (TB).

Note: Patients in whom TB is proved or strongly suspected should have treatment initiated with isoniazid, rifampin, pyrazinamide, and ethambutol for the initial 2 months. A repeat smear and culture should be performed when 2 months of treatment has been completed. If cavities were seen on the initial chest radiograph or the acid-fast smear is positive at completion of 2 months of treatment, the continuation phase of treatment should consist of isoniazid and rifampin daily or twice weekly for 4 months to complete a total of 6 months of treatment. If cavitation was present on the initial chest radiograph and the culture at the time of completion of 2 months of therapy is positive, the continuation phase should be lengthened to 7 months (total of 9 months of treatment). If the patient has HIV infection and the CD+ cell count is <100/μL (<100 × 10⁶/L), the continuation phase should consist of daily or three-times-weekly isoniazid and rifampin. In HIV-uninfected patients having no cavitation on chest radiograph and negative acid-fast smears at completion of 2 months of treatment, the continuation phase may consist of either once-weekly isoniazid and rifapentine, or daily or twice-weekly isoniazid and rifampin, to complete a total of 6 months (bottom). Patients receiving isoniazid and rifapentine, and whose 2-month cultures are positive, should have treatment extended by an additional 3 months (total of 9 months). (CXR, chest radiograph; EMB, ethambutol; INH, isoniazid; PZA, pyrazinamide; RIF, rifampin; RPT, rifapentine.)

aEMB may be discontinued when results of drug susceptibility testing indicate no drug resistance. bPZA may be discontinued after it has been taken for 2 months (56 doses). cRPT should not be used in HIV-infected patients with tuberculosis or in patients with extrapulmonary tuberculosis. dTherapy should be extended to 9 months if the 2-month culture is positive.

(Reproduced from Treatment of tuberculosis. MMWR Recomm Rep 2003;52(RR-11):1–77. A Joint Statement of the American Thoracic Society (ATS), the Centers for Disease Control and Prevention (CDC) and Infectious Diseases Society of America.)

TABLE 49-4 Drug Regimens for Culture-Positive Pulmonary TB Caused by Drug-Susceptible Organisms

Regimen	Drugs	Initial Phase — Interval and Dose[c] (Minimal Duration)	Continuation Phase — Drugs	Continuation Phase — Interval and Doses[c,d] (Minimal Duration)	Range of Total Doses (Minimal Duration)	Rating[a] (Evidence)[b] HIV−	Rating[a] (Evidence)[b] HIV+
1	Isoniazid, rifampin, pyrazinamide, ethambutol	Seven days per week for 56 doses (8 weeks) or 5 days/wk for 40 doses (8 weeks)[e]	Isoniazid/rifampin	Seven days per week for 126 doses (18 weeks) or 5 days/wk for 90 doses (18 weeks)[e]	182–130 (26 weeks)	A (I)	A (II)
			Isoniazid/rifampin	Twice weekly for 36 doses (18 weeks)	92–76 (26 weeks)	A (I)	A (II)[f]
			Isoniazid/rifapentine[g]	Once weekly for 18 doses (18 weeks)	74–58 (26 weeks)	B (I)	E (I)
2	Isoniazid, rifampin, pyrazinamide, ethambutol	Seven days per week for 14 doses (2 weeks), then twice weekly for 12 doses (6 weeks) or 5 days/wk for 10 doses (2 weeks),[e] and then twice weekly for 12 doses (6 weeks)	Isoniazid/rifampin	Twice weekly for 36 doses (18 weeks)	62–58 (26 weeks)	A (II)	B (I)[f]
			Isoniazid/rifapentine[g]	Once weekly for 18 doses (18 weeks)	44–40 (26 weeks)	B (I)	E (I)

	Initial phase		Continuation phase		Total doses (range in days)	Rating (evidence) HIV–	Rating (evidence) HIV+
3	Isoniazid, rifampin, pyrazinamide, ethambutol	Three times weekly for 24 doses (8 weeks)	Isoniazid/rifampin	Three times weekly for 54 doses (18 weeks)	78 (26 weeks)	B (I)	B (II)
4	Isoniazid, rifampin, ethambutol	Seven days per week for 56 doses (8 weeks) or 5 days/wk for 40 doses (8 weeks)[e]	Isoniazid/rifampin	Seven days per week for 217 doses (31 weeks) or 5 days/wk for 155 doses (31 weeks)[e]	273–195 (39 weeks)	C (I)	C (II)
			Isoniazid/rifampin	Twice weekly for 62 doses (31 weeks)	118–102 (39 weeks)	C (I)	C (II)

[a]Ratings: A, preferred; B, acceptable alternative; C, offer when A and B cannot be given.

[b]Evidence ratings: I, randomized clinical trial; II, data from clinical trials that were not randomized or were conducted in other populations; III, expert opinion.

[c]When directly observed therapy is used, drugs may be given 5 days/wk, and the necessary number of doses adjusted accordingly. Although there are no studies that compare five with seven daily doses, extensive experience indicates this would be an effective practice.

[d]Patients with cavitation on initial chest radiograph and positive cultures at completion of 2 months of therapy should receive a 7-month (31-week; either 217 doses [daily] or 62 doses [twice weekly]) continuation phase.

[e]Five-day-a-week administration is always given by directly observed therapy. Rating for 5-day-per-week regimens is A (III).

[f]Not recommended for HIV-infected patients with CD4+ cell counts <100 cells/μL (<100 × 10⁶/L).

[g]Should be used only in HIV-negative patients who have negative sputum smears at the time of completion of 2 months of therapy and who do not have cavitation on initial chest radiograph (see text). For patients started on this regimen and found to have a positive culture from the 2-month specimen, treatment should be extended an extra 3 months.

Adapted from *Treatment of tuberculosis. MMWR Recomm Rep 2003;52(RR-11):1–77. A Joint Statement of the American Thoracic Society (ATS), the Centers for Disease Control and Prevention (CDC) and Infectious Diseases Society of America.*

TABLE 49–5 Doses[a] of Antituberculosis Drugs for Adults and Children[b,c]

Drug	Preparation	Adults/Children	Typical Doses			
			Daily	1× Per Week	2× Per Week	3× Per Week
First-line drugs						
Isoniazid	Tablets (50, 100, 300 mg); elixir (50 mg/5 mL); aqueous solution (100 mg/mL) for IV or intramuscular injection	Adults[c]	5 mg/kg	15 mg/kg	15 mg/kg	15 mg/kg
		Children[c]	10–15 mg/kg		20–30 mg/kg	—
Rifampin	Capsule (150, 300 mg); powder may be suspended for oral administration; aqueous solution for IV injection	Adults[d,c]	10 mg/kg		10 mg/kg	10 mg/kg
		Children[c]	10–20 mg/kg		10–20 mg/kg	
Rifabutin	Capsule (150 mg)	Adult[d,c]	5 mg/kg		5 mg/kg	5 mg/kg
		Children	Appropriate dosing for children is unknown	Appropriate dosing for children is unknown	Appropriate dosing for children is unknown	Appropriate dosing for children is unknown
Rifapentine	Tablet (150 mg, film coated)	Adults[c]		10 mg/kg (continuation phase) (600 mg usual adult dose)		
		Children	The drug is not approved for use in children	The drug is not approved for use in children	The drug is not approved for use in children	The drug is not approved or use in children
Pyrazinamide	Tablet (500 mg, scored)	Adults[c]	40–55 kg: 1000 mg 56–75 kg: 1500 mg 76–90 kg: 2000 mg		40–55 kg: 2000 mg 56–75 kg: 3000 mg 76–90 kg: 4000 mg	40–55 kg: 1500 mg 56–75 kg: 2500 mg 76–90 kg: 3000 mg
		Children[c]	15–30 mg/kg		50 mg/kg	
Ethambutol	Tablet (100, 400 mg)	Adults[c]	40–55 kg: 800 mg 56–75 kg: 1200 mg 76–90 kg: 1600 mg		40–55 kg: 2000 mg 56–75 kg: 2800 mg 76–90 kg: 4000 mg	40–55 kg: 1200 mg 56–75 kg: 2000 mg 76–90 kg: 2400 mg
		Children[d,c]	15–20 mg/kg daily		50 mg/kg	—

(continued)

Second-line drugs

Drug	Preparation	Patient	Dose			
Cycloserine	Capsule (250 mg)	Adults^c	10–15 mg/kg/day, usually 500–750 mg/day in two doses^e	No data	No data	No data
		Children^c	10–15 mg/kg/day	—	—	—
Ethionamide	Tablet (250 mg)	Adults^f,c	15–20 mg/kg/day, usually 500–750 mg/day in a single daily dose or two divided doses^f	No data	No data	No data
		Children^c	15–20 mg/kg/day	No data	No data	g
Streptomycin	Aqueous solution (1-g vials) for IV or intramuscular administration	Adults^c	15 mg/kg/day^g	g	g	—
		Children^c	20–40 mg/kg/day	—	20 mg/kg	g
Amikacin/ kanamycin	Aqueous solution (500-mg and 1-g vials) for IV or intramuscular administration	Adults^c	15 mg/kg/day^g	g	15–30 mg/kg	—
		Children^c	15–30 mg/kg/day IV or intramuscular as a single daily dose			
Capreomycin	Aqueous solution (1-g vials) for IV or intramuscular administration	Adults^c	15 mg/kg/day^g	g	15–30 mg/kg	g
		Children^c	15–30 mg/kg/day as a single daily dose	—	—	—
p-Aminosalicylic acid (PAS)	Granules (4-g packets) can be mixed with food; tablets (500 mg) are still available in some countries, but not in the United States; a solution for IV administration is available in Europe	Adults^c	8–12 g/day in two or three doses	No data	No data	No data
		Children^c	200–300 mg/kg/day in two to four divided doses	No data	No data	No data

TABLE 49-5 Doses[a] of Antituberculosis Drugs for Adults and Children[b,c] *(Continued)*

Drug	Preparation	Adults/ Children	Typical Doses			
			Daily	1× Per Week	2× Per Week	3× Per Week
Levofloxacin	Tablets (250, 500, 750 mg); aqueous solution (500-mg vials) for IV injection	Adults[c] Children[c]	500–1000 mg daily [h]	No data [h]	No data [h]	No data [h]
Moxifloxacin	Tablets (400 mg); aqueous solution (400 mg/250 mL) for IV injection	Adults[c] Children[c]	400 mg daily [i]	No data [i]	No data [i]	No data [i]

Higher doses of rifampin and rifapentine are being studied. Rifabutin dose may need to be adjusted when there is concomitant use of protease inhibitors or non-nucleoside reverse transcriptase inhibitors.

[a]Dose per weight is based on ideal body weight. Children weighing more than 40 kg should be dosed as adults.

[b]For purposes of this document, adult dosing begins at age 15 years.

[c]The authors of this chapter do not agree with the use of maximum doses, since this arbitrarily caps doses for patients who otherwise might need larger doses. These maximum doses were not based on prospective studies in large or overweight individuals, and do not consider patients with documented malabsorption of their medications. Clinical judgment should be used in such circumstances.

[d]The drug can likely be used safely in older children but should be used with caution in children younger than 5 years, in whom visual acuity cannot be monitored. In younger children, ethambutol at the dose of 15 mg/kg/day can be used if there is suspected or proven resistance to isoniazid or rifampin.

[e]It should be noted that, although this is the dose recommended generally, most clinicians with experience using cycloserine indicate that it is unusual for patients to be able to tolerate this amount. Serum concentration measurements are often useful in determining the optimal dose for a given patient.

[f]The single daily dose can be given at bedtime or with the main meal.

[g]Dose: 15 mg/kg/day (1 g), and 10 mg/kg in persons older than 59 years (750 mg). Usual dose: 750 to 1000 mg administered intramuscularly or IV, given as a single dose 5–7 days/wk and reduced to two or three times per week after the first 2 to 4 months or after culture conversion, depending on the efficacy of the other drugs in the regimen.

[h]The long-term (more than several weeks) use of levofloxacin in children and adolescents has not been approved because of concerns about effects on bone and cartilage growth. However, most experts agree that the drug should be considered for children with tuberculosis caused by organisms resistant to both isoniazid and rifampin. The optimal dose is not known.

[i]The long-term (more than several weeks) use of moxifloxacin in children and adolescents has not been approved because of concerns about effects on bone and cartilage growth. The optimal dose is not known.

Adapted from Treatment of tuberculosis. MMWR Recomm Rep 2003;52(RR-11):1–77. A Joint Statement of the American Thoracic Society (ATS), the Centers for Disease Control and Prevention (CDC) and Infectious Diseases Society of America.

DRUG RESISTANCE

- If the organism is drug resistant, the aim is to introduce two or more active agents that the patient has not received previously. With MDR-TB, no standard regimen can be proposed. It is critical to avoid monotherapy or adding only a single drug to a failing regimen.
- Drug resistance should be suspected in the following situations:
  ✓ Patients who have received prior therapy for TB
  ✓ Patients from geographic areas with a high prevalence of resistance (South Africa, Mexico, Southeast Asia, the Baltic countries, and the former Soviet states)
  ✓ Patients who are homeless, institutionalized, IV drug abusers, and/or infected with HIV
  ✓ Patients who still have acid-fast bacilli–positive sputum smears after 2 months of therapy
  ✓ Patients who still have positive cultures after 2 to 4 months of therapy
  ✓ Patients who fail therapy or relapse after retreatment
  ✓ Patients known to be exposed to MDR-TB cases

SPECIAL POPULATIONS

Tuberculous Meningitis and Extrapulmonary Disease

- In general, **isoniazid, pyrazinamide, ethionamide**, and **cycloserine** penetrate the cerebrospinal fluid readily. Patients with CNS TB are often treated for longer periods (9–12 months). Extrapulmonary TB of the soft tissues can be treated with conventional regimens. TB of the bone is typically treated for 9 months, occasionally with surgical debridement.

Children

- TB in children may be treated with regimens similar to those used in adults, although some physicians still prefer to extend treatment to 9 months. Pediatric doses of drugs should be used.

Pregnant Women

- The usual treatment of pregnant women is isoniazid, rifampin, and ethambutol for 9 months.
- Women with TB should be cautioned against becoming pregnant, as the disease poses a risk to the fetus as well as to the mother. Isoniazid or ethambutol is relatively safe when used during pregnancy. Supplementation with B vitamins is particularly important during pregnancy. **Rifampin** has been rarely associated with birth defects, but those seen are occasionally severe, including limb reduction and CNS lesions. **Pyrazinamide** has not been studied in a large number of pregnant women, but anecdotal information suggests that it may be safe. **Ethionamide** may be associated with premature delivery, congenital deformities, and Down syndrome when used during pregnancy, so it cannot be recommended in pregnancy. **Streptomycin** has been associated with hearing impairment in the newborn, including complete deafness and must be reserved for critical situations where alternatives do not exist. **Cycloserine** is not recommended during pregnancy. Fluoroquinolones should be avoided in pregnancy and during nursing.

Renal Failure

- In nearly all patients, isoniazid and rifampin do not require dose modifications in renal failure. Pyrazinamide and ethambutol typically require a reduction in dosing frequency from daily to three times weekly (Table 49–6).

EVALUATION OF THERAPEUTIC OUTCOMES AND PATIENT MONITORING

- The most serious problem with TB therapy is nonadherence to the prescribed regimen. The most effective way to ensure adherence is with directly observed therapy.
- Patients who are AFB smear positive should have sputum samples sent for acid-fast bacilli stains every 1 to 2 weeks until two consecutive smears are negative. Once on

TABLE 49–6	Dosing Recommendations for Adult Patients with Reduced Renal Function and for Adult Patients Receiving Hemodialysis	
Drug	**Change in Frequency?**	**Recommended Dose and Frequency for Patients with Creatinine Clearance <30 mL/min (<0.50 mL/s)or for Patients Receiving Hemodialysis[a,b,c,d]**
Isoniazid	No change	300 mg once daily, or 900 mg three times per week
Rifampin	No change	600 mg once daily, or 600 mg three times per week
Pyrazinamide	Yes	25–35 mg/kg per dose three times per week (not daily)
Ethambutol	Yes	15–25 mg/kg per dose three times per week (not daily)
Levofloxacin	Yes	750–1000 mg per dose three times per week (not daily)
Cycloserine	Yes	250 mg once daily, or 500 mg/dose three times per week[e]
Ethionamide	No change	250–500 mg/dose daily
p-Aminosalicylic acid	No change	4 g/dose, twice daily
Streptomycin	Yes	12–15 mg/kg per dose two or three times per week (not daily)
Capreomycin	Yes	12–15 mg/kg per dose two or three times per week (not daily)
Kanamycin	Yes	12–15 mg/kg per dose two or three times per week (not daily)
Amikacin	Yes	12–15 mg/kg per dose two or three times per week (not daily)

[a]Standard doses are given unless there is intolerance.
[b]The medications should be given after hemodialysis on the day of hemodialysis.
[c]Monitoring of serum drug concentrations should be considered to ensure adequate drug absorption, without excessive accumulation, and to assist in avoiding toxicity.
[d]Data currently are not available for patients receiving peritoneal dialysis. Until data become available, begin with doses recommended for patients receiving hemodialysis and verify adequacy of dosing, using serum concentration monitoring.
[e]The appropriateness of 250-mg daily doses has not been established. There should be careful monitoring for evidence of neurotoxicity.
Adapted from Treatment of tuberculosis. MMWR Recomm Rep 2003;52(RR-11):1–77. A Joint Statement of the American Thoracic Society (ATS), the Centers for Disease Control and Prevention (CDC) and Infectious Diseases Society of America.

maintenance therapy, patients should have sputum cultures performed monthly until negative, which generally occurs over 2 to 3 months. If sputum cultures continue to be positive after 2 months, drug susceptibility testing should be repeated, and serum drug concentrations should be checked.

• Patients should have blood urea nitrogen, serum creatinine, aspartate transaminase or alanine transaminase, and a complete blood count determined at baseline and periodically, depending on the presence of other factors that may increase the likelihood of toxicity (advanced age, alcohol abuse, and possibly pregnancy). Hepatotoxicity should be suspected in patients whose transaminases exceed five times the upper limit of normal or whose total bilirubin exceeds 3 mg/dL (51.3 μmol/L). At this point, the offending agent(s) should be discontinued and alternatives selected.

See Table 49–7 for drug monitoring recommendations.

TABLE 49–7	Antituberculosis Drug Monitoring Table	
Drug	**Adverse Effects**	**Monitoring**
Isoniazid	Asymptomatic elevation of aminotransferases, clinical hepatitis, fatal hepatitis, peripheral neurotoxicity, CNS effects, lupus-like syndrome, hypersensitivity, monoamine poisoning, diarrhea	LFT monthly in patients who have preexisting liver disease or who develop abnormal liver function that does not require discontinuation of drug; dosage adjustments may be necessary in patients receiving anticonvulsants or warfarin
Rifampin	Cutaneous reactions, GI reactions (nausea, anorexia, abdominal pain), flu-like syndrome, hepatotoxicity, severe immunologic reactions, orange discoloration of bodily fluids (sputum, urine, sweat, tears), drug interactions due to induction of hepatic microsomal enzymes	Liver enzymes and interacting drugs as needed (eg, warfarin)
Rifabutin	Hematologic toxicity, uveitis, GI symptoms, polyarthralgias, hepatotoxicity, pseudojaundice (skin discoloration with normal bilirubin), rash, flu-like syndrome, orange discoloration of bodily fluids (sputum, urine, sweat, tears)	Drug interactions are less problematic than rifampin
Rifapentine	Similar to those associated with rifampin	Drug interactions are being investigated and are likely similar to rifampin
Pyrazinamide	Hepatotoxicity, GI symptoms (nausea, vomiting), nongouty polyarthralgia, asymptomatic hyperuricemia, acute gouty arthritis, transient morbilliform rash, dermatitis	Serum uric acid can serve as a surrogate marker for adherence; LFTs in patients with underlying liver disease
Ethambutol	Retrobulbar neuritis, peripheral neuritis, cutaneous reactions	Baseline visual acuity testing and testing of color discrimination; monthly testing of visual acuity and color discrimination in patients taking >15–20 mg/kg, having renal insufficiency, or receiving the drug for >2 months
Streptomycin	Ototoxicity, neurotoxicity, nephrotoxicity	Baseline audiogram, vestibular testing, Romberg's testing, and SCr. Monthly assessments of renal function and auditory or vestibular symptoms

(continued)

TABLE 49–7	Antituberculosis Drug Monitoring Table (*Continued*)	
Drug	**Adverse Effects**	**Monitoring**
Amikacin/kanamycin	Ototoxicity, nephrotoxicity	Baseline audiogram, vestibular testing, Romberg's testing, and SCr; monthly assessments of renal function and auditory or vestibular symptoms
Capreomycin	Nephrotoxicity, ototoxicity	Baseline audiogram, vestibular testing, Romberg's testing, and SCr Monthly assessments of renal function and auditory or vestibular symptoms Baseline and monthly serum K^+ and Mg^{2+}
p-Aminosalicylic acid	Hepatotoxicity, GI distress, malabsorption syndrome, hypothyroidism, coagulopathy	Baseline LFTs and TSH TSH every 3 months
Moxifloxacin	GI disturbance, neurologic effects, cutaneous reactions	No specific monitoring recommended

(CNS, central nervous system; GI, gastrointestinal; LFT, liver function test; SCr, serum creatinine; TSH, thyroid-stimulating hormone.)
Adapted from Treatment of tuberculosis. MMWR Recomm Rep 2003;52(RR-11):1–77. A Joint Statement of the American Thoracic Society (ATS), the Centers for Disease Control and Prevention (CDC) and Infectious Diseases Society of America.

See Chapter 112, Tuberculosis, authored by Rocsanna Namdar, Michael Lauzardo, and Charles A. Peloquin, for a more detailed discussion of this topic.

50   Urinary Tract Infections

- Infections of the urinary tract represent a wide variety of clinical syndromes including urethritis, cystitis, prostatitis, and pyelonephritis.
- A *urinary tract infection* (UTI) is defined as the presence of microorganisms in the urine that cannot be accounted for by contamination. The organisms have the potential to invade the tissues of the urinary tract and adjacent structures.
- Lower tract infections include cystitis (bladder), urethritis (urethra), prostatitis (prostate gland), and epididymitis. Upper tract infections involve the kidney and are referred to as *pyelonephritis.*
- Uncomplicated UTIs are not associated with structural or neurologic abnormalities that may interfere with the normal flow of urine or the voiding mechanism. Complicated UTIs are the result of a predisposing lesion of the urinary tract, such as a congenital abnormality or distortion of the urinary tract, stone, indwelling catheter, prostatic hypertrophy, obstruction, or neurologic deficit that interferes with the normal flow of urine and urinary tract defenses.
- Recurrent UTIs, two or more UTIs occurring within 6 months or three or more within 1 year, are characterized by multiple symptomatic episodes with asymptomatic periods occurring between these episodes. These infections are due to reinfection or to relapse. Reinfections are caused by a different organism and account for the majority of recurrent UTIs. Relapse represents the development of repeated infections caused by the same initial organism.

ETIOLOGY

- The most common cause of uncomplicated UTIs is *Escherichia coli*, accounting for more than 80% to 90% of community-acquired infections. Additional causative organisms are *Staphylococcus saprophyticus, Klebsiella pneumoniae, Proteus* spp., *Pseudomonas aeruginosa*, and *Enterococcus* spp.
- The urinary pathogens in complicated or nosocomial infections may include *E. coli*, which accounts for less than 50% of these infections, *Proteus* spp., *K. pneumoniae, Enterobacter* spp., *P. aeruginosa*, staphylococci, and enterococci. Enterococci represent the second most frequently isolated organisms in hospitalized patients.
- Most UTIs are caused by a single organism; however, in patients with stones, indwelling urinary catheters, or chronic renal abscesses, multiple organisms may be isolated.

CLINICAL PRESENTATION

- The typical symptoms of lower and upper UTIs are presented in Table 50–1.
- Symptoms alone are unreliable for the diagnosis of bacterial UTIs. The key to the diagnosis of a UTI is the ability to demonstrate significant numbers of microorganisms present in an appropriate urine specimen to distinguish contamination from infection.
- Elderly patients frequently do not experience specific urinary symptoms, but they will present with altered mental status, change in eating habits, or gastrointestinal (GI) symptoms.
- A standard urinalysis should be obtained in the initial assessment of a patient. Microscopic examination of the urine should be performed by preparation of a Gram stain of unspun or centrifuged urine. The presence of at least one organism per oil-immersion field in a properly collected uncentrifuged specimen correlates with greater than 100,000 colony-forming units (CFU)/mL (10^5 CFU/mL) ($>10^8$ CFU/L) of urine.
- Criteria for defining significant bacteriuria are listed in Table 50–2.

TABLE 50–1	CLINICAL PRESENTATION: Urinary Tract Infections in Adults

Signs and Symptoms
- Lower UTI: Dysuria, urgency, frequency, nocturia, and suprapubic heaviness
- Gross hematuria
- Upper UTI: Flank pain, fever, nausea, vomiting, and malaise

Physical Examination
- Upper UTI: Costovertebral tenderness

Laboratory Tests
- Bacteriuria
- Pyuria (WBC count more than 10/mm^3 [more than 10×10^6/L])
- Nitrite-positive urine (with nitrite reducers)
- Leukocyte esterase-positive urine
- Antibody-coated bacteria (upper UTI)

- The presence of pyuria (>10 white blood cells/mm^3 [10×10^6/L]) in a symptomatic patient correlates with significant bacteriuria. A count of 5 to 10 WBC/mm^3 (5×10^6 to 10×10^6/L) is accepted as the upper limit of normal.
- The nitrite test can be used to detect the presence of nitrate-reducing bacteria in the urine (eg, *E. coli*). The leukocyte esterase test is a rapid dipstick test to detect pyuria.
- The most reliable method of diagnosing UTIs is by quantitative urine culture. Patients with infection usually have more than 10^5 bacteria/mL [10^8/L] of urine, although as many as one third of women with symptomatic infection have less than 10^5 bacteria/mL [10^8/L].

TREATMENT

- The goals of treatment for UTIs are to eradicate the invading organisms, prevent or treat systemic consequences of infection, prevent recurrence of infection, and to decrease the potential for collateral damage with too broad of antimicrobial therapy.
- The management of a patient with a UTI includes initial evaluation, selection of an antibacterial agent and duration of therapy, and follow-up evaluation.
- The initial selection of an antimicrobial agent for the treatment of UTI is primarily based on the severity of the presenting signs and symptoms, the site of infection, and whether the infection is determined to be complicated or uncomplicated.

PHARMACOLOGIC TREATMENT

- The ability to eradicate bacteria from the urinary tract is directly related to the sensitivity of the organism and the achievable concentration of the antimicrobial agent in the urine.
- The therapeutic management of UTIs is best accomplished by first categorizing the type of infection: acute uncomplicated cystitis, symptomatic abacteriuria, asymptomatic bacteriuria, complicated UTIs, recurrent infections, or prostatitis.

TABLE 50–2	Diagnostic Criteria for Significant Bacteriuria

≥10^2 CFU coliforms/mL (≥10^5 CFU/L) or ≥10^5 CFU noncoliforms/mL (≥10^8 CFU/L) in a symptomatic female
≥10^4 CFU bacteria/mL (≥10^7 CFU/L) in a symptomatic male
≥10^5 CFU bacteria/mL (≥10^8 CFU/L) in asymptomatic individuals on two consecutive specimens
Any growth of bacteria on suprapubic catheterization in a symptomatic patient
≥10$^{2-5}$ CFU bacteria/mL (≥10$^{5-8}$ CFU/L) in a catheterized patient

(CFU, colony-forming unit.)

- Most *E. coli* remain susceptible to amoxicillin and ampicillin, and trimethoprim-sulfamethoxazole, although resistance is increasing.
- Table 50–3 lists the most common agents used in the treatment of UTIs, along with comments concerning their general use.
- Table 50–4 presents an overview of various therapeutic options for outpatient therapy for UTI.
- Table 50–5 describes empiric treatment regimens for specific clinical situations.

Acute Uncomplicated Cystitis

- These infections are predominantly caused by *E. coli*, and antimicrobial therapy should be directed against this organism initially. Because the causative organisms and their susceptibilities are generally known, a cost-effective approach to management is recommended that includes a urinalysis and initiation of empiric therapy without a urine culture (Fig. 50–1).
- Short-course therapy (3-day therapy) with **trimethoprim–sulfamethoxazole** or a **fluoroquinolone** (eg, **ciprofloxacin** or **levofloxacin**, but not moxifloxacin) is superior to single-dose therapy for uncomplicated infection. Fluoroquinolones should be reserved for patients with suspected or possible pyelonephritis due to the collateral damage risk. Instead, a 3-day course of trimethoprim–sulfamethoxazole, a 5-day course of nitrofurantoin, or a one-time dose of fosfomycin should be considered as first-line therapy. In areas where there is more than 20% resistance of *E. coli* to trimethoprim–sulfamethoxazole, nitrofurantoin or fosfomycin should be utilized. Amoxicillin or ampicillin is not recommended because the high incidence of resistant *E. coli*. Follow-up urine cultures are not necessary in patients who respond.

Complicated Urinary Tract Infections

ACUTE PYELONEPHRITIS

- The presentation of high-grade fever (>38.3°C [100.9°F]) and severe flank pain should be treated as acute pyelonephritis, and aggressive management is warranted. Severely ill patients with pyelonephritis should be hospitalized and IV drugs administered initially. Milder cases may be managed with oral antibiotics in an outpatient setting.
- At the time of presentation, a Gram stain of the urine should be performed, along with urinalysis, culture, and sensitivities.
- In the mild to moderately symptomatic patient for whom oral therapy is considered, an effective agent should be administered for 7 to 14 days, depending on the agent used. Fluoroquinolones (ciprofloxacin or levofloxacin) orally for 7 to 10 days are the first-line choice in mild to moderate pyelonephritis. Other options include trimethoprim–sulfamethoxazole for 14 days. If a Gram stain reveals gram-positive cocci, *Streptococcus faecalis* should be considered and treatment directed against this pathogen (**ampicillin**).
- In the seriously ill patient, the traditional initial therapy is an IV fluoroquinolone, an aminoglycoside with or without **ampicillin**, or an extended-spectrum cephalosporin with or without an aminoglycoside.
- If the patient has been hospitalized in the last 6 months, has a urinary catheter, or is in a nursing home, the possibility of *P. aeruginosa* and *enterococci* infection, as well as multiple-resistant organisms, should be considered. In this setting, **ceftazidime, ticarcillin–clavulanic acid, piperacillin, aztreonam, meropenem**, or **imipenem**, in combination with an aminoglycoside, is recommended. If the patient responds to initial combination therapy, the aminoglycoside may be discontinued after 3 days.
- Follow-up urine cultures should be obtained 2 weeks after the completion of therapy to ensure a satisfactory response and to detect possible relapse.

URINARY TRACT INFECTIONS IN MEN

- The conventional view is that therapy in men requires prolonged treatment (Fig. 50–2).
- A urine culture should be obtained before treatment, because the cause of infection in men is not as predictable as in women.

TABLE 50–3 Commonly Used Antimicrobial Agents in the Treatment of UTIs

Drug	Adverse Drug Reactions	Monitoring Parameters	Comments
Oral therapy			
Trimethoprim–sulfamethoxazole	Rash, Stevens–Johnson Syndrome, renal failure, photosensitivity, hematologic (neutropenia, anemia, etc.)	Serum creatinine, BUN, electrolytes, signs of rash, and CBC	This combination is highly effective against most aerobic enteric bacteria except *P. aeruginosa*. High urinary tract tissue concentrations and urine concentrations are achieved, which may be important in complicated infection treatment. Also effective as prophylaxis for recurrent infections
Nitrofurantoin	GI intolerance, neuropathies, and pulmonary reactions	Baseline serum creatinine and BUN	This agent is effective as both a therapeutic and prophylactic agent in patients with recurrent UTIs. Main advantage is the lack of resistance even after long courses of therapy
Fosfomycin trometamol	Diarrhea, headache, and angioedema	No routine tests recommended	Single-dose therapy for uncomplicated infections, low levels of resistance, use with caution in patients with hepatic dysfunction
Fluoroquinolones			
Ciprofloxacin Levofloxacin	Hypersensitivity, photosensitivity, GI symptoms, dizziness, confusion, and tendonitis (black box warning)	CBC, baseline serum creatinine, and BUN	The fluoroquinolones have a greater spectrum of activity, including *P. aeruginosa*. These agents are effective for pyelonephritis and prostatitis. Avoid in pregnancy and children. Moxifloxacin should not be used owing to inadequate urinary concentrations
Penicillins			
Amoxicillin–clavulanate	Hypersensitivity (rash, anaphylaxis), diarrhea, superinfections, and seizures	CBC, signs of rash, or hypersensitivity	Due to increasing *E. coli* resistance, amoxicillin–clavulanate is the preferred penicillin for uncomplicated cystitis
Cephalosporins			
Cefaclor Cefpodoxime-proxetil	Hypersensitivity (rash, anaphylaxis), diarrhea, superinfections, and seizures	CBC, signs of rash, or hypersensitivity	There are no major advantages of these agents over other agents in the treatment of UTIs, and they are more expensive. These agents are not active against enterococci

Parenteral therapy

Aminoglycosides

Gentamicin Tobramycin Amikacin	Ototoxicity, nephrotoxicity	Serum creatinine and BUN, serum drug concentrations, and individual pharmacokinetic monitoring	These agents are renally excreted and achieve good concentrations in the urine. Amikacin generally is reserved for multidrug-resistant bacteria

Penicillins

Ampicillin–sulbactam Piperacillin–tazobactam	Hypersensitivity (rash, anaphylaxis), diarrhea, superinfections, and seizures	CBC, signs of rash, or hypersensitivity	These agents generally are equally effective for susceptible bacteria. The extended-spectrum penicillins are more active against *P. aeruginosa* and enterococci and often are preferred over cephalosporins. They are very useful in renally impaired patients or when an aminoglycoside is to be avoided

Cephalosporins

Ceftriaxone Ceftazidime Cefepime	Hypersensitivity (rash, anaphylaxis), diarrhea, superinfections, and seizures	CBC, signs of rash, or hypersensitivity	Second- and third-generation cephalosporins have a broad spectrum of activity against gram-negative bacteria, but are not active against enterococci and have limited activity against *P. aeruginosa*. Ceftazidime and cefepime are active against *P. aeruginosa*. They are useful for nosocomial infections and urosepsis due to susceptible pathogens

Carbapenems/monobactams

Imipenem–cilastatin Meropenem Doripenem Ertapenem Aztreonam	Hypersensitivity (rash, anaphylaxis), diarrhea, superinfections, and seizures	CBC, signs of rash, or hypersensitivity	Carbapenems have a broad spectrum of activity, including gram-positive, gram-negative, and anaerobic bacteria. Imipenem, meropenem, and doripenem are active against *P. aeruginosa* and enterococci, but ertapenem is not. Aztreonam is a monobactam that is only active against gram-negative bacteria, including some strains of *P. aeruginosa*. Generally useful for nosocomial infections when aminoglycosides are to be avoided and in penicillin-sensitive patients

Fluoroquinolones

Ciprofloxacin Levofloxacin	Hypersensitivity, photosensitivity, GI symptoms, dizziness, confusion, and tendonitis (black box warning)	CBC, baseline serum creatinine, and BUN	These agents have broad-spectrum activity against both gram-negative and gram-positive bacteria. They provide urine and high-tissue concentrations and are actively secreted in reduced renal function

(BUN, blood urea nitrogen; CBC, complete blood count; GI, gastrointestinal; UTIs, urinary tract infections.)

TABLE 50–4 Overview of Outpatient Antimicrobial Therapy for Lower Tract Infections in Adults

Indications	Antibiotic	Dose	Interval	Duration
Lower tract infections				
Uncomplicated	Trimethoprim–sulfamethoxazole	1 DS tablet	Twice a day	3 days
	Nitrofurantoin monohydrate	100 mg	Twice a day	5 days
	Fosfomycin trometamol	3 g	Single dose	1 day
	Ciprofloxacin	250 mg	Twice a day	3 days
	Levofloxacin	250 mg	Once a day	3 days
	Amoxicillin–clavulanate	500 mg	Every 8 hours	5–7 days
	Pivmecillinam	400 mg	Twice a day	3 days
Complicated	Trimethoprim–sulfamethoxazole	1 DS tablet	Twice a day	7–10 days
	Ciprofloxacin	250–500 mg	Twice a day	7–10 days
	Levofloxacin	250 mg	Once a day	10 days
		750 mg	Once a day	5 days
	Amoxicillin–clavulanate	500 mg	Every 8 hours	7–10 days
Recurrent infections	Nitrofurantoin	50 mg	Once a day	6 months
	Trimethoprim–sulfamethoxazole	1/2 SS tablet	Once a day	6 months
Acute pyelonephritis	Trimethoprim–sulfamethoxazole	1 DS tablet	Twice a day	14 days
	Ciprofloxacin	500 mg	Twice a day	14 days
		1000 mg ER	Once a day	7 days
	Levofloxacin	250 mg	Once a day	10 days
		750 mg	Once a day	5 days
	Amoxicillin–clavulanate	500 mg	Every 8 hours	14 days

(DS, double strength; SS, single strength.)
Dosing intervals for normal renal function.

TABLE 50-5	Evidence-Based Empirical Treatment of UTIs and Prostatitis		
Diagnosis	**Pathogens**	**Treatment Recommendation**	**Comments**
Acute uncomplicated cystitis	Escherichia coli, Staphylococcus saprophyticus	1. Nitrofurantoin × 5 days (A,I)[a] 2. Trimethoprim–sulfamethoxazole × 3 days (A,I)[a] 3. Fosfomycin trometamol × 1 dose (A,I)[a] 4. Fluoroquinolone × 3 days (A,I)[a] 5. β-Lactams × 3–7 days (B,I)[a] 6. Pivmecillinam × 3–7 days (A,I)	Short-course therapy more effective than single dose Reserve fluoroquinolones as alternatives to development of resistance (A-III)[a] β-Lactams as a group are not as effective in acute cystitis then trimethoprim–sulfamethoxazole or the fluoroquinolones, do not use amoxicillin or ampicillin[a] Pivmecillinam not available in United States
Pregnancy	As above	1. Amoxicillin–clavulanate × 7 days 2. Cephalosporin × 7 days 3. Trimethoprim–sulfamethoxazole × 7 days	Avoid trimethoprim–sulfamethoxazole during the third trimester
Acute pyelonephritis			
Uncomplicated	E. coli	1. Quinolone × 7 days (A,I)[a] 2. Trimethoprim–sulfamethoxazole (if susceptible) × 14 days (A,I)[a]	Can be managed as outpatient
	Gram-positive bacteria	1. Amoxicillin or amoxicillin–clavulanic acid × 14 days	
Complicated	E. coli P. mirabilis K. pneumoniae P. aeruginosa Enterococcus faecalis	1. Quinolone × 14 days 2. Extended-spectrum penicillin plus aminoglycoside	Severity of illness will determine duration of IV therapy; culture results should direct therapy Oral therapy may complete 14 days of therapy
Prostatitis	E. coli K. pneumoniae Proteus spp. P. aeruginosa	1. Trimethoprim–sulfamethoxazole × 4–6 weeks 2. Quinolone × 4–6 weeks	Acute prostatitis may require IV therapy initially Chronic prostatitis may require longer treatment periods or surgery

(UTI, urinary tract infection.)

[a]Strength of recommendations: A, good evidence for; B, moderate evidence for; C, poor evidence for and against; D, moderate against; E, good evidence against. Quality of evidence: I, at least one proper randomized, controlled study; II, one well-designed clinical trial; III, evidence from opinions, clinical experience, and expert committees.

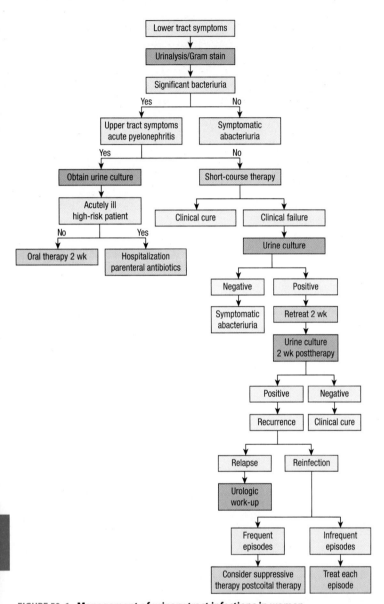

FIGURE 50-1. Management of urinary tract infections in women.

- If gram-negative bacteria are presumed, trimethoprim–sulfamethoxazole or a fluoroquinolone is a preferred agent. Initial therapy is for 10 to 14 days. For recurrent infections in men, cure rates are much higher with a 6-week regimen of trimethoprim–sulfamethoxazole.

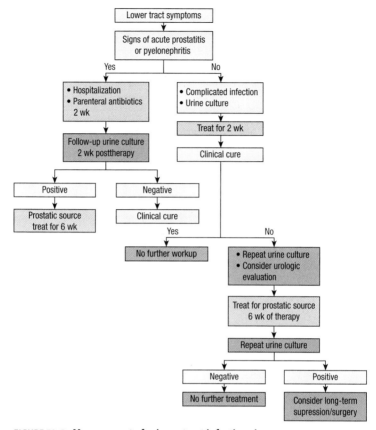

FIGURE 50–2. Management of urinary tract infections in men.

Recurrent Infections

- Recurrent episodes of UTI (reinfections and relapses) account for a significant portion of all UTIs. These patients are most commonly women and can be divided into two groups: those with fewer than two or three episodes per year and those who develop more frequent infections.
- In patients with infrequent infections (ie, fewer than three infections per year), each episode should be treated as a separately occurring infection. Short-course therapy should be used in symptomatic female patients with lower tract infection.
- In patients who have frequent symptomatic infections, long-term prophylactic antimicrobial therapy may be instituted (see Table 50–4). Therapy is generally given for 6 months, with urine cultures followed periodically.
- In women who experience symptomatic reinfections in association with sexual activity, voiding after intercourse may help prevent infection. Also, self-administered, single-dose prophylactic therapy with **trimethoprim–sulfamethoxazole** taken after intercourse significantly reduces the incidence of recurrent infection in these patients.
- Women who relapse after short-course therapy should receive a 2-week course of therapy. In patients who relapse after 2 weeks, therapy should be continued for another 2 to 4 weeks. If relapse occurs after 6 weeks of treatment, urologic examination should be performed, and therapy for 6 months or even longer may be considered.

SPECIAL CONDITIONS

Urinary Tract Infection in Pregnancy

- In patients with significant bacteriuria, symptomatic or asymptomatic treatment is recommended to avoid possible complications during the pregnancy. Therapy should consist of an agent with a relatively low adverse-effect potential (**cephalexin, amoxicillin, or amoxicillin/clavulanate**) administered for 7 days.
- Tetracyclines should be avoided because of teratogenic effects and sulfonamides should not be administered during the third trimester because of the possible development of kernicterus and hyperbilirubinemia. Also, the fluoroquinolones should not be given because of their potential to inhibit cartilage and bone development in the newborn.

Catheterized Patients

- When bacteriuria occurs in the asymptomatic, short-term catheterized patient (<30 days), the use of systemic antibiotic therapy should be withheld and the catheter removed as soon as possible. If the patient becomes symptomatic, the catheter should again be removed, and treatment as described for complicated infections should be started.
- The use of prophylactic systemic antibiotics in patients with short-term catheterization reduces the incidence of infection over the first 4 to 7 days. In long-term catheterized patients, however, antibiotics only postpone the development of bacteriuria and lead to emergence of resistant organisms.

See Chapter 116, Urinary Tract Infections and Prostatitis, authored by Elizabeth A. Coyle and Randall A. Prince, for a more detailed discussion of this topic.

51 Vaccines, Toxoids, and Other Immunobiologics

- *Vaccines* are substances administered to generate a protective immune response. They can be live attenuated or killed.
- *Toxoids* are inactivated bacterial toxins. They retain the ability to stimulate the formation of antitoxins, which are antibodies directed against the bacterial toxin.
- *Adjuvants* are inert substances, such as aluminum salts (ie, alum), which enhance vaccine antigenicity by prolonging antigen absorption.
- *Immune sera* are sterile solutions containing antibody derived from human (immunoglobulin [Ig]) or equine (antitoxin) sources.

VACCINE AND TOXOID RECOMMENDATIONS

- The childhood, adolescent, and adult immunization schedules are updated frequently and published annually. Recommendations for the use of influenza vaccine are issued annually. Healthcare providers involved in primary care and immunization delivery must keep themselves abreast of these changes in a systematic way. Electronic newsletters and browsing reliable Websites are efficient methods for obtaining information (Table 51–1).
- In general, killed vaccines can be administered simultaneously at separate sites. Killed and live-attenuated vaccines may be administered simultaneously at separate sites. If they cannot be administered simultaneously, they can be administered at any interval between doses with the exception of cholera (killed) and yellow fever (live) vaccines, which should be given at least 3 weeks apart. If live vaccines are not administered simultaneously, their administration should be separated by at least 4 weeks.
- Administration of live vaccines, such as rubella or varicella, are deferred until postpartum and are routinely recommended for new mothers who do not have evidence of immunity prior to hospital discharge. These live vaccines can be administered without regard to administration of Rho(D) Ig (RDIg) in the postpartum period. Additionally, Tdap is recommended for all new mothers who have not received a Tdap before because household contacts are frequently implicated as the source of pertussis infection in a young infant.
- In general, severely immunocompromised individuals should not receive live vaccines.
- Patients with chronic conditions that cause limited immunodeficiency (eg, renal disease, diabetes, liver disease, and asplenia) and who are not receiving immunosuppressants may receive live-attenuated and killed vaccines, as well as toxoids.
- Patients with active malignant disease may receive killed vaccines or toxoids but should not be given live vaccines. Live virus vaccines may be administered to persons with leukemia who have not received chemotherapy for at least 3 months.
- If a person has been receiving high-dose corticosteroids or has had a course lasting longer than 2 weeks, then at least 1 month should pass before immunization with live virus vaccines.
- Responses to live and killed vaccines generally are suboptimal for human immune deficiency virus (HIV)–infected patients and decrease as the disease progresses.
- General contraindications to vaccine administration include a history of anaphylactic reaction to a previous dose or an unexplained encephalopathy occurring within 7 days of a dose of pertussis vaccine. Immunosuppression and pregnancy are temporary contraindications to live vaccines.
- Whenever possible, transplant patients should be immunized before transplantation. Live vaccines generally are not given after transplantation.

TABLE 51–1	Web Resources for Vaccine Information
Recommended internet sites for vaccine information	
http://www.cdc.gov/vaccines/	Vaccines & Immunizations Centers for Disease Control and Prevention
www.immunize.org	Immunization Action Coalition
www.nfid.org/	National Foundation for Infectious Diseases
www.cdc.gov/mmwr/	Morbidity and Mortality Weekly Report
http://iom.nationalacademies.org/	Institute of Medicine of the National Academies
http://www.hrsa.gov/vaccinecompensation/	Vaccine Injury Compensation Program
http://www.chop.edu/service/vaccine-education-center/	Vaccine Education Center Children's Hospital of Philadelphia
http://vaers.hhs.gov/index	Vaccine Adverse Event Reporting System
Recommended electronic newsletters	
www.immunize.org/express	The Immunization Action Coalition's newsletter
www.cdc.gov/mmwr/	Morbidity and Mortality Weekly Report

DIPHTHERIA TOXOID ADSORBED AND DIPHTHERIA ANTITOXIN

- Two strengths of diphtheria toxoid are available: pediatric (D) and adult, which contains less antigen. Primary immunization with D is indicated for children older than 6 weeks. Generally, D is given along with tetanus and acellular pertussis (DTaP) vaccines at 2, 4, and 6 months of age, and then at 15 to 18 months and 4 to 6 years of age.
- For nonimmunized adults, a complete three-dose series of diphtheria toxoid should be administered, with the first two doses given at least 4 weeks apart and the third dose 6 to 12 months after the second. One dose in the series should be Tdap. The combined preparation, tetanus–diphtheria (Td), is recommended in adults because it contains less diphtheria toxoid than DTaP, with fewer reactions seen from the diphtheria preparation. Booster doses are given every 10 years.
- Adverse effects to diphtheria toxoid include mild to moderate tenderness, erythema, and induration at the injection site.

TETANUS TOXOID, TETANUS TOXOID ADSORBED, AND TETANUS IMMUNOGLOBULIN

- In children, primary immunization against tetanus is usually done in conjunction with diphtheria and pertussis vaccination using DTaP or a combination vaccine that includes other antigens. A 0.5-mL dose is recommended at 2, 4, 6, and 15 to 18 months of age.
- In children 7 years and older and in adults who have not been previously immunized, a series of three 0.5 mL doses of Td are administered intramuscularly (IM) initially. The first two doses are given 1 to 2 months apart and the third dose 6 to 12 months later. Boosters are recommended every 10 years.
- Tetanus toxoid may be given to immunosuppressed patients if indicated.
- Tetanus Ig (TIg) is used to provide passive tetanus immunization after the occurrence of traumatic wounds in nonimmunized or suboptimally immunized persons (Table 51–2). A dose of 250 to 500 units is administered IM. When administered with tetanus toxoid, separate sites for administration should be used.

TABLE 51–2	Tetanus Prophylaxis			
Vaccination History	**Clean, Minor**		**All Other**	
	Td[a]	TIG	Td[a]	TIG
Unknown or fewer than three doses	Yes	No	Yes	Yes
Three or more doses	No[a,b]	No	No[a,c]	No

[a]A single dose of Tdap should be used for the next dose of tetanus-diphtheria toxoid for individuals aged >10 years.
[b]Yes, if more than 10 years since last dose.
[c]Yes, if more than 5 years since last dose.

- TIg also used for the treatment of tetanus. In this setting, a single dose of 3000 to 6000 units is administered IM.

HAEMOPHILUS INFLUENZAE TYPE B VACCINES

- *Haemophilus influenzae* type b (Hib) vaccines currently in use are conjugate products, consisting of either a polysaccharide or oligosaccharide of polyribosylribitol phosphate (PRP) covalently linked to a protein carrier.
- Hib conjugate vaccines are indicated for routine use in all infants and children younger than 5 years.
- The primary series of Hib vaccination consists of 0.5-mL IM doses at 2, 4, and 6 months of age. If PRP-OMP (PRP conjugated to an outer membrane protein) is used, it should be given at ages 2 and 4 months. A booster dose is recommended at age 12 to 15 months.
- For infants 7 to 11 months of age who have not been vaccinated, three doses of Hib vaccine should be given: two doses spaced 4 weeks apart and then a booster dose at age 12 to 15 months (but at least 8 weeks since the second dose). For unvaccinated children ages 12 to 14 months, two doses should be given, with an interval of 2 months between doses. In a child older than 15 months, a single dose of any of the four conjugate vaccines is indicated.

HEPATITIS VACCINES

- Information on hepatitis vaccines can be found in Chap. 40.

HUMAN PAPILLOMAVIRUS VACCINE

- The vaccines are recommended for adolescents aged 11 to 12 years and for all females aged 13 to 26 years. Males should be immunized routinely up to age 21 years. Males who have sex with males and the immunocompromised should be immunized through age 26 years. The vaccine is administered as a three-dose series (0, 1–2, and 6 months).
- The vaccine is well tolerated, with injection site reactions and headache and fatigue occurring as commonly as in placebo groups.

INFLUENZA VIRUS VACCINE

- See Chap. 41 for information regarding influenza vaccination.

MEASLES VACCINE

- Measles vaccine is a live-attenuated vaccine that is administered for primary immunization to persons 12 to 15 months of age or older, usually as a combination of measles, mumps, and rubella (MMR). A second dose is recommended at 4 to 6 years of age.

- The vaccine should not be given to immunosuppressed patients (except those infected with HIV) or pregnant women. HIV-infected persons who have never had measles or have never been vaccinated should be given measles-containing vaccine unless there is evidence of severe immunosuppression.
- The vaccine should not be given within 1 month of any other live vaccine unless the vaccine is given on the same day (as with the MMR vaccine).
- Measles vaccine is indicated in all persons born after 1956 or in those who lack documentation of wild virus infection by either history or antibody titers.

MENINGOCOCCAL POLYSACCHARIDE VACCINE

- There are two meningococcal conjugate vaccines: Menactra is licensed for individuals 9 months to 55 years old and Menveo for those 12 to 55 years old. They are recommended for all children 11 to 12 years old with a second dose at 16 years of age. The vaccine is indicated in high-risk populations such as those exposed to the disease, those in the midst of uncontrolled outbreaks, travelers to an area with epidemic hyperendemic meningococcal disease, and individuals who have terminal complement deficiencies or asplenia. Reimmunization at 5-year intervals is recommended for individuals who are at high risk. The polysaccharide vaccine should be reserved for those older than 55 years who require immunization.
- The polysaccharide vaccine is administered subcutaneously as a single 0.5-mL dose, and the conjugate vaccine is administered by IM injection.

MUMPS VACCINE

- The vaccine (usually given in conjunction with measles and rubella, MMR) is given beginning at age 12 to 15 months, with a second dose prior to entry into elementary school.
- Two doses of mumps vaccine are recommended for school-age children, international travelers, college students, and healthcare workers born after 1956.
- Postexposure vaccination is of no benefit.
- Mumps vaccine should not be given to pregnant women or immunosuppressed patients. The vaccine should not be given within 6 weeks (preferably 3 months) of administration of Ig.

PERTUSSIS VACCINE

- Acellular pertussis vaccine is usually administered in combination with diphtheria and tetanus toxoids (as DTaP).
- The primary immunization series for pertussis vaccine consists of four doses given at ages 2, 4, 6, and 15 to 18 months. A booster dose is recommended at age 4 to 6 years. Pertussis vaccine is administered in combination with diphtheria and tetanus (DTaP). Administration of an acellular pertussis-containing vaccine is also recommended for adolescents once between ages 11 and 18 years. In addition, adolescents should receive a pertussis-containing vaccine with their next dose of Td toxoids.
- Systemic reactions, such as moderate fever, occur in 3% to 5% of those receiving vaccines. Very rarely, high fever, febrile seizures, persistent crying spells, and hypotonic hyporesponsive episodes occur after vaccination.
- There are only two contraindications to pertussis administration: (1) an immediate anaphylactic reaction to a previous dose and (2) encephalopathy within 7 days of a previous dose, with no evidence of other cause.

PNEUMOCOCCAL VACCINES

- Pneumococcal polysaccharide vaccine is a mixture of capsular polysaccharides from 23 of the 83 most prevalent types of *Streptococcus pneumoniae* seen in the United States (PPV23).

- Pneumococcal vaccine (PPV23) is recommended for the following immunocompetent persons:
  - ✓ Persons 65 years or older. If an individual received vaccine more than 5 years earlier and was younger than 65 at the time of administration, revaccination should be given.
  - ✓ Persons ages 2 to 64 years with chronic illness
  - ✓ Persons ages 2 to 64 years with functional or anatomical asplenia. When splenectomy is planned, pneumococcal vaccine should be given at least 2 weeks before surgery.
  - ✓ Persons ages 2 to 64 years living in environments where the risk of invasive pneumococcal disease or its complications is increased. This does not include daycare center employees and children.
  - ✓ Persons aged 19 to 64 years who smoke cigarettes or have asthma.
  - ✓ Persons with cochlear implants.
- Pneumococcal vaccination (PPV23) is recommended for immunocompromised persons 2 years of age or older with
  - ✓ HIV infection
  - ✓ Leukemia, lymphoma, Hodgkin disease, or multiple myeloma
  - ✓ Generalized malignancy
  - ✓ Chronic renal failure of nephritic syndrome
  - ✓ Patients receiving immunosuppressive therapy
  - ✓ Organ or bone marrow transplant recipients
- Because children younger than 2 years do not respond adequately to the pneumococcal polysaccharide vaccine, a pneumococcal conjugate vaccine was created.
- PCV 13 valent, (PCV13) is administered as a 0.5-mL IM injection at 2, 4, and 6 months of age and between 12 and 15 months of age. A single dose of PCV13 should be administered to children aged 6 to 18 with sickle cell disease or splenic dysfunction, HIV infection, immunocompromising conditions, cochlear implant, or cerebral spinal fluid leak should be immunized. It is also licensed for individuals aged 50 years and older.

POLIOVIRUS VACCINES

- Two types of trivalent poliovirus vaccines are currently licensed for distribution in the United States: an enhanced inactivated poliovirus vaccine (IPV) and a live-attenuated, oral poliovirus vaccine (OPV). IPV is the recommended vaccine for the primary series and booster dose for children in the United States, whereas OPV is recommended in areas of the world that have circulating poliovirus.
- IPV is given to children ages 2, 4, and 6 to 18 months and 4 to 6 years. Primary poliomyelitis immunization is recommended for all children and young adults up to age 18 years. Allergies to any component of IPV, including streptomycin, polymyxin B, and neomycin, are contraindications to vaccine use.
- The routine use of OPV in the United States has been discontinued.

RUBELLA VACCINE

- The vaccine is given with measles and mumps vaccines (MMR) at 12 to 15 months of age, then at 4 to 6 years.
- The vaccine should not be given to immunosuppressed individuals, although MMR vaccine should be administered to young children with HIV without severe immunosuppression as soon as possible after their first birthday. The vaccine should not be given to individuals with anaphylactic reaction to neomycin.
- Although the vaccine has not been associated with congenital rubella syndrome, its use in pregnancy is contraindicated. Women should be counseled not to become pregnant for 4 weeks after vaccination.

VARICELLA VACCINE

- Varicella virus vaccine is recommended for all children 12 to 18 months of age, with a second dose prior to entering school between 4 and 6 years of age. It is also recommended for persons above this age if they have not had chickenpox. Persons ages 13 years and older should receive two doses separated by 4 to 8 weeks.
  - ✓ The vaccine is contraindicated in immunosuppressed or pregnant patients.
  - ✓ Children with asymptomatic or mildly symptomatic HIV should receive two doses of varicella vaccine 3 months apart.

VARICELLA ZOSTER VACCINE

- The zoster vaccine is recommended for immunocompetent individuals older than 60 years. It should not be used in immunocompromised individuals, including those with HIV or malignancies or in pregnant women.
- Administration of varicella zoster Ig is by the IM route (never IV).

IMMUNOGLOBULIN

- Ig is available as both IM (IGIM) and IV (IGIV) preparations.
- Table 51–3 lists the suggested dosages for IGIM in various disease states.
- The uses for IGIV are as follows:
  - ✓ Primary immunodeficiency states, including both antibody deficiencies and combined deficiencies
  - ✓ Idiopathic thrombocytopenic purpura
  - ✓ Chronic lymphocytic leukemia in patients who have had a serious bacterial infection
  - ✓ Kawasaki disease (mucocutaneous lymph node syndrome)
  - ✓ Pediatric HIV infection
  - ✓ Allogeneic bone marrow transplant
  - ✓ Chronic inflammatory demyelinating polyneuropathy and multifocal motor neuropathy
  - ✓ Kidney transplantation involving a recipient with high antibody concentrations of and ABO incompatible donor

RHO(D) IMMUNOGLOBULIN

- Rho(D) Ig (RDIg) suppresses the antibody response and formation of anti-Rho(D) in Rho(D)-negative, D^u-negative women exposed to Rho(D)-positive blood and prevents the future chance of erythroblastosis fetalis in subsequent pregnancies with a Rho(D)-positive fetus.
- RDIg, when administered IM within 72 hours of delivery of a full-term infant, reduces active antibody formation from 1% to 0.2%.

TABLE 51–3	Indications and Dosage of Intramuscular Immunoglobulin in Infectious Diseases
Primary immunodeficiency states	1.2 mL/kg IM then 0.6 mL/kg every 2-4 weeks
Hepatitis A exposure	0.02 mL/kg IM within 2 weeks if <1 year or >39 years of age
Hepatitis A prophylaxis	0.02 mL/kg IM for exposure <3 months' duration 0.06 mL/kg IM for exposure up to 5 months' duration
Hepatitis B exposure	0.06 mL/kg (HBIG preferred in known exposures)
Measles exposure	0.25 mL/kg (maximum dose 15 mL) as soon as possible 0.5 mL/kg (maximum dose 15 mL) as soon as possible for immunocompromised individuals

- RDIg is also used in the case of a premenopausal woman who is Rho(D) negative and has inadvertently received Rho(D)-positive blood or blood products.
- RDIg may be used after abortion, miscarriage, amniocentesis, or abdominal trauma.

See Chapter 125, Vaccines, Toxoids, and Other Immunobiologics, authored by Mary S. Hayney, for a more detailed discussion of this topic.

CHAPTER

52 | Alzheimer Disease

- *Alzheimer disease* (AD), which accounts for about 60% of dementias, is a progressive and eventually fatal dementia of unknown cause characterized by loss of cognitive and physical functioning, commonly with behavior symptoms.

PATHOPHYSIOLOGY

- Dominantly inherited forms of AD are fewer than 1% of cases. More than half of young-onset, dominantly inherited cases are attributed to alterations on chromosomes 1, 14, or 21. Genetic susceptibility to late-onset AD is primarily linked to the apolipoprotein E (APOE) genotype, but an interaction of multiple genes with the environment may be at play.
- Risk factors associated with AD include age, decreased reserve capacity of the brain, head injury, Down syndrome, depression, mild cognitive impairment, and risk factors for vascular disease, including hypertension, elevated homocysteine, elevated low-density lipoprotein cholesterol, low high-density lipoprotein cholesterol, obesity, metabolic syndrome, and diabetes.
- Signature findings include intracellular neurofibrillary tangles (NFTs), extracellular amyloid plaques in the cortex and medial temporal lobe, degeneration of neurons and synapses, and cortical atrophy. Density of NFTs correlates with severity of dementia.
- Proposed mechanisms for these changes include: (1) β-amyloid protein aggregation, leading to formation of plaques; (2) hyperphosphorylation of tau protein, leading to NFTs; (3) synaptic failure and depletion of neurotrophin and neurotransmitters; (4) mitochondrial dysfunction; and (5) oxidative stress. The amyloid cascade hypothesis states that there is an imbalance between production and clearance of β-amyloid, with aggregation and accumulation of β-amyloid leading to AD. Whether this is the primary pathology in most forms of AD remains to be shown.
- Of neurotransmitter deficits, loss of cholinergic activity is most prominent, and it correlates with AD severity. Cholinergic cell loss seems to be a consequence of AD pathology, not the cause of it.
- Other neurotransmitter considerations include: (1) Serotonergic neurons of the raphe nuclei and noradrenergic cells of the locus ceruleus are lost; (2) monoamine oxidase type B activity is increased; (3) glutamate pathways of the cortex and limbic structures are abnormal; and (4) excitatory neurotransmitters, including glutamate, may be neurotoxic.

CLINICAL PRESENTATION

- Cognitive decline is gradual and includes memory loss, aphasia, apraxia, agnosia, disorientation, and impaired executive function. Other symptoms include depression, psychotic symptoms, aggression, motor hyperactivity, uncooperativeness, wandering, and combativeness. Patients become increasingly unable to care for themselves. Table 52–1 shows the stages of AD.

TABLE 52-1	Stages of Alzheimer Disease
Mild (MMSE score 26–21)	Patient has difficulty remembering recent events. Ability to manage finances, prepare food, and carry out other household activities declines. May get lost while driving. Begins to withdraw from difficult tasks and to give up hobbies. May deny memory problems
Moderate (MMSE score 20–10)	Patient requires assistance with activities of daily living. Frequently disoriented with regard to time (date, year, and season). Recall for recent events is severely impaired. May forget some details of past life and names of family and friends. Functioning may fluctuate from day to day. Patient generally denies problems. May become suspicious or tearful. Loses ability to drive safely. Agitation, paranoia, and delusions are common
Severe (MMSE score 9–0)	Patient loses ability to speak, walk, and feed self. Incontinent of urine and feces. Requires care 24 hours a day, 7 days a week

(MMSE, Mini-Mental State Examination.)

DIAGNOSIS

- The National Institute on Aging and the Alzheimer's Association view AD as a spectrum beginning with an asymptomatic preclinical phase progressing to the symptomatic preclinical phase and then to the dementia phase. AD is a clinical diagnosis, based largely on identified symptoms and difficulty with activities of daily living revealed by patient and caregiver interviews.
- In the future, improved brain imaging and validated biomarkers of disease will enable a more sophisticated diagnosis with identified cognitive strengths and weaknesses and neuroanatomic localization of deficits.
- Patients with suspected AD should have a history and physical examination with appropriate laboratory tests (serum B_{12}, folate, thyroid panel, blood cell counts, serum electrolytes, and liver function tests), and computed tomography or magnetic resonance imaging may aid diagnosis. To exclude other diagnoses, cerebrospinal fluid analysis or an electroencephalogram can occasionally be justified.
- Obtain information on medication use; alcohol or other substance use; family medical history; and history of trauma, depression, or head injury. Rule out medication use (eg, anticholinergics, sedatives, hypnotics, opioids, antipsychotics, and anticonvulsants) as contributors to dementia symptoms. Rule out medications that could contribute to delirium (eg, digoxin, nonsteroidal anti-inflammatory drugs [NSAIDs], histamine 2 [H_2] receptor antagonists, amiodarone, antihypertensives, and corticosteroids).
- The Folstein Mini-Mental State Examination (MMSE) can help establish a history of deficits in two or more areas of cognition at baseline against which to evaluate change in severity over time. The average expected decline in an untreated patient is 2 to 4 points per year.

TREATMENT

- <u>Goals of Treatment</u>: The goal of treatment in AD is to maintain cognitive functioning and activities of daily living as long as possible, with a secondary goal to treat the psychiatric and behavioral symptoms.
- For mild to moderate AD, consider use of a cholinesterase inhibitor, and titrate to maintenance dose. For moderate to severe AD, consider adding memantine, and titrate to maintenance dose. Alternatively, consider memantine or cholinesterase

inhibitor alone. Treat behavioral symptoms with support and behavioral interventions, and use pharmacological management only if necessary.

NONPHARMACOLOGIC THERAPY

- Sleep disturbances, wandering, urinary incontinence, agitation, and aggression should be managed with behavioral and environmental interventions whenever possible, for example, redirecting the patient's attention and removing stressors and triggers.
- On initial diagnosis, the patient and caregiver should be educated on the course of illness, available treatments, legal decisions, changes in lifestyle that will become necessary, and other quality-of-life issues.

PHARMACOTHERAPY OF COGNITIVE SYMPTOMS

- Primary prevention of AD may include smoking cessation, increasing physical activity, and reducing midlife obesity, hypertension, and diabetes. Also adherence to the Mediterranean Diet or Dietary Approaches to Stop Hypertension Diet may reduce the risk of cognitive impairment or decline.
- Reasonable expectations of treatment may be a slowed decline in abilities and delayed long-term care placement.
- Those who respond to treatment may lose the benefits when medication is stopped.

Cholinesterase Inhibitors

- Table 52–2 summarizes dosing of the cholinesterase inhibitors and **memantine**.
- No comparative trials have assessed the effectiveness of one agent over another. **Donepezil**, **rivastigmine**, and **galantamine** are indicated in mild to moderate AD; donepezil is also indicated for severe AD.
- MMSE is practical to use in the clinical setting to measure changes in cognitive function. Successful treatment would show a decline in MMSE score of less than 2 points per year.
- The three cholinesterase inhibitors have similar efficacy in mild to moderate AD, and duration of benefit lasts 3 to 24 months. Because of their short half-lives, if rivastigmine or galantamine treatment is interrupted for several days or longer, retitrate starting at the lowest dose. Gradual dose titration over several months improves tolerability.
- The most frequent adverse effects include mild to moderate gastrointestinal (GI) symptoms (nausea, vomiting, and diarrhea), urinary incontinence, dizziness, headache, syncope, bradycardia, muscle weakness, salivation, and sweating. Abrupt discontinuation can cause worsening of cognition and behavior in some patients. Table 52–3 shows side effects and monitoring parameters.

Other Drugs

- **Memantine** (Namenda) blocks glutamatergic neurotransmission by antagonizing N-methyl-D-aspartate receptors, which may prevent excitotoxic reactions. It is used as monotherapy and in combination with a cholinesterase inhibitor. It is indicated for treatment of moderate to severe AD, but not for mild AD. It is not metabolized by the liver but is primarily excreted unchanged in the urine. Dosing must be adjusted in patients with renal impairment. It is usually well tolerated; side effects include constipation, confusion, dizziness, and headache.
- Trials do not support the use of **estrogen** to prevent or treat dementia.
- **Vitamin E** is under investigation for prevention of AD and is not recommended for treatment of AD.
- Because of the incidence of side effects and a lack of supporting evidence, neither **NSAIDs** nor **prednisone** is recommended for treatment or prevention of AD.
- Trials of *statin* drugs have not shown significant benefit in prevention or treatment of AD.

TABLE 52-2	Dosing of Drugs Used for Cognitive Symptoms				
Drug	Brand Name	Initial Dose	Usual Range	Special Population Dose	Other
Cholinesterase inhibitors					
Donepezil	Aricept, Aricept ODT	5 mg daily in the evening	5–10 mg daily in mild to moderate AD 10–23 mg daily in moderate to severe AD	No dosage adjustments recommended	Available as: tablet, ODT Can be taken with or without food Weight loss associated with 23 mg daily dose
Rivastigmine	Exelon, Exelon Patch	1.5 mg twice daily (capsule, oral solution) 4.6 mg/day (transdermal patch)	3–6 mg twice a day (capsule, oral solution) 9.5–13.3 mg/day (transdermal patch)	Capsule/oral solution: Renal impairment, hepatic impairment, or low body weight (≤50 kg [<110 lb]): Patients may be able to only tolerate lower doses Transdermal patch: Mild to moderate hepatic impairment or low body weight: consider maximum daily dose of 4.6 mg every 24 hours	Available as: capsule, oral solution, transdermal patch Take with meals Also indicated for Parkinson disease dementia Application of multiple transdermal patches at same time associated with hospitalization and death
Galantamine	Razadyne, Razdyne ER	4 mg twice daily (tablet, oral solution) 8 mg daily in the morning (extended-release capsule)	8–12 mg twice a day (tablet, oral solution) 16–24 mg (extended-release capsule)	Moderate renal or hepatic impairment: maximum daily dose of 16 mg Severe renal or hepatic impairment: not recommended	Available as: tablet, oral solution, extended-release capsule Take with meals

N-methyl-D-aspartate (NMDA) receptor antagonist

Memantine	Namenda, Namenda XR	5 mg daily 7 mg daily (extended-release capsule)	10 mg twice daily 28 mg daily (extended-release capsule)	Severe renal impairment: recommended maintenance dose of 5 mg twice daily (tablet, oral solution) or 14 mg daily (extended-release capsule) Severe hepatic impairment: administer with caution	Available as: tablet, oral solution, extended-release capsule Can be taken with or without food Can open extended-release capsule and sprinkle contents on applesauce for ease of administration

Cholinesterase inhibitor + NMDA receptor antagonist

Memantine + Donepezil	Namzaric	28 mg/10 mg	14–28 mg/10 mg daily	Severe renal impairment: 14 mg/10 mg daily	Available as: memantine extended-release and donepezil capsule Can be taken with or without food Can open capsule and sprinkle contents on applesauce for ease of administration

(ODT, orally disintegrating tablet.)

TABLE 52-3 Monitoring Drug Therapy for Cognitive Symptoms

Drug	Adverse Drug Reaction	Monitoring Parameter	Comments
Galantamine	Serious skin reactions (Stevens-Johnson syndrome and acute generalized exanthematous pustulosis)	Appearance of skin rash	Discontinue galantamine at first sign of skin rash, unless clearly not drug-related If signs/symptoms are suggestive of a serious reaction, consider alternative treatment and do not rechallenge
Rivastigmine	Allergic dermatitis	Application site reaction spread beyond patch size, evidence of a more intense local reaction (increasing erythema, edema, papules, vesicles), and if symptoms do not improve within 48 hours of patch removal	Discontinue rivastigmine if evidence of disseminated allergic dermatitis appears Patients sensitized by exposure to the transdermal patch may not be able to take rivastigmine by mouth either; allergy testing and close medical supervision recommended
Cholinesterase inhibitors	Dizziness, syncope, bradycardia, atrial arrhythmias, myocardial infarction, angina, seizures, sinoatrial and atrioventricular block	Report of dizziness or falls, pulse, blood pressure, and postural blood pressure change	Dizziness is usually mild, transient, and not related to cardiovascular problems Routine pulse checks at baseline, monthly during titration, and every 6 months thereafter
Cholinesterase inhibitors	Nausea, vomiting, diarrhea, anorexia, and weight loss	Weight and GI complaints	Take with food to decrease GI upset Usually transient, dose-related GI adverse effects seen with drug initiation, dosage titration, or drug switch Debilitated patients or those weighing <55 kg (<121 lb) may be more likely to experience GI adverse effects and significant weight loss, particularly when rivastigmine is prescribed or when titrating to donepezil 23 mg GI adverse effects less prominent with transdermal versus oral rivastigmine

Cholinesterase inhibitors	Peptic ulcer disease, GI bleeding	Signs or symptoms of active or occult GI bleeding	Of particular concern for patients at increased risk of developing ulcers, such as those with a history of ulcer disease or concurrently taking NSAIDs
Cholinesterase inhibitors	Insomnia, vivid/abnormal dreams, nightmares	Complaints of sleep disturbances, daytime drowsiness	Donepezil can be taken in the morning to decrease risk of sleep disturbances
Memantine	Headache, confusion, dizziness, hallucinations	Report of dizziness or falls, hallucinations	Confusion may be observed during dose titration and is usually transient
Memantine			Memantine may mitigate GI adverse effects associated with cholinesterase inhibitor therapy
Memantine	Constipation	GI complaints	

(NSAIDs, nonsteroidal antiinflammatory drugs.)

- Because of limited efficacy data, the potential for adverse effects (eg, nausea, vomiting, diarrhea, headache, dizziness, restlessness, weakness, and hemorrhage), and poor standardization of herbal products, **ginkgo biloba** is not recommended for prevention or treatment of AD.
- Do not use ginkgo biloba in individuals taking anticoagulants or antiplatelet drugs, and use cautiously in those taking **NSAIDs**.
- **Huperzine A** has not been adequately evaluated and is not currently recommended for treatment of AD.

PHARMACOTHERAPY OF NONCOGNITIVE SYMPTOMS

- Pharmacotherapy for noncognitive symptoms targets psychotic symptoms, inappropriate or disruptive behavior, and depression.
- General guidelines include the following: (1) Use environmental interventions first and pharmacotherapy only when necessary; (2) identify and correct underlying causes of disruptive behaviors when possible; (3) start with reduced doses and titrate slowly; (4) monitor closely; (5) periodically attempt to taper and discontinue medication; and (6) document carefully.
- Avoid anticholinergic psychotropic medications as they may worsen cognition.

Cholinesterase Inhibitors and Memantine

- **Cholinesterase inhibitors** and **memantine**, individually or in combination, have shown modest improvement of behavioral symptoms over time, but may not significantly reduce acute agitation.

Antipsychotics

- Antipsychotic medications have traditionally been used for disruptive behaviors and neuropsychiatric symptoms, but the risks and benefits must be carefully weighed.
- A meta-analysis found that only 17% to 18% of dementia patients showed a modest treatment response with atypical antipsychotics. Adverse events (eg, somnolence, extrapyramidal symptoms, abnormal gait, worsening cognition, cerebrovascular events, and increased risk of death [see black-box warning]) offset advantages. Another systematic review and meta-analysis found small but significant improvement in behavioral symptom scores in patients treated with **aripiprazole**, **olanzapine**, and **risperidone**.
- Typical antipsychotics may also produce a small increased risk of death, and more severe extrapyramidal effects and hypotension than the atypicals.
- Antipsychotic treatment in AD patients should rarely be continued beyond 12 weeks.

Antidepressants

- Depression and dementia share many symptoms, and the diagnosis of depression can be difficult, especially later in the course of AD.
- **A selective serotonin reuptake inhibitor** (SSRI) is usually given to depressed patients with AD, and the best evidence is for **sertraline** and **citalopram**. **Tricyclic antidepressants** are usually avoided.

Miscellaneous Therapies

- Use of **benzodiazepines** is not advised except on an "as needed" basis for infrequent episodes of agitation.
- **Carbamazepine**, **valproic acid**, and **gabapentin** may be alternatives for agitation, but evidence is conflicting.

EVALUATION OF THERAPEUTIC OUTCOMES

- At baseline interview both patient and caregiver to identify target symptoms; define therapeutic goals; and document cognitive status, physical status, functional performance, mood, thought processes, and behavior.

- Use the MMSE for cognition, Bristol Activities of Daily Living Scale for activities of daily living, and Neuropsychiatric Inventory Questionnaire for assessment of behavioral disturbances to quantify changes in symptoms and functioning.
- Observe the patient carefully for potential side effects. The specific side effects to be monitored and the method and frequency of monitoring should be documented.
- Assess for drug effectiveness, side effects, adherence to regimen, and need for dosage adjustment or change in treatment after 1 month and at least every 6 months thereafter. Several months to 1 year of treatment may be required to determine whether medications for cognition are beneficial.

See Chapter 54, Alzheimer Disease, authored by Emily P. Peron, Patricia W. Slattum, Kacie E. Powers, and Sarah E. Hobgood, for a more detailed discussion of this topic.

53 Epilepsy

- *Epilepsy* is defined by the occurrence of at least two unprovoked seizures with or without convulsions (ie, violent, involuntary contraction[s] of the voluntary muscles) separated by at least 24 hours, often with neurobiological, cognitive, psychological, and social consequences. A seizure results from an excessive discharge of cortical neurons and is characterized by changes in electrical activity as measured by the electroencephalogram (EEG).

PATHOPHYSIOLOGY

- Seizures result from excessive excitation or from disordered inhibition of neurons. Initially, a small number of neurons fire abnormally. Normal membrane conductances and inhibitory synaptic currents then break down, and excitability spreads locally (focal seizure) or more widely (generalized seizure). Epileptic seizures result only when there is also synchronization of excessive neuronal firing.
- Mechanisms that may contribute to synchronous hyperexcitability include (1) alterations of ion channels in neuronal membranes, (2) biochemical modifications of receptors, (3) modulation of second messaging systems and gene expression, (4) changes in extracellular ion concentrations, (5) alterations in vesicle trafficking and neurotransmitter release, (6) alterations in neurotransmitter uptake and metabolism, and (7) modification in the ratio and function of inhibitory circuits.

CLINICAL PRESENTATION

- Table 53–1 shows the International League Against Epilepsy (ILAE) classification of electroclinical syndromes and other epilepsies. Figure 53–1 shows the ILAE terminology for classification of seizures.
- Many patients, particularly those with focal onset seizures with dyscognitive features or generalized tonic-clonic (GTC) seizures, are amnestic to the actual seizure event.

SYMPTOMS AND SIGNS

- Symptoms depend on seizure type and where the abnormal firing occurs. Although seizures can vary between patients, they tend to be stereotyped within an individual.
- Focal seizures (ie, partial seizures) begin in one hemisphere of the brain, and unless they become secondarily generalized (ie, evolve to a bilateral convulsive seizure), result in an asymmetric seizure. Focal seizures manifest as alterations in motor functions (eg, twitching or shaking), sensory (eg, numbness or tingling) or somatosensory symptoms, aberrations in behavior, or automatisms. Focal seizures without dyscognitive features (formerly called simple partial seizures) are associated with no impairment of consciousness. In focal seizures with dyscognitive features (formerly called complex partial seizures), there is impairment of consciousness and awareness and no memory of the event.
- Absence seizures generally occur in young children or adolescents and exhibit a sudden onset, interruption of ongoing activities, a blank stare, and possibly a brief upward rotation of the eyes. There is only a very brief (seconds) period of altered consciousness. Absence seizures have a characteristic two to four cycles per second spike and slow-wave EEG pattern.
- GTC seizures are major convulsive episodes and are always associated with a loss of consciousness. Motor symptoms are bilateral. GTC seizures may be preceded by premonitory symptoms (ie, an aura). A tonic-clonic seizure that is preceded by an aura is likely a focal seizure that is secondarily generalized. Tonic-clonic seizures begin with a short tonic contraction of muscles followed by a period of rigidity and clonic movements. The patient may lose sphincter control, bite the tongue, or become cyanotic. The episode is frequently followed by a deep sleep.

TABLE 53–1	2010 ILAE Electroclinical Syndromes and Other Epilepsies

I. **Electroclinical Syndromes** (and common examples arranged by age at onset)
Infancy:
   West Syndrome
   Dravet Syndrome
Childhood:
   Febrile Seizure Plus (FS+)
   Lennox-Gastaut Syndrome
   Childhood Absence Epilepsy
Adolescent-Adult:
   Juvenile Myoclonic Epilepsy (JME)
   Progressive Myoclonic Epilepsy (PME—including Lafora)
   Epilepsy with Generalized Tonic-Clonic Seizures Alone

II. **Distinctive Constellations** (and common example):
Mesial Temporal Lobe Epilepsy with Hippocampal Sclerosis

III. **Epilepsies Attributed to and Organized by Structural-Metabolic Causes** (and common examples):
Malformations of Cortical Development
Tuberous Sclerosis
Tumor
Trauma
Strokes

IV. **Epilepsies of Unknown Cause**

- Interictally (between seizure episodes), there are typically no objective, pathognomonic signs of epilepsy.
- Myoclonic seizures are brief shock-like muscular contractions (jerks) of the face, trunk, and extremities. They may be isolated events or rapidly repetitive. There is no alteration of consciousness.
- In atonic seizures (the hallmark of Lennox-Gastaut Syndrome), there is a sudden loss of muscle tone that may be described as a head drop, dropping of a limb, or slumping to the ground.

DIAGNOSIS

- Ask the patient and family to characterize the seizure for signs/symptoms, triggers, frequency, duration, precipitating factors, time of occurrence, presence of an aura, impairment of consciousness, ictal activity, and postictal state.
- Physical and neurologic examination and laboratory examination may identify an etiology.
- According to ILAE, a person is considered to have epilepsy if they have (1) at least 2 unprovoked (or reflex) seizures occurring greater than 24 hours apart; (2) one unprovoked (or reflex) seizure and a probability of further seizures of at least 60% after 2 unprovoked seizures, occurring over the next 10 years; or (3) a diagnosis of an epilepsy syndrome.

LABORATORY TESTS

- In some cases, particularly following GTC seizures, serum prolactin levels may be transiently elevated. A serum prolactin level obtained within 10 to 20 minutes of a tonic-clonic seizure can help differentiate seizure activity from pseudoseizure activity but not from syncope.
- Laboratory tests (SMA-20 [sequential multichannel analysis], complete blood cell count, urinalysis, and special blood chemistries) may be done to rule out treatable causes of seizures (hypoglycemia, altered serum electrolyte concentrations, infections, etc.) that do not represent epilepsy. A lumbar puncture may be indicated if there is fever.

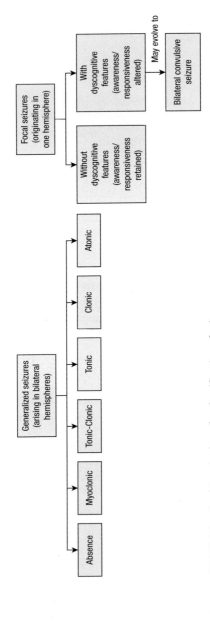

FIGURE 53−1. 2010 ILAE revised terminology for classification of seizures.

OTHER DIAGNOSTIC TESTS

• EEG is very useful in the diagnosis of various seizure disorders, but epileptiform activity is found in only about 50% of patients with epilepsy.
• Although magnetic resonance imaging is very useful (especially imaging of the temporal lobes), computed tomography typically is not helpful except in the initial evaluation for a brain tumor, cerebral bleeding, or gross anatomic injury.

TREATMENT

• <u>Goals of Treatment</u>: The goals are to control or reduce the frequency and severity of seizures, minimize side effects, and ensure compliance, allowing the patient to live as normal a life as possible. Complete suppression of seizures must be balanced against tolerability of side effects, and the patient should be involved in defining the balance. Side effects and comorbidities (eg, anxiety and depression) as well as social issues (eg, driving, job security, relationships, and social stigma) have significant impact on quality of life.

GENERAL APPROACH

• Drug selection depends on the seizure type and epilepsy classification (Table 53–2), drug-specific adverse effects, patient characteristics, and insurance coverage. Figure 53–2 is a suggested algorithm for treatment of epilepsy.
• Begin with monotherapy. About 65% of patients can be maintained on one antiseizure drug (ASD), although not necessarily seizure free.
• Up to 60% of patients with epilepsy are noncompliant; this is the most common reason for treatment failure.
• Some initiate ASDs after one unprovoked seizure, other do so after one unprovoked seizure with an abnormal epileptiform EEG. Others wait until a second unprovoked seizure has occurred. Patients who have had two or more seizures should generally be started on ASDs.
• Provide the patient with a seizure and side effect diary.
• Initiate ASD with a low dose, and titrate gradually to a moderate dose. If seizures continue, titrate to a maximum dose. If the first ASD is ineffective or causes intolerable side effects, add a second ASD (preferably with a different mechanism of action), and then taper and discontinue the ineffective or intolerable drug. If the second ASD is ineffective, then polytherapy may be indicated.
• Start at a lower dose and titrate more slowly in elderly patients.
• Factors favoring successful withdrawal of ASDs include a seizure-free period of 2 to 4 years, complete seizure control within 1 year of onset, an onset of seizures after age 2 years and before age 35 years, and a normal EEG and neurologic examination. Factors favoring an unsuccessful withdrawal of ASDs include a history of a high frequency of seizures, repeated episodes of status epilepticus, a combination of seizure types, and development of abnormal mental functioning. According to the American Academy of Neurology Guidelines, discontinuation of ASDs may be considered in patients seizure free for 2 to 5 years, if there is a single type of focal seizure or primary generalized seizures, if the neurologic examination and IQ are normal, and if the EEG normalized with treatment. Always withdraw ASDs gradually.

MECHANISM OF ACTION

• The mechanism of action of most ASDs includes effects on ion channel (sodium and Ca) kinetics, augmentation of inhibitory neurotransmission (increasing CNS GABA), and modulation of excitatory neurotransmission (decreasing or antagonizing glutamate and aspartate). ASDs effective against GTC and focal seizures probably work by delaying recovery of sodium channels from activation. Drugs that reduce corticothalamic T-type Ca currents are effective against generalized absence seizures.

TABLE 53–2	Drugs of Choice for Specific Seizure Disorders		
Seizure Type	**Effective Drugs[a]**	**Alternative Drugs[b]**	**Comments**
Focal onset seizures (newly diagnosed)			
US Guidelines	*Adults and adolescents:* Carbamazepine Gabapentin Oxcarbazepine Phenobarbital Phenytoin Topiramate Valproic acid		*FDA approved:* Carbamazepine Lacosamide Phenobarbital Phenytoin Topiramate Valproic acid
ILAE Guidelines	*Adults:* Carbamazepine Phenytoin* Valproic acid* Levetiracetam Zonisamide *Children:* Oxcarbazepine *Elderly:* Gabapentin Lamotrigine	*Adults:* Gabapentin Lamotrigine Oxcarbazepine Phenobarbital Topiramate Vigabatrin *Children:* Phenobarbital Phenytoin Topiramate Valproic acid Carbamazepine *Elderly:* Carbamazepine	*Potentially efficacious* Carbamazepine Primidone *side effects make these ASDs unpopular first choices *Potentially efficacious* Clonazepam Clobazam Lamotrigine Vigabatrin Zonisamide *Potentially efficacious:* Topiramate Valproic acid
U.S. Expert Panel 2005	Carbamazepine Lamotrigine Oxcarbazepine	Levetiracetam	
Focal onset seizures (refractory monotherapy)			
US Guidelines	Lamotrigine Oxcarbazepine Topiramate		*FDA approved:* Carbamazepine Lamotrigine Oxcarbazepine Phenobarbital Phenytoin Topiramate Valproic acid
Focal onset seizures (refractory adjunct)			
US Guidelines	*Adults:* Gabapentin Lamotrigine Levetiracetam Oxcarbazepine Tiagabine Topiramate Zonisamide *Children:* Gabapentin Lamotrigine Oxcarbazepine Topiramate		*FDA approved:* Carbamazepine Gabapentin Lamotrigine Levetiracetam Oxcarbazepine Phenobarbital Phenytoin Pregabalin Tiagabine Valproic acid Vigabatrin Zonisamide

(continued)

TABLE 53–2	Drugs of Choice for Specific Seizure Disorders *(Continued)*		
Seizure Type	**Effective Drugs[a]**	**Alternative Drugs[b]**	**Comments**
Generalized seizures absence (newly diagnosed)			
US Guidelines	Lamotrigine		*FDA approved:* Ethosuximide Valproic acid
ILAE Guidelines	Ethosuximide Valproic acid	Lamotrigine	Gabapentin is ineffective
US Expert Panel 2005	Ethosuximide Valproic acid	Lamotrigine	
Generalized onset (tonic-clonic)			
US Guidelines	Topiramate		*FDA approved:* Lamotrigine Levetiracetam Topiramate Perampanel
ILAE Guidelines	*Adults* None	*Adults:* Carbamazepine* Lamotrigine Oxcarbazepine Phenobarbital Phenytoin* Topiramate Valproic acid *Children:* Carbamazepine* Phenobarbital Phenytoin* Topiramate Valproic acid	*may precipitate other generalized seizures—use w/caution *Potential Efficacy:* Oxcarbazepine *may precipitate other generalized seizures—use w/caution
US Expert Panel 2005		Lamotrigine Topiramate	
Juvenile myoclonic epilepsy			
ILAE Guidelines	None	Clonazepam Lamotrigine Levetiracetam Valproic acid Zonisamide	
US Expert Panel 2005	Valproic acid	Levetiracetam Topiramate Zonisamide	

(ILAE, International League Against Epilepsy.)
[a]Includes probably effective drugs based on Level A or B evidence.
[b]Includes possibly effective drugs based on less than Level A or B evidence.

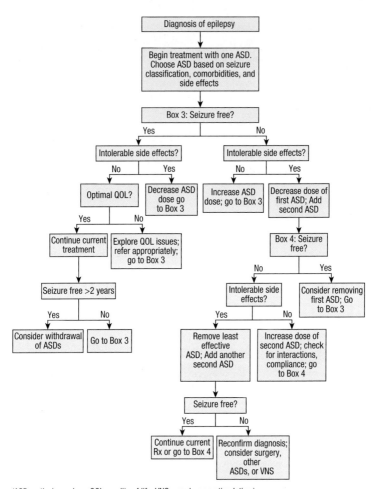

(ASD, antiseizure drug; QOL, quality of life; VNS, vagal nerve stimulation.)

FIGURE 53-2. Algorithm for the treatment of epilepsy.

SPECIAL CONSIDERATIONS IN THE FEMALE PATIENT

- **Estrogen** has a seizure-activating effect, whereas **progesterone** has a seizure-protective effect. Enzyme-inducing ASDs (eg, **phenobarbital**, **phenytoin**, **carbamazepine**, **topiramate**, **oxcarbazepine**, and perhaps **rufinamide**, **lamotrigine**, **clobazam**, and **felbamate**) may cause treatment failures in women taking **oral contraceptives**; a supplemental form of birth control is advised if breakthrough bleeding occurs. It is suggested that women taking these ASDs should take twice the usual dose of emergency contraception.
- For catamenial epilepsy (seizures just before or during menses) or seizures that occur at the time of ovulation, conventional ASDs should be tried first, but intermittent supplementation with higher-dose ASDs or benzodiazepines should be considered. **Acetazolamide** has been used with limited success. **Progestational agents** may also be effective.

- Seizures often improve in frequency at menopause.
- Women with epilepsy who are seizure free for 9 to 12 months before becoming pregnant have an 84% to 92% chance of being seizure free during pregnancy. Fluctuations in ASD serum concentrations during pregnancy may be due to reduced gastric motility, nausea and vomiting, increased drug distribution, increased renal elimination, altered hepatic enzyme activity, or changes in protein binding.
- ASD monotherapy is preferred in pregnancy. Clearance of **phenytoin**, **carbamazepine**, **lamotrigine**, **oxcarbazepine**, and **levetiracetam**, increases during pregnancy, and protein binding may be reduced. Serum concentrations of **phenobarbital**, **primidone**, **ethosuximide**, and **valproic** acid may also fluctuate during pregnancy. Serum concentrations of ASDs, especially **lamotrigine**, should be monitored closely during pregnancy. There is a higher incidence of adverse pregnancy outcomes in women taking ASDs, including an increased risk of major congenital malformations (MCMs).
- **Valproic acid** is associated with a risk of MCMs 3.5 to 4 times that of offspring of nonepileptic women. There is also an increased risk of neurodevelopmental effects including effects on cognition in children exposed to valproic acid in utero. **Valproic** acid should not be used in pregnancy, but when it is used, doses should not exceed 500 to 600 mg/day.
- **Topiramate** use during pregnancy has been associated with cleft palate and possibly low birth weight and hypospadias.
- Teratogenic effects may possibly be prevented by adequate folate intake, although strong evidence is lacking. Prenatal vitamins with folic acid (0.4–5 mg/day) are recommended for women of child-bearing potential taking ASDs. Higher folate doses should be used in women who have previously delivered a child with a neural tube defect and women who are taking **valproic** acid.
- ASDs with low protein binding will accumulate in breast milk.
- Other adverse outcomes of maternal seizures are growth, psychomotor, and mental retardation. **Vitamin K**, 10 mg/day orally, given to the woman during the last month of pregnancy may prevent neonatal hemorrhagic disorder. Alternatively, parenteral vitamin K can be given to the newborn at delivery.

PHARMACOKINETICS AND SPECIAL POPULATIONS

- ASD pharmacokinetic data are summarized in Table 53–3. For populations known to have altered plasma protein binding, measure free rather than total serum concentrations if the ASD is highly protein bound. Conditions altering ASD protein binding include chronic renal failure, liver disease, hypoalbuminemia, burns, pregnancy, malnutrition, displacing drugs, and age (neonates and the elderly). Unbound concentration monitoring is especially useful for **phenytoin**.
- Neonates and infants display decreased efficiency in renal elimination and may metabolize drugs more slowly, but by age 2 or 3 years children may metabolize drugs more rapidly than adults. Thus, neonates and infants require lower doses of ASD, but children require higher doses of many ASDs than adults.
- Lower doses of ASDs are often required in the elderly due to compromised renal or hepatic function. Some elderly patients have increased receptor sensitivity to CNS drugs, making the accepted therapeutic range invalid. The elderly often take many medications, and thus are more prone to experience neurocognitive effects and drug–drug interactions involving ASDs that affect the CPY450 system (eg, **carbamazepine**, **phenytoin**, **valproic acid**, and **phenobarbital**). Hypoalbuminemia is common in the elderly, and highly bound ASDs (eg, **valproic acid**) can be problematic. They also experience body mass changes which can affect elimination half-life and volume of distribution. **Lamotrigine** is often considered a drug of choice for elderly patients with focal onset seizures because of effectiveness and tolerability.

TABLE 53-3	Antiseizure Drug Pharmacokinetic Data					
ASD	$t_{1/2}$ (Hours)	Time to Steady State (Days)	Unchanged (%)	V_D (L/kg)	Clinically Important Metabolite	Protein Binding (%)
Carbamazepine	12 M; 5–14 Co	21–28 for completion of autoinduction	<1	1–2	10,11-epoxide	40–90
Clobazam	36–42	7–14	3	1.4	N-desmethylclobazam	80–90
Eslicarbazepine	13–20	4–5	67%	0.87	oxcarbazepine	<40
Ethosuximide	A 60; C 30	6–12	10–20	0.67	No	0
Ezogabine	7–11	3–4	36%	2–3	n-Acetyl metabolite	80
Felbamate	16–22	5–7	50	0.73–0.82	No	~25
Gabapentin[a]	5–40[b]	1–2	100	0.65–1.04	No	0
Lacosamide	13	3	40	0.6	No	<15
Lamotrigine	25.4 M	3–15	10	1.28	No	40–50
Levetiracetam	7–10	2		0.7	No	<10
Oxcarbazepine	3–13	2		0.7	10-Hydroxycarbazepine	40
Perampanel	105	14–21	74–80	77 L	No	95%–96%
Phenobarbital	A 46–136; C 37–73	14–21	20–40	0.6	No	50
Phenytoin	A 10–34; C 5–14	7–28	<5	0.6–8.0	No	90
Pregabalin	A 6–7[b]	1–2	90	0.5	No	0
Primidone	A 3.3–19; C 4.5–11	1–4	40	0.43–1.1	PB	20
Rufinamide	6–10	2	4	0.8–1.2	No	26–35

Tiagabine	5–13		Negligible		No	95
Topiramate	18–21	4–5	50–70	0.55–0.8 (male); 0.23–0.4 (female)	No	15
Valproic acid	A 8–20; C 7–14	1–3	<5	0.1–0.5	May contribute to toxicity	90–95 binding saturates
Vigabatrin	5–8	N/A	80	0.8	No	0
Zonisamide	24–60	5–15	35	0.8–1.6	No	40–60

(A, adult; ASD, antiseizure drug; C, child; Co, combination therapy; M, monotherapy; N/A, not applicable since effect depends on inhibiting enzyme; PB, phenobarbital; V_d, volume of distribution.)

[a]The bioavailability of gabapentin is dose-dependent.

[b]Half-life depends on renal function.

THE ROLE OF SERUM CONCENTRATION MONITORING

- Table 53–4 shows dosing and target serum concentration ranges for ASDs. Seizure control may occur before the "minimum" of the therapeutic serum range is reached, and some patients may need serum concentrations beyond the "maximum." The therapeutic range for ASDs may be different for different seizure types (eg, higher for focal seizures with dyscognitive features than for GTC seizures). Clinicians should determine the optimal serum concentration for each patient. Serum concentration determinations can be useful to document lack of or loss of efficacy, establish noncompliance, and guide therapy in patients with renal and/or hepatic disease and patients taking multiple drugs, as well as in women who are pregnant or taking **oral contraceptives**.

EFFICACY

- Many newer ASDs have been tested only as adjunctive therapy, but many providers will use them off-label as monotherapy.
- Evidence for comparable effectiveness is mostly available for older agents and for a few newer ones. In general, the newer ASDs appear to have comparable efficacy to the older drugs, and some may be better tolerated.
- **Carbamazepine, ethosuximide, gabapentin, levetiracetam, oxcarbazepine, phenytoin valproic acid**, and **zonisamide** have strong enough evidence to be labeled efficacious or effective or as probably efficacious or effective as initial monotherapy in certain seizure types.
- Some ASDs may possibly precipitate or aggravate certain seizure types, and it is suggested that they be used with caution in those patients. Examples are **carbamazepine, gabapentin, oxcarbazepine, phenytoin, tiagabine**, and **vigabatrin** in children with absence or juvenile myoclonic epilepsy.
- After 12 months of treatment, the percentage who are seizure free is highest for those with only GTC seizures (48%–55%), lowest for those who have only focal seizures (23%–26%), and intermediate for those with mixed seizure types (25%–32%).
- Drug resistance is defined as failure of adequate trials of two tolerated and appropriately chosen and used ASD schedules (whether as monotherapies or in combination) to achieve sustained seizure freedom.

ADVERSE EFFECTS

- ASD side effects and monitoring are shown in Table 53–5. Concentration-dependent side effects can often be alleviated by decreasing the dose or avoided by increasing the dose very slowly.
- CNS side effects are frequent and include sedation, dizziness, blurred vision, poor concentration and ataxia.
- **Barbiturates** can cause more cognitive impairment than other ASDs, but in children, they can cause paradoxical excitement. In general, the newer agents have less effect on cognition, except topiramate.
- The most widely recognized idiosyncratic reactions are ASD-induced drug rashes, which can progress to Stevens-Johnson Syndrome/toxic epidermal necrolysis. Others are hepatitis, blood dyscrasias, and acute organ failure.
- When acute organ failure occurs, it usually happens within the first 6 months of ASD therapy.
- Studies have found that there is a strong association between the presence of an inherited variant of the HLA-B gene, HLA-B*1502, in Asians and south Asians, and the risk of developing Stevens–Johnson syndrome as well as toxic epidermal necrolysis with **carbamazepine** (and possibly **phenytoin, lamotrigine**, and **oxcarbazepine**). This variant is found in up to 15% of individuals of Asian, southeast Asian, and south Asian origin. Patients with this variant should generally avoid these drugs. Also, the HLA genotype HLA-A*3101 is associated with carbamazepine-induced skin reactions in Chinese, Japanese, and European people.

TABLE 53-4	Antiseizure Drug Dosing and Target Serum Concentration Ranges			
Drug	Brand Name	Initial or Starting Dose	Usual Range or Maximum Dose	Comments Target Serum Concentration Range
Barbiturates				
Phenobarbital	Various	1–3 mg/kg/day (10–20 mg/kg LD)	180–300 mg	10–40 mcg/mL[a] (43–172 μmol/L)
Primidone	Mysoline	100–125 mg/day	750–2000 mg	5–10 mcg/mL (23–46 μmol/L)
Benzodiazepines				
Clobazam	Onfi	≤30 kg 5 mg/day; >30 kg 10 mg/day	≤30 kg up to 20 mg; >30 kg up to 40 mg	0.03–0.3 ng/mL (0.1–1.0 nmol/L)
Clonazepam	Klonopin	1.5 mg/day	20 mg	20–70 ng/mL (67–233 pmol/L)
Diazepam	Valium	PO: 4–40 mg IV: 5–10 mg	PO: 4–40 mg IV: 5–30 mg	100–1000 ng/mL (0.4–3.5 μmol/L)
Lorazepam	Ativan	PO: 2–6 mg IV: 0.05 mg/kg IM: 0.05 mg/kg	PO: 10 mg IV: 0.05 mg/kg	10–30 ng/mL (31–93 nmol/L)
Hydantoin				
Phenytoin	Dilantin	PO: 3–5 mg/kg (200–400 mg) (15–20 mg/kg LD)	PO: 300–600 mg	Total: 10–20 mcg/mL (40–79 μmol/L) Unbound: 0.5–3 mcg/mL (2–12 μmol/L)
Succinimide				
Ethosuximide	Zarontin	500 mg/day	500–2000 mg	40–100 mcg/mL (282–708 μmol/L)
Other				
Carbamazepine	Tegretol Tegretol XR	400 mg/day	400–2400 mg	4–12 mcg/mL (17–51 μmol/L)
Eslicarbazepine	Aptiom	400 mg/day	800–1600 mg	Not defined
Ezogabine	Potiga	300 mg/day	1200 mg	Not defined

(continued)

TABLE 53-4 Antiseizure Drug Dosing and Target Serum Concentration Ranges (Continued)

Drug	Brand Name	Initial or Starting Dose	Usual Range or Maximum Dose	Comments Target Serum Concentration Range
Felbamate	Felbatol	1200 mg/day	3600 mg	30–60 mcg/mL (126–252 μmol/L)
Gabapentin	Neurontin	300–900 mg/day	4800 mg	2–20 mcg/mL (12–117 μmol/L)
Lacosamide	Vimpat	100 mg/day	400 mg	Not defined
Lamotrigine	Lamictal Lamictal XR	25 mg every other day if on VPA; 25–50 mg/day if not on VPA	100–150 mg if on VPA; 300–500 mg if not on VPA	4–20 mcg/dL (16–78 μmol/L)
Levetiracetam	Keppra Keppra XR	500–1000 mg/day	3000–4000 mg	12–46 mcg/mL (70–270 μmol/L)
Oxcarbazepine	Trileptal Oxtellar XR	300–600 mg/day	1200–2400 mg	3–35 mcg/mL (MHD) (12–139 μmol/L)
Perampanel	Fycompa	2 mg/day	8–12 mg	Not defined
Pregabalin	Lyrica	150 mg/day	600 mg	Not defined
Rufinamide	Banzel	400–800 mg/day	3200 mg	Not defined
Tiagabine	Gabitril	4–8 mg/day	80 mg	0.02–0.2 mcg/mL (0.05–0.5 μmol/L)
Topiramate	Topamax Trokendi XR	25–50 mg/day	200–1000 mg	5–20 mcg/mL (15–59 μmol/L)
Valproic acid	Depakene Depakote DR/ER Depacon	15 mg/kg (500–1000 mg)	60 mg/kg (3000–5000 mg)	50–100 mcg/mL (347–693 μmol/L)
Vigabatrin	Sabril	1000 mg/day	3000 mg	0.8–36 mcg/mL (6–279 μmol/L)
Zonisamide	Zonegran	100–200 mg/day	600 mg	10–40 mcg/mL (47–188 μmol/L)

(IM, intramuscular; LD, loading does; MHD, 10-monohydroxy-derivative; PO, orally; VPA, valproic acid.)
[a]Units mcg/mL and mg/L are numerically equivalent, and units of ng/mL and mcg/L are numerically equivalent.

TABLE 53-5 Antiseizure Drug Side Effects and Monitoring

Drug	Concentration Dependent	Idiosyncratic	Chronic Side Effects
Carbamazepine	Diplopia Dizziness Drowsiness Nausea Unsteadiness Lethargy	Blood dyscrasias Rash (HLA antigen testing may be relevant to avoid Stevens-Johnson or toxic epidermal necrolysis)	Hyponatremia Metabolic bone disease (monitor Vit D and serum calcium)
Clobazam	Somnolence Sedation Pyrexia Ataxia	Drooling Aggression Irritability Constipation	
Eslicarbazepine	Dizziness Ataxia Somnolence/fatigue Cognitive changes Visual changes	Rash	Hyponatremia
Ethosuximide	Ataxia Drowsiness GI distress (avoid by multiple daily dosing) Unsteadiness Hiccoughs	Blood dyscrasias Rash	Behavior changes Headache

(continued)

TABLE 53-5 Antiseizure Drug Side Effects and Monitoring *(Continued)*

| Drug | Adverse Drug Reaction Acute Side Effects | | Chronic Side Effects |
	Concentration Dependent	Idiosyncratic	
Ezogabine	Dizziness Somnolence Fatigue Confusion Vertigo Tremors Blurred vision	Urinary retention QT prolongation (get baseline ECG and during treatment) Euphoria	Blue gray skin discoloration Retinal abnormalities
Felbamate	Anorexia Nausea Vomiting Insomnia Headache	Aplastic anemia (follow CBC) Acute hepatic failure (follow liver enzymes)	Not established
Gabapentin	Dizziness Fatigue Somnolence Ataxia	Pedal edema	Weight gain
Lacosamide	Dizziness Vertigo Headache Nausea Vomiting PR interval increase (get baseline ECG and during treatment)	Liver enzyme elevation	Not established
Lamotrigine	Diplopia Dizziness Unsteadiness Headache	Rash (slower titration of dose may decrease chance of occurrence)	Not established

Epilepsy | CHAPTER 53

Levetiracetam	Sedation Behavioral disturbance	Psychosis (rare but more common in elderly or persons with mental illness)	Not established
Oxcarbazepine	Sedation Dizziness Ataxia Nausea	Rash	Hyponatremia
Perampanel	Severe behavior changes Dizziness Ataxia/falls Somnolence/fatigues	Rash	Weight gain
Phenobarbital	Ataxia Hyperactivity Headache Unsteadiness Sedation Nausea	Blood dyscrasias Rash	Behavior changes Connective tissue disorders Intellectual blunting Metabolic bone disease Mood change Sedation
Phenytoin	Ataxia Nystagmus Behavior changes Dizziness Headache Incoordination Sedation Lethargy Cognitive impairment Fatigue Visual blurring	Blood dyscrasias Rash (HLA antigen testing may be relevant to avoid Stevens-Johnson or toxic epidermal necrolysis) Immunologic reaction	Behavior changes Cerebellar syndrome (occurs high serum levels) Connective tissue changes Skin thickening Folate deficiency Gingival hyperplasia Hirsutism Coarsening of facial features Acne Cognitive impairment Metabolic bone disease (monitor Vit D and serum calcium) Sedation

(continued)

TABLE 53–5 Antiseizure Drug Side Effects and Monitoring (*Continued*)

Drug	Adverse Drug Reaction Acute Side Effects			Chronic Side Effects
	Concentration Dependent	Idiosyncratic		
Pregabalin	Dizziness Somnolence Incoordination Dry mouth Blurred vision	Pedal edema Creatine kinase elevation Decreased platelets		Weight gain
Primidone	Behavior changes Headache Nausea Sedation Unsteadiness	Blood dyscrasias Rash		Behavior change Connective tissue disorders Cognitive impairment Sedation
Rufinamide	Dizziness Nausea Vomiting Somnolence	Multiorgan hypersensitivity Status epilepticus Leukopenia QT shortening		Not established
Tiagabine	Dizziness Fatigue Difficulties concentrating Nervousness Tremor Blurred vision Depression Weakness	Spike-wave stupor		Not established

Topiramate	Difficulties concentrating Psychomotor slowing Speech or language problems Somnolence, fatigue Dizziness Headache	Metabolic acidosis Acute angle glaucoma Oligohydrosis	Kidney stones Weight loss
Valproic acid	GI upset Sedation Unsteadiness Tremor Thrombocytopenia	Acute hepatic failure Acute pancreatitis Alopecia	Polycystic ovary-like syndrome (increase incidence in females <20 years or overweight) Weight gain Hyperammonemia Menstrual cycle irregularities
Vigabatrin	Permanent vision loss Fatigue Somnolence Weight gain Tremor Blurred vision	Abnormal MRI brain signal changes (infants with infantile spasms) Peripheral neuropathy Anemia	Permanent vision loss (greater frequency, adults vs. children vs. infants)
Zonisamide	Sedation Dizziness Cognitive impairment Nausea	Rash (is a sulfa drug) Metabolic acidosis Oligohydrosis	Kidney stones Weight loss

- Any patient taking ASDs who complains of lethargy, vomiting, fever, or rash should have a laboratory assessment, including white blood cell counts and liver function tests.
- A side effect of long-term use of ASDs is osteomalacia or osteoporosis. It is hypothesized that **phenytoin**, **phenobarbital**, **carbamazepine**, **oxcarbazepine**, **felbamate**, and **valproic acid** may interfere with vitamin D metabolism. Patients taking these drugs should receive vitamin D supplementation and calcium and bone mineral density testing if other risk factors for osteoporosis are present. Laboratory tests may reveal elevated bone-specific alkaline phosphatase and decreased serum Ca and 25-OH vitamin D, as well as intact parathyroid hormone.

DRUG–DRUG INTERACTIONS

- Table 53–6 shows ASD elimination pathways and major effects on hepatic enzymes. Use caution when ASDs are added to or discontinued from a drug regimen. Pharmacokinetic interactions are common complicating factor in ASD selection.
- **Phenobarbital**, **phenytoin**, **primidone**, and **carbamazepine** are potent inducers of cytochrome P450 (CYP450), epoxide hydrolase, and uridine diphosphate glucuronosyltransferase enzyme systems. **Valproic acid** inhibits many hepatic enzyme systems and displaces some drugs from plasma albumin.
- **Felbamate** and **topiramate** can act as inducers with some isoforms and inhibitors with others.

CLINICAL APPLICATION

- ASD dosing is shown in Table 53–4. Tables 53–3, 53–5, and 53–6 show ASD pharmacokinetics, side effects and monitoring, and elimination pathways, respectively.
- Usually dosing is initiated at one-fourth to one-third of the anticipated maintenance dose and gradually increased over 3 to 4 weeks to an effective dose.

Carbamazepine

- Food, especially fat, may enhance the bioavailability of **carbamazepine**.
- Controlled- and sustained-release preparations dosed every 12 hours are bioequivalent to immediate-release preparations dosed every 6 hours. The sustained-release capsule can be opened and sprinkled on food.
- Hyponatremia occurs less frequently than with oxcarbazepine, but periodic serum sodium concentrations are recommended, especially in the elderly.
- Leukopenia is the most common hematologic side effect (up to 10%) but is usually transient. It may be persistent in 2% of patients. Carbamazepine may be continued unless the white blood cell count drops to less than 2500/mm^3 (2.5×10^9/L) and the absolute neutrophil count drops to less than 1000/mm^3 (1×10^9/L).
- Rashes may occur in 10% of patients. Other side effects include nausea, hepatitis, osteomalacia, cardiac conduction defects, and lupus-like reactions.
- Carbamazepine may interact with other drugs by inducing their metabolism. **Valproic acid** increases concentrations of the 10,11-epoxide metabolite without affecting the concentration of carbamazepine. The interaction of **erythromycin** and **clarithromycin** (CYP3A4 inhibition) with carbamazepine is particularly significant. Autoinduction of its own metabolism starts 3–5 days after initiating and is complete in 21 to 28 days. Reversal of autoinduction is rapid after discontinuation.
- Extended-release preparations can be dosed twice daily, but immediate-release preparations must be given four times daily.
- Compared to other first generation ASDs, it causes minimal cognitive impairment.

Clobazam

- Abrupt discontinuation can cause a withdrawal syndrome (eg, behavioral disorder, tremor, anxiety, dysphoria, insomnia, convulsions, and psychosis).
- As an inducer of CYP3A4, **clobazam** may lower serum levels of some oral contraceptives. It is an inhibitor of CYP2D6. In the elderly and poor metabolizers of CYP2C19, initiate dosing as in patients weighing less than 30 kg. Many patients develop some tolerance.

TABLE 53-6 Antiseizure Drug Elimination Pathways and Major Effects on Hepatic Enzymes

Antiepileptic Drugs	Major Hepatic Enzymes	Renal Elimination (%)	Induced	Inhibited
Carbamazepine	CYP3A4; CYP1A2; CYP2C8	<1	CYP1A2; CYP2C; CYP3A; GT	None
Clobazam	CYP3A4; CYP2C19; CYP2B6	0	CYP3A4 (weak)	CYP2D6
Eslicarbazepine	Undergoes hydrolysis	<90% parent drug >60% active metabolite	GT (mild)	CYP2C19
Ethosuximide	CYP3A4	12–20	None	None
Ezogabine	GT; acetylation	85	None	None
Felbamate	CYP3A4; CYP2E1; other	50	CYP3A4	CYP2C19; β-oxidation
Gabapentin	None	Almost completely	None	None
Lacosamide	CYP2C19	70	None	None
Lamotrigine	GT	10	GT	None
Levetiracetam	None (undergoes nonhepatic hydrolysis)	66	None	None
Oxcarbazepine (MHD is active oxcarbazepine metabolite)	Cytosolic system	1 (27 as MHD)	CYP3A4; CYP3A5; GT	CYP2C19
Perampanel	CYP3A4/5; CYP1A2; CYP2B6	Undefined	CYP3A4/5;GT	CYPA3A4/5
Phenobarbital	CYP2C9; other	25	CYP3A; CYP2C; GT	None
Phenytoin	CYP2C9; CYP2C19	5	CYP3A; CYP2C; GT	None
Pregabalin	None	100	None	None
Rufinamide	Hydrolysis	2	CYP3A4 (weak)	CYP2E1 (weak)
Tiagabine	CYP3A4	2	None	None
Topiramate	Not known	70	CYP3A (dose dependent)	CYP2C19
Valproate	GT; β-oxidation	2	None	CYP2C9; GT epoxide hydrolase
Vigabatrin	None	Almost completely	CYP2C9	None
Zonisamide	CYP3A4	35	None	None

(CYP, cytochrome P450 isoenzyme system; GT, glucuronyltransferase.)

- It is more effective than clonazepam for Lennox–Gastaut syndrome but less effective than clonazepam for myoclonic jerks and absence seizures. It is adjunctive treatment for seizures of Lennox–Gastaut syndrome.

Eslicarbazepine

- **Eslicarbazepine** acetate is a prodrug that undergoes hydrolysis to S-licarbazepine, the major active metabolite of oxcarbazepine. It is FDA approved for monotherapy or adjunctive therapy of focal onset seizures.
- It is mostly renally excreted, and dosage adjustment is needed when creatinine clearance is less than 50 mL/min (0.8 mL/s). It may increase the PR interval on the ECG. It causes less hyponatremia than oxcarbazepine.
- It inhibits CYP2C19, and its metabolism is induced by **carbamazepine**, **phenytoin**, **phenobarbital**, and **primidone**.
- It can be dosed once daily.

Ethosuximide

- Titration over 1 to 2 weeks to maintenance doses of 20 mg/kg/day usually produces therapeutic serum concentrations. It is usually given in two equal doses daily.
- There is some evidence for nonlinear metabolism at higher serum concentrations.
- Valproic acid may inhibit metabolism of **ethosuximide**, but only if the metabolism of ethosuximide is near saturation.

Ezogabine

- **Ezogabine** is approved for adjunctive treatment of focal onset seizures, and is recommended only after several alternative drugs have been tried.
- Lower doses are recommended in the elderly.
- It can cause urinary retention and QT prolongation.
- Alcohol may increase systemic exposure to **ezogabine** with an increase in side effects. It can increase **lamotrigine** clearance and reduce digoxin clearance.
- It may cause falsely elevated results on urine and serum bilirubin laboratory tests.
- It must be taken three times daily.

Felbamate

- **Felbamate** is approved as adjunctive treatment for seizures of Lennox–Gastaut syndrome and is effective as monotherapy or adjunctive therapy for focal onset seizures as well. Because of reports of aplastic anemia (1 in 3000 patients) and hepatitis (1 in 10,000 patients), felbamate is recommended only for patients refractory to other ASDs. Risk factors for aplastic anemia may include a history of cytopenia, ASD allergy or toxicity, viral infection, and/or immunologic problems.

Gabapentin

- **Gabapentin** is a second-line agent for patients with focal onset seizures.
- Binding is saturable, causing dose dependent bioavailability. It is eliminated exclusively renally, and dosage adjustment is necessary in patients with impaired renal function.
- Dosing is initiated at 300 mg at bedtime and increased to 300 mg twice daily on the second day and 300 mg three times daily on the third day. Further titrations are then made. When the total daily dose is 3600 mg/day or greater, divide the daily dose into at least four doses.

Lacosamide

- **Lacosamide** is a schedule V controlled substance approved as adjunctive therapy in patients 17 years old or greater with focal onset seizures.
- There is a linear relationship between daily doses and serum concentrations up to 800 mg/day. Moderate hepatic and renal impairment both increase systemic drug exposure by up to 40%.

- Lacosamide can cause a small increase in the median PR interval.
- The starting dose is 100 mg/day in two divided doses, with dose increase by 100 mg/day every week until a daily dose of 200 to 400 mg has been reached.

Lamotrigine

- **Lamotrigine** is useful as both adjunctive therapy and monotherapy for partial seizures and can be considered first- or second-line therapy. It is also approved for primary GTC seizures, and for primary generalized seizure of Lennox-Gastaut Syndrome.
- Rashes are usually generalized, erythematous, and morbilliform, but Stevens–Johnson reaction has also occurred. The incidence of the more serious rashes appears to be increased in patients who are also receiving **valproic acid** and who have rapid dosage titration. Valproic acid substantially inhibits the metabolism of lamotrigine and alters dosing (see Table 53–4).

Levetiracetam

- Renal elimination of unchanged drug accounts for 66% of **levetiracetam** clearance, and the dose should be adjusted for impaired renal function. It is metabolized in blood by nonhepatic enzymatic hydrolysis.
- It is effective in the adjunctive treatment of focal onset seizures in patients one month of age and older, myoclonic seizures in patients 12 years and older, and primary GTC seizures in patients 6 years and older.
- Adverse effects include sedation, fatigue, coordination difficulties, agitation, irritability, and lethargy. It is generally well tolerated.
- The recommended initial adult dose is 500 mg orally twice daily. In some intractable seizure patients, the oral dose has been titrated rapidly over 3 days up to 3000 mg/day (1500 mg twice daily). It can be loaded orally or intravenously.

Oxcarbazepine

- The relationship between dose and serum concentration is linear. It does not autoinduce its own metabolism.
- It is indicated for use as adjunctive therapy for partial seizures in patients 6 years and older.
- It generally has fewer side effects than **phenytoin**, **valproic acid**, or **carbamazepine**. Hyponatremia is reported in up to 25% of patients and is more likely in the elderly. About 25% to 30% of patients who have had a rash with carbamazepine will have a similar reaction with oxcarbazepine.
- Concurrent use of oxcarbazepine with **ethinyl estradiol** and **levonorgestrel**-containing contraceptives may render these agents less effective. Oxcarbazepine may increase serum concentrations of **phenytoin** and decrease serum concentrations of **lamotrigine** (induction of uridine diphosphate glucuronosyltransferase).
- In patients converted from carbamazepine, the typical maintenance doses of oxcarbazepine are 1.5 times the carbamazepine dose or less if patients are on larger carbamazepine doses. See manufacturer's recommendations for dosing by weight.

Perampanel

- **Perampanel** has a half-life of approximately 100 hours, and its clearance in increased two- to threefold by enzyme inducing ASDs.
- It has a boxed warning pertaining to monitoring for psychiatric, behavioral, mood, and personality change which may be life threatening.
- It is FDA approved for adjunctive therapy of focal onset seizures in patients 12 years and older and as adjunctive therapy for primary GTC in patients 12 years and older.

Phenobarbital

- **Phenobarbital**, a potent enzyme inducer, interacts with many drugs. **Valproic acid**, **felbamate**, **oxcarbazepine**, and **phenytoin** may inhibit its metabolism.

- Phenobarbital impairs cognitive performance. In children, paradoxical hyperactivity can occur.
- Long-term use is associated with osteomalacia, megaloblastic anemia, and folate deficiency.

Phenytoin

- **Phenytoin** is a first-line ASD for many seizure types, and is FDA approved for focal onset seizures and GTC seizures. It may exacerbate seizures in generalized epilepsies. It has many acute and long-term side effects (see **Table 53–5**).
- Absorption may be saturable at higher doses (above 400 mg). Do not change brands without careful monitoring. The intramuscular route is best avoided, as absorption is erratic. Fosphenytoin can safely be administered IV and intramuscularly. Equations are available to normalize the phenytoin concentration in patients with hypoalbuminemia or renal failure.
- Zero-order kinetics occurs within the usual therapeutic range, so any change in dose may produce disproportional changes in serum concentrations.
- It can be loaded orally, but in nonacute situations, phenytoin may be initiated in adults at oral doses of 100 mg three times daily. Subsequent dosage adjustments should be done cautiously because of nonlinearity in elimination. Most adult patients can be maintained on a single-daily dose, but children often require more frequent administration. Only extended-release preparations should be used for single-daily dosing.
- One author suggested that if the phenytoin serum concentration is less than 7 mcg/mL (28 μmol/L), the daily dose should be increased by 100 mg; if the concentration is 7 to 12 mcg/mL (28–48 μmol/L), the daily dose can be increased by 50 mg; and if the concentration is greater than 12 mcg/mL (48 μmol/L), the daily dose can be increased by 30 mg or less.
- At concentrations greater than 50 mcg/mL (200 μmol/L), phenytoin can exacerbate seizures.
- Phenytoin is prone to many drug interactions. If protein-binding interactions are suspected, free rather than total phenytoin serum concentrations are a better therapeutic guide.
- Phenytoin decreases **folic acid** absorption, but folic acid replacement enhances phenytoin clearance and can result in loss of efficacy. Phenytoin tablets and suspension contain phenytoin acid, whereas the capsules and parenteral solution are phenytoin sodium. Ninety-two mg of phenytoin acid is approximately equal to 100 mg of phenytoin sodium. Caution: There are two different strengths of phenytoin suspension and capsules.

Pregabalin

- **Pregabalin**, a schedule V controlled substance. It is FDA approved as adjunctive therapy for adults with focal onset seizures. It is considered a second-line agent for those who have failed initial treatment.
- It is eliminated unchanged primarily by renal excretion; dosage adjustment is required in patients with significant renal dysfunction.
- Drug interactions are unlikely.

Rufinamide

- **Rufinamide** is an adjunctive agent used for seizures of Lennox–Gastaut syndrome in patients 1 year and older and in adults. Reserve rufinamide for patients who have failed other ASDs.
- Children may have a higher clearance of rufinamide than adults.
- It is dosed twice daily because of slow absorption and a short half-life.
- Multiorgan hypersensitivity has occurred within 4 weeks of dose initiation in children younger than 12 years.
- Drug interactions are common.

Tiagabine

- **Tiagabine** is adjunctive therapy for patients 12 years and older with focal onset seizures who have failed initial therapy.
- Side effects are usually transient and can be diminished by taking it with food. It has a potential to cause seizures and status epilepticus in some patients.
- Tiagabine is displaced from protein by **naproxen**, **salicylates**, and **valproate**.
- Minimal effective adult dosing level is 30 mg/day, but those taking enzyme inducing drugs may require up to 50 to 60 mg/day.

Topiramate

- **Topiramate** is a first-line ASD for patients with partial seizures as an adjunct or for monotherapy. It is also approved for tonic-clonic seizures in primary generalized epilepsy and for generalized seizures in Lennox–Gestaut syndrome.
- Approximately 50% of the dose is excreted renally as unchanged drug, and tubular reabsorption may be prominently involved. The dose should be adjusted in renally impaired patients.
- Nephrolithiasis occurs in 1.5% of patients. It has also been associated with word-finding difficulties and metabolic acidosis.
- Enzyme inducers may decrease topiramate serum levels. It increases the clearance of ethinyl estradiol.
- Dose increments may occur every 1 or 2 weeks. For patients on other ASDs, doses greater than 400 mg/day do not appear to lead to improved efficacy and may increase side effects.

Valproic Acid and Divalproex Sodium

- The free fraction may increase as the total serum concentration increases, and monitoring free concentrations may be more useful than total concentrations, especially at higher serum concentrations and in patients with hypoalbuminemia.
- At least 10 metabolites have been identified, and some may be active. One may account for hepatotoxicity (4-*ene*-valproic acid), and it is increased by enzyme-inducing drugs. Most hepatotoxicity deaths were in children with intellectual disability who were younger than 2 years and receiving multiple drug therapy.
- It is first-line therapy for primary generalized seizures, such as absence, myoclonic, and atonic seizures, and is approved for adjunctive and monotherapy treatment of focal onset seizures. It can also be useful in mixed seizure disorders.
- GI complaints may be minimized with the enteric-coated formulation or by giving with food. Thrombocytopenia is common. Pancreatitis is rare.
- Although **carnitine** supplementation may partially ameliorate hyperammonemia, it is expensive and is not generally supported.
- Valproic acid is an enzyme inhibitor that increases serum concentrations of concurrently administered **phenobarbital**, carbamazepine 10,11-epoxide (without affecting concentrations of the parent drug), and **lamotrigine**. **Carbapenems** and combination **oral contraceptives** may lower serum levels of valproic acid.
- Once-daily dosing is possible with the extended-release divalproex, but more frequent dosing is the norm due to reports of breakthrough seizures on once-daily dosing.
- The enteric-coated tablet **divalproex sodium** causes fewer GI side effects. It is metabolized in the gut to valproic acid. When switching from Depakote to Depakote-ER, the dose should be increased by 14% to 20%.

Vigabatrin

- **Vigabatrin** is monotherapy for infantile spasms in infants 1 month to 2 years of age, and a third-line adjunctive agent for refractory complex partial seizures in patients 10 years and older.
- It is excreted unchanged in the urine. Dosage adjustment is necessary in pediatric and renally impaired patients.

- It can cause permanent bilateral concentric visual field constriction and reduce visual acuity. Vision should be checked at baseline and every 3 months for up to 6 months after discontinuation. It may aggravate myoclonic and absence seizures.
- Vigabatrin induces CYP2C9 and decreases phenytoin plasma levels by ~20%.

Zonisamide

- **Zonisamide,** a broad-spectrum **sulfonamide** ASD, is approved as adjunctive therapy for partial seizures, in adults.
- Word-finding difficulties can occur. Symptomatic kidney stones may occur in 2.6% of patients. As hypersensitivity reactions may occur in 0.02% of patients, use it cautiously (if at all) in patients with a history of sulfonamide allergy.
- Start dosing in adults at 100 mg/day and increase by 100 mg/day every 2 weeks. It is suitable for once- or twice-daily dosing, but once-daily dosing may cause more side effects.

EVALUATION OF THERAPEUTIC OUTCOMES

- Monitor long term for seizure control, side effects, social adjustment including quality of life, drug interactions, compliance, and side effects. Clinical response is more important than serum drug concentrations.
- Screen periodically for psychiatric disorders (eg, anxiety and depression).
- Ask patients and caregivers to record severity and frequency of seizures.

See Chapter 56, Epilepsy, authored by Viet-Huong V. Nguyen, Christine B. Baca, Jack J. Chen, and Susan J. Rogers, for a more detailed discussion of this topic.

CHAPTER 54

Headache: Migraine and Tension-Type

MIGRAINE HEADACHE

- *Migraine*, a common, recurrent, primary headache of moderate to severe intensity, interferes with normal functioning and is associated with gastrointestinal (GI), neurologic, and autonomic symptoms. In migraine with aura, focal neurologic symptoms precede or accompany the attack.

PATHOPHYSIOLOGY

- Activation of trigeminal sensory nerves triggers the release of vasoactive neuropeptides, including calcitonin gene-related peptide, neurokinin A, and substance P from perivascular axons. Vasodilation of dural blood vessels may occur with extravasation of dural plasma resulting in inflammation.
- Twin studies suggest 50% heritability of migraine, with a multifactorial polygenic basis. Migraine triggers may be modulators of the genetic set point that predisposes to migraine headache.
- Specific populations of serotonin (5-HT) receptors appear to be involved in the pathophysiology and treatment of migraine headache. **Ergot alkaloids** and **triptan** derivatives are agonists of vascular and neuronal 5-HT_1 receptors, resulting in vasoconstriction and inhibition of vasoactive neuropeptide release.

CLINICAL PRESENTATION AND DIAGNOSIS

- Migraine headache is characterized by recurring episodes of throbbing head pain, frequently unilateral.
- Approximately 12% to 79% of migraineurs have premonitory symptoms (not to be confused with aura) in the hours or days before headache onset. Neurologic symptoms (phonophobia, photophobia, hyperosmia, and difficulty concentrating) are most common, but psychological (anxiety, depression, euphoria, irritability, drowsiness, hyperactivity, and restlessness), autonomic (eg, polyuria, diarrhea, and constipation), and constitutional (eg, stiff neck, yawning, thirst, food cravings, and anorexia) symptoms may also occur.
- A migraine aura is experienced by approximately 25% of migraineurs. Aura evolves over 5 to 20 minutes and lasts less than 60 minutes. Headache usually occurs within 60 minutes of the end of the aura. Visual auras can include both positive features (eg, scintillations, photopsia, teichopsia, and fortification spectrum) and negative features (eg, scotoma and hemianopsia). Sensory symptoms such as paresthesias or numbness of the arms and face, dysphasia or aphasia, weakness, and hemiparesis may also occur.
- Migraine headache may occur at any time but usually occurs in the early morning. Pain is usually gradual in onset, peaking in intensity over minutes to hours and lasting 4 to 72 hours. Pain is typically in the frontotemporal region and is moderate to severe. Headache is usually unilateral and throbbing with GI symptoms (eg, nausea and vomiting) almost invariably accompanying the headache. Other systemic symptoms include anorexia, constipation, diarrhea, abdominal cramps, nasal stuffiness, blurred vision, diaphoresis, facial pallor, and localized facial, scalp, or periorbital edema. Sensory hyperacuity (photophobia, phonophobia, or osmophobia) is frequent. Many patients seek a dark, quiet place.
- Once the headache pain wanes, a resolution phase characterized by exhaustion, malaise, and irritability ensues.
- A comprehensive headache history is essential and includes age at onset; frequency, timing, and duration of attacks; possible triggers; ameliorating factors; description and characteristics of symptoms; associated signs and symptoms; treatment history; and family and social history.

- Neuroimaging should be considered in patients with unexplained abnormal neurologic examination or atypical headache history.
- Onset of migraine headaches after age 50 suggests an organic etiology, such as a mass lesion, cerebrovascular disease, or temporal arteritis.

TREATMENT

- <u>Goals of Treatment</u>: The goal is to achieve consistent, rapid headache relief with minimal adverse effects and symptom recurrence, and minimal disability and emotional distress, enabling the patient to resume normal activities. Ideally, patients should be able to manage their headaches without emergency department or physician office visits.

Nonpharmacologic Treatment

- Apply ice to the head and recommend periods of rest or sleep, usually in a dark, quiet environment.
- Identify and avoid triggers of migraine attacks (Table 54–1).
- Behavioral interventions (relaxation therapy, biofeedback, and cognitive therapy) may help patients who prefer nondrug therapy or when drug therapy is ineffective or not tolerated.

Pharmacologic Treatment of Acute Migraine

- Administer acute migraine therapies at the onset of migraine (Table 54–2 and Fig. 54–1).
- Pretreatment with an antiemetic (eg, **metoclopramide**, **chlorpromazine**, or **prochlorperazine**) 15 to 30 minutes before oral or nonoral migraine treatments (rectal suppositories, nasal spray, or injections) may be advisable when nausea and vomiting are severe. In addition to its antiemetic effects, metoclopramide helps reverse gastroparesis and enhances absorption of oral medications.

TABLE 54–1	Commonly Reported Triggers of Migraine

Food triggers
Alcohol
Caffeine/caffeine withdrawal
Chocolate
Fermented and pickled foods
Monosodium glutamate (eg, in Chinese food, seasoned salt, and instant foods)
Nitrate-containing foods (eg, processed meats)
Saccharin/aspartame (eg, diet foods or diet sodas)
Tyramine-containing foods

Environmental triggers
Glare or flickering lights
High altitude
Loud noises
Strong smells and fumes
Tobacco smoke
Weather changes

Behavioral–physiologic triggers
Excess or insufficient sleep
Fatigue
Menstruation, menopause
Sexual activity
Skipped meals
Strenuous physical activity (eg, prolonged overexertion)
Stress or post-stress

TABLE 54-2 Dosing of Acute Migraine Therapies[a]

Drug	Dose	Usual Range/Comments
Analgesics		
Acetaminophen (Tylenol)	1000 mg at onset; repeat every 4–6 hours as needed	Max. daily dose is 4 g
Acetaminophen 250 mg/aspirin 250 mg/caffeine 65 mg (Excedrin Migraine)	2 tablets at onset and every 6 hours	Available over-the-counter as Excedrin Migraine
Nonsteroidal anti-inflammatory drugs		
Aspirin	500–1000 mg every 4–6 hours	Max. daily dose is 4 g
Ibuprofen (Motrin)	200–800 mg every 6 hours	Avoid doses >2.4 g/day
Naproxen sodium (Aleve, Anaprox)	550–825 mg at onset; can repeat 220 mg in 3–4 hours	Avoid doses >1.375 g/day
Diclofenac (Cataflam, Voltaren)	50–100 mg at onset; can repeat 50 mg in 8 hours	Avoid doses >150 mg/day
Ergotamine tartrate		
Oral tablet (1 mg) with caffeine 100 mg (Cafergot)	2 mg at onset; then 1–2 mg every 30 minutes as needed	Max. dose is 6 mg/day or 10 mg/wk; consider pretreatment with an antiemetic
Sublingual tablet (2 mg) (Ergomar)		
Rectal suppository (2 mg) with caffeine 100 mg (Cafergot, Migergot)	Insert 1/2 to 1 suppository at onset; repeat after 1 hour as needed	Max. dose is 4 mg/day or 10 mg/wk; consider pretreatment with an antiemetic
Dihydroergotamine		
Injection 1 mg/mL (D.H.E. 45)	0.25–1 mg at onset IM, IV or subcutaneous; repeat every hour as needed	Max. dose is 3 mg/day or 6 mg/wk
Nasal spray 4 mg/mL (Migranal)	One spray (0.5 mg) in each nostril at onset; repeat sequence 15 minutes later (total dose is 2 mg or 4 sprays)	Max. dose is 3 mg/day; prime sprayer 4 times before using; do not tilt head back or inhale through nose while spraying; discard open ampules after 8 hours

(continued)

TABLE 54–2 Dosing of Acute Migraine Therapies[a] (Continued)

Drug	Dose	Usual Range/Comments
Serotonin agonists (triptans)		
Sumatriptan (Imitrex)		
Injection	6 mg subcutaneous at onset; can repeat after 1 hour if needed	Max. daily dose is 12 mg
Oral tablets	25, 50, 85 or 100 mg at onset; can repeat after 2 hours if needed	Optimal dose is 50–100 mg; max. daily dose is 200 mg; combination product with naproxen, 85 mg/500 mg
Nasal spray	5, 10, or 20 mg at onset; can repeat after 2 hours if needed	Optimal dose is 20 mg; max. daily dose is 40 mg; single-dose device delivering 5 or 20 mg; administer one spray in one nostril
Zolmitriptan (Zomig, Zomig-ZMT)		
Oral tablets	2.5 or 5 mg at onset as regular or orally disintegrating tablet; can repeat after 2 hours if needed	Optimal dose is 2.5 mg; max. dose is 10 mg/day Do not divide ODT dosage form
Nasal spray	5 mg (one spray) at onset; can repeat after 2 hours if needed	Max. daily dose is 10 mg/day
Naratriptan (Amerge)	1 or 2.5 mg at onset; can repeat after 4 hours if needed	Optimal dose is 2.5 mg; max. daily dose is 5 mg
Rizatriptan (Maxalt, Maxalt-MLT)	5 or 10 mg at onset as regular or orally disintegrating tablet; can repeat after 2 hours if needed	Optimal dose is 10 mg; max. daily dose is 30 mg; onset of effect is similar with standard and orally disintegrating tablets; use 5-mg dose (15 mg/day max.) in patients receiving propranolol
Almotriptan (Axert)	6.25 or 12.5 mg at onset; can repeat after 2 hours if needed	Optimal dose is 12.5 mg; max. daily dose is 25 mg
Frovatriptan (Frova)	2.5 or 5 mg at onset; can repeat in 2 hours if needed	Optimal dose 2.5–5 mg; max. daily dose is 7.5 mg (3 tablets)
Eletriptan (Relpax)	20 or 40 mg at onset; can repeat after 2 hours if needed	Max. single dose is 40 mg; max. daily dose is 80 mg
Miscellaneous		
Metoclopramide (Reglan)	10 mg IV at onset	Useful for acute relief in the office or emergency department setting
Prochlorperazine (Compazine)	10 mg IV or IM at onset	Useful for acute relief in the office or emergency department setting

(ODT, orally disintegrating tablet.)

[a]Limit use of symptomatic medications to fewer than 10 days/mo when possible to avoid medication-overuse headache.

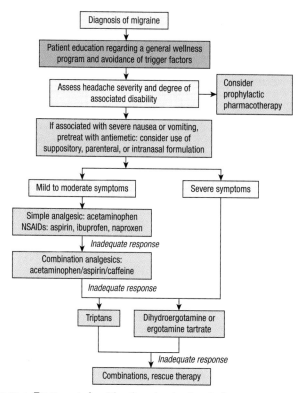

FIGURE 54–1. Treatment algorithm for migraine headaches.

- Prochlorperazine (IM or IV), metoclopramide (IV), as well as parenteral chlorpromazine and **droperidol** have been used for refractory migraine.
- Frequent or excessive use of acute migraine medications can result in increasing headache frequency and drug consumption known as medication-overuse headache. This occurs commonly with overuse of simple or combination analgesics, **opiates**, **ergotamine tartrate**, and **triptans**. Limit use of acute migraine therapies to 2 or 3 days per week or 10 days per month.

ANALGESICS AND NONSTEROIDAL ANTI-INFLAMMATORY DRUGS

- **Simple analgesics** and **nonsteroidal anti-inflammatory drugs (NSAIDs)** are first-line treatments for mild to moderate migraine attacks; some severe attacks are also responsive. **Aspirin**, **diclofenac**, **ibuprofen**, **ketorolac**, **naproxen sodium**, **tolfenamic acid**, and the combination of **acetaminophen** plus **aspirin** and **caffeine** are effective.
- NSAIDs appear to prevent neurogenically mediated inflammation in the trigemino-vascular system by inhibiting prostaglandin synthesis.
- Rectal suppositories and IM **ketorolac** are options for patients with severe nausea and vomiting.
- The combination of **acetaminophen**, **aspirin**, and **caffeine** is approved in the United States for relieving migraine pain.
- Aspirin and acetaminophen are also available by prescription in combination with a short-acting barbiturate (**butalbital**). No randomized, placebo-controlled studies support the efficacy of butalbital-containing formulations for migraine.

ERGOT ALKALOIDS AND DERIVATIVES

- **Ergot alkaloids** are useful for moderate to severe migraine attacks. They are nonselective $5HT_1$ receptor agonists that constrict intracranial blood vessels and inhibit the development of neurogenic inflammation in the trigeminovascular system. Venous and arterial constriction occurs.
- **Ergotamine tartrate** is available for oral, sublingual, and rectal administration. Oral and rectal preparations contain **caffeine** to enhance absorption and potentiate analgesia. Titrate to an effective dose that is not nauseating.
- **Dihydroergotamine (DHE)** is available for intranasal and parenteral (IM, IV, or subcutaneous [SC]) administration. Patients can self-administer IM or SC DHE.
- Nausea and vomiting are common with ergotamine derivatives, so consider antiemetic pretreatment. Other common side effects include abdominal pain, weakness, fatigue, paresthesias, muscle pain, diarrhea, and chest tightness. Symptoms of severe peripheral ischemia (ergotism) include cold, numb, painful extremities; continuous paresthesias; diminished peripheral pulses; and claudication. Gangrenous extremities, myocardial infarction (MI), hepatic necrosis, and bowel and brain ischemia have occurred rarely with ergotamine. Do not use **ergotamine derivatives** and **triptans** within 24 hours of each other.
- Contraindications to use of ergot derivatives include renal and hepatic failure; coronary, cerebral, or peripheral vascular disease; uncontrolled hypertension; sepsis; and women who are pregnant or nursing.
- DHE does not appear to cause rebound headache, but dosage restrictions for ergotamine tartrate should be strictly observed to prevent this complication.

SEROTONIN RECEPTOR AGONISTS (TRIPTANS)

- The **triptans** (Table 54–3) are appropriate first-line therapies for patients with mild to severe migraine or as rescue therapy when nonspecific medications are ineffective.

TABLE 54–3	Pharmacokinetic Characteristics of Triptans		
Drug	**Half-Life (hours)**	**Time to Maximal Concentration (t_{max})**	**Bioavailability (%)**	**Elimination**
Almotriptan	3–4	1.4–3.8 hours	80	MAO-A, CYP3A4, CYP2D6
Eletriptan	4–5	1–2 hours	50	CYP3A4
Frovatriptan	25	2–4 hours	24–30	Mostly unchanged, CYP1A2
Naratriptan	5–6	2–3 hours	63–74	Largely unchanged, CYP450 (various isoenzymes)
Rizatriptan	2–3		45	MAO-A
Oral tablets		1–1.2 hours		
Disintegrating tablets		1.6–2.5 hours		
Sumatriptan	2			MAO-A
SC injection		12–15 minutes	97	
Oral tablets		2.5 hours	14	
Nasal spray		1–2.5 hours	17	
Zolmitriptan	3		40–48	CYP1A2, MAO-A
Oral		2 hours		
Disintegrating		3.3 hours		
Nasal		4 hours		

(CYP, cytochrome P450; MAO-A, monoamine oxidase type A.)

- They are selective agonists of the $5HT_{1B}$ and $5HT_{1D}$ receptors. Relief of migraine headache results from (1) normalization of dilated intracranial arteries, (2) inhibition of vasoactive peptide release, and (3) inhibition of transmission through second-order neurons ascending to the thalamus.
- **Sumatriptan** SC injection is packaged as an autoinjector device for self-administration. Compared with the oral formulation, SC administration offers enhanced efficacy and more rapid onset of action. Intranasal sumatriptan also has a faster onset of effect than the oral formulation and produces similar rates of response.
- Second-generation triptans (all except sumatriptan) have higher oral bioavailability and longer half-lives than oral sumatriptan, which could theoretically reduce headache recurrence. However, comparative clinical trials are necessary to determine their relative efficacy. **Frovatriptan** and **naratriptan** have the longest half-lives, slowest onset of action, and less headache recurrence.
- Pharmacokinetic characteristics of the triptans are shown in Table 54–3.
- Lack of response to one triptan does not preclude effective therapy with another triptan.
- Side effects of triptans include paresthesias, fatigue, dizziness, flushing, warm sensations, and somnolence. Minor injection site reactions are reported with SC use, and taste perversion and nasal discomfort may occur with intranasal administration. Up to 25% of patients report chest tightness; pressure; heaviness; or pain in the chest, neck, or throat. The mechanism of these symptoms is unknown, but a cardiac source is unlikely in most patients. Isolated cases of MI and coronary vasospasm with ischemia have been reported.
- Contraindications include ischemic heart disease, uncontrolled hypertension, cerebrovascular disease, hemiplegic and basilar migraine, and pregnancy. Do not give triptans within 24 hours of ergotamine derivative administration or within 2 weeks of therapy with monoamine oxidase inhibitors. Concomitant use of triptans with selective serotonin reuptake inhibitors or serotonin–norepinephrine reuptake inhibitors can cause serotonin syndrome, a potentially life-threatening condition.
- Use triptans cautiously in patients at risk for unrecognized coronary artery disease. Do a cardiovascular assessment before giving triptans to postmenopausal women, men over 40 years of age, and patients with uncontrolled risk factors, and administer the first dose under medical supervision.

OPIOIDS

- Reserve **opioids** and derivatives (eg, **meperidine**, **butorphanol**, **oxycodone**, and **hydromorphone**) for patients with moderate to severe infrequent headaches in whom conventional therapies are contraindicated or as rescue medication after failure to respond to conventional therapies. Closely supervise opioid therapy.

Pharmacologic Prophylaxis of Migraine

- Prophylactic therapies (Table 54–4 and Fig. 54–2) are administered daily to reduce the frequency, severity, and duration of attacks, and to increase responsiveness to acute therapies.
- Consider prophylaxis in the setting of recurring migraines that produce significant disability; frequent attacks requiring symptomatic medication more than twice per week; symptomatic therapies that are ineffective, contraindicated, or produce serious side effects; uncommon migraine variants that cause profound disruption or risk of neurologic injury; and patient preference to limit the number of attacks.
- Preventive therapy may also be given intermittently when headaches recur in a predictable pattern (eg, exercise-induced or menstrual migraine).
- Because efficacy of various prophylactic agents appears to be similar, drug selection is based on side effect profiles and comorbid conditions. Response to an agent is unpredictable, and a 2- to 3-month trial is necessary to achieve clinical benefit.
- Only **propranolol, timolol, divalproex sodium**, and **topiramate** are Food and Drug Administration (FDA) approved for migraine prevention.

TABLE 54–4 Dosing of Prophylactic Migraine Therapies

Drug	Initial Dose	Usual Range	Comments
β-Adrenergic antagonists			
Atenolol[a] (Tenormin)	50 mg/day	50–200 mg/day	
Metoprolol[b] (Toprol, Toprol XL)	100 mg/day in divided doses	100–200 mg/day in divided doses	Dose short-acting 4 times a day and long-acting 2 times a day; available as extended release
Nadolol[a] (Corgard)	40–80 mg/day	80–240 mg/day	
Propranolol[b] (Inderal, Inderal LA)	40 mg/day in divided doses	40–160 mg/day in divided doses	Dose short-acting 2–3 times a day and long-acting 1–2 times a day; available as extended release
Timolol[b] (Blocadren)	20 mg/day in divided doses	20–60 mg/day in divided doses	
Antidepressants			
Amitriptyline[a] (Elavil)	10 mg at bedtime	20–50 mg at bedtime	
Venlafaxine[a] (Effexor, Effexor-XR)	37.5 mg/day	75–150 mg/day	Available as extended release; increase dose after 1 week
Anticonvulsants			
Topiramate[b] (Topamax)	25 mg/day	50–200 mg/day in divided doses	As effective as amitriptyline, propranolol or valproate; increase by 25 mg/wk
Valproic acid/divalproex sodium[b] (Depakene, Depakote, Depakote ER)	250–500 mg/day in divided doses, or daily for extended release	500–1500 mg/day in divided doses, or daily for extended release	Monitor levels if compliance is an issue
Nonsteroidal anti-inflammatory drugs			
Ibuprofen[a] (Motrin)	400–1200 mg/day in divided doses	Same as initial dose	Use intermittently, such as for menstrual migraine prevention; daily or prolonged use may lead to medication-overuse headache and is limited by potential toxicity
Ketoprofen[a] (Orudis)	150 mg/day in divided doses	Same as initial dose	
Naproxen sodium[a] (Aleve, Anaprox)	550–1100 mg/day in divided doses	Same as initial dose	

Serotonin agonists (triptans)

Frovatriptan[b] (Frova)	2.5 mg/day or 5 mg/day in divided doses	Same as initial dose	Taken in the perimenstrual period to prevent menstrual migraine
Naratriptan[a] (Amerge)	2 mg/day in divided doses	Same as initial dose	
Zolmitriptan[a] (Zomig)	5–7.5 mg/day in divided doses	Same as initial dose	
Miscellaneous			
Histamine[a] (Histatrol)	1–10 ng two times/wk	Same as initial dose	May cause transient itching and burning at injection site
Magnesium[a]	400 mg/day	800 mg/day in divided doses	May be more helpful in migraine with aura and menstrual migraine
MIG-99[a] (feverfew)	10–100 mg/day in divided doses	Same as initial dose	Withdrawal may be associated with increased headaches
Petasites[b]	100–150 mg/day in divided doses	150 mg/day in divided doses	Use only commercial preparations, plant is carcinogenic
Riboflavin[a]	400 mg/day in divided doses	400 mg/day in divided doses	Benefit only after 3 months

[a]Level B—probably effective (1 Class I or 2 Class II studies).
[b]Level A—established efficacy (≥2 Class I studies).
(Data from Silberstein SD, Holland S, et al. Neurology 2012;78:1337–1345; Holland S, Silberstein SD, et al. Neurology 2012;78:1346–1353. Copyright © the American Academy of Neurology.)

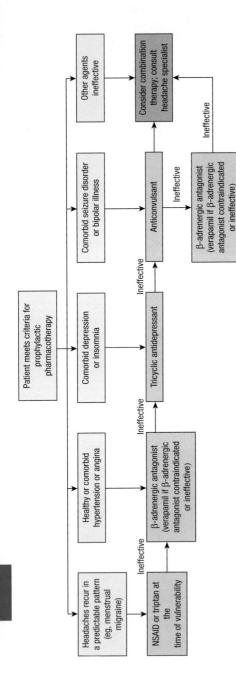

(NSAID, nonsteroidal anti-inflammatory drug.)

FIGURE 54–2. Treatment algorithm for prophylactic management of migraine headaches.

- Initiate prophylaxis with low doses, and advance slowly until a therapeutic effect is achieved or side effects become intolerable.
- Continue prophylaxis for at least 6 to 12 months after headache frequency and severity have diminished, and then gradual tapering or discontinuation may be reasonable.

β-ADRENERGIC ANTAGONISTS

- **Propranolol**, **timolol**, and **metoprolol** reduce the frequency of migraine attacks by 50% in more than 50% of patients. **Atenolol** and **nadolol** are probably also effective.
- Side effects include drowsiness, fatigue, sleep disturbances, vivid dreams, memory disturbance, depression, sexual dysfunction, bradycardia, and hypotension.
- Use with caution in patients with heart failure, peripheral vascular disease, atrioventricular conduction disturbances, asthma, depression, and diabetes.

ANTIDEPRESSANTS

- The tricyclic antidepressants (TCAs) **amitriptyline** and **venlafaxine** are probably effective for migraine prophylaxis. There are insufficient data to support or refute the efficacy of other antidepressants.
- Their beneficial effects in migraine prophylaxis are independent of antidepressant activity and may be related to downregulation of central $5HT_2$ receptors, increased synaptic norepinephrine, and enhanced opioid receptor actions.
- TCAs are usually well tolerated at the doses used for migraine prophylaxis, but anticholinergic effects may limit use, especially in elderly patients or those with benign prostatic hyperplasia or glaucoma. Evening doses are preferred because of sedation. Increased appetite and weight gain can occur. Orthostatic hypotension and slowed atrioventricular conduction are occasionally reported.

ANTICONVULSANTS

- **Valproic acid**, **divalproex sodium** (a 1:1 molar combination of valproate sodium and valproic acid), and **topiramate** can reduce the frequency, severity, and duration of headaches.
- Side effects of valproic acid and divalproex sodium include nausea (less common with divalproex sodium and gradual dosing titration), tremor, somnolence, weight gain, hair loss, and hepatotoxicity (the risk of hepatotoxicity appears to be low in patients older than 10 years on monotherapy). Obtain baseline liver function tests. The extended-release formulation of divalproex sodium is administered once daily and is better tolerated than the enteric-coated formulation. Valproate is contraindicated in pregnancy and patients with a history of pancreatitis or chronic liver disease.
- Fifty percent of patients respond to **topiramate**. Paresthesias (~50% of patients) and weight loss (9%–12% of patients) are common. Other side effects include fatigue, anorexia, diarrhea, difficulty with memory, language problems, taste perversions, and nausea. Use topiramate cautiously or avoided in those with a history of kidney stones or cognitive impairment.
- **Carbamazepine** is possibly effective.

NONSTEROIDAL ANTI-INFLAMMATORY DRUGS

- **Nonsteroidal anti-inflammatory drugs (NSAIDs)** are modestly effective for reducing the frequency, severity, and duration of migraine attacks, but potential GI and renal toxicity limit daily or prolonged use.
- They may be used intermittently to prevent headaches that recur in a predictable pattern (eg, menstrual migraine). Initiate up to one week before the time of headache vulnerability, and continue until vulnerability is passed.
- For migraine prevention, evidence for efficacy is strongest for naproxen and weakest for aspirin.

OTHER DRUGS

- **Verapamil** has been widely used, but evidence for efficacy is inadequate.
- **Frovatriptan** is effective for prophylaxis of menstrual migraine, and **naratriptan** and **zolmitriptan** are probably effective.

- Other medications that may be effective include **Petasites, riboflavin (vitamin B$_2$), extract of feverfew, magnesium**, subcutaneous **histamine, lisinopril, candesartan, clonidine, guanfacine**, and **coenzyme Q10**, but additional research is needed to confirm efficacy.

TENSION-TYPE HEADACHE

- Tension-type headache, the most common type of primary headaches, is more common in women than men. Pain is usually mild to moderate and nonpulsatile. Episodic headaches may become chronic in some patients.

PATHOPHYSIOLOGY

- Pain is thought to originate from myofascial factors and peripheral sensitization of nociceptors. Central mechanisms are also involved. Mental stress, nonphysiologic motor stress, a local myofascial release of irritants, or a combination of these may be the initiating stimulus.

CLINICAL PRESENTATION

- Premonitory symptoms and aura are absent, and pain is usually mild to moderate, bilateral (having a hatband pattern), and nonpulsatile.
- Mild photophobia or phonophobia may occur. Pericranial or cervical muscles may have tender spots or localized nodules in some patients.

TREATMENT

- Nonpharmacologic therapies include reassurance and counseling, stress management, relaxation training, and biofeedback. Evidence supporting physical therapeutic options (eg, heat or cold packs, ultrasound, electrical nerve stimulation, massage, acupuncture, trigger point injections, and occipital nerve blocks) has been inconsistent.
- **Simple analgesics** (alone or in combination with caffeine) and **NSAIDs** are the mainstay of acute therapy. **Acetaminophen, aspirin, diclofenac, ibuprofen, naproxen, ketoprofen,** and **ketorolac** are effective.
- The combination of aspirin or acetaminophen with **butalbital**, or rarely, **codeine** are effective options, but avoid the use of butalbital and codeine combinations when possible.
- Give acute medication for episodic headache no more often than 3 days (butalbital-containing), 9 days (combination analgesics), or 15 days (NSAIDs) per month to prevent the development of chronic tension-type headache.
- There is no evidence to support the efficacy of muscle relaxants.
- Consider preventive treatment if headache frequency is more than two per week, duration is longer than 3 to 4 hours, or severity results in medication overuse or substantial disability.
- The **TCAs** are used most often for prophylaxis of tension headache, but **venlafaxine, mirtazapine, gabapentin, topiramate, and tizanidine** may also be effective.

EVALUATION OF THERAPEUTIC OUTCOMES

- Monitor for frequency, intensity, and duration of headaches and for any change in the headache pattern. Encourage patients to keep a headache diary to document frequency, duration, and severity of headaches, headache response, and potential triggers of migraine headaches.
- Monitor patients taking abortive therapy for frequency of use of prescription and nonprescription medications and for side effects.
- Document patterns of abortive medication used to establish the need for prophylactic therapy. Monitor prophylactic therapies closely for adverse reactions, abortive therapy needs, adequate dosing, and compliance.

See Chapter 61, Headache Disorders, authored by Deborah S. Minor and Marion T. Kristopher Harrell, for a more detailed discussion of this topic.

CHAPTER 55

Pain Management

- *Pain* is a subjective, unpleasant, sensory, and emotional experience associated with actual or potential tissue damage or abnormal functioning of nerves. It may be classified as acute, chronic, or cancer pain.

PHYSIOLOGY AND PATHOPHYSIOLOGY

ADAPTIVE (PHYSIOLOGIC) PAIN

- Nociceptive (eg, from touching something too hot, too cold, or sharp) and inflammatory pain (eg, trauma or surgery) are both adaptive and protective.
- The steps in processing pain are:
  - ✓ Transduction—stimulation of nociceptors.
    - ❖ Nociceptors found in both somatic and visceral structures, are activated by mechanical, thermal, and chemical stimuli. Noxious stimuli may cause release of cytokines and chemokines that sensitize and/or activate nociceptors.
  - ✓ Conduction—Receptor activation leads to action potentials that continue along afferent fibers to the spinal cord. Stimulation of large-diameter, sparsely myelinated fibers evokes sharp, well-localized pain. Stimulation of small-diameter, unmyelinated fibers produces aching, poorly localized pain.
  - ✓ Transmission—Afferent nociceptive fibers synapse in the spinal cord's dorsal horn, releasing excitatory neurotransmitters (eg, glutamate and substance P). The spinothalamic tract and other pathways bring the signal to the brain's higher cortical structures.
  - ✓ Perception—The experience of pain occurs when signals reach higher cortical structures. Relaxation, meditation, and distraction can lessen pain, and anxiety and depression can worsen pain.
  - ✓ Modulation—Possible modulating factors include glutamate, substance P, endogenous opioids, γ-aminobutyric acid (GABA), norepinephrine, and serotonin.
- The interface between neurons and immune cells in the central nervous system (CNS) may facilitate maintenance of chronic pain.

MALADAPTIVE (PATHOPHYSIOLOGIC) PAIN

- Pathophysiologic pain (eg, postherpetic neuralgia, diabetic neuropathy, fibromyalgia, irritable bowel syndrome, and chronic headaches) is often described as chronic pain. It results from damage or abnormal functioning of nerves in the CNS or peripheral nervous system (PNS). Pain circuits sometimes rewire themselves anatomically and biochemically, resulting in chronic pain, hyperalgesia, or allodynia.

CLINICAL PRESENTATION

GENERAL

- Patients may be in acute distress or display no noticeable suffering.

SYMPTOMS

- Acute pain can be sharp or dull, burning, shock-like, tingling, shooting, radiating, fluctuating in intensity, varying in location, and occurring in a temporal relationship with an obvious noxious stimulus. Chronic pain can present similarly and often occurs without a temporal relationship to a noxious stimulus. Over time, the chronic pain presentation may change (eg, sharp to dull).

SIGNS

- Acute pain can cause hypertension, tachycardia, diaphoresis, mydriasis, and pallor. These signs are seldom present in chronic pain. In chronic noncancer pain, depression, sleep disturbances, anxiety, and employment and family instability tend to dominate.

- In acute pain, outcomes of treatment are generally predictable. In chronic pain, comorbid conditions are often present, and treatment outcomes are often unpredictable. For chronic noncancer pain, an interdisciplinary approach (eg, pain clinic) is preferred.

DIAGNOSIS

- Pain is always subjective; thus pain is best diagnosed based on patient description, history, and physical examination. A baseline description of pain can be obtained by accessing PQRST characteristics (*p*alliative and *p*rovocative factors, *q*uality, *r*adiation, *s*everity, and *t*emporal factors). Mental factors may lower the pain threshold (eg, anxiety and depression). Behavioral, cognitive, social, and cultural factors may also affect the pain experience.

TREATMENT

- Goals of Treatment:
  - ✓ Acute pain: pain relief that allows for attainment of defined functional goals.
  - ✓ Chronic or noncancer pain: improve level of functioning, decrease pain, reduce medication use if possible, and improve quality of life.
  - ✓ Cancer pain: pain relief that enables patients to tolerate diagnostic and therapeutic manipulations and preserves function as much as possible while minimizing adverse effects.
- Figures 55–1 and 55–2 are algorithms for management of acute pain and pain in oncology patients, respectively.

NONOPIOID AGENTS

- Initiate treatment with the most effective analgesic with the fewest side effects. See Table 55–1 for adult dosages of Food and Drug Administration (FDA)–approved nonopioid analgesics.
- Acetaminophen and nonsteroidal anti-inflammatory drugs (NSAIDS) are often preferred over the opioids for mild to moderate pain. The **NSAIDs** reduce prostaglandins, decreasing the number of pain impulses received by the CNS.
- **NSAIDs** may be particularly useful for cancer-related bone pain and chronic low back pain. An adequate trial of an NSAID is about 1 month in duration. Chronic use may cause gastrointestinal (GI), cardiac, and renal toxicities. Topical NSAIDs may have similar efficacy as oral NSAIDs with improved safety when treating small or superficial joint arthritis.
- **Acetaminophen** has analgesic and antipyretic activity but little anti-inflammatory action. It is highly hepatotoxic on overdose, and its efficacy has been questioned.

OPIOID AGENTS

- Very limited data support the safety and efficacy of opioids for chronic noncancer pain. If opioids are used in this setting, carefully select patients and identify risks (eg, misuse and abuse) before initiating opioid therapy, and employ treatment agreements outlining responsibilities. At baseline and throughout treatment, assess aberrant behaviors and risks for misuse, abuse, and addiction (eg, history of abuse, misuse, diversion, or addiction; family history of substance abuse; and underlying psychiatric diagnosis). Random drug screens and pill counts may be useful.
- The onset of action of oral **opioids** is about 45 minutes, and peak effect usually is seen in about 1 to 2 hours.
- Addiction is characterized by impaired control over drug use, compulsive use, continued use despite harm, and craving. For definitions of physical dependence, substance abuse, substance dependence, tolerance, and withdrawal, see Chapter 71.
- Equianalgesic doses, histamine-releasing characteristics, dosing guidelines and major adverse effects are shown in Tables 55–2, 55–3, and 55–4. Equianalgesic doses are only a guide, and doses must be individualized. Exercise caution in the use of (or avoid altogether) the opioids shown in Table 55–5.

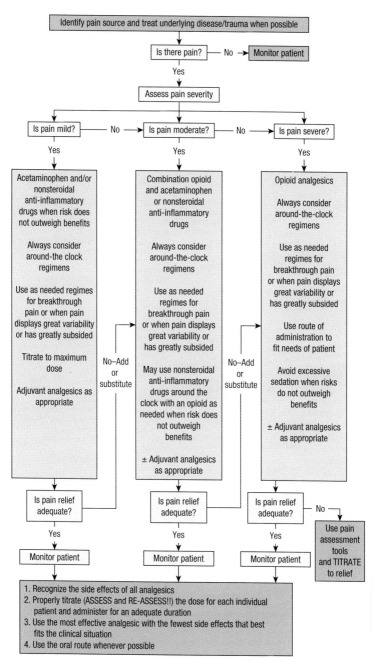

FIGURE 55–1. Algorithm for management of acute pain. (Data modified from Omnicare, Inc, Acute Pain Pathway.)

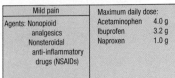

Mild pain	Maximum daily dose:	Principles of therapy

Mild pain

Agents: Nonopioid analgesics
Nonsteroidal anti-inflammatory drugs (NSAIDs)

Maximum daily dose:
- Acetaminophen 4.0 g
- Ibuprofen 3.2 g
- Naproxen 1.0 g

Principles of therapy
1. Assess the frequency/duration/occurrence/etiology of the pain on a routine basis.
2. If bone pain is present, consideration of an NSAID should be routine.
3. Always dose a medication to its maximum before reverting to the next step, unless pain is totally out of control.
4. If pain is constant or recurring, always dose around-the-clock (ATC).
5. Some authors suggest a lower maximum dose of acetaminophen.

Response

Good — Continue

Poor / Not tolerated
GI: Take with food/milk/antacid
Switch to acetaminophen (unless bone pain)
Oral: Rectal acetaminophen

Mild/moderate pain

Agents: Acetaminophen or NSAID combinations with opioids
Adjuncts: Tricyclic antidepressants
Anticonvulsants
Radiopharmaceuticals (Bone pain)

Maximum daily dose:
- Acetaminophen (See above)
- Opioids Titrate
- Amitriptyline 300 mg
- Imipramine 300 mg
- NSAIDs (See above)
- Gabapentin (Neurontin) 3.6 g

Principles of therapy
1. Assess the frequency/duration/occurrence/etiology of the pain on a routine basis.
2. Whenever bone pain is present, consideration of an NSAID with opioid should be routine.
3. Pain management needs to take precedence over other therapies.
4. Fulminating sites of pain, especially in bone, need to be evaluated quickly for alternate therapy such as radiation/radiopharmaceuticals.
5. Accurate assessment and history of reported opiate allergies are important. A differentiation between allergy, sensitivity, and side effect needs to be made.
6. Always dose to the maximum of each agent when possible.
7. If pain is constant or recurring, always dose ATC.
8. Consider adjunct therapy when appropriate.
9. When using opioids, prevent constipation with a GI stimulant laxative.

Response

Good — Continue

Poor / Not tolerated
GI: Take with food/milk/antacid
Delete NSAID (unless bone pain)
Oral: See below

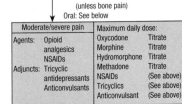

Moderate/severe pain

Agents: Opioid analgesics
NSAIDs
Adjuncts: Tricyclic antidepressants
Anticonvulsants

Maximum daily dose:
- Oxycodone Titrate
- Morphine Titrate
- Hydromorphone Titrate
- Methadone Titrate
- NSAIDs (See above)
- Tricyclics (See above)
- Anticonvulsant (See above)

Principles of therapy
1. Assess the frequency/duration/occurrence/etiology of the pain on a routine basis.
2. Morphine is often the choice in this category: (1) multiple products available; (2) multiple route of administration options, such as oral, rectal, IM, SC, IV, epidural, and intrathecal; and (3) a known equipotency between these routes that allows a much easier transition.
3. No real practical dosage limits with opioids mentioned; can be titrated to patient response. If myoclonic jerking occurs, consider switching to alternative opioid.
4. Management should be ATC dosing, with sustained-release product and an immediate-release product as for breakthrough pain.
5. Utilize all possible adjuncts to minimize increases in dose.
6. Initial control may require doses higher than those needed in maintenance.
7. A fentanyl patch placed every 72 h may provide a more convenient dosing regimen when patients are on a stable oral dosing program.

Response

Good — Continue to titrate

Poor / Not tolerated

Nerve block
Epidural
Intrathecal

Change route of administration (see note 2)
Change opioid (see note 12)

8. Special situations of sudden-onset/sudden-resolution pain, especially along a nerve track, or neuralgias, may require an adjunct of an anticonvulsant and/or tricyclic antidepressant.
9. Any time nonpharmacologic options of radiation, chemotherapy, surgical debulking, or neurologic interventions
10. When using opioids, prevent constipation with a GI stimulant laxative.
11. Any new report of pain requires reevaluation.
12. If patient does not tolerate an opioid, consider switching to another opioid.

FIGURE 55–2. Algorithm for pain management in oncology patients. (Data modified from the Kaiser Permanente Algorithm for Pain Management in Patients with Advanced Malignant Disease. Hooten WM, Timming R, Belgrade M, et al. Institute for Clinical Systems Improvement. Assessment and Management of Chronic Pain. Updated November 2013.)

TABLE 55–1 Adult Doses of Nonopioid Analgesics (Includes Only FDA-Approved Agents for Pain)

Class and Generic Name (Brand Name)	Approximate Half-Life (h)	Usual Dosage Range (mg)	Maximal Dose (mg/day)
Salicylates			
Acetylsalicylic acid[a]—aspirin (various)	0.25	325–1000 every 4–6 h	4000
Choline and magnesium trisalicylate (various)	9–17	1000–1500 every 12 h 750 every 8 h (elderly)	3000
Diflunisal (Dolobid, various)	8–12	500–1000 initial 250–500 every 8–12 h	1500
Salsalate (various)	1	1000 every 12 h or 500 every 6 h	3000
Para-aminophenol			
Acetaminophen[a] (Oral—Tylenol, various; Parenteral—Ofirmev)	2–3	325–1000 every 4–6 h	4000[b] Dosing for peds lower based on weight
Fenamates			
Meclofenamate (various)	0.8–3.3	50–100 every 4–6 h	400
Mefenamic acid (Ponstel)	2	Initial 500, 250 every 6 h (max. 7 days)	1000[c]
Pyranocarboxylic acid			
Etodolac (various) (immediate release)	7.3	200–400 every 6–8 h	1000 with immediate release product; 1200 with extended release product
Acetic acid			
Diclofenac potassium (Cataflam, various, Flector [patch] Voltaren Gel, Pennsaid [solution])	1.9	In some patients, initial 100, 50 three times per day Patch available—to be applied twice daily to painful area (intact skin only). Gel and solution dosing joint specific	150[d]
Propionic acids			
Ibuprofen[a] (Motrin, Caldolor, various)	2–2.5	200–400 every 4–6 h Injectable, 400–800 every 6 h (infused over 30 min)	3200[e] 2400[e] 1200[f]
Fenoprofen (Nalfon, various)	3	200 every 4–6 h	3200
Ketoprofen (various)	2	25–50 every 6–8 h	300 200 with extended-release product

(continued)

TABLE 55-1	Adult Doses of Nonopioid Analgesics (Includes Only FDA-Approved Agents for Pain) (Continued)		
Class and Generic Name (Brand Name)	Approximate Half-Life (h)	Usual Dosage Range (mg)	Maximal Dose (mg/day)
Naproxen (Naprosyn, Anaprox, various)	12–17	500 initial 500 every 12 h or 250 every 6–8 h	1000[c]
Naproxen sodium[a] (Aleve, various, combined with esomeprazole [Vimovo])	12–17	In some patients, 440 initial[f] 220 every 8–12 h[f]	660[f]
Pyrrolizine carboxylic acid			
Ketorolac—parenteral (Toradol, various)	5–6	30[g]–60 (single IM dose only) 15[g]–30 (single IV dose only) 15[g]–30 every 6 h (IV dose) (max. 5 days)	30[g]–60 15[g]–30 60[g]–120
Ketorolac—oral, indicated for continuation with parenteral only (various)	5–6	10 every 4–6 h (max. 5 days, which includes parenteral doses) In nonelderly patients, initial oral dose of 20	40
Ketorolac—nasal spray, indicated for acute, moderate to moderately severe pain		1 spray (15.75 mg) in each nostril every 6–8 h in adults < 65 yr and weight ≥ 50 kg	126
Pyrazoles			
Celecoxib (Celebrex)	11	Initial 400 followed by another 200 on first day, then 200 twice daily (note some recommend maintenance doses of 200 mg/day due to cardiovascular concerns)	400

(FDA, Food and Drug Administration; h, hours; IM, intramuscular; IV, intravenous.)

[a]Available both as an over-the-counter preparation and as a prescription drug.

[b]Some experts believe 4000 mg may be too high. OTC max dose 3000 mg daily, lower with weight based dosing in pediatric patients.

[c]Up to 1250 mg on the first day.

[d]Up to 200 mg on the first day.

[e]Some individuals may respond better to 3200 mg as opposed to 2400 mg, although well-controlled trials show no better response; consider risk versus benefits when using 3200 mg/day.

[f]Over-the-counter dose.

[g]Dose for elderly and those under 50 kg (110 lb).

TABLE 55–2 Opioid Analgesics, Central Analgesics, Opioid Antagonist

Class and Generic Name (Brand Name)	Chemical Source	Relative Histamine Release	Route*	Equianalgesic Dose in Adults (mg)	Approximate Onset (min)/Half-Life (h)
Phenanthrenes (morphine-like agonists)					
Morphine (Embeda¹ various)	Naturally occurring	+++	IM/IV	10	10–20/2
			PO	30	
Hydromorphone (Dilaudid, Exalgo, various)	Semisynthetic	+	IM	1.5	10–20/2–3
			PO	7.5	
Oxymorphone (Numorphan, Opana)	Semisynthetic	+	IM	1	10–20/2–3
			PO	10	
Levorphanol (various)	Semisynthetic	+	IM	Variable	10–20/12–16
			PO	Variable	
Codeine (various)	Naturally occurring	+++	IM	15–30ᵃ	10–30/3
			PO	15–30ᵃ	
Hydrocodone (available as combination, single entity extended release—Hysingla ER, Zohydro ER)	Semisynthetic	N/A	PO	5–10ᵃ	30–60/4
Oxycodone (OxyContin¹, Oxecta¹, Xtampza, Xartemis XR [oxycodone & acetaminophen])	Semisynthetic	+	PO	15–30ᵇ	30–60/2–3

(continued)

TABLE 55–2	Opioid Analgesics, Central Analgesics, Opioid Antagonist (*Continued*)				
Class and Generic Name (Brand Name)	Chemical Source	Relative Histamine Release	Route*	Equianalgesic Dose in Adults (mg)	Approximate Onset (min)/Half-Life (h)
Phenylpiperidines (meperidine-like agonists)					
Meperidine (Demerol, various)	Synthetic	+++	IM/IV	75	10–20/3–5
			PO	300[b]; not recommended	
Fentanyl (Sublimaze, Duragesic, Lazanda, Abstral, Fentora, Subsys, OTFC, Ionsys, various)	Synthetic	+	IM	0.125[c]	7–15/3–4
			Transdermal Buccal, transmucosal, sublingual, nasal inhaled	Variable[d] Variable[d]	
Diphenylheptanes (methadone-like agonists)					
Methadone	Synthetic	+	IM/IV	Variable[e] (acute)	30–60/12–190
(Dolophine, various)			PO	Variable[e] (acute)	
			IM	Variable[e] (chronic)	
			PO	Variable[e] (chronic)	
Agonist–antagonist derivatives					
Pentazocine (Talwin, various)	Synthetic	N/A	IM	Not recommended	15–30/2–3
			PO	50[a]	
Butorphanol (Stadol, various)	Synthetic	N/A	IM	2	10–20/3–4
			Intranasal	1[a] (one spray)	
Nalbuphine (Nubain, various)	Synthetic	N/A	IM/IV	10	<15/5

Buprenorphine (Buprenex, Butrans, Suboxone, Belbuca, Subutex, various)	Synthetic	N/A	IM Transdermal Sublingual	0.3 Variable Variable	10–20/2–3
Antagonist					
Naloxone (Narcan, various)	Synthetic	N/A	IV	0.4–2[f]	1–2 (IV), 2–5 (IM)/0.5–1.3
Methylnaltrexone (Relistor)	Synthetic	N/A	SC	Variable	
Naltrexone (Revia)	Synthetic	N/A	PO		
Alvimopan (Entereg)	Synthetic	N/A	PO	12 mg QD–Q12 h	
Naloxegol (Movantik)	Synthetic	N/A	PO	12.5–25 mg QD	120/6–11
Central analgesics					
Tramadol (Ultram, Rybix, Ryzolt, ConZip, various)	Synthetic	N/A	PO	50–100[a,g,h]	<60/5–7
Tapentadol (Nucynta)	Synthetic	N/A	PO	50–100[a,g,h]	Within 60/4

(IM, intramuscular; IV, intravenous; N/A, not available; PO, oral.)

*The IM route should be avoided whenever possible —produces significant pain with administration and rate and extent of absorption is highly variable. If IV route is unavailable then administer subcutaneously (SC).

[a]Starting dose only (equianalgesia not shown).

[b]Starting doses lower (oxycodone 5–10 mg, meperidine 50–150 mg).

[c]Equivalent PO morphine dose = variable.

[d]For breakthrough pain only. Equianalgesic dose conversion should be avoided for Transmucosal Immediate Release Fentanyl (TIRF) products.

[e]The equianalgesic dose of methadone when compared with other opioids will decrease progressively the higher the previous opioid dose. Caution should be exercised when initiating in opioid naive patients.

[f]Starting doses to be used in cases of opioid overdose.

[g]First day of dosing may administer second dose 1 hour after first dose.

[h]Onset of action may differ for long-acting formulations. Ceiling dose recommendations exist and may differ from immediate release dosing recommendations.

[i]FDA approved as abuse-deterrent formulation.

TABLE 55–3 Dosing Guidelines

Agent(s)	Doses (Use Lowest Effective Dose, Titrate Up or Down Based on Patient Response, Opioid Tolerant Patients May Need Dose Modification)	Notes
NSAIDs/acetaminophen/aspirin	Use lowest effective dose for the shortest duration possible	Used in mild-to-moderate pain May use in conjunction with opioid agents to decrease doses of each Regular alcohol use and acetaminophen may result in liver toxicity Care must be exercised to avoid overdose when combination products containing these agents are used Underlying renal impairment, hypovolemia, and heart failure may predispose to nephrotoxicity
Morphine	PO 5–30 mg every 4 h[a] IM 5–20 mg every 4 h[a] IV 5–15 mg every 4 h[a] SR 15–30 mg every 12 h (may need to be every 8 h in some patients) Rectal 10–20 mg every 4 h[a]	Drug of choice in severe pain Use immediate-release product with SR product to control breakthrough pain in cancer patients Typical patient controlled analgesia IV dose is 1 mg with a 10-minute lock out interval Every 24-hour products available; use caution in renally-compromised patients
Hydromorphone	PO 2–4 mg every 4–6 h[a] XR 8 mg to 64 mg every 24 h IM 1–2 mg every 4–6 h[a] IV 0.5–2 mg every 4 h[a] Rectal 3 mg every 6–8 h[a]	Use in severe pain More potent than morphine; otherwise, no advantages Typical patient controlled analgesia IV dose is 0.2 mg with a 10-minute lock out interval Every 24-hour product (Exalgo) available
Oxymorphone	IM 1–1.5 mg every 4–6 h[a] IV 0.5 mg every 4–6 h[a] PO immediate-release 5–10 mg every 4–6 h[a]	Use in severe pain No advantages over morphine Use immediate-release product with controlled-release product to control breakthrough pain in cancer or chronic pain patients

Drug	Dosing	Notes
	PO extended-release 5–10 mg every 12 h[a]	Manufacturer recommends 5 mg every 12 h in opioid-naïve patients Take ER on empty stomach
Levorphanol	PO 2–3 mg every 6–8 h[a] (Levo-Dromoran) PO 2 mg every 3–6 h[a] (Levorphanol Tartrate) IM 1–2 mg every 6–8 h[a] IV 1 mg every 3–6 h[a]	Use in severe pain Extended half-life useful in cancer patients In chronic pain, wait 3 days between dosage adjustments
Codeine	PO 15–60 mg every 4–6 h[a] IM 15–60 mg every 4–6 h[a]	Use in mild to moderate pain Weak analgesic; analgesic prodrug
Hydrocodone	PO 5–10 mg every 4–6 h[a]	Use in moderate/severe pain
Oxycodone	PO 5–15 mg every 4–6 h[a] Controlled release 10–20 mg every 12 h	Use in moderate/severe pain Use immediate-release product with controlled-release product to control breakthrough pain in cancer or chronic pain patients CR reformulated to deter abuse
Meperidine	IM 50–150 mg every 3–4 h[a] IV 5–10 mg every 5 min prn[a]	Use in severe pain Oral not recommended Do not use in renal failure May precipitate tremors, myoclonus, and seizures Monoamine oxidase inhibitors can induce hyperpyrexia and/or seizures or opioid overdose symptoms
Fentanyl	IV 25–50 mcg/h IM 50–100 mcg every 1–2 h[a] Transdermal 25 mcg/h every 72 h Transmucosal (Actiq/OTFC Lozenge and Onsolis buccal film) 200 mcg may repeat × 1, 30 min after first dose is started, then titrate	Used in severe pain **Do not use transdermal in acute pain** Transmucosal for breakthrough cancer pain in patients already receiving or tolerant to opioids **Always start with lowest dose despite daily opioid intake. Product specific titration recommendations exist**

(continued)

579

TABLE 55–3 Dosing Guidelines (Continued)

Agent(s)	Doses (Use Lowest Effective Dose, Titrate Up or Down Based on Patient Response, Opioid Tolerant Patients May Need Dose Modification)	Notes
	Transmucosal (Fentora Buccal Tablet) 100 mcg, may repeat × 1, 30 min after first dose is started, then titrate Intranasal (Lazanda Spray) 100 mcg (one spray) in one nostril. Wait 2 h prior to redosing Sublingual (Subsys Spray) 100 mcg (1 spray). Wait 4 h prior to redosing Sublingual (Abstral Tablet) 100 mcg tablets placed sublingually. Must wait 2 h prior to redosing	
Methadone	PO 2.5–10 mg every 8–12 h[a] IM 2.5–10 mg every 8–12 h[a]	Effective in severe chronic pain Some chronic pain patients can be dosed every 12 h Equianalgesic dose of methadone when compared with other opioids will decrease progressively the higher the previous opioid dose. Avoid dose titrations more frequently than weekly in chronic pain maintenance
Pentazocine	PO 50–100 mg every 3–4 h[b] (max. 600 mg daily, for those 50 mg tablet containing 0.5 mg of naloxone) PO 25 mg every 4 h[b] (max. 150 mg daily, for those 25 mg tablet containing 325 mg of acetaminophen)	Second-line agent for moderate-to-severe pain May precipitate withdrawal in opiate-dependent patients Parenteral doses not recommended
Butorphanol	IM 1–4 mg every 3–4 h[b] IV 0.5–2 mg every 3–4 h[b] Intranasal 1 mg (1 spray) every 3–4 h[b] If inadequate relief after initial spray, may repeat in other nostril × 1 in 60–90 min Max. 2 sprays (one per nostril) every 3–4 h[b]	Second-line agent for moderate-to-severe pain May precipitate withdrawal in opiate-dependent patients

Drug	Dosing	Notes
Nalbuphine	IM/IV 10 mg every 3–6 h[b] (max. 20 mg dose, 160 mg daily)	Second-line agent for moderate-to-severe pain May precipitate withdrawal in opiate-dependent patients Used frequently in low doses to treat/prevent opioid-induced pruritus
Buprenorphine	IM 0.3 mg every 6 h[b] Slow IV 0.3 mg every 6 h[b]	Second-line agent for moderate-to-severe pain May precipitate withdrawal in opiate-dependent patients Transdermal delivery systems (5, 7.5, 10, 15, 20 mcg/h) available for every 7 day administration. Detailed manufacturer dosing conversion recommendations exist Naloxone may not be effective in reversing respiratory depression
Naloxone	May repeat × 1, 30–60 min after initial dose IV IM 0.4–2 mg	When reversing opiate side effects in patients needing analgesia, dilute and titrate (0.1–0.2 mg every 2–3 min) so as not to reverse analgesia
Tramadol	PO 50–100 mg every 4–6 h[a] If rapid onset not required, start 25 mg/day and titrate over several days Extended release PO 100 mg every 24 h	Maximum dose for nonextended-release, 400 mg/24 h; maximum for extended release, 300 mg/24 h Decrease dose in patient with renal impairment and in the elderly
Tapentadol	PO 50–100 mg every 4–6 h[a]	First day of therapy may administer second dose after the first within 1 h; maximum dose first day 700 mg, max. dose thereafter 600 mg (max. dose for CR 500 mg)

(CR, controlled release; ER, extended release; IM, intramuscular; IV, intravenous; NSAID, nonsteroidal antiinflammatory drug; PO, oral; prn, as needed; SR, sustained release; HCL, hydrochloride.)

[a]May start with an around-the-clock regimen and switch to prn if/when the painful signal subsides or is episodic.
[b]May reach a ceiling analgesic effect.

TABLE 55–4	Major Adverse Effects of the Opioid Analgesics
Effect	**Manifestation**
Mood changes	Dysphoria, euphoria
Somnolence	Sedation, inability to concentrate
Stimulation of chemoreceptor trigger zone	Nausea, vomiting
Respiratory depression	Decreased respiratory rate
Decreased gastrointestinal motility	Constipation
Increase in sphincter tone	Biliary spasm, urinary retention (varies among agents)
Histamine release	Urticaria, pruritus, rarely exacerbation of asthma due to bronchospasm (varies among agents)
Tolerance	Larger doses for same effect
Dependence	Withdrawal symptoms upon abrupt discontinuation
Addiction	Genetic predisposition leads to loss of control of drug use, continued use despite harm, compulsion to use, cravings
Hypogonadism	Fatigue, depression, loss of analgesia, sexual dysfunction, amenorrhea (women)
Sleep	Disrupts sleep-wake cycle, causes dose-dependent rapid eye movement (REM) suppression

TABLE 55–5	Opioids to Avoid/Exercise Caution	
Drug	**Caution**	**Notes**
Codeine	Do not use—especially in children and breastfeeding	Codeine is a prod rug, must be converted by CYP 2D6 to morphine to produce analgesia. High degree of polymorphism of 2D6, ultra-rapid metabolism = toxicity, poor metabolism = no analgesia
Meperidine	Do not use	Short duration of analgesia requiring frequent dosing Produces non-analgesic, toxic metabolite normeperidine, accumulation results in seizures, risk of accumulation increased in renal insufficiency
Agonist/Antagonist agents	Caution	Can produce opioid withdrawal in patients chronically taking opioid. Higher rate of psychomimetic reactions compared to other opioids
Tramadol	Caution—especially in elderly or in renal dysfunction	Tramadol is a pro-drug, must be converted by CYP 2D6 to desmethyl-tramadol (M1) to produce analgesia. High degree of polymorphism of 2D6, ultra-rapid metabolism = toxicity, poor metabolism = no analgesia Risk of seizure, risk of serotonin syndrome, risk of hypoglycemia

- Partial agonists and antagonists (eg, **nalbuphine**) compete with agonists for opioid receptor sites and exhibit mixed agonist–antagonist activity. They may produce analgesia with fewer side effects.
- Initially give analgesics around-the-clock for acute pain. As pain subsides, as-needed schedules can be used. Around-the-clock administration is also useful for management of chronic pain.
- Patients with severe pain may receive high doses of opioids with no unwanted side effects, but as pain subsides, patients may not tolerate even low doses.
- Most opioid-related itching or rash is due to histamine release from cutaneous mast cells, and is not a true allergic response.
- When opioid allergies occur, an opioid from a different structural class may be cautiously tried. For these purposes, the mixed agonist–antagonist class behaves most like the morphine-like agonists.
- With patient-controlled analgesia (PCA), patients self-administer preset amounts of IV opioids via a syringe pump electronically interfaced with a timing device. PCA provides better pain control, improved patient satisfaction, and relatively few differences in side effects compared to traditional as needed administration.
- Administration of opioids directly into the CNS (see Table 55–6) (eg, epidural and intrathecal/subarachnoid routes) is commonly used by anesthesiology pain consult services for acute pain, chronic noncancer pain, and cancer pain. These methods require very careful monitoring as marked sedation, respiratory depression, pruritus, vomiting, urinary retention, and hypotension can occur. **Naloxone** is used to reverse respiratory depression, but continuous infusion may be required. Monitor respiratory function for at least 24 hours after a single dose of intrathecal or epidural morphine with standing orders for naloxone if needed.
- All agents administered directly into the CNS should be preservative-free.

Morphine and Congeners (Phenanthrenes)

- Many clinicians consider **Morphine** the first-line agent for moderate to severe pain. It is often considered the opioid of choice for pain associated with myocardial infarction, as it decreases myocardial oxygen demand.
- In patients with head trauma who are not ventilated, morphine-induced respiratory depression can increase intracranial pressure and cloud the neurologic examination results.
- Respiratory depression often manifests as decreased respiratory rate, but tidal exchange and minute volume are also affected, and the cough reflex is depressed. Patients with underlying pulmonary dysfunction are at increased risk for respiratory depression, which can be reversed by **naloxone**.

TABLE 55–6	Intraspinal Opioids			
Agent	Single Dose (mg)	Onset of Pain Relief (min)	Duration of Pain Relief (h)	Continual Infusion Dose (mg/h)
Epidural route				
Morphine	1–6	30	6–24	0.1–1
Hydromorphone	0.8–1.5	5–8	4–8	0.1–0.3
Fentanyl	0.025–0.1	5	2–8	0.025–0.1
Sufentanil	0.01–0.06	5	2–4	0.01–0.05
Subarachnoid route				
Morphine	0.1–0.3	15	8–34	–
Fentanyl	0.005–0.025	5	3–6	–

Note: Doses above should not be interpreted as equianalgesic doses for conversion to or from the specific opioid or route of administration.

- Combining opioid analgesics with alcohol or other CNS depressants amplifies CNS depression and is potentially lethal.
- Hypovolemic patients are at particular risk for **morphine**-induced orthostatic hypotension.
- Most clinicians avoid morphine in renally compromised patients (i.e., creatinine clearance less than or equal to 30 mL/min [0.5 mL/s]).
- Counsel patients to take the extended release **oxymorphone** without food, as high-fat meals can greatly increase absorption, increasing risk of toxicity.
- **Codeine**, alone or combined with other analgeics (eg, acetaminophen) is commonly used for mild to moderate pain. **Oxycodone** is useful for moderate to severe pain, especially when combined with nonopioids.

Meperidine and Congeners (Phenylpiperidines)

- **Meperidine** is less potent and has a shorter duration of action than morphine.
- With high doses or in patients with renal failure, the metabolite normeperidine accumulates, causing tremor, muscle twitching, and possibly seizures. In most settings, meperidine offers no advantages over morphine. Do not use it long term, and avoid its use in the elderly and in those with renal dysfunction.
- Do not combine meperidine with monoamine oxidase inhibitors because severe respiratory depression or excitation, delirium, hyperpyrexia, and convulsions may occur.
- **Fentanyl**, often used as an adjunct to general anesthesia, is more potent and faster acting than meperidine. It is used for breakthrough cancer pain (see Table 55–3).

Methadone and Congeners (Diphenylheptanes)

- **Methadone** has extended duration of action. Studies show a growing number of methadone-related deaths. High doses cause cardiac arrhythmias. Do not titrate more frequently than every 5 to 7 days. Although effective for acute pain, it is used for chronic cancer pain.
- There is a growing number of methadone-related deaths. The equianalgesic dose of methadone may decrease with higher doses of the previous opioid.

Opioid Agonist–Antagonist Derivatives

- This analgesic class may cause less respiratory depression than opioids and may have lower abuse potential than morphine. However, psychotomimetic responses (eg, hallucinations and dysphoria), a limited analgesic effect, and the propensity to initiate withdrawal in opioid-dependent patients have limited their use.

Opioid Antagonists

- **Naloxone**, a pure opioid antagonist that binds competitively to opioid receptors, does not produce analgesia or opioid side effects. It reverses the toxic effects of agonist and agonist–antagonist opioids. In some states in the United States, pharmacists are assuming greater roles in administering or dispensing naloxone for patients who have experienced opioid overdoses.

Central Analgesic

- **Tramadol** and **tapentadol** are centrally acting analgesics. Tramadol, indicated for moderate to moderately severe pain, binds to μ opiate receptors and inhibits norepinephrine and serotonin reuptake. Tapentadol, for moderate to severe acute pain and diabetic peripheral neuropathy, binds to the same receptor and inhibits norepinephrine.
- They have side-effect profiles similar to those of other opioid analgesics. They may increase the risk of seizures. Tramadol may be useful for chronic pain, especially neuropathic pain. Tapentadol, a schedule II controlled substance, may be useful for acute pain.

COANALGESICS

- Chronic pain with a neuropathic component (eg, diabetic neuropathy) often requires coanalgesic therapy, such as antidepressants (eg, **nortriptyline**, **duloxetine**, **venlafaxine**),

TABLE 55–7	Local Anesthetics[a]	
Agent (Brand Name)	Onset (min)	Duration (h)
Esters		
Procaine (Novocain, various)	2–5	0.25–1
Chloroprocaine (Nesacaine, various)	6–12	0.5
Tetracaine (Pontocaine)	≤15	2–3
Amides		
Mepivacaine (Polocaine, various)	3–5	0.75–1.5
Bupivacaine (Marcaine, various)	5	2–4
Bupivacaine liposomal (Exparel—wound infiltration only)	Variable	24 local 96 systemic
Lidocaine (Xylocaine, various)	<2	0.5–1
Prilocaine (Citanest)	<2	1–2
Ropivacaine[b] (Naropin)	10–30	0.5–6

[a]Unless otherwise indicated, values are for infiltrative anesthesia.
[b]Epidural administration.

anticonvulsants (**gabapentin**, **pregabalin**), or topically applied local anesthetics. For cancer bone pain, **strontium-89**, **samarium**, **corticosteroids**, and **bisphosphonates** are useful coanalgesics.

REGIONAL ANALGESIA

• Regional analgesia with **local anesthetics** (Table 55–7) is useful for both acute and chronic pain. Anesthetics can be positioned by injection (eg, in the joints, epidural or intrathecal space, nerve plexus, or along nerve roots), or applied topically.

• High plasma concentrations of local anesthetics can cause dizziness, tinnitus, drowsiness, seizures, and respiratory arrest. Cardiovascular effects include myocardial depression, heart block, hypotension, bradycardia, and cardiac arrest. Skillful application, frequent administration, and specialized follow-up are required.

SPECIAL POPULATIONS

• The elderly and young are at higher risk of undertreatment. In these populations, it is important to monitor signs (eg, heart rate) and to talk with parents or caregivers.

• Those with chronic, debilitating, and life threatening illnesses need specialized pain control and palliative care.

• Pharmacologic therapy of cancer pain (see Fig. 55–2) should be coupled with psychological, surgical, and supportive therapies using an interdisciplinary approach. Continuous assessment of pain response, side effects, and behavior are required.

• Do not give aspirin-like compounds to children or teenagers with viral illnesses (eg, influenza or chickenpox), as Reye syndrome may result.

EVALUATION OF THERAPEUTIC OUTCOMES

- Pain intensity, pain relief, and medication side effects must be assessed regularly. The frequency of assessment depends on the type of pain, analgesic used, route of administration, and concomitant medications. Postoperative pain and acute exacerbations of cancer pain may require hourly assessment. Chronic nonmalignant pain may need only daily (or less frequent) monitoring. Quality of life must be assessed regularly.
- The four A's (eg, *a*nalgesia, *a*ctivity, *a*berrant drug behavior, and *a*dverse effects) are key assessment measures for patients with chronic pain.
- Patients taking opioids should be counseled on proper intake of fluids and fiber, and a stimulant laxative should be added with chronic opioid use.

See Chapter 60, Pain Management, authored by Chris M. Herndon, Jennifer M. Strickland, and James B. Ray, for a more detailed discussion of this topic.

56 Parkinson Disease

- *Parkinson disease* (PD) has highly characteristic neuropathologic findings and a clinical presentation, including motor deficits and, in some cases, mental deterioration.

PATHOPHYSIOLOGY

- Two hallmark features in the substantia nigra pars compacta are loss of neurons and presence of Lewy bodies. The degree of nigrostriatal dopamine loss correlates positively with severity of motor symptoms.
- Reduced activation of dopamine$_1$ and dopamine$_2$ receptors results in greater inhibition of the thalamus and reduced activation of the motor cortex. Clinical improvement may be tied to restoring activity more at the dopamine$_2$ receptor than at the dopamine$_1$ receptor.

CLINICAL PRESENTATION

- PD develops insidiously and progresses slowly over many years.
- Initial symptoms may be sensory, but as the disease progresses, one or more classic primary features present (eg, resting tremor, rigidity, bradykinesia, and postural instability that may lead to falls).
- Resting tremor is often the sole presenting complaint. However, only two thirds of PD patients have tremor on diagnosis, and some never develop this sign. Tremor is present most commonly in the hands, often begins unilaterally, and sometimes has a characteristic "pill-rolling" quality. Resting tremor is usually abolished by volitional movement and is absent during sleep.
- Muscular rigidity involves increased muscular resistance to passive range of motion and can be cogwheel in nature. It commonly affects both upper and lower extremities; neck and facial muscles may be affected.
- Intellectual deterioration is not inevitable, but some patients deteriorate in a manner indistinguishable from Alzheimer disease.
- Nonmotor symptoms are common and must be identified, treated, and monitored (Table 56–1).

DIAGNOSIS

- A diagnosis of PD can be made with a high level of confidence when there is bradykinesia (along with resting tremor and/or rigidity), prominent asymmetry, and a positive response to dopaminergic medication.
- Other symptoms may include: decreased dexterity, difficulty arising from a chair, postural instability, festinating gait, dysarthria, difficulty swallowing, reduced facial expression, freezing at initiation of movement, hypophonia, micrographia, overactive bladder, constipation, blood pressure changes, dementia, anxiety, depression, sleepiness, insomnia, obstructive sleep apnea.
- Exclude other conditions, such as medication-induced Parkinsonism (eg, induced by antipsychotics, phenothiazine antiemetics, or metoclopramide), essential tremor, corticobasal ganglionic degeneration, multiple system atrophy, and progressive supranuclear palsy.

TREATMENT

- <u>Goals of Treatment</u>: The goals of treatment are to minimize symptoms, disability, and side effects while maintaining quality of life. Education of patients and caregivers, exercise, and proper nutrition are essential.

TABLE 56–1	Nonmotor Symptoms and Possible Treatments
Symptom	**Possible Treatments**
Anxiety	Cognitive behavioral therapy, selective serotonin reuptake inhibitors, venlafaxine, minimize "off" times.
Cognitive impairment	Eliminate anticholinergic agents. Add cholinesterase inhibitor.
Constipation	Fiber, hydration, exercise, laxatives, stool softeners.
Daytime sleepiness	Proper night time sleep hygiene, reduce dose of dopamine agonist, referral to sleep specialist to rule out apnea and sleep disorders.
Depression	Selective serotonin reuptake inhibitor, newer-generation serotonin norepinephrine reuptake inhibitor, cognitive behavioral therapy.
Drooling	Local injection of botulinum toxin, atropine sublingual drop, glycopyrrolate, ipratropium sublingual spray.
Dysphagia	Referral to speech therapist, dysphagia diet, avoid anti-cholinergic medications, manage dry mouth.
Fatigue	Caffeine, armodafinil, modafinil, proper night time sleep hygiene, referral to sleep specialist to rule out sleep disorder.
Falling	Referral to physical therapy; assistance with ambulation, minimize risk for bone fractures, treat osteoporosis.
Hallucinations/psychosis	Eliminate adjunctive medications, especially anticholinergic agents and dopamine agonists. Add clozapine, quetiapine, pimavanserin.
Impulse control disorder	Discontinue dopamine agonist or add clozapine, quetiapine, or naltrexone
Insomnia	Nonbenzodiazepine $GABA_A$ agonists, trazodone.
Orthostatic hypotension	Reduce dose of alpha-blockers, dopamine agonist, diuretics, vasodilators. Abdominal compression, add salt and water to diet, water boluses, fludrocortisone, midodrine, droxidopa, pyridostigmine.
Overactive bladder	Behavioral therapies (eg, bladder training, fluid management, pelvic floor muscle exercises), antimuscarinic agents, mirabegron, intradetrusor injections of botulinum toxin.
Pain	Treatment as per type of pain (eg, dystonic, musculoskeletal, neuropathic), minimize "off" times, appropriate referral to orthopedics, physical therapy, pain specialist, rheumatology.
REM sleep behavior disorder	Clonazepam, melatonin.
Restless legs syndrome	Dopamine agonist at bedtime; gabapentin.

(GABA, γ-aminobutyric acid; REM, rapid eye movement.)

PHARMACOLOGIC THERAPY

General Approach

- An algorithm for management of early to advanced PD is shown in **Fig. 56–1**. **Table 56–2** is a summary of available antiparkinson medications and their dosing, and **Table 56–3** shows side effect monitoring.

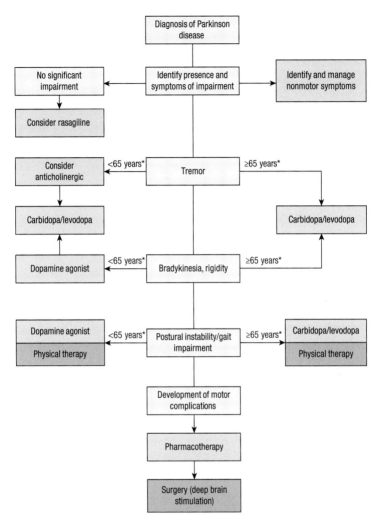

*Age is not the sole determinant for drug choice. Other factors such as cognitive function and overall tolerability of drug (especially in the elderly) should be considered.

FIGURE 56–1. General approach to the management of early to advanced Parkinson disease.

- Monotherapy usually begins with a **monoamine oxidase-B (MAO-B) inhibitor**.
- Consider addition of a **catechol-*O*-methyltransferase (COMT) inhibitor** if motor fluctuations develop to extend L-**dopa** duration of activity. Alternatively, consider addition of an MAO-B inhibitor or **dopamine agonist**.
- For management of L-dopa-induced peak-dose dyskinesias, consider addition of **amantadine**.

TABLE 56-2	Dosing of Drugs Used in Parkinson Disease[a]			
Generic Name	Trade Name	Starting Dose[b] (mg/day)	Maintenance Dose[b] (mg/day)	Dosage Forms (mg)
Anticholinergic drugs				
Benztropine	Cogentin	0.5–1	1–6	0.5, 1, 2
Trihexyphenidyl	Artane	1–2	6–15	2, 5, 2/5 mL
Carbidopa/Levodopa products				
Carbidopa/L-dopa	Sinemet	300[c]	300–2000[c]	10/100, 25/100, 25/250
Carbidopa/L-dopa ODT	Parcopa	300[c]	300–2000[c]	10/100, 25/100, 25/250
Carbidopa/L-dopa CR	Sinemet CR	400[c]	400–2000[c]	25/100, 50/200
Carbidopa/L-dopa IR/ER	Rytary	435[c]	435–2450[c]	23.75/95, 36.25/145, 48.75/195, 61.25/245[d]
Carbidopa/L-dopa enteral suspension	Duopa	1000[c]	1000–2000[c]	4.63/20 per mL
Carbidopa/L-dopa/ entacapone	Stalevo	600[e]	600–1600[e]	12.5/50/200, 18.75/75/200, 25/100/200, 31.25/125/200, 37.5/150/200, 50/200/200
Carbidopa	Lodosyn	25	25–75	25
Dopamine agonists				
Apomorphine	Apokyn	1–3	3–12	30/3 mL[f]
Bromocriptine	Parlodel	2.5–5	15–40	2.5, 5
Pramipexole	Mirapex	0.125	1.5–4.5	0.125, 0.25, 0.5, 1, 1.5
Pramipexole ER	Mirapex ER	0.375	1.5–4.5	0.375, 0.75, 1.5, 3, 4.5
Ropinirole	Requip	0.75	9–24	0.25, 0.5, 1, 2, 3, 4, 5
Ropinirole XL	Requip XL	2	8–24	2, 4, 6, 8, 12
Rotigotine	Neupro	2	2–8	1, 2, 3, 4, 6, 8
COMT inhibitors				
Entacapone	Comtan	200–600	200–1600	200
Tolcapone	Tasmar	300	300–600	100, 200
MAO-B inhibitors				
Rasagiline	Azilect	0.5–1	0.5–1	0.5, 1
Selegiline	Eldepryl	5–10	5–10	5
Selegiline ODT	Zelapar	1.25	1.25–2.5	1.25, 2.5
Miscellaneous				
Amantadine	Symmetrel	100	200–300	100, 50/5 mL

(COMT, catechol-O-methyltransferase; CR, controlled release; IR/ER, immediate-release/extended-release; MAO, monoamine oxidase; ODT, orally disintegrating tablet.)
[a]Marketed in the United States for Parkinson disease.
[b]Dosages may vary.
[c]Dosages expressed as L-dopa component.
[d]Dosages of Rytary were developed to avoid confusion with other oral carbidopa/L-dopa products that contain L-dopa in multiples of 50 mg.
[e]Dosages expressed as entacapone component.
[f]Sterile solution of subcutaneous injection with supplied pen injector.

TABLE 56–3	Monitoring of Potential Adverse Reactions to Drug Therapy for Parkinson Disease		
Generic Name	Adverse Drug Reaction	Monitoring Parameter	Comments
Amantadine	Confusion	Mental status; renal function	Reduce dosage; adjust dose for renal impairment
	Livedo reticularis	Lower extremity examination; ankle edema	Reversible upon drug discontinuation
Benztropine	Anticholinergic effects, confusion, drowsiness	Dry mouth, mental status, constipation, urinary retention, vision	Reduce dosage; avoid in elderly and in those with a history of constipation, memory impairment, urinary retention
Trihexyphenidyl	See benztropine	See benztropine	See benztropine
Carbidopa/L-dopa	Drowsiness	Mental status	Reduce dose
	Dyskinesias	Abnormal involuntary movements	Reduce dose; add amantadine
	Nausea	Nausea	Take with food
COMT Inhibitors			
Entacapone	Augmentation of L-dopa side effects; also diarrhea	See carbidopa/L-dopa; also bowel movements	Reduce dose of L-dopa; antidiarrheal agents
Tolcapone	See entacapone; also liver toxicity	See carbidopa/L-dopa; also ALT/AST	See carbidopa/L-dopa; also at start of therapy and for every dose increase, ALT and AST levels at baseline and every 2–4 weeks for the first 6 months of therapy; afterward monitor based on clinical judgment.
Dopamine Agonists			
Apomorphine	Drowsiness	Mental status	Reduce dose
	Nausea	Nausea	Premedicate with trimethobenzamide
	Orthostatic hypotension	Blood pressure, dizziness upon standing	Reduce dose
Bromocriptine	See pramipexole; also pulmonary fibrosis	Mental status; also chest radiograph	Reduce dose; chest radiograph at baseline and once yearly

(continued)

591

TABLE 56–3 Monitoring of Potential Adverse Reactions to Drug Therapy for Parkinson Disease *(Continued)*

Generic Name	Adverse Drug Reaction	Monitoring Parameter	Comments
Pramipexole	Confusion	Mental status	Reduce dose
	Drowsiness	Mental status	Reduce dose
	Edema	Lower extremity swelling	Reduce dose or discontinue medication
	Hallucinations/delusions	Behavior, mental status	Reduce dose or discontinue medication
	Impulsivity	Behavior	Discontinue medication
	Nausea	Nausea	Titrate dose upward slowly; take with food
	Orthostatic hypotension	Blood pressure, dizziness upon standing	Reduce dose
Ropinirole	See pramipexole	See pramipexole	See pramipexole
Rotigotine	See pramipexole; also skin irritation at site of patch application	See pramipexole; also skin examination	See pramipexole; rotate patch application site
MAO-B Inhibitors			
Rasagiline	Nausea	Nausea	Take with food
Selegiline	Agitation/confusion	Mental status	Reduce dose
	Insomnia	Sleep	Administer dose earlier in day
	Hallucinations	Behavior, mental status	Reduce dose
	Orthostatic hypotension	Blood pressure, dizziness upon standing	Reduce dose

(ALT, alanine aminotransferase; AST, aspartate aminotransferase; COMT, catechol-O-methyltransferase; MAO, monoamine oxidase.)

Anticholinergic Medications

- Anticholinergic drugs can improve tremor and sometimes dystonic features in some patients, but they rarely substantially improve bradykinesia or other disabilities. They can be used as monotherapy or in conjunction with other antiparkinson drugs.
- Anticholinergic side effects include dry mouth, blurred vision, constipation, and urinary retention. More serious reactions include forgetfulness, confusion, sedation, depression, and anxiety (see Table 56–3). Patients with preexisting cognitive deficits and the elderly are at greater risk for central anticholinergic side effects.

Amantadine

- Amantadine often provides modest benefit for tremor, rigidity, and bradykinesia, but is most often used for L-dopa-induced dyskinesia.
- Adverse effects include sedation, dry mouth, hallucinations, dizziness, and confusion. Livedo reticularis (a diffuse mottling of the skin in the upper or lower extremities) is a common but reversible side effect.
- Doses should be reduced in patients with renal dysfunction (100 mg/day with creatinine clearances of 30–50 mL/min [0.50–0.84 mL/s], 100 mg every other day for creatinine clearances of 15–29 mL/min [0.25–0.49 mL/s], and 200 mg every 7 days for creatinine clearances less than 15 mL/min [0.25 mL/s]) and those on hemodialysis.

L-Dopa and Carbidopa/L-Dopa

- L-**dopa**, the most effective drug available, is a precursor of dopamine. Unlike **dopamine**, **carbidopa**, and **benserazide**, it crosses the blood-brain barrier. Ultimately, all PD patients will require L-dopa.
- In the central nervous system (CNS) and peripherally, L-dopa is converted by L-amino acid decarboxylase (L-AAD) to dopamine. In the periphery, carbidopa or benserazide can block L-AAD, thus increasing CNS penetration of administered L-dopa and decreasing dopamine adverse effects (eg, nausea, cardiac arrhythmias, postural hypotension, and vivid dreams). Benserazide is unavailable in the United States.
- The usual maximal dose of L-dopa tolerated is approximately 1000 to 1500 mg/day.
- About 75 mg of carbidopa is required to effectively block peripheral L-AAD, but some patients need more. Carbidopa/L-dopa 25/100 mg tablet three times daily is the usual initial maintenance dose. Also available are the 25/250 mg and 10/100 mg dosage forms. Controlled-release preparations of carbidopa/L-dopa are also available (Table 56–2). For patients with difficulty swallowing, an orally disintegrating tablet is available, and a capsule containing beads is available which can be sprinkled on food (Rytary).
- After oral L-dopa administration, time to peak plasma concentrations varies intra- and intersubject. Meals delay gastric emptying, but antacids promote gastric emptying. L-dopa is absorbed primarily in the proximal duodenum via a saturable large neutral amino acid transport system, thus high-protein meals can interfere with bioavailability.
- L-dopa is not bound to plasma proteins, and the elimination half-life is approximately 1 hour. Adding carbidopa or benserazide can extend the half-life to 1.5 hours, and adding a COMT inhibitor (eg, **entacapone**) can extend it to approximately 2 to 2.5 hours.
- Sinemet CR and Rytary are 70% and 75% bioavailable compared to the standard immediate release carbidopa/L-dopa formulation.
- Long-term, L-dopa-associated motor complications can be disabling. The most common of these are "end-of-dose wearing off" and "peak-dose dyskinesias." The risk of developing motor fluctuations or dyskinesias is approximately 10% per year of L-dopa therapy. However, motor complications can occur 5 to 6 months after starting L-dopa, especially when excessive doses are used initially. Table 56–4 shows these motor complications and suggests management strategies.

TABLE 56–4	Common Motor Complications and Possible Initial Treatments
Effect	**Possible Treatments**
End-of-dose "wearing off" (motor fluctuation)	Increase frequency of carbidopa/L-dopa doses; add either COMT inhibitor or MAO-B inhibitor or dopamine agonist; add or switch to extended release carbidopa/L-dopa (ie, Rytary)
"Delayed on" or "no on" response	Give carbidopa/L-dopa on empty stomach; use carbidopa/L-dopa ODT; avoid carbidopa/L-dopa SR; use apomorphine subcutaneous
Start hesitation ("freezing")	Increase carbidopa/L-dopa dose; add a dopamine agonist or MAO-B inhibitor; utilize physical therapy along with assistive walking devices or sensory cues (eg, rhythmic commands, stepping over objects)
Peak-dose dyskinesia	Provide smaller doses of carbidopa/L-dopa; reduce dose of adjunctive dopamine agonist; add amantadine

(COMT, catechol-O-methyltransferase; MAO, monoamine oxidase; ODT, orally disintegrating tablet; SR, sustained release.)

- "End-of-dose wearing off" is related to the increasing loss of neuronal dopamine storage capability and the short half-life of L-dopa. Bedtime administration of a dopamine agonist or a sustained-release formulation product (eg, carbidopa/L-dopa CR, **ropinirole XL**, **rotigotine transdermal patch**, or **pramipexole ER**) may help reduce nighttime off episodes and improve morning functioning. Administration of Rytary may also be useful, as therapeutic levels of L-dopa are rapidly achieved and maintained for 4 to 5 hours (see Table 56–4).
- "Delayed-on" or "no-on" can result from delayed gastric emptying or decreased absorption in the duodenum. Chewing or crushing carbidopa/L-dopa tablets and taking with a glass of water or using the orally disintegrating tablet on an empty stomach may help. Subcutaneous apomorphine may be used as rescue therapy.
- "Freezing," episodic inhibition of lower extremity motor function, may be worsened by anxiety and may increase falls.
- Dyskinesias, involuntary choreiform movements usually involving the neck, trunk, and extremities, are usually associated with peak striatal dopamine levels. Less commonly, dyskinesias can develop during the rise and fall of L-dopa effects (the dyskinesias-improvement-dyskinesias or diphasic pattern of response).
- "Off-period dystonia," muscle contractions most commonly in distal lower extremities (eg, feet or toes) occurs often in the early morning. Consider bedtime administration of sustained-release products, use of baclofen, or selective denervation with botulinum toxin. If dystonia occurs as part of an L-dopa peak dose effect, management is similar to that of dyskinesias.

Monoamine Oxidase B Inhibitors

- At therapeutic doses, **selegiline** and **rasagiline**, selective, irreversible inhibitors of MAO-B, are unlikely to induce a "cheese reaction" (hypertension, headache) unless excessive amounts of dietary tyramine are ingested. However, combining MAO-B inhibitors with meperidine and other opioid analgesics is contraindicated because of a small risk of serotonin syndrome.
- Selegiline blocks dopamine breakdown and can extend the on time of L-dopa up to 1 hour. It often permits reduction of the L-dopa dose by as much as one half.
- Selegiline also increases the peak effects of L-dopa and can worsen preexisting dyskinesias or psychiatric symptoms, such as delusions. Metabolites of selegiline are L-methamphetamine and L-amphetamine. The oral disintegrating tablet may provide improved response and fewer side effects than the conventional formulation.

- Rasagiline also enhances L-dopa effects and is modestly beneficial as monotherapy. Early initiation may be associated with better long-term outcomes.
- Rasagiline may provide 1 hour of extra "on" time during the day. It is considered a first-line agent (as is entacapone) for managing motor fluctuations of L-dopa.
- There is no firm evidence that selegiline or rasagiline slow neurodegeneration.

Catechol-O-Methyltransferase Inhibitors

- **Tolcapone** and **entacapone** are used in conjunction with carbidopa/L-dopa to prevent the peripheral conversion of L-dopa to dopamine (increasing the area under the curve of L-dopa by approximately 35%). Thus, "on" time is increased by approximately 1 to 2 hours, and dosage requirements of L-dopa are decreased. Avoid concomitant use of nonselective MAO inhibitors to prevent inhibition of the pathways for normal catecholamine metabolism.
- Tolcapone's use is limited by the potential for fatal liver toxicity, requiring strict monitoring of liver function. Reserve tolcapone for patients with fluctuations unresponsive to other therapies.
- Because entacapone has a shorter half-life, 200 mg is given with each dose of carbidopa/L-dopa up to eight times a day. Dopaminergic adverse effects may occur and are managed by reducing the carbidopa/L-dopa dose. Brownish orange urine discoloration may occur (as with tolcapone), but hepatotoxicity is not reported with entacapone.

Dopamine Agonists

- The ergot derivative **bromocriptine** and the nonergots **pramipexole**, **rotigotine**, and **ropinirole** are beneficial adjuncts in patients experiencing fluctuation in response to L-dopa. They decrease the frequency of "off" periods and provide an L-dopa-sparing effect.
- Titrate the dose of dopamine agonists slowly to enhance tolerability, and find the least dose that provides optimal benefit (see Table 56–2).
- The nonergots are safer and are effective as monotherapy in mild to moderate PD and as adjuncts to L-dopa in patients with motor fluctuations.
- There is less risk of developing motor complications from monotherapy with dopamine agonists than from L-dopa. Because younger patients are more likely to develop motor fluctuations, dopamine agonists are preferred in this population. Older patients are more likely to experience psychosis and orthostatic hypotension from dopamine agonists; therefore, carbidopa/L-dopa may be the best initial medication in elderly patients. For patients with cognitive problems or dementia, dopamine agonists are best avoided.
- Common side effects of dopamine agonists are shown in Table 56–3. Other side effects include vivid dreams and sleep attacks. When added to L-dopa, dopamine agonists may worsen dyskinesias. Hallucinations or delusions should be managed by dosage reduction or discontinuation and if needed addition of an atypical antipsychotic, such as clozapine, quetiapine, or pimavanserin.
- **Bromocriptine** is not commonly used because of its safety profile, which includes a risk of pulmonary fibrosis.
- **Pramipexole** is primarily renally excreted, and the initial dose must be adjusted in renal insufficiency. A once-daily extended-release formulation is available.
- **Ropinirole** is metabolized by cytochrome P4501A2; **fluoroquinolones** and smoking may alter ropinirole clearance. A once-daily formulation is available.
- **Rotigotine** patch provides continuous release over 24 hours, and disposition is not affected by hepatic or renal impairment.
- **Apomorphine** is a nonergot dopamine agonist given as a subcutaneous "rescue" injection. For patients with advanced PD with intermittent "off" episodes despite optimized therapy, subcutaneous apomorphine triggers an "on" response within 20 minutes, and duration of effect is up to 100 mins. Most patients require 0.06 mg/kg. Prior to injection, patients should be premedicated with the antiemetic **trimethobenzamide**. It is contraindicated with the serotonin-3-receptor blockers (eg, **ondansetron**).

EVALUATION OF THERAPEUTIC OUTCOMES

- Comprehensive monitoring is essential to achieve desired outcomes. Educate patients and caregivers about recording medication doses and administration times and duration of "on" and "off" periods.
- Monitor symptoms, side effects, and activities of daily living, and individualize therapy. Concomitant medications that may worsen motor symptoms, memory, falls, or behavioral symptoms should be discontinued if possible.

See Chapter 59, Parkinson Disease, authored by Jack J. Chen and Khashayar Dashtipour, for a more detailed discussion of this topic.

57 Status Epilepticus

- *Status epilepticus* (SE) is any seizure lasting more than 30 minutes, whether or not consciousness is impaired or recurrent seizures without an intervening period of consciousness. SE is a medical emergency, and aggressive treatment of seizures that last 5 minutes or more is strongly recommended. Seizure duration of greater than 30 minutes is associated with increasing risk of long-term consequences. **Table 57–1** shows the classification of SE. This chapter focuses on generalized convulsive status epilepticus (GCSE), the most common and severe form.
- The four stages of GCSE are (1) impending, (2) established, (3) refractory, and (4) superrefractory.

PATHOPHYSIOLOGY

- Seizure initiation is likely caused by an imbalance between excitatory (eg, glutamate, calcium, sodium, substance P, and neurokinin B) and inhibitory (γ-aminobutyric acid [GABA], adenosine, potassium, neuropeptide Y, opioid peptides, and galanin) neurotransmission.
- GCSE is largely caused by glutamate acting on postsynaptic N-methyl-D-aspartate (NMDA) and α-amino-3-hydroxy-5-methylisoxazole-4-propionate (AMPA)/kainate receptors. Sustained depolarization can result in neuronal death.
- $GABA_A$ receptors may become less responsive to endogenous GABA and GABA agonists.
- During phase I of GCSE, each seizure produces marked increases in plasma epinephrine, norepinephrine, and steroid concentrations that may cause hypertension, tachycardia, and cardiac arrhythmias. Muscle contractions and hypoxia can cause acidosis, hypotension, shock, rhabdomyolysis, and secondary hyperkalemia, and acute tubular necrosis may ensue.
- In phase II, beginning 30 minutes into the seizure, the patient begins to decompensate and may become hypotensive with compromised cerebral blood flow. Serum glucose may be normal or decreased, and hyperthermia, respiratory deterioration, hypoxia, and ventilatory failure may develop.
- In prolonged seizures, motor activity may cease, but electrical seizures may persist.

MORBIDITY AND MORTALITY

- Younger children, the elderly, and those with preexisting epilepsy have a higher propensity for sequelae.
- Recent estimates suggest a mortality rate up to 16% in children, 20% in adults, and 38% in the elderly. Neonates have a higher mortality and more neurologic sequelae.
- Variables affecting outcome are (1) the time between onset of GCSE and the initiation of treatment and (2) the duration of the seizure. The mortality rate is 2.6%, 19%, and 32% for those with seizures lasting 10 to 29 minutes, longer than 30 minutes, and longer than 60 minutes, respectively.

CLINICAL PRESENTATION

- Symptoms: impaired consciousness (eg, ranging from lethargy to coma); disorientation (once GCSE is controlled); and pain associated with injuries.
- Early signs: generalized convulsions; acute injuries; central nervous system (CNS) insults that cause extensor or flexor posturing; hypothermia or fever suggestive of intercurrent illnesses (eg, sepsis or meningitis); incontinence; normal blood pressure or hypotension; and respiratory compromise.

TABLE 57–1	International Classification of Status Epilepticus		
Convulsive		**Nonconvulsive**	
International	**Traditional terminology**	**International**	**Traditional terminology**
Generalized SE • Tonic–Clonic[a,b] • Tonic[c] • Clonic[c] • Myoclonic[b] • *Erratic*[d]	Grand mal, epilepticus convulsivus	Absence[c]	Petit mal, spike-and-wave stupor, spike and-slow-wave or 3/s spike-and-wave, epileptic fugue, epilepsia minora continua, epileptic twilight, minor SE
Secondary generalized SE[a,b] • Tonic • Partial seizures with secondary generalization		Partial SE[a,b] Simple partial Somatomotor Dysphasic Other types Complex partial	Focal motor, focal sensory, epilepsia partialis continua, adversive SE Elementary Temporal lobe, psychomotor, epileptic fugue state, prolonged epileptic stupor, prolonged epileptic confusional state, continuous epileptic twilight state

(SE, status epilepticus.)
[a]Most common in older children.
[b]Most common in adolescents and adults.
[c]Most common in infants and young children.
[d]Most common in neonates.

- Late signs: clinical seizures may or may not be apparent; pulmonary edema with respiratory failure; cardiac failure (dysrhythmias, arrest, or cardiogenic shock); hypotension or hypertension; disseminated intravascular coagulation or multisystem organ failure; rhabdomyolysis; and hyperpyrexia.

DIAGNOSIS

- Assess: language; cognitive abilities; motor, sensory, and reflex abnormalities; pupillary response; injuries; asymmetry; and posturing.
- Initial laboratory tests: complete blood count (CBC) with differential; serum chemistry profile (eg, electrolytes, calcium, magnesium, glucose, serum creatinine, alanine aminotransferase [ALT], and aspartate aminotransferase [AST]); urine drug/alcohol screen; albumin, hepatic function; renal function; blood cultures; arterial blood gases (ABGs); and serum drug concentrations if previous anticonvulsant use is suspected or known.
- Other potential diagnostic tests: spinal tap if CNS infection suspected; obtain electroencephalogram (EEG) immediately and once clinical seizures are controlled; computed tomography (CT) with and without contrast; magnetic resonance imaging (MRI); and radiograph if indicated to diagnose fractures.

TREATMENT

- <u>Goals of Treatment</u>: (1) identify GCSE subtype and precipitating factors; (2) terminate clinical and electrical seizure activity as soon as possible, and preserve cardiorespiratory function; (3) minimize side effects; (4) prevent recurrent seizures; and (5) avoid pharmacoresistant epilepsy and/or neurologic sequelae.
- For any tonic-clonic seizure that does not stop automatically or when doubt exists regarding the diagnosis, treatment of GCSE should begin during the diagnostic workup. **Figure 57–1** is an algorithm for treatment of GCSE. **Table 57–2** shows doses used in the pharmacologic management of GCSE, and **Table 57–3** shows the adverse drug reactions and monitoring of patients being treated with these drugs.

PREHOSPITAL CARE
- Monitor Vital signs (HR, RR)
- PR diazepam (0.2–0.5 mg/kg)
- Consider IN midazolam (0.15–0.3 mg/kg) or IM midazolam (0.2 mg/kg up to 10 mg)
- Transport to hospital if seizures persist

INITIAL HOSPITAL CARE
- Time from seizure onset
- Assess and control airway and cardiac function; pulse oximetry
- 100% oxygen
- Place IV catheter; Intraosseous if unable to IV and patient is younger than 6 years
- Begin IV fluids; blood pressure support as needed
- Thiamine 100 mg (adult)
- Pyridoxine 50–100 mg (infant)
- Glucose (adult: 50 mL of 50%; children: 1 mL/kg of 10%) if serum glucose is <60 mg/dL (<3.3 mmol/L)
- Naloxone 0.1 mg/kg for suspected narcotic overdose
- Antibiotics if infection suspected
- Treat hyperthermia

LABORATORY STUDIES
- CBC with differential
- Serum chemistry profile (eg, electrolytes, glucose, renal/hepatic function, calcium, magnesium)
- Arterial blood gas
- Blood cultures
- Serum anticonvulsant concentration
- Urine drug/alcohol screen
- EEG as needed

IMPENDING GSCE (0–30 minutes)
- IV lorazepam (0.1 mg/kg over 30–60 seconds up to 6 mg) may repeat in 5 minutes if no response or IN midazolam (0.5–0.3 mg/kg) or IM midazolam (0.2 mg/kg up to 10 mg)
- Additional therapies may not be required if seizure stops

ESTABLISHED GSCE (30–60 minutes)
First-line
  Phenytoin (IV): 18–20 mg/kg over 20 minutes (<1 mg/kg/min; max 50 mg/min); may give an additional 5 mg/kg as needed or Fosphenytoin (IV or IM): 18–20 mg PE/kg (<3 mg PE/kg/min; max <150 mg PE/min)
Second-line
  Phenobarbital (IV): 15–20 mg/kg over 20 minutes (<100 mg/min)
  Valproate (IV): 25–30 mg/kg over 5–15 minutes (<3 mg/kg/min up to 200 mg/min) followed by an infusion of 1-mg/kg/h
Third-line
  Lacosamide (IV): 50–400 mg; 200 mg given over 15 minutes
  Levetiracetam (IV): 40–60 mg/kg, maximum 3000 mg (administer 2–5 mg/kg/min)

REFRACTORY GSCE (>120 minutes)
Implement continuous EEG monitoring
Assure patient is normovolemic
Assure cerebral perfusion pressure is >70 mm Hg (>9.3 kPa)
Administer volume as stated above and then begin vasopressors to achieve adequate mean arterial pressure (>120 mm Hg [>16.0 kPa]). Continuous ECG monitoring if on propofol
First-line
- Midazolam: 0.2–0.4 mg/kg bolus at a rate of 2 mg/min followed by 0.05–2 mg/kg/h
- Pentobarbital: 10–20 mg/kg bolus at a rate of ≤50 mg/min followed by 1–5 mg/kg/h
- Propofol: 1–2 mg/kg bolus followed by <4 mg/kg/min children; larger dose may be used in adults

SUPER-REFRACTORY GSCE (>24 hours)
Implement continuous EEG monitoring
Assure patient is normovolemic
Assure cerebral perfusion pressure is >70 mm Hg (>9.3 kPa)
Administer volume as stated above and then begin vasopressors to achieve adequate mean arterial pressure (>120 mm Hg [>16.0 kPa])

- Ketamine
- Hypothermia
- Lidocaine
- Topiramate
- Inhaled Anesthetics
- Immunomodulating therapies
- Ketogenic diet
- Vagus Nerve Stimulator

[a]Because variability exists in dosing, monitor serum concentration.
[b]If seizure is controlled, begin maintenance doses and optimize using serum concentration monitoring.

(BP, blood pressure; CBC, complete blood count; EEG, electroencephalogram; GCSE, generalized convulsive status epilepticus; HR, heart rate; PR, per rectum; RR, respiratory rate.)

FIGURE 57–1. Algorithm for the treatment of GCSE.

TABLE 57–2	Dosing of Medications Used in the Initial Treatment of GCSE			
Drug (Route)	Brand name	Initial Dose (Maximum Dose)	Maintenance Dose	Comments
Diazepam (IV)	Valium plus generic			
Adult		0.25 mg/kg[a,b,c] (20 mg)	Not used	Given IV at a rate not to exceed 5 mg/min
Pediatric		0.25–0.5 mg/kg[a,c] (20 mg)	Not used	
Fosphenytoin (IV)	Cerebyx plus generic			
Adult		20–25 mg PE/kg	4–5 mg PE/kg/day	Given IV at a rate not to exceed 150 mg
Pediatric		20–25 mg PE/kg	5–10 mg PE/kg/day	PE/min in adults and 3 mg PE/kg/min in pediatric patients
Lorazepam (IV)	Ativan plus generic			
Adult		4 mg[b,c] (6 mg)	Not used	Given IV at a rate not to exceed 2 mg/min in
Pediatric		0.1 mg/kg[a,c] (6 mg)	Not used	adult and pediatric patients
Midazolam (IV, IM)	Versed plus generic			
Adult		200 mcg/kg[a,d] (10mg)	50–500 mcg/kg/h[e]	Given IV at a rate 0.5–1 mg/min in
Pediatric		150 mcg/kg[a,d] (10 mg)	60–120 mcg/kg/h[e]	adults and over 2–3 minutes in pediatric patients
Phenobarbital (IV)	Generic			
Adult		10–20 mg/kg[e]	1–4 mg/kg/day[e]	Given IV at a rate not to exceed 100 mg/
Pediatric		15–20 mg/kg[e]	3–5 mg/kg/day[e]	min in adults and 30 mg/min in pediatric patients
Phenytoin (IV)	Dilantin plus generic			
Adult		20–25 mg/kg[f]	4–5 mg/kg/day[e]	Given IV at a rate not to exceed 50 mg/min[g] in
Pediatric		20–25 mg/kg[f]	5–10 mg/kg/day[e]	adults and 3 mg/kg/min (max 50 mg/min) in pediatric patients

(GCSE, generalized convulsive status epilepticus; PE, phenytoin equivalents.)
[a]Doses can be repeated every 10 to 15 minutes until the maximum dosage is given.
[b]Initial doses in the elderly are 2 to 5 mg.
[c]Larger doses can be required if patients chronically on a benzodiazepine (eg, clonazepam).
[d]Can be given by the intramuscular, rectal, or buccal routes.
[e]Titrate dose as needed.
[f]Administer additional loading dose based on serum concentration.
[g]The rate should not exceed 25 mg/min in elderly patients and those with known atherosclerotic cardiovascular disease.

TABLE 57–3 Adverse Drug Reactions and Monitoring of Patients Receiving Drugs for GCSE

Drug	Adverse Drug Reaction	Monitoring Parameters	Comments
Diazepam	Hypotension and cardiac arrhythmias	Vital signs and ECG during administration	Propylene glycol causes hypotension and cardiac arrhythmias when administered too rapidly; hypotension may occur with large doses
Fosphenytoin	Hypotension and cardiac arrhythmias; paresthesia, pruritus	Vital signs and ECG during administration	Hypotension is less than that noted with phenytoin, as this product does not contain propylene glycol; pruritus generally involves the face and groin areas, is dose and rate related, and subsides 5–10 minutes after infusion
Lidocaine	Fasciculations, visual disturbances, tinnitus, seizures		Occur at serum concentrations between 6 and 8 mg/L (25.6–34.1 μmol/L); seizures >8 mg/L (>34.1 μmol/L)
Lorazepam	Apnea, hypotension, bradycardia, cardiac arrest, respiratory depression, metabolic acidosis, and renal toxicity	Vital signs and ECG during administration; HCO_3 and serum creatinine; cumulative dose of propylene glycol	Accumulation of propylene glycol during prolong continuous infusions may cause acidosis
Pentobarbital	Hypotension	Vital signs and ECG during administration	Rate of infusion should be slower or dopamine should be added if hypotension occurs
Phenytoin	Hypotension and cardiac arrhythmia; nystagmus	Vital signs and ECG during administration	Propylene glycol causes hypotension and cardiac arrhythmias when administered too rapidly. Large loading doses are generally not given to elderly individuals with preexisting cardiac disease or in critically ill patients with marginal blood pressure. The infusion rate should be slowed if the QT interval widens or if hypotension or arrhythmias develop; horizontal nystagmus suggests serum concentration above the reference range and toxicity; if a serum phenytoin concentration validates this, the dose should be decreased

(continued)

TABLE 57-3	Adverse Drug Reactions and Monitoring of Patients Receiving Drugs for GCSE (Continued)		
Drug	Adverse Drug Reaction	Monitoring Parameters	Comments
Phenobarbital	Hypotension, respiratory and CNS depression	Vital signs and mental status; EEG if used in anesthesia doses	Contains propylene glycol; if hypotension occurs, slow the rate of administration or begin dopamine; apnea and hypopnea can be more profound in patients treated initially with benzodiazepines
Propofol	Progressive metabolic acidosis, hemodynamic instability, and bradyarrhythmias	Vital signs, ECG, osmolar gap; EEG if used in anesthesia doses	Referred to as propofol-related infusion syndrome, which can be fatal
Topiramate	Metabolic acidosis	Acid base status (serum bicarbonate)	Extremely rare

(CNS, central nervous system; ECG, electrocardiogram; EEG, electroencephalogram.)

- Maintain normal to high blood pressure. Aggressively treat hyperthermia (eg, rectal acetaminophen; cooling blankets).
- Give **thiamine** (100 mg IV) prior to IV glucose (see Fig. 57–1).
- Assess metabolic and/or respiratory acidosis with frequent ABG measurements to determine pH, partial pressure of oxygen (Pao_2), partial pressure of carbon dioxide ($Paco_2$), and HCO_3. If pH is less than 7.2 secondary to metabolic acidosis, give sodium bicarbonate. Use assisted ventilation to correct respiratory acidosis.

BENZODIAZEPINES

- Give a **benzodiazepine** as soon as possible if the patient is actively seizing. Generally, one or two IV doses stops seizures within 2 to 3 minutes. Diazepam, lorazepam, and midazolam are equally effective.
- IV **diazepam** is extremely lipophilic and quickly distributed into the brain, but it redistributes rapidly into body fat, causing a very short duration of effect (<0.5 hour). Therefore, give a longer-acting anticonvulsant (eg, **phenytoin** or **phenobarbital**) immediately after the diazepam.
- IV **lorazepam** is currently considered the benzodiazepine of choice by most practitioners. It takes longer to reach peak brain levels than diazepam but has a longer duration of action (12–24 h). Propylene glycol, which is in the vehicle of diazepam and lorazepam, can cause dysrhythmia and hypotension if administered too rapidly. They are also irritating to veins and must be diluted with an equal volume of compatible diluent before administration.
- IV **midazolam** is water soluble and diffuses rapidly into the CNS but has a very short half-life. Maintenance doses must be given by continuous infusion. There is increasing interest in giving it buccally, intramuscularly, and intranasally when IV access cannot be obtained readily. Buccal midazolam may be more effective than rectal diazepam in children.
- With benzodiazepine administration, a brief period of cardiorespiratory depression (<1 min) may occur and can necessitate assisted ventilation or require intubation, especially if the benzodiazepine is used with a barbiturate. Hypotension may occur with high doses of benzodiazepines.

PHENYTOIN

- **Phenytoin** is the second-line agent for GCSE that is unresponsive to the benzodiazepines or in seizures that recur after successful treatment with benzodiazepines.
- Phenytoin has a 20 to 36 hour half-life, but it cannot be delivered fast enough to be a first-line agent. It takes longer to control seizures than the benzodiazepines because it enters the brain more slowly. It causes less respiratory depression and sedation than the **benzodiazepines** or **phenobarbital**, but its vehicle (propylene glycol) is associated with administration-related hypotension and cardiac arrhythmias, which are more likely with large loading doses and in critically ill patients with marginal blood pressure.
- Phenytoin should be diluted to 5 mg/mL or less in normal saline. See Tables 57–2 and 57–3 for dosing, rates of administration, cautions, and monitoring. Maintenance doses should be started within 12 to 24 hours of the loading dose.
- In determining a loading dose, consider whether the patient was taking phenytoin prior to admission and the phenytoin serum concentration if known. A larger loading dose is required in obese patients.
- Phenytoin is associated with pain and burning during infusion. Phlebitis may occur with chronic infusion, and tissue necrosis is likely on infiltration. Intramuscular administration is not recommended.

FOSPHENYTOIN

- **Fosphenytoin**, the water-soluble phosphate ester of phenytoin, is a phenytoin prodrug. See Table 57–3 for adverse effects and monitoring.
- The dose of fosphenytoin sodium is expressed as phenytoin sodium equivalents (PE). Do not give the loading dose intramuscularly (IM) unless IV access is impossible.
- Serum phenytoin concentrations should not be obtained for at least 2 hours after IV and 4 hours after IM administration.

PHENOBARBITAL

- **Phenobarbital** continues to be given after a benzodiazepine plus phenytoin has failed.
- Estimated lean body mass should be used to calculate the dose in obese patients.
- Peak brain concentrations occur 12 to 60 minutes after IV dosing. Usually, seizures are controlled within minutes of the loading dose.
- See Table 57–2 for dosing and Table 57–3 for adverse effects, cautions, and monitoring. If the initial loading dose does not stop the seizures within 20 to 30 minutes, an additional 10 to 20 mg/kg dose may be given. If seizures continue, a third 10 mg/kg load may be given. When necessary, larger loading doses (eg, 30 mg/kg) have been used in neonates. There is no maximum dose beyond which further doses are likely to be ineffective. Once seizures are controlled, start the maintenance dose within 12 to 24 hours.

REFRACTORY GENERALIZED CONVULSIVE STATUS EPILEPTICUS

- When adequate doses of a benzodiazepine, hydantoin, or phenobarbital have failed, the condition is termed refractory. Approximately 10% to 15% of patients will develop refractory GCSE. Doses of agents used to treat refractory GCSE are given in **Table 57–4.**
- Most clinicians recommend anesthetic doses of **midazolam**, **pentobarbital**, or **propofol**, but other options include a **benzodiazepine**, **valproate**, **lacosamide**, **levetiracetam**, or **topiramate**.

Benzodiazepines

- Some clinicians recommend anesthetic doses of **midazolam** as the first-line treatment for refractory GCSE (see Table 57–4). Most patients respond within an hour. Successful discontinuation is enhanced by maintaining serum **phenytoin** concentrations greater than 20 mg/L (79 μmol/L) and **phenobarbital** concentrations greater than 40 mg/L (172 μmol/L). Hypotension and poikilothermia can occur and may require supportive therapies.

Pentobarbital

- If response to high doses of **midazolam** is inadequate, anesthetizing is recommended. Intubation and respiratory support are mandatory during **barbiturate** coma, and continuous EEG and monitoring of vital signs are essential. A short-acting barbiturate (eg, **pentobarbital** or **thiopental**) is preferred (see Fig. 57–1).
- Give a loading dose of **Pentobarbital** to provide serum concentration (40 mg/L; 177 μmol/L) sufficient to induce an isoelectric EEG. Usual duration of coma is 2 to 3 days. To avoid complications, discontinue pentobarbital as soon as possible. Other anticonvulsants should be at therapeutic levels before pentobarbital is withdrawn. As pentobarbital is a hepatic enzyme inducer, maintenance doses of most anticonvulsants need to be higher than usual.

Valproate

- For dosing **valproate** see Table 57–4. The IV dosage form is not FDA approved for GCSE.
- One study suggested that the maintenance infusion rate should be adjusted as follows: (1) if no metabolic enzyme inducers are present, infuse at 1 mg/kg/h; (2) if one or more inducers are present (eg, phenobarbital and phenytoin), infuse at 2 mg/kg/h; and (3) if inducers and pentobarbital coma are present, infuse at 4 mg/kg/h.
- There are no reports of respiratory depression; hemodynamic instability is rare, but vital signs should be monitored closely for hypotension during the loading dose.

Levetiracetam

- IV **levetiracetam** is not hepatically metabolized and is minimally protein bound. Doses above 3000 mg/day do not add additional efficacy. A meta-analysis reported that there is sufficient evidence to support use of levetiracetam as first line therapy in those refractory to benzodiazepines.

TABLE 57–4 Dosing of Medications Used to Treat Refractory or Super-Refractory GCSE

Drug (Brand Name)	Initial Dose (Maximum Dose)	Maintenance Dose	Comments
Ketamine (generics)			
Adult	1–4 mg	1–5 mg/kg/h	
Pediatric	0.5–2 mg/kg	1–10 mg/kg/h	
Lacosamide (Vimpat)			
Adult	200–400 mg	200 mg bid	Administer IV over 15 minutes, monitor serum concentrations
Pediatric	4–6 mg/kg	6–8 mg/kg/day, given in two doses	
Levetiracetam (Keppra plus generics)			
Adult	2000–3000 mg	1000 mg thrice a day	Administer IV over 5–15 minutes
Pediatric	40–60 mg/kg	40–60 mg/kg/day, given in two or three doses	
Lidocaine (generics)			
Adult	50–100 mg	1.5–3.5 mg/kg/h	Administer IV in ≤2 minutes
Pediatric	1 mg/kg (maximum 3–5 mg/kg in the first hour)	1.2–3 mg/kg/h	
Midazolam (Versed plus generic)			
Adult	200 mcg/kg[a]	50–500 mcg/kg/h[b]	Initial dose may be given IM; administer IV over 0.5–1 mg/min; continuous-infusion rate should be increased every 15 minutes in those who do not respond and should be guided by EEG response; development of tachyphylaxis can require frequent increases in dose; decrease dose by 1 mcg/kg/min every 2 hours once GCSE is controlled
pediatric	150 mcg/kg[a]	60–120 mcg/kg/h[b]	

(continued)

TABLE 57–4 Dosing of Medications Used to Treat Refractory or Super-Refractory GCSE (*Continued*)

Drug (Brand Name)	Initial Dose (Maximum Dose)	Maintenance Dose	Comments
Pentobarbital (generics)			
Adult	10–20 mg/kg	1–5 mg/kg/h[b]	Over 1–2 hours, rate of infusion should be slowed or dopamine should be added if hypotension occurs; gradually titrate dose upward until there is evidence of burst suppression on EEG (ie, isoelectric EEG) or prohibitive adverse effects occur. Twelve hours after a burst suppression is obtained, the rate should be titrated downward every 2–4 hours
Pediatric	15–20 mg/kg	1–5 mg/kg/h[b]	
Propofol (Diprivan plus generic)			
Adult	2 mg/kg	5–10 mg/kg/h[b]	Over 10 seconds in adults and 20–30 seconds in pediatric patients
Pediatric	3 mg/kg	2–4 mg/kg/h[c]	
Topiramate (Topamax plus generic)			
Adult	300–500 mg	400–1620 mg/day	Given orally in divided dose every 12 hours. Doses as large as 25 mg/kg/day for 2–5 days have been used in children. Monitor serum bicarbonate levels and serum concentrations
Pediatric	5–10 mg/kg	5–10 mg/kg/day, given in three doses	
Valproate (Depacon plus generic)			
Adult	15–30 mg/kg	1–4 mg/kg/h[b]	Administer at 3 mg/kg/min; and follow by a continuous or intermittent infusion; larger doses may be required in those on hepatic enzyme inducers, monitor serum concentrations
Pediatric	20–25 mg/kg	1–4 mg/kg/h[b], or give every 4–6 hour	

(EEG, electroencephalogram; GCSE, generalized convulsive status epilepticus; IM, intramuscular; IV, intravenous.)

[a]Doses can be repeated twice at 10 to 15 minute intervals until the maximum dosage is given.

[b]Titrate dose as needed.

[c]Generally recommended not to exceed a dose of 4 mg/kg/h and a duration of 48 hours.

Propofol

- **Propofol** is very lipid soluble and has a large volume of distribution and a rapid onset of action. It has comparable efficacy to midazolam for refractory GCSE. Adverse effects and monitoring are shown in Table 57–3 and dosing is shown in Table 57–4. Once EEG burst suppression is achieved, the dose should be reduced.
- Prolonged infusions greater than 4 mg/kg/h have been associated with propofol-related infusion syndrome (PRIS). Symptoms include metabolic acidosis, hemodynamic instability, and refractory bradyarrhythmias with or without hepatosplenomegaly, rhabdomyolysis, or lipemia.

SUPER-REFRACTORY GENERALIZED CONVULSIVE STATUS EPILEPTICUS

Ketamine

- **Ketamine** appears to be a reasonable option to consider in refractory GCSE that has failed inhaled analgesics. An advantage of ketamine is its ability to maintain arterial blood pressure, pulse, and cardiac output, but it may cause hallucinations upon awakening, increased salivation, and increased intraocular and intracranial pressures.

Topiramate

- **Topiramate** tablets can be crushed, dissolved in a small amount of water, and given orally or nasogastrically. Response tends to be delayed hours to days. If metabolic acidosis occurs, it can be treated with citrates, with a goal of maintaining a serum bicarbonate level of at least 20 mEq/L (mmol/L).

Lidocaine

- IV **lidocaine** is not recommended unless other agents have failed. Serum concentrations should be monitored to avoid drug accumulation and toxicity.

Inhaled Anesthetics

- **Inhaled anesthetics** are not used until other approaches fail. **Halothane, isoflurane,** and other inhaled anesthetics are difficult to administer outside the operating room, and an anesthesiologist is required. They have no proven advantages over traditional anticonvulsants, and they can increase intracranial pressure.
- Isoflurane can induce hypotension, so close hemodynamic monitoring is necessary.
- In the absence of contraindications, a trial of large doses of steroids (eg, 1 g/day of IV **prednisolone** for 3 days, followed by 1 mg/kg/day in four divided doses) should be used in patients with unidentified etiology for superrefractory GCSE. Responders should continue long-term steroids, IV immunoglobulins, and other immunomodulatory agents, such as **cyclophosphamide** or **rituximab**.

EVALUATION OF THERAPEUTIC OUTCOMES

- An EEG allows practitioners to determine when abnormal electrical activity has ceased and may assist in determining which anticonvulsant was effective. Monitor vital signs during drug loading and the infusion. Assess the infusion site for evidence of infiltration before and during administration of phenytoin.

See Chapter 57, Status Epilepticus, authored by Stephanie J. Phelps and James W. Wheless, for a more detailed discussion of this topic.

CHAPTER 58 Obesity

- *Obesity* occurs when there is an imbalance between energy intake and energy expenditure over time, resulting in increased energy storage.

PATHOPHYSIOLOGY

- The etiology of obesity is usually unknown, but it is likely multifactorial and related to varying contributions from genetic, environmental, and physiologic factors.
- Genetic factors appear to be the primary determinants of obesity in some individuals, whereas environmental factors are more important in others. The total number and identity of contributing genes are still being determined.
- Environmental factors include reduced physical activity or work, abundant food supply, relatively sedentary lifestyles, increased availability of high-fat foods, and cultural factors and religious beliefs.
- Medical conditions including Cushing disease and growth hormone deficiency or genetic syndromes such as Prader–Willi syndrome can be associated with weight gain.
- Medications associated with unintended weight gain include insulin, corticosteroids, some antidepressants, antipsychotics, and several anticonvulsants.
- Many neurotransmitters and neuropeptides stimulate or depress the brain's appetite network, impacting total calorie intake.
- The degree of obesity is determined by the net balance of energy ingested relative to energy expended over time. The single largest determinant of energy expenditure is metabolic rate, which is expressed as *resting energy expenditure* or *basal metabolic rate*. Physical activity is the other major factor that affects total energy expenditure and is the most variable component.
- Major types of adipose tissue are (1) white adipose tissue, which manufactures, stores, and releases lipid; and (2) brown adipose tissue, which dissipates energy via uncoupled mitochondrial respiration. Adrenergic stimulation activates lipolysis in fat cells and increases energy expenditure in adipose tissue and skeletal muscle.

CLINICAL PRESENTATION

- Obesity is associated with serious health risks and increased mortality. Central obesity reflects high levels of intraabdominal or visceral fat that is associated with the development of hypertension, dyslipidemia, type 2 diabetes, and cardiovascular disease. Other obesity comorbidities are osteoarthritis and changes in the female reproductive system.
- Body mass index (BMI) and waist circumference (WC) are recognized, acceptable markers of excess body fat that independently predict disease risk (**Table 58–1**).
- BMI is calculated as weight (kg) divided by the square of the height (m^2).
- WC, the most practical method of characterizing central adiposity, is the narrowest circumference between the last rib and the top of the iliac crest.

TREATMENT

- <u>Goals of Treatment</u>: Weight management goals may include losing a predefined amount of weight, decreasing the rate of weight gain, or maintaining a weight-neutral status, depending on the clinical situation.

TABLE 58–1	Classification of Overweight and Obesity by Body Mass Index, Waist Circumference, and Associated Disease Risk			
			Disease Risk[a] (Relative to Normal Weight and Waist Circumference)	
	BMI (kg/m²)	Obesity Class	Men ≤40 in (≤102 cm) Women ≤35 in (≤89 cm)	>40 in (>102 cm) >35 in (>89 cm)
Underweight	<18.5		—	—
Normal weight[b]	18.5–24.9		—	High
Overweight	25.0–29.9		Increased	High
Obesity	30.0–34.9	I	High	Very high
	35.0–39.9	II	Very high	Very high
Extreme obesity	≥40	III	Extremely high	Extremely high

(BMI, body mass index.)
[a]Disease risk for type 2 diabetes, hypertension, and cardiovascular disease.
[b]Increased waist circumference can also be a marker for increased risk even in persons of normal weight.
Data from Obesity: Preventing and Managing the Global Epidemic. Report of a WHO Consultation on Obesity, Geneva, 1997; Explore Overweight and Obesity, National Institutes of Health, National Heart, Lung and Blood Institute.

GENERAL APPROACH

- Nonpharmacologic therapy, including reduced caloric intake, increased physical activity, and behavior modification is the mainstay of obesity management (Fig. 58–1). Measures of success not only include pounds lost but also improvement in comorbid conditions, including blood pressure, blood glucose, and lipids.
- Current adult guidelines recommend reduced caloric intake through adherence to a low-calorie diet. Adherence to this type of diet has been shown to result in an average weight loss of 8% over 6 months.
- The primary aim of behavior modification is to help patients choose lifestyles conducive to safe and sustained weight loss. Behavioral therapy is based on principles of human learning, which use stimulus control and reinforcement to substitute desirable behaviors for learned, undesirable habits.
- Bariatric surgery, which reduces the stomach volume or absorptive surface of the alimentary tract, remains the most effective intervention for obesity. Surgery should be reserved for those with extreme obesity (BMI ≥40 kg/m²) or BMI >35 kg/m² with significant comorbidities such as hypertension, type 2 diabetes, or obstructive sleep apnea.

PHARMACOLOGIC THERAPY

- The debate regarding the role of pharmacotherapy remains heated, fueled by the need to treat a growing epidemic and by the fallout from the removal of several agents from the market because of adverse reactions.
- Long-term pharmacotherapy may have a role for patients who have no contraindications to approved drug therapy (Table 58–2). Current guidelines recommend consideration of pharmacotherapy in adults with BMI ≥30 kg/m² or BMI ≥27 kg/m² with at least one weight-related comorbidity.
- **Orlistat** (180 or 360 mg in three divided doses/day) is a lipase inhibitor that induces weight loss by lowering dietary fat absorption; it also improves lipid profiles, glucose control, and other metabolic markers. Soft stools, abdominal pain or colic, flatulence, fecal urgency, and/or incontinence occur in 80% of individuals using prescription

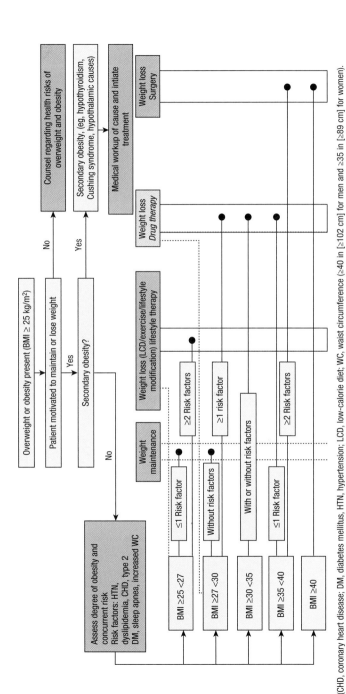

(CHD, coronary heart disease; DM, diabetes mellitus; HTN, hypertension; LCD, low-calorie diet; WC, waist circumference.)

FIGURE 58-1. Treatment algorithm. Candidates for pharmacotherapy are selected on the basis of body mass index and waist circumference criteria along with consideration of concurrent risk factors. Medication therapy is always used as an adjunct to a comprehensive weight-loss program that includes diet, exercise, and behavioral modification.

TABLE 58-2 FDA-Approved Pharmacotherapeutic Agents for Weight Loss

Drug	Brand Name	Initial Dose	Usual Range	Special Population Dose	Comment
Gastrointestinal lipase inhibitor					
Orlistat	Xenical	120 mg three times daily with each main meal containing fat	120 mg three times daily with each main meal containing fat		Approved for long-term use Take during or up to 1 hour after the meal Omit dose if meal is occasionally missed or contains no fat
Orlistat	Alli[a]	60 mg three times daily with each main meal containing fat	60 mg three times daily with each main meal containing fat		Same as Xenical
Serotonin 2C receptor agonist					
Lorcaserin	Belviq	10 mg twice daily	10 mg twice daily	Use with caution in moderate renal impairment and severe hepatic impairment; not recommended in patients with end state renal disease	Approved for long-term use Controlled substance: C–IV
Phentermine–topiramate combination					
Phentermine and topiramate extended release	Qsymia	3.75 mg of phentermine and 23 mg of topiramate once daily for 14 days; then increase to 7.5 mg of phentermine and 46 mg of topiramate once daily	7.5 mg of phentermine and 46 mg of topiramate once daily to a maximum dose of phentermine 15 mg and topiramate 92 mg once daily	Maximum dose for patients with moderate or severe renal impairment or patients with moderate hepatic impairment is 7.5 mg of phentermine and 46 mg of topiramate	Approved for long-term use Take dose in the morning to avoid insomnia Controlled substance: C–IV

Naltrexone-bupropion combination

Bupropion and naltrexone extended release	Contrave	8 mg naltrexone/90 mg bupropion (1 tablet) once daily in the morning for 1 week; then 8 mg naltrexone/90 mg bupropion twice daily (morning and evening) for 1 week; then 16 mg naltrexone/180 mg bupropion in the morning and 8 mg naltrexone/90 mg bupropion in the evening for 1 week; then 16 mg naltrexone/180 mg bupropion twice daily (morning and evening)	16 mg naltrexone and 180 mg bupropion (2 tablets) twice daily	Maximum dose for patients with moderate or severe renal impairment is 8 mg naltrexone/90 mg bupropion (1 tablet) twice daily Maximum dose for patients with hepatic impairment is 8 mg naltrexone/90 mg bupropion (1 tablet) once daily in the morning	Approved for long-term use Do not take dose with high-fat meal

Glucagon-like peptide-1 antagonist

Liraglutide	Saxenda	0.6 mg once daily for 1 week 1.2 mg once daily for 1 week 1.8 mg once daily for 1 week 2.4 mg once daily for 1 week 3.0 mg once daily for 1 week * administered by subcutaneous injection	3 mg once daily	Use with caution in mild, moderate, and severe renal and hepatic impairment	Approved for long-term use Inject subcutaneously in the abdomen, thigh, or upper arm Administer at any time of day without regard to the timing of meals

(continued)

TABLE 58–2 FDA-Approved Pharmacotherapeutic Agents for Weight Loss (*Continued*)

Drug	Brand Name	Initial Dose	Usual Range	Special Population Dose	Comment
Noradrenergic agents					
Phendimetrazine	Bontril PDM; Bontril Slow-Release	Conventional tablet: start at 17.5 mg two or three times daily, given 1 hour before meals Extended-release capsule: 105 mg once daily 30–60 minutes before morning meal	70–105 mg/day	Use caution in patients with renal impairment	Approved for short-term monotherapy Controlled substance: C–III Prescriptions should be written for the smallest quantity to minimize possibility of overdose
Phentermine	Adipex-P, Suprenza	Orally disintegrating tablet: 15 or 30 mg once every morning Phentermine hydrochloride: 15–37.5 mg/day given in one or two divided doses; administer before breakfast or 1–2 hours after breakfast	Orally disintegrating tablet: 15 or 30 mg once every morning Phentermine hydrochloride: 15–37.5 mg/day given in one or two divided doses; administer before breakfast or 1–2 hours after breakfast	Use with caution in patients with renal impairment	Approved for short-term monotherapy Controlled substance: C–IV Prescriptions should be written for the smallest quantity to minimize possibility of overdose Individualize to achieve adequate response with lowest effective dose
Diethylpropion	Tenuate, Tenuate Dospan	Immediate release: 25 mg three times daily administered 1 hour before meals Controlled release: 75 mg once daily administered at midmorning	75 mg/day	Use with caution in patients with renal impairment	Approved for short-term monotherapy Dose should not be administered in the evening or at bedtime Controlled substance: C–IV

a Available without a prescription.

strength, are mild to moderate in severity, and improve after 1 to 2 months of therapy. Orlistat is approved for long-term use. It interferes with the absorption of fat-soluble vitamins, **cyclosporine**, **levothyroxine**, and **oral contraceptives**. A nonprescription formulation is also available.

- **Lorcaserin** is a selective serotonin receptor agonist (5-HT$_{2c}$) approved for chronic weight management. Activation of central 5-HT$_{2c}$ receptors results in appetite suppression leading to modest weight loss as compared with placebo. Discontinue lorcaserin if 5% weight loss is not achieved by week 12. Common adverse effects include headache, dizziness, constipation, fatigue, and dry mouth.
- **Phentermine** in combination with **topiramate extended release** is indicated for chronic weight management. Doses are gradually titrated from phentermine 3.75 to 15 mg and topiramate 23 to 92 mg over 4 months but the drug should be stopped after 12 weeks if 5% weight loss is not achieved. Common adverse effects include constipation, dry mouth, paraesthesia, dysgeusia, and insomnia.
- **Naltrexone** in combination with **bupropion extended release** is indicated for chronic weight management. Doses are gradually increased over 4 weeks, starting with one tablet daily (8 mg naltrexone/90 mg bupropion) to a maintenance dose of two tablets twice daily. Patients should avoid taking their dose with a high-fat meal. Common adverse effects include nausea, constipation, headache, vomiting, dizziness, insomnia, dry mouth, and diarrhea. Discontinue treatment if 5% weight loss is not achieved after 12 weeks.
- **Liraglutide** is a glucagon-like peptide-1 receptor agonist indicated for chronic weight management at a dose of 3 mg daily. It is administered subcutaneously and is available in prefilled, multidose pens. A 5-week dose escalation schedule is recommended to improve tolerability of GI adverse events, beginning with 0.6 mg daily and increasing weekly by 0.6 mg increments to a maintenance dose of 3 mg daily. Common adverse effects include nausea, diarrhea, constipation, vomiting, dyspepsia, hypoglycemia, and abdominal pain. Discontinue liraglutide if weight loss of at least 4% is not achieved after 16 weeks of therapy.
- **Amphetamines** should generally be avoided because of their powerful stimulant effects and addictive potential.
- Many complementary and alternative therapy products are promoted for weight loss. Regulation of dietary supplements is less rigorous than that of prescription and over-the-counter drug products; manufacturers do not have to prove safety and effectiveness prior to marketing.

EVALUATION OF THERAPEUTIC OUTCOMES

- Assess progress once or twice monthly for 1 to 2 months, then monthly. Each encounter should document weight, WC, BMI, blood pressure, medical history, and patient assessment of tolerability of drug therapy.
- Discontinue medication therapy after 3 months if the patient has failed to demonstrate weight loss or maintenance of prior weight.
- Diabetic patients require more intense medical monitoring and self-monitoring of blood glucose. Weekly healthcare visits for 1 to 2 months may be necessary until the effects of diet, exercise, and weight loss medication become more predictable.
- Monitor patients with hyperlipidemia or hypertension to assess effects of weight loss on appropriate end points.

See Chapter 144, Obesity, authored by Amy Heck Sheehan, Judy T. Chen, Jack A. Yanovski, and Karim Anton Calis, for a more detailed discussion of this topic.

- Malnutrition is a consequence of nutrient imbalance resulting from inadequate intake, absorption, or utilization of protein and energy. Undernutrition can result in changes in subcellular, cellular, or organ function that increase the individual's risks of morbidity and mortality.
- For information on overnutrition or obesity, see Chap. 58.
- Nutrition screening provides a systematic way to identify individuals in any care environment who need a detailed nutrition assessment.
- Nutrition assessment is the first step in developing a nutrition care plan. Goals of nutrition assessment are to identify the presence of factors associated with an increased risk of developing undernutrition and complications, estimate nutrition needs, and establish baseline parameters for assessing the outcome of therapy.
- This assessment should include a nutrition-focused history, a physical exam including anthropometrics, and laboratory measurements.

CLINICAL EVALUATION

- Medical and dietary history should include weight changes within 6 months, dietary intake changes, gastrointestinal (GI) symptoms, functional capacity, and disease states.
- Physical examination should focus on assessment of lean body mass (LBM) and physical findings of vitamin, trace element, and essential fatty acid deficiencies.

ANTHROPOMETRIC MEASUREMENTS

- Anthropometric measurements are physical measurements of the size, weight, and proportions of the human body used to compare an individual with normative population standards. The most common measurements are weight, stature, head circumference (for children younger than 3 years of age) waist circumference, and measurements of limb size (eg, skinfold thickness and midarm muscle and wrist circumferences), along with bioelectrical impedance analysis (BIA).
- Interpretation of actual body weight (ABW) should consider ideal weight (IBW) for height, usual body weight (UBW), fluid status, and age. Change over time can be calculated as the percentage of UBW. Unintentional weight loss, especially rapid weight loss (5% of UBW in one month or 10% of UBW in 6 months), increases risk of poor clinical outcome in adults.
- The best indicator of adequate nutrition in children is appropriate growth. Weight, stature, and head circumference should be plotted on the appropriate growth curve and compared with usual growth velocities. Average weight gain for newborns is 10 to 20 g/kg/day (24–35 g/day for term infants and 10–25 g/day for preterm infants).
- Body mass index (BMI) is another index of weight-for-height that is highly correlated with body fat. Interpretation of BMI should include consideration of gender, frame size, and age. BMI values greater than 25 kg/m^2 are indicative of overweight, and values less than 18.5 kg/m^2 are indicative of undernutrition. BMI is calculated as follows:
  Body weight (kg)/[height (m)]^2 or [Body weight (lbs) × 703]/[height (in)]^2
- Measurements of skinfold thickness estimate subcutaneous fat, midarm muscle circumference estimates skeletal muscle mass, and waist circumference estimates abdominal fat content.
- BIA is a simple, noninvasive, and relatively inexpensive way to assess LBM, TBW, and water distribution. It is based on differences between fat tissue and lean tissue's resistance to conductivity. Hydration status should be considered in interpretation of BIA results.

TABLE 59–1	Visceral Proteins Used for Assessment of Lean Body Mass			
Serum Protein	Half-Life (Days)	Function	Factors Resulting in Increased Values	Factors Resulting in Decreased Values
Albumin	18–20	Maintains plasma oncotic pressure; transports small molecules	Dehydration, anabolic steroids, insulin, infection	Fluid overload; edema; kidney dysfunction; nephrotic syndrome; poor dietary intake; impaired digestion; burns; heart failure; cirrhosis; thyroid, adrenal, or pituitary hormones; trauma; sepsis
Transferrin	8–9	Binds Fe in plasma; transports Fe to bone	Fe deficiency, pregnancy, hypoxia, chronic blood loss, estrogens	Chronic infection, cirrhosis, burns, enteropathies, nephrotic syndrome, cortisone, testosterone
Prealbumin	2–3	Binds T_3 and, to a lesser extent, T_4; retinol-binding protein carrier	Kidney dysfunction	Cirrhosis, hepatitis, stress, surgery, inflammation, hyperthyroidism, cystic fibrosis, burns, zinc deficiency

(T_3, triiodothyronine; T_4, thyroxine.)

BIOCHEMICAL AND IMMUNE FUNCTION STUDIES

• LBM can be assessed by measuring serum visceral proteins (Table 59–1). They are of greatest value for assessing uncomplicated starvation and recovery, and less useful for assessing status during acute stress. Interpret visceral proteins relative to overall clinical status because they are affected by factors other than nutrition.
• Nutrition affects immune status both directly and indirectly. Total lymphocyte count and delayed cutaneous hypersensitivity reactions are immune function tests useful in nutrition assessment, but their lack of specificity limits their usefulness as nutrition status markers.
• Delayed cutaneous hypersensitivity is commonly assessed using antigens to which the patient was likely previously sensitized. The recall antigens used most frequently are mumps and *Candida albicans*. Anergy is associated with severe malnutrition, and immune response is restored with nutrition repletion.

SPECIFIC NUTRIENT DEFICIENCIES

• Biochemical assessment of trace element, vitamin, and essential fatty acid deficiencies should be based on the nutrient's function, but few practical methods are available. Therefore, most assays measure serum concentrations of the individual nutrient.
• Clinical syndromes are associated with deficiencies of the following trace elements: zinc, copper, manganese, selenium, chromium, iodine, fluoride, molybdenum, and iron.
• Single vitamin deficiencies are uncommon; multiple vitamin deficiencies more commonly occur with undernutrition. For information on iron deficiency and other anemias, see Chap. 33.

- Essential fatty acid deficiency is rare but can occur with prolonged lipid-free parenteral nutrition, very-low-fat enteral formulas or diets, severe fat malabsorption, or severe malnutrition. The body can synthesize all fatty acids except for linoleic and α-linolenic acid.
- Carnitine can be synthesized from lysine and methionine, but synthesis is decreased in premature infants. Low carnitine levels can occur in premature infants receiving parenteral nutrition or carnitine-free diets.

ASSESSMENT OF NUTRIENT REQUIREMENTS

- Assessment of nutrient requirements must be made in the context of patient-specific factors (eg, age, gender, size, disease state, clinical condition, nutrition status, and physical activity).
- To replace recommended dietary allowances, the Food and Nutrition Board created the dietary reference intakes made up of seven nutrient groups.
- Adults should consume 45% to 65% of total calories from carbohydrates, 20% to 35% from fat, and 10% to 35% from protein. Recommendations are similar for children, except that infants should consume 40% to 50% of total calories from fat.

ENERGY REQUIREMENTS

- Energy requirements of individuals can be estimated using published, validated equations or directly measured, depending on factors including severity of illness and resources available. The simplest method is to use population estimates of calories required per kilogram of body weight.
- Healthy adults with normal nutrition status and minimal illness severity require an estimated 20 to 25 kcal ABW/kg/day (84–105 kJ ABW/kg/day). Daily energy requirements for children are approximately 150% of basal metabolic rate with additional calories to support activity and growth. Consult references for equations used to estimate energy expenditure in adults and children.
- Energy requirements for all ages increase with fever, sepsis, major surgery, trauma, burns, long-term growth failure, and chronic conditions (eg, bronchopulmonary dysplasia, congenital heart disease, and cystic fibrosis).

PROTEIN, FLUID, AND MICRONUTRIENT REQUIREMENTS

Protein

- Protein requirements are based on age, gender, nutrition status, disease state, and clinical condition. The usual recommended daily protein allowances are 0.8 g/kg for adults, 1.5 g/kg for adults over 60 years of age, 1.5 to 2 g/kg for patients with metabolic stress (eg, infection, trauma, and surgery), and 2.5 to 3 g/kg for patients with burns.

Fluid

- Daily adult fluid requirements are approximately 30 to 35 mL/kg, 1 mL/kcal (or per every 4.18 kJ) ingested, or 1500 mL/m^2.
- Daily fluid requirements for children and preterm infants who weigh less than 10 kg are at least 100 mL/kg. An additional 50 mL/kg should be provided for each kilogram of body weight between 11 and 20 kg, and 20 mL/kg for each kilogram greater than 20 kg.
- Examples of factors that result in increased fluid requirements include gastrointestinal (GI) losses, fever, sweating, and increased metabolism, whereas kidney or cardiac failure and hypoalbuminemia with starvation are examples of factors that result in decreased fluid requirements.
- Assess fluid status by monitoring urine output and specific gravity, serum electrolytes, and weight changes. An hourly urine output of at least 1 mL/kg for children and 40 to 50 mL for adults is needed to ensure tissue perfusion.

Micronutrients

- Requirements for micronutrients (ie, electrolytes, trace elements, and vitamins) vary with age, gender, route of administration, and underlying clinical conditions.
- Sodium, potassium, magnesium, and phosphorus requirements are typically decreased in patients with kidney failure, whereas calcium requirements are increased (see Chaps. 73 and 74).

DRUG–NUTRIENT INTERACTIONS

- Concomitant drug therapy can alter serum concentrations of vitamins (Table 59–2), minerals, and electrolytes.

TABLE 59–2	Drug and Nutrient Interactions
Drug	**Effect**
Antacids	Thiamine deficiency
Antibiotics	Vitamin K deficiency
Aspirin	Folic acid deficiency; increased vitamin C excretion
Cathartics	Increased requirements for vitamins D, C, and B_6
Cholestyramine	Vitamins A, D, E, and K and β-carotene malabsorption
Colestipol	Vitamins A, D, E, and K and β-carotene malabsorption
Corticosteroids	Decreased vitamins A, D, and C
Diuretics (loop)	Thiamine deficiency
Efavirenz	Vitamin D deficiency caused by increased metabolism of 25(OH)-vitamin D and 1,25-(OH)$_2$-vitamin D
Histamine$_2$ antagonists	Vitamin B_{12} malabsorption (reduced acid results in impaired release of B_{12} from food)
Isoniazid	Vitamin B_6 and niacin deficiency
Isotretinoin	Vitamin A increases toxicity
Mercaptopurine	Niacin deficiency
Methotrexate	Folic acid inhibits effect
Orlistat	Vitamins A, D, E, and K malabsorption caused by fat malabsorption
Pentamidine	Folic acid deficiency
Phenobarbital	Increased vitamin D metabolism
Phenytoin	Increased vitamin D metabolism, decreased folic acid concentrations
Primidone	Folic acid deficiency
Protease inhibitors	Vitamin D deficiency (impaired renal hydroxylation)
Proton pump inhibitors	Vitamin B_{12} malabsorption (reduced acid results in impaired release of B_{12} from food)
Sulfasalazine	Folic acid malabsorption
Trimethoprim	Folic acid depletion
Warfarin	Vitamin K inhibits effect; vitamins A, C, and E may affect prothrombin time
Valproic acid	Zinc
Zidovudine	Folic acid and B_{12} deficiencies increase myelosuppression

- Some drug delivery vehicles contain nutrients. For example, the vehicle for propofol is 10% lipid emulsion, and most IV therapies include dextrose or sodium.

NUTRITION SUPPORT

- The primary objective of nutrition support therapy is to promote positive clinical outcomes of an illness and improve quality of life.

ENTERAL NUTRITION

- Enteral nutrition (EN) delivers nutrients by tube or mouth into the GI tract; we will focus on delivery through a feeding tube.
- EN is indicated for the patient who cannot or will not eat enough to meet nutritional requirements and who has a functioning GI tract and a method of enteral access. Potential indications include neoplastic disease, organ failure, hypermetabolic states, GI disease, and neurologic impairment.
- Distal mechanical intestinal obstruction, bowel ischemia, active peritonitis, uncorrectable coagulopathy, and necrotizing enterocolitis are contraindications to EN. Conditions that challenge the success of EN include severe diarrhea, protracted vomiting, enteric fistulas, severe GI hemorrhage, hemodynamic instability, and intestinal dysmotility.
- EN has replaced parenteral nutrition (PN) as the preferred method for the feeding of critically ill patients requiring specialized nutrition support. Advantages of EN over PN include maintaining GI tract structure and function; fewer metabolic, infectious, and technical complications; and lower costs.
- The timing of initiation of EN in the critically ill patients is of clinical significance. Initiation within 24 to 72 hours of admission appears to attenuate the stress response and reduce infectious complications and mortality. If patients are only mildly to moderately stressed and well nourished, EN initiation can be delayed until oral intake is inadequate for 5 to 7 days.

ACCESS

- EN can be administered through four routes, which have different indications, tube placement options, advantages, and disadvantages (Table 59-3). The choice depends on the anticipated duration of use and the feeding site (ie, stomach vs small bowel).
- The stomach is generally the least expensive and least labor-intensive access site; however, patients who have impaired gastric emptying are at risk for aspiration and pneumonia.
- Long-term access should be considered when EN is anticipated for more than 4 to 6 weeks.

ADMINISTRATION METHODS

- EN can be administered by continuous, cyclic, bolus, and intermittent methods. The choice depends on the location of the feeding tube tip, patient's clinical condition, intestinal function, and tolerance to tube feeding.
- Continuous EN is preferred for initiation and has the advantage of being well tolerated. Disadvantages include cost and inconvenience associated with pump and administration sets.
- Cyclic EN has the advantage of allowing breaks from the infusion system, thereby increasing mobility, especially if EN is administered nocturnally.
- Bolus EN is most commonly used in patients in the home or long-term care setting who have a gastrostomy. Advantages include short administration time (eg, 5–10 min) and minimal equipment (eg, a syringe). Bolus EN has the potential disadvantages of causing cramping, nausea, vomiting, aspiration, and diarrhea.
- Intermittent EN is similar to bolus EN except that the feeding is administered over 20 to 60 minutes, which improves tolerability but requires more equipment

TABLE 59–3	Options and Considerations in the Selection of Enteral Access			
Access	**EN Duration/Patient Characteristics**	**Tube Placement Options**	**Advantages**	**Disadvantages**
Nasogastric or orogastric	Short term Intact gag reflex Normal gastric emptying	Manually at bedside	Ease of placement Allows for all methods of administration Inexpensive Multiple commercially available tubes and sizes	Potential tube displacement Potential increased aspiration risk
Nasojejunal or orojejunal	Short term Impaired gastric motility or emptying High risk of GER or aspiration	Manually at bedside Fluoroscopically Endoscopically	Potential reduced aspiration risk Allows for early postinjury or postoperative feeding Multiple commercially available tubes and sizes	Manual transpyloric passage requires greater skill Potential tube displacement or clogging Bolus or intermittent feeding not tolerated
Gastrostomy	Long term Normal gastric emptying	Surgically Endoscopically Radiologically Laparoscopically	Allows for all methods of administration Low-profile buttons available Large-bore tubes less likely to clog Multiple commercially available tubes and sizes	Attendant risks associated with each type of procedure Potential increased aspiration risk Risk of stoma site complications
Jejunostomy	Long term Impaired gastric motility or gastric emptying High risk of GER or aspiration	Surgically Endoscopically Radiologically Laparoscopically	Allows for early postinjury or postoperative feeding Potential reduced aspiration risk Multiple commercially available tubes and sizes Low-profile buttons available	Attendant risks associated with each type of procedure Bolus or intermittent feeding not tolerated Risk of stoma site complications

(EN, enteral nutrition; GER, gastroesophageal reflux.)

(eg, reservoir bag and infusion pump). Like bolus EN, intermittent EN mimics normal eating patterns.

- Protocols outlining initiation and advancement criteria are a useful strategy to optimize achievement of nutrient goals based on GI tolerance. Clinical signs of intolerance include abdominal distention or cramping, high gastric residual volumes, aspiration, and diarrhea.
- Continuous EN feedings are typically started in adults at 20 to 50 mL/hour and advanced by 10 to 25 mL/hour every 4 to 8 hours until the goal is achieved. Intermittent EN feedings are started at 120 mL every 4 hours and advanced by 30 to 60 mL every 8 to 12 hours.
- EN feedings are typically started in children at 1 to 2 mL/kg/hour for continuous feeding or 2 to 4 mL/kg per bolus with advancement by similar amounts every 4 to 24 hours. Feedings are started at lower rates or volumes in premature infants, usually 10 to 20 mL/kg/day.

FORMULATIONS

- Historically, EN formulations were created to provide essential nutrients, including macronutrients (eg, carbohydrates, fats, and proteins) and micronutrients (eg, electrolytes, trace elements, vitamins, and water).
- Over time, formulations have been enhanced to improve tolerance and meet specific patient needs. For example, nutraceuticals or pharmaconutrients are added to modify the disease process or improve clinical outcome; however, these health claims are not regulated by the FDA.
- The molecular form of the protein source determines the amount of digestion required for absorption within the small bowel. The carbohydrate component usually provides the major source of calories; polymeric entities are preferred over elemental sugars. Vegetable oils rich in polyunsaturated fatty acids are the most common sources of fat in EN formulations.
- Soluble and insoluble fiber has been added to several EN formulations. Potential benefits of soluble fiber include trophic effects on colonic mucosa, promotion of sodium and water absorption, and regulation of bowel function.
- Osmolality is a function of the size and quantity of ionic and molecular particles primarily related to protein, carbohydrate, electrolyte, and mineral content. The osmolality of EN formulations for adults ranges from 300 to 900 mOsm/kg (mmol/kg), and an osmolality less than 450 mOsm/kg (mmol/kg) is recommended for children. Osmolality is commonly thought to affect GI tolerability, but there is a lack of supporting evidence.

CLASSIFICATION OF ENTERAL FEEDING FORMULATIONS

- EN formulations are classified by their composition and intended patient population (Table 59–4). Formularies should focus on clinically significant characteristics of available products, avoid duplicate formulations, and include only specialty formulations with evidence-based indications.

COMPLICATIONS AND MONITORING

- Monitor patients for metabolic, GI, and mechanical complications of EN (Table 59–5).
- Metabolic complications associated with EN are similar to those of parenteral nutrition (PN), but the occurrence is lower.
- GI complications include nausea, vomiting, abdominal distention, cramping, aspiration, diarrhea, and constipation. Gastric residual volume is thought to increase the risk of vomiting and aspiration.
- Mechanical complications include tube occlusion or malposition and inadvertent nasopulmonary intubation. Techniques for clearing occluded tubes include pancreatic enzymes in sodium bicarbonate and using a declogging device. Techniques for

TABLE 59–4 Adult Enteral Feeding Formulation Classification System

Category	Features	Indications
Standard polymeric	Isotonic 1–1.2 kcal/mL (4.2–5 kJ/mL) NPC:N 125:1–150:1 May contain fiber	Designed to meet the needs of the majority of patients Patients with functional GI tract Not suitable for oral use
High protein	NPC:N <125:1 May contain fiber	Patients with protein requirements >1.5 g/kg/day, such as trauma patients and those with burns, pressure sores, or wounds Patients receiving propofol
High caloric density	1.5–2 kcal/mL (6.3–8.4 kJ/mL) Lower electrolyte content per calorie Hypertonic	Patients requiring fluid and/or electrolyte restriction, such as kidney insufficiency
Elemental	High proportion of free amino acids Low in fat	Patients who require low fat Use has generally been replaced by peptide-based formulations
Peptide-based	Contains dipeptides and tripeptides Contains MCTs	Indications/benefits not clearly established Trial may be warranted in patients who do not tolerate intact protein due to malabsorption
Disease specific		
Kidney	Caloric dense Protein content varies Low electrolyte content	Alternative to high caloric density formulations, but generally more expensive
Liver	Increased branched-chain and decreased aromatic amino acids	Patients with hepatic encephalopathy
Lung	High fat, low carbohydrate Antiinflammatory lipid profile and antioxidants	Patients with ARDS and severe ALI
Diabetes mellitus	High fat, low carbohydrate	Alternative to standard, fiber-containing formulation in patients with uncontrolled hyperglycemia

(continued)

TABLE 59–4 Adult Enteral Feeding Formulation Classification System (*Continued*)

Category	Features	Indications
Immune-modulating	Supplemented with glutamine, arginine, nucleotides, and/or omega-3 fatty acids	Patients undergoing major elective GI surgery, trauma, burns, head and neck cancer, and critically ill patients on mechanical ventilation Use with caution in patients with sepsis Select nutrients may be beneficial or harmful in subgroups of critically ill patients
Oral supplement	Sweetened for taste Hypertonic	Patients who require supplementation to an oral diet

(ALI, acute lung injury; ARDS, acute respiratory distress syndrome; MCT, medium-chain triglyceride; NPC:N, nonprotein calorie-to-nitrogen ratio.)

TABLE 59–5 Suggested Monitoring for Patients on Enteral Nutrition

Parameter	During Initiation of EN Therapy	During Stable EN Therapy
Vital signs	Every 4–6 hours	As needed with suspected change (ie, fever)
Clinical assessment		
Weight	Daily	Weekly
Length/height (children)	Weekly-monthly	Monthly
Head circumference (<3 years of age)	Weekly-monthly	Monthly
Total intake/output	Daily	As needed with suspected change in intake/output
Tube-feeding intake	Daily	Daily
Enterostomy tube site assessment	Daily	Daily
GI tolerance		
Stool frequency/volume	Daily	Daily
Abdomen assessment	Daily	Daily
Nausea or vomiting	Daily	Daily
Gastric residual volumes	Every 4–8 hours (varies)	As needed when delayed gastric emptying suspected
Tube placement	Prior to starting, then ongoing	Ongoing
Laboratory		
Electrolytes, blood urea nitrogen/serum creatinine, glucose	Daily until stable, then 2–3 times/week	Every 1–3 months
Calcium, magnesium, phosphorus	Daily until stable, then 2–3 times/week	Every 1–3 months
Liver function tests	Weekly	Every 1–3 months
Trace elements, vitamins	If deficiency/toxicity suspected	If deficiency/toxicity suspected

(EN, enteral nutrition.)

maintaining patency include flushing with at least 15 to 30 mL of water before and after medication administration and intermittent feedings and at least every 8 hours during continuous feeding.

DRUG DELIVERY VIA FEEDING TUBE

• Administering drugs via tube feeding is a common practice. If the drug is a solid that can be crushed (eg, *not* a sublingual, sustained-release, or enteric-coated formulation) or is a capsule, mix with 15 to 30 mL of water or other appropriate solvent and administer. Otherwise, a liquid dosage preparation should be used. Administer multiple medications separately, each followed by flushing the tube with 5 to 15 mL of water.

- Mixing of liquid medications with EN formulations can cause physical incompatibilities that inhibit drug absorption and clog small-bore feeding tubes. Incompatibility is more common with formulations containing intact (vs hydrolyzed) protein and medications formulated as acidic syrups. Mixing of liquid medications and EN formulations should be avoided whenever possible.
- The most significant drug–nutrient interactions result in reduced bioavailability and suboptimal pharmacologic effect (Table 59–6). Continuous feeding requires interruption for drug administration, and medications should be spaced between bolus feedings.

PARENTERAL NUTRITION

- Parenteral nutrition (PN) provides macro- and micronutrients by central or peripheral venous access to meet specific nutritional requirements of the patient.
- PN should be considered when a patient cannot meet nutritional requirements through use of the GI tract. Consider PN after suboptimal nutritional intake for 1 day in preterm infants, 2 to 3 days in term infants, 3 to 5 days in critically injured children, 5 to 7 days in other children, and 7 to 14 days in older children and adults.

COMPONENTS OF PARENTERAL NUTRITION

- Macronutrients (ie, water, protein, dextrose, and fat) are used for energy (dextrose and fat) and as structural substrates (protein and fat).
- Protein is provided as crystalline amino acids (CAAs). When oxidized, 1 g of protein yields 4 calories (~17 J). Including the caloric contribution from protein in calorie calculations is controversial; therefore, PN calories can be calculated as either total or nonprotein calories.
- Standard CAA products contain a balanced profile of essential, semi-essential, and nonessential L-amino acids and are designed for patients with "normal" organ function and nutritional requirements. Standard CAA products differ in protein concentration, total nitrogen, and electrolyte content but have similar effects on protein markers.
- The primary energy source in PN solutions is carbohydrate, usually as dextrose monohydrate, which is available in concentrations ranging from 5% to 70%. When oxidized, 1 g of hydrated dextrose provides 3.4 kcal (14.2 kJ).
- Commercially available intravenous fat emulsions (IVFEs) provide calories and essential fatty acids. These products differ in triglyceride source, fatty acid content, and essential fatty acid concentration.
- When oxidized, 1 g of fat yields 9 kcal (38 kJ). Because of the caloric contribution from egg phospholipid and glycerol, caloric content of IVFE is 1.1 kcal/mL (4.6 kJ/mL) for the 10%, 2 kcal/mL (8.4 kJ/mL) for the 20%, and 3 kcal/mL (12.6 kJ/mL) for the 30% emulsions.
- Essential fatty acid deficiency can be prevented by giving IVFE, 0.5 to 1 g/kg/day for neonates and infants and 100 g/wk for adults.
- IVFE 10% and 20% products can be administered by a central or peripheral vein, added directly to PN solution as a total nutrient admixture (TNA) or three-in-one system (lipids, protein, glucose, and additives), or co-infused with a CAA and dextrose solution, commonly referred to as a two-in-one solution. IVFE 30% is approved only for TNA preparation.
- Micronutrients (ie, vitamins, trace elements, and electrolytes) support metabolic activities for cellular homeostasis such as enzyme reactions, fluid balance, and regulation of electrophysiologic processes.
- Multivitamin products have been formulated to comply with guidelines for adults, children, and infants. These products contain 13 essential vitamins, including vitamin K.
- Requirements for trace elements depend on the patient's age and clinical condition.
- Chromium, copper, manganese, selenium, and zinc are considered essential and available as single- or multiple-entity products for addition to PN solutions.

TABLE 59–6 Medications with Special Considerations for Enteral Feeding Tube Administration

Drug	Interaction	Comments
Phenytoin	Reduced bioavailability in the presence of tube feedings Possible phenytoin binding to calcium caseinates or protein hydrolysates in enteral feeding	To minimize interaction, holding tube feedings 1–2 hours before and after administration has been suggested; this has no proven benefit Adjust tube-feeding rate to account for time held for phenytoin administration Monitor phenytoin serum concentration and clinical response closely Consider switching to IV phenytoin if unable to reach therapeutic serum concentration
Fluoroquinolones Tetracyclines	Potential for reduced bioavailability because of complexation of drug with divalent and trivalent cations found in enteral feeding	Consider holding tube feeding 1 hour before and after administration Avoid jejunal administration of ciprofloxacin Monitor clinical response
Warfarin	Decreased absorption of warfarin because of enteral feeding; therapeutic effect antagonized by vitamin K in enteral formulations	Adjust warfarin dose based on INR Anticipate need to increase warfarin dose when enteral feedings are started and decrease dose when enteral feedings are stopped Consider holding tube feeding 1 hour before and after administration
Omeprazole Lansoprazole	Administration via feeding tube complicated by acid-labile medication within delayed-release, base-labile granules	Granules become sticky when moistened with water and may occlude small-bore tubes Granules should be mixed with acidic liquid when given via a gastric feeding tube An oral liquid suspension can be extemporaneously prepared for administration via a feeding tube

(INR, International normalized ratio.)

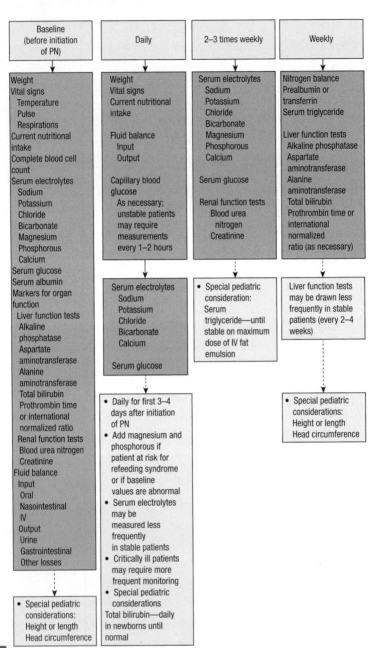

FIGURE 59–1. Monitoring strategy for patients receiving parenteral nutrition (PN).

- Sodium, potassium, calcium, magnesium, phosphorus, chloride, and acetate are necessary components of PN for maintenance of numerous cellular functions.
- Electrolyte requirements depend on the patient's age, disease state, organ function, previous and current drug therapy, nutrition status, and extrarenal losses.

SPECIFICS OF PARENTERAL NUTRITION

- The patient's clinical condition determines whether PN is administered through a peripheral or central vein.
- Peripheral parenteral nutrition (PPN) candidates do not have large nutritional requirements, are not fluid restricted, and are expected to regain GI tract function within 10 to 14 days. Solutions for PPN have lower final concentrations of amino acid (3%–5%), dextrose (5%–10%), and micronutrients as compared with central parenteral nutrition (CPN).
- Primary advantages of PPN include a lower risk of infectious, metabolic, and technical complications.
- CPN is useful in patients who require PN for more than 7 to 14 days and who have large nutrient requirements, poor peripheral venous access, or fluctuating fluid requirements.
- CPN solutions are highly concentrated hypertonic solutions that must be administered through a large central vein. The choice of venous access site depends on factors including patient age and anatomy. Peripherally inserted central catheters (PICCs) are often used for both short- and long-term central venous access in acute or home care settings.
- Disadvantages include risks associated with catheter insertion, use, and care. Central venous access has a greater potential for infection.
- PN regimens for adults can be based on formulas computer programs, or standardized order forms. Order forms are popular because they help educate practitioners and foster cost-efficient nutrition support by minimizing errors in ordering, compounding, and administering.
- Pediatric PN regimens typically require an individualized approach because practice guidelines often recommend nutrient intake based on weight. Labeling should reflect "amount per day" and also "amount per kilogram per day."

EVALUATION OF THERAPEUTIC OUTCOMES

- Assessing the outcome of EN includes monitoring objective measures of body composition, protein and energy balance, and subjective outcome for physiologic muscle function and wound healing.
- Measures of disease-related morbidity include length of hospital stay, infectious complications, and patient's sense of well-being. Ultimately, the successful use of EN avoids the need for PN.
- Outcomes with PN are determined through routine assessment of the clinical condition of the patient, with a focus on nutritional and metabolic effects of the PN regimen.
- Biochemical and clinical parameters should be monitored routinely in patients receiving PN (Fig. 59–1).

See Chapter 141, Assessment of Nutrition Status and Nutrition Requirements, authored by Katherine Hammond Chessman and Vanessa J. Kumpf; Chapter 142, Parenteral Nutrition, authored by Todd W. Mattox and Catherine M. Crill; and Chapter 143, Enteral Nutrition, authored by Vanessa J. Kumpf and Katherine Hammond Chessman, for a more detailed discussion of this topic.

CHAPTER 60

Breast Cancer

- *Breast cancer* is a malignancy originating from breast tissue. Disease confined to a localized breast lesion is referred to as *early, primary, localized*, or *curable*. Disease detected clinically or radiologically in sites distant from the breast is referred to as *advanced* or *metastatic breast cancer* (MBC), which is usually incurable.

EPIDEMIOLOGY

- Two variables most strongly associated with occurrence of breast cancer are gender and advancing age. Additional risk factors include endocrine factors (eg, early menarche, nulliparity, late age at first birth, and hormone replacement therapy), genetic factors (eg, personal and family history, mutations of tumor suppresser genes [*BRCA1* and *BRCA2*]), and environmental and lifestyle factors (eg, radiation exposure).
- Breast cancer cells often spread undetected by contiguity, lymph channels, and through the blood early in the course of the disease, resulting in metastatic disease after local therapy. The most common metastatic sites are lymph nodes, skin, bone, liver, lungs, and brain.

PREVENTION OF BREAST CANCER

- SERMs and AIs are being studied for pharmacologic risk reduction of breast cancer.
- The most clinical information is available for the SERMs, **tamoxifen** and **raloxifene**, which reduce the rates of invasive breast cancer in women at high risk for developing the disease. Rates of endometrial cancer and deep vein thromboses are higher in patients receiving tamoxifen, but the overall quality of life is similar between the two agents.
- **Exemestane** taken for 5 years significantly reduced the rates of invasive breast cancers with tolerable adverse events.
- Risk reduction strategies include mastectomy, oophorectomy, and pharmacologic agents. Clinical guidelines recommend the use of tamoxifen, raloxifene, or exemestane for postmenopausal women at high risk and tamoxifen for premenopausal women at high risk based on the woman's wishes.

CLINICAL PRESENTATION

- A painless, palpable lump is the initial sign of breast cancer in most women. The typical malignant mass is solitary, unilateral, solid, hard, irregular, and nonmobile. Nipple changes are less commonly seen. More advanced cases present with prominent skin edema, redness, warmth, and induration.
- Symptoms of MBC depend on the site of metastases but may include bone pain, difficulty breathing, abdominal pain or enlargement, jaundice, and mental status changes.
- Many women first detect some breast abnormalities themselves, but it is increasingly common for breast cancer to be detected during routine screening mammography in asymptomatic women.

DIAGNOSIS

- Initial workup should include a careful history, physical examination of the breast, three-dimensional mammography, and, possibly, other breast imaging techniques, such as ultrasound and magnetic resonance imaging (MRI).
- Breast biopsy is indicated for a mammographic abnormality that suggests malignancy or for a palpable mass on physical examination.

STAGING

- Stage (anatomical extent of disease) is based on primary tumor extent and size (T_{1-4}), presence and extent of lymph node involvement (N_{1-3}), and presence or absence of distant metastases (M_{0-1}). The staging system determines prognosis and assists with treatment decisions. Simplistically stated, these stages may be represented as follows:
  - ✓ *Early breast cancer*
    - ❖ Stage 0: Carcinoma in situ or disease that has not invaded the basement membrane
    - ❖ Stage I: Small primary invasive tumor without lymph node involvement
    - ❖ Stage II: Involvement of regional lymph nodes
  - ✓ *Locally advanced breast cancer*
    - ❖ Stage III: Usually a large tumor with extensive nodal involvement in which the node or tumor is fixed to the chest wall; also includes inflammatory breast cancer, which is rapidly progressive
  - ✓ *Advanced or metastatic breast cancer*
    - ❖ Stage IV: Metastases in organs distant from the primary tumor

PATHOLOGIC EVALUATION

- Development of malignancy is a multistep process involving preinvasive (or noninvasive) and invasive phases. The goal of treatment for noninvasive carcinomas is to prevent the development of invasive disease.
- Pathologic evaluation of breast lesions establishes the histologic diagnosis and confirms the presence or absence of prognostic factors.
- Most breast carcinomas are adenocarcinomas and are classified as ductal or lobular.

PROGNOSTIC FACTORS

- The ability to predict prognosis is used to design treatment recommendations to maximize quantity and quality of life.
- Age at diagnosis and ethnicity are patient characteristics that may affect prognosis.
- Tumor size and presence and number of involved axillary lymph nodes are primary factors in assessing the risk for breast cancer recurrence and subsequent metastatic disease. Other disease characteristics that provide prognostic information are histologic subtype, nuclear or histologic grade, lymphatic and vascular invasion, and proliferation indices.
- Hormone receptors [estrogen (ER) and progesterone (PR)] are not strong prognostic markers but are used clinically to predict response to endocrine therapy.
- HER2/*neu* (HER2) overexpression is associated with transmission of growth signals that control aspects of normal cell growth and division. Overexpression of HER2 is associated with increased tumor aggressiveness, rates of recurrence, and mortality.
- Genetic profiling tools provide additional prognostic information to aid in treatment decisions for subgroups of patients with otherwise favorable prognostic features.

TREATMENT

- <u>Goals of Treatment</u>: Adjuvant therapy for early and locally advanced breast cancer is administered with curative intent. Neoadjuvant therapy is given to eradicate micrometastatic disease, determine prognosis, and potentially conserve breast tissue for a better cosmetic result. Palliation is the desired therapeutic outcome in the treatment of MBC.

- Treatment is rapidly evolving. Specific information regarding the most promising interventions can be found only in the primary literature.
- Treatment can cause substantial toxicity, which differs depending on the individual agent, administration method, and combination regimen. A comprehensive review of toxicities is beyond the scope of this chapter; consult appropriate references.

EARLY BREAST CANCER

Local-Regional Therapy

- Surgery alone can cure most patients with in situ cancers, 70% to 80% of stage I cancers, and approximately one half of those with stage II cancers.
- Breast-conserving therapy (BCT) is often primary therapy for stage I and stage II disease; it is preferable to modified radical mastectomy because it produces equivalent survival rates with cosmetically superior results. BCT includes removal of part of the breast, surgical evaluation of axillary lymph nodes, and radiation therapy (RT) to prevent local recurrence.
- RT is administered to the entire breast over 3 to 5 weeks to eradicate residual disease after BCT. Reddening and erythema of the breast tissue with subsequent shrinkage of total breast mass are minor complications associated with RT.
- Simple or total mastectomy involves removal of the entire breast without dissection of underlying muscle or axillary nodes. This procedure is used for carcinoma in situ where the incidence of axillary node involvement is only 1% or with local recurrence following BCT.
- Axillary lymph nodes should be sampled for staging and prognostic information. Lymphatic mapping with sentinel lymph node biopsy is a less invasive alternative to axillary dissection.

Systemic Adjuvant Therapy

- Systemic adjuvant therapy is the administration of systemic therapy following definitive local therapy (surgery, radiation, or in combination) when there is no evidence of metastatic disease but a high likelihood of disease recurrence. The goal of such therapy is cure.
- Administration of chemotherapy, endocrine therapy, targeted therapy, or some combination of these agents results in improved disease-free survival (DFS) and/or overall survival (OS) for all treated patients.
- The National Comprehensive Cancer Network (NCCN) practice guidelines are updated at least annually and should be consulted for treatment recommendations.
- Genetic tests are being prospectively validated as decision-support tools for adjuvant chemotherapy in ER-positive, node-negative, invasive breast cancer to identify primary tumor characteristics that may predict for the likelihood of distant recurrence and/or death.

ADJUVANT CHEMOTHERAPY

- Early administration of effective combination chemotherapy at a time of low tumor burden should increase the likelihood of cure and minimize emergence of drug-resistant tumor cell clones. Combination regimens have historically been more effective than single-agent chemotherapy (Table 60–1).
- Anthracycline-containing regimens (eg, **doxorubicin** and **epirubicin**) reduce the rate of recurrence and death as compared with regimens that contain **cyclophosphamide**, **methotrexate**, and **fluorouracil**.
- The addition of taxanes, **docetaxel** and **paclitaxel**, to adjuvant regimens comprised of the drugs listed above resulted in reduced risk of distant recurrence, any recurrence, and overall mortality compared with a nontaxane regimen in node-positive breast cancer patients. The use of taxane-containing regimens in node-negative patients remains controversial.
- Initiate chemotherapy within 12 weeks of surgical removal of the primary tumor. Optimal duration of adjuvant treatment is unknown but appears to be 12 to 24 weeks, depending on the regimen used.

TABLE 60–1 Selected Adjuvant Chemotherapy Regimens for Breast Cancer

AC

Doxorubicin 60 mg/m² IV, day 1

Cyclophosphamide 600 mg/m² IV, day 1

Repeat cycles every 21 days for 4 cycles

FAC

Fluorouracil 500 mg/m² IV, days 1 and 4

Doxorubicin 50 mg/m² IV continuous infusion over 72 hours

Cyclophosphamide 500 mg/m² IV, day 1

Repeat cycles every 21–28 days for 6 cycles

AC → Paclitaxel

Doxorubicin 60 mg/m² IV, day 1

Cyclophosphamide 600 mg/m² IV, day 1

Repeat cycles every 21 days for 4 cycles

Followed by:

Paclitaxel 80 mg/m² IV weekly

Repeat cycles every 7 days for 12 cycles

FEC

Fluorouracil 500 mg/m² IV, day 1

Epirubicin 100 mg/m² IV bolus, day 1

Cyclophosphamide 500 mg/m² IV, day 1

Repeat cycle every 21 days for 6 cycles

TC

Docetaxel 75 mg/m² IV, day 1

Cyclophosphamide 600 mg/m² IV, day 1

Repeat cycles every 21 days for 4 cycles

TAC

Docetaxel 75 mg/m² IV, day 1

Doxorubicin 50 mg/m² IV bolus, day 1

Cyclophosphamide 500 mg/m² IV, day 1 (doxorubicin should be given first)

Repeat cycles every 21 days for 6 cycles (must be given with growth factor support)

Paclitaxel → FAC

Paclitaxel 80 mg/m² per week IV over 1 hour every week for 12 weeks

Followed by:

Fluorouracil 500 mg/m² IV, days 1 and 4

Doxorubicin 50 mg/m² IV continuous infusion over 72 hours

Cyclophosphamide 500 mg/m² IV, day 1

Repeat cycles every 21–28 days for 4 cycles

CEF

Cyclophosphamide 75 mg/m² per day orally on days 1–14

Epirubicin 60 mg/m² IV, days 1 and 8

Fluorouracil 600 mg/m² IV, days 1 and 8

Repeat cycles every 21 days for 6 cycles (requires prophylactic antibiotics or growth factor support)

CMF

Cyclophosphamide 100 mg/m² per day orally, days 1–14

Methotrexate 40 mg/m² IV, days 1 and 8

Fluorouracil 600 mg/m² IV, days 1 and 8

Repeat cycles every 28 days for 6 cycles

Or

Cyclophosphamide 600 mg/m² IV, day 1

Methotrexate 40 mg/m² IV, day 1

Fluorouracil 600 mg/m² IV, days 1 and 8

Repeat cycles every 21 days for 6 cycles

Dose-Dense AC → Paclitaxel

Doxorubicin 60 mg/m² IV bolus, day 1

Cyclophosphamide 600 mg/m² IV, day 1

Repeat cycles every 14 days for 4 cycles (must be given with growth factor support)

Followed by:

Paclitaxel 175 mg/m² IV over 3 hours

Repeat cycles every 14 days for 4 cycles (must be given with growth factor support)

[AC, Adriamycin (doxorubicin), Cytoxan (cyclophosphamide); CAF, Cytoxan (cyclophosphamide), Adriamycin (doxorubicin), 5-fluorouracil; CEF, cyclophosphamide, epirubicin, 5-fluorouracil; CMF, cyclophosphamide, methotrexate, 5-flourouracil; FAC, 5-fluorouracil, Adriamycin (doxorubicin), cyclophosphamide; FEC, 5-fluorouracil, epirubicin, cyclophosphamide; TAC, Taxotere (docetaxel), Adriamycin (doxorubicin), cyclophosphamide; TC, Taxotere (docetaxel), cyclophosphamide].

- *Dose intensity* refers to the amount of drug administered per unit of time, which can be achieved by increasing dose, decreasing time between doses, or both. *Dose density* is one way of achieving dose intensity by decreasing time between treatment cycles.
- Dose-dense adjuvant regimens for node-positive breast cancer resulted in prolonged DFS and OS. No benefit in DFS or OS was shown for sequential versus concurrent chemotherapy but sequential therapy appears to be less toxic.
- Concomitant or sequential administration of a taxane with an anthracycline-based regimen is standard of care in node-positive breast cancer.
- Dose increases in standard regimens appear to not be beneficial and may be harmful.
- Avoid dose reductions in standard regimens unless necessitated by severe toxicity.
- Short-term toxicities of adjuvant chemotherapy are generally well tolerated, especially with the availability of serotonin-antagonist and substance P/neurokinin 1–antagonist antiemetics and myeloid growth factors.
- Survival benefit for adjuvant chemotherapy in stage I and II breast cancer is modest. The absolute reduction in mortality at 10 years is 5% in node-negative and 10% in node-positive disease.

ADJUVANT BIOLOGIC THERAPY

- **Trastuzumab** in combination with or sequentially after adjuvant chemotherapy is indicated in patients with early stage, *HER*2-positive breast cancer. The risk of recurrence was reduced up to 50% in clinical trials.
- Unanswered questions with the use of adjuvant trastuzumab include optimal concurrent chemotherapy, optimal dose, schedule and duration of therapy, and use of other concurrent therapeutic modalities.

ADJUVANT ENDOCRINE THERAPY

- Tamoxifen, **toremifene**, oophorectomy, ovarian irradiation, luteinizing hormone–releasing hormone (LHRH) agonists, and aromatase inhibitors (AI) are hormonal therapies used in the treatment of primary or early-stage breast cancer. Tamoxifen was the gold standard adjuvant hormonal therapy for three decades and is generally considered the adjuvant hormonal therapy of choice for premenopausal women. It has both estrogenic and antiestrogenic properties, depending on the tissue and gene in question.
- Tamoxifen 20 mg daily, beginning soon after completing chemotherapy and continuing for 5 years, reduces the risk of recurrence and mortality. It is usually well tolerated; however, symptoms of estrogen withdrawal (hot flashes and vaginal bleeding) may occur but decrease in frequency and intensity over time. Tamoxifen reduces the risk of hip radius and spine fractures. It increases the risks of stroke, pulmonary embolism, deep vein thrombosis, and endometrial cancer, particularly in women age 50 years or older. Administration of tamoxifen for 10 years in patients with a higher risk of recurrence is supported by recent studies.
- Premenopausal women benefit from ovarian ablation with LHRH agonists (eg, **goserelin**) in the adjuvant setting, either with or without concurrent tamoxifen. Trials are ongoing to further define the role of LHRH agonists.
- Guidelines recommend incorporation of AIs into adjuvant hormonal therapy for postmenopausal, hormone-sensitive breast cancer. Experts believe that **anastrozole**, **letrozole**, and exemestane have similar antitumor efficacy and toxicity profiles. Adverse effects with AIs include bone loss/osteoporosis, hot flashes, myalgia/arthralgia, vaginal dryness/atrophy, mild headaches, and diarrhea.
- The optimal drug, dose, sequence, and duration of administration of AIs in the adjuvant setting are not known.

LOCALLY ADVANCED BREAST CANCER (STAGE III)

- Neoadjuvant or primary chemotherapy is the initial treatment of choice. Benefits include rendering inoperable tumors resectable and increasing the rate of BCT.
- Primary chemotherapy with an anthracycline- and taxane-containing regimen is recommended. The use of trastuzumab and **pertuzumab** with chemotherapy is appropriate for patients with *HER*2-positive tumors.

- Surgery followed by chemotherapy and adjuvant RT should be administered to minimize local recurrence.
- Cure is the primary goal of therapy for most patients with stage III disease.

METASTATIC BREAST CANCER (STAGE IV)

- The choice of therapy for MBC is based on the extent of disease involvement and the presence or absence of certain tumor or patient characteristics, as described below.
- The most important factors predicting response to therapy are the presence of *HER2*, estrogen, and progesterone receptors in the primary tumor tissue.
- Consider adding bone-modifying agents (eg, **pamidronate**, **zoledronic acid**, or **denosumab**) to treat breast cancer patients with metastases to the bone to decrease rates of skeletal-related events and the need for radiation to the bones or surgery.

Biologic or Targeted Therapy

- Four anti-*HER2* agents are available: trastuzumab, **lapatinib**, pertuzumab, and **ado-trastuzumab emtansine**. Addition of trastuzumab to chemotherapy increases progression-free (PFS), time-to-progression (TTP) and overall response rate benefits in patients with *HER2*-positive MBC.
- Consider combination endocrine plus *HER2*-directed therapy when chemotherapy is not tolerated or after achieving maximal response with chemotherapy-*HER2* therapy approach.
- HER2-targeted therapies are cardiotoxic with the type of toxicity differing among agents. The incidence of heart failure is ~5% with single-agent trastuzumab and unacceptably high in combination with an anthracycline.
- HER2-targeted regimens for MBC are summarized in Table 60–2.
- Other targeted agents including mTOR inhibitors (eg, **everolimus**) and cell cycle regulators (eg, **palbociclib**) are used in combination with endocrine agents to improve outcomes.

Endocrine Therapy

- Endocrine therapy is the treatment of choice for patients who have hormone receptor–positive metastases in soft tissue, bone, pleura, or, if asymptomatic, viscera. Compared with chemotherapy, endocrine therapy has an equal probability of response and a better safety profile.
- Patients are sequentially treated with endocrine therapy until their tumors cease to respond, at which time chemotherapy can be given.
- No one endocrine therapy has clearly superior survival benefit. Choice of agent is based primarily on mechanism of action, toxicity, and patient preference (Table 60–3).
- AIs are generally first line therapy in postmenopausal women. AIs reduce circulating and target organ estrogens by blocking peripheral conversion from an androgenic precursor, the primary source of estrogens in postmenopausal women. The third-generation aromatase inhibitors anastrozole, letrozole, and exemestane are more selective and have an improved toxicity profile. When compared with tamoxifen, patients receiving AIs had similar response rates as well as lower incidence of thromboembolic events and vaginal bleeding.
- Tamoxifen, a selective estrogen receptor modulator (SERM) is the preferred initial agent when metastases are present in premenopausal women except when metastases occur within 1 year of adjuvant tamoxifen. In addition to the side effects described for adjuvant therapy, tumor flare or hypercalcemia occurs in approximately 5% of patients with MBC.
- **Toremifene**, also a SERM, has similar efficacy and tolerability as tamoxifen and is an alternative to tamoxifen in postmenopausal patients. **Fulvestrant** is a second-line intramuscular agent with similar efficacy and safety when compared with anastrozole or exemestane in patients who progressed on tamoxifen.

TABLE 60–2   Selected Regimens for *HER2*-Positive Metastatic Breast Cancer

Selected chemotherapy/biologic regimens

Docetaxel + Trastuzumab + Pertuzumab
Docetaxel 75 mg/m² IV day 1
Trastuzumab 8 mg/kg IV day 1 followed by 6 mg/kg IV
Pertuzumab 840 mg IV day 1 followed by 420 mg IV
Repeat cycle every 21 days

Paclitaxel + Trastuzumab + Pertuzumab
Paclitaxel 80 mg/m² IV days 1, 8, 15
Trastuzumab 8 mg/kg IV day 1 followed by 6 mg/kg IV
Pertuzumab 840 mg IV day 1 followed by 420 mg IV
Repeat cycle every 21 days

Selected endocrine therapy/biologic therapy regimens

Trastuzumab + Lapatinib
Lapatinib 1000 mg orally daily continuously
Trastuzumab 8 mg/kg IV day 1 followed by 6 mg/kg IV day 1
Repeat cycle every 21 days **OR**
Trastuzumab 4 mg/kg IV day 1 followed by 2 mg/kg IV day 1
Repeat cycle weekly

Lapatinib + Capecitabine
Lapatinib 1250 mg orally daily continuously
Capecitabine 1000 mg/m² twice daily × 14 days
Repeat cycle every 21 days

Ado-trastuzumab emtansine (T-DM1)
Ado-Trastuzumab Emtansine 3.6 mg/kg IV day 1
Repeat cycle every 21 days

Trastuzumab + chemotherapy
Trastuzumab 8 mg/kg IV day 1 followed by 6 mg/kg IV day 1
Repeat cycle every 21 days (for Q 21 day chemotherapy) **OR**
Trastuzumab 4 mg/kg IV day 1 followed by 2 mg/kg IV day 1
Repeat cycle weekly (for weekly chemotherapy)
Chemotherapy may include any one of the following:
Paclitaxel, docetaxel, protein-bound paclitaxel, capecitabine, vinorelbine, gemcitabine

Trastuzumab + Anastrozole
Anastrozole 1 mg orally daily continuously
Trastuzumab 8 mg/kg IV day 1 followed by 6 mg/kg IV day 1
Repeat cycle every 21 days **OR**
Trastuzumab 4 mg/kg IV day 1 followed by 2 mg/kg IV day 1
Repeat cycle weekly

Lapatinib + Letrozole
Lapatinib 1500 mg orally daily continuously
Letrozole 2.5 mg orally daily continuously

1. NCCN Clinical Practice Guidelines in Oncology (NCCN Guidelines®) for *Breast Cancer* V.3.2015 © National Comprehensive Cancer Network, Inc 2015. Last accessed, September 1, 2015.
2. Giordano SH, Temin S, Kirshner JJ, et al. Systemic therapy for patients with advanced human epidermal growth factor receptor 2-positive breast cancer: American Society of Clinical Oncology clinical practice guideline. *J Clin Oncol* 2014;32:2078-2099.
3. Herceptin (trastuzumab) product information. 2015 April 2015 [cited 2015 12/2/15]; Product information. Available from: http://www.gene.com/download/pdf/herceptin_prescribing.pdf.
4. Tykerb (lapatinib) product information. 2015 March 2015 [cited 2015 December 2]; Tykerb prescribing information]. Available from: http://www.pharma.us.novartis.com/product/pi/pdf/tykerb.pdf.

TABLE 60–3 Therapies Used for HR-Positive Metastatic Breast Cancer

Drug	Brand Name	Initial Dose	Usual Range	Special Population Dose	Comments
Aromatase inhibitors: Nonsteroidal					
Anastrozole	Arimidex, generic	1 mg orally daily			
Letrozole	Femara, generic	2.5 mg orally daily		Caution in severe liver impairment[a]	
Aromatase inhibitor: Steroidal					
Exemestane	Aromasin, generic	25 mg orally daily			Take after meals
Antiestrogens: SERMs					
Tamoxifen	Nolvadex, generic	20 mg orally daily		See text regarding CYP2D6	See text regarding CYP2D6
Toremifene	Fareston	60 mg orally daily			
Antiestrogen: SERD					
Fulvestrant	Faslodex	500 mg IM every 28 days (after loading days 1, 15, 29)	250–500 mg (see text for details)	Moderate liver impairment[a] administer 250 mg IM every 28 days (after loading days 1, 15, 29)	
LHRH agonists					
Goserelin	Zoladex	3.6 mg SC every 28 days		Premenopausal women only	
Leuprolide	Lupron (IM), generic	3.75 mg IM every 28 days	Other formulations and doses are not used for breast cancer	Premenopausal women only	Not FDA approved for breast cancer, other formulations are administered differently
Triptorelin	Trelstar	3.75 mg IM every 28 days		Premenopausal women only	Not FDA-approved for breast cancer

(continued)

TABLE 60-3 Therapies Used for HR-Positive Metastatic Breast Cancer (Continued)

Drug	Brand Name	Initial Dose	Usual Range	Special Population Dose	Comments
Progestins					
Megestrol acetate	Megace, generic	40 mg orally 4 times a day	80 mg twice daily also appropriate		Absorption maybe increased when taken with food
Medroxyprogesterone	DepoProvera, generic	400 mg IM every week	400–1000 mg IM every week	May need to decrease dose in severe liver impairment[a]	
Androgens					
Fluoxymesterone	Androxy, generic	10 mg orally twice a day	10–20/day in divided doses	Avoid in severe renal or liver impairment[a]	
Estrogens					
Ethinyl estradiol	Multiple generics	1 mg orally 3 times a day	Lower doses not effective	Avoid in jaundice or "marked" liver disease	Take with food
Conjugated estrogens	Premarin	2.5 mg orally 3 times a day	Lower doses not effective	Avoid in jaundice or "marked" liver disease	Take with food
Biologic/targeted therapies					
Everolimus (+ Exemestane)	Afinitor	10 mg orally daily	2.5–10 mg daily	Adjust dose in mild, moderate and severe liver impairment; also monitor for myelosuppression, hyperglycemia, dyslipidemia, renal dysfunction. May need to adjust dose with concomitant CYP3A4 inhibitors/inducers	Do not split tablets
Palbociclib (+ Letrozole or Fulvestrant)	Ibrance	125 mg orally daily × 21 days, followed by 7 days off, repeated every 28 days	75–125 mg daily	Adjust dose for myelosuppression. Avoid concomitant strong inhibitors of CYP3A4 and moderate/severe inducers of CYP3A4	Do not split tablets

(IM, intramuscular; LHRH, luteinizing hormone-releasing hormone; SC, subcutaneous; SERD, selective estrogen receptor downregulator SERM, selective estrogen receptor modulator)
[a]Severe liver impairment: Child-Pugh class C; moderate liver impairment: Child-Pugh class B; minor liver impairment: Child-Pugh class A.

- Surgical or chemical ovarian ablation is considered by some to be the endocrine therapy of choice in premenopausal women and produces similar overall response rates as tamoxifen. Medical castration with an LHRH analogue (**goserelin**, **leuprolide**, or **triptorelin**) is a reversible alternative to surgery.
- Progestins are generally reserved for third-line therapy. They cause weight gain, fluid retention, and thromboembolic events.

Chemotherapy

- Chemotherapy is used as initial therapy for women with hormone receptor–negative tumors; with triple negative tumors; and after failure of endocrine therapy.
- The choice of treatment depends on patient characteristics, expected toxicities, and previous exposure to chemotherapy. Single agents are associated with lower response rates than combination therapy, but time to progression and OS are similar. Single agents are better tolerated, an important consideration in the palliative metastatic setting (Table 60–4).
- Treatment with sequential single agents is recommended over combination regimens unless the patient has rapidly progressive disease, life-threatening visceral disease, or the need for rapid symptom control.
- Most patients experience partial responses to chemotherapy, but complete disappearance of disease occur in less than 10% of patients. The median duration of response is highly variable, ranging from 5 to 18 months; the median OS is 14 to 33 months. A specific chemotherapy regimen is continued until there is unequivocal evidence of progressive disease or intolerable side effects.
- **Anthracyclines** and **taxanes** produce response rates of 50% to 60% when used as first-line therapy for MBC. Single-agent **capecitabine**, **vinorelbine**, and **gemcitabine** have response rates of 20% to 25% when used after an anthracycline and a taxane.
- **Ixabepilone**, a microtubule stabilizing agent, is indicated as monotherapy or in combination with capecitabine. **Eribulin** is a second antimicrotubule agent approved as monotherapy in patients who have received at least two prior chemotherapy regimens for MBC.

Radiation Therapy

- Commonly used to treat painful bone metastases or other localized sites of disease, including brain and spinal cord lesions. Pain relief is seen in approximately 90% of patients who receive RT.

EVALUATION OF THERAPEUTIC OUTCOMES

EARLY BREAST CANCER

- The goal of adjuvant therapy in early-stage disease is cure. Because there is no clinical evidence of disease when adjuvant therapy is administered, assessment of this goal cannot be fully evaluated for years after initial diagnosis and treatment.
- Adjuvant chemotherapy can cause significant toxicity. Optimize supportive care measures such as antiemetics and growth factors to maintain dose intensity.

LOCALLY ADVANCED BREAST CANCER

- The goal of neoadjuvant chemotherapy in locally advanced breast cancer is cure. Complete pathologic response, determined at the time of surgery, is the desired end point.

METASTATIC BREAST CANCER

- Palliation is the therapeutic end point in the treatment of patients with MBC. Optimizing quality of life is an important therapeutic end point. Valid and reliable tools are available for objective assessment of quality of life in patients with breast cancer.

TABLE 60–4 Selected Chemotherapy Regimens for *HER2*-Negative Metastatic Breast Cancer

Single-Agent Chemotherapy

Paclitaxel[a,b]
Paclitaxel 175 mg/m^2 IV over 3 hours
Repeat cycles every 21 days
or
Paclitaxel 80 mg/m^2/wk IV over 1 hour
Repeat dose every 7 days

Docetaxel[d,e]
Docetaxel 60–100 mg/m^2 IV over 1 hour
Repeat cycles every 21 days
or
Docetaxel 30–35 mg/m^2/wk IV over 30 minutes
Repeat dose every 7 days

Protein-bound paclitaxel[g,h]
Protein-bound Paclitaxel 260 mg/m^2 IV over 30 minutes
Repeat cycles every 21 days
or
Protein-bound paclitaxel 100–150 mg/m^2 IV over 30 minutes on days 1, 8, and 15
Repeat cycle every 28 days

Capecitabine[j]
Capecitabine 2000–2500 mg/m^2 per day orally, divided twice daily for 14 days
Repeat cycles every 21 days

Vinorelbine[c]
Vinorelbine 30 mg/m^2 IV, days 1 and 8
Repeat cycles every 21 days
or
Vinorelbine 25–30 mg/m^2/wk IV
Repeat cycles every 7 days (adjust dose based on absolute neutrophil count; see product information)

Gemcitabine[f]
Gemcitabine 600–1000 mg/m^2/wk IV, days 1, 8, and 15
Repeat cycles every 28 days (may need to hold day 15 dose based on blood counts)

Ixabepilone[i]
Ixabepilone 40 mg/m^2 IV over 3 hours
Repeat cycles every 21 days

Eribulin[k]
Eribulin 1.4 mg/m^2/dose IV over 2–5 minutes on days 1 and 8
Repeat dose every 21 days

Liposomal doxorubicin[l]
Liposomal doxorubicin 30–50 mg/m^2 IV over variable duration
Repeat cycles every 28 days

Combination Chemotherapy Regimens

Gemcitabine + Carboplatin[m]

Gemcitabine 1000 mg/m² IV, days 1 & 8
Carboplatin AUC 2 IV, day 1 & 8
Repeat cycles every 21 days

Ixabepilone + Capecitabine[i]

Ixabepilone 40 mg/m² IV over 3 hours, day 1
Capecitabine 1750–2000 mg/m²/day orally divided twice daily for 14 days
Repeat cycles every 21 days

Paclitaxel + Gemcitabine[n]

Paclitaxel 175 mg/m² IV over 3 hours, day 1
Gemcitabine 1250 mg/m² IV days 1 and 8
Repeat cycles every 21 days

Paclitaxel + Bevacizumab[o]

Paclitaxel 90 mg/m² IV over 1 hour, days 1, 8, and 15
Bevacizumab 10 mg/kg IV over 30–90 minutes, days 1 and 15
Repeat cycles every 28 days

[a] From Taxol (paclitaxel) product information. Princeton, NJ: Bristol-Myers Squibb, July 2007.

[b] From Perez EA, Vogelci, Irwin DH, et al. Multicenter phase II trial of weekly paclitaxel in women with metastatic breast cancer. *Clin Oncol* 2001;19:4216.

[c] From Zelek L, Barthier S, Riofrio M, et al. Weekly vinorelbine is an effective palliative regimen after failure with anthracyclines and taxanes in metastatic breast carcinoma. *Cancer* 2001;92:2267.

[d] From Taxotere (docetaxel) product information. *Bridgewater*, NJ: Sanofi-Aventis, 2008.

[e] From Hainsworth JD, Burris HA 3rd, Erlaud JB, et al. Phase I trial of docetaxel administered by weekly infusion in patients with advanced refractory cancer. *J Clin Oncol* 1998;16:164.

[f] From Carmichael J, Possinger K, Philip P, et al. Advanced breast cancer: a phase II trial with gemcitabine. *J Clin Oncol* 1995;13:2731.

[g] From Abraxane (paclitaxel protein-bound particles for injectable suspension) product information. *Bridgewater*, NJ: Abraxis Bioscience, September 2009.

[h] From Gradishar WJ, Krasnojon D, Cheporov S, et al. Significantly longer progression-free survival with nab-paclitaxel compared with docetaxel as first-line therapy for metastatic breast cancer. *J Clin Oncol* 2009;27:3611-3619.

[i] From Boehnke Michaud L. The optimal therapeutic use of ixabepilone in patients with locally advanced or metastatic breast cancer. *J Oncol Pharm Pract* 2009;15(2):95-106.

[j] From Gralow, JR. Optimizing the treatment of metastatic breast cancer. *Breast Cancer Res Treat* 2005;89(Suppl 1):S9-S15.

[k] From Halaven (eribulin) product information. *Woodcliff Lake*, NJ: Eisai Inc., February 2012.

[l] From O'Brien ME, Wigler N, Inbar M, et al. Reduced cardiotoxicity and comparable efficacy in a phase III trial of pegylated liposomal doxorubicin HCl (CAELYX/Doxil) versus conventional doxorubicin for first-line treatment of metastatic breast cancer. *Ann Oncol* 2004;15(3):440-449.

[m] From O'Shaughnessy J, Schwartzberg LS, Danso MA, et al. A randomized phase III study of iniparib (BSI-201) in combination with gemcitabine/carboplatin (G/C) in metastatic triple-negative breast cancer (TNBC). [abstract]. *J Clin Oncol* 2011;29(Suppl 15):Abstract 1007.

[n] From Gemzar (gemcitabine) product information. *Indianapolis*, IN: Eli Lilly and Co, May 2007.

[o] From Miller K, Wang M, Gralow J, et al. Paclitaxel plus bevacizumab versus paclitaxel alone for metastatic breast cancer. *N Engl J Med* 2007;357(26):2666-2676.

- The least toxic therapies are used initially, with increasingly aggressive therapies applied in a sequential manner that does not significantly compromise quality of life.
- Tumor response is measured by changes in laboratory tests, diagnostic imaging, or physical examination.

See Chapter 128, Breast Cancer, authored by Chad M. Barnett, Bonnie Lin Boster, and Laura Boehnke Michaud for a more detailed discussion of this topic.

Colorectal Cancer

- *Colorectal cancer* (CRC) is a malignant neoplasm involving the colon, rectum, and anal canal.

PATHOPHYSIOLOGY

- Development of a colorectal neoplasm is a multistep process of genetic and phenotypic alterations of normal bowel epithelium structure and function leading to dysregulated cell growth, proliferation, and tumor development.
- Features of colorectal tumorigenesis include genomic instability, activation of oncogene pathways, mutational inactivation or silencing of tumor-suppressor genes, DNA mismatch repairs, and activation of growth factor pathways.
- Adenocarcinomas account for about 85% of tumors of the large intestine.

PREVENTION AND SCREENING

- Primary prevention is aimed at preventing CRC in an at-risk population. Trials with celecoxib in people with familial adenomatous polyposis (FAP) showed reduction in size and number of polyps after 6 to 9 months of treatment, but there is a lack of long-term benefit.
- Secondary prevention is aimed at preventing malignancy in a population that has already manifested an initial disease process. Secondary prevention includes procedures ranging from colonoscopic removal of precancerous polyps detected during screening colonoscopy to total colectomy for high-risk individuals (eg, FAP)
- Current US guidelines for average-risk individuals include annual occult fecal blood testing starting at age 50 years and examination of the colon every 5 or 10 years, depending on the procedure.

CLINICAL MANIFESTATIONS

- Signs and symptoms of CRC can be extremely varied, subtle, and nonspecific. Early-stage CRC is often asymptomatic and detected by screening procedures.
- Blood in the stool is the most common sign; however, any change in bowel habits, vague abdominal discomfort, or abdominal distention may be a warning sign. Less common signs and symptoms include nausea, vomiting, and, if anemia is severe, fatigue.
- Twenty percent of patients present with metastatic disease most commonly in the liver, lung, and bones.

DIAGNOSIS

- Perform a physical examination and obtain a careful personal and family history. Evaluate entire large bowel by colonoscopy.
- Obtain baseline laboratory tests: complete blood cell count, international normalized ratio (INR), activated partial thromboplastin time, liver and renal function tests, and serum carcinoembryonic antigen (CEA). Serum CEA serves as a marker for monitoring CRC response to treatment, but it is too insensitive and nonspecific to be used as a screening test for early-stage CRC.
- Radiographic imaging studies may include chest radiographs, bone scan, chest and abdominal computed tomography scans, positron emission tomography, ultrasonography, and magnetic resonance imaging.
- Determine CRC stage at diagnosis to predict prognosis and develop treatment options. Stage is based on size of the primary tumor (T_{1-4}), presence and extent of lymph node involvement (N_{0-2}), and presence or absence of distant metastases (M).

✓ Stage I disease involves tumor invasion of the submucosa (T_1) or muscularis propria (T_2) and negative lymph nodes.

✓ Stage II disease involves tumor invasion through the muscularis propria into pericolorectal tissues (T_3), or penetration to the surface of the visceral peritoneum (T_{4a}), or directly invades or is adherent to other organs or structures (T_{4b}), and negative lymph nodes.

✓ Stage III disease includes T_{1-4} and positive regional lymph nodes.

✓ Stage IV disease includes any T, any N, and distant metastasis.

PROGNOSIS

• Stage at diagnosis is the most important independent prognostic factor for survival and disease recurrence. Five-year relative survival is approximately 90% for those with localized tumor as compared with 13% for those with metastatic disease.

• Poor prognostic clinical factors at diagnosis include bowel obstruction or perforation, high preoperative CEA level, distant metastases, and location of the primary tumor in the rectum or rectosigmoid area.

• Molecular markers, particularly MSI, 18q/*DCC* mutation or LOH, *BRAF* V600E mutation, and *KRAS* mutations are also associated with CRC prognosis.

TREATMENT

• <u>Goals of Treatment</u>: The goals include cure for stages I, II, and III; the intent is to eradicate micrometastatic disease. Most stage IV disease is incurable; palliative treatment is given to control cancer growth, reduce symptoms, improve quality of life, and extend survival. Twenty to thirty percent of patients with metastatic disease may be cured if their metastases are resectable.

• Treatment modalities are surgery, radiation therapy (RT), chemotherapy, and biomodulators.

OPERABLE DISEASE

Surgery

• Complete surgical resection of the primary tumor with regional lymphadenectomy is a curative approach for patients with operable CRC.

• The preferred surgical procedure for rectal cancer is a total excision of the mesorectum that includes tissue containing perirectal fat and draining lymph nodes.

• Common complications of colorectal surgery include infection, anastomotic leakage, obstruction, adhesions, sexual dysfunction, and malabsorption syndromes.

Adjuvant Therapy for Colon Cancer

• Adjuvant therapy is administered after complete tumor resection to eliminate residual micrometastatic disease. Adjuvant therapy is not indicated for stage I CRC because more than 90% of patients are cured by surgical resection alone.

• Results of adjuvant chemotherapy studies in patients with stage II disease are conflicting. Despite a lack of consensus among practitioners, the approach to treatment of high-risk stages II and III disease is similar.

• Adjuvant chemotherapy is the standard of care for stage III colon cancer.

Adjuvant Radiation Therapy

• Adjuvant radiation therapy (RT) has a limited role in colon cancer because most recurrences are extrapelvic and occur in the abdomen.

Adjuvant Chemotherapy

• Standard adjuvant regimens include a fluoropyrimidine (**fluorouracil** [with **leucovorin**] or **capecitabine**) as a single agent or in combination with **oxaliplatin**. Leucovorin enhances cytotoxic activity of fluorouracil.

- Administration method affects clinical activity and toxicity. In most common combination regimens, fluorouracil is administered by both IV bolus injection and by continuous IV infusion. No one treatment schedule is superior for overall patient survival.
- Continuous IV infusion of fluorouracil is generally well tolerated but is associated with palmar-plantar erythrodysesthesia (hand–foot syndrome) and stomatitis. IV bolus administration is associated with leukopenia, which is dose limiting and can be life threatening. Both administration methods are associated with a similar incidence of mucositis, diarrhea, nausea and vomiting, and alopecia.
- In rare cases, patients deficient in dihydropyrimidine dehydrogenase, responsible for the catabolism of fluorouracil, develop severe toxicity, including death, after fluorouracil administration.
- National guidelines recommend oxaliplatin-based regimens as the first-line option for patients with stage III colon cancer who can tolerate combination therapy. It is commonly administered with fluorouracil/leucovorin. Oxaliplatin is associated with both acute and persistent neuropathies, including rare, acute pharyngolaryngeal dysesthesia, neutropenia, and gastrointestinal (GI) toxicity.
- Selection of an adjuvant regimen (Table 61–1) is based on patient-specific factors, including performance status, comorbid conditions, and patient preference based on lifestyle factors. Age should also be considered as subset analysis of large clinical trials has shown that patients older than 70 years may not benefit from adjuvant oxaliplatin.
- Fluorouracil/leucovorin regimens currently have limited use but are acceptable options in patients who cannot receive oxaliplatin and are unable to tolerate oral capecitabine.

Adjuvant Therapy for Rectal Cancer

- Rectal cancer is more difficult to resect with wide margins, so local recurrences are more frequent than with colon cancer. Adjuvant RT plus chemotherapy is considered the standard of care for stages II and III rectal cancer.
- RT reduces the risk of local tumor recurrence in patients undergoing surgery for rectal cancer. RT is given prior to surgery to decrease tumor size, making it more resectable.
- Preoperative (neoadjuvant) chemoradiation shrinks rectal tumors prior to surgical resection, improving sphincter preservation. Preoperative infusional fluorouracil-based regimens or oral capecitabine plus RT are recommended. Patients should receive adjuvant chemotherapy following surgery to total 6 months of chemotherapy.

METASTATIC DISEASE

Initial Therapy

- Patients with metastatic colorectal cancer (MCRC) are considered to have resectable, potentially resectable, or unresectable metastatic disease. Multimodality therapy is indicated for resectable or potentially resectable metastases. Chemotherapy is for disseminated disease and the primary treatment modality for unresectable MCRC.
- Determine mutation status with tumor *RAS* genotyping at diagnosis. Epidermal growth factor receptor (EGFR) inhibitors should be considered only in patients with tumors with wild-type *RAS*.

RESECTABLE OR POTENTIALLY RESECTABLE MCRC

- Surgical resection of metastases with curative intent is the primary goal. Five-year overall survival (OS) rates are improved to 20% to 70% with resection. Best candidates are patients with no significant medical risk factors, fewer than four hepatic lesions, CEA less than 200 ng/mL (mcg/L), small tumor size, lack of extrahepatic tumor, and adequate surgical margins. Adjuvant systemic chemotherapy is recommended.
- Neoadjuvant or conversional chemotherapy is administered to increase complete resection rates with resectable and potentially resectable liver or lung lesions (Table 61–2). Chemotherapy with or without biologic agents is given over 2 to 3 months pre-op. Adjuvant chemotherapy is always administered.

TABLE 61–1	Chemotherapy Regimens for the Adjuvant Treatment of Colorectal Cancer	
Regimen	Agents	Comments
The historical standard		
FOLFOX4	Oxaliplatin 85 mg/m^2 IV day 1 Leucovorin 200 mg/m^2 per day IV over 2 hours days 1 and 2 Fluorouracil 400 mg/m^2 IV bolus, after leucovorin, then 600 mg/m^2 CIV over 22 hours days 1 and 2 Repeat every 2 weeks	Improved OS and DFS as compared with infusional fluorouracil-leucovorin–based regimens
The current standard		
mFOLFOX6	Oxaliplatin 85 mg/m^2 IV on day 1 Leucovorin 400 mg/m^2 IV on day 1 Fluorouracil 400 mg/m^2 IV bolus, after leucovorin on day 1, then 1200 mg/m^2/day × 2 days CIV (total 2400 mg/m^2 over 46–48 hours) Repeat every 2 weeks	Easier administration and better tolerated as compared to FOLFOX4; common toxicities: sensory neuropathy, neutropenia. A preferred regimen for adjuvant colon and rectal therapy
Alternative regimens		
Capecitabine	Capecitabine 1250 mg/m^2 PO twice daily on days 1 through 14 Each cycle lasts 14 days and is repeated every 3 weeks × 24 weeks	Equivalent DFS as compared with the Mayo Clinic regimen with improved tolerability; hand-foot syndrome common, useful for patients without vascular access or have difficulties with travel to infusion center
CapOx	Oxaliplatin 130 mg/m^2 IV day 1 Capecitabine 850–1000 mg/m^2 twice daily orally days 1 through 14 Each cycle lasts 3 weeks × 24 weeks	Improved DFS in patients with stage III colon cancer compared to capecitabine alone; common dose-limiting toxicities: neuropathies and hand–foot syndrome. A preferred regimen for adjuvant rectal therapy.

Regimen	Dosing	Comments
de Gramont regimen	Leucovorin 200 mg/m² per day IV over 2 hours, days 1 and 2 Fluorouracil 400 mg/m² per day IV bolus, followed by 600 mg/m² CIV over 22 hours, days 1 and 2 for 2 consecutive days after leucovorin Repeat every 2 weeks	Improved safety as compared with the Mayo Clinic regimen; hand–foot syndrome common
FLOX	Oxaliplatin 85 mg/m² IV administered on weeks 1, 3, and 5 Fluorouracil 500 mg/m² IV bolus weekly × 6 Leucovorin 500 mg/m² IV weekly × 6 Each cycle lasts 8 weeks and is repeated for 3 cycles	Improved DFS as compared with bolus fluorouracil-leucovorin–based regimens. Increased toxicity (diarrhea and neuropathies) compared to FOLFOX4
Mayo Clinic regimen	Leucovorin 20 mg/m² per day IV, days 1 to 5 Fluorouracil 425 mg/m² per day IV, days 1 to 5 after leucovorin Repeat every 4 to 5 weeks	Leukopenia common dose-limiting toxicity, diarrhea, and stomatitis common
Roswell Park Regimen	Leucovorin 500 mg/m² IV day 1 over 2 hours Fluorouracil 500 mg/m² IV day 1 after leucovorin Repeat weekly for 6 of 8 weeks × 4 cycles	Leukopenia common dose-limiting toxicity, diarrhea, and stomatitis common
Simplified Biweekly	Leucovorin 400 mg/m² per day IV Fluorouracil 400 mg IV bolus, after leucovorin, then 1200 mg/m²/day days 1 and 2 (total 2400 mg/m² over 46–48 hours) for 2 consecutive days Repeat every 2 weeks	Hand-foot syndrome common

(CIV, continuous intravenous infusion; DFS, disease-free survival; OS, overall survival; PO, by mouth.)

TABLE 61–2 Initial Chemotherapeutic Regimens for Metastatic Colorectal Cancer

Regimen	Agents	Major–Dose Limiting Toxicities	Comments
Patients appropriate for intensive therapy with _RAS_ mutations			
mFOLFOX4+/– bevacizumab	Oxaliplatin 85 mg/m² IV day 1 Leucovorin 400 mg/m² IV day 1 Fluorouracil 400 mg/m² IV bolus, after leucovorin day 1, then 1200 mg/m²/day × 2 days CIV (total 2400 mg/m² over 46–48 hours) Repeat every 2 weeks +/– Bevacizumab 5 mg/kg IV day 1 before mFOLFOX6 Repeat cycle every 2 weeks	mFOLFOX4: Sensory neuropathy, neutropenia Bevacizumab: hypertension, thrombosis, proteinuria	Easier administration as compared with original FOLFOX
CapeOX +/– bevacizumab	Oxaliplatin 130 mg/m² IV day 1 Capecitabine 850–1000 mg/m² orally twice a day, days 1 to 14 Repeat cycle every 3 weeks +/– Bevacizumab 7.5 mg/kg IV day 1 Repeat cycle every 3 weeks	CapeOX: Diarrhea, hand–foot syndrome, neuropathies Bevacizumab: hypertension, thrombosis, proteinuria	Reduced capecitabine dose better tolerated; patient must be able to be adherent and report side effects a timely fashion
FOLFIRI+/– bevacizumab	Irinotecan 180 mg/m² IV day 1 Leucovorin 400 mg/m² IV day 1 Fluorouracil 400 mg/m² IV bolus, after leucovorin day 1, then 1200 mg/m²/day × 2 days CIV (total 2400 mg/m² over 46–48 hours) +/– Bevacizumab 5 mg/kg IV day prior to FOLFIRI Repeat cycle every 2 weeks	FOLFIRI: Diarrhea, mucositis, neutropenia Bevacizumab: hypertension, thrombosis, proteinuria	May be preferred in patients who have preexisting neuropathy or those in which neuropathy may be debilitating to their line of work (eg, musician)

Regimen	Dosing	Toxicities	Comments
Fluorouracil/leucovorin +/– bevacizumab	See Table 107-X for fluorouracil/leucovorin regimen options +/– Bevacizumab 5 mg/kg IV day prior to fluorouracil and leucovorin Repeat cycle every 2 weeks	Fluorouracil/Leucovorin: diarrhea, hand–foot syndrome, mucositis, neutropenia Bevacizumab: hypertension, thrombosis, proteinuria	Infusional fluorouracil/leucovorin regimen preferred to bolus fluorouracil regimen. Infusional regimens tend to have more hand–foot syndrome and stomatitis; weekly or bimonthly schedule of leucovorin plus fluorouracil (either bolus or continuous infusion) may be more convenient for the patient in terms of fewer scheduled clinic appointments, less interference with work schedules, and ease of dose adjustments based on toxicity
Capecitabine +/– bevacizumab	Capecitabine 850–1250 mg/m² orally twice a day, days 1–14 +/– Bevacizumab 7.5 mg/kg IV day 1 Repeat cycle every 3 weeks	Capecitabine: Hand–foot syndrome, diarrhea, hyperbilirubinemia Bevacizumab: hypertension, thrombosis, proteinuria	May be preferred in those without a port or limited venous access; patient must be able to be adherent and report side effects a timely fashion
FOLFOXIRI +/– bevacizumab	Irinotecan 165 mg/m² IV day 1 prior to oxaliplatin Oxaliplatin 85 mg/m² IV day 1 prior to leucovorin day 1 Leucovorin 400 mg/m² IV day 1 prior to fluorouracil Fluorouracil 1600 mg/m²/day × 2 days CIV (total 3200 mg/m² over 48 hours) Repeat cycle every 2 weeks +/– Bevacizumab 5 mg/kg IV day 1 before FOLFOXIRI Repeat cycle every 2 weeks	FOLFOXIRI: Neutropenia, diarrhea, stomatitis, peripheral neurotoxicity, thrombocytopenia Bevacizumab: hypertension, thrombosis, proteinuria	More neutropenia and peripheral neurotoxicity compared to FOLFIRI; often used in medically fit individuals with diffuse aggressive disease to palliate symptoms and as potential conversion therapy

(continued)

TABLE 61–2 Initial Chemotherapeutic Regimens for Metastatic Colorectal Cancer *(Continued)*

Regimen	Agents	Major-Dose Limiting Toxicities	Comments
Patients appropriate for intensive therapy with *RAS* wild type			
mFOLFOX4 + cetuximab or panitumumab	mFOLFOX4 regimen + Cetuximab (400 mg/m² IV loading dose, then cetuximab 250 mg/m² IV weekly thereafter OR cetuximab 500 mg/m² IV every 2 weeks) IV before mFOLFOX 4 OR Panitumumab 6 mg/kg IV day 1 before mFOLFOX6 Repeat cycle every 2 weeks	mFOLFOX4: Sensory neuropathy, neutropenia Cetuximab: Papulopustular and follicular rash, asthenia, constipation, diarrhea, allergic reactions, hypomagnesemia Panitumumab: rash, diarrhea, hypomagnesemia	Only *RAS* wild-type tumor
FOLFIRI + cetuximab or panitumumab	FOLFIRI + Cetuximab (400 mg/m² IV loading dose, then cetuximab 250 mg/m² IV weekly thereafter OR cetuximab 500 mg/m² IV every 2 weeks) IV before FOLFIRI OR Panitumumab 6 mg/kg IV day 1 before FOLFIRI Repeat cycle every 2 weeks	FOLFIRI: Diarrhea, mucositis, neutropenia Cetuximab: papulopustular and follicular rash, asthenia, constipation, diarrhea, allergic reactions, hypomagnesemia Panitumumab: Rash, diarrhea, hypomagnesemia	Only *RAS* wild-type tumor; preferred for patients with pre existing neuropathy or those in which neuropathy may be debilitating to their line of work (eg, musician)

Patients NOT appropriate for intensive therapy with *RAS* mutations

Infusional fluorouracil + leucovorin +/− bevacizumab	Fluorouracil 400 mg/m² IV bolus, after leucovorin on day 1, then 1200 mg/m²/day × 2 days CIV (total 2400 mg/m² over 46–48 hours) Repeat cycle every 2 weeks +/− Bevacizumab 5 mg/kg IV day 1 prior to fluorouracil and leucovorin Repeat cycle every 2 weeks	Infusional fluorouracil/leucovorin: neutropenia, diarrhea Bevacizumab: hypertension, bleeding, proteinuria	Infusional fluorouracil/leucovorin regimen preferred to bolus fluorouracil regimen

Patients NOT appropriate for intensive therapy with *RAS* wild type

Cetuximab	Cetuximab 400 mg/m² IV loading dose, then cetuximab 250 mg/m² IV weekly thereafter Or Cetuximab 500 mg/m² IV every 2 weeks	Papulopustular and follicular rash, asthenia, constipation, diarrhea, allergic reactions, hypomagnesemia	Only *RAS* wild-type tumor
Panitumumab	6 mg/kg IV over 60 minutes every 2 weeks	Rash, hypomagnesemia, rare allergic reactions	Only *RAS* wild-type tumor

- Consider hepatic-directed therapy in addition to or as an alternative to surgical resection in patients with liver-only or liver-predominant MCRC. Hepatic artery infusion (HAI) delivers chemotherapy (eg, **floxuridine** and **fluorouracil**) through the hepatic artery directly into the liver. Tumor ablation uses radiofrequency ablation or microwave energy to generate heat to destroy tumor cells. Cryoablation is also used. These strategies are less successful than surgical interventions.

UNRESECTABLE MCRC

- Systemic chemotherapy palliates symptoms and improves survival in patients with unresectable disease. RT may control localized symptoms. Most MCRCs are incurable; however, randomized trials confirm that chemotherapy prolongs life and improves quality of life.

- Consider goals of therapy, history of prior chemotherapy, tumor *RAS* mutation status, and risk of drug-related toxicities to determine a management strategy. Regimens are the same for metastatic cancer of the colon and rectum.

- Accepted initial chemotherapy regimens consist of oxaliplatin-containing regimens (FOLFOX, CapOx), **irinotecan**-containing regimens (FOLFIRI), oxaliplatin plus irinotecan plus fluorouracil plus leucovorin (FOLFOXIRI), infusional fluorouracil plus leucovorin alone, and capecitabine alone (see Table 61–2).

- Irinotecan is a topoisomerase I inhibitor. Tumor response rates, time to progression, and OS are improved when irinotecan is administered with fluorouracil plus leucovorin as initial therapy. Early- and late-onset diarrhea and neutropenia are dose-limiting toxicities of irinotecan. Decrease incidence of late-onset diarrhea with aggressive antidiarrheal intervention.

- Oxaliplatin in combination with infusional fluorouracil plus leucovorin results in higher response rates and improved progression-free survival (PFS), with variable effects on OS. It is approved for first-line and salvage therapy.

- **Capecitabine** monotherapy is suitable for first-line therapy in patients not likely to tolerate IV chemotherapy. Available for oral administration, it is converted to fluorouracil and is a suitable replacement for infusional fluorouracil in combination with oxaliplatin (CapOx).

- Guidelines recommend addition of **bevacizumab** to FOLFOX, CapOx, FOLFIRI, infusional fluorouracil plus leucovorin, and capecitabine alone. Bevacizumab is a humanized monoclonal antibody directed against vascular endothelial growth factor (VEGF). Addition of bevacizumab to fluorouracil-based regimens increases PFS and OS as compared to chemotherapy alone.

- Hypertension is common with bevacizumab and easily managed with oral antihypertensive agents. Other safety concerns include bleeding, thrombocytopenia, and proteinuria. GI perforation is a rare but potentially fatal complication necessitating prompt evaluation of abdominal pain associated with vomiting or constipation. Bevacizumab can interfere with wound healing; schedule surgery at least 6 weeks after the last dose of bevacizumab and wait at least 6 to 8 weeks after surgery to restart.

- **Cetuximab** is an EGFR inhibitor indicated for use in patients with wild-type *RAS* tumors in combination with FOLFOX, or FOLFIRI or administered alone. Common adverse events include acne-like skin rash, asthenia, lethargy, malaise, and fatigue.

- **Panitumumab**, an EGFR inhibitor, can be combined with either FOLFOX or FOLFIRI in patients with wild-type *RAS* tumors.

- Patients may receive consecutive regimens; the sequence of drugs appears less important than exposure to all active agents in the course of chemotherapy treatments.

Second-Line Therapy

- The selection of second-line chemotherapy is primarily based on the type of and response to prior therapy received, site and extent of disease, and patient factors and treatment preferences. The optimal sequence of regimens has not been established (Table 61–3).

TABLE 61–3	Second-line and Salvage Chemotherapy Regimens for Metastatic Colorectal Cancer

Disease Progression with First-Line Regimen	Comments
First-line therapy: Oxaliplatin-based regimen ± Bevacizumab (ie, FOLFOX, CapeOX)	
Second-line options	
1. FOLFIRI ± bevacizumab or ziv-afilbercept or ramucirumab	Bevacizumab is preferred antiangiogenic agent based on toxicity and cost
2. Irinotecan ± bevacizumab or ziv-afilbercept or ramucirumab	Bevacizumab is preferred antiangiogenic agent based on toxicity and cost
3. Single agent cetuximab or panitumumab	Only if *RAS* wild-type; cetuximab improved OS compared to best supportive care
4. FOLFIRI ± cetuximab or panitumumab	Only if *RAS* wild type; increased PFS compared to FOLFIRI alone
First-line therapy: Irinotecan-based regimen ± Bevacizumab (ie, FOLFIRI)	
Second-line options	
1. FOLFOX or CapOx ± bevacizumab	Bevacizumab FDA-approved to continue with second-line options
2. Irinotecan ± cetuximab or panitumumab	Only if *RAS* wild-type; response rates with combination greater than cetuximab monotherapy
3. Single-agent cetuximab or panitumumab	Only if *RAS* wild type
First-line therapy: Fluorouracil-based regimen ± Bevacizumab (ie, Fluorouracil/ Leucovorin, Capecitabine)	
Second-line options	
1. FOLFOX or CapOx ± bevacizumab or ziv-afilbercept or ramucirumab	Bevacizumab has least toxicity and lower cost of antiangiogenic agents
2. Irinotecan + oxaliplatin (IROX) ± bevacizumab or ziv-afilbercept or ramucirumab	Bevacizumab has least toxicity and lower cost of antiangiogenic agents
3. Irinotecan ± bevacizumab or ziv-afilbercept or ramucirumab	Bevacizumab has least toxicity and lower cost of antiangiogenic agents
4. FOLFIRI ± bevacizumab or ziv-afilbercept or ramucirumab	Bevacizumab has least toxicity and lower cost of antiangiogenic agents
Therapy after second progression or third progression	
1. Regorafenib	Can be given without regard to *RAS* genotype
2. Irinotecan ± cetuximab or panitumumab	Only if *RAS* wild type; response rates with combination greater than cetuximab monotherapy
3. FOLFOX or CapeOX	Only after second-line irinotecan regimens
4. Cetuximab or panitumumab	Only if *RAS* wild-type and for patients unable to tolerate combination therapy
5. Trifluridine/tipiracil	Only after treatment with fluoropyrimidine-, oxaliplatin-, and irinotecan-based chemotherapy, anti-VEGF biologic product, and anti EGFR-monoclonal antibody if *RAS* wild type
6. Clinical trial	If available and only if patient eligible
7. Best supportive care	Appropriate for patients who do not want to pursue treatment or quality of life is expected to decrease

(CapOx, capecitabine plus oxaliplatin; EGFR, endothelial growth factor receptor; FOLFIRI, fluorouracil plus leucovorin plus irinotecan; FOLFOX, fluorouracil plus leucovorin plus oxaliplatin; OS, overall survival; PFS, profession-free survival; VEGF, vascular-endothelial growth factor.)

- Cetuximab, either alone or in combination with irinotecan, can be used in patients with disease progression on irinotecan. Response rates are greater with combination therapy.
- Panitumumab monotherapy or in combination with irinotecan-containing regimens may be used as second or subsequent lines of therapy inpatients with *RAS* wild type.
- Neither panitumumab nor cetuximab should be used in the second-line setting if used in the initial regimen.
- Angiogenesis inhibitors including VEGF inhibitors bevacizumab, **ramucircumab**, and **ziv-aflibercept** and the oral multikinase inhibitor **regorafenib** may be used in patients with progressive disease.
- No conclusive survival advantage has been demonstrated for palliative HAI.

Personalized Pharmacotherapy

- Tumor and patient pharmacogenetic factors and molecular markers assist with drug therapy individualization, and may predict prognosis and/or response to therapies.
- Tumors should be genotyped for *RAS* and *BRAF* mutations at diagnosis of stage IV disease.
- High-frequency microsatellite instability (MSI-H) confers a good prognosis for stage II CRC and these patients do not benefit from adjuvant single-agent fluoropyrimidine.

Evaluation of Therapeutic Outcomes

- Goals of monitoring are to evaluate benefit of treatment and detect recurrence.
- Patients who undergo curative surgical resection, with or without adjuvant therapy, require routine follow-up. Consult practice guidelines for specifics.
- Evaluate patients for anticipated side effects such as loose stools or diarrhea, nausea or vomiting, mouth sores, fatigue, and fever.
- Patients should be closely monitored for side effects that require prompt intervention, such as irinotecan-induced diarrhea, bevacizumab-induced GI perforation, hypertension and proteinuria, oxaliplatin-induced neuropathy, and cetuximab and panitumumab-induced skin rash.
- Less than one half of patients develop symptoms of recurrence, such as pain syndromes, changes in bowel habits, rectal or vaginal bleeding, pelvic masses, anorexia, and weight loss. Recurrences in asymptomatic patients may be detected because of increased serum CEA levels.
- Monitor quality-of-life indices, especially in patients with metastatic disease.

See Chapter 130, Colorectal Cancer, authored by Lisa M. Holle, Jessica M. Clement, and Lisa E. Davis for a more detailed discussion of this topic.

62 Lung Cancer

- *Lung cancer* is a solid tumor originating from the bronchial epithelial cells. This chapter distinguishes between non–small-cell lung cancer (NSCLC) and small-cell lung cancer (SCLC) because they have different natural histories and responses to therapy.

PATHOPHYSIOLOGY

- Lung carcinomas arise from normal bronchial epithelial cells that have acquired multiple genetic lesions and are capable of expressing a variety of phenotypes.
- Activation of proto-oncogenes, inhibition or mutation of tumor suppressor genes, and production of autocrine growth factors contribute to cellular proliferation and malignant transformation. Molecular changes, such as overexpression of c-KIT in SCLC and epidermal growth factor receptor (EGFR) in NSCLC, also affect disease prognosis and response to therapy.
- Cigarette smoking is responsible for approximately 80% of lung cancer cases. Other risk factors are exposure to environmental respiratory carcinogens (eg, asbestos, benzene, and arsenic), genetic risk factors, and history of other lung diseases (eg, chronic obstructive pulmonary disease [COPD] and asthma).
- The major cell types are SCLC (~15% of all lung cancers), adenocarcinoma (~50%), squamous cell carcinoma (<30%), and large cell carcinoma. The last three types are grouped together and referred to as NSCLC.

CLINICAL PRESENTATION

- The most common initial signs and symptoms are cough, dyspnea, chest pain, or discomfort, with or without hemoptysis. Many patients also exhibit systemic symptoms such as anorexia, weight loss, and fatigue.
- Disseminated disease can cause neurologic deficits from CNS metastases, bone pain, or pathologic fractures secondary to bone metastases, or liver dysfunction from hepatic involvement.
- Paraneoplastic syndromes may be the first sign of an underlying malignancy; examples include hypercalcemia, syndrome of inappropriate antidiuretic hormone secretion, and hypercoagulable state.

DIAGNOSIS

- Chest radiographs, endobronchial ultrasound, computed tomography (CT) scan, and positron emission tomography (PET) scan are the most valuable diagnostic tests. Integrated CT–PET technology appears to improve diagnostic accuracy in staging NSCLC over CT or PET alone.
- Pathologic confirmation is established by examination of sputum cytology and/or tumor biopsy by bronchoscopy, mediastinoscopy, percutaneous needle biopsy, or open-lung biopsy.
- All patients must have a thorough history and physical examination to detect signs and symptoms of the primary tumor, regional spread of the tumor, distant metastases, paraneoplastic syndromes, and ability to withstand aggressive surgery or chemotherapy.

STAGING

- The World Health Organization has established a TNM staging classification for NSCLC based on primary tumor size and extent (T), regional lymph node involvement (N), and presence or absence of distant metastases (M).

- A simpler system is commonly used to compare treatments. Stage I includes tumors confined to the lung without lymphatic spread, Stage II includes large tumors with ipsilateral peribronchial or hilar lymph node involvement, Stage III includes other lymph node and regional involvement, and Stage IV includes any tumor with distant metastases.
- A two-stage classification is widely used for SCLC. Limited disease is confined to one hemithorax and can be encompassed by a single radiation port. All other disease is classified as extensive.

TREATMENT

NON–SMALL-CELL LUNG CANCER

- Goals of Treatment: Definitive cure is the desired outcome with early stage disease. Prolongation of survival is desired in patients with advanced stage disease.
- The stage of NSCLC and the patient's comorbidities and performance status (ie, the ability to perform activities of daily living) determine which treatment modalities will be used. The intent of treatment—curative or palliative—influences the aggressiveness of therapy.

Recommendations for Chemotherapy, Radiation Therapy, and Surgery

- Local disease (stages IA and IB) is associated with a favorable prognosis. Surgery is the mainstay of treatment and may be used alone or with radiation therapy (RT) and/or chemotherapy. The adjuvant treatment regimen of choice is not clear.
- Stages IIA and IIB disease is primarily treated with surgery followed by adjuvant chemotherapy (Table 62–1). Chemoradiotherapy is recommended for stage II medically inoperable patients. Platinum-based regimens are preferred and should be given concurrently rather than sequentially with RT.
- Optimal outcomes with resectable stage IIIA disease are achieved with chemotherapy plus either radiation or surgery, depending on patient and tumor features.
- A majority of patients present with unresectable stage IIIB or IV NSCLC. Chemotherapy is administered to select patients with intent to palliate symptoms, improve quality of life, and increase duration of survival.
- Historically a platinum doublet has been used as first-line therapy regardless of tumor histology. Translation of tumor genetics to practice has led to personalized

TABLE 62–1	Common Chemotherapy Regimens used in the Adjuvant Treatment of Non–Small-Cell Lung Cancer	
Regimen	**Drugs and Doses**	**Frequency and Number of Cycles**
Cisplatin/etoposide	Cisplatin 100 mg/m^2 IV day 1 Etoposide 100 mg/m^2 IV daily on days 1, 2, and 3	Every 28 days for 4 cycles
Cisplatin/vinorelbine	Cisplatin 50 mg/m^2 IV days 1 and 8 Vinorelbine 25 mg/m^2 IV days 1, 8, 15, and 22	Every 28 days for 4 cycles
	Cisplatin 100 mg/m^2 IV day 1 Vinorelbine 30 mg/m^2 IV days 1, 8, 15, and 22	Every 28 days for 4 cycles
Carboplatin/paclitaxel	Carboplatin AUC 6 IV day 1 Paclitaxel 200 mg/m^2 IV day 1	Every 21 days for 4 cycles
Cisplatin/pemetrexed	Cisplatin 75 mg/m^2 IV day 1 Pemetrexed 500 mg/m^2 IV day 1	Every 21 days for 4 cycles (for nonsquamous histology only)

medicine for advanced NSCLC with four patient categories: (1) squamous histology, (2) EGFR mutated, (3) ALK positive (EML4-ALK rearrangement), or (4) nonsquamous with wild-type EGFR and ALK. Select treatments for each group are outlined in Table 62–2.

- First line therapy for advanced-stage *squamous cell lung cancer* continues to be four to six cycles of a platinum doublet, either **carboplatin-paclitaxel** or **cisplatin-gemcitabine**. **Necitumumab** combined with cisplatin and gemcitabine is approved for first-line treatment; six cycles are given of the 3-drug regimen but the necitumumab continues until progression. Non–platinum-based doublets (eg, gemcitabine–paclitaxel and gemcitabine–**docetaxel**) are recommended as first-line therapy of advanced NSCLC in patients with a contraindication to a platinum agent.

- The efficacy of docetaxel for second-line therapy is improved with the addition of **ramucirumab**, a VEGFR2 inhibitor.

- The immune checkpoint inhibitors **nivolumab** and **pembrolizumab** (PD-1 inhibitors) are approved as second-line therapy for advanced stage squamous histology (nivolumab) or all NSCLC histologies (pembrolizumab). Both increased progression-free survival in study populations. Median time-to-response is 10 to 12 weeks.

- Genetic testing is recommended for patients with advanced *nonsquamous* disease to determine the treatment plan based on histology.

  (1) Patients with a tumor that harbors a *mutation in the EGFR receptor* should receive first-line EGFR tyrosine kinase inhibitors: **afatinib**, **erlotinib**, or **gefitinib**. The most effective agent has not been determined in randomized, head-to-head comparisons. Second-line treatment with an EGFR tyrosine kinase inhibitor is recommended after failure of first-line therapy. Platinum doublet chemotherapy is also a second-line option.

  (2) Patients with a tumor with an *ALK rearrangement* should receive **crizotinib**, an ALK tyrosine kinase inhibitor that was found to be superior to chemotherapy in a phase III trial. Second-line options include two other ALK tyrosine kinase inhibitors **ceritinib** and **alectinib** or chemotherapy.

  (3) Patients with a tumor with *no EGFR or ALK aberration* should receive four to six cycles of a platinum doublet as first-line treatment. **Bevacizumab**, a recombinant, humanized monoclonal antibody, neutralizes vascular endothelial growth factor, and is of most benefit when combined with carboplatin and paclitaxel. Use of bevacizumab is restricted to patients with no history of hemoptysis, no CNS metastasis, and not receiving therapeutic anticoagulation. Cisplatin and pemetrexed is an option in patients with a contraindication to bevacizumab. Patients may receive continuation or switch maintenance therapy after completion of four to six cycles of first-line treatment. Numerous options are available for second-line therapy.

SMALL-CELL LUNG CANCER

- Goals of Treatment: The goals include cure or prolonged survival, which requires aggressive combination chemotherapy.

Limited Disease

- Use of surgery in SCLC is limited to solitary nodules without evidence of metastasis to lymph nodes.
- SCLC is very radiosensitive. Radiation is given concurrently with chemotherapy and the regimen of choice is **etoposide** and cisplatin (EP regimen).
- Radiotherapy is used to prevent and treat brain metastases, a frequent occurrence with SCLC. Prophylactic cranial irradiation (PCI) is used in patients with limited or extensive disease to reduce the risk of brain metastases.

Extensive Disease

- The EP regimen is the regimen of choice to treat extensive-stage SCLC, with **irinotecan** and cisplatin as an acceptable alternative. Concurrent radiotherapy is not routinely used in extensive disease.

TABLE 62–2 Common Chemotherapy Regimens Used to Treat Advanced Stage Lung Cancer

Place in Therapy	Small-Cell Lung Cancer		Non-squamous EGFR and ALK WT		Squamous Cell		EGFR Mutation Positive		ALK Rearrangement Positive	
	Regimen	Dosage Schedule	Regimen	Drugs, Doses, Frequency	Regimen	Drugs, Doses, Frequency	Regimen	Drugs, Doses, Frequency	Regimen	Drugs, Doses, Frequency
First Line	Etoposide/cisplatin (EP)	Cisplatin 80 mg/m² IV on day 1 Etoposide 100 mg/m² IV on days 1–3; repeat cycle every 3 weeks or Cisplatin 60 mg/m² IV on day 1 Etoposide 120 mg/m² IV on days 1–3; repeat cycle every 3 weeks	Carboplatin/paclitaxel/bevacizumab	Carboplatin AUC 6 IV mg/mL/min on day 1 Paclitaxel 200 mg/m² IV on day 1 Bevacizumab 15 mg/kg IV on day 1 Repeat cycle every 3 weeks × 6 cycles—continue bevacizumab until progression	Gemcitabine/cisplatin (GC)	Gemcitabine 1000 mg/m² IV on days 1, 8, and 15 Cisplatin 100 mg/m² IV on day 1 repeat cycle every 28 days	Erlotinib	Erlotinib 150 mg (one 150 mg capsule) po daily on an empty stomach	Crizotinib	Crizotinib 250 mg (one 250 mg capsule) po bid without regard to meals

	Regimen	Dosing
Cisplatin/irinotecan (IP)		Cisplatin 60 mg/m² IV on day 1 Irinotecan 60 mg/m² IV on days 1, 8, and 15; repeat cycle every 4 weeks Or Cisplatin 30 mg/m² IV on day 1 Irinotecan 65 mg/m² IV on days 1 and 8; repeat cycle every 3 weeks
	Carboplatin/pemetrexed	Carboplatin AUC 5 mg/mL/min IV on day 1 Pemetrexed 500 mg/m² IV on day 1 Repeat cycle every 3 weeks
	Gemcitabine/cisplatin/Necitumumab	Gemcitabine 1250 mg/m² IV on days 1 and 8 Cisplatin 75 mg/m² IV on day 1 Necitumumab 800 mg IV on day 1 and 8 Repeat cycle every 21 days
	Afatinib	Afatinib 40 mg (one 40 mg tablet) po daily on an empty stomach
Second Line	Topotecan	Topotecan 1.5 mg/m²/day IV days 1–5 Repeat every 21 days
	Docetaxel/Ramucirumab[3]	Docetaxel 75 mg/m² IV day 1 Ramucirumab 10 mg/kg IV day 1 Repeat every 21 days
	Nivolumab	Nivolumab 3 mg/kg IV day 1 Repeat every 2 weeks
	Pembrolizumab	Pembrolizumab 2 mg/kg IV day 1 Repeat every 3 weeks
	Osimertinib	Osimertinib 80 mg (one 80 mg tablet) po daily without regard to meals
	Ceritinib	Ceritinib 750 mg (five 150 mg capsules) po daily on an empty stomach
	Alectinib	Alectinib 600 mg (four 150 mg capsules) po twice daily with food

Recurrent Disease

- Recurrent SCLC is usually less sensitive to chemotherapy. **Topotecan** (IV and oral) is the only FDA-approved second-line therapy for SCLC. If recurrence occurs in more than 3 months, national guidelines recommend single-agent topotecan, gemcitabine, irinotecan, paclitaxel, docetaxel, oral etoposide, **temozolomide**, and **vinorelbine**; CAV regimen (**cyclophosphamide, doxorubicin**, and **vincristine**); and participation in a clinical trial.
- SCLC that recurs within 3 months of first-line chemotherapy is considered refractory to chemotherapy and unlikely to respond to a second-line regimen. Patients should receive best supportive care or be enrolled in a clinical trial.

EVALUATION OF THERAPEUTIC OUTCOMES

- Evaluate tumor response to chemotherapy for NSCLC at the end of the second or third cycle and at the end of every second cycle thereafter. Patients with stable disease, objective response, or measurable decrease in tumor size should continue treatment until four to six cycles have been administered. Consider maintenance therapy with pemetrexed in responding patients with nonsquamous histology.
- Evaluate efficacy of first-line therapy for SCLC after two or three cycles of chemotherapy. If there is no response or progressive disease, therapy can be discontinued or changed to a non–cross-resistant regimen. If responsive to chemotherapy, the induction regimen should be administered for four to six cycles. Responding patients benefit from the addition of PCI following initial therapy.
- Intensive therapeutic monitoring is required for all patients with lung cancer to avoid drug-related and radiotherapy-related toxicities. These patients frequently have numerous concurrent medical problems requiring close attention.
- References should be consulted for management of common toxicities associated with the aggressive chemotherapy regimens used for lung cancer.

See Chapter 129, Lung Cancer, authored by Val R. Adams and Sarah Scarpace Peters, for a more detailed discussion of this topic.

- *Lymphomas* are a heterogeneous group of malignancies that arise from malignant transformation of immune cells residing predominantly in lymphoid tissues. Differences in histology have led to the classification of Hodgkin and non-Hodgkin lymphoma (HL and NHL, respectively), which are addressed separately in this chapter.

HODGKIN LYMPHOMA

PATHOPHYSIOLOGY

- B-cell transcriptional processes are disrupted during malignant transformation, preventing expression of B-cell surface markers and production of immunoglobulin messenger RNA. Alterations in the normal apoptotic pathways favor cell survival and proliferation.
- Malignant Reed–Sternberg cells overexpress nuclear factor-κ B, which is associated with cell proliferation and antiapoptotic signals. Infections with viral and bacterial pathogens upregulate nuclear factor-κ B. Epstein–Barr virus is found in many, but not all, HL tumors.

CLINICAL PRESENTATION

- Most patients with HL present with a painless, rubbery, enlarged lymph node in the supradiaphragmatic area and commonly have mediastinal nodal involvement. Asymptomatic adenopathy of the inguinal and axillary regions may also be present.
- Constitutional, or "B," symptoms (eg, fever, drenching night sweats, and weight loss) are present at diagnosis in approximately 25% of patients with HL.

DIAGNOSIS AND STAGING

- Diagnosis requires the presence of Reed–Sternberg cells in the lymph node biopsy.
- Staging is performed to provide prognostic information and to guide therapy. Clinical staging is based on noninvasive procedures such as history, physical examination, laboratory tests, and radiography, including positron emission tomography (PET). Pathologic staging is based on biopsy findings of strategic sites (eg, bone marrow, spleen, and abdominal nodes) using an invasive procedure (eg, laparoscopy).
- At diagnosis, approximately half of patients have localized disease (stages I, II, and IIE) and the others have advanced disease, of which 10% to 15% is stage IV.
- Prognosis predominantly depends on age and amount of disease; patients older than 65 to 70 years have a lower cure rate than younger patients. Patients with limited stage disease (stages I and II) have a 90% to 95% cure rate, whereas those with advanced disease (stages III and IV) have a 60% to 80% cure rate.

TREATMENT

- <u>Goals of Treatment</u>: The goal is to maximize curability while minimizing short- and long-term treatment-related complications.
- Treatment options include radiation therapy (RT), chemotherapy, or both (combined-modality therapy). The therapeutic role of surgery is limited, regardless of stage.
- RT is an integral part of treatment and can be used alone for select patients with early-stage disease, although most patients will receive chemotherapy and radiation.
- Long-term complications of RT, chemotherapy, and chemoradiotherapy include gonadal dysfunction, secondary malignancies (eg, lung, breast, and GI tract, as well as leukemia), and cardiac disease.

Initial Chemotherapy

- Treat all stages and risk-groups of HL with 8 to 12 weeks of chemotherapy and then obtain a restaging PET-CT (Table 63–1). Most patients with unfavorable disease will require radiation therapy.

TABLE 63-1	Combination Chemotherapy Regimens for Hodgkin Lymphoma		
Drug	**Dosage (mg/m²)**	**Route**	**Days**
MOPP			
Mechlorethamine	6	IV	1, 8
Vincristine	1.4	IV	1, 8
Procarbazine	100	Oral	1–14
Prednisone	40	Oral	1–14
Repeat every 21 days			
ABVD			
Doxorubicin (Adriamycin®)	25	IV	1, 15
Bleomycin	10	IV	1, 15
Vinblastine	6	IV	1, 15
Dacarbazine	375	IV	1, 15
Repeat every 28 days			
MOPP/ABVD			
Alternating months of MOPP and ABVD			
MOPP/ABV hybrid			
Mechlorethamine	6	IV	1
Vincristine	1.4	IV	1
Procarbazine	100	Oral	1–7
Prednisone	40	Oral	1–14
Doxorubicin	35	IV	8
Bleomycin	10	IV	8
Vinblastine	6	IV	8
Repeat every 28 days			
Stanford V			
Doxorubicin	25	IV	Weeks 1, 3, 5, 7, 9, 11
Vinblastine	6	IV	Weeks 1, 3, 5, 7, 9, 11
Mechlorethamine	6	IV	Weeks 1, 5, 9
Etoposide	60	IV	Weeks 3, 7, 11
Vincristine	1.4ᵃ	IV	Weeks 2, 4, 6, 8, 10, 12
Bleomycin	5	IV	Weeks 2, 4, 6, 8
Prednisone	40	Oral	Every other day for 12 weeks; begin tapering at week 10
One course (12 weeks)			
BEACOPP (standard-dose)			
Bleomycin	10	IV	8
Etoposide	100	IV	1–3
Adriamycin (doxorubicin)	25	IV	1
Cyclophosphamide	650	IV	1
Oncovin® (vincristine)	1.4ᵃ	IV	8
Procarbazine	100	Oral	1–7
Prednisone	40	Oral	1–14
Repeat every 21 days			

(*continued*)

TABLE 63–1	Combination Chemotherapy Regimens for Hodgkin Lymphoma (*Continued*)		
Drug	**Dosage (mg/m²)**	**Route**	**Days**
BEACOPP (escalated-dose)			
Bleomycin	10	IV	8
Etoposide	200	IV	1–3
Adriamycin (doxorubicin)	35	IV	1
Cyclophosphamide	1250	IV	1
Oncovin® (vincristine)	1.4[a]	IV	8
Procarbazine	100	Oral	1–7
Prednisone	40	Oral	1–14
Granulocyte colony-stimulating factor		Subcutaneously	8+
Repeat every 21 days			

[a]Vincristine dose capped at 2 mg.

Salvage Chemotherapy

- Response to salvage therapy depends on the extent and site of recurrence, previous therapy, and duration of first remission. Choice of salvage therapy should be guided by response to initial therapy and a patient's ability to tolerate therapy.
- Patients who relapse after an initial complete response can be treated with the same regimen, a non–cross-resistant regimen, RT, or high-dose chemotherapy and autologous hematopoietic stem cell transplantation (HSCT).
- Lack of complete remission after initial therapy or relapse within 1 year after completing initial therapy is associated with a poor prognosis. Patients with these prognostic factors are candidates for high-dose chemotherapy and HSCT.

NON-HODGKIN LYMPHOMA

PATHOPHYSIOLOGY

- NHLs are derived from monoclonal proliferation of malignant B or T lymphocytes and their precursors. Current classification schemes characterize NHLs according to cell of origin, clinical features, and morphologic features.
- World Health Organization (WHO) classification uses *grade* to refer to histologic parameters such as cell and nuclear size, density of chromatin, and proliferation fraction, and *aggressiveness* to denote clinical behavior of a tumor.

CLINICAL PRESENTATION

- Patients present with a variety of symptoms, which depend on site of involvement and whether it is nodal or extranodal.
- Adenopathy can be localized or generalized. Involved nodes are painless, rubbery, and discrete and usually located in the cervical and supraclavicular regions. Mesenteric or GI involvement can cause nausea, vomiting, obstruction, abdominal pain, palpable abdominal mass, or GI bleeding. Bone marrow involvement can cause symptoms related to anemia, neutropenia, or thrombocytopenia.
- Forty percent of patients with NHL present with B symptoms—fever, drenching night sweats, and weight loss.

DIAGNOSIS AND STAGING

- Diagnosis is established by biopsy of an involved lymph node. Diagnostic workup of NHL is generally similar to that of HL.
- NHL classification systems continue to evolve. Slow-growing or indolent lymphomas are favorable (untreated survival measured in years), whereas rapid-growing or aggressive lymphomas are unfavorable (untreated survival measured in weeks to months).

- Prognosis depends on histologic subtype and clinical risk factors (eg, age >60 years, performance status of two or more, abnormal lactate dehydrogenase, extranodal involvement, and stage III or IV disease). These risk factors are used to calculate the International Prognostic Index (IPI) that is most useful in patients with aggressive lymphomas.
- A newer prognostic index for patients with indolent (follicular) lymphomas uses similar risk factors except that poor performance status is replaced with low hemoglobin (<12 g/dL [<120 g/L; 7.45 mmol/L]). Current research is focused on prognostic importance of phenotypic and molecular characteristics of NHL.

TREATMENT

- <u>Goals of Treatment</u>: The goals are to relieve symptoms and, whenever possible, cure the patient of disease while minimizing the risk of serious toxicity.

General Principles

- Appropriate therapy for NHL depends on many factors, including patient age, histologic type, stage and site of disease, presence of adverse prognostic factors, and patient preference.
- Treatment is divided into two categories: limited disease (eg, localized disease; Ann Arbor stages I and II) and advanced disease (eg, Ann Arbor stage III or IV and stage II patients with poor prognostic features).
- Treatment options include RT, chemotherapy, and biologic agents. RT is used for remission induction with early stage, localized disease and, more commonly, as a palliative measure in advanced disease.
- Effective chemotherapy ranges from single-agent therapy for indolent lymphomas to aggressive, complex combination regimens for aggressive disease.

Indolent Lymphomas

- Follicular lymphomas occur in older adults, with a majority having advanced disease that includes the chromosomal translocation t(14;18). Clinical course is generally indolent, with median survival of 8 to 10 years. The natural history of follicular lymphoma is unpredictable, with spontaneous regression of objective disease seen in 20% to 30% of patients.

LOCALIZED FOLLICULAR LYMPHOMA

- Options for stage I and II follicular lymphoma include locoregional RT and immunotherapy (ie, **rituximab**) with or without chemotherapy or RT.
- RT is the standard treatment and is usually curative. Chemotherapy is not recommended, unless the patient has high-risk, stage II disease.

ADVANCED FOLLICULAR LYMPHOMA

- Management of stages II Bulky, III and IV indolent lymphoma is controversial because standard approaches are not curative. Median time to relapse is only 18 to 36 months. After relapse, response can be reinduced; however, response rates and durations decrease with each retreatment.
- Therapeutic options are diverse and include watchful waiting, RT, single-agent chemotherapy, combination chemotherapy, biologic therapy, radioimmunotherapy, and combined-modality therapy. Immediate aggressive therapy does not improve survival compared with conservative therapy (ie, watchful waiting followed by single-agent chemotherapy, **rituximab**, or RT, when treatment is needed).
- Oral alkylating agents **chlorambucil** or **cyclophosphamide**, used alone or in combination with **prednisone**, are the mainstay of treatment. These single agents are as effective as combination regimens and produce minimal toxicity, but secondary acute leukemia is a concern. **Bendamustine** is an IV alkylating agent approved for relapsed or refractory indolent NHL.

TABLE 63-2	CHOP Regimen		
Drug	**Dose**	**Route**	**Treatment Days**
Cyclophosphamide	750 mg/m^2	IV	1
Doxorubicin	50 mg/m^2	IV	1
Vincristine[a]	1.4 mg/m^2	IV	1
Prednisone	100 mg	Oral	1–5
One cycle is 21 days			

Another name for doxorubicin is hydroxydaunorubicin.
[a]Vincristine dose is typically capped at 2 mg.

- **Fludarabine** is an adenosine analogue that produces high response rates in previously untreated and relapsed advanced follicular lymphoma. Fludarabine is associated with prolonged myelosuppression and profound immunosuppression, increasing the risk of opportunistic infections.
- Rituximab, a chimeric monoclonal antibody directed at the CD20 molecule on B cells, is one of the most widely used therapies for follicular lymphoma. It is approved for first-line therapy either alone or combined with chemotherapy and as maintenance therapy for patients with stable disease or with partial or complete response following induction chemotherapy.
- The most common chemotherapy regimen used with rituximab is the CHOP regimen (Table 63–2). Practice guidelines list rituximab maintenance for up to 2 years as an option in both first- and second-line therapy.
- Rituximab adverse effects are usually infusion related, especially after the first infusion, and consist of fever, chills, respiratory symptoms, fatigue, headache, pruritus, and angioedema. Pretreatment with oral **acetaminophen**, 650 mg, and **diphenhydramine**, 50 mg, 30 minutes before the infusion is recommended.
- ^{90}**Y-ibritumomab tiuxetan** is an anti-CD20 radioimmunoconjugate, linking mouse antibodies to radioisotopes. Radiation is selectively delivered to tumor cells expressing the CD20 antigen and to adjacent tumor cells that do not express it.
- Radioimmunotherapy was initially used as salvage therapy and is being evaluated as first-line therapy in combination with CHOP.
- Radioimmunotherapy is generally well tolerated. Toxicities include infusion-related reactions, myelosuppression, and possibly myelodysplastic syndrome or acute myelogenous leukemia.
- High-dose chemotherapy followed by HSCT is an option for relapsed follicular lymphoma. The recurrence rate is lower after allogeneic than after autologous HSCT, but the benefit is offset by increased treatment-related mortality.

Aggressive Lymphomas

- Diffuse large B-cell lymphomas (DLBCLs) are the most common lymphoma in patients of all ages but most commonly seen in the seventh decade. Extranodal disease is present at diagnosis in 30% to 40% of patients. IPI score correlates with prognosis. Diffuse aggressive lymphomas are sensitive to chemotherapy, with cure achieved in some patients.

TREATMENT OF LOCALIZED DISEASE

- Stage I and nonbulky stage II should be treated with three or four cycles of rituximab and CHOP (R-CHOP) followed by locoregional RT.
- Patients with at least one adverse risk factor should receive six cycles of R-CHOP followed by locoregional RT.

TREATMENT OF ADVANCED DISEASE

- Bulky stage II and stages III and IV lymphoma should be treated with R-CHOP or rituximab and CHOP-like chemotherapy until achieving complete response (usually four cycles). Two or more additional cycles should be given following complete response for a total of six to eight cycles. Maintenance therapy following a complete response does not improve survival.
- Consider high-dose chemotherapy with autologous HSCT in high-risk patients who respond to standard chemotherapy and meet HSCT criteria.
- Although historically elderly adults have lower complete response and survival rates than younger patients, full-dose R-CHOP is recommended as initial treatment for aggressive lymphoma in the elderly.

TREATMENT OF REFRACTORY OR RELAPSED DISEASE

- Approximately one third of patients with aggressive lymphoma will require salvage therapy at some point. Salvage therapy is more likely to induce response if the response to initial chemotherapy was complete (chemosensitivity) than if it was primarily or partially resistant to chemotherapy.
- High-dose chemotherapy with autologous HSCT is the therapy of choice for younger patients with chemosensitive relapse.
- Salvage regimens incorporate drugs not used as initial therapy. Commonly used regimens include DHAP (**dexamethasone, cytarabine**, and **cisplatin**), ESHAP (**etoposide, methylprednisolone,** cytarabine, and cisplatin), and MINE (**mesna, ifosfamide, mitoxantrone,** and **etoposide**). None is clearly superior to the others.
- Rituximab is being evaluated in combination with many salvage regimens.

NON-HODGKIN LYMPHOMA IN ACQUIRED IMMUNODEFICIENCY SYNDROME

- Patients with AIDS have more than a 100-fold increased risk of developing NHL, which is usually aggressive (eg, Burkitt or DLBCL).
- Treatment of AIDS-related lymphoma is difficult because underlying immunodeficiency increases the risk of treatment-related myelosuppression.
- Standard combination regimens (eg, CHOP) yield disappointing results. Newer approaches, including dose-adjusted EPOCH (etoposide, prednisone, vincristine, cyclophosphamide, and doxorubicin), appear promising. The role of rituximab in the treatment of AIDS-related DLBCL is not clear.
- Prophylactic antibiotics should be continued during chemotherapy, but the optimal timing for highly active antiretroviral therapy (HAART) is not clear in patients with AIDS-related lymphoma.

EVALUATION OF THERAPEUTIC OUTCOMES

- The primary outcome to be identified is tumor response, which is based on physical examination, radiologic evidence, PET/computed tomography (CT) scanning, and other baseline findings.
- Patients are evaluated for response at the end of four cycles or, if treatment is shorter, at the end of treatment.

See Chapter 132, Lymphomas, authored by Alexandre Chan and Jolynn Sessions, for a more detailed discussion of this topic.

64 | Prostate Cancer

- *Prostate cancer* is a malignant neoplasm that arises from the prostate gland. Prostate cancer has an indolent course; localized prostate cancer is curable by surgery or radiation therapy, but advanced prostate cancer is not yet curable.

PATHOPHYSIOLOGY

- The normal prostate is composed of acinar secretory cells that are altered when invaded by cancer. The major pathologic cell type is adenocarcinoma (>95% of cases).
- Prostate cancer can be graded. Well-differentiated tumors grow slowly, whereas poorly differentiated tumors grow rapidly and have a poor prognosis.
- Metastatic spread can occur by local extension, lymphatic drainage, or hematogenous dissemination. Skeletal metastases from hematogenous spread are the most common sites of distant spread. The lung, liver, brain, and adrenal glands are the most common sites of visceral involvement, but these organs are not usually involved initially.
- The rationale for hormone therapy is based on the effect of androgens on the growth and differentiation of the normal prostate (Fig. 64–1).
- The testes and the adrenal glands are the major sources of androgens, specifically dihydrotestosterone (DHT).
- Luteinizing hormone–releasing hormone (LHRH) from the hypothalamus stimulates the release of luteinizing hormone (LH) and follicle-stimulating hormone (FSH) from the anterior pituitary gland.
- LH complexes with receptors on the Leydig cell testicular membrane, stimulating the production of testosterone and small amounts of estrogen.
- FSH acts on testicular Sertoli cells to promote maturation of LH receptors and produce an androgen-binding protein.
- Circulating testosterone and estradiol influence the synthesis of LHRH, LH, and FSH by a negative-feedback loop at the hypothalamic and pituitary level.

CHEMOPREVENTION

- The risk of prostate cancer was reduced approximately 25% in patients taking **finasteride** for treatment of benign prostatic hypertrophy (BPH), but prostate cancer diagnosed in patients on finasteride is more aggressive.
- Current guidelines do not recommend the use of finasteride or **dutasteride** for prostate cancer chemoprevention. Although finasteride reduces the prevalence of prostate cancer, the impact on prostate cancer morbidity or mortality has not been demonstrated.

SCREENING

- Screening for prostate cancer is controversial. The American Urologic Association does not recommend routine screening in men between the ages of 40 and 54 years of average risk. They recommend that men aged 55 to 69 years discuss the risks and benefits of prostate cancer screening. Men who elect screening should do so no more than every 2 years; a recent study suggests that screening every 5 years may be adequate.
- PSA is a glycoprotein produced and secreted by prostate epithelial cells. Acute urinary retention, acute prostatitis, and BPH influence PSA, thereby limiting the usefulness of PSA alone for early detection, but it is a useful marker for monitoring response to therapy.

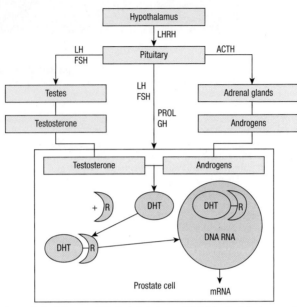

(ACTH, adrenocorticotropic hormone; DHT, dihydrotestosterone; FSH, follicle-stimulating hormone; GH, growth hormone; LH, luteinizing hormone; LHRH, luteinizing hormone–releasing hormone; mRNA, messenger RNA; PROL, prolactin; R, receptor.)

FIGURE 64-1. Hormonal regulation of the prostate gland.

CLINICAL PRESENTATION

- Localized prostate cancer is usually asymptomatic.
- Locally invasive prostate cancer is associated with ureteral dysfunction or impingement, such as alterations in micturition (eg, urinary frequency, hesitancy, and dribbling).
- Advanced disease commonly presents with back pain and stiffness due to osseous metastases. Untreated spinal cord lesions can lead to cord compression. Lower extremity edema can occur as a result of lymphatic obstruction. Anemia and weight loss are nonspecific signs of advanced disease.

TREATMENT

- <u>Goals of Treatment</u>: In early-stage prostate cancer, the goal is to minimize morbidity and mortality. Surgery and radiation therapy are curative but also associated with significant morbidity and mortality. In advanced prostate cancer, treatment focuses on providing symptom relief and maintaining quality of life.

GENERAL APPROACH

- Initial treatment depends on disease stage, Gleason score, presence of symptoms, and patient's life expectancy. The most appropriate therapy for early-stage prostate cancer is unknown. See Table 64-1 for management recommendations based on risk of recurrence.
- Initial treatment modality for advanced prostate cancer is androgen ablation (eg, orchiectomy or LHRH agonists with or without antiandrogens). After disease progression, secondary hormonal manipulations, cytotoxic chemotherapy, and supportive care are used.

TABLE 64–1 Initial Management of Prostate Cancer Based on Expected Survival and Recurrence Risk

Recurrence Risk	Expected Survival (Years)	Initial Therapy
Very Low		
T$_{1c}$	Less than 20	Observation
T$_{1c}$	20 or more	Observation
		or
		Radical prostatectomy with or without pelvic lymph node dissection
		or
		Radiation therapy
Low		
T$_1$–T$_{2a}$ and Gleason 2–6 and PSA less than 10 ng/mL (10 mcg/L) and less than 5% tumor in specimen	10 or more	Observation
		or
		Radical prostatectomy with or without pelvic lymph node dissection or radiation therapy
	Less than 10	Observation
Intermediate		
T$_{2b}$–T$_{2c}$ or Gleason 7 or PSA 10–20 ng/mL (10–20 mcg/L)	10 or less	Observation
		or
		Radical prostatectomy with pelvic lymph node dissection
		or
		Radiation therapy with or without 4–6 months of neoadjuvant androgen deprivation therapy with or without brachytherapy
T$_{2b}$–T$_{2c}$ or Gleason 7 or PSA 10–20 ng/mL (10–20 mcg/L)	10 or more	Radical prostatectomy with pelvic lymph node dissection
		or
		Radiation therapy with or without 4–6 months of neoadjuvant androgen deprivation therapy with or without brachytherapy

(continued)

TABLE 64–1	Initial Management of Prostate Cancer Based on Expected Survival and Recurrence Risk (*Continued*)	
Recurrence Risk	**Expected Survival (Years)**	**Initial Therapy**
High		
T$_{3a}$, Gleason 8–10, PSA greater than 20 ng/mL (20 mcg/L)		Radiation therapy and ADT[a] (2–3 years) with or without brachytherapy *or* Radical prostatectomy and pelvic lymph node dissection
Very High		
T$_{3b}$–T$_4$		Radiation therapy and ADT (2–3 years) with or without brachytherapy *or* Radical prostatectomy and pelvic lymph node dissection *or* ADT
Very High		
Any T, N$_1$		ADT (2–3 years) *or* Radiation therapy and ADT (2–3 years)
Any T, Any N, M$_1$		ADT with Orchiectomy *or* LHRH agonist[b] + 7 days antiandrogen therapy *or* LHRH agonist + antiandrogen *or* LHRH agonist

ADT, androgen deprivation therapy; LHRH, luteinizing hormone-releasing hormone; PSA, prostate-specific antigen.
[a]Androgen deprivation therapy to achieve serum testosterone levels less than 50 ng/dL (1.7 nmol/L)
[b]LHRH agonist, medical castrations, or surgical are equivalent.

NONPHARMACOLOGIC THERAPY

Observation

- Observation or watchful waiting involves monitoring the course of disease and initiating treatment if the cancer progresses. PSA and digital rectal exam (DRE) are performed every 6 months.
- Advantages include avoiding adverse effects of definitive therapies and minimizing risk of unnecessary therapies. The major disadvantage is the risk of cancer progression requiring more intense therapy.

Surgery and Radiation Therapy

- Bilateral orchiectomy rapidly reduces circulating androgens to castrate levels. Many patients are not surgical candidates due to advanced age, and other patients find this procedure psychologically unacceptable. Orchiectomy is the preferred initial treatment for patients with impending spinal cord compression or ureteral obstruction.
- Radical prostatectomy and radiation therapy are potentially curative therapies but are associated with complications that must be weighed against expected benefit. Consequently, many patients postpone therapy until symptoms develop.
- Complications of radical prostatectomy include blood loss, stricture formation, incontinence, lymphocele, fistula formation, anesthetic risk, and impotence. Nerve-sparing techniques facilitate return of sexual potency after prostatectomy.
- Acute complications of radiation therapy include cystitis, proctitis, hematuria, urinary retention, penoscrotal edema, and impotence.
- Chronic complications of radiation therapy include proctitis, diarrhea, cystitis, enteritis, impotence, urethral stricture, and incontinence.

PHARMACOLOGIC THERAPY

Drug Treatments of First Choice

LUTEINIZING HORMONE–RELEASING HORMONE AGONISTS

- LHRH agonists are a reversible method of androgen ablation and are as effective as orchiectomy.
- There are no comparative trials of LHRH agonists, so the choice is usually based on cost and patient and physician preference for a dosing schedule (Table 64–2). **Leuprolide acetate**, **leuprolide depot, leuprolide implant, triptorelin depot, triptorelin implant,** and **goserelin acetate implant** are currently available. Dosing intervals range from once monthly to every 16 weeks. Leuprolide implant is a mini-osmotic pump that delivers daily doses for 1 year.
- The most common adverse effects of LHRH agonists include disease flare-up during the first week of therapy (eg, increased bone pain or urinary symptoms), hot flashes, erectile impotence, decreased libido, and injection-site reactions. Use of an antiandrogen (eg, **flutamide, bicalutamide,** or **nilutamide**) prior to initiation of LHRH therapy and for 2 to 4 weeks after is a strategy to minimize initial tumor flare.
- Decreases in bone mineral density complicate androgen deprivation therapy (ADT), resulting in increased risk of osteoporosis, osteopenia, and skeletal fractures. Calcium and vitamin D supplements and a baseline bone mineral density are recommended. Consider administering an antiresorptive agent (eg, denosumab or zoledronic acid) to reduce the risk of skeletal-related events.
- Screen patients receiving ADT for cardiovascular disease and diabetes due to increased risk of metabolic effects.

GONADOTROPIN-RELEASING HORMONE ANTAGONISTS

- The gonadotropin-releasing hormone (GnRH) antagonist **degarelix** binds reversibly to GnRH receptors in the pituitary gland, reducing the production of testosterone to castrate levels in 7 days or less. A major advantage of degarelix over LHRH agonists is the lack of tumor flare.

TABLE 64-2	Hormonal Therapies for Prostate Cancer					
Drug (Brand Name)	**Usual Dose**	**Toxicities**	**Hepatic/Renal Adjustments**	**Monitoring Parameters**	**Drug Interactions**	**Administration**
Antiandrogens						
Flutamide (Eulexin)	750 mg/day	Gynecomastia Hot flashes Gastrointestinal disturbances (diarrhea) Loss of libido LFT abnormalities Breast tenderness Methemoglobinemia	Contraindicated in patients with hepatic impairment No dosage adjustment necessary in chronic renal impairment	Serum transaminases should be monitored prior to start of therapy and monthly for first 4 months, then periodically thereafter Monitor for tumor reduction, testosterone/estrogen, and phosphatase serum levels	Substrate of CYP1A2 and CYP3A4	Administered orally in three divided doses; capsule may be opened into applesauce, pudding, or other soft foods
Bicalutamide (Casodex)	50 mg/day (up to 150 mg/day—unlabeled use)	Gynecomastia Hot flashes Gastrointestinal disturbances (diarrhea) Decrease libido LFT abnormalities Breast tenderness	Discontinue if ALT >2 times upper limit of normal or patient develops jaundice	Serum transaminases should be monitored prior to start of therapy and monthly for first 4 months, then periodically thereafter Periodic monitoring of CBC, EKG, echocardiograms, serum testosterone, luteinizing hormone, and PSA	Inhibits CYP3A4 May increase concentration of vitamin K antagonists	May be taken with or without food

| Nilutamide (Nilandron) | 300 mg/day for first month then 150 mg/day | Gynecomastia Hot flashes Gastrointestinal Disturbances (constipation) LFT abnormalities Breast tenderness Visual disturbances (impaired dark adaptation) Alcohol intolerance Interstitial pneumonitis | Contraindicated in patients with hepatic impairment Discontinue if ALT >2 times upper limit of normal or patient develops jaundice | Serum transaminases should be monitored prior to start of therapy and monthly for first 4 months, then periodically thereafter Chest x-ray at baseline and consideration of pulmonary function testing (at baseline) | Substrate of CYP2C19 and weak inhibitor of CYP2C19 | May be taken with or without food |
| Enzalutamide (Xtandi) | 160 mg/day | Gastrointestinal disturbances (diarrhea) Musculoskeletal disorders (back pain, arthralgias, muscle pain, weakness) Asthenia Peripheral edema CNS (headache, dizziness) Seizures LFT abnormalities | No adjustment necessary for renal or hepatic impairment | Complete blood counts baseline and periodically LFTs baseline and periodically | Strong CYP3A4 and moderate CYP2C9 and CYP2C19 inducer; avoid CYP3A4, CYP2C9 and CYP2C19 sensitive substrates. CYP2C8 substrate, avoid strong inducers and inhibitors of CYP2C8 If vitamin K antagonists necessary, conduct additional INR monitoring | May be taken with or without food |

(continued)

TABLE 64-2 Hormonal Therapies for Prostate Cancer (*Continued*)

Drug (Brand Name)	Usual Dose	Toxicities	Hepatic/Renal Adjustments	Monitoring Parameters	Drug Interactions	Administration
Androgen synthesis inhibitor						
Abiraterone acetate (Zytiga)	1000 mg/day + prednisone 5 mg BID	Gastrointestinal disturbances (diarrhea) Edema Hypokalemia Hypophosphatemia LFT abnormalities Hypertriglyceridemia	250 mg daily for Child Pugh Class B; avoid use in Child Pugh Class C Withhold treatment if LFTs >5 times the ULN or bilirubin >3 ULN	Serum transaminases should be monitored prior to start of therapy, every 2 weeks for 3 months, then monthly thereafter Monitor for signs and symptoms of adreno-corticoid insufficiency; monthly for hypertension, hypokalemia, and fluid retention	Substrate of CYP3A4. Use with caution with CYP3A4 inhibitors and inducers. Inhibits CYP1A2, CYP2C19, CYP2C8, CYP2C9, CYP2D6, CYP3A4, and P-glycoprotein Use sensitive substrates with caution	Administer on an empty stomach, at least 1 hour before and 2 hours after food
Luteinizing-hormone agonists						
Leuprolide (Lupron)	7.5 mg IM every month 22.5 mg IM every 3 months 30 mg IM every 4 months 45 mg IM every 6 months	Hot flashes Decreased libido Gynecomastia Osteoporosis Fatigue Weight gain	No adjustment necessary for renal or hepatic impairment	Serum testosterone ~4 weeks after initiation, PSA, blood glucose, and HgbA$_{1c}$ prior to initiation and periodically thereafter	May diminish the effects of antidiabetic agents	Vary injection site

Drug	Dose	Adverse Effects	Dosing Adjustments	Monitoring	Drug Interactions	Counseling
Goserelin (Zoladex)	3.6 mg SQ implant every month; 10.8 mg SQ implant every 3 months	Hot flashes, Decreased libido, Gynecomastia, Osteoporosis, Fatigue, Weight gain	No adjustment necessary for renal or hepatic impairment	Monitor bone mineral density, serum calcium, and cholesterol/lipids	May diminish the effects of antidiabetic agents	Vary injection site
Triptorelin (Trelstar)	3.75 mg IM every month; 11.25 mg IM every 3 months; 22.5 mg IM every 6 months	Hot flashes, Decreased libido, Gynecomastia, Osteoporosis, Fatigue, Weight gain	No adjustment necessary for renal or hepatic impairment	Monitor serum testosterone levels and prostate specific antigen	May diminish the effects of antidiabetic agents	Vary injection site
Gonadotropin-releasing hormone antagonists						
Degarelix (Firmagon)	240 mg SQ loading dose; 80 mg SQ every 28 days (following 28 days after loading dose)	Hot flashes, Decreased libido, Gynecomastia, Osteoporosis, Fatigue, Weight gain	Use with caution with CL_{cr} <50 mL/min (<0.83 mL/s); Do not use in patients with severe hepatic impairment	Prostate-specific antigen periodically, serum testosterone monthly until castration achieved then every other month, LFTs at baseline in addition to serum electrolytes and bone mineral density	Use with caution with agents that may increase QTC interval	Vary injection site

(ALT, alanine aminotransferase; BID, twice daily; CBC, complete blood count; CL_{cr}, creatinine clearance; CNS, central nervous system; CYP, cytochrome P450; EKG, electrocardiogram; HgbA1c, hemoglobin A1c; IM, intramuscular injection; INR, international normalized ratio; LFT, liver function test; PSA, prostate-specific antigen; SQ, subcutaneous injection; ULN, upper limit of normal.)

- Degarelix is administered as a subcutaneous injection every 28 days. Injection site reactions are the most frequently reported adverse effects and include pain, erythema, swelling, induration, and nodules. Osteoporosis may develop, and calcium and vitamin D supplementation should be considered.

ANTIANDROGENS

- Monotherapy with flutamide, bicalutamide, and nilutamide is no longer recommended due to decreased efficacy as compared with patients treated with LHRH agonist therapy. Antiandrogens are indicated for advanced prostate cancer only when combined with an LHRH agonist (flutamide and bicalutamide]) or orchiectomy (nilutamide). In combination, antiandrogens can reduce the LHRH agonist–induced flare.
- **Enzalutamide** is approved as a single agent in metastatic castrate-resistant prostate cancer patients. It may be used in the first line setting to delay the initiation of chemotherapy.
- Adverse effects of antiandrogens are summarized in Table 64–2.

COMBINED ANDROGEN BLOCKADE

- The role of combined androgen blockade (CAB), also referred to as *maximal androgen deprivation* or *total androgen blockade*, continues to be evaluated. The combination of LHRH agonists or orchiectomy with antiandrogens is the CAB approach most extensively studied.
- Some clinicians consider CAB to be the initial hormone therapy of choice for newly diagnosed patients because the major benefit is seen in patients with minimal disease. Some argue that treatment should not be delayed because combined androgen deprivation trials demonstrate a survival advantage for young patients with good performance status and minimal disease who were initially treated with hormone therapy.

ALTERNATIVE DRUG TREATMENTS

- Selection of salvage therapy depends on what was used as initial therapy. Radiotherapy can be used after failed radical prostatectomy. Androgen ablation can be used after progression of disease after radiation therapy or radical prostatectomy.
- An antiandrogen or orchiectomy may be indicated if testosterone levels are not suppressed (ie, >20 ng/dL [0.7 nmol/L]) after initial LHRH agonist therapy. If testosterone levels are suppressed, the disease is considered androgen independent and palliative androgen-independent salvage therapy can be used.
- Androgen withdrawal should be attempted if initial therapy consists of CAB with an LHRH agonist and antiandrogen. Mutations of the androgen receptor may allow antiandrogens to become agonists. Androgen withdrawal produces responses lasting 3 to 14 months in up to 35% of patients.
- Androgen synthesis inhibitors provide symptomatic but brief relief in approximately 50% of patients. **Aminoglutethimide** causes adverse effects in 50% of patients, such as lethargy, ataxia, dizziness, and self-limiting rash. The adverse effects of **ketoconazole** include GI intolerance, transient increases in liver and renal function tests, and hypoadrenalism. **Abiraterone** targets CYP17A1 resulting in decreased circulating levels of testosterone (Table 64–2). Review medication profiles for potential drug interactions because abiraterone is an inhibitor of CYP2D6.

CHEMOTHERAPY

- **Docetaxel,** 75 mg/m^2 every 3 weeks, combined with **prednisone**, 5 mg twice daily, improves survival in castrate-refractory prostate cancer. The most common adverse events include nausea, alopecia, and myelosuppression.
- **Cabazitaxel** 25 mg/m^2 every 3 weeks with prednisone 10 mg daily significantly improves progression-free and overall survival. Neutropenia, febrile neutropenia, neuropathy, and diarrhea are the most significant toxicities.

IMMUNOTHERAPY

- **Sipuleucel-T** is a novel autologous cellular immunotherapy indicated for asymptomatic or minimally symptomatic metastatic hormone-refractory prostate cancer. Use is controversial because trials have not been done to compare it to standard second-line hormonal interventions.

EVALUATION OF THERAPEUTIC OUTCOMES

- Monitor primary tumor size, involved lymph nodes, and tumor marker response such as PSA with definitive, curative therapy. PSA level is checked every 6 months for the first 5 years, then annually.
- With metastatic disease, clinical benefit can be documented by evaluating performance status, weight, quality of life, analgesic requirements, and PSA or DRE at 3-month intervals.

See Chapter 131, Prostate Cancer, authored by LeAnn B. Norris and Jill M. Kolesar, for a more detailed discussion of this topic.

CHAPTER

65 Glaucoma

- *Glaucomas* are ocular disorders that lead to an optic neuropathy characterized by changes in the optic nerve head (optic disc) that is associated with loss of visual sensitivity and field.

PATHOPHYSIOLOGY

- There are two major types of glaucoma: primary open-angle glaucoma (POAG) or ocular hypertension, which accounts for most cases and is therefore the focus of this chapter, and primary angle closure glaucoma (PACG). Either type can be a primary inherited disorder, congenital, or secondary to disease, trauma, or drugs.
- In POAG, the specific cause of optic nerve damage is unknown. Increased intraocular pressure (IOP) was historically considered to be the sole cause. Additional contributing factors include increased susceptibility of the optic nerve to ischemia, excitotoxicity, autoimmune reactions, and other abnormal physiologic processes.
- Although IOP is a poor predictor of which patients will have visual field loss, the risk of visual field loss increases with increasing IOP. IOP is not constant; it changes with pulse, blood pressure, forced expiration or coughing, neck compression, and posture. IOP demonstrates diurnal variation with a minimum pressure around 6 PM and a maximum pressure upon awakening.
- The balance between the inflow and outflow of aqueous humor determines IOP. Inflow is increased by β-adrenergic agents and decreased by $α_2$- and β-adrenergic blockers, dopamine blockers, carbonic anhydrase inhibitors (CAIs), meltatonin-1 agonists, and adenylate cyclase stimulators. Outflow is increased by cholinergic agents (eg, pilocarpine), which contract the ciliary muscle and open the trabecular meshwork, and by prostaglandin analogues and β- and $α_2$-adrenergic agonists, which affect uveoscleral outflow.
- Secondary OAG has many causes, including exfoliation syndrome, pigmentary glaucoma, systemic diseases, trauma, surgery, ocular inflammatory diseases, and drugs. Secondary glaucoma can be classified as pretrabecular (normal meshwork is covered and prevents outflow of aqueous humor), trabecular (meshwork is altered or material accumulates in the intertrabecular spaces), or posttrabecular (episcleral venous blood pressure is increased).
- Many drugs can increase IOP (Table 65–1). The potential to induce or worsen glaucoma depends on the type of glaucoma and on whether it is adequately controlled.
- PACG occurs when there is a physical blockage of the trabecular meshwork, resulting in increased IOP.

CLINICAL PRESENTATION

- POAG is slowly progressive and is usually asymptomatic until onset of substantial visual field loss. Central visual acuity is maintained, even in late stages.
- Patients with PACG typically experience intermittent prodromal symptoms (eg, blurred or hazy vision with halos around lights and, occasionally, headache). Acute episodes produce symptoms associated with a cloudy, edematous cornea; ocular pain; nausea, vomiting, and abdominal pain; and diaphoresis.

TABLE 65-1	Drugs That May Induce or Potentiate Increased Intraocular Pressure

Open-angle glaucoma
  Ophthalmic corticosteroids (high risk)
  Systemic corticosteroids
  Nasal/inhaled corticosteroids
  Fenoldopam
  Ophthalmic anticholinergics
  Succinylcholine
  Vasodilators (low risk)
  Cimetidine (low risk)

Closed-angle glaucoma
  Topical anticholinergics
  Topical sympathomimetics
  Systemic anticholinergics
  Heterocyclic antidepressants
  Low-potency phenothiazines
  Antihistamines
  Ipratropium
  Benzodiazepines (low risk)
  Theophylline (low risk)
  Vasodilators (low risk)
  Systemic sympathomimetics (low risk)
  CNS stimulants (low risk)
  Serotonin-selective reuptake inhibitors
  Imipramine
  Venlafaxine
  Topiramate
  Tetracyclines (low risk)
  Carbonic anhydrase inhibitors (low risk)
  Monoamine oxidase inhibitors (low risk)
  Topical cholinergics (low risk)

DIAGNOSIS

- POAG is confirmed by the presence of characteristic optic disc changes and visual field loss, with or without increased IOP. *Normal tension glaucoma* refers to disc changes, visual field loss, and IOP less than 21 mm Hg (2.8 kPa). *Ocular hypertension* refers to IOP greater than 21 mm Hg (2.8 kPa) without disc changes or visual field loss.
- PACG is usually visualized by gonioscopy. IOP is generally markedly elevated (eg, 40–90 mm Hg [5.3–12 kPa]) when symptoms are present. Additional signs include hyperemic conjunctiva, cloudy cornea, shallow anterior chamber, and occasionally edematous and hyperemic optic disc.

TREATMENT OF OCULAR HYPERTENSION AND OPEN-ANGLE GLAUCOMA

- <u>Goal of Treatment</u>: The goal is to preserve visual function by reducing IOP to a level at which no further optic nerve damage occurs.
- Treat ocular hypertension if the patient has a significant risk factor such as IOP greater than 25 mm Hg (3.3 kPa), vertical cup:disc ratio greater than 0.5, or central

corneal thickness less than 555 μm. Additional risk factors to be considered include family history of glaucoma, black race, severe myopia, and presence of only one eye. The goal of therapy is to lower IOP by 20% to 30% from baseline to decrease the risk of optic nerve damage.

- Treat all patients with elevated IOP and characteristic optic disc changes or visual field defects. An initial target IOP reduction of 25% to 30% is desired in patients with POAG.
- Initiate drug therapy in a stepwise manner (Fig. 65–1), starting with lower concentrations of a single well-tolerated topical agent (Table 65–2). Historically, β-blockers (eg, **timolol**) were the treatment of choice provided no contraindications existed.
- Newer agents are also suitable for first-line therapy. Prostaglandin analogs (eg, **latanoprost, bimatoprost,** and **travoprost**) offer once-daily dosing, better IOP reduction, good tolerance, and, recently, availability of lower-cost generics. **Brimonidine** and topical CAIs are also suitable for first-line therapy.
- **Pilocarpine** and **dipivefrin**, a prodrug of **epinephrine**, are used as third-line therapies because of adverse events or reduced efficacy as compared with newer agents.
- **Carbachol**, topical cholinesterase inhibitors, and oral CAIs (eg, **acetazolamide**) are used as last-resort options after failure of less toxic options.
- Surgical procedures such as laser trabeculoplasty or surgical trabeculectomy can be considered when drug therapy fails, is not tolerated or is excessively complicated. Antiproliferative agents such as **fluorouracil** and **mitomycin C** are used to modify the healing process and maintain patency.

TREATMENT OF CLOSED-ANGLE GLAUCOMA

- Acute ACG with high IOP requires rapid reduction in IOP. Iridectomy is the definitive treatment producing a hole in the iris that permits aqueous humor flow to move directly from the posterior to the anterior chamber.
- Drug therapy of an acute attack typically consists of a miotic (eg, pilocarpine), secretory inhibitor (eg, β-blocker, α_2-agonist, **latanoprost**, or CAI), or prostaglandin agonist.
- Osmotic agents are used to rapidly decrease IOP. Examples include oral **glycerin**, 1 to 2 g/kg, and **mannitol**, 1 to 2 g/kg IV.
- Topical corticosteroids can be used to reduce ocular inflammation and synechiae.

EVALUATION OF THERAPEUTIC OUTCOMES

- Successful outcomes require identifying an effective, well-tolerated regimen; closely monitoring therapy; and patient adherence. Whenever possible, therapy for open-angle glaucoma should be started as a single agent in one eye to facilitate evaluation of drug efficacy and tolerance. Many drugs or combinations may need to be tried before the optimal regimen is identified.
- Monitoring therapy for POAG should be individualized. Assess IOP response every 4 to 6 weeks initially, every 3 to 4 months after IOPs become acceptable, and more frequently if therapy is changed. Visual field and disc changes are monitored annually, unless glaucoma is unstable or worsening.
- Monitor patients for loss of control of IOP (tachyphylaxis), especially with β-blockers or **apraclonidine**. Treatment can be temporarily discontinued to monitor benefit.
- There is no specific target IOP because the correlation between IOP and optic nerve damage is poor. Typically, a reduction of 25% to 30% is desired.
- The target IOP also depends on disease severity and is generally less than 21 mm Hg (2.8 kPa) for early visual field loss or optic disc changes, with progressively lower

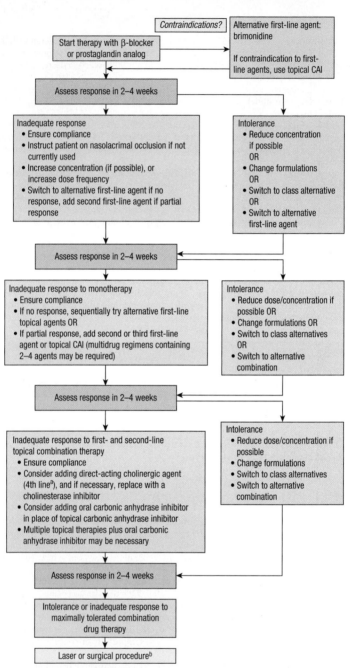

Contraindications?

Start therapy with β-blocker or prostaglandin analog

Alternative first-line agent: brimonidine

If contraindication to first-line agents, use topical CAI

Assess response in 2–4 weeks

Inadequate response
• Ensure compliance
• Instruct patient on nasolacrimal occlusion if not currently used
• Increase concentration (if possible), or increase dose frequency
• Switch to alternative first-line agent if no response, add second first-line agent if partial response

Intolerance
• Reduce concentration if possible
  OR
• Change formulations
  OR
• Switch to class alternative
  OR
• Switch to alternative first-line agent

Assess response in 2–4 weeks

Inadequate response to monotherapy
• Ensure compliance
• If no response, sequentially try alternative first-line topical agents OR
• If partial response, add second or third first-line agent or topical CAI (multidrug regimens containing 2–4 agents may be required)

Intolerance
• Reduce dose/concentration if possible OR
• Change formulations OR
• Switch to class alternatives OR
• Switch to alternative combination

Assess response in 2–4 weeks

Inadequate response to first- and second-line topical combination therapy
• Ensure compliance
• Consider adding direct-acting cholinergic agent (4th line[a]), and if necessary, replace with a cholinesterase inhibitor
• Consider adding oral carbonic anhydrase inhibitor in place of topical carbonic anhydrase inhibitor
• Multiple topical therapies plus oral carbonic anhydrase inhibitor may be necessary

Intolerance
• Reduce dose/concentration if possible
• Change formulations
• Switch to class alternatives
• Switch to alternative combination

Assess response in 2–4 weeks

Intolerance or inadequate response to maximally tolerated combination drug therapy

Laser or surgical procedure[b]

[a]Fourth-line agents not commonly used any longer.
[b]Most clinicians believe the laser procedure should be performed earlier (eg, after three-drug maximum or with a poorly adherent patient). (CAI, carbonic anhydrase inhibitor.)

FIGURE 65–1. Algorithm for the pharmacotherapy of open-angle glaucoma.

684

TABLE 65–2 Topical Drugs Used in the Treatment of Open-Angle Glaucoma

Drug	Pharmacologic Properties	Common Brand Names	Dose Form	Strength (%)	Usual Dose[a]	Mechanism of Action
β-Adrenergic blocking agents						
Betaxolol	Relative β₁-selective	Generic	Solution	0.5	One drop twice a day	All reduce aqueous production of ciliary body
		Betoptic-S	Suspension	0.25	One drop twice a day	
Carteolol	Nonselective, intrinsic sympathomimetic activity	Generic	Solution	1	One drop twice a day	
Levobunolol	Nonselective	Betagan	Solution	0.25, 0.5	One drop twice a day	
Metipranolol	Nonselective	OptiPranolol	Solution	0.3	One drop twice a day	
Timolol	Nonselective	Timoptic, Betimol, Istalol	Solution	0.25, 0.5	One drop every day—one to two times a day	
		Timoptic-XE	Gelling solution	0.25, 0.5	One drop every day[a]	
Adrenergic agonists						
Non-specific adrenergic agent						
Dipivefrin**	Epinephrine prodrug	Propine	Solution	0.1	One drop twice a day	Increased aqueous humor outflow
α₂-Adrenergic Agonists						
Apraclonidine	Specific α₂-agonists	Iopidine	Solution	0.5 (U.D.), 1	One drop two to three times a day	Both reduce aqueous humor production; brimonidine known to also increase uveoscleral outflow; only brimonidine has primary indication
Brimonidine		Alphagan P	Solution	0.2 (generic) 0.15 (brand/generic), 0.1	One drop two to three times a day	

(continued)

TABLE 65–2 Topical Drugs Used in the Treatment of Open-Angle Glaucoma (*Continued*)

Drug	Pharmacologic Properties	Common Brand Names	Dose Form	Strength (%)	Usual Dose[a]	Mechanism of Action
Cholinergic agonists direct acting						
Carbachol**	Irreversible	Carboptic, Isopto Carbachol	Solution	1.5, 3	One drop two to three times a day	All increase aqueous humor outflow through trabecular meshwork
Pilocarpine	Irreversible	Isopto Carpine, Pilocar	Solution	0.5, 1, 2, 4, 6	One drop two to three times a day	
		Pilopine HS**	Gel	4	One drop four times a day Every 24 hours at bedtime	
Cholinesterase inhibitors						
Echothiophate**		Phospholine Iodide	Solution	0.125	Once or twice a day	
Carbonic anhydrase inhibitors						
Topical						
Brinzolamide	All carbonic anhydrase inhibition	Azopt	Suspension	1	Two to three times a day	All reduce aqueous humor production of ciliary body
Dorzolamide		Trusopt Generic	Solution	2	Two to three times a day	
Systemic						
Acetazolamide		Generic	Tablet	125 mg, 250 mg	125–250 mg two to four times a day	
		Injection Diamox Sequels	500 mg/vial Capsule	250–500 mg 500 mg	500 mg twice a day	
Methazolamide		Generic	Tablet	25 mg, 50 mg	25–50 mg two to three times a day	

Prostaglandin analogs

Drug	Class	Brand	Form	Concentration	Dose	Mechanism
Latanoprost	Prostanoid agonist	Xalatan	Solution	0.005	One drop every night	Increases aqueous uveoscleral outflow and to a lesser extent trabecular outflow
Bimatoprost	Prostamide agonist	Lumigan	Solution	0.01, 0.03	One drop every night	
Travoprost	Prostanoid agonist	Travatan Z	Solution	0.004	One drop every night	
Tafluprost	Prostanoid agonist	Zioptan	Preservative free solution	0.0015	One drop every night	
Combinations						
Timolol–dorzolamide		Cosopt Generic	Solution	Timolol 0.5 dorzolamide 2	One drop twice daily	Reduce aqueous production
Timolol–brimonidine		Combigan	Solution	Timolol 0.5 brimonidine 0.2	One drop twice daily	Reduce aqueous production and increase uveoscleral outflow
Brinzolamide–brimonidine		Simbrinza		Brinzolamide 1 brimonidine 0.2	One drop three times daily	Reduce aqueous production and increase uveoscleral outflow
Timolol-latanoprost***		Xalacom	Solution	Timolol 0.5 latanoprost 0.005	One drop every night	All reduce aqueous production and increase uveoscleral outflow
Timolo-travoprost***		Duotrav	Solution	Timolol 0.5 travoprost 0.004	One drop every night	
Timolol-bimatoprost***		Ganfort	Solution	Timolol 0.5 Bimatoprost 0.03	One drop every night	

aUse of eyelid closure (ELC) technique for 5 minutes will increase the drug availability and reduce potential for local and systemic side effects.
**Often used as fourth-line agents; limited or no commerical availability.
***Not available in U.S.

targets for greater levels of glaucomatous damage. Targets as low as less than 10 mm Hg (1.3 kPa) are desired for very advanced disease, continued damage at higher IOPs, normal-tension glaucoma, and pretreatment pressures in the low to middle teens.

• Monitor medication adherence because it is commonly inadequate and a cause of therapy failure.

See Chapter 94, Glaucoma, authored by Richard G. Fiscella, Timothy S. Lesar, Ohoud A. Owaidhah, and Deepak P. Edward, for a more detailed discussion of this topic.

66 | Generalized Anxiety Disorder, Panic Disorder, and Posttraumatic Stress Disorder

CHAPTER

- In anxiety disorders (eg, generalized anxiety disorder and panic disorder), the most prominent features are anxiety and avoidance which are irrational or that impair functioning. In posttraumatic stress disorder, there is previous exposure to trauma and intrusive, avoidant, and hyperarousal symptoms.

PATHOPHYSIOLOGY

- *Noradrenergic model.* This model suggests that the autonomic nervous system of anxious patients is hypersensitive and overreacts to various stimuli. The locus ceruleus (LC) may have a role in regulating anxiety, as it activates norepinephrine release and stimulates the sympathetic and parasympathetic nervous systems. Chronic noradrenergic overactivity downregulates α_2-adrenoreceptors in patients with generalized anxiety disorder (GAD) and posttraumatic stress disorder (PTSD). This receptor is hypersensitive in some patients with panic disorder. Drugs with anxiolytic or antipanic effects (eg, **benzodiazepines** and **antidepressants**) inhibit LC firing, decrease noradrenergic activity, and block the effects of anxiogenic drugs. Hyperactive noradrenergic signaling in patients with PTSD is a consistent research finding.
- *γ-Aminobutyric acid (GABA) receptor model.* GABA is the major inhibitory neurotransmitter in the central nervous system (CNS). Many antianxiety drugs target the $GABA_A$ receptor. **Benzodiazepines** enhance the inhibitory effects of GABA, which regulates or inhibits serotonin (5-hydroxytryptamine; 5-HT), norepinephrine, and dopamine activity. The number of $GABA_A$ receptors can change with alterations in the environment, and GABA receptor subunit expression can be altered by hormonal changes. Abnormal functioning of several neurotransmitter systems, including norepinephrine, GABA, glutamate, dopamine, and 5-HT may affect manifestations of anxiety and PTSD.
- *5-HT model.* Abnormalities in serotonergic functioning may play a role in anxiety disorders. Preclinical models suggest that greater 5-HT function facilitates avoidance behavior; but primate studies show that reducing 5-HT increases aggression. GAD symptoms may reflect excessive 5-HT transmission or overactivity of the stimulatory 5-HT pathways. The selective serotonin reuptake inhibitors (**SSRIs**) increase 5-HT levels at the synapse and are efficacious in blocking manifestations of panic and anxiety.
- Patients with PTSD hypersecrete corticotropin-releasing factor, but have subnormal levels of cortisol at the time of trauma and chronically. Cortisol reduces the stress response by tempering the sympathetic reaction. Dysregulation of the hypothalamic-pituitary-adrenal axis may be a risk factor for eventual development of PTSD.
- Neuroimaging studies support the role of the amygdala, anterior cingulate cortex, and insula in the pathophysiology of anxiety. In GAD, there is an abnormal increase in the brain's fear circuitry and increased activity in the prefrontal cortex. Patients with panic disorder have abnormalities of midbrain structures. In PTSD, the amygdala plays a role in the persistence of traumatic memory. Hypofunctioning in the ventromedial prefrontal cortex is theorized to prevent extinction in patients with PTSD and is inversely correlated with severity of symptoms. Low hippocampal volumes in patients with PTSD are likely a precursor for vulnerability for subsequent development of PTSD.

TABLE 66–1	Clinical Presentation of Generalized Anxiety Disorder
Psychological and Cognitive Symptoms	**Physical Symptoms**
• Excessive anxiety • Worries that are difficult to control • Feeling keyed up or on edge • Trouble concentrating or mind going blank	• Restlessness • Fatigue • Muscle tension • Sleep disturbance • Irritability

- Glutamate signaling abnormalities may result in distortion of amygdala-dependent emotional processing under stress. Dysregulation of the processing of sensory input and memories may contribute to the dissociative and hypervigilant symptoms in PTSD.

CLINICAL PRESENTATION

GENERALIZED ANXIETY DISORDER

- The diagnosis of GAD requires excessive anxiety and worry most days about a number of matters for at least 6 months. Anxiety and worry are associated with at least three of the following: restlessness, fatigue, difficulty concentrating, irritability, muscle tension, and sleep disturbance (Table 66–1).
- Significant distress or impairment in functioning is present, and the disturbance is not caused by a substance or another medical condition.
- Women are twice as likely as men to have GAD. The illness has a gradual onset at an average age of 21 years. The course is chronic, with multiple exacerbations and remissions.

PANIC DISORDER

- Recurrent unexpected panic attacks. At least one attack has been followed by at least one month of either or both (1) persistent worry about having another panic attack or their consequences or (2) maladaptive change in behavior related to the attacks.
- Symptoms of a panic attack are shown in Table 66–2. During an attack, there must be at least four symptoms in addition to intense fear or discomfort. Symptoms reach a peak within 10 minutes and usually last no more than 20 or 30 minutes.

TABLE 66–2	Clinical Presentation of Panic Attack

Psychological Symptoms

- Depersonalization (being detached from oneself)
- Derealization (feelings of being detached from one's environment)
- Fear of losing control, going crazy, or dying

Physical Symptoms

- Abdominal distress
- Chest pain or discomfort
- Chills
- Dizziness or light-headedness
- Feeling of choking
- Heat sensations
- Nausea
- Palpitations
- Paresthesias
- Sensations of shortness of breath or smothering
- Sweating
- Tachycardia
- Trembling or shaking

TABLE 66-3	Clinical Presentation of Posttraumatic Stress Disorder

Intrusion Symptoms
- Recurrent, intrusive distressing memories of the trauma
- Recurrent, disturbing dreams of the event
- Feeling that the traumatic event is recurring (eg, dissociative flashbacks)
- Physiologic reaction to or psychological distress from reminders of the trauma

Avoidance Symptoms
- Avoidance of conversations, thoughts, or feelings about the trauma
- Avoidance of people, places, or activities that are reminders of the event

Persistent Negative Alterations in Thinking and Mood
- Inability to recall an important aspect of the trauma
- Anhedonia
- Estrangement from others
- Restricted affect
- Negative beliefs about oneself
- Distorted beliefs causing one to blame others or themselves for the trauma
- Negative mood state

Hyperarousal Symptoms
- Decreased concentration
- Easily startled
- Self-destructive behavior
- Hypervigilance
- Insomnia
- Irritability or anger outbursts

Specifiers
- Dissociative symptoms: depersonalization or derealization
- With delayed expression: full criteria are not met until at least 6 months posttrauma

- Up to 50% of panic disorder patients eventually develop agoraphobia, which is marked fear or anxiety about being in at least 2 situations where escape could be difficult or help unavailable (eg, being in crowded places or crossing bridges) where they fear a panic attack might occur. Patients may become homebound.

POSTTRAUMATIC STRESS DISORDER

- In adults and children older than 6, there is exposure to actual or threatened death, serious injury, or sexual violence, either directly, or by witnessing the event(s) happening to others, learning about the event(s) happening to someone close, or experiencing repeated or extreme exposure to details of the event(s).
- Duration of intrusive, avoidance, alterations in thinking and mood, and hyperarousal symptoms (Table 66–3) must be present longer than 1 month and cause significant distress or impairment. There must be at least one intrusive symptom, one symptom of avoidance of stimuli associated with the trauma, at least two symptoms of negative alterations in thinking and mood, and at least two symptoms of increased arousal. PTSD co-occurs with mood, anxiety, and substance use disorders.

DIAGNOSIS

- Evaluation of the anxious patient requires a physical and mental status examination; complete psychiatric diagnostic exam; appropriate laboratory tests; and a medical, psychiatric, and drug history.
- Anxiety symptoms may be associated with medical illnesses (Table 66–4) or drug therapy (Table 66–5), and they may be present in several major psychiatric illnesses (eg, mood disorders, schizophrenia, organic mental syndromes, and substance withdrawal).

TABLE 66–4	Common Medical Illnesses Associated with Anxiety Symptoms

Cardiovascular

Angina, arrhythmias, cardiomyopathy, congestive heart failure, hypertension, ischemic heart disease, mitral valve prolapse, myocardial infarction

Endocrine and metabolic

Cushing disease, diabetes, hyperparathyroidism, hyperthyroidism, hypothyroidism, hypoglycemia, hyponatremia, hyperkalemia, pheochromocytoma, vitamin B_{12} or folate deficiencies

Gastrointestinal

Crohn disease, irritable bowel syndrome, ulcerative colitis, peptic ulcer disease

Neurologic

Migraine, seizures, stroke, neoplasms, poor pain control

Respiratory system

Asthma, chronic obstructive pulmonary disease, pulmonary embolism, pneumonia

Others

Anemias, cancer, systemic lupus erythematosus, vestibular dysfunction

TREATMENT

GENERALIZED ANXIETY DISORDER

- Goals of Treatment: The goals are to reduce severity, duration, and frequency of symptoms and improve functioning. The long-term goal is minimal or no anxiety symptoms, no functional impairment, prevention of recurrence, and improved quality of life.
- Nonpharmacologic modalities include psychotherapy, short-term counseling, stress management, psychoeducation, meditation, and exercise. Ideally, patients with GAD

TABLE 66–5	Drugs Associated with Anxiety Symptoms

Anticonvulsants: Carbamazepine, phenytoin

Antidepressants: Bupropion, selective serotonin reuptake inhibitors, serotonin–norepinephrine reuptake inhibitors

Antihypertensives: Clonidine, felodipine

Antibiotics: Quinolones, isoniazid

Bronchodilators: Albuterol, theophylline

Corticosteroids: Prednisone

Dopamine agonists: Amantadine, levodopa

Herbals: Ma huang, ginseng, ephedra

Illicit substances: Ecstasy, marijuana

Nonsteroidal antiinflammatory drugs: Ibuprofen, indomethacin

Stimulants: Amphetamines, caffeine, cocaine, methylphenidate, nicotine

Sympathomimetics: Pseudoephedrine, phenylephrine

Thyroid hormones: Levothyroxine

Toxicity: Anticholinergics, antihistamines, digoxin

should have psychological therapy, alone or in combination with antianxiety drugs. Cognitive behavioral therapy (CBT), though not widely available, is the most effective psychological therapy. Patients should avoid caffeine, nicotine, stimulants, excessive alcohol, and diet pills.

- A treatment algorithm from the International Psychopharmacology Algorithm Project (IMAP) is shown in **Fig. 66–1**.
- Drug choices for GAD and panic disorder are shown in **Table 66–6**, and non-benzodiazepine antianxiety agents for GAD and their dosing are shown in **Table 66–7**.
- **Hydroxyzine**, often used in primary care, is considered a second-line agent.
- **Pregabalin** produced anxiolytic effects similar to **lorazepam, alprazolam**, and **venlafaxine** in acute trials. Sedation and dizziness were the most common adverse effects.
- **Quetiapine** extended release, 150 mg/day was superior to placebo and as effective as **paroxetine** 20 mg/day and **escitalopram** 10 mg/day, but with earlier onset of action. Quetiapine is not FDA approved for GAD.

Antidepressants

- **Antidepressants** are efficacious for acute and long-term management of GAD (Table 66–7). They are the treatment of choice for long-term management of chronic anxiety, especially in the presence of depressive symptoms. **Venlafaxine extended-release, duloxetine, paroxetine**, and **escitalopram** are FDA-approved for GAD, and **imipramine** is considered a second-line agent. Antianxiety response requires 2 to 4 weeks or longer. See Chap. 68 for additional information on antidepressants.
- **Selective serotonin reuptake inhibitors (SSRIs), extended-release venlafaxine**, and **duloxetine** are effective in acute therapy (response rates of 60%–68%). In a meta-analysis, **fluoxetine** was found most likely to achieve remission of GAD symptoms, sertraline was best tolerated.
- Common side effects and monitoring parameters for patients taking medications used for anxiety disorders are shown in **Table 66–8**.
- Some patients require small initial doses of antidepressants for the first week to limit the development of transient increased anxiety, also known as jitteriness syndrome.
- The Food and Drug Administration (FDA) has established a link between anti-depressant use and suicidality (suicidal thinking and behaviors) in children, adolescents, and young adults less than 25 years. All antidepressants carry a black box warning advising caution in using antidepressants in this population, and the FDA also recommends specific monitoring parameters (consult the FDA-approved labeling or the FDA website).

Benzodiazepine Therapy

- The **benzodiazepines** are the most effective and frequently prescribed drugs for the treatment of acute anxiety (Table 66–9). About 65% to 75% of patients with GAD have a marked to moderate response, and most of the improvement occurs in the first 2 weeks of therapy. They are more effective for somatic and autonomic symptoms of GAD, whereas antidepressants are more effective for the psychic symptoms (eg, apprehension and worry).
- The dose must be individualized. The elderly are more sensitive to benzodiazepines and may experience falls when taking them.

BENZODIAZEPINE PHARMACOKINETICS

- Benzodiazepine pharmacokinetic properties are shown in **Table 66–10**. **Diazepam** and **clorazepate** have high lipophilicity and are rapidly absorbed and distributed into the CNS. They have rapid antianxiety effects, but a shorter duration of effect after a single dose than would be predicted based on half-life, as they are rapidly distributed to the periphery.
- **Lorazepam** and **oxazepam** are less lipophilic, have a slower onset, but a longer duration of action. They are not recommended for immediate relief of anxiety.

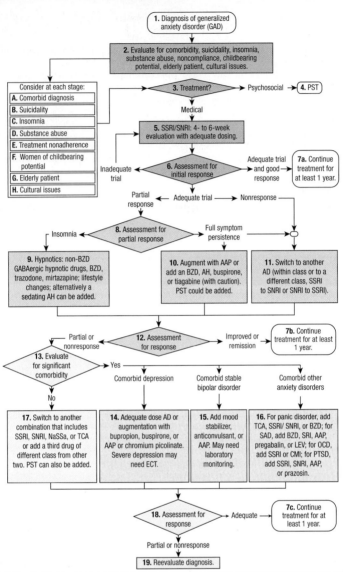

Dark blue, first-line treatment (nodes 2, 3, 5, 6); medium blue, second-line treatment (nodes 8–12); light blue, third-line treatment, no comorbidity (nodes 13, 17, 18, 19); gray, third-line treatment, with comorbidity (nodes 14–16). Levels of evidence used in development of the flowchart were: 1, more than one placebo-controlled trial with sample sizes over 30; 2, one placebo-controlled trial (or active vs active drug comparison) with sample size of 30 or greater; 3, one or small ($n < 30$) placebo-controlled trial; 4, case reports or open-label trials; and 5, expert consensus without published evidence. (*Used by permission of The International Psychopharmacology Algorithm Project. IPAP—Generalized Anxiety Disorder Algorithm. http://www.ipap.org/gad/index.php, accessed December 22, 2015.*)

(AAP, atypical antipsychotic; AD, antidepressant; AH, antihistamine; BZD, benzodiazepine; CMI, clomipramine; ECT, electroconvulsive therapy; GAD, generalized anxiety disorder; LEV, levetiracetam; NaSSa, noradrenergic and selective serotonergic antidepressant; PST, psychosocial treatment; SAD, social anxiety disorder; SNRI, serotonin-norepinephrine reuptake inhibior; SRI, serotonin reuptake inhibitor; SSRI, selective serotonin reuptake inhibitor; TCA, tricyclic antidepressant.)

FIGURE 66–1. International Psychopharmacology Algorithm Project (IPAP) generalized anxiety disorder (GAD) algorithm flowchart.

- **Avoid intramuscular (IM) diazepam** and **IM chlordiazepoxide** because of variability in rate and extent of absorption. **IM lorazepam** provides rapid and complete absorption.
- **Clorazepate**, a prodrug, is converted to **desmethyldiazepam** in the stomach through a pH-dependent process that may be impaired by concurrent antacid use. Several other benzodiazepines are also converted to desmethyldiazepam, which has a long half-life and can accumulate, especially in the elderly and others with impaired oxidation.
- Intermediate- or short-acting benzodiazepines are preferred for chronic use in the elderly and those with liver disorders because of minimal accumulation and achievement of steady state within 1 to 3 days.

ADVERSE EVENTS

- The most common side effect of benzodiazepines is CNS depression. Tolerance usually develops to this effect. Other side effects are disorientation, psychomotor impairment, confusion, aggression, excitement, ataxia, and anterograde amnesia (see Table 66–8).

ABUSE, DEPENDENCE, WITHDRAWAL, AND TOLERANCE

- Those with a history of drug abuse should not receive benzodiazepines. Those with GAD and panic disorder are at high risk for dependence because of the chronicity of the illnesses.
- Benzodiazepine dependence is defined by appearance of a withdrawal syndrome (ie, anxiety, insomnia, agitation, muscle tension, irritability, nausea, diaphoresis, nightmares, depression, hyperreflexia, tinnitus, delusions, hallucinations, and seizures) upon abrupt discontinuation.

BENZODIAZEPINE DISCONTINUATION

- After benzodiazepines are abruptly discontinued, three events can occur: (1) rebound symptoms are an immediate but transient return of original symptoms with an increased intensity compared with baseline; (2) recurrence or relapse is the return of original symptoms at the same intensity as before treatment; or (3) withdrawal is the emergence of new symptoms and a worsening of preexisting symptoms.
- The onset of withdrawal symptoms is within 24 to 48 hours after discontinuation of short-elimination half-life benzodiazepines and 3 to 8 days after discontinuation of long-elimination half-life drugs.
- Discontinuation strategies include:
  ✓ A 25% per week reduction in dosage until 50% of the dose is reached, and then reduce by one eighth every 4 to 7 days. If therapy duration exceeds 8 weeks, a taper over 2 to 3 weeks is recommended, but if duration of treatment is 6 months, a taper over 4 to 8 weeks is reasonable. Longer durations of treatment may require a 2- to 4-month taper.
  ✓ Adjunctive use of **pregabalin** can help to reduce withdrawal symptoms during the benzodiazepine taper.

BENZODIAZEPINE DRUG INTERACTIONS

- Combining **benzodiazepines** with **alcohol** or other **CNS depressants** may be fatal.
- Addition of **nefazodone**, **ritonavir**, or **ketoconazole** (CYP3A4 inhibitors) can increase the blood levels of **alprazolam** and **diazepam.**
- Consult the drug interaction literature for more information on benzodiazepine drug interactions.

DOSING AND ADMINISTRATION

- Start with low doses, and adjust weekly (see Table 66–9).
- Treatment of acute anxiety generally should not exceed 4 weeks. Manage persistent symptoms with antidepressants.

TABLE 66–6	Drug Choices for Anxiety Disorders		
Anxiety Disorder	**First-Line Drugs**	**Second-Line Drugs**	**Alternatives**
Generalized anxiety disorder	Duloxetine Escitalopram Paroxetine Sertraline Venlafaxine XR	Benzodiazepines Buspirone Imipramine Pregabalin	Hydroxyzine Quetiapine
Panic disorder	SSRIs Venlafaxine XR	Alprazolam Citalopram Clomipramine Clonazepam Imipramine	Phenelzine

(SSRI, selective serotonin reuptake inhibitor; XR, extended-release.)

- Long half-life benzodiazepines may be dosed once daily at bedtime, providing nighttime hypnotic and next day anxiolytic effects.
- Use low doses of short-elimination half-life agents in the elderly.

Buspirone Therapy

- **Buspirone** is a 5-HT$_{1A}$ partial agonist that lacks anticonvulsant, muscle relaxant, sedative-hypnotic, motor impairment, and dependence-producing properties.
- It is a second-line agent for GAD because of inconsistent reports of long-term efficacy, delayed onset of effect, and lack of efficacy for potentially comorbid depressive and anxiety disorders. It is an option for patients who fail other anxiolytic therapies or patients with a history of alcohol or substance abuse. It does not provide rapid or "as needed" antianxiety effects. It is effective for the psychic symptoms of anxiety.
- It has a mean t$_{1/2}$ of 2.5 hours, and it is dosed two to three times daily (see Table 66–7).

DRUG INTERACTIONS

- **Buspirone** may elevate blood pressure in patients taking a monoamine oxidase inhibitor (MAOI).
- **Verapamil, itraconazole,** and **fluvoxamine** can increase buspirone levels, and **rifampin** reduces buspirone blood levels 10-fold.

DOSING AND ADMINISTRATION

- Buspirone can be titrated in increments of 5 mg/day every 2 or 3 days as needed.
- The onset of anxiolytic effects requires 2 weeks or more; maximum benefit may require 4 to 6 weeks. Improvement in psychic symptoms precedes improvement in somatic symptoms.
- It may be less effective in patients who have previously taken benzodiazepines.

Evaluation of Therapeutic Outcomes

- Initially, monitor anxious patients every two weeks for reduction in anxiety symptoms, improvement in functioning, and side effects. The Hamilton Rating Scale for Anxiety or the Sheehan Disability Scale can help measure drug response.

PANIC DISORDER

- <u>Goals of Treatment</u>: The goals are complete resolution of panic attacks, marked reduction in anticipatory anxiety, elimination of phobic avoidance, and no functional impairment.

TABLE 66–7 Nonbenzodiazepine Antianxiety Agents for Generalized Anxiety Disorder

Drug	Brand Name	Initial Dose	Usual Range (mg/day)[a]	Comments
Antidepressants				
Duloxetine	Cymbalta	30 or 60 mg/day	60–120	FDA-approved
Escitalopram	Lexapro	10 mg/day	10–20	FDA-approved, available generically
Imipramine	Tofranil	50 mg/day	75–200	Available generically
Paroxetine	Paxil Pexeva	20 mg/day	20–50	FDA-approved, available generically, avoid in pregnancy
Sertraline	Zoloft	50 mg/day	50–200	Available generically
Venlafaxine XR	Effexor XR	37.5 or 75 mg/day	75–225[b]	FDA-approved, available generically
Vilazodone	Viibryd	10 mg/day	20–40[b]	During concomitant use of a strong CYP3A4 inhibitor (eg, itraconazole, clarithromycin, voriconazole), dose should not exceed 20 mg once daily
Vortioxetine	Brintellix	5 mg/day	5–20	
Azapirone				
Buspirone	BuSpar	7.5 mg twice daily	15–60[b]	FDA-approved, available generically
Diphenylmethane				
Hydroxyzine	Vistaril	25 or 50 mg four times daily (adult)	200–400	FDA-approved, available generically, also approved for children with anxiety and tension
Anticonvulsant				
Pregabalin	Lyrica	50 mg three times daily	150–600	Dosage adjustment required in renal impairment
Atypical antipsychotic				
Quetiapine XR	Seroquel XR	50 mg at bedtime	150–300	

(XR, extended-release.)
[a]Elderly patients are usually treated with approximately one half of the dose listed.
[b]No dosage adjustment is required in elderly patients.

General Approach

- **SSRIs** or **venlafaxine XR** are first-line agents for panic disorder (Table 66–11), but **benzodiazepines** (second-line agents) are the most commonly used drugs. **Imipramine** is considered second-line. FDA-approved drugs include **fluoxetine**, **paroxetine**, **sertraline**, **venlafaxine**, **alprazolam**, and **clonazepam**. An algorithm for drug therapy of panic disorder is shown in Fig. 66–2.

TABLE 66–8   Monitoring of Adverse Effects Associated with Medications Used for Anxiety Disorders

Medication Class/Drug	Adverse Drug Reaction	Monitoring Parameter	Comments
SSRIs			
	Jitteriness syndrome	Patient interview	
	Suicidality	Patient interview	Monitor weekly in first few weeks in patients with comorbid depression and patients under age 25
	Nausea, diarrhea	Patient interview	Typically transient
	Headache	Patient interview	Typically transient
	Weight gain	Body weight, BMI, waist circumference	Paroxetine may be more likely to cause weight gain
	Sexual dysfunction	Patient interview	Significant reason for nonadherence
	Hyponatremia	Basic metabolic panel	Monitor at baseline and periodically thereafter. More frequent monitoring required in high-risk groups, especially the elderly (>65 years)
	Thrombocytopenia	Complete blood count	Reported with citalopram
	Teratogenicity	Pregnancy test at baseline	Avoid paroxetine in pregnancy; Pregnancy Category D
	QT prolongation	ECG	Before starting citalopram, consider ECG and measurement of QT interval in patients with cardiac disease
	Discontinuation syndrome	Patient interview	Avoid abrupt discontinuation in all but fluoxetine
SNRIs			
	Jitteriness syndrome	Patient interview	
	Suicidality	Patient interview	Monitor weekly in first few weeks in patients with comorbid depression and patients under age 25
	Nausea, diarrhea	Patient interview	Typically transient
	Headache	Patient interview	Typically transient
	Elevated blood pressure	Blood pressure	Monitor blood pressure on initiation and regularly during treatment
	Sexual dysfunction	Patient interview	Significant reason for nonadherence
	Discontinuation syndrome	Patient interview	Avoid abrupt discontinuation

TCAs	Jitteriness syndrome	Patient interview	Monitor weekly in first few weeks in patients with comorbid depression and patients under age 25
	Suicidality	Patient interview	
	Anticholinergic effects	Patient interview	Contraindicated with narrow-angle glaucoma, prostatic hypertrophy, and urinary retention
	Weight gain	Body weight, BMI, waist circumference	
	Sexual dysfunction	Patient interview	Significant reason for nonadherence
	Sedation	Patient interview	Administer dosage at bedtime when feasible
	Arrhythmia	ECG	At baseline and periodically in children and patients >40 years of age
	Orthostatic hypotension	Blood pressure with position changes	
	Cholinergic rebound	Patient interview	Avoid abrupt discontinuation; taper doses
Benzodiazepines	Drowsiness, fatigue	Patient interview	Avoid operating large machinery; tolerance to sedation develops after repeated dosing
	Anterograde amnesia and memory impairment	Patient interview	Risk of anterograde amnesia is worsened with concomitant intake of alcohol
	Dependence	Patient interview; Prescription Monitoring Program	Monitor for early refills or escalation of dosage
	Withdrawal symptoms	Physical examination; patient interview	Taper doses on discontinuation
	Respiratory depression	Respiratory rate	Avoid administering with other CNS depressants (ie, opioids, alcohol)
	Psychomotor impairment	Physical examination	Increased risk of falls
	Paradoxical disinhibition	Physical examination; family report	Increase in anxiety, irritability, or agitation may be seen in the elderly or children

(continued)

TABLE 66–8 Monitoring of Adverse Effects Associated with Medications Used for Anxiety Disorders (*Continued*)

Medication Class/Drug	Adverse Drug Reaction	Monitoring Parameter	Comments
Other drugs			
Buspirone	Nausea, abdominal pain	Patient interview	Typically transient
	Drowsiness, dizziness	Patient interview	Typically transient
Phenelzine	Jitteriness syndrome	Patient interview	
	Suicidality	Patient interview	Monitor weekly in first few weeks in patients with comorbid depression and patients under age 25
	Hypertensive crisis	Blood pressure	Tyramine-free diet and avoidance of drug interactions required
	Orthostatic hypotension	Blood pressure with position changes	Fasting labs at baseline and then periodically
Pregabalin	Dizziness, somnolence	Patient interview	
	Peripheral edema	Physical examination	
	Thrombocytopenia	Complete blood count	
	Weight gain	Body weight	
	Sedation	Patient interview	
Quetiapine	Metabolic syndrome	Body weight, BMI, waist circumference, fasting lipids and glucose	Fasting labs at baseline and then periodically
	Akathisia	Patient interview	
	Tardive dyskinesia	Abnormal Involuntary Movement Scale	
	Orthostatic hypotension	Blood pressure with position changes	

(BMI, body mass index; ECG, electrocardiogram; SNRI, serotonin–norepinephrine reuptake inhibitor; SSRIs, selective serotonin reuptake inhibitors; TCAs, tricyclic antidepressants.)

TABLE 66–9	Benzodiazepine Antianxiety Agents				
Drug	Brand Name	Approved Dosage Range (mg/day)	Maximum Dosage for Geriatric Patients (mg/day)	Approximate Equivalent Dose (mg)	Comments
Alprazolam[a]	Niravam,[b] Xanax	0.75–4	2	0.5	Associated with interdose rebound anxiety
	Xanax XR	1–10[c]			
Chlordiazepoxide[a]	Librium	25–400	40	10	
Clonazepam[a]	Klonopin Klonopin Wafer[b]	1–4[c]	3	0.25–0.5	
Clorazepate[a]	Tranxene	7.5–60	30	7.5	
Diazepam[a]	Valium	2–40	20	5	
Lorazepam[a]	Ativan	0.5–10	3	1	Preferred in elderly
Oxazepam[a]	Serax	30–120	60	30	Preferred in elderly

(XR, extended-release.)
[a]Available generically.
[b]Orally disintegrating formulation.
[c]Panic disorder dose.

- Most patients without agoraphobia improve with pharmacotherapy alone, but if agoraphobia is present, cognitive behavioral therapy (CBT) typically is initiated concurrently. Adding psychosocial treatment to pharmacotherapy may reduce likelihood of relapse when drug therapy is stopped.
- Educate patient to avoid **caffeine**, nicotine, alcohol, drugs of abuse, and stimulants.
- If pharmacotherapy is used, antidepressants, especially the **SSRIs**, are preferred in elderly patients and youth. The **benzodiazepines** are second line in these patients because of potential problems with disinhibition.
- Usually patients are treated for 12 to 24 months before discontinuation is attempted over 4 to 6 months. Many patients require long-term therapy. Single weekly doses of **fluoxetine** have been used for maintenance.

Antidepressants

- Stimulatory side effects (eg, anxiety, insomnia, and jitteriness) can occur in up to 40% of **tricyclic antidepressant (TCA)**- and **SSRI**-treated patients. This may hinder compliance and dose escalation. Low initial doses and gradual dose titration may eliminate these effects (see Table 66–11).
- **Imipramine** blocks panic attacks within 4 weeks in 75% of patients, but reducing anticipatory anxiety and phobic avoidance requires 8 to 12 weeks.
- 25% of panic disorder patients discontinue **TCAs** because of side effects.
- **SSRIs** eliminate panic attacks in 60% to 80% of patients within about 4 weeks, but some patients require 8 to 12 weeks.
- **Venlafaxine extended release** is superior to placebo and similar in efficacy to **paroxetine** in relieving panic attacks, anticipatory anxiety, fear and avoidance.

TABLE 66-10	Pharmacokinetics of Benzodiazepine Antianxiety Agents				
Drug	Time to Peak Plasma Level (Hours)	Elimination Half-Life, Parent (Hours)	Metabolic Pathway	Clinically Significant Metabolites	Protein Binding (%)
Alprazolam	1–2	12–15	Oxidation	–	80
Chlordiazepoxide	1–4	5–30	N-Dealkylation Oxidation	Desmethyl chlordiazepoxide Demoxepam DMDZ[a]	96
Clonazepam	1–4	30–40	Nitroreduction	–	85
Clorazepate	1–2	Prodrug	Oxidation	DMDZ	97
Diazepam	0.5–2	20–80	Oxidation	DMDZ Oxazepam	98
Lorazepam	2–4	10–20	Conjugation	–	85
Oxazepam	2–4	5–20	Conjugation	–	97

[a]Desmethyldiazepam (DMDZ) half-life 50–100 hours.

TABLE 66-11 Drugs Used in the Treatment of Panic Disorder

Class/Generic Name	Brand Name	Starting Dose	Antipanic Dosage Range (mg)	Comments
SSRIs				
Citalopram	Celexa	10 mg/day	20–40	Dosage used in clinical trials; maximum dose limited by QT prolongation; available generically
Escitalopram	Lexapro	5 mg/day	10–20	Dosage used in clinical trials; available generically
Fluoxetine	Prozac	5 mg/day	10–30	Available generically
Fluvoxamine	Luvox	25 mg/day	100–300	Available generically
Paroxetine	Paxil Pexeva	10 mg/day	20–60	FDA-approved; available generically
	Paxil CR	12.5 mg/day	25–75	
Sertraline	Zoloft	25 mg/day	50–200	FDA-approved; available generically
SNRI				
Venlafaxine XR	Effexor XR	37.5 mg/day	75–225	FDA-approved; available generically
Benzodiazepines				
Alprazolam	Xanax	0.5 mg three times a day	4–10	FDA-approved; available generically
	Xanax XR	0.5–1 mg/day	3–10	
Clonazepam	Klonopin	0.25 mg once or twice per day	1–4	FDA-approved; available generically
Diazepam	Valium	2–5 mg three times a day	5–20	Dosage used in clinical trials; available generically
Lorazepam	Ativan	0.5–1 mg three times a day	2–8	Dosage used in clinical trials; available generically
TCA				
Imipramine	Tofranil	10 mg/day	75–250	Dosage used in clinical trials; available generically
MAOI				
Phenelzine	Nardil	15 mg/day	45–90	Dosage used in clinical trials

(CR, controlled release; MAOI, monoamine oxidase inhibitor; SNRI, serotonin–norepinephrine reuptake inhibitor; SSRIs, selective serotonin reuptake inhibitors; TCA, tricyclic antidepressant; XR, extended release.)

Benzodiazepines

• **Benzodiazepines** are second-line agents for panic disorder except when rapid response is essential. Avoid benzodiazepine monotherapy in patients with panic disorder who are depressed or have a history of depression. Avoid benzodiazepines in patients with a history of **alcohol** or drug abuse. They are often used concomitantly with antidepressants in the first 4 to 6 weeks to achieve a more rapid antipanic response.
• Relapse rates of 50% or higher are common despite slow drug tapering.

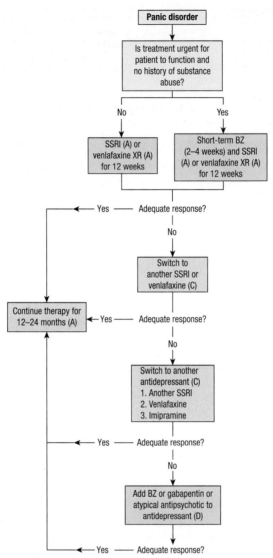

Strength of recommendations: A, directly based on category I evidence (ie, meta-analysis of randomized controlled trials [RCT] or at least one RCT); B, directly based on category II evidence (ie, at least one controlled study without randomization or one other type of quasi-experimental study); C, directly based on category III evidence (ie, nonexperimental descriptive studies); D, directly based on category IV evidence (ie, expert committee reports or opinions and/or clinical experience of respected authorities).

(BZ, benzodiazepine; SSRI, selective serotonin reuptake inhibitor.)

FIGURE 66–2. **Algorithm for the pharmacotherapy of panic disorder.**

• **Alprazolam** and **clonazepam** are the preferred benzodiazepines for panic disorder. Therapeutic response typically occurs within 1 to 2 weeks. With alprazolam, there may be breakthrough symptoms between doses. The use of extended-release alprazolam or clonazepam avoids this problem.

DOSING AND ADMINISTRATION

- The starting dose of **clonazepam** is 0.25 mg once or twice daily, with a dose increase of 0.25 to 0.5 mg every 3 days to 4 mg/day if needed.
- The starting dose of **alprazolam** is 0.25 three times daily (or 0.5 mg once daily of extended-release alprazolam), slowly increasing over several weeks as needed. Most patients require 3 to 6 mg/day.

EVALUATION OF THERAPEUTIC OUTCOMES

- Evaluate patients with panic disorder every 1 to 2 weeks during the first few weeks to fine-tune dosing and to monitor side effects. Once stabilized, they can be seen every 2 months. The Panic Disorder Severity Scale (with a remission goal of three or less with no or mild agoraphobic avoidance, anxiety, disability, or depressive symptoms) and the Sheehan Disability Scale (with a goal of less than or equal to one on each item) can be used to measure disability. During drug discontinuation, the frequency of appointments should be increased.

POSTTRAUMATIC STRESS DISORDER

- <u>Goals of Treatment</u>: The goals are to decrease core symptoms, disability, and comorbidity and improve quality of life.
- Immediately after the trauma, patients should receive treatment individualized to their presenting symptoms (eg, **nonbenzodiazepine hypnotic** or short courses of CBT). Brief courses of CBT in close proximity to the trauma can help prevent PTSD.
- If symptoms persist for 3 to 4 weeks, and there is social or occupational impairment, patients can receive pharmacotherapy or psychotherapy, or both.
- Psychotherapies for PTSD include stress management, eye movement desensitization and reprocessing (EMDR), and psychoeducation. Trauma-focused CBT (TFCBT) and EMDR are more effective than stress management or group therapy to reduce PTSD symptoms.
- **Figure 66–3** shows an algorithm for the pharmacotherapy of PTSD.
- The **SSRIs** and **venlafaxine** are first-line pharmacotherapy for PTSD (**Table 66–12**). The **TCAs** and **MAOIs** also can be effective, but side effects can be problematic.
- **Sertraline** and **paroxetine** are approved for acute treatment of PTSD, and sertraline is approved for long-term management.
- Antiadrenergics and atypical antipsychotics can be used as augmenting agents.

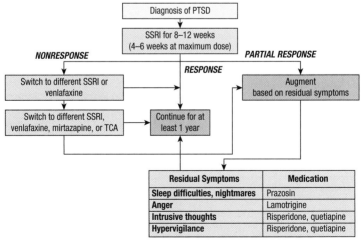

FIGURE 66–3. Algorithm for the pharmacotherapy of posttraumatic stress disorder (PTSD).

TABLE 66–12	Dosing of Antidepressants in the Treatment of PTSD			
Drug	Brand Name	Initial Dose	Usual Range (mg/day)	Comments
SSRIs				
Fluoxetine[a]	Prozac®	10 mg/day	10–40[b]	
Paroxetine[a]	Paxil®, Pexeva®	10–20 mg/day	20–40	Maximum dose is 50 mg/day[c]
Sertraline[a]	Zoloft®	25 mg/day	50–100	Maximum dose is 200 mg/day[c]
Other Agents				
Amitriptyline[a]	Elavil®	25 or 50 mg/day	75–200[b]	
Imipramine[a]	Tofranil®	25 or 50 mg/day	75–200[b]	
Mirtazapine[a]	Remeron®	15 mg/night	30–60[b]	
Phenelzine[a]	Nardil®	15 or 30 mg every night	45–90[b]	
Venlafaxine extended-release[a]	Effexor XR®	37.5 mg/day	75–225[b]	

(PTSD, posttraumatic stress disorder; SSRIs, selective serotonin reuptake inhibitors.)
[a]Available generically.
[b]Dosage used in clinical trials but not FDA approved.
[c]Dosage is FDA approved.

- Large prospective studies document the effectiveness of **sertraline** and **paroxetine** in acute management of PTSD. Long-term use of SSRIs (9–12 months) was effective in preventing relapse.
- In a 12-week trial comparing **venlafaxine XR** and **sertraline**, venlafaxine XR was effective in reducing the avoidance/numbing and hyperarousal cluster, whereas sertraline improved all PTSD symptom clusters.
- **Mirtazapine** was effective in doses up to 45 mg/day and is a second-line agent. **Amitriptyline and imipramine**, are also second-line drugs. **Phenelzine** is considered a third-line drug.
- If there is no improvement in the acute stress response 3 to 4 weeks following trauma, SSRIs should be started in a low dose with slow titration upward toward antidepressant doses. Eight to 12 weeks is an adequate duration of treatment to determine response.
- Responders to drug therapy should continue treatment for at least 12 months. When discontinued, drug therapy should be tapered slowly over 1 month or more to reduce the likelihood of relapse.
- **Prazosin**, in daily doses of 1 to 4 mg, can be useful in some patients with PTSD. It may be particularly helpful for nightmares and insomnia.
- **Risperidone, quetiapine, α_1-adrenergic antagonists**, **antidepressants**, **mood stabilizers**, and **anticonvulsants** may be used as augmenting agents in partial responders.

EVALUATION OF THERAPEUTIC OUTCOMES

- See patients frequently for the first 3 months, then monthly for 3 months. In months 6 to 12, patients can be seen every 2 months.
- Monitor for symptom response, suicidal ideation, disability, side effects, and treatment adherence. The Clinician-Administered PTSD Scale (CAPS) can be useful to assess symptom severity.

See Chapter 70, Anxiety Disorders: Generalized Anxiety, Panic, and Social Anxiety Disorders, authored by Sarah T. Melton and Cynthia K. Kirkwood, and Chapter 71, Posttraumatic Stress Disorder and Obsessive-Compulsive Disorder, authored by Cynthia K. Kirkwood, Sarah T. Melton, and Barbara G. Wells, for a more detailed discussion of this topic.

67 Bipolar Disorder

- Bipolar disorder is a common, lifelong, often severe cyclic mood disorder characterized by recurrent fluctuations in mood, energy, and behavior. The mania or hypomania is neither substance-related nor caused by any other medical condition or psychiatric disorder.
  - ✓ *Bipolar I disorder*: At least one manic episode, which may have been preceded by and may be followed by hypomanic or major depressive episode(s).
  - ✓ *Bipolar II disorder*: At least one hypomanic episode and a current or past major depressive episode.
- *Cyclothymic disorder*: Chronic fluctuations between subsyndromal depressive and hypomanic episodes.

PATHOPHYSIOLOGY

- Medical conditions, medications, and treatments that may induce mania are shown in Table 67–1.
- Bipolar disorder is influenced by developmental, genetic, neurobiological, and psychological factors. Probably multiple gene loci are involved in heredity.

CLINICAL PRESENTATION

- Different types of episodes may occur sequentially with or without a period of normal mood (euthymia) between. There can be mood fluctuations that continue for months or after one episode, there can be years without recurrence of any type of mood episode (Table 67–2).

DIAGNOSIS

- The *Diagnostic and Statistical Manual of Mental Disorders*, 5th edition classifies bipolar disorders as (1) bipolar I, (2) bipolar II, (3) cyclothymic disorder, (4) other specified bipolar and related disorder, and (5) unspecified bipolar and related disorder. See Table 67–2 for diagnostic criteria for major depressive episode, manic episode, and hypomanic episode.
- A medical, psychiatric, and medication history; physical examination; and laboratory testing are necessary to rule out organic causes of mania or depression.
- Delusions, hallucinations, and suicide attempts are more common in bipolar depression than in unipolar depression.
- Acute mania usually begins abruptly, and symptoms increase over several days. Bizarre behavior, hallucinations, and paranoid or grandiose delusions may occur. There is marked impairment in functioning. Manic episodes may be precipitated by stressors, sleep deprivation, antidepressants, central nervous system (CNS) stimulants, or bright light.
- In hypomanic episodes, there is no marked impairment in social or occupational functioning, no delusions, and no hallucinations. Some patients may be more productive than usual, but 5% to 15% of patients may rapidly switch to a manic episode.

COURSE OF ILLNESS

- Childhood onset is associated with more mood episodes, rapid cycling, and comorbid psychiatric conditions.
- Rapid cyclers, 20% of bipolar patients, have four or more episodes per year (major depressive, manic, or hypomanic). Rapid cycling is associated with frequent and severe episodes of depression and a poorer long-term prognosis.

TABLE 67-1	Secondary Causes of Mania

Medical conditions that induce mania
- CNS disorders (brain tumor, strokes, head injuries, subdural hematoma, multiple sclerosis, systemic lupus erythematosus, temporal lobe seizures, Huntington disease)
- Infections (encephalitis, neurosyphilis, sepsis, human immunodeficiency virus)
- Electrolyte or metabolic abnormalities (calcium or sodium fluctuations, hyperglycemia or hypoglycemia)
- Endocrine or hormonal dysregulation (Addison disease, Cushing disease, hyperthyroidism or hypothyroidism, menstrual-related or pregnancy-related or perimenopausal mood disorders)

Medications or drugs that induce mania
- Alcohol intoxication
- Drug withdrawal states (alcohol, α_2-adrenergic agonists, antidepressants, barbiturates, benzodiazepines, opiates)
- Antidepressants (MAOIs, TCAs, 5-HT and/or NE and/or DA reuptake inhibitors, 5-HT antagonists)
- DA-augmenting agents (CNS stimulants: amphetamines, cocaine, sympathomimetics; DA agonists, releasers, and reuptake inhibitors)
- Hallucinogens (LSD, PCP)
- Marijuana intoxication precipitates psychosis, paranoid thoughts, anxiety, and restlessness
- NE-augmenting agents (α_2-adrenergic antagonists, β-agonists, NE reuptake inhibitors)
- Steroids (anabolic, adrenocorticotropic hormone, corticosteroids)
- Thyroid preparations
- Xanthines (caffeine, theophylline)
- Nonprescription weight loss agents and decongestants (ephedra, pseudoephedrine)
- Herbal products (St. John wort)

Somatic therapies that induce mania
- Bright light therapy
- Deep brain stimulation
- Sleep deprivation

(CNS, central nervous system; DA, dopamine; 5-HT, serotonin; LSD, lysergic acid diethylamide; MAOI, monoamine oxidase inhibitor; NE, norepinephrine; PCP, phencyclidine; TCA, tricyclic antidepressant.)

- Women are more likely to have depressive symptoms, older age of onset, better adherence, and thyroid abnormalities. Men may have more manic episodes and substance use.
- Suicide attempts occur in up to 50% of patients with bipolar disorder, and ~10% to 19% of individuals with bipolar I disorder commit suicide. Patients with bipolar II disorder may have a higher rate of suicide attempts.
- With aging, episodes may become longer in duration and more frequent.

TREATMENT

- Goals of Treatment: Table 67–3.

GENERAL APPROACH

- Table 67–4 shows an algorithmic approach to treating acute episodes including refractory episodes in adults.
- Adherence to treatment is the most important factor in achieving goals.
- Bipolar patients should remain on a mood stabilizer (eg, lithium, valproate, carbamazepine) lifelong.

TABLE 67–2	Evaluation and Diagnosis of Mood Episodes	
Diagnosis Episode	**Impairment of Functioning or Need for Hospitalization[a]**	**DSM-5 Criteria[b]**
Major depressive	Yes	At least 2 week period of either depressed mood or loss of interest or pleasure in normal activities, associated with at least five of the following symptoms: • Depressed, sad mood (adults); can be irritable mood in children • Decreased interest and pleasure in normal activities • Decreased or increased appetite, weight loss or weight gain • Insomnia or hypersomnia • Psychomotor retardation or agitation • Decreased energy or fatigue • Feelings of excessive guilt or worthlessness • Impaired concentration or indecisiveness • Recurrent thoughts of death, suicidal thoughts or attempts
Manic	Yes	At least 1-week period of abnormally and persistently elevated mood (expansive or irritable) and energy, associated with at least three of the following symptoms (four if the mood is only irritable): • Inflated self-esteem (grandiosity) • Decreased need for sleep • Increased talking (pressure of speech) • Racing thoughts (flight of ideas) • Distractibility (poor attention) • Increased goal-directed activity (socially, at work, or sexually) or psychomotor agitation • Excessive involvement in activities that are pleasurable but have a high risk for serious consequences (buying sprees, sexual indiscretions, poor judgment in business ventures)
Hypomanic	No	At least 4 days of abnormally and persistently elevated mood (expansive or irritable) and energy, associated with at least three of the following symptoms (four if the mood is only irritable): • Inflated self-esteem (grandiosity) • Decreased need for sleep • Increased talking (pressure of speech) • Racing thoughts (flight of ideas) • Distractibility (poor attention) • Increased goal-directed activity (socially, at work, or sexually) or psychomotor agitation • Excessive involvement in activities that are pleasurable but have a high risk for serious consequences (buying sprees, sexual indiscretions, poor judgment in business ventures)

[a]Impairment in social or occupational functioning; may include need for hospitalization because of potential self-harm, harm to others, or psychotic symptoms.
[b]The disorder is not caused by a medical condition (eg, hypothyroidism) or substance-induced disorder (eg, antidepressant treatment, medications, drugs of abuse). Numerous specifiers are available to further characterize episodes (eg, with mixed features, with anxious distress, with rapid cycling, with melancholic features).

TABLE 67–3	General Principles for the Management of Bipolar Disorder

Goals of treatment
- Eliminate mood episode with complete remission of symptoms (ie, acute treatment)
- Prevent recurrences or relapses of mood episodes (ie, continuation phase treatment)
- Return to baseline psychosocial functioning
- Maximize adherence with therapy
- Minimize adverse effects
- Use medications with the best tolerability and fewest drug interactions
- Treat comorbid substance use and abuse
- Eliminate alcohol, marijuana, cocaine, amphetamines, and hallucinogens
- Minimize nicotine use and stop caffeine intake at least 8 hours prior to bedtime
- Avoidance of stressors or substances that precipitate an acute episode

Monitor for
- Mood episodes: Document symptoms on a daily mood chart (document life stressors, type of episode, length of episode, and treatment outcome); monthly and yearly life charts are valuable for documenting patterns of mood cycles
- Medication adherence (missing doses of medications is a primary reason for nonresponse and recurrence of episodes)
- Adverse effects, especially sedation and weight gain (manage rapidly and vigorously to avoid noncompliance)
- Suicidal ideation or attempts (suicide completion rates with bipolar I disorder are 10%–15%; suicide attempts are primarily associated with depressive episodes, mixed episodes with severe depression, or presence of psychosis)

NONPHARMACOLOGIC THERAPY

- Nonpharmacologic approaches may include: (1) psychotherapy, interpersonal therapy, and/or cognitive behavioral therapy, (2) stress reduction techniques, relaxation therapy, massage, and yoga, (3) sleep (regular bedtime and awake schedule; avoid alcohol or caffeine intake prior to bedtime), (4) nutrition (regular intake of protein-rich foods or drinks and essential fatty acids; supplemental vitamins and minerals), and (5) exercise at least three times a week.

PHARMACOLOGIC THERAPY

- See Table 67–5 for product and dosing information on medications for bipolar disorder.
- See Table 67–6 for guidelines for laboratory monitoring of patients on mood stabilizers.
- **Lithium, divalproex sodium (valproate), extended-release carbamazepine, aripiprazole, asenapine, cariprazine, olanzapine, quetiapine, risperidone**, and **ziprasidone** are currently approved by the U.S. Food and Drug administration (FDA) for treatment of acute mania. **Lithium, aripiprazole, olanzapine**, and **lamotrigine** are approved for maintenance treatment.
- **Quetiapine** and **lurasidone** are the only FDA-approved monotherapy antipsychotics for bipolar depression.
- Combination therapies (see Table 67–4) can provide better acute response and long-term prevention of relapse and recurrence than monotherapy in some bipolar patients.
- Useful guidelines include the following: Canadian Network for Mood and Anxiety Treatments (CANMAT); International Society for Bipolar Disorders Guidelines; and International Task Force of the World Federation of Societies of Biological Psychiatry (WFSBP).

TABLE 67–4 Algorithm and Guidelines for the Acute Treatment of Mood Episodes in Patients with Bipolar I Disorder

Acute Manic or Mixed Episode	Acute Depressive Episode
General guidelines Assess for secondary causes of mania or mixed states (eg, alcohol or drug use) Discontinue antidepressants Taper off stimulants and caffeine if possible Treat substance abuse Encourage good nutrition (with regular protein and essential fatty acid intake), exercise, adequate sleep, stress reduction, and psychosocial therapy	**General guidelines** Assess for secondary causes of depression (eg, alcohol or drug use) Taper off antipsychotics, benzodiazepines, or sedative–hypnotic agents if possible Treat substance abuse Encourage good nutrition (with regular protein and essential fatty acid intake), exercise, adequate sleep, stress reduction, and psychosocial therapy
Hypomania **First**, optimize current mood stabilizer or initiate mood-stabilizing medication: lithium,[a] valproate,[a] carbamazepine,[a] or SGAs Consider adding a benzodiazepine (lorazepam or clonazepam) for short-term adjunctive treatment of agitation or insomnia if needed Alternative medication treatment options: oxcarbazepine **Mania** **First**, two- or three-drug combinations (lithium,[a] valproate,[a] or SGA) **plus** a benzodiazepine (lorazepam or clonazepam) and/or antipsychotic for short-term adjunctive treatment of agitation or insomnia; lorazepam is recommended for catatonia Do not combine antipsychotics Alternative medication treatment options: carbamazepine[a]; if patient does not respond or tolerate, consider oxcarbazepine	**Mild to moderate depressive episode** **First**, initiate and/or optimize mood-stabilizing medication: lithium,[a] quetiapine, lurasidone Alternative anticonvulsants: lamotrigine,[b] valproate[a]; antipsychotics: fluoxetine/olanzapine combination **Severe depressive episode** **First**, optimize current mood stabilizer or initiate mood-stabilizing medication: lithium[a] or quetiapine or lurasidone Alternative fluoxetine/olanzapine combination If psychosis is present, initiate an antipsychotic in combination with above Do not combine antipsychotics Alternative anticonvulsants: lamotrigine,[b] valproate[a]

(continued)

TABLE 67–4 Algorithm and Guidelines for the Acute Treatment of Mood Episodes in Patients with Bipolar I Disorder *(Continued)*

Acute Manic or Mixed Episode	Acute Depressive Episode
Second, if response is inadequate, consider a two-drug combination: Lithium[a] **plus** an anticonvulsant or an SGA — Anticonvulsant **plus** an anticonvulsant or SGA — **Second,** if response is inadequate, consider a three-drug combination: Lithium[a] **plus** an anticonvulsant **plus** an antipsychotic — Anticonvulsant **plus** an anticonvulsant **plus** an antipsychotic — **Third,** if response is inadequate, consider ECT for mania with psychosis or catatonia,[d] or add clozapine for treatment-refractory illness	**Second,** if response is inadequate, consider carbamazepine[c] or adding antidepressant — **Third,** if response is inadequate, consider a three-drug combination: Lithium **plus** lamotrigine[b] **plus** an antidepressant — Lithium **plus** quetiapine[c] **plus** antidepressant[c] — **Fourth,** if response is inadequate, consider ECT for treatment-refractory illness and depression with psychosis or catatonia[d]

(ECT, electroconvulsive therapy; SGA, second-generation antipsychotic.)

[a]Use standard therapeutic serum concentration ranges if clinically indicated; if partial response or breakthrough episode, adjust dose to achieve higher serum concentrations without causing intolerable adverse effects; valproate is preferred over lithium for mixed episodes and rapid cycling; lithium and/or lamotrigine is preferred over valproate for bipolar depression.

[b]Lamotrigine is not approved for the acute treatment of depression, and the dose must be started low and slowly titrated up to decrease adverse effects if used for maintenance therapy of bipolar I disorder. Lamotrigine may be initiated during acute treatment with plans to transition to this medication for long-term maintenance. A drug interaction and a severe dermatologic rash can occur when lamotrigine is combined with valproate (ie, lamotrigine doses must be halved from standard dosing titration).

[c]Controversy exists concerning the use of antidepressants, and they are often considered third line in treating acute bipolar depression, except in patients with no recent history of severe acute mania or potentially in bipolar II patients.

[d]ECT is used for severe mania or depression during pregnancy and for mixed episodes; prior to treatment, anticonvulsants, lithium, and benzodiazepines should be tapered off to maximize therapy and minimize adverse effects.

TABLE 67-5 Products, Dosage and Administration, and Clinical Use of Agents Used in the Treatment of Bipolar Disorder

Drug "Brand name"	Initial Dosing	Usual Dosing; Special Population Dosing	Comments
Lithium salts: FDA-approved for bipolar disorder			
Lithium carbonate[a,b] "Eskalith" "Eskalith CR" "Lithobid" Lithium citrate[a,b] "Cibalith-S"	300 mg twice daily	900–2400 mg/day in two to four divided doses, preferably with meals Renal impairment: lower doses required with frequent serum monitoring There is wide variation in the dosage needed to achieve therapeutic response and trough serum lithium concentration (ie, 0.6–1.2 mEq/L [mmol/L] for maintenance therapy and 0.8–1.2 mEq/L [mmol/L] for acute mood episodes taken 12 hours after the last dose)	Use alone or in combination with other medications (eg, valproate, carbamazepine, antipsychotics) for the acute treatment of mania and for maintenance treatment
Anticonvulsants: FDA-approved for bipolar disorder			
Divalproex sodium[a] "Depakote" "Depakote ER" Valproic acid[a] "Stavzor"	250–500 mg twice daily A loading dose of divalproex (20–30 mg/kg/day) can be given	750–3000 mg/day (20–60 mg/kg/day) given once daily or in divided doses Titrate to clinical response Dose adjustment needed with hepatic impairment	Use alone or in combination with other medications (eg, lithium, carbamazepine, antipsychotics) for the acute treatment of mania and for maintenance treatment Use caution when combining with lamotrigine because of potential drug interaction
Lamotrigine[b] "Lamictal"	25 mg daily	50–400 mg/day in divided doses. Dosage should be slowly increased (eg, 25 mg/day for 2 weeks, then 50 mg/day for weeks 3 and 4, and then 50-mg/day increments at weekly intervals up to 200 mg/day) Dose adjustment needed with hepatic impairment and in those taking valproate	Use alone or in combination with other medications (eg, lithium, carbamazepine) for long-term maintenance treatment for bipolar I disorder

(continued)

TABLE 67–5	Products, Dosage and Administration, and Clinical Use of Agents Used in the Treatment of Bipolar Disorder *(Continued)*		
Drug	Initial Dosing	Usual Dosing; Special Population Dosing	Comments
Carbamazepine "Equetro"	200 mg twice daily	200–1800 mg/day in two to four divided doses Titrate to clinical response Dose adjustment needed with hepatic impairment	Use alone or in combination with other medications (eg, lithium, valproate, antipsychotics) for the acute and long-term maintenance treatment of mania or mixed episodes for bipolar I disorder. APA guidelines recommend reserving it for patients unable to tolerate or who have inadequate response to lithium or valproate Extended-release tablets should be swallowed whole and not be broken or chewed
Anticonvulsants: not FDA-approved for bipolar disorder			
Carbamazepine "Tegretol" "Epitol" "Tegretol-XR" "Carbatrol"	200 mg twice daily	200–1800 mg/day in two to four divided doses Titrate to clinical response Dose adjustment needed with hepatic impairment	"Carbatrol" capsules can be opened and contents sprinkled over food
Valproic acid "Depakene" Valproate sodium "Depacon"	250–500 mg twice daily A loading dose of divalproex (20–30 mg/kg/day) can be given	750–3000 mg/day (20–60 mg/kg/day) given once daily or in divided doses Titrate to clinical response Dose adjustment needed with hepatic impairment	Use caution when combining with lamotrigine because of potential drug interaction
Oxcarbazepine "Trileptal"	300 mg twice daily	300–1200 mg/day in two divided doses Titrate based on clinical response Dose adjustment required with severe renal impairment	Use after patients have failed treatment with carbamazepine or have intolerable side effects May have fewer adverse effects and be better tolerated than carbamazepine

Bipolar Disorder | CHAPTER 67

Atypical antipsychotics: FDA-approved for bipolar disorder

Drug	Dose
Aripiprazole[a,b] "Abilify"	10–15 mg daily	10–30 mg/day once daily
Asenapine[a] "Saphris"	5–10 mg twice daily sublingually	5–10 mg twice daily sublingually
Cariprazine[a] "Vraylar"	1.5 mg daily	3–6 mg daily
Lurasidone[c] "Latuda"	20 mg daily	20–120 mg daily with food
Olanzapine[a,b] "Zyprexa" "Zyprexa Zydis"	2.5–5 mg twice daily	5–20 mg/day once daily or in divided doses
Olanzapine and fluoxetine[c] "Symbyax"	6 mg olanzapine and 25 mg fluoxetine daily	6–12 mg olanzapine and 25–50 mg fluoxetine daily
Quetiapine[a,c] "Seroquel"	50 mg twice daily	50–800 mg/day in divided doses or once daily when stabilized
Risperidone[a] "Risperdal" "Risperdal M-Tab"	0.5–1 mg twice daily	0.5–6 mg/day once daily or in divided doses
Ziprasidone[a] "Geodon"	40–60 mg twice daily	40–160 mg/day in divided doses
Benzodiazepines	Dosage should be slowly adjusted up and down according to response and adverse effects	Use in combination with other medications (eg, antipsychotics, lithium, valproate) for the acute treatment of mania or mixed episodes Use as a short-term adjunctive sedative–hypnotic agent

FDA-approved agents may be used as monotherapy in various phases of the illness as noted in table footnotes.[a,b,c]
[a]FDA-approved for acute mania.
[b]FDA-approved for maintenance.
[c]FDA-approved for acute bipolar depression.

715

TABLE 67–6 Guidelines for Baseline and Routine Laboratory Tests and Monitoring for Patients with Bipolar Disorder Taking Mood Stabilizers

	Baseline: Physical Examination and General Chemistry[a]	Hematologic Tests[b]		Metabolic Tests[c]		Liver Function Tests[d]		Renal Function Tests[e]		Thyroid Function Tests[f]		Serum Electrolytes[g]		Dermatologic[h]	
	Baseline	Baseline	6–12 months	Baseline	6–12 months	Baseline	6–12 months	Baseline	6–12 months	Baseline	6–12 months	Baseline	6–12 months	Baseline	6–12 months
SGAs[i]	X			X	X										
Carbamazepine[j]	X	X	X			X	X	X					X	X	X
Lamotrigine[k]	X													X	X
Lithium[l]	X	X	X	X				X	X	X	X	X	X	X	X
Oxcarbazepine[m]	X											X	X		
Valproate[n]	X	X	X	X		X	X							X	X

(SGAs, second-generation antipsychotics.)

[a]Screen for drug abuse and serum pregnancy.

[b]Complete blood count (CBC) with differential and platelets.

[c]Fasting glucose, serum lipids, and weight.

[d]Lactate dehydrogenase, aspartate aminotransferase, alanine aminotransferase, total bilirubin, and alkaline phosphatase.

[e]Serum creatinine, blood urea nitrogen, urinalysis, and specific gravity.

[f]Triiodothyronine, total thyroxine, thyroxine uptake, and thyroid-stimulating hormone.

[g]Serum sodium.

[h]Rashes, hair thinning, and alopecia.

[i]Second-generation antipsychotics: Monitor for increased appetite with weight gain (primarily in patients with initial low or normal body mass index); monitor closely if rapid or significant weight gain occurs during early therapy; cases of hyperlipidemia and diabetes reported.

[j]Carbamazepine: Manufacturer recommends CBC and platelets (and possibly reticulocyte counts and serum iron) at baseline, and that subsequent monitoring be individualized by the clinician (eg, CBC, platelet counts, and liver function tests every 2 weeks during the first 2 months of treatment, and then every 3 months if normal). Monitor more closely if patient exhibits hematologic or hepatic abnormalities or if the patient is receiving a myelotoxic drug; discontinue if platelets are $<100,000/mm^3$ ($<100 \times 10^9/L$), if white blood cell (WBC) count is $<3000/mm^3$ ($<3 \times 10^9/L$), or if there is evidence of bone marrow suppression or liver dysfunction. Serum electrolyte levels should be monitored in the elderly or those at risk for hyponatremia. Carbamazepine interferes with some pregnancy tests.

[k]Lamotrigine: If renal or hepatic impairment, monitor closely and adjust dosage according to manufacturer's guidelines. Serious dermatologic reactions have occurred within 2 to 8 weeks of initiating treatment and are more likely to occur in patients receiving concomitant valproate, with rapid dosage escalation, or using doses exceeding the recommended titration schedule.

[l]Lithium: Obtain baseline electrocardiogram for patients older than 40 years or if preexisting cardiac disease (benign, reversible T-wave depression can occur). Renal function tests should be obtained every 2 to 3 months during the first 6 months, and then every 6 to 12 months; if impaired renal function, monitor 24-hour urine volume and creatinine every 3 months; if urine volume >3 L/day, monitor urinalysis, osmolality, and specific gravity every 3 months. Thyroid function tests should be obtained once or twice during the first 6 months, and then every 6 to 12 months; monitor for signs and symptoms of hypothyroidism; if supplemental thyroid therapy is required, monitor thyroid function tests and adjust thyroid dose every 1 to 2 months until thyroid function indices are within normal range, and then monitor every 3 to 6 months.

[m]Oxcarbazepine: Hyponatremia (serum sodium concentrations <125 mEq/L [mmol/L]) has been reported and occurs more frequently during the first 3 months of therapy; serum sodium concentrations should be monitored in patients receiving drugs that lower serum sodium concentrations (eg, diuretics or drugs that cause inappropriate antidiuretic hormone secretion) or in patients with symptoms of hyponatremia (eg, confusion, headache, lethargy, and malaise). Hypersensitivity reactions have occurred in approximately 25% to 30% of patients with a history of carbamazepine hypersensitivity and require immediate discontinuation.

[n]Valproate: Weight gain reported in patients with low or normal body mass index. Monitor platelets and liver function during first 3 to 6 months if evidence of increased bruising or bleeding. Monitor closely if patients exhibit hematologic or hepatic abnormalities or in patients receiving drugs that affect coagulation, such as aspirin or warfarin; discontinue if platelets are <100,000/mm^3/L (<100 × 10^9/L) or if prolonged bleeding time. Pancreatitis, hyperammonemic encephalopathy, polycystic ovary syndrome, increased testosterone, and menstrual irregularities have been reported; not recommended during first trimester of pregnancy due to risk of neural tube defects.

Lithium

- **Lithium** is a first-line agent for acute mania, acute bipolar depression, and maintenance treatment of bipolar I and II disorders.
- Lithium is rapidly absorbed, neither protein bound nor metabolized, and excreted unchanged in the urine and other body fluids.
- It may require 6 to 8 weeks to show antidepressant efficacy. It is more effective for elated mania and less effective for mania with psychotic features, mixed episodes, rapid cycling, and when alcohol and drug abuse are present. It produces a prophylactic response in up to two thirds of patients and reduces suicide risk.
- Abrupt discontinuation or noncompliance with lithium therapy can increase the risk of relapse.
- Lithium augmentation of **carbamazepine**, **lamotrigine**, and **valproate** can improve response in bipolar I patients, but it may increase the risk of sedation, weight gain, gastrointestinal (GI) complaints, and tremor.
- Initial GI and central nervous system (CNS) side effects are often dose related and are worse at peak serum concentrations (1–2 hours postdose). Lowering the dose, taking smaller doses with food, using extended-release products, and once-daily dosing at bedtime may help. Diarrhea can sometimes be improved by switching to a liquid formulation.
- Muscle weakness and lethargy occur in ~40% to 50% of patients and is usually transient.
- A fine hand tremor occurs in up to 50% of patients and usually resolves with continued treatment. It may be treated by switching to a long-acting preparation, lowering the dose, or adding **propranolol**, 20 to 120 mg/day.
- Polydipsia with polyuria with or without nephrogenic diabetes insipidus (DI) can occur. About 30% to 50% of patients will develop nephrogenic DI soon after initiating lithium, and it persists in about 10% to 25% of patients. It is typically reversible with continued lithium dosing. Nocturia is common and is managed by changing to once-daily dosing at bedtime.
- Lithium reduces the kidneys' ability to concentrate urine and may cause a nephrogenic DI with low urine-specific gravity and low osmolality polyuria (urine volume >3 L/day). This may be treated with **loop** or **thiazide diuretics** or **triamterene**. If a thiazide diuretic is used, lithium doses should be decreased by 50% and lithium and potassium levels monitored. **Amiloride** has weaker natriuretic effects and seems to have little effect on lithium clearance.
- Long-term lithium therapy is associated with a 10% to 20% risk of morphologic renal changes.
- Hypothyroidism can occur in 1% to 4% of lithium-treated patients (more common in women) and does not require discontinuation of lithium. Exogenous thyroid hormone (ie, levothyroxine) can be added to the regimen. If lithium is discontinued, the need for the levothyroxine should be reassessed, as hypothyroidism can be reversible.
- Lithium may cause cardiac effects including T-wave flattening or inversion (up to 30% of patients), atrioventricular block, and bradycardia. In patients with significant cardiac disease, an ECG and consultation with a cardiologist is recommended at baseline and periodically during therapy.
- Other late-appearing lithium side effects are benign reversible leukocytosis, acne, alopecia, exacerbation of psoriasis, folliculitis, and weight gain.
- Lithium toxicity can occur with serum levels greater than 1.5 mEq/L (mmol/L), but the elderly may have toxic symptoms at therapeutic levels. Severe toxic symptoms (eg, vomiting, diarrhea, incontinence, incoordination, impaired cognition, arrhythmias, seizures, permanent neurologic impairment, and kidney damage) may occur with serum concentrations above 2 mEq/L (mmol/L).
- Factors predisposing to lithium toxicity include sodium restriction, dehydration, vomiting, diarrhea, age greater than 50 years, heart failure, drug interactions that decrease lithium clearance, heavy exercise, sauna baths, hot weather, and fever. Tell patients to maintain adequate sodium and fluid intake and to avoid alcohol and excessive caffeine-containing beverages.

- If lithium toxicity is suspected, discontinue lithium and send the patient immediately to the emergency room.
- Consider intermittent hemodialysis in these situations:
  ✓ In lithium naive patients, when lithium serum concentrations are at least 4 mEq/L (mmol/L).
  ✓ In patients previously taking lithium, when lithium serum concentrations are 2.5 mEq/L (mmol/L) or greater and moderate-to-severe neurologic toxicity is present or as clinically indicated.
- Continue hemodialysis until serum lithium concentration is below 2 mEq/L (mmol/L) when drawn 8 hours after the last dialysis.
- **Thiazide diuretics, nonsteroidal anti-inflammatory drugs, angiotensin-converting enzyme inhibitors**, and salt-restricted diets can elevate lithium levels. Neurotoxicity can occur when lithium is combined with antipsychotics, methyldopa, metronidazole, phenytoin, and verapamil. Combining lithium with **calcium channel blockers** is not recommended because of reports of neurotoxicity. **Acetaminophen** or **aspirin** and **loop diuretics** are less likely to interfere with lithium clearance. Caffeine and theophylline can enhance renal elimination of lithium.
- Lithium is usually initiated with 600 mg/day for prophylaxis and 900 to 1200 mg/day for acute mania. Give immediate-release preparations two or three times daily and extended-release products once or twice daily. After patients are stabilized, many patients can switch to once-daily dosing.
- Lithium levels are considered to be at steady state after approximately 5 days. Initially, check serum lithium concentrations once or twice weekly. After a desired serum concentration is achieved, check levels in 2 weeks, and when stable, check them every 3 to 6 months.
- Lithium clearance increases by 50% to 100% during pregnancy. Monitor serum levels monthly during pregnancy and weekly the month before delivery. At delivery, reduce dose to prepregnancy levels and maintain hydration.
- A reasonable therapeutic trial in outpatients is at least 4 to 6 weeks with lithium serum concentrations of 0.6 to 1.2 mEq/L (mmol/L). Patients with serum concentrations between 0.8 and 1 mEq/L (mmol/L) may have fewer relapses than those with lower serum concentrations. Acutely manic patients can require serum concentrations of 1 to 1.2 mEq/L (mmol/L), and some need up to 1.5 mEq/L (mmol/L). Draw lithium levels 12 hours postdose. For bipolar prophylaxis in elderly patients, serum concentrations of 0.4 to 0.6 mEq/L (mmol/L) are recommended.

Anticonvulsants

- For more in-depth information on the side effects, pharmacokinetics, and drug interactions of anticonvulsants, refers to Chap. 53.

Valproate Sodium and Valproic Acid

- **Divalproex sodium** (**sodium valproate**), approved for acute manic or mixed episodes, is the most prescribed mood stabilizer in the United States. It is as effective as **lithium** and **olanzapine** for pure mania, and it can be more effective than lithium for rapid cycling, mixed states, and bipolar disorder with substance abuse. It reduces the frequency of (or prevents) recurrent manic, depressive, and mixed episodes.
- **Lithium, carbamazepine, antipsychotics**, or **benzodiazepines** can augment the antimanic effects of valproate. Valproate can be added to lithium to achieve synergistic effects in patients who are treatment refractory and are rapid cyclers or have mixed features, and the combination is effective as maintenance therapy of bipolar I disorder. The potential for drug interactions necessitate blood level monitoring of both agents. **Second-generation antipsychotics (SGA)** can be added to valproate for breakthrough mania, but they can increase the risk of sedation and weight gain. Combining valproate with lamotrigine increases the risk of rashes, ataxia, tremor, sedation, and fatigue.

- The most frequent dose-related side effects of valproate are GI complaints, fine tremor, and sedation. Giving it with food, reducing the initial dose and making gradual increases, or switching to the extended release formulation can help alleviate the GI complaints. Reducing the dose or adding a β-blocker may alleviate tremors. Giving the total dose at bedtime can minimize daytime sedation. Other side effects are ataxia, lethargy, alopecia, pruritus, prolonged bleeding, transient increases in liver enzymes, weight gain, and hyperammonemia. Lowering valproate dose may restore platelet counts to normal levels. Fatal necrotizing hepatitis is rare and idiosyncratic, occurring in children on multiple anticonvulsants. Life-threatening pancreatitis has been reported.
- For healthy patients with acute mania, a loading dose of 20 to 30 mg/kg/day of divalproex can be given over 12 hours. The daily dose is adjusted by 250 to 500 mg every 1 to 3 days based on response and tolerability. The maximum dose is 60 mg/kg/day (see Table 67–5).
- For outpatients who are hypomanic or euthymic, or for elderly patients, the initial dose is generally lower (5–10 mg/kg/day in divided doses) and gradually titrated to avoid side effects.
- After establishing the optimal dose, the dose can be given twice daily or at bedtime if tolerated.
- Extended-release divalproex can be given once daily, but bioavailability can be 15% lower than that of immediate release products.
- Most clinicians seek a serum concentration range of 50 to 125 mcg/mL (347–866 μmol/L) measured 12 hours after the last dose. Patients with cyclothymia or bipolar II disorder respond at lower blood levels, while patients with more severe forms may require up to 150 mcg/mL (1040 μmol/L). Serum levels are most useful when assessing for compliance or toxicity.

Carbamazepine

- **Carbamazepine** is usually reserved for use after treatment failure with lithium or divalproex sodium. Only the extended-release formulation is FDA approved for bipolar disorder in the United States.
- It has acute antimanic effects, but its long-term effectiveness is less clear. It may be less effective than lithium for maintenance therapy and for bipolar depression.
- The combination of carbamazepine with **lithium, valproate**, and antipsychotics is often used for manic episodes in treatment-resistant patients.
- Adverse effects of carbamazepine are summarized in Chap. 56.
- Carbamazepine induces the hepatic metabolism of antidepressants, anticonvulsants, antipsychotics, and many other medications. Women taking **oral contraceptives** who receive carbamazepine should be counseled to use a nonhormonal method of contraception.
- Certain medications that inhibit CYP3A4 (eg, **cimetidine, diltiazem, erythromycin, fluoxetine, fluvoxamine, itraconazole, ketoconazole, nefazodone**, and **verapamil**) added to carbamazepine therapy may cause carbamazepine toxicity. When carbamazepine is combined with valproate, reduce the carbamazepine dose, as its free levels can be increased. Do not combine **clozapine** and carbamazepine because of possible additive bone marrow suppression.
- For inpatients in an acute manic episode, doses can be started at 400 to 600 mg/day in divided doses with meals and increased by 200 mg/day every 2 to 4 days up to 10 to 15 mg/kg/day. Outpatients should be started at lower doses and titrated upward more slowly to avoid side effects. Many patients tolerate once-daily dosing after stabilization.
- During the first month of therapy, serum concentrations may decrease because of autoinduction of cytochrome P450 3A4 enzymes, requiring a dose increase.
- Carbamazepine serum levels are usually obtained every 1 or 2 weeks during the first 2 months, then every 3 to 6 months during maintenance. Serum samples are drawn 10 to 12 hours postdose and at least 4 to 7 days after dosage initiation or change. Most clinicians attempt to maintain levels between 6 and 10 mcg/mL (25–42 μmol/L), but some patients may require 12 to 14 mcg/mL (51–59 μmol/L).

- Use of carbamazepine in patients of Asian ancestry requires genetic testing for human leukocyte antigen (HLA) allele, HLA-B 1502, to help detect a higher risk of Stevens-Johnson syndrome and toxic epidermal necrolysis.

Oxcarbazepine

- **Oxcarbazepine** is not FDA approved for treatment of bipolar disorder in the United States. Guidelines typically recommend it as a third-line option for mania, a third- or fourth-line option for maintenance treatment, and it is not recommended for treatment of bipolar depression.
- It does not autoinduce its own metabolism. Discontinue oxcarbazepine at the first sign of a skin reaction, as severe dermatologic reactions have been reported (eg, Stevens-Johnson syndrome). Other adverse effects may include impaired cognitive or psychomotor performance, somnolence, fatigue, incoordination, and hyponatremia. It causes more hyponatremia than carbamazepine.
- It is a CYP 2C19 inhibitor and a 3A3/4 inducer. It induces the metabolism of **oral contraceptives**, necessitating use of alternative contraception measures.

Lamotrigine

- **Lamotrigine** has both antidepressant and mood-stabilizing effects. It may have augmenting properties when combined with **lithium** or **valproate**. It has a low rate of switching patients to mania. Although it is less effective for acute mania compared with lithium and valproate, it may be beneficial for the maintenance therapy of treatment-resistant bipolar I and II disorders. It seems most effective for prevention of bipolar depression.
- Common adverse effects include headache, nausea, dizziness, ataxia, diplopia, drowsiness, tremor, maculopapular rash, and pruritus. Although most rashes resolve with continued therapy, some progress to life-threatening Stevens–Johnson syndrome. Discontinue lamotrigine if the rash is diffuse, involves mucous membranes, and is accompanied by fever or sore throat. The incidence of rash is greatest with concomitant administration of **valproate**, rapid dose escalation of lamotrigine, and higher than recommended lamotrigine initial doses.
- In patients taking valproate, dose lamotrigine at about one half the standard doses, and titrate upward more slowly than usual.
- For maintenance treatment of bipolar disorder, the usual dosage range of lamotrigine is 50 to 300 mg/day. The target dose is generally 200 mg/day (100 mg/day when combined with **valproate** and 400 mg/day when combined with **carbamazepine**). For patients not taking medications that affect lamotrigine's clearance, the dose is 25 mg/day for the first 2 weeks, then 50 mg/day for weeks 3 and 4, 100 mg/day for the next week, then 200 mg/day. Patients who stop dosing for more than a few days should restart the dose escalation schedule.

Antipsychotics

- First- and second-generation antipsychotics, such as **aripiprazole, asenapine, haloperidol, olanzapine, quetiapine, risperidone**, and **ziprasidone** are effective as monotherapy or as add-on therapy for acute mania. Long-term antipsychotics can be needed for some patients, but the risks versus benefits must be weighed in view of long-term side effects (eg, obesity, type 2 diabetes, hyperlipidemia, hyperprolactinemia, and tardive dyskinesia).
- Both first- and second-generation antipsychotics are effective in ~70% of patients with acute mania associated with agitation, aggression, and psychosis.
- Clinical trials support the use of **quetiapine** and **lurasidone** as monotherapy and adjunctive treatment for bipolar depression. Data also support use of combined fluoxetine/olanzapine for bipolar depression.
- **Haloperidol decanoate, fluphenazine decanoate**, and **risperidone, aripiprazole, quetiapine, and olanzapine long-acting injection** are monotherapy options for maintenance therapy of bipolar disorder with noncompliance or treatment resistance.

- Controlled studies in acute mania suggest that **lithium** or **valproate** plus an antipsychotic is more effective than any of these agents alone.
- **Clozapine** monotherapy has acute and long-term mood stabilizing effects in refractory bipolar disorder, but requires regular white blood cell monitoring for agranulocytosis.
- Higher initial doses of antipsychotics (eg, 20 mg/day of **olanzapine**) can be required for acute mania. After mania is controlled (usually 7–28 days), the antipsychotic can be gradually tapered and discontinued, and the mood stabilizer monotherapy maintained.
- For more information on the side effects, pharmacokinetics, and drug interactions of specific antipsychotics, refer to Chap. 69.

Alternative Medication Treatment

- High-potency benzodiazepines (eg, **clonazepam** and **lorazepam**) are commonly used alternatives to (or adjuncts to) antipsychotics for acute mania, agitation, anxiety, panic, and insomnia or in those who cannot take mood stabilizers. **Intramuscular (IM) lorazepam** may be used for acute agitation. A relative contraindication for long-term benzodiazepines is a history of drug or alcohol abuse or dependency.
- Many clinicians consider adjunctive antidepressants third-line for acute bipolar depression, except in those with no history of severe and/or recent mania or potentially in bipolar II patients. The rate of mood switching from depression to mania with **tricyclic antidepressants** and **venlafaxine** is higher than the rate associated with use of selective serotonin reuptake inhibitors. Before initiating an antidepressant, be sure the patient has a therapeutic dose or blood level of a primary mood stabilizer. Be cautious in using antidepressants in those with a history of mania after a depressive episode, and those with frequent cycling. Generally, the antidepressant should be withdrawn 2 to 6 months after remission.

Special Populations

- The occurrence of Epstein anomaly in infants exposed to **lithium** during the first trimester is estimated to be between 1 and 10.78:1000, and the risk of neural tube defects is 13.4:1000.
- When **lithium** is used during pregnancy, use the lowest effective dose to prevent relapse, thus lessening the risk of "floppy" infant syndrome, hypothyroidism, and nontoxic goiter in the infant. Monitor closely and adjust dose as appropriate.
- Breast-feeding is usually discouraged for women taking lithium.
- When **valproate, carbamazepine**, and **lamotrigine** are taken during the first trimester, the risk of neural tube defects is ~4%, ~3%, and ~ 2%, respectively. Administration of folic acid can reduce the risk of neural tube defects.
- Women taking valproate may breast-feed, but mother and infant should have identical laboratory monitoring.
- **First generation antipsychotics** seem to have little teratogenic risk when used during pregnancy. Data on the **SGAs** are more limited. Risk to benefit ratio must be considered before using antipsychotics during pregnancy.
- **Lithium, valproic acid**, and **carbamazepine** are used in pediatric bipolar disorder, but data are limited. **Aripiprazole** and **risperidone** are FDA approved for bipolar mania in adolescents 13 to 17 years. Quetiapine is approved as monotherapy or adjunctive therapy to lithium or **divalproex** in manic patients aged 10 to 17 years. **Olanzapine** is approved for manic or mixed episodes in patients aged 13 to 17 years.
- Lithium is FDA approved as a mood stabilizer for children older than 12 years.
- A guideline for treatment of children and adolescents with bipolar disorder is *Practice Parameters for the Assessment and Treatment of Children and Adolescents with Bipolar Disorder.*
- The elimination half-life of **lithium** and **valproate** increases with age. Elderly patients can have many medical comorbidities and increased sensitivity to side effects of mood stabilizers and antipsychotics.

EVALUATION OF THERAPEUTIC OUTCOMES

- Monitoring parameters are shown in Table 67–3.
- Patients with partial response or nonresponse to therapy should be reassessed for accurate diagnosis, concomitant medical or psychiatric conditions, medication adherence, and use of medications or substances that exacerbate mood symptoms.
- Involve patients and family members in treatment to monitor target symptom response and side effects and to enhance adherence and reduce stressors. Standardized rating scales may be useful in monitoring for response.

See Chapter 69, Bipolar Disorder, authored by Shannon J. Drayton and Christopher S. Fields, for a more detailed discussion of this topic.

Major Depressive Disorder

- The essential feature of *major depressive disorder* (MDD) is a clinical course characterized by one or more major depressive episodes without a history of manic or hypomanic episodes.
- The reader is referred to the Practice Guideline for the Treatment of Patients with Major Depressive Disorder developed by the American Psychiatric Association and the guideline of the British Association of Psychopharmacology.

PATHOPHYSIOLOGY

- *Biogenic amine hypothesis:* Decreased brain levels of the neurotransmitters norepinephrine, serotonin (5-HT), and dopamine may cause depression.
- *Postsynaptic changes in receptor sensitivity:* Studies have demonstrated that desensitization or downregulation of norepinephrine or 5-HT_{1A} receptors may relate to onset of antidepressant effects.
- *Dysregulation hypothesis:* This theory emphasizes a failure of homeostatic regulation of neurotransmitter systems, rather than absolute increases or decreases in their activities.
- *5-HT/norepinephrine link hypothesis:* This theory suggests that 5-HT and norepinephrine activities are linked, and that both the serotonergic and noradrenergic systems are involved in antidepressant response.
- *The role of dopamine:* Evidence suggests that dopamine transmission is decreased in depression and that increased dopamine activity in the mesolimbic pathway contributes to antidepressant activity.
- Disruption of brain derived neurotrophic factor expression in the hippocampus may be associated with depression.

CLINICAL PRESENTATION

- *Emotional symptoms:* diminished ability to experience pleasure, loss of interest in usual activities, sadness, pessimism, crying, hopelessness, anxiety, guilt, and psychotic features (eg, auditory hallucinations and delusions).
- *Physical symptoms:* fatigue, pain (especially headache), sleep disturbance, decreased or increased appetite, loss of sexual interest, and gastrointestinal (GI) and cardiovascular complaints (especially palpitations).
- *Intellectual or cognitive symptoms:* decreased ability to concentrate, poor memory for recent events, confusion, and indecisiveness.
- *Psychomotor disturbances:* psychomotor retardation (slowed physical movements, thought processes, and speech) or psychomotor agitation.

DIAGNOSIS

- Major depressive disorder is characterized by one or more major depressive episodes, as defined by the *Diagnostic and Statistical Manual of Mental Disorders*, 5th ed. Five or more of the following must have been present nearly every day during the same 2-week period and cause significant distress or impairment (NOTE: depressed mood or loss of interest or pleasure must be present in adults [or irritable mood in children and adolescents]): depressed mood; diminished interest or pleasure in almost all activities; weight loss or gain; insomnia or hypersomnia; psychomotor agitation or retardation; fatigue or loss of energy; feelings of worthlessness or excessive guilt; diminished concentration or indecisiveness; recurrent thoughts of death, suicidal ideation without a specific plan, suicide attempt, or a plan for committing suicide.

The depressive episode must not be attributable to physiological effects of a substance or medical condition. Lastly, there must not be a history of manic-like or hypomanic-like episodes unless they were induced by a substance or medical condition.

- Diagnosis requires a medication review, physical examination, mental status examination, a complete blood count with differential, thyroid function tests, and electrolyte determination.
- Many chronic illnesses (eg, stroke, Parkinson disease, traumatic brain injury, hypothyroidism) and substance abuse and dependence disorders are associated with depression. Medications associated with depression include many antihypertensives, oral contraceptives, isotretinoin, interferon-β_{1a}, and many others.

TREATMENT

- <u>Goals of Treatment</u>: Resolution of current symptoms (ie, remission) and the prevention of further episodes of depression (ie, relapse or recurrence).

NONPHARMACOLOGIC TREATMENT

- Psychotherapy (eg, cognitive therapy, behavioral therapy, or interpersonal psychotherapy) may be first-line therapy for mild to moderately severe major depressive episode. The efficacy of psychotherapy and antidepressants is considered to be additive. Psychotherapy alone is not recommended for acute treatment of severe and/or psychotic MDD. For uncomplicated, nonchronic MDD, combined treatment may provide no unique advantage.
- Electroconvulsive therapy (ECT) may be considered when a rapid response is needed, risks of other treatments outweigh potential benefits, there is history of a poor response to drugs, and the patient prefers ECT. A rapid therapeutic response (10–14 days) has been reported.
- Repetitive transcranial magnetic stimulation has demonstrated efficacy and does not require anesthesia as does ECT.

PHARMACOLOGIC THERAPY
General Approach

- Figure 68–1 shows an algorithm for treatment of uncomplicated MDD. Table 68–1 guides adult dosing of antidepressants.
- Antidepressants are equal in efficacy in groups of patients when administered in comparable doses.
- Choice of antidepressant is influenced by the patient's or family member's history of response, concurrent medical conditions, medications the patient is taking, presenting symptoms, potential for drug–drug interactions, side effect profiles, patient preference, and drug cost.
- 50% to 60% of patients with varying types of depression improve with drug therapy.
- A 6-week trial of an antidepressant at maximum dosage is considered an adequate trial of that medication.
- The acute phase of treatment lasts 6 to 12 weeks, and the goal is remission (ie, absence of symptoms). The continuation phase (4–9 months after remission) seeks to eliminate residual symptoms or prevent relapse. The maintenance phase (12–36 months or more) seeks to prevent recurrence of a new episode of depression.
- Give elderly patients one half of the initial dose given to younger adults, and increase the dose more slowly. The elderly may require 6 to 12 weeks of treatment to achieve the desired antidepressant response.
- Some clinicians recommend lifelong therapy for persons younger than 40 years with two or more prior episodes and for all persons with three or more prior episodes.
- Educate patients and their support systems about the delay in antidepressant response (typically 2–4 weeks) and the importance of adherence before starting therapy and throughout treatment.

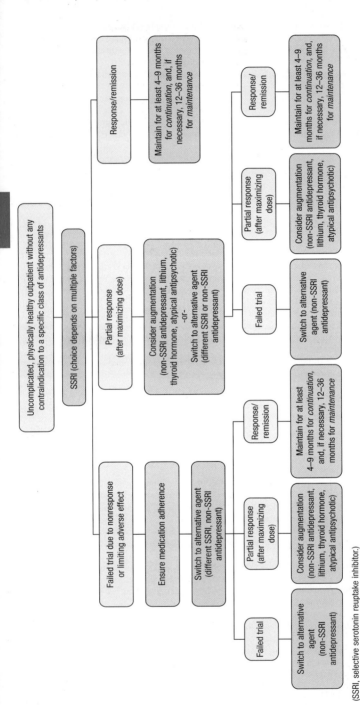

(SSRI, selective serotonin reuptake inhibitor.)

FIGURE 68–1. Suggested algorithm for treatment of uncomplicated MDD. Note: both the BAP guidelines and the STAR*D trial suggest that switching and augmentation strategies are supported by stronger evidence compared to dose increases (among poor antidepressant responders).

TABLE 68–1 Adult Dosing Guidance for Currently Available Antidepressant Medications

Drug (Brand Name)	Initial Dose (mg/day)	Usual Dosage Range (mg/day)	Comments (eg, Maximum Daily Dosage, Suggested Therapeutic Plasma Concentration)ᵃ
Selective serotonin reuptake inhibitors (SSRIs)			
Citalopram (Celexa)	20	20–40	Doses >40 mg/day not recommended due to QT prolongation risk; maximum 20 mg/day for CYP2C19 poor metabolizers or coadministration with CYP2C19 inhibitors; 20 mg/day recommended for patients older than 60 years of age
Escitalopram (Lexapro)	10	10–20	Maximum 20 mg/day; dose may be increased to maximum daily dose after at least 1 week if needed; 5 mg tablet available for unique circumstances
Fluoxetine (Prozac)	20	20–60	Maximum 80 mg/day; dose may be increased in 20 mg increments; doses of 5 or 10 mg/day have been used as initial therapy; doses >20 mg/day may be given in a single daily dose or divided twice daily
Fluvoxamine (Luvox)	50	50–300	Maximum 300 mg/day; daily doses >100 mg total dose should be divided twice daily, with the larger dose given at night Maximum 300 mg/day (ER formulation)
Paroxetine (Paxil)	20	20–50	Maximum 50 mg/day (IR formulation); titrate 10 mg/day increments weekly Maximum 62.5 mg/day (CR formulation); titrate 12.5 mg/day increments weekly
Sertraline (Zoloft)	50	50–200	Maximum 200 mg/day; titrate 25 mg/day increments weekly
Serotonin–Norepinephrine reuptake inhibitors (SNRIs)			
Newer-generation SNRIs			
Desvenlafaxine (Pristiq)	50	50	Doses up to 400 mg/day have been studied; however, AEs are increased and no additional benefit has been shown at doses exceeding 50 mg/day. Dose reductions or discontinuation may be required if sustained hypertension occurs
Duloxetine (Cymbalta)	30	30–90	Maximum 120 mg/day (given once or twice daily); doses exceeding 60 mg/day not shown to provide increased efficacy for the treatment of MDD

(continued)

TABLE 68–1 Adult Dosing Guidance for Currently Available Antidepressant Medications (Continued)

Drug (Brand Name)	Initial Dose (mg/day)	Usual Dosage Range (mg/day)	Comments (eg, Maximum Daily Dosage, Suggested Therapeutic Plasma Concentration)[a]
Venlafaxine (Effexor)	37.5–75	75–225	Maximum 375 mg/day (IR); maximum 225 mg/day (ER); may increase in increments up to 75 mg/day at a minimum of every 4 days. Dose reductions or discontinuation may be required if sustained hypertension occurs
Levomilnacipran (Fetzima)	20	40–120	Initial dose (20 mg) for 2 days before dose increases are recommended at intervals of two or more days. Dose adjustment or discontinuation may be required if sustained elevated heart rate or hypertension occurs
Tricyclic antidepressants (TCAs)			
Amitriptyline (Elavil)	25	100–200	Maximum 300 mg/day for MDD; depending on the total dose, it may be given as a single daily dose at bedtime or in divided doses throughout the day; Therapeutic serum level 100–250 ng/mL (mcg/L; 370–925 nmol/L); parent drug plus metabolite (ie, nortriptyline)
Desipramine (Norpramin)	25	100–200	Maximum 300 mg/day; Suggested therapeutic concentration range for combined imipramine + desipramine: 150–300 ng/mL (mcg/L; 550–1100 nmol/L)
Doxepin (Sinequan)	25	100–200	Maximum 300 mg/day; may be given in a single daily dose at bedtime (if tolerated) or in divided doses throughout the day; a single dose should not exceed 150 mg
Imipramine (Tofranil)	25	100–200	Maximum 300 mg/day; may be given in a single daily dose at bedtime (if tolerated) or in divided doses throughout the day; Suggested therapeutic concentration range for combined imipramine + desipramine: 150–300 ng/mL (mcg/L; 550–1100 nmol/L)
Nortriptyline (Pamelor)	25	50–150	Maximum 150 mg/day; total daily may be given as a single daily dose (if tolerated) or 25 mg doses given three to four times daily; Therapeutic serum level 50–150 ng/mL (mcg/L; 190–570 nmol/L)
Norepinephrine and dopamine reuptake inhibitor (NDRI)			
Bupropion (Wellbutrin)	150 (75 mg given twice daily)	150–300	Please see text for proper dosing, which can help decrease seizure risk; Maximum 450 mg/day (IR, ER), 400 mg/day (SR); ER dosed once daily; SR dosed once or twice daily; IR may be dosed up to three times daily

Mixed serotonergic effects (Mixed 5-HT)

Nefazodone (Serzone)	100	200–400	Maximum 600 mg/day; daily doses should be divided twice daily
Trazodone (Desyrel; Oleptro)	50	150–300	Maximum 600 mg/day; IR daily dose should be divided three times daily and may increase by 50 mg/day increments every 3–7 days; ER dose titration initiated at 150 mg at bedtime and can be increased 75 mg/day every 3 days
Vilazodone (Viibryd)	10	20–40	Target dose 20–40 mg/day unless coadministered with CYP3A4 inhibitor (dose not to exceed 20 mg/day). Dose titration: 10 mg/day for 7 days, 20 mg/day for 7 days, and then may increase to 40 mg/day. Dose must be taken with food to ensure adequate drug absorption and bioavailability.
Vortioxetine (Brintellix)	10	20	Maximum 20 mg/day; US studies demonstrated better treatment effects at the higher dose

Serotonin and α₂-adrenergic antagonist

Mirtazapine (Remeron)	15	15–45	Maximum 45 mg/day; may increase dose no more frequently than every 1–2 weeks; dose adjustment may be required for renal impairment

Monoamine oxidase inhibitors (MAOIs)

Phenelzine (Nardil)	15	30–90	Early phase recommended dosing: 15 mg three times daily; dosing may be increased to 90 mg/day based on tolerance and response; Maintenance phase: dose should be reduced over several weeks to a daily dose as low as 15 mg/day or 15 mg every other day
Selegiline (transdermal) (Emsam)	6	6–12	Not to exceed 12 mg/24 hours; dose may be increased by 3 mg/day increments every 2 weeks; transdermal delivery system designed to deliver dose continuously over a 24-hour period
Tranylcypromine (Parnate)	10	20–40	Maximum 60 mg/day; divided dosing; if no response after 2 weeks, increase by 10 mg increments at 1- to 3-week intervals; Medication cross-taper; allow at least 1 medication-free week, then initiate tranylcypromine at 50% of usual starting dose for at least 1 week

(AE, adverse effects; CR, continuous release; ER, extended release; IR, immediate release; MDD, major depressive disorder; SR, sustained release.)
ªSI conversion for cases where reference ranges are for a mixture of parent drug and active metabolite is calculated based on a 1:1 ratio.

Drug Classification

- **Table 68–2** shows antidepressant potency and relative selectivity for inhibition of norepinephrine and 5-HT reuptake and side-effect profiles.
- The **selective serotonin reuptake inhibitors** (SSRIs) inhibit the reuptake of 5-HT into the presynaptic neuron. They are generally chosen as first-line antidepressants because of their relative safety in overdose and improved tolerability compared with earlier agents. Evidence suggests escitalopram and sertraline have the best efficacy/ side effect profile compared to other newer-generation antidepressants.
- **Tricyclic antidepressant** (TCA) use has diminished because of the availability of equally effective therapies that are safer on overdose and better tolerated. They inhibit the reuptake of norepinephrine and 5-HT and have affinity for adrenergic, cholinergic, and histaminergic receptors.
- The monoamine oxidase inhibitors (MAOIs) **phenelzine** and **tranylcypromine** increase the concentrations of norepinephrine, 5-HT, and dopamine within the neuronal synapse through inhibition of monoamine oxidase (MAO). They are nonselective inhibitors of MAO-A and MAO-B. Table 68–3 shows dietary and medication restrictions for patients taking phenelzine or tranylcypromine. **Selegiline**, available as a transdermal patch for treatment of major depression, inhibits brain MAO-A and MAO-B but has reduced effects on MAO-A in the gut.
- The triazolopyridines **trazodone** and **nefazodone** antagonize the 5-HT_2 receptor and inhibit the reuptake of 5-HT. They can also enhance 5-HT_{1A} neurotransmission. Trazodone blocks α_1-adrenergic and histaminergic receptors increasing dizziness and sedation.
- Other antidepressants with mixed serotonin effects are vilazodone and vortioxetine. Vilazodone may be particularly useful for depressed patients with anxiety, and vortioxetine may be helpful for depressed patients with cognitive difficulties.
- The serotonin–norepinephrine reuptake inhibitors include **venlafaxine, desvenlafaxine, duloxetine, and levomilnacipran.** Some studies suggest a slight efficacy advantage for venlafaxine compared to other antidepressants.
- **Mirtazapine** enhances central noradrenergic and serotonergic activity by antagonizing central presynaptic α_2-adrenergic autoreceptors and heteroreceptors. It also antagonizes 5-HT_2 and 5-HT_3 receptors and blocks histamine receptors. It may be an option for patients who experience sexual dysfunction taking other antidepressants.
- **St. John's wort**, an herb containing hypericum, may be effective for mild to moderate depression. It is associated with several drug–drug interactions. All antidepressant regimens should be overseen by a trained healthcare professional.

Adverse Effects

- See **Table 68–2** for adverse effect profiles and Table 68–4 for adverse effects and monitoring parameters of new-generation antidepressants.
- Early in treatment, all antidepressants can increase suicidal thinking and behavior in children, adolescents, and young adults less than 25 years of age.
- Any antidepressant that enhances serotonergic activity can be associated with serotonin syndrome characterized by mental status changes, autonomic instability, and neuromuscular abnormalities.

Tricyclic Antidepressants and Other Heterocyclics

- TCAs cause anticholinergic side effects (eg, dry mouth, blurred vision, constipation, urinary retention, tachycardia, memory impairment, and delirium) and sedation. Additional adverse effects include weight gain, orthostatic hypotension, cardiac conduction delay, and sexual dysfunction.
- **Desipramine** carries an increased risk of death in patients with a family history of sudden cardiac death, cardiac dysrhythmias, or cardiac conduction disturbances.
- Abrupt withdrawal of **TCAs** (especially high doses) may result in cholinergic rebound (eg, dizziness, nausea, diarrhea, insomnia, and restlessness).
- **Maprotiline**, a tetracyclic drug, causes seizures at a higher incidence than do standard TCAs and is contraindicated in patients with a history of seizure disorder.

TABLE 68-2 Relative Potencies of Norepinephrine and Serotonin Reuptake Blockade and Selected Side Effect Profile of Antidepressants

	Reuptake Antagonism		ACh Effects	Sedation	OH	Seizures[a]	Conduction Changes[a]
	NE	5-HT					
Selective serotonin reuptake inhibitors (SSRIs)							
Citalopram	0	++++	0	+	0	++	++
Escitalopram	0	++++	0	0	0	0	0
Fluoxetine	+	++++	0	0	0	++	0
Fluvoxamine	0	++++	0	+	0	++	0
Paroxetine	++	++++	+	+	0	++	0
Sertraline	0	++++	0	0	0	++	0
Serotonin–Norepinephrine reuptake inhibitors (SNRIs)							
Duloxetine[b]	+++	++++	+	0	+	0	0
Levomilnacipran[c]	++++	+++	+	0	0	0	0
Venlafaxine[d] and desvenlafaxine	+++	++++	+	+	0	++	+
Tricyclic antidepressants (TCAs)							
Amitriptyline	++	++++	++++	++++	+++	++	++
Desipramine	++++	++	++	++	++	++	++++
Doxepin	++	++	+++	++++	++	+++	++
Imipramine	++	++++	+++	+++	++++	+++	+++
Nortriptyline	++++	++	++	++	+	++	++

(continued)

TABLE 68-2 Relative Potencies of Norepinephrine and Serotonin Reuptake Blockade and Selected Side Effect Profile of Antidepressants (*Continued*)

	Reuptake Antagonism		ACh Effects	Sedation	OH	Seizures[a]	Conduction Changes[a]
	NE	5-HT					
Mixed serotonergic (mixed 5-HT)							
Nefazodone	0	++	0	+++	+++	++	+
Trazodone	0	++	0	++++	+++	++	+
Vilazodone	0	++++	0	+	0	++	0
Norepinephrine and dopamine reuptake inhibitor (NDRI)							
Bupropion[e]	+	0	+	0	0	++++	+
Serotonin and α_2-receptor antagonist							
Mirtazapine	0	0	+	++	++	0	+

++++, high; +++, moderate; ++, low; +, very low; 0, absent or not adequately studied.
(Ach, anticholinergic; OH, orthostatic hypotension.)
[a]These are uncommon side effects of antidepressant drugs, particularly when used at normal therapeutic doses; they may be dose-dependent, resulting in corresponding dose restrictions. (eg, citalopram 40 mg/day maximum due to QTc prolongation concerns.)
[b]Duloxetine: balanced 5-HT and NE reuptake inhibition.
[c]Levomilnacipran: greater potency at NE reuptake inhibition compared to 5-HT.
[d]Venlafaxine: primarily 5-HT at lower doses, NE at higher doses, and DA at very high doses.
[e]Bupropion: also blocks dopamine reuptake.

TABLE 68-3	Dietary and Medication Restrictions for Patients Taking Monoamine Oxidase Inhibitors[a]

Foods

Aged cheese[b]	Liver (chicken or beef, more than 2 days old)
Sour cream[c]	Raisins
Yogurt[c]	Pods of broad beans (fava beans)
Cottage cheese[c]	Yeast extract and other yeast products
American cheese[c]	Soy sauce
Mild Swiss cheese[c]	Chocolate[e]
Wine[d] (especially Chianti and sherry)	Coffee[e]
Beer	Ripe avocado
Sardines	Sauerkraut
Canned, aged, or processed meats	Licorice
Monosodium glutamate	

Medications

Amphetamines	Levodopa
Appetite suppressants	Local anesthetics containing sympathomimetic vasoconstrictors
Asthma inhalants	
Buspirone	Meperidine
Carbamazepine	Methyldopa
Cocaine	Methylphenidate
Cyclobenzaprine	Other antidepressants[f]
Decongestants (topical and systemic)	Other MAOIs
Dextromethorphan	Reserpine
Dopamine	Rizatriptan
Ephedrine	Stimulants
Epinephrine	Sumatriptan
Guanethidine	Sympathomimetics
	Tryptophan

[a]According to the FDA-approved prescribing information for the transdermal selegiline patch, patients receiving the 6-mg/24-hour dose are not required to modify their diet. However, patients receiving the 9- or 12-mg/24-hour dose are still required to follow the dietary restrictions similar to the other MAOIs.
[b]Clearly warrants absolute prohibition (eg, English Stilton, blue, Camembert, and cheddar).
[c]Up to 2 oz (~60 g) daily is acceptable.
[d]Three ounce white wine or a single cocktail is acceptable.
[e]Up to 2 oz (~60 mL) daily is acceptable: larger amounts of decaffeinated coffee are acceptable.
[f]Tricyclic antidepressants may be used with caution by experienced clinicians in treatment-resistant populations.

Serotonin-Norepinephrine Reuptake Inhibitors

• **Venlafaxine** may cause a dose-related increase in diastolic blood pressure. Dosage reduction or discontinuation may be necessary if sustained hypertension occurs. Side effects are similar to those of SSRIs, except nausea and vomiting may be worse with venlafaxiine. There may be higher side-effect-related discontinuation rates with venlafaxine and duloxetine than with the SSRIs.
• **Levomilnacipran** may increase blood pressure and heart rate.
• The most common side effects of **duloxetine** are nausea, dry mouth, constipation, decreased appetite, insomnia, and increased sweating.

Selective Serotonin Reuptake Inhibitors

• SSRIs produce fewer sedative, anticholinergic, and cardiovascular adverse effects than the TCAs and are less likely to cause weight gain. The primary adverse effects are nausea, vomiting, diarrhea, headache, insomnia, fatigue, and sexual dysfunction.

TABLE 68-4	Adverse Drug Reactions and Monitoring Parameters Associated with Select New-Generation Antidepressants		
Drug	ADR(s)	Monitoring	Comments
Antidepressants from each pharmacologic class			
Common to all antidepressants			
	Suicidality	Behavioral changes Mental status	(US boxed warning) for all antidepressants; caregivers should be alerted to monitor for acute changes in behavior (especially early in treatment)
Selective serotonin reuptake inhibitors (SSRIs)			
Common to all SSRIs			
	Anxiety or nervousness	Assess severity and impact on patient functioning and quality of life	Most prominent on initial treatment; generally subsides over time as antidepressant causes neurochemical adaptations
	Insomnia	Sleep patterns	Among SSRI class: fluoxetine may be more activating; fluvoxamine and paroxetine may be more sedating
	Nausea	Frequency and severity	
	Serotonin syndrome	Autonomic function (eg, pulse, temperature); neuromuscular function	Criteria include mental status change, clonus, hyperthermia, diaphoresis, and tachycardia
	Sexual dysfunction	Assess severity and impact on patient functioning and quality of life	Spontaneous self-reporting may be low; clinician should assess symptoms; reversible on drug discontinuation
SSRI-specific			
Citalopram (possibly escitalopram)	QT interval prolongation	Electrocardiogram; electrolytes (eg, potassium, magnesium)	Caution use in "at-risk" patients (eg, electrolyte disturbance); discontinue if QTc persistently >500 milliseconds
Fluoxetine	Anorexia	Weight (over time)	SSRIs are generally considered weight neutral
Fluvoxamine	Somnolence	Mental status	May be less tolerable than other SSRIs
Paroxetine	Anticholinergic effects	Symptoms: dry mouth, constipation, urinary retention, mental status	Paroxetine possesses relatively more anticholinergic effects than other SSRIs

Serotonin–Norepinephrine reuptake inhibitors (SNRIs)

Common to all SNRIs

Cardiovascular changes	Increases in blood pressure; heart rate	Possibly less likely with duloxetine; may need to lower/discontinue dose
Insomnia	Sleep patterns	Possibly less likely with duloxetine
Nausea	Frequency and severity	
Serotonin syndrome	Autonomic function (eg, pulse temperature); neuromuscular function	Criteria include mental status changes, clonus, hyperthermia, diaphoresis, and tachycardia
Sexual dysfunction	Assess severity and impact on patient functioning and quality of life	Spontaneous self-reporting may be low; clinicians should assess symptoms; reversible on drug discontinuation

SNRI-specific

Desvenlafaxine	Dose-related hyperlipidemia	Lipid profile	Elevations in total cholesterol, low-density lipoproteins, and triglycerides
Duloxetine	Orthostatic hypotension	Blood pressure, pulse	Initial treatment or on dose increase
Venlafaxine	Dose-related hypertension	Blood pressure, pulse	May need to lower dose or discontinue

Mixed serotonergic effects (Mixed 5-HT)

Nefazodone	Liver toxicity	Liver function tests	Nefazodone use is extremely limited in the United States due to concerns about liver toxicity
Trazodone	Orthostatic hypotension	Blood pressure, pulse	May be more severe than with other antidepressants; rate-limiting side effect
	Priapism	Patient report of sexual side effects, especially painful erection	Patient should seek medical attention for prolonged erection (ie, >4 hours)

TABLE 68-4 Adverse Drug Reactions and Monitoring Parameters Associated with Select New-Generation Antidepressants (*Continued*)

Drug	ADR(s)	Monitoring	Comments
Vilazodone	Serotonin syndrome	Autonomic function (eg, pulse temperature); neuromuscular function	Criteria include mental status changes, clonus, hyperthermia, diaphoresis, and tachycardia
Serotonin and α₂-adrenergic antagonist			
Mirtazapine	Weight gain	Body weight	Frequently occurring and significant (>7%) weight gain among adults
Norepinephrine and dopamine reuptake inhibitor (NDRI)			
Bupropion	Seizure activity	Electroencephalogram	See text for proper dosing, which can help decrease seizure risk; caution use in patients with eating disorders or alcohol use disorders

A few patients have anxiety symptoms early in treatment. Citalopram has been linked to an increase in QT interval at doses above 40 mg/day (see **Table 68–1**). This may also occur with escitalopram.

Mixed Serotonergic Medications

- **Trazodone** and **nefazodone** cause minimal anticholinergic effects. Sedation, dizziness, and cognitive slowing are the most frequent dose limiting side effects with trazodone. Common side effects with nefazodone are dizziness, orthostatic hypotension, and somnolence.
- Priapism occurs rarely with trazodone (1 in 6000 male patients). Surgical intervention may be required, and impotence may result.
- Nefazodone carries a black box warning for life-threatening liver failure. Do not initiate nefazodone in individuals with active liver disease or elevated serum transaminases.
- Vilazodone is associated with nausea, diarrhea, dizziness, insomnia, and decreased libido, especially in men.
- Vortioxetine causes nausea and constipation and sexual dysfunction in men at the highest dose (20 mg/day).

Aminoketone

- The occurrence of seizures with **bupropion** is dose related and may be increased by predisposing factors (eg, history of head trauma or central nervous system [CNS] tumor). At the ceiling dose (450 mg/day), the incidence of seizures is 0.4%. Other side effects are nausea, vomiting, tremor, insomnia, dry mouth, and skin reactions. It is contraindicated in patients with bulimia or anorexia nervosa, as these patients have a higher risk for seizures. It causes less sexual dysfunction than SSRIs.

Mirtazapine

- **Mirtazapine**'s most common adverse effects are somnolence, weight gain, dry mouth, and constipation.

Monoamine Oxidase Inhibitors

- The most common adverse effect of MAOIs is postural hypotension (more likely with **phenelzine** than **tranylcypromine**), which can be minimized by divided-daily dosing. Phenelzine is mildly to moderately sedating, but tranylcypromine is often stimulating, and the last dose of the day is administered in the early afternoon. Sexual dysfunction in both genders is common. Phenelzine has been associated with hepatocellular damage and weight gain.
- Hypertensive crisis is a potentially fatal reaction that can occur when MAOIs are taken concurrently with certain foods, especially those high in tyramine, and with certain drugs (see **Table 68–3**). Symptoms of hypertensive crisis include occipital headache, stiff neck, nausea, vomiting, sweating, and sharply elevated blood pressure. Hypertensive crisis may be treated with agents such as captopril. Education of patients taking MAOIs regarding dietary and medication restrictions is critical. Patients taking transdermal selegiline patch doses greater than 6-mg/24 hours must follow the dietary restrictions.

Pharmacokinetics

- The pharmacokinetics of the antidepressants is summarized in Table 68–5.
- Metabolism of the **TCAs** appears to be linear within the usual dosage range. Dose-related kinetics cannot be ruled out in the elderly. Factors reported to influence TCA plasma concentrations include renal or hepatic dysfunction, genetics, age, cigarette smoking, and concurrent drug administration.
- The SSRIs, with the possible exceptions of **citalopram** and **sertraline**, may have a nonlinear pattern of drug accumulation with chronic dosing. Hepatic impairment, renal impairment, and age can influence the pharmacokinetics of **SSRIs**
- **Mirtazapine** and **levomilnacipran** are primarily eliminated in the urine.

TABLE 68-5 Pharmacokinetic Properties of Antidepressants

Generic Name	Elimination Half-Life[a]	Time of Peak Plasma Concentration (Hours)	Plasma Protein Binding (%)	Percentage Bioavailable	Clinically Important Metabolites
Selective serotonin reuptake inhibitors (SSRIs)					
Citalopram	33 hours	2–4	80	≥80	None
Escitalopram	27–32 hours	5	56	80	None
Fluoxetine	4–6 days[b]	4–8	94	95	Norfluoxetine
Fluvoxamine	15–26 hours	2–8	77	53	None
Paroxetine	24–31 hours	5–7	95		None
Sertraline	27 hours	6–8	99	36[c]	None
Serotonin–Norepinephrine reuptake inhibitors (SNRIs)					
Desvenlafaxine	11 hours	7.5	30	80	None
Duloxetine	12 hours	6	90	50	None
Levomilnacipran	12 hours	6–8	22	92	None
Venlafaxine	5 hours	2	27–30	45	O-Desmethyl-venlafaxine
TCAs					
Amitriptyline	9–46 hours	1–5	90–97	30–60	Nortriptyline
Desipramine	11–46 hours	3–6	73–92	33–51	2-Hydroxy-desipramine
Doxepin	8–36 hours	1–4	68–82	13–45	Desmethyl-doxepin
Imipramine	6–34 hours	1.5–3	63–96	22–77	Desipramine
Nortriptyline	16–88 hours	3–12	87–95	46–70	10-Hydroxy-nortriptyline
Mixed serotonergic (mixed 5-HT)					
Nefazodone	2–4 hours	1	99	20	meta-Chlorophenyl-piperazine

	Half-life	Time to peak	Protein binding (%)	Bioavailability (%)	Active metabolites
Trazodone	6–11 hours	1–2	92	[d]	meta-Chlorophenyl-piperazine
Vilazodone	25 hours	4–5	>95	72[e]	
Vortioxetine	66 hours	7–11	98	75	
Norepinephrine/dopamine reuptake inhibitor (NDRI)					
Bupropion	10–21 hours	3	82–88	[d]	Hydroxy-bupropion Threohydro-bupropion Erythrohydro-bupropion
Serotonin and α₂-adrenergic antagonists					
Mirtazapine	20–40 hours	2	85	50	None

[a] Biologic half-life in slowest phase of elimination.
[b] Four to 6 days with chronic dosing; norfluoxetine, 4–16 days.
[c] Increases 30%–40% when taken with food.
[d] No data available.
[e] Take with food to increase area under the curve concentrations by greater than 60%.

- In acutely depressed patients, there is a correlation between antidepressant effect and plasma concentrations for some **TCAs (eg, amitriptyline, nortriptyline, imipramine, and desipramine). Table 68–1** shows suggested therapeutic plasma concentration ranges. The best-established therapeutic range is for **nortriptyline**, and data suggest a therapeutic window.
- Some indications for TCA plasma level monitoring include inadequate response; relapse; serious or persistent adverse effects; use of higher than standard doses; suspected non-adherence; toxicity; pharmacokinetic interactions; elderly, pediatric, and adolescent patients; pregnant patients; patients of African or Asian descent (because of slower metabolism); cardiac disease; and changing brands. Plasma concentrations should be obtained at steady state, usually after a minimum of 1 week at constant dosage, during the elimination phase, and usually in the morning 12 hours after the last dose.

Drug–Drug Interactions

- **TCAs** may interact with other drugs that modify hepatic cytochrome P450 (CYP450) enzyme activity or hepatic blood flow. TCAs also are involved in interactions through displacement from protein-binding sites.
- Increased plasma concentrations of TCAs and symptoms of toxicity may occur when **fluoxetine** or **paroxetine** (both inhibitors of CYP2D6) are added.
- The very slow elimination of **fluoxetine** and **norfluoxetine** makes it critical to ensure a 5-week washout after fluoxetine discontinuation before starting an **MAOI**. Potentially fatal reactions may occur when any **SSRI** or **TCA** is coadministered with an MAOI. TCAs and MAOIs can be combined in refractory patients by experienced clinicians with careful monitoring.
- Combining an SSRI with another 5-HT augmenting agent can lead to the serotonin syndrome characterized by clonus, hyperthermia, and mental status changes.
- The ability of any antidepressant to inhibit or induce the CYP450 enzymes can be a significant factor determining its capability to cause a pharmacokinetic drug–drug interaction. If an SSRI is added to a regimen which includes drugs known to interact with SSRIs, the SSRI starting dose should be low and slowly titrated.
- Table 68–6 compares second- and third-generation antidepressants for their effects on CYP450 enzymes. CYP2D6 and 3A4 are responsible for the metabolism of more than 80% of currently marketed drugs. Mirtazapine, venlafaxine, duloxetine, and

TABLE 68–6	Second- and Third-Generation Antidepressants and Cytochrome (CYP) P450 Enzyme Inhibitory Potential			
	CYP Enzyme			
Drug	1A2	2C	2D6	3A4
Bupropion	0	0	+	0
Citalopram	0	0	+	NA
Duloxetine	0	0	+++	0
Escitalopram	0	0	+	0
Fluoxetine	0	++	++++	++
Fluvoxamine	++++	++	0	+++
Mirtazapine	0	0	0	0
Nefazodone	0	0	0	++++
Paroxetine	0	0	++++	0
Sertraline	0	++	+	+
(des)-Venlafaxine	0	0	0/+	0

++++, high; +++, moderate; ++, low; +, very low; 0, absent.

bupropion have relatively little inhibition on CYP450 enzymes; thus their drug interactions are largely pharmacodynamic, not pharmacokinetic.
• Consult the drug interaction literature for detailed information concerning any real or potential psychotherapeutic drug interactions.

SPECIAL POPULATIONS

Elderly Patients

• In the elderly, depressed mood may be less prominent than other symptoms, such as loss of appetite, cognitive impairment, sleeplessness, fatigue, physical complaints, and loss of interest in usual activities.
• The **SSRIs** are often considered first-choice antidepressants for elderly patients. **Bupropion, venlafaxine, and mirtazapine** are also effective and well tolerated.

Pediatric Patients

• Symptoms of depression in childhood include boredom, anxiety, failing adjustment, and sleep disturbance.
• Data supporting efficacy of antidepressants in children and adolescents are sparse. **Fluoxetine** and escitalopram are the only FDA approved antidepressants for patients below 18 years of age.
• The FDA has established a link between antidepressant use and suicidality (suicidal thinking and behaviors) in children, adolescents, and young adults less than 25 years old. All antidepressants carry a black box warning for caution when using antidepressants in this population, and the FDA recommends specific monitoring parameters. Consult the FDA-approved labeling or the FDA website for additional information.
• Several cases of sudden death have been reported in children and adolescents taking **desipramine**. A baseline electrocardiogram (ECG) is recommended before initiating a TCA in children and adolescents, and an additional ECG is advised when steady-state plasma concentrations are achieved. TCA plasma concentration monitoring is critical to ensure safety.

Pregnancy

• As a general rule, if effective, nondrug approaches are preferred when treating depressed pregnant patients. For those with history of relapse after antidepressant discontinuation, the antidepressant can be continued throughout pregnancy. One study showed that pregnant women who discontinued antidepressants were five times more likely to relapse during pregnancy than women who continued treatment.
• There is a possible association of **SSRIs** with low birth weight and respiratory distress. Another study reported a sixfold greater likelihood of persistent pulmonary hypertension in newborn infants exposed to an SSRI after the twentieth week of gestation.
• Consider risks of untreated depression in pregnancy, including low birth weight, maternal suicidality, potential for hospitalization or marital discord, poor prenatal care, and difficulty caring for other children.

Relative Resistance and Treatment-Resistant Depression

• Most "treatment-resistant" depressed patients have received inadequate therapy. In patients who have not responded to treatment, consider the following: (1) Is the diagnosis correct? (2) Does the patient have a psychotic depression? (3) Has the patient received an adequate dose and duration of treatment? (4) Do adverse effects preclude adequate dosing? (5) Has the patient adhered to the prescribed regimen? (6) Was treatment outcome measured adequately? (7) Is there a coexisting or pre-existing medical or psychiatric disorder? (8) Was a stepwise approach to treatment used? (9) Are there other factors that interfere with treatment?
• The STAR*D study showed that one in three depressed patients who did not achieve remission with an antidepressant became symptom-free when an additional medication (eg, **sustained-release bupropion**) was added, and one in four achieved remission after switching to a different antidepressant (eg, **extended-release venlafaxine**).

- The current antidepressant may be stopped and a trial initiated with different agent (eg, **mirtazapine** or **nortriptyline**).
- Alternatively, the current antidepressant may be augmented (potentiated) by addition of another agent (eg, **lithium** or **triiodothyronine [T₃]**), or another antidepressant can be added. An atypical antipsychotic (eg, aripiprazole, quetiapine, brexpiprazole) can be used to augment antidepressant response.
- The practice guideline of the American Psychiatric Association recommends that after 6 to 8 weeks of antidepressant treatment, partial responders should consider changing the dose, augmenting the antidepressant, or adding psychotherapy or ECT. For those with no response, options include changing to another antidepressant or the addition of psychotherapy or ECT. **Figure 68–1** is an algorithm for treatment of depression including refractory patients.

EVALUATION OF THERAPEUTIC OUTCOMES

- Several monitoring parameters, in addition to plasma concentrations, are useful. Monitor regularly for adverse effects (see **Table 68–4**), remission of target symptoms, and changes in social or occupational functioning. Assure regular monitoring for several months after discontinuation of antidepressants.
- Regularly monitor blood pressure of patients given serotonin-norepinephrine reuptake inhibitors.
- Order a pretreatment ECG before starting TCA therapy in children, adolescents, and patients over 40 years of age, and perform follow-up ECGs periodically.
- Monitor for emergence of suicidal ideation after initiation of any antidepressant, especially in the first few weeks of treatment.
- In addition to the clinical interview, use psychometric rating instruments to rapidly and reliably measure the nature and severity of depressive and associated symptoms.

See Chapter 68, Major Depressive Disorder, authored by Christian J. Teter, Judith C. Kando, and Barbara G. Wells, for a more detailed discussion of this topic.

- *Schizophrenia* is characterized by delusions, hallucinations, disorganized thinking and speech, abnormal motor behavior, inappropriate affect, negative symptoms, and impaired psychosocial functioning.

PATHOPHYSIOLOGY

- Increased ventricular size and decreased gray matter, have been reported.
- Schizophrenia causation theories include genetic predisposition, obstetric complications with hypoxia, increased neuronal pruning, immune system abnormalities, neurodevelopmental disorders, neurodegenerative theories, dopamine receptor defect, and regional brain abnormalities including hyper- or hypo-activity of dopaminergic processes in specific brain regions.
- Positive symptoms may be more closely associated with dopamine receptor hyperactivity in the mesocaudate, whereas negative and cognitive symptoms may be most closely related to dopamine receptor hypofunction in the prefrontal cortex.
- *Glutamatergic dysfunction.* A deficiency of glutamatergic activity produces symptoms similar to those of dopaminergic hyperactivity and possibly schizophrenic symptoms.

CLINICAL PRESENTATION

- Symptoms of the acute episode may include: being out of touch with reality; hallucinations (especially hearing voices); delusions (fixed false beliefs); ideas of influence (actions controlled by external influences); disconnected thought processes (loose associations); illogical conversation (alogia), ambivalence (contradictory thoughts); flat, inappropriate, or labile affect; autistic thinking (withdrawn and inwardly directed thinking); uncooperativeness, hostility, and verbal or physical aggression; impaired self-care skills; and disturbed sleep and appetite.
- After the acute psychotic episode has resolved, typically there are residual features (eg, anxiety, suspiciousness, lack of motivation, poor insight, impaired judgment, social withdrawal, difficulty in learning from experience, and poor self-care skills). Comorbid substance abuse and nonadherence with medications are common.
- Positive symptoms—delusions, disorganized speech (association disturbance), hallucinations, behavior disturbance (disorganized or catatonic), and illusions.
- Negative symptoms—alogia (poverty of speech), avolition, flat affect, anhedonia, and social isolation.
- Cognitive dysfunction—impaired attention, working memory, and executive function.

DIAGNOSIS

- The *Diagnostic and Statistical Manual of Mental Disorders*, 5th ed. (*DSM-5*), specifies the following diagnostic criteria:
  ✓ Continuous symptoms that persist for at least 6 months with at least one month of active phase symptoms (Criterion A) and may include prodromal or residual symptoms.
    ❖ Criterion A: For at least 1 month, there must be at least two of the following present for a significant portion of time: delusions, hallucinations, disorganized speech, grossly disorganized or catatonic behavior, and negative symptoms. At least one symptom must be delusions, hallucinations, or disorganized speech.
    ❖ Criterion B: Significantly impaired functioning.

TREATMENT

- <u>Goals of Treatment</u>: The goal is to alleviate target symptoms, avoid side effects, improve psychosocial functioning and productivity, achieve compliance with the prescribed regimen, integrate the patient back into the community, prevent relapse, and involve the patient in treatment planning.

- Before treatment, perform a mental status examination, physical and neurologic examination, complete family and social history, psychiatric diagnostic interview, and laboratory workup (complete blood count [CBC], electrolytes, hepatic function, renal function, electrocardiogram [ECG], fasting serum glucose, serum lipids, thyroid function, and urine drug screen).

GENERAL APPROACH

- Available antipsychotics and dosage ranges are shown in **Table 69–1**. Second-generation antipsychotics (SGAs) may have superior efficacy for negative symptoms and cognition, but this is controversial.
- SGAs are said to cause few or no acutely occurring extrapyramidal side effects, and to have enhanced efficacy for negative and cognitive symptoms, minimal or no propensity to cause tardive dyskinesia (TD), and less effect on serum prolactin than the first-generation antipsychotics (FGAs) (typical antipsychotics). **Clozapine** is the only SGA that fulfills all these criteria.
- SGAs have less neurologic side effects, especially effects on movement, but they have increased risk for metabolic side effects, including weight gain, hyperlipidemias, and diabetes mellitus.
- The Clinical Antipsychotic Trials of Intervention Effectiveness (CATIE) study showed that olanzapine, compared with quetiapine, risperidone, ziprasidone, and perphenazine, has modest (but statistically nonsignificant) superiority in persistence of maintenance therapy but more metabolic side effects.
- Base antipsychotic selection on (1) the need to avoid certain side effects, (2) concurrent medical or psychiatric disorders, and (3) patient or family history of response. **Figure 69–1** is an algorithm for management of schizophrenia. Clozapine has superior efficacy for suicidal behavior.
- In first-episode schizophrenia, initiate antipsychotic dosing at the lower end of the dosing range. Long-acting risperidone injection is more effective than oral risperidone in preventing relapse over a 1-year period.
- In stage 4 of **Fig. 69–1**, adding ziprasidone 80 mg/day to clozapine may improve general psychopathology including negative symptoms. Based on limited evidence, an additional antipsychotic, mood stabilizer, or electroconvulsive therapy (ECT) may also be used to augment clozapine in stage 4, but these approaches are controversial.
- Predictors of good antipsychotic response include prior good response to the drug selected, absence of alcohol or drug abuse, acute onset and short duration of illness, precipitating factors, later age of onset, affective symptoms, family history of affective illness, medication compliance, employment, and good premorbid adjustment. Negative symptoms are generally less responsive to antipsychotic therapy.
- An initial dysphoric response, that is, a dislike of the medication or feeling worse, combined with anxiety or akathisia, portends a poor drug response, adverse effects, and nonadherence.

PHARMACOKINETICS

- Pharmacokinetic parameters and major metabolic pathways of antipsychotics are summarized in **Table 69–2**.
- Antipsychotics, highly lipophilic and highly bound to membranes and plasma proteins, have large volumes of distribution and are largely metabolized by cytochrome P450 (CYP) pathways (except ziprasidone).
- **Risperidone**, and its active metabolite 9-OH-resperidone, **fluphenazine**, and **perphenazine** are metabolized by CYP2D6. Polymorphic metabolism should be considered in those with side effects at low doses. CYP2D6 is also a major pathway for aripiprazole, brexpiprazole, and iloperidone. Polymorphism in CYP1A2 can decrease (and smoking can increase) metabolism of **clozapine**. Eating or drinking within 10 minutes of **asenapine** sublingual administration reduces its bioavailability.

TABLE 69–1	Available Antipsychotics and Dosage Ranges			
Generic Name	Trade Name	Starting Dose (mg/day)	Usual Dosage Range (mg/day)	Comments
First-generation antipsychotics				
Chlorpromazine	Thorazine	50–150	300–1000	Most weight gain among FGAs
Fluphenazine	Prolixin	5	5–20	
Haloperidol	Haldol	2–5	2–20	Higher dropout rate in first episode
Loxapine	Loxitane	20	50–150	
Loxapine inhaled	Adasuve	10	10	Maximum 10 mg per 24 hours Approved REMS program only
Perphenazine	Trilafon	4–24	16–64	
Thioridazine	Mellaril	50–150	100–800	Significant QTc prolongation
Thiothixene	Navane	4–10	4–50	
Trifluoperazine	Stelazine	2–5	5–40	
Second-generation antipsychotics				
Aripiprazole	Abilify	5–15	15–30	
Asenapine	Saphris	5	10–20	Sublingual only, no food or drink for 10 minutes after administration of the dose
Brexpiprazole	Rexulti	1	2–4	
Cariprazine	Vraylar	1.5	1.5–6	Due to long half-life, steady-state is not reached for several weeks
Clozapine	Clozaril	25	100–800	Check plasma level before exceeding 600 mg
Iloperidone	Fanapt	1–2	6–24	Care with dosing in CYP2D6 slow metabolizers
Lurasidone	Latuda	20–40	40–120	Take with food; ≥350 calories (≥1460 J)
Olanzapine	Zyprexa	5–10	10–20	Avoid in first episode because of weight gain
Paliperidone	Invega	3–6	3–12	Bioavailability increased when administered with food
Quetiapine	Seroquel	50	300–800	
Quetiapine XR	Seroquel XR	300 mg	400–800	
Risperidone	Risperdal	1–2	2–8	
Ziprasidone	Geodon	40	80–160	Take with food, ≥500 calories (≥2100 J)

Note: In first-episode patients, starting dose and target dose should generally be 50% of the usual dose range. See Long-Acting Injectable Antipsychotics in text for dosing of these agents.

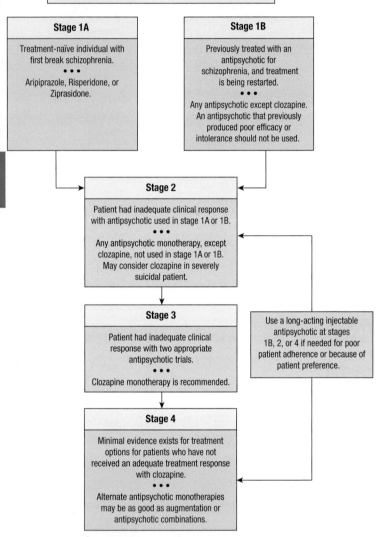

FIGURE 69–1. Suggested pharmacotherapy algorithm for treatment of schizophrenia. Schizophrenia should be treated in the context of an interprofessional model that addresses the psychosocial needs of the patient, necessary psychiatric pharmacotherapy, psychiatric co-occurring mental disorders, treatment adherence, and any medical problems the patient may have.

- Most antipsychotics have half-lives of elimination of 24 or more, except quetiapine and ziprasidone. After dosage stabilization, most antipsychotics (except **quetiapine** and **ziprasidone**) can be dosed once daily.
- A 12-hour postdose **clozapine** serum concentration of at least 350 ng/mL (1.07 μmol/L) is associated with efficacy. Monitor serum concentrations of clozapine

TABLE 69-2 Pharmacokinetic Parameters of Selected Antipsychotics

Drug	Bioavailability (%)	Half-Life	Major Metabolic Pathways	Active Metabolites
Selected first-generation antipsychotics (FGAs)				
Chlorpromazine	10–30	8–35 hours	FMO3, CYP3A4	7-Hydroxy, others
Fluphenazine	20–50	14–24 hours	CYP2D6	?
Fluphenazine decanoate		14.2 ± 2.2ª days	CYP2D6	
Haloperidol	40–70	12–36 hours	CYP1A2, CYP2D6, CYP3A4	Reduced haloperidol
Haloperidol decanoate		21 days	CYP1A2, CYP2D6, CYP3A4	Reduced haloperidol
Perphenazine	20–25	8.1–12.3 hours	CYP2D6	7-OH-perphenazine
Second-generation antipsychotics (SGAs)				
Aripiprazole	87	48–68 hours	CYP2D6, CYP3A4	Dehydroaripiprazole
Aripiprazole Lauroxil		29.2–34.9 days	CYP2D6, CYP3A4	Dehydroaripiprazole
Aripiprazole Monohydrate		29.9–46.5 days	CYP2D6, CYP3A4	Dehydro-aripiprazole
Asenapine	<2 orally 35 SL Nonlinear	13–39 hours	UGT1A4, CYP1A2	None known
Brexpiprazole	95	91 hours	CYP2D6, CYP3A4	DM-3411
Cariprazine		2–4 days, DDCAR 1–3 weeks	CYP2D6, CYP3A4	Desmethyl cariprazine [DCAR], Didesmethyl cariprazine [DDCAR]
Clozapine	12–81	11–105 hours	CYP1A2, CYP3A4, CYP2C19	Desmethylclozapine
Iloperidone	96	18–33 hours	CYP2D6, CYP3A4	P88
Lurasidone	10–20	18 hours	CYP3A4	ID-14233 and ID-14326

(continued)

TABLE 69–2 Pharmacokinetic Parameters of Selected Antipsychotics (*Continued*)

Drug	Bioavailability (%)	Half-Life	Major Metabolic Pathways	Active Metabolites
Olanzapine	80	20–70 hours	CYP1A2, CYP3A4, FMO3	N-Glucuronide; 2-OH-methyl; 4-N-oxide
Olanzapine LAI		30 days	CYP1A2, CYP3A4, FMO3	N-Glucuronide; 2-OH-methyl; 4-N-oxide
Paliperidone ER	28	23 hours	Renal unchanged (59%) CYP3A4 and multiple pathways	None known
Paliperidone palmitate		25–49 days	Renal unchanged (59%) CYP3A4 and multiple pathways	None known
Paliperidone Palmitate ER		84–89 days (deltoid) 118–139 days (gluteal)	Renal unchanged (59%) CYP3A4 and multiple pathways	None known
Quetiapine	9 ± 4	6.88 hours	CYP3A4	N-desalkylquetiapine
Quetiapine XR		7 hours	CYP3A4	N-desalkylquetiapine
Risperidone	68	3–24 hours	CYP2D6	9-OH-risperidone
Risperidone Consta		3–6 days	CYP2D6	9-OH-risperidone
Ziprasidone	59	4–10 hours	Aldehyde oxidase, CYP3A4	None

(UGT, UDP glucuronosyltransferases genes; FMO3, flavin containing monooxygenase 3 gene; SL, sublingual.)
aBased on multiple-dose data. Single-dose data indicate a β-half-life of 6–10 days.

before exceeding 600 mg daily, in patients with unusual or severe adverse effects, in those concomitantly taking potentially interacting medications, in those with age or pathophysiologic changes suggesting altered kinetics, and in those suspected of medication nonadherence.

INITIAL THERAPY

- The goals during the first 7 days are decreased agitation, hostility, anxiety, and aggression and normalization of sleep and eating. Average doses are about at the middle of the ranges shown in **Table 69–1**. For first episode psychosis, the dose range is about one half of that of chronically ill patients.
- Titrate over the first few days to an average effective dose. Titrate iloperidone and clozapine more slowly due to risk of hypotension. If there is no improvement within 2 weeks at a therapeutic dose, then an alternative antipsychotic should be considered (ie, move to the next treatment stage in **Fig. 69–1**).
- In partial responders who are tolerating the antipsychotic well, it may be reasonable to titrate above the usual dose range for 2 to 4 weeks with close monitoring.
- Rapid titration of antipsychotic dose is not recommended.
- Intramuscular (IM) antipsychotic administration (eg, aripiprazole 5.25–9.75 mg, ziprasidone 10–20 mg, olanzapine 2.5–10 mg, or haloperidol 2–5 mg) can be used to calm agitated patients. However, this approach does not improve the extent of response, time to remission, or length of hospitalization. IM **lorazepam**, 2 mg, as needed for agitation added to the maintenance antipsychotic is a rational alternative to an injectable antipsychotic. Combining IM lorazepam with **olanzapine** or **clozapine** is not recommended because of the risk of hypotension, central nervous system (CNS) depression, and respiratory depression.
- Inhaled loxapine powder, FDA approved for acute agitation associated with schizophrenia or bipolar I disorder in adults, can be administered only in a health-care facility and through the FDA-approved Risk Evaluation and Mitigation Strategy (REMS). Use is limited to one 10 mg inhaled dose per 24 hours. Patients with any lung disease associated with bronchospasm (eg, asthma, chronic obstructive pulmonary disease, other) are excluded. It may offer no advantage over IM and oral products.

STABILIZATION THERAPY

- During weeks 2 and 3, the goal is to improve socialization, self-care, and mood. Improvement in formal thought disorder may require an additional 6 to 8 weeks.
- Dose titration may continue every 1 to 2 weeks as long as the patient has no side effects.
- If the patient begins to show an adequate response at a particular dose, then continue at that dosage as long as symptoms continue to improve.

MAINTENANCE THERAPY

- Avoidance of relapses is the goal of maintenance therapy.
- Continue medication for at least 12 months after remission of the first psychotic episode. After remission of the first psychotic episode, many experts recommend treatment for at least 5 years. Lifetime pharmacotherapy at the lowest effective dose is necessary in most schizophrenic patients.
- Antipsychotics (especially FGAs and **clozapine**) should be tapered slowly before discontinuation to avoid cholinergic rebound.
- In general, when switching from one antipsychotic to another, the first should be tapered and discontinued over at least 1 to 2 weeks while the second antipsychotic is initiated and tapered upward.

Long-Acting Injectable Antipsychotics

- Table 69–3 summarizes the long-acting injectable antipsychotics (LAIs). A LAI antipsychotic should be considered for patients with poor adherence, and some clinicians recommend LAIs earlier in treatment before a pattern of nonadherence develops.

TABLE 69-3	Summary of Available Long Acting Injectable (LAI) Antipsychotics									
Medication Name Parameter	**Fluphenazine Decanoate**	**Haloperidol Decanoate**	**Risperidone LAI Risperdal Consta**	**Paliperidone Palmitate**			**Olanzapine Pamoate Zyprexa Relprevv**	**Aripiprazole Monohydrate Abilify Maintena**	**Aripiprazole Lauroxil Aristada**
				Invega Sustenna	**Invega Trinza**				
FDA Approved Indication	Schizophrenia	Schizophrenia	Schizophrenia Bipolar I Disorder maintenance	Schizophrenia Schizoaffective Disorder	Schizophrenia		Schizophrenia	Schizophrenia	Schizophrenia
Dose Range (mg)	12.5–100	20–450	12.5–50	39–234	273–819		150–405	160–400	441–882
PO Overlap	None	4 weeks (none if loading); use PO dose patient was taking prior to injection	3 weeks after first injection Use PO dose patient was taking prior to injection	None	None		None	2 weeks PO dose ranges from 10 to 20 mg/day	21 days PO overlap after first injection
Recommended maximum dose	100 mg every 2–3 weeks	450 mg every 4 weeks	50 mg every 2 weeks	234 mg every 4 weeks	819 mg every 3 months		300 mg every 2 weeks or 405 mg every 4 weeks	400 mg monthly	882 mg monthly
Initiation or Loading	Can Load	Can Load	None	Initiation required	None required, dose used depends on last Invega Sustenna dose as follows: If 78 mg give 273 mg If 117 mg give 410 mg If 156 mg give 546 mg If 234 mg give 819 mg		Initiation required	None	None required, dose depends on PO dose as follows: If 10 mg/day PO give 441 mg per month IM If 15 mg/day PO give 662 mg per month IM If 20 mg PO give 882 mg per month IM

Time to peak	8–24 hours	4–11 days	4–5 weeks	13 days	30–33 days	<1 week	5–7 days	5–6 days
T_{ss}	2–3 months	2–3 months	6–8 weeks	36 days		3 months	3–4 months	4 months
Injection Site — Gluteal	Yes	Yes	Yes	Yes after 2nd dose	Yes	Yes	Yes	Yes for all dose strengths
Injection Site — Deltoid	Yes	Yes	Yes	Yes	Yes	No	No	Yes, but only 441 mg dose
Injection Method/Technique		Z-Track				Standard		
Notes			A starting dose of 12.5 mg is recommended in patients with hepatic or renal impairment	Avoid use in patients with moderate to severe renal impairment (CrCl <50 mL/min [<0.83 mL/s])	Requires at least a 4 month trial with Invega Sustenna. Not recommended in patients with moderate or severe renal impairment (CrCl <50 mL/min [<0.83 mL/s])	Monitor for PDSS. Subject to REMS	Maintenance dose reduced to 300 mg if patient experiences adverse events. Dose adjustment needed in CYP2D6 slow metabolizers. Avoid use in patients taking CYP 3A4 inhibitors >14 days	May require up to 2 weeks of PO trial to establish tolerability to aripiprazole before initiating LAI. Avoid use of strong CYP2D6 and 3A4 inhibitors in patients taking 662 mg and 882 mg dose, no adjustment needed for 441mg dose

(PO, Oral; T_{ss}, Time to steady-state; CrCl, Creatine Clearance; IM, intramuscular; LAI, Long Acting Injectable.)

- Conversion from oral antipsychotics to depot formulations:
  ✓ Stabilize on an oral dosage form of the same agent (or at least a short trial of 3–7 days) to ensure adequate tolerance.
- **Risperidone Consta** is started at 25 mg. Usual dosing range is 25 to 50 mg deep IM every 2 weeks. Oral medication must be administered for at least 3 weeks after beginning injections. Make dose adjustments no more often than every 4 weeks.
- Olanzapine pamoate monohydrate is administered every 2 or 4 weeks by deep gluteal injection. The initial dose varies from 210 mg to 405 mg. About 2% of patients have a postinjection sedation/delirium syndrome (boxed warning), and it must be administered in a registered healthcare facility with patient observation by a professional for at least 3 hours postdose.
- Paliperidone palmitate (Invega Sustenna) is initiated with 234 mg and 156 mg a week later. Then monthly doses are titrated within a range of 39 to 234 mg. An every 3 month formulation (Invega Trinza) requires patients to be treated for at least 4 months with Invega Sustenna prior to initiation of Invega Trinza at a dose shown in **Table 69–3**.
- Aripiprazone LAI is available as Abilify Maintena and Aristada. See **Table 69–3** and manufacturers prescribing information for dosing.
- For **haloperidol decanoate**, the first dose should be 10 to 20 times the oral daily dose. The initial injection should be limited to 100 mg followed by the remaining balance of the first monthly dose given 3 to 7 days later. An oral haloperidol overlap is recommended for the first month. The maintenance dose is typically 10 to 15 times the oral daily dose given once monthly.

MANAGEMENT OF TREATMENT-RESISTANT SCHIZOPHRENIA

- Only **clozapine** has shown superiority over other antipsychotics in randomized trials for treatment-resistant schizophrenia. Improvement with clozapine often occurs slowly in resistant patients; as high as 60% of patients may improve if clozapine is used for up to 6 months.
- Because of the risk of orthostatic hypotension, clozapine is usually titrated more slowly than other antipsychotics. If a 12.5-mg test dose does not produce hypotension, then 25 mg of clozapine at bedtime is recommended, increased to 25 mg twice daily after 3 days, then increased in 25 to 50 mg/day increments every 3 days until a dose of at least 300 mg/day is reached.
- Augmentation therapy involves the addition of a nonantipsychotic drug to an antipsychotic in a poorly responsive patient, whereas combination treatment involves using two antipsychotics simultaneously.
- Mood stabilizers (eg, **lithium, valproic acid**, and **carbamazepine**) may improve labile affect and agitation. A placebo-controlled trial supports faster symptom improvement when **divalproex** is combined with either **olanzapine** or **risperidone**. The 2009 Schizophrenia Patient Outcomes Research Team (PORT) recommendations do not endorse mood stabilizer augmentation in resistant patients.
- **Selective serotonin reuptake inhibitors (SSRIs)** may improve obsessive-compulsive symptoms that worsen or arise during **clozapine** treatment.
- Combining a FGA and SGA and combining different SGAs have been suggested, but no data support or refute these strategies, and the 2009 PORT recommendations do not support their use. If a series of antipsychotic monotherapies fails, a time-limited combination antipsychotic trial may be attempted. If there is no improvement within 6 to 12 weeks, discontinue one of the drugs.

ADVERSE EFFECTS

- Table 69–4 shows relative incidence of antipsychotic side effects.

Anticholinergic Effects

- Anticholinergic side effects, most likely to occur with low potency FGA, clozapine, and olanzapine, include impaired memory, dry mouth, constipation, tachycardia, blurred vision, inhibition of ejaculation, and urinary retention. Elderly patients are especially sensitive to these side effects.

TABLE 69–4	Relative Side Effect Incidence of Commonly Used Antipsychotics[a,b]					
	Sedation	EPS	Anticholinergic	Orthostasis	Weight Gain	Prolactin
Aripiprazole	+	+	+	+	+	+
Asenapine	+	++	±	++	+	+
Brexpiprazole	+	+	+	+	+	+
Chlorpromazine	++++	+++	+++	++++	++	+++
Clozapine	++++	+	++++	++++	++++	+
Fluphenazine	+	++++	+	+	+	++++
Haloperidol	+	++++	+	+	+	++++
Iloperidone	+	±	++	+++	++	+
Lurasidone	+	+	+	+	±	±
Olanzapine	++	++	++	++	++++	+
Paliperidone	+	++	+	++	++	++++
Perphenazine	++	++++	++	+	+	++++
Quetiapine	++	+	+	++	++	+
Risperidone	+	++	+	++	++	++++
Thioridazine	++++	+++	++++	++++	+	+++
Thiothixene	+	++++	+	+	+	++++
Ziprasidone	++	++	+	+	+	+

(EPS, extrapyramidal side effects. Relative side effect risk: ±, negligible; +, low; ++, moderate; +++, moderately high; ++++, high.)
[a]Side effects shown are relative risk based on doses within the recommended therapeutic range.
[b]Individual patient risk varies depending on patient-specific factors.

Central Nervous System

EXTRAPYRAMIDAL SYSTEM

Dystonia

- Dystonias are prolonged tonic muscle contractions, (occurring usually within 24–96 hours of dosage initiation or dosage increase); they may be life threatening (eg, pharyngeal-laryngeal dystonias). Other dystonias are trismus, glossospasm, tongue protrusion, blepharospasm, oculogyric crisis, torticollis, and retrocollis. Risk factors include younger patients (especially male) and use of FGA, high-potency agents, and high dose.
- Treatment includes IM or IV anticholinergics (Table 69–5) or **benzodiazepines**. **Benztropine** 2 mg, or **diphenhydramine** 50 mg, may be given IM or IV, or **diazepam**, 5 to 10 mg slow IV push, or **lorazepam**, 1 to 2 mg IM, may be given. Relief usually occurs within 15 to 20 minutes of IM injection or 5 minutes of IV administration.
- Prophylactic anticholinergic medications (but not amantadine) are reasonable when using high-potency FGAs (eg, **haloperidol** and **fluphenazine**), in young men, and in patients with a prior dystonia.
- Dystonias can be minimized by using lower initial doses of FGAs and by using SGAs instead of FGAs.

Akathisia

- Akathisia occurs in 20% to 40% of patients treated with high potency FGA. Symptoms include subjective complaints (feelings of inner restlessness) and/or objective symptoms (pacing, shifting, shuffling, or tapping feet).

TABLE 69–5	Agents Used to Treat Extrapyramidal Side Effects	
Generic Name	**Equivalent Dose (mg)**	**Daily Dosage Range (mg)**
Antimuscarinics		
Benztropine[a]	1	1–8[b]
Biperiden[a]	2	2–8
Trihexyphenidyl	2	2–15
Antihistaminic		
Diphenhydramine[a]	50	50–400
Dopamine Agonist		
Amantadine	NA	100–400
Benzodiazepines		
Lorazepam[a]	NA	1–8
Diazepam	NA	2–20
Clonazepam	NA	2–8
β-Blockers		
Propranolol	NA	20–160

(NA, Not applicable.)
[a]Injectable dosage form can be given intramuscularly for relief of acute dystonia.
[b]In treatment-refractory cases, dosage can be titrated to 12 mg/day with careful monitoring; nonlinear pharmacokinetics have been reported.

- Treatment with anticholinergics is disappointing. Reduction in antipsychotic dose may be the best intervention, but not always feasible. Alternatively, switch to an SGA. Although akathisia occasionally occurs with the SGAs, particularly **aripiprazole** and **risperidone, quetiapine** and **clozapine** appear to have the lowest risk. **Benzodiazepines** may be used, but not in patients with a history of substance abuse. **Propranolol** (up to 160 mg/day), **nadolol** (up to 80 mg/day), and **metoprolol** (up to 100 mg/day) are reported to be effective. Emerging literature suggests that agents with antagonist activity at the 5-HT$_2$ receptor (**cyproheptadine**, **mirtazapine**, and **trazodone**) may be protective against akathisia.

Pseudoparkinsonism

- Patients with pseudoparkinsonism may have any of four cardinal symptoms:
  ✓ Akinesia, bradykinesia, or decreased motor activity, including mask-like facial expression, micrographia
  ✓ Tremor—predominantly at rest; decreasing with movement
  ✓ Rigidity—stiffness; cogwheel rigidity is seen as the patient's limbs yield in jerky, ratchet-like fashion when moved passively by the examiner
  ✓ Postural abnormalities—stooped, unstable posture and slow, shuffling, or festinating gait
- Risk factors—FGAs (especially in high dose), increasing age, and possibly female gender.
- Accessory symptoms—seborrhea, sialorrhea, hyperhidrosis, fatigue, weakness, dysphagia, and dysarthria.
- Usually symptoms start 1 to 2 weeks after initiation of antipsychotic therapy or dose increase. The risk of pseudoparkinsonism with SGAs is low except with **risperidone** in doses greater than 6 mg/day.
- **Benztropine** has a half-life that allows once- to twice-daily dosing. Typical dosing is 1 to 2 mg twice daily up to a maximum of 8 mg daily. Diphenhydramine produces more sedation (see **Table 69–5**). All of the anticholinergics have been abused for euphoriant effects.
- **Amantadine** is as efficacious as anticholinergics with less effect on memory. **Rotigotine** is effective at doses from 2 to 8 mg daily.
- Attempt to taper and discontinue these agents 6 weeks to 3 months after symptoms resolve.

Tardive Dyskinesia

- ***Tardive Dyskinesia*** (TD), characterized by abnormal involuntary movements, occurs with chronic antipsychotic therapy.
- The classic presentation is buccolingual-masticatory (BLM) or orofacial movements. If severe, symptoms may interfere with chewing, wearing dentures, speech, respiration, or swallowing. Facial movements include frequent blinking, brow arching, grimacing, upward deviation of the eyes, and lip smacking. Restless choreiform and athetotic movements of the limbs occur in later stages. Movements may worsen with stress, decrease with sedation, and disappear with sleep.
- Screen at baseline and at least quarterly using the Abnormal Involuntary Movement Scale (AIMS) and the Dyskinesia Identification System: Condensed User Scale (DISCUS) to detect TD.
- Dosage reduction or discontinuation may reduce symptoms, and some patients may have complete disappearance of symptoms if implemented early in the course of TD.
- Prevention of TD—(1) use SGAs as first-line agents; (2) use the DISCUS or other scales to assess for early signs of TD at least quarterly; and (3) discontinue antipsychotics or switch to SGAs at the earliest symptoms of TD, if possible.
- Risk factors for TD—duration of antipsychotic therapy, higher dose, possibly cumulative dose, possibly female gender, increasing age, occurrence of acute extrapyramidal symptoms, poor antipsychotic response, and diagnosis of organic mental disorder, diabetes mellitus, and mood disorders. With FGAs the prevalence of TD ranges from 20% to 50%. With SGAs, the risk of TD is ~3.0% per year in nonelderly adults compared to 7.7% per year for FGAs.
- The American Academy of Neurology guideline recommends short-term treatment of TD with **clonazepam** or **ginkgo biloba**.
- The FDA recently approved valbenazine (Ingrezza®) for the treatment of adults with TD. It is a selective vesicular monoamine transporter 2 inhibitor. Side effects include sedation and QT interval prolongation (see FDA approved labeling for contraindications and cautions). Initial dose is 40 mg once daily, to be increased to 80 mg once daily after 1 week.

SEDATION AND COGNITION

- Administration of most or the entire antipsychotic daily dose at bedtime can decrease daytime sedation and may eliminate the need for hypnotics.
- Some clinicians believe SGAs have cognitive benefits compared to FGAs.

SEIZURES

- All patients treated with antipsychotics have an increased risk of seizures. The highest risk for antipsychotic-induced seizures is with **chlorpromazine** or **clozapine**. Seizures are more likely with initiation of treatment, higher doses, and rapid dose increases.
- When an isolated seizure occurs, a dosage decrease is recommended, and anticonvulsant therapy is usually not recommended.
- If a change in antipsychotic therapy is required, **risperidone, thioridazine, haloperidol, pimozide, trifluoperazine**, and **fluphenazine** may be considered.

THERMOREGULATION

- In temperature extremes, patients (especially the elderly) taking antipsychotics may experience their body temperature adjusting to ambient temperature (poikilothermia). Hyperpyrexia can lead to heat stroke. Hypothermia is also a risk. These problems are more common with the use of low-potency FGAs and can occur with the more anticholinergic SGAs.

NEUROLEPTIC MALIGNANT SYNDROME

- Neuroleptic malignant syndrome (NMS) occurs in 0.5% to 1% of patients taking FGAs. NMS can occur with SGAs, including **clozapine**, but is less frequent.

- Symptoms develop rapidly over 24 to 72 hours (eg, body temperature exceeding 38°C (100.4°F), altered level of consciousness, autonomic dysfunction (tachycardia, labile blood pressure, diaphoresis, and tachypnea), and rigidity.
- Myoglobinuria, leukocytosis, increases in creatine kinase (CK), aspartate aminotransferase (AST), alanine aminotransferase (ALT), and lactate dehydrogenase (LDH) are common.
- Discontinue antipsychotics, and provide supportive care. **Bromocriptine** reduces rigidity, fever, or CK levels in up to 94% of patients. **Amantadine** has been used successfully in up to 63% of patients. **Dantrolene** has been used with favorable effects on temperature, heart rate, respiratory rate, and CK in up to 81% of patients.
- Rechallenge with the lowest effective dose of SGA or low potency FGA may be considered only for patients in need of reinstitution of antipsychotics following observation for at least 2 weeks without antipsychotics. Monitor carefully and titrate the dose slowly.

Endocrine System

- Antipsychotic-induced elevations in serum prolactin with associated galactorrhea, gynecomastia, decreased libido, and menstrual irregularities are common. Prolactin elevations are especially likely with FGAs, **risperidone**, and **paliperidone**. Possible management strategies for galactorrhea include switching to an antipsychotic with lower risk for causing prolactin elevations (eg, **asenapine, iloperidone,** or **lurasidone**).
- Weight gain, frequent with antipsychotic therapy, may be most likely with **olanzapine, clozapine, risperidone, quetiapine,** and **iloperidone**. Ziprasidone, aripiprazole, asenapine, and lurasidone cause minimal weight gain.
- Schizophrenics have a higher prevalence of type 2 diabetes than nonschizophrenics. Antipsychotics may adversely affect glucose levels in diabetic patients. **Olanzapine** and **clozapine** have the highest risk of causing new-onset diabetes, followed by **risperidone** and **quetiapine**. The risk with **aripiprazole** and **ziprasidone** is likely less than with other SGA. The 2009 PORT do not recommend **olanzapine** as first-line therapy.

Cardiovascular System

- The incidence of orthostatic hypotension (defined as >20 mm Hg drop in systolic pressure upon standing) is greatest with low-potency FGAs, **clozapine, iloperidone, quetiapine,** and combination antipsychotics. Diabetics with cardiovascular disease and the elderly are predisposed. Reducing the dose or changing to an antipsychotic with less α-adrenergic blockade may help, and tolerance may develop within 2 to 3 months.
- The low-potency piperidine phenothiazines (**thioridazine**), **clozapine, iloperidone,** and **ziprasidone** are the most likely to cause ECG changes, including increased heart rate, flattened T waves, ST-segment depression, and prolongation of QT and PR intervals. Thioridazine prolongs the QTc on average about 20 milliseconds longer than **haloperidol, risperidone, olanzapine,** or **quetiapine**. For thioridazine, the effect is dose related, and the drug's labeling carries a boxed warning for torsades de pointes and sudden death.
- **Ziprasidone** prolonged the QTc interval about one half as much as **thioridazine. Iloperidone** prolongs the QTc in a dose related manner, especially in CYP2D6 slow metabolizers. High IV doses of **haloperidol** also can prolong the QTc, and it also carries a boxed warning.
- It has been recommended to discontinue a medication associated with QTc prolongation if the interval consistently exceeds 500 milliseconds. A recent review suggests that QTc intervals greater than or equal to 450 milliseconds and/or a 30 millisecond increase from baseline are predictors of a drug's risk to cause Torsades. Torsades rarely happens in the absence of additional risk factors (eg, age greater than 60, female gender, preexisting cardiac or cerebrovascular disease, hepatic impairment, hypokalemia, hypomagnesemia, additional meds that prolong the QTc interval, metabolic inhibition by another medication, or preexisting QTc prolongation).
- In patients older than 50 years, pretreatment ECG and serum potassium and magnesium levels are recommended.
- Those taking FGAs or SGAs have twice the risk of sudden cardiac death that nonusers have. Use of antipsychotics was associated with a 1.53 fold increase in ventricular arrhythmia or sudden cardiac death.

Lipid Effects

- Some SGAs and phenothiazines cause elevations in serum triglycerides and cholesterol. The risk for this effect may be less with **risperidone**, **ziprasidone**, **aripiprazole**, **asenapine**, **iloperidone**, and **lurasidone**. Weight gain, diabetes, and lipid abnormalities during antipsychotic therapy is consistent with development of metabolic syndrome.
- Metabolic syndrome consists of raised triglycerides (≥150 mg/dL [1.70 mmol/L]), low high-density lipoprotein cholesterol (≤40 mg/dL [1.03 mmol/L] for males, ≤50 mg/dL [1.29 mmol/L] for females), elevated fasting glucose (≥100 mg/dL [5.6 mmol/L]), blood pressure elevation (≥130/85 mm Hg), and weight gain (abdominal circumference >102 cm [40 in] for males, >89 cm [35 in] for females.

Psychiatric Side Effects

- Akathisia, akinesia, and dysphoria can result in apathy, withdrawal, and pseudo-depression (behavioral toxicity).
- Chronic confusion and disorientation can occur in the elderly.
- Delirium and psychosis may occur with high doses of FGAs or combinations of FGAs with anticholinergics.

Ophthalmologic Effects

- Exacerbation of narrow-angle glaucoma can occur with use of antipsychotics and/or anticholinergics.
- Opaque deposits in the cornea and lens may occur with chronic phenothiazine treatment, especially **chlorpromazine**. Although visual acuity is not usually affected, periodic slit-lamp examinations are recommended with long-term phenothiazine use. Baseline and periodic slit-lamp examinations are also recommended for **quetiapine**-treated patients because of cataract development in animal studies.
- **Thioridazine** doses greater than 800 mg daily (the recommended maximum dose) can cause retinitis pigmentosa with permanent visual impairment or blindness.

Genitourinary System

- Urinary hesitancy and retention are common, especially with low-potency FGAs and **clozapine**, and in men with benign prostatic hypertrophy.
- Urinary incontinence may result from α-blockade, and among the SGA, it is especially problematic with **clozapine**.
- **Risperidone** produces at least as much sexual dysfunction as FGAs, but other SGAs (which have a weaker effect of prolactin) pose less risk.

Hematologic System

- Antipsychotics can cause transient leukopenia, but it usually does not progress to clinical significance. **Clozapine**, **chlorpromazine**, and **olanzapine** have the highest risk for neutropenia.
- Agranulocytosis reportedly occurs in 0.01% of patients receiving FGAs, and it may occur more frequently with **chlorpromazine** and **thioridazine**. The onset is usually within the first 8 weeks of therapy.
- Agranulocytosis can manifest as sore throat, leukoplakia, erythema, and ulcerated pharynx. Patients with these symptoms taking antipsychotics should have an absolute neutrophil count (ANC). If he ANC is less than 500/μL (0.5×10^9/L), discontinue the antipsychotic with close monitoring for secondary infection.
- The risk of developing neutropenia or agranulocytosis with **clozapine** is approximately 3% and 0.8%, respectively. Increasing age and female gender increase risk. The greatest risk is between 1 and 6 months of initiating treatment. The baseline ANC must be at least 1500/μL (1.5×10^9/L) in order to start clozapine. Weekly ANC monitoring for the first 6 months is FDA mandated. After this time, if the ANC remains greater than 1500/μL (1.5×10^9/L), ANC monitoring can be decreased to every 2 weeks for the next 6 months. Subsequently, if all ANCs remain greater than 1500/μL (1.5×10^9/L) ANC monitoring can be decreased to monthly. If at any time the ANC drops to less than 500/μL (0.5×10^9/L), clozapine must be discontinued and the ANC monitored daily until it is

greater than 1500/μL (1.5×10^9/L). Refer to the product labeling for more detailed information regarding ANC monitoring, including monitoring for mild and moderate leukopenia.

Dermatologic System

- Allergic reactions are rare and usually occur within 8 weeks of initiating therapy. They manifest as maculopapular, erythematous, or pruritic rashes.
- Contact dermatitis, on the skin or oral mucosa, may occur. Swallowing of the FGA oral concentrates quickly may decrease rashes on the oral mucosa.
- **Ziprasidone** can cause a rare but fatal skin reaction called Drug Reaction with Eosinophilia and Systemic Symptoms (DRESS).
- Both FGAs and SGAs can cause photosensitivity with severe sunburns. Educate patients to use maximal blocking sunscreens, hats, protective clothing, and sunglasses when in the sun.
- Blue-gray or purplish discoloration of skin exposed to sunlight may occur with higher doses of low-potency phenothiazines (especially **chlorpromazine**) given long term. This may occur with concurrent corneal or lens pigmentation.

USE IN PREGNANCY AND LACTATION

- There is a slightly increased risk of birth defects, including cardiovascular defects, with in utero exposure to low-potency FGAs.
- No relationship between **haloperidol** use and teratogenicity has been found.
- A meta-analysis found a greater risk of birth defects and preterm births with first trimester exposure to SGA, but no specific abnormality was identified. Large, well-controlled studies are needed to clarify the safety of SGA during pregnancy.
- Schizophrenic women taking FGAs have a greater than two-fold increased risk of preterm birth compared with unaffected mothers not taking antipsychotics.
- There is nearly twofold greater odds of gestational diabetes in women taking antipsychotics during pregnancy.
- The FDA requires the pregnancy section of antipsychotic labeling to highlight the potential risk for extrapyramidal symptoms and withdrawal symptoms in newborns whose mothers received antipsychotics during the third trimester.
- Antipsychotics appear in breast milk, with milk:plasma ratios of 0.5:1, however, 1-week postdelivery **clozapine** milk concentrations were found to be 279% of serum concentrations. Use of clozapine during breast-feeding is not recommended.
- **Aripiprazole, quetiapine, haloperidol, perphenazine**, and **trifluoperazine** are generally considered safe for the mother to take during breastfeeding. Infants exposed to **chlorpromazine** in breast milk have been reported to be drowsy and lethargic. Co-administration of chlorpromazine and **haloperidol** to breastfeeding mothers may cause developmental delays in infants at 12 to 18 months of age.

DRUG INTERACTIONS

- Antipsychotic drug interactions often involve additive hypotensive, anticholinergic, or sedative effects.
- Antipsychotic pharmacokinetics can be significantly affected by concomitantly administered enzyme inducers or inhibitors. Smoking is a potent inducer of hepatic enzymes and may increase antipsychotic clearance by as much as 50%. **Asenapine**, an inhibitor of CPY2D6, is the only antipsychotic found to significantly affect the pharmacokinetics of other medications. **Fluvoxamine**, an inhibitor of CYP1A2, increases **clozapine** serum concentrations by twofold to threefold or more. **Ketoconazole** profoundly decreases lurasidone metabolism, and it is recommended that they not be used concomitantly. **Carbamazepine** reportedly decreases **aripiprazole** serum concentrations. Reduce the **iloperidone** dose by 50% when used with CYP2D6 inhibitors such as **fluoxetine** or **paroxetine**. Consult the published literature for antipsychotic drug interactions.

EVALUATION OF THERAPEUTIC OUTCOMES

- Table 69–6 summarizes antipsychotic adverse effects and patient monitoring parameters. Before starting antipsychotic therapy, at baseline take a family history

TABLE 69–6 Antipsychotic Adverse Effects and Monitoring Parameters

Adverse Reaction	Monitoring Parameter	Frequency	Comments
Adverse effect monitoring parameters for all antipsychotic medications			
Akathisia	Ask about restless or anxiety. Observe patient for restlessness. Barnes Akathisia Scale can also be used	Every visit	
Anticholinergic side effects	Ask patient about constipation, blurry vision, urinary retention, or unusually dry mouth	Every visit	
Glucose intolerance	FBS or HbA1c	At baseline, after 3 months, and if normal, then annually	
Hyperlipidemia	Lipid profile	At baseline, after 3 months, and if normal, then annually	
Orthostatic hypotension	Ask patient about dizziness on standing. If present, check BP and HR in sitting and standing positions	Every visit	The degree of orthostatic change in BP to produce symptoms varies. In general, a BP change of 20 mm Hg or more is significant
Hyperprolactinemia	In women, ask about expression of milk from the breast and menstrual irregularities. In men, ask about breast enlargement or expression of milk from nipples. If symptoms present, check serum prolactin level	Every visit	In the absence of symptoms, there is no need to monitor serum prolactin
Sedation	Ask patient about unusual sedation or sleepiness	Every visit	
Sexual dysfunction	Ask patient about decreased sexual desire, difficulty being aroused, or problems with orgasm	Every visit	Patients with schizophrenia have more sexual dysfunction than the normal population. Compare symptoms with medication-free state
Tardive dyskinesia	Standardized rating scale such as the AIMS or the DISCUS	At baseline, and then every 3 months for FGAs and every 6 months for SGAs	

(continued)

TABLE 69-6 Antipsychotic Adverse Effects and Monitoring Parameters (*Continued*)

Adverse Reaction	Monitoring Parameter	Frequency	Comments
Weight gain	Measure body weight, BMI, and waist circumference	At baseline, monthly for the first 3 months, and then quarterly	Waist circumference is the single best predictor of cardiac morbidity
Adverse effect monitoring parameters for specific antipsychotics			
Agranulocytosis	White blood cell (WBC) and absolute neutrophil counts (ANC)	At baseline, weekly for 6 months, then every 2 weeks for 6 months, and then monthly	Clozapine only
Sialorrhea or excess drooling	Ask patient about problems with excess drooling, waking in the morning with a wet ring on his or her pillow. Visual observation of the patient for drooling	Every visit	Clozapine only
Bronchospasm, respiratory distress, respiratory depression, respiratory arrest	Before administration, patients must be screened for a history of asthma, chronic obstructive pulmonary disease, or other lung disease associated with bronchospasm. Monitor patient every 15 minutes for a minimum of 1 hour after drug administration for signs and symptoms of bronchospasm (ie, vital signs and chest auscultation). Only one 10 mg dose can be given every 24 hours	Every dose administration	Inhaled loxapine only. Can only be administered in approved healthcare facilities registered in REMS program
Postinjection sedation/delirium syndrome	Observation of the patient for at least 3 hours after drug administration. Monitor for possible sedation, altered level of consciousness, coma, delirium, confusion, disorientation, agitation, anxiety, or other cognitive impairment	Every dose administration	Long-acting olanzapine pamoate monohydrate only. Can only be administered in approved healthcare facilities registered in REMS program

of response, and measure weight, height, body mass index, waist circumference, blood pressure, fasting plasma glucose, and fasting lipid profile. Do a follow up check of these parameters after beginning or changing SGAs. Measure body weight monthly for 3 months, then quarterly. Assess the other parameters after 3 months, then annually.

• The four-item Positive Symptom Rating Scale and the Brief Negative Symptom Assessment are brief enough to be useful in the outpatient setting to measure changes in symptomatology. Patient-rated self-assessments can also be useful, as they engage the patient in treatment and can open the door for patient education and addressing misconceptions. Clinicians should be assertive in attempting to achieve symptom remission.

See Chapter 67, Schizophrenia, authored by M. Lynn Crismon, Rania S. Kattura, and Peter F. Buckley, for a more detailed discussion of this topic.

- The *Diagnostic and Statistical Manual of Mental Disorders*, 5th ed., category of sleep-wake disorders encompasses insomnia, hypersomnolence, narcolepsy, breathing-related sleep disorders, circadian rhythm sleep-wake disorders, nonrapid eye movement (NREM) sleep arousal disorders, nightmare disorder, rapid eye movement (REM) sleep behavior disorder, restless legs syndrome, and substance/medication-induced sleep disorder.

SLEEP PHYSIOLOGY

- Humans typically have four to six cycles of NREM and REM sleep each night, each cycle lasting 70 to 120 minutes. Usually, there is progression through the four stages of NREM sleep before the first REM period.
- Stage 1 of NREM is the stage between wakefulness and sleep. Stages 3 and 4 sleep are called *delta sleep* (ie, slow-wave sleep).
- In REM sleep, there is a low-amplitude, mixed-frequency electroencephalogram, increased electrical and metabolic activity, increased cerebral blood flow, muscle atonia, poikilothermia, vivid dreaming, and fluctuations in respiratory and cardiac rate.
- The elderly have lighter more fragmented sleep with more arousals and gradual reduction in slow-wave sleep.
- REM sleep is turned on by cholinergic cells. Dopamine has an alerting effect. Neurochemicals involved in wakefulness include norepinephrine and acetylcholine in the cortex and histamine and neuropeptides (eg, substance P and corticotropin-releasing factor) in the hypothalamus.
- Polysomnography (PSG) measures multiple electrophysiologic parameters simultaneously during sleep (eg, electroencephalogram, electrooculogram of each eye, electrocardiogram, electromyogram, air thermistors, abdominal and thoracic strain belts, and oxygen saturation) to characterize sleep and diagnose sleep disorders.

INSOMNIA

CLINICAL PRESENTATION AND DIAGNOSIS

- Patients with insomnia complain of difficulty falling asleep, maintaining sleep, or experiencing nonrestorative sleep.
- Transient (two or three nights) and short-term (less than 3 months) insomnia is common. Chronic insomnia (more than 3 months duration) occurs in 9% to 12% of adults and in up to 20% of the elderly.
- Causes of insomnia include stress; jet lag or shift work; pain or other medical problems; mood or anxiety disorders; substance withdrawal; stimulants, steroids, or other medications.
- In patients with chronic disturbances, a diagnostic evaluation includes physical and mental status examinations, routine laboratory tests, and medication and substance abuse histories.

TREATMENT

- <u>Goals of Treatment</u>: Correct the underlying sleep complaint, improve daytime functioning, and avoid adverse drug effects.

General Approach

- Behavioral and educational interventions that may help include short-term cognitive behavioral therapy, relaxation therapy, stimulus control therapy, cognitive therapy, sleep restriction, paradoxical intention, and sleep hygiene education (Table 70–1).

| TABLE 70–1 | Nonpharmacologic Recommendations for Management of Insomnia |

Stimulus control procedures

1. Establish regular times to wake up and to go to sleep (including weekends).
2. Sleep only as much as necessary to feel rested.
3. Go to bed only when sleepy. Avoid long periods of wakefulness in bed. Use the bed only for sleep or intimacy; do not read or watch television in bed.
4. Avoid trying to force sleep; if you do not fall asleep within 20–30 minutes, leave the bed and perform a relaxing activity (eg, read, listen to music) until drowsy. Repeat this as often as necessary.
5. Avoid blue spectrum light from television, smart phones, tablets, and other mobile devices.
6. Avoid daytime naps.
7. Schedule worry time during the day. Do not take your troubles to bed.

Sleep hygiene recommendations

1. Exercise routinely (three to four times weekly) but not close to bedtime because this can increase wakefulness.
2. Create a comfortable sleep environment by avoiding temperature extremes, loud noises, and illuminated clocks in the bedroom.
3. Discontinue or reduce the use of alcohol, caffeine, and nicotine.
4. Avoid drinking large quantities of liquids in the evening to prevent nighttime trips to the restroom.
5. Do something relaxing and enjoyable before bedtime.

- Management includes identifying the cause of insomnia, educating about sleep hygiene, managing stress, monitoring for mood symptoms, and eliminating unnecessary pharmacotherapy.
- Transient and short-term insomnia should be treated with good sleep hygiene and careful use of sedative-hypnotics if necessary. Chronic insomnia calls for careful assessment for a medical cause, nonpharmacologic treatment, and careful use of sedative-hypnotics if necessary (**Fig. 70–1**).
- **Antihistamines** (eg, **diphenhydramine, doxylamine**, and **pyrilamine**) are less effective than **benzodiazepines**, but side effects are usually minimal. Their anticholinergic side effects may be problematic, especially in the elderly.
- Antidepressants are good alternatives for patients who should not receive benzodiazepines, especially those with depression, pain, or a history of substance abuse.
- **Amitriptyline, doxepin**, and **nortriptyline** are effective, but side effects include sedation, anticholinergic effects, adrenergic blockade effects, and cardiac conduction prolongation.
- Low-dose doxepin is approved for sleep maintenance insomnia.
- Mirtazapine many improve sleep, but may cause daytime sedation and weight gain.
- **Trazodone**, 25 to 100 mg at bedtime, is often used for insomnia induced by selective serotonin reuptake inhibitors or bupropion and in patients prone to substance abuse. Side effects include serotonin syndrome (when used with other serotonergic drugs), oversedation, α-adrenergic blockade, dizziness, and rarely, priapism.
- **Suvorexant** (an orexinA and orexinB antagonist) turns off wake signaling. Doses of 10 to 20 mg at bedtime are indicated for difficulty initiating or maintaining sleep. Side effects include sedation and rarely narcolepsy-like symptoms.
- **Ramelteon** is a melatonin receptor agonist selective for the MT_1 and MT_2 receptors. The dose is 8 mg at bedtime. It is well tolerated, but side effects include headache, dizziness, and somnolence. It is not a controlled substance. It is effective for patients with chronic obstructive pulmonary disease and sleep apnea.
- **Valerian**, an herbal product, is available without a prescription. The recommended dose is 300 to 600 mg. Purity and potency concerns are an issue. It may cause daytime sedation.

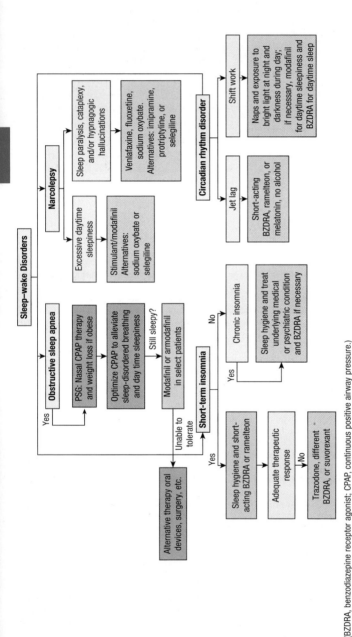

(BZDRA, benzodiazepine receptor agonist; CPAP, continuous positive airway pressure.)

FIGURE 70–1. Algorithm for treatment of dyssomnias. *(Used with permission from Jermaine DM. Sleep Disorders. In: Carter BL, Angaran DM, Lake KD, Raebel MA, eds. Pharmacotherapy Self-Assessment Program, 2nd ed. Neurology and Psychiatry. Kansas City: American College of Clinical Pharmacy, 1995;139–154.)*

- The benzodiazepine receptor agonists are the most commonly used drugs for insomnia. They carry a caution regarding anaphylaxis, facial angioedema, complex sleep behaviors (eg, sleep driving, phone calls, and sleep eating). They include the newer nonbenzodiazepine γ-aminobutyric acid$_A$ (GABA$_A$) agonists and the traditional benzodiazepines, which also bind to GABA$_A$ (Table 70–2).

Nonbenzodiazepine GABA$_A$ Agonists

- In general, the nonbenzodiazepine hypnotics do not have significant active metabolites, and they are associated with less withdrawal, tolerance, and rebound insomnia than the benzodiazepines.
- **Zolpidem** is comparable in effectiveness to benzodiazepine hypnotics, and it has little effect on sleep stages. Its duration is approximately 6 to 8 hours. Common side effects are drowsiness, amnesia, dizziness, headache, and gastrointestinal (GI) complaints. It appears to have minimal effects on next-day psychomotor performance. The usual dose is 5 mg in women, the elderly, and those with liver impairment, and 5 to 10 mg in men. Sleep eating has been reported. It should be taken on an empty stomach.
- **Zaleplon** has a rapid onset, a half-life of ~1 hour, and no active metabolites. It decreases time to sleep onset, but does not reduce nighttime awakenings or increase the total sleep time. It does not appear to cause next-day psychomotor impairment. The most common side effects are dizziness, headache, and somnolence. The recommended dose is 10 mg (5 mg in the elderly).
- **Eszopiclone** has a rapid onset and duration of action of up to 6 hours. The most common adverse effects are somnolence, unpleasant taste, headache, and dry mouth. It may be taken nightly for up to 6 months.

Benzodiazepine Hypnotics

- The pharmacokinetics and dosing of benzodiazepine receptor agonists are summarized in **Table 70–2**.
- Benzodiazepines have sedative, anxiolytic, muscle relaxant, and anticonvulsant properties. They increase stage 2 sleep and decrease REM and delta sleep.
- Overdose fatalities are rare unless benzodiazepines are taken with other central nervous system (CNS) depressants.
- **Triazolam** is distributed quickly because of its high lipophilicity, and it has a short duration of effect. **Erythromycin, nefazodone, fluvoxamine**, and **ketoconazole** reduce the clearance of triazolam and increase plasma concentrations.
- The effects of **flurazepam** and **quazepam** are long because of active metabolites.

BENZODIAZEPINE ADVERSE EFFECTS

- Side effects include drowsiness, psychomotor incoordination, decreased concentration, cognitive deficits, and anterograde amnesia which are minimized by using the lowest dose possible.
- Tolerance to daytime CNS effects (eg, drowsiness, decreased concentration) may develop in some individuals.
- Rebound insomnia is minimized by using the lowest effective dose and tapering the dose upon discontinuation.
- Long elimination half-life benzodiazepines are associated with falls and hip fractures; thus, **flurazepam**, and **quazepam** should be avoided in the elderly.

SLEEP APNEA

- Apnea is repetitive episodes of cessation of breathing during sleep followed by blood oxygen desaturation.

OBSTRUCTIVE SLEEP APNEA

- Obstructive sleep apnea (OSA) is potentially life threatening and characterized by repeated episodes of nocturnal breathing cessation. It is caused by occlusion of the upper airway, and blood oxygen (O_2) desaturation can occur. Episodes may be caused by obesity or fixed upper airway lesions, enlarged tonsils, amyloidosis,

TABLE 70–2 Pharmacokinetics of Benzodiazepine-Receptor Agonists

Generic Name (Brand Name)	t_{max} (hours)[a]	Half-Life[b] (hours)	Daily Dose Range (mg)	Metabolic Pathway	Clinically Significant Metabolites
Estazolam (ProSom)	2	12–15	1–2	Oxidation	—
Eszopiclone (Lunesta)	1–1.5	6	2–3	Oxidation Demethylation	—
Flurazepam (Dalmane)	1	8	15–30	Oxidation N-dealkylation	Hydroxyethylflurazepam, Flurazepam aldehyde N-desalkylflurazepam[c]
Quazepam (Doral)	2	39	7.5–15	Oxidation, N-dealkylation	2-Oxo-quazepam, N-desalkylflurazepam[c]
Temazepam (Restoril)	1.5	10–15	15–30	Conjugation	—
Triazolam (Halcion)	1	2	0.125–0.25	Oxidation	—
Zaleplon (Sonata)	1	1	5–10	Oxidation	—
Zolpidem (Ambien; Intermezzo)	1.6	2–2.6	1.75–10[d]	Oxidation	—

[a]Time to peak plasma concentration.
[b]Half-life of parent drug.
[c]N-desalkylflurazepam, mean half-life 47 to 100 hours.
[d]Oral and sublingual dosing 5 to 10 mg; sublingual tablets for middle-of-the night dosing 1.75 to 3.5 mg (1.75 for women, 3.5 mg for men).

and hypothyroidism. OSA is associated with motor vehicle accidents, depression, increased cancer risk, stroke, arrhythmias, hypertension, cor pulmonale, and sudden death.

- Heavy snoring, severe gas exchange disturbances, respiratory failure, and gasping occur in severe episodes. Patients with OSA usually complain of excessive daytime sleepiness (EDS). Other symptoms are morning headache, poor memory, and irritability.
- The apneic episode is terminated by a reflex action in response to the fall in blood O_2 saturation that causes an arousal with resumed breathing.

Treatment

- <u>Goal of Treatment</u>: The goal is to alleviate sleep-disordered breathing and prevent complications (**Fig. 70–1**).
- Nonpharmacologic approaches are the treatments of choice (eg, weight loss [for all overweight patients], tonsillectomy, nasal septal repair, and nasal positive airway pressure [PAP], which may be continuous (CPAP) or bilevel). Other surgical therapies, such as uvulopalatopharyngoplasty and tracheostomy, may be necessary in severe cases.
- Management parameters are published by the American Academy of Sleep Medicine. Avoid all CNS depressants and drugs that promote weight gain. **Angiotensin-converting enzyme (ACE) inhibitors** can also worsen sleep-disordered breathing.
- **Modafinil** and **armodafinil** are approved by the FDA to improve wakefulness in those with residual daytime sleepiness. They should be used only in patients without cardiovascular disease who are using optimal PAP therapy.

CENTRAL SLEEP APNEA

- Central sleep apnea (CSA), less frequent than OSA, is characterized by repeated episodes of apnea caused by temporary loss of respiratory effort during sleep. It may be caused by autonomic nervous system lesions, neurologic diseases, high altitudes, opioid use, and congestive heart failure.

Treatment

- PAP with or without supplemental O_2 improves CSA.
- **Acetazolamide** (which causes metabolic acidosis that stimulates respiratory drive) and theophylline have been studied, but have minimal effects.

NARCOLEPSY

- The narcolepsy tetrad includes EDS, cataplexy, hallucinations, and sleep paralysis. Patients complain of EDS, sleep attacks that last up to 30 minutes, fatigue, impaired performance, and disturbed nighttime sleep.
- Cataplexy, which occurs in 70% to 80% of narcoleptics, is sudden bilateral loss of muscle tone with collapse. It is often precipitated by highly emotional situations.
- Dysfunction of the hypocretin/orexin neurotransmitter system may play a central role in narcolepsy. An autoimmune process may cause destruction of hypocretin-producing cells.

TREATMENT

- <u>Goals of Treatment</u>: The goal is to maximize alertness during waking hours and improve quality of life (**Fig. 70–1**).
- Encourage good sleep hygiene and two or more daytime naps daily (as little as 15 min).
- Pharmacotherapy (**Table 70–3**) focuses on EDS and REM sleep abnormalities.
- **Modafinil**, the standard for treatment of EDS, and **armodafinil** (the active R-isomer) are FDA approved. They do not treat cataplexy. Evidence suggests no risk of tolerance, withdrawal, or risk of abuse. Side effects include headache, nausea, nervousness, and insomnia.

TABLE 70–3 Dosing of Drugs Used to Treat Narcolepsy

Generic Name	Brand Name	Initial Dose (mg)	Usual dose (mg)	Comments
Excessive daytime somnolence				
Dextroamphetamine	Dexedrine	5–10	5–60	Concurrent use of amphetamines and acidic foods may reduce amphetamine absorption
Dextroamphetamine/ Amphetamine salts[a]	Adderall	5–20	5–60	See above
Methamphetamine[b]	Desoxyn	5–15	5–15	See above
Lisdexamfetamine	Vyvanse	20–30	20–70	Prodrug of dextroamphetamine
Methylphenidate	Ritalin	10–40	30–80	May increase risk of bleeding with concomitant warfarin therapy
Modafinil	Provigil	100–200	200–400	May reduce effectiveness of hormonal contraceptives
Armodafinil	Nuvigil	150	150–250	May reduce effectiveness of hormonal contraceptives
Sodium oxybate[c]	Xyrem	4.5/night	4.5–9 g/night	Do not use with other CNS depressants
Agents for cataplexy				
Fluoxetine	Prozac	10–20	20–80	Will see cataplexy benefits sooner than antidepressant benefits
Imipramine	Tofranil	50–100	50–250	Anticholinergic side effects
Nortriptyline	Aventyl, Pamelor	50–100	50–200	Anticholinergic side effects
Protriptyline	Vivactil	5–10	5–30	
Venlafaxine	Effexor	37.5	37.5–225	May increase blood pressure
Selegiline	Eldepryl	5–10	20–40	Doses <10 mg per day do not require dietary tyramine restrictions

(CNS, central nervous system).

[a]Dextroamphetamine sulfate, dextroamphetamine saccharate, amphetamine aspartate, and amphetamine sulfate.

[b]Not available in some states.

[c]Also is effective at treating cataplexy.

- **Amphetamines** and **methylphenidate** have a fast onset of effect and durations of 3 to 4 hours and 6 to 10 hours, respectively, for EDS. Amphetamines have more risk of abuse and tolerance. Side effects include insomnia, hypertension, palpitations, and irritability.
- The most common treatments for cataplexy are the **tricyclic antidepressants, serotonin norepinephrine reuptake inhibitors, and selective serotonin reuptake inhibitors. Imipramine, protriptyline, clomipramine, fluoxetine**, and **nortriptyline** are effective in approximately 80% of patients. **Selegiline** improves hypersomnolence and cataplexy.
- **Sodium oxybate** (γ-**hydroxybutyrate**) improves EDS and decreases episodes of sleep paralysis, cataplexy, and hypnagogic hallucinations. Give at bedtime and repeat 2.5 to 4 hours later. Side effects include nausea, somnolence, confusion, dizziness, and incontinence.

EVALUATION OF THERAPEUTIC OUTCOMES

- Assess patients with short-term or chronic insomnia after 1 week of therapy for drug effectiveness, adverse events, and adherence to nonpharmacologic recommendations. Patients should maintain a daily recording of awakenings, medications taken, naps, and an index of sleep quality.
- Assess patients with OSA after 1 to 3 months of treatment for improvement in alertness, daytime symptoms, weight reduction, and compliance with PAP therapy. Bed partners can report on snoring and gasping.
- Patients with narcolepsy should keep a diary of frequency and severity of core symptoms. Pharmacotherapy monitoring parameters include reduction in daytime sleepiness, cataplexy, hypnagogic and hypnopompic hallucinations, and sleep paralysis. Assess patients regularly during medication titration, then every 6 to 12 months for side effects (eg, hypertension, sleep disturbances, and cardiovascular abnormalities).

See Chapter 72, Sleep-Wake Disorders, authored by John M. Dopp and Bradley G. Phillips, for a more detailed discussion of this topic.

Substance-Related Disorders

- The *Diagnostic and Statistical Manual of Mental Disorders*, 5th edition (DSM-5) divides substance-related disorders (encompassing 10 separate classes of drugs) into (1) substance use disorders and (2) substance-induced disorders (eg, intoxication, withdrawal, and substance-induced mental disorders).
- The diagnosis of substance use disorder is based on a pathologic pattern of behaviors related to use of the substance. Diagnostic criteria fall into the categories of (1) impaired control, (2) social impairment, (3) risky use, and (4) pharmacological criteria, including tolerance and withdrawal.
- DSM-5 does not separate the diagnoses of substance abuse and substance dependence. Criteria are provided for substance use disorder, accompanied by criteria for intoxication, withdrawal, substance-induced disorders, and unspecified substance-related disorders in some cases.
- *Addiction:* A primary chronic neurobiologic disease characterized by one or more of the following five Cs: chronicity, impaired control over drug use, compulsive use, continued use despite harm, and craving.
- *Intoxication:* Development of a substance-specific syndrome after recent ingestion and presence in the body of a substance; it is associated with maladaptive behavior during the waking state caused by effects of the substance on the central nervous system (CNS).
- *Physical dependence:* A state of adaptation manifested by a drug class–specific withdrawal syndrome that can be produced by abrupt cessation, rapid dose reduction, decreasing blood level of the drug, and/or administration of an antagonist.
- *Substance dependence:* The characteristic feature is a continued maladaptive pattern of substance use in spite of repeated adverse consequences related to the repeated use.
- *Tolerance:* A state of adaptation in which exposure to a drug induces changes that result in a diminution of one or more of the drug's effects over time.
- *Withdrawal:* A substance-specific syndrome occurring after cessation of or reduction in intake of a substance that was used regularly.

CENTRAL NERVOUS SYSTEM DEPRESSANTS

ALCOHOL

- Table 71–1 relates the effects of **alcohol** to the blood alcohol concentration (BAC).
- Signs and symptoms of alcohol intoxication include euphoria, slurred speech, ataxia, incoordination, sedation, nystagmus, impaired judgment, impaired memory, unconsciousness, nausea, vomiting, respiratory depression, and coma. Signs and symptoms of alcohol withdrawal include tachycardia, diaphoresis, hyperthermia, hallucinations, delirium, and seizures.
- Alcohol withdrawal includes (1) a history of cessation or reduction in heavy and prolonged alcohol use and (2) the presence of two or more of the symptoms of alcohol withdrawal.
- There is 14 g of alcohol in 12 oz of beer, 5 oz of wine, or 1.5 oz (one shot) of 80-proof whiskey. This amount will increase the BAC by approximately 20 to 25 mg/dL (4.3–5.4 mmol/L) in a healthy 70 kg (154 lb) man. Deaths generally occur when BACs are greater than 400 to 500 mg/dL (87–109 mmol/L).
- Absorption of alcohol begins in the stomach within 5 to 10 minutes of ingestion. Peak concentrations are usually achieved 30 to 90 minutes after finishing the last drink.
- Alcohol is metabolized by alcohol dehydrogenase to acetaldehyde, which is metabolized to carbon dioxide and water by aldehyde dehydrogenase. Catalase and the microsomal alcohol oxidase system are also involved.
- Most clinical laboratories report BAC in milligrams per deciliter. In legal cases, results are reported in percentage (grams of alcohol per 100 mL of whole blood). Thus, a BAC of 150 mg/dL = 0.15% = 34 mmol/L.

TABLE 71-1	Specific Effects of Alcohol Related to BAC
BAC (%)ª (mmol/L)	**Effect**
0.02–0.03 (4–8)	No loss of coordination, slight euphoria, and loss of shyness
0.04–0.06 (9–14)	Feeling of well-being, relaxation, lower inhibitions, sensation of warmth. Euphoria. Some minor impairment of reasoning and memory, lowering of caution
0.07–0.09 (15–21)	Slight impairment of balance, speech, vision, reaction time, and hearing. Euphoria. Judgment and self-control are reduced, and caution, reason, and memory are impaired. It is illegal to operate a motor vehicle in some states at this level
0.10–0.125 (22–27)	Significant impairment of motor coordination and loss of good judgment. Speech can be slurred; balance, vision, reaction time, and hearing impaired. Euphoria. It is illegal to operate a motor vehicle at this level of intoxication
0.13–0.15 (28–34)	Gross motor impairment and lack of physical control. Blurred vision and major loss of balance. Euphoria is reduced, and dysphoria is beginning to appear
0.16–0.20 (35–43)	Dysphoria (anxiety, restlessness) predominates; nausea can appear. The drinker has the appearance of a "sloppy drunk"
0.25 (54)	Needs assistance in walking; total mental confusion. Dysphoria with nausea and some vomiting
0.30 (65)	Loss of consciousness
≥0.40 (>87)	Onset of coma, possible death caused by respiratory arrest

(BAC, blood alcohol concentration.)
ªGrams of ethyl alcohol per 100 mL of whole blood.

BENZODIAZEPINES AND OTHER SEDATIVE-HYPNOTICS

- Emergency department visits involving benzodiazepines outnumber those involving any other psychotherapeutic agent.
- **Benzodiazepine** intoxication is manifested as slurred speech, poor coordination, swaying, drowsiness, hypotension, nystagmus, and confusion.
- Likelihood and severity of withdrawal are a function of dose and duration of exposure. Gradual tapering of dosage is necessary to minimize withdrawal and rebound anxiety.
- Signs and symptoms of benzodiazepine withdrawal are similar to those of alcohol withdrawal, including dizziness, flu-like symptoms, impaired memory and concentration, nausea, vomiting, nightmares, visual disturbances, convulsions, muscle pain, anxiety, agitation, restlessness, confusion, irritability, hallucinations, delirium, seizures, and cardiovascular collapse. Withdrawal from short-acting benzodiazepines (eg, **oxazepam, lorazepam**, and **alprazolam**) has an onset within 12 to 24 hours of the last dose. **Diazepam, chlordiazepoxide**, and **clorazepate** have elimination half-lives (or active metabolites with elimination half-lives) of 24 to more than 100 hours. Thus, withdrawal may be delayed for up to 7 days after their discontinuation.
- **Flunitrazepam** (Rohypnol) is most commonly ingested orally, frequently in conjunction with alcohol or other drugs. Often called a *date-rape drug*, it has been given to women (without their knowledge) to lower their inhibitions.
- Zolpidem is suggested to have little liability for physical dependence, but tolerance and withdrawal have been reported.

CARISOPRODOL

- **Carisoprodol** is used for muscle spasms and back pain. **Meprobamate** is one of its metabolites.

- It can cause drowsiness, dizziness, vertigo, ataxia, tremor, irritability, headache, syncope, insomnia, tachycardia, postural hypotension, nausea, agitation, depression, weakness, and confusion.
- Overdose can cause stupor, coma, respiratory depression, and death.

OPIATES

- Deaths from prescription opioids have reached epidemic levels.
- Signs and symptoms of opioid intoxication include euphoria, dysphoria, slurred speech, miosis, apathy, sedation, and attention impairment. Signs and symptoms of withdrawal include lacrimation, mydriasis, piloerection, diaphoresis, diarrhea, yawning, muscle aches, and insomnia. The onset of withdrawal ranges from a few hours after stopping heroin to 3 to 5 days after stopping methadone. Duration of withdrawal ranges from 3 to 14 days. Occurrence of delirium suggests withdrawal from another drug (eg, **alcohol**).
- **Heroin** can be snorted, smoked, and given IV. Complications of heroin use include overdoses, anaphylactic reactions to impurities, nephrotic syndrome, septicemia, endocarditis, and acquired immunodeficiency.
- **Hydrocodone** is the most widely abused pharmaceutical controlled substance in the United States.
- **Fentanyl** is a synthetic short-acting opioid which is 50 to 100 times more potent than morphine and approved for management of acute or chronic pain associated with advanced cancer. Most fentanyl-related morbidity and mortality have been linked to illicitly manufactured fentanyl and fentanyl analogs. It is often mixed with heroin or cocaine, with or without the user's knowledge. Several states have reported spikes in overdose deaths due to fentanyl and its analogs (eg, carfentanil).
- **Opiates** are commonly combined with stimulants (eg, **cocaine** [speedball]) or **alcohol**.
- **Methadone** has caused an increased number of deaths in recent years. Converting to methadone from other opioid agonists can be tricky, and lethal when done improperly. Peak respiratory depressant effects occur later and last longer than peak analgesic effects.
- **Dextromethorphan,** an over-the-counter drug, causes depressant and mild hallucinogenic effects in high doses and significant hallucinations and CNS depression in excessive doses. Acute overdoses are treated with naloxone.

CENTRAL NERVOUS SYSTEM STIMULANTS

COCAINE

- **Cocaine** may be the most behaviorally reinforcing of all drugs. Ten percent of people who begin to use the drug "recreationally" go on to heavy use.
- It blocks reuptake of catecholamine neurotransmitters.
- The hydrochloride salt is inhaled or injected. The high from snorting lasts 15 to 30 minutes. Smoking cocaine base (crack or rock) is almost instantly absorbed and causes intense euphoria. The high from smoking lasts 5 to 10 minutes. Tolerance to the "high" develops quickly. The elimination half-life of cocaine is 1 hour.
- In the presence of alcohol, cocaine is metabolized to cocaethylene, a longer-acting compound than cocaine with a greater risk for causing death.
- Adverse events include ulceration of nasal mucosa and nasal septal collapse, tachycardia, heart failure, hyperthermia, shock, seizures, psychosis (similar to paranoid schizophrenia), and sudden death.
- Signs and symptoms of cocaine intoxication include agitation, euphoria, loquacity, sweating or chills, nausea, tachycardia, arrhythmias, respiratory depression, mydriasis, altered blood pressure, and seizures.
- Withdrawal symptoms begin within hours of discontinuation and last up to several days. Signs and symptoms of withdrawal include fatigue, sleep disturbances, nightmares, depression, drug craving, changes in appetite, bradyarrhythmias, myocardial infarction (MI), and tremors.

METHAMPHETAMINE

- **Methamphetamine** (known as speed, meth, and crank) can be taken orally, rectally, intranasally, by IV injection, and by smoking.
- Systemic effects of methamphetamine are similar to those of cocaine. Inhalation or IV injection results in an intense rush that lasts a few minutes. Methamphetamine has a longer duration of effect than cocaine. Intoxication may present as increased wakefulness, increased physical activity, decreased appetite, dental caries, increased respiration, hyperthermia, euphoria, irritability, insomnia, confusion, tremors, anxiety, paranoia, aggressiveness, convulsions, increased heart rate and blood pressure, stroke, and death.
- Individuals in withdrawal may exhibit depression, cognitive impairment, drug craving, dyssomnia, and fatigue, but they are usually not in acute distress. Duration of withdrawal ranges from 2 days to several months. Occurrence of delirium suggests withdrawal from another drug (eg, **alcohol**).
- **Ephedrine** and **pseudoephedrine** can be extracted from cold and allergy tablets and converted to methamphetamine. In the United States, federal law now requires that pseudoephedrine-containing products be kept behind a counter and that identification be shown at the time of purchase.

OTHER DRUGS OF ABUSE

NICOTINE

- Cigarette smoking is the leading cause of preventable morbidity and mortality in the United States. It increases the risks of cardiovascular diseases, lung cancer, other cancers, and nonmalignant respiratory diseases.
- **Nicotine** is a ganglionic cholinergic-receptor agonist with dose-dependent pharmacologic effects, including stimulation and depression in the central and peripheral nervous systems; respiratory stimulation; skeletal muscle relaxation; catecholamine release by the adrenal medulla; peripheral vasoconstriction; and increased blood pressure, heart rate, cardiac output, and oxygen consumption. Low doses produce increased alertness and improved cognitive functioning. Higher doses stimulate the "reward" center in the brain.
- Abrupt cessation results in withdrawal symptoms usually within 24 hours, including anxiety, cravings, difficulty concentrating, frustration, irritability, hostility, insomnia, and restlessness.

ECSTASY (MDMA)

- **3,4-methylenedioxymethamphetamine** (MDMA; Ecstasy) is usually taken by mouth as a tablet, capsule, or powder, but it can also be smoked, snorted, or injected; if taken by mouth, effects last 4 to 6 hours.
- MDMA stimulates the CNS, causes euphoria and relaxation, and produces a mild hallucinogenic effect. It can cause muscle tension, nausea, impaired memory, impaired attention and reasoning, impaired incidental learning, chills, sweating, panic, anxiety, depression, hallucinations, convulsions, and paranoid thinking. It increases heart rate and blood pressure and destroys serotonin (5-HT)–producing neurons in animals. It is considered to be neurotoxic in humans.

SYNTHETIC CATHINONES (BATH SALTS)

- **Bath salts** (schedule I controlled substances) are synthetic, sympathomimetic, designer drugs that can cause intoxication, dependence, and death. They are known collectively as cathinones. They are CNS stimulants that can cause MI, esophagitis, gastritis, oral keratotic lesions, and liver failure. The pharmacology of the various cathinones and related drugs is not well studied.
- **Flakka** is a new very potent cathinone that has become very popular in some counties in Florida.
- Adverse effects of bath salts include tachycardia, hypertension, diabetic ketoacidosis, paranoid psychosis, hyperthermia, agitation, headache, hyponatremia, and suicide.

MARIJUANA

- **Marijuana** (known as reefer, pot, grass, and weed) is the most commonly used illicit drug. The principal psychoactive component is Δ^9-**tetrahydrocannabinol (THC)**. **Hashish**, the dried resin of the top of the plant, is more potent than the plant itself. Pharmacologic effects begin immediately and last 1 to 3 hours. One in 10 marijuana users become addicted (one in six among adolescents).
- Initial effects of marijuana use include increased heart rate, dilated bronchial passages, and bloodshot eyes. Subsequent effects include euphoria, dry mouth, hunger, tremor, sleepiness, anxiety, fear, distrust, panic, incoordination, poor recall, amotivation, and toxic psychosis. Other physiologic effects include sedation, difficulty in performing complex tasks, and disinhibition. Endocrine effects include amenorrhea, decreased testosterone production, and inhibition of spermatogenesis. Recent findings suggest a neurotoxic effect on the adolescent brain.
- Cannabis use impairs driving performance, and is associated with increased risk of motor vehicle crashes.
- After abrupt discontinuation, heavy users may have a withdrawal syndrome characterized by irritability, anger, aggression, anxiety, depressed mood, restlessness, sleep difficulty, decreased appetite, or weight loss.
- During 2012 to 2013, approximately 30% of people who used marijuana in the United States in the past year met the criteria for marijuana use disorder as defined by the DSM-5.
- In chronic users, THC is detectable on toxicologic screening for up to 4 to 5 weeks after cessation of use.

SYNTHETIC CANNABINOIDS

- Over 100 compounds are cannabinoid receptor agonists called **synthetic marijuana** (spice, K2, dream, red X dawn, and others). The product is inert dry plant material sprayed with these compounds. Toxic symptoms are similar to the effects of marijuana plus sympathomimetic effects, including agitation, anxiety, tachycardia, hypertension, nausea and vomiting, muscle spasms, seizures, tremors, paranoid behavior, nonresponsiveness, diaphoresis, hallucinations, and suicidal thoughts and behaviors.

LYSERGIC ACID DIETHYLAMIDE (LSD)

- Signs and symptoms of **LSD** intoxication include mydriasis, tachycardia, diaphoresis, palpitations, blurred vision, tremor, incoordination, dizziness, weakness, and drowsiness; psychiatric signs and symptoms include perceptual intensification, depersonalization, derealization, illusions, psychosis, synesthesia, and flashbacks. It produces tolerance but is not addictive. There is no withdrawal syndrome.
- LSD can cause either agonist or antagonist effects on 5-HT activity.
- It is sold as tablets, capsules, a liquid, and on squares of decorated paper.

INHALANTS

- Organic solvents inhaled by abusers include **gasoline, glue, aerosols, amyl nitrite, butyl nitrite, typewriter correction fluid, lighter fluid, cleaning fluids, paint products, nail polish remover, waxes,** and **varnishes**. Chemicals in these products include **nitrous oxide, toluene, benzene, methanol, methylene chloride, acetone, methylethyl ketone, methylbutyl ketone, trichloroethylene,** and **trichloroethane**.
- Physiologic effects include CNS depression, headache, nausea, anxiety, hallucinations, and delusions. With chronic use, the drugs are toxic to virtually all organ systems. Death may occur from arrhythmias or suffocation by plastic bags.

TREATMENT

- <u>Goals of Treatment</u>: The goals include cessation of use of the drug, termination of drug-seeking behaviors, and return to normal functioning. The goals of treatment of withdrawal include prevention of progression to life-threatening severity, thus enabling comfort and functionality conducive to participation in a treatment program.

INTOXICATION

- In treating acute intoxications, drug therapy should be avoided when possible, but it may be indicated if patients are agitated, combative, or psychotic (Table 71–2).
- When toxicology screens are desired, blood or urine should be collected immediately upon arrival for treatment.
- *Benzodiazepine overdose*: **Flumazenil** is not indicated in all cases, and it is contraindicated when cyclic antidepressant use is known or suspected because of seizure risk. Use with caution when benzodiazepine physical dependence is suspected, as it may precipitate withdrawal.
- *Opiate intoxication*: **Naloxone** may revive unconscious patients with respiratory depression, but it may precipitate physical withdrawal in dependent patients.
- **Stimulants**, including **Cocaine** *intoxication*: Treat pharmacologically only if the patient is agitated or psychotic. Injectable **lorazepam** 2 to 4 mg IM every 30 minutes to 6 hours can be used for agitation. Low-dose antipsychotics can be used short term for psychosis. Treat seizures supportively, but IV lorazepam or **diazepam** can be used for status epilepticus.
- Many patients with **hallucinogen** intoxication respond to reassurance, but short-term antianxiety and/or antipsychotic therapy can be used.

TABLE 71–2	Pharmacologic Treatment of Substance Intoxication		
Drug Class	**Nonpharmacologic Therapy**	**Pharmacologic Therapy**	**Level of Evidence[a,b]**
Benzodiazepines	Support vital functions	Flumazenil 0.2 mg/min IV initially, repeat up to 3 mg max.	AI
Alcohol, barbiturates, and sedative-hypnotics (nonbenzodiazepines)	Support vital functions	None	B3
Opiates	Support vital functions	Naloxone 0.4–2 mg IV every 3 minutes	A1
Cocaine and other CNS stimulants	Monitor cardiac function	Lorazepam 2–4 mg IM every 30 minutes to 6 hours as needed for agitation	B2
		Haloperidol 2–5 mg (or other antipsychotic agent) every 30 minutes to 6 hours as needed for psychotic behavior	B3
Hallucinogens, marijuana, and inhalants	Reassurance; "talk-down therapy"; support vital functions	Lorazepam and/or haloperidol as above	B3
Phencyclidine	Minimize sensory input	Lorazepam and/or haloperidol as above	B3

[a]Strength of recommendations, evidence to support recommendation, A, good; B, moderate; C, poor.
[b]Quality of evidence: 1, evidence from more than 1 properly randomized, controlled trial; 2, evidence from more than one well-designed clinical trial with randomization, from cohort or case-controlled analytic studies or multiple time series; or dramatic results from uncontrolled experiments; 3, evidence from opinions of respected authorities, based on clinical experience, descriptive studies, or reports of expert communities.

WITHDRAWAL

- Treatment of withdrawal from some common drugs of abuse is summarized in Table 71–3.

Alcohol

- Most clinicians agree that symptom-triggered treatment with **benzodiazepines** is the standard of care for **alcohol** detoxification.
- **Lorazepam** is preferred by many clinicians because it can be administered IV, intramuscularly, or orally with predictable results (Table 71–4). Address fluid, electrolyte, and vitamin deficiencies as in **Table 71–4**.
- With symptom-triggered therapy, medication is given only if symptoms emerge, resulting in shorter treatment duration and avoidance of oversedation compared to a fixed-dose schedule. A typical regimen would be lorazepam 2 mg administered every hour as needed when a structured assessment scale (eg, Clinical Institute Withdrawal Assessment–Alcohol, Revised [CIWA-AR]) indicates that symptoms are moderate to severe.
- Alcohol withdrawal seizures do not require anticonvulsant drug treatment unless they progress to status epilepticus. Treat patients with seizures supportively. An increase in the dosage and slowing of the tapering schedule of the **benzodiazepine** used for detoxification or a single injection of a benzodiazepine may be necessary to prevent further seizure activity.

Benzodiazepines

- For benzodiazepine withdrawal, use the same drugs and dosages that are used for alcohol withdrawal (see **Table 71–3**).
- The onset of withdrawal from long-acting benzodiazepines may be up to 7 days after discontinuation of the drug. Initiate treatment at usual doses and maintain this dose for 5 days. Then taper over 5 days. Alprazolam withdrawal may require a more gradual taper of the benzodiazepine used for detoxification.

Opiates

- Avoid unnecessary detoxification with drugs if possible (eg, if symptoms are tolerable). **Heroin** withdrawal reaches a peak within 36 to 72 hours of discontinuation and may last for 7 to 10 days, and the **methadone** withdrawal peaks at 72 hours, but can last for 2 weeks or longer.
- Conventional drug therapy for opiate withdrawal has been **methadone**, a synthetic opiate. Usual starting doses of 20 to 40 mg/day. Some clinicians use discontinuation schedules over 30 days or over 180 days.
- Other detoxification regimens (eg, adrenergic agonists) also are effective. Regardless of detoxification strategy, most heroin users relapse to heroin use.
- A rapid opioid detoxification technique has been developed to shorten detoxification by precipitating withdrawal through administration of opioid antagonists such as naloxone or naltrexone. This rapid detoxification minimizes the risk of relapse and initiates treatment more quickly with naltrexone maintenance and psychosocial interventions.
- In the United States, **Buprenorphine** is available in three formulations (i.e., single-ingredient tablet, buprenorphine plus naloxone tablet, and buprenorphine plus naloxone mucoadhesive film). All three are assigned to schedule III, and are available for office-based management of opioid dependence by qualified clinicians.
- Medically supervised withdrawal with buprenorphine consists of an induction phase and a dose reduction phase. The Substance Abuse and Mental Health Services Administration (SAMHSA) provides evidence-based recommendations for use of buprenorphine for opioid addiction (Treatment Improvement Protocols 40 (TIP 40).
- Patients dependent on short-acting opioids (eg, heroin, hydrocodone, and oxycodone) should be inducted directly onto buprenorphine/naloxone tablets. The use of buprenorphine, either as monotherapy or as combination therapy, to taper off of long-acting opioids should be used only for patients who have evidence of sustained medical and psychosocial stability, and this treatment should be part of an overall opioid treatment program.

TABLE 71-3	Treatment of Withdrawal from Some Common Drugs of Abuse	
Drug or Drug Class	**Pharmacologic Therapy**	**Level of Evidence[a,b]**
Benzodiazepines		
Short to intermediate acting	Lorazepam 2 mg three to four times a day; taper over 5–7 days	A1
Long-acting	Lorazepam 2 mg three to four times a day; taper over additional 5–7 days	A1
Barbiturates	Pentobarbital tolerance test; initial detoxification at upper limit of tolerance test; decrease dosage by 100 mg every 2–3 days	B3
Opiates	Methadone 20–80 mg orally daily; taper by 5–10 mg daily or buprenorphine 4–32 mg orally daily, or clonidine 2 mcg/kg three times a day × 7 days; taper over additional 3 days	A1 (methadone and buprenorphine) B1 (clonidine)
Mixed-substance withdrawal		
Drugs are cross-tolerant	Detoxify according to treatment for longer-acting drug used	B3
Drugs are not cross-tolerant	Detoxify from one drug while maintaining second drug (cross-tolerant drugs), then detoxify from second drug	B3
CNS stimulants	Supportive treatment only; pharmacotherapy often not used; bromocriptine 2.5 mg three times a day or higher may be used for severe craving associated with cocaine withdrawal	B2

[a]Strength of recommendations, evidence to support recommendation, A, good; B, moderate; C, poor.
[b]Quality of evidence: 1, evidence from more than 1 properly randomized, controlled trial; 2, evidence from more than one well-designed clinical trial with randomization, from cohort or case-controlled analytic studies or multiple time series; or dramatic results from uncontrolled experiments; 3, evidence from opinions of respected authorities, based on clinical experience, descriptive studies, or reports of expert communities.

- Treatment with buprenorphine for opioid addiction has three phases: induction, stabilization, and maintenance. Induction helps patients switch from the opioid of abuse to buprenorphine, and the goal is to find the minimum dose of buprenorphine at which the patient discontinues or markedly diminishes use of the opioid of abuse and experiences no withdrawal symptoms, minimal or no side effects, and no craving. The buprenorphine/naloxone combination will be used for induction, stabilization, and maintenance for most patients. The initial induction doses should be administered as observed treatment. Patients who are transferring from long-acting opioids (methadone, sustained-release morphine, and sustained-release oxycodone) to buprenorphine should be inducted using buprenorphine monotherapy, but switched to buprenorphine/naloxone soon thereafter. Refer to the SAMHSA treatment protocols.
- The stabilization phase starts when the patient is experiencing no withdrawal symptoms, is having minimal or no side effects, and no longer has uncontrollable cravings. The maintenance phase may be indefinite, and should focus on psychosocial and family issues.
- Buprenorphine can be abused, but the film is less likely to be abused than the tablet formulations.

TABLE 71–4 Dosing and Monitoring of Pharmacologic Agents Used in the Treatment of Alcohol Withdrawal

Drug	Dose Per Day (Unless Otherwise Stated)	Indication	Monitoring	Duration of Dosing	Level of Evidence for Efficacy[a]
Multivitamin	1 tablet	Malnutrition	Diet	At least until eating a balanced diet at caloric goal	B3
Thiamine	50–100 mg	Deficiency	CBC, WBC, nystagmus	Empiric × 5 days. More if evidence of deficiency	B2
Crystalloid fluids (typically D5–0.45 NS with 20 mEq (20 mmol) of KCl per liter)	50–100 mL/hour	Dehydration	Weight, electrolytes urine output, nystagmus if dextrose	Until intake and outputs stabilize and oral intake is adequate	A3
Clonidine oral (Catapres)	0.05–0.3 mg Consider dose reduction in the elderly	Autonomic tone rebound and hyperactivity	Shaking, tremor, sweating, blood pressure	3 days or less	B2
Clonidine transdermal (Catapres-TTS)	TTS-1 to TTS-3 Consider dose reduction in the elderly	Autonomic tone rebound and hyperactivity	Shaking, tremor, sweating, blood pressure	1 week or less. One patch only	B3
Labetalol	20 mg IV every 2 hours as needed; dosage reduction (eg, by about 50% for oral dosage) is advised in patients with hepatic impairment	Hypertensive urgencies and above	Blood pressure target	Individual doses as needed	B3
Antipsychotics, haloperidol (Haldol)	2.5–5 mg every 4 hours	Agitation unresponsive to benzodiazepines, hallucinations (tactile, visual, auditory, or otherwise), or delusions	Subjective response plus rating scale (CIWA-AR or equivalent)	Individual doses as needed	B1

Drug	Dosage	Indication	Monitoring	Comments	Recommendation
Antipsychotics, atypical Quetiapine (Seroquel)	25–200 mg; dosage adjustment is necessary in hepatic impairment	Agitation unresponsive to benzodiazepines, hallucinations, or delusions in patients intolerant of conventional antipsychotics	Subjective response plus CIWA-AR rating scale or equivalent	Individual doses as needed in addition to scheduled antipsychotic	C3
Aripiprazole (Abilify)	5–15 mg				
Benzodiazepines Lorazepam (Ativan) Chlordiazepoxide (Librium) Clonazepam (Klonopin) Diazepam (Valium)	0.5–2 mg 5–100 mg 0.5–2 mg 2.5–10 mg	Tremor, anxiety, diaphoresis, tachypnea, dysphoria, seizures	Subjective response plus CIWA-AR rating scale or equivalent	Individual doses as needed. Underdosing is more common than overdosing	A2
Alcohol oral		Prevent withdrawal	Subjective signs of withdrawal	Wide variation	C3
Alcohol IV		Prevent withdrawal	Subjective signs of withdrawal	Wide variation	C3

(CBC, complete blood count; CIWA-AR, Clinical Institute Withdrawal Assessment for Alcohol, Revised; D5, dextrose 5%; KCl, potassium chloride; NS, normal saline; WBC, white blood cell count.)

[a]Strength of recommendations, evidence to support recommendation: A, good; B, moderate; C, poor.

Quality of evidence: 1, evidence from more than one properly randomized controlled trial; 2, evidence from more than one well-designed clinical trial with randomization, from cohort or case–control analytic studies or multiple time series, or dramatic results from uncontrolled experiments; 3, evidence from opinions of respected authorities, based on clinical experience, descriptive studies, or reports of expert communities.

SUBSTANCE USE DISORDERS

- Treatment of drug dependence or addiction is primarily behavioral. The goal is complete abstinence, and treatment is a lifelong process. Most drug-dependence treatment programs embrace treatment based on the Alcoholics Anonymous approach (ie, a 12-step model).

Alcohol Dependence

- **Disulfiram** deters a patient from drinking by producing an aversive reaction if the patient drinks. It inhibits aldehyde dehydrogenase in the pathway for alcohol metabolism, allowing acetaldehyde to accumulate, resulting in flushing, vomiting, headache, palpitations, tachycardia, fever, and hypotension. Severe reactions include respiratory depression, arrhythmias, MI, seizures, and death. Inhibition of the enzyme continues for as long as 2 weeks after stopping disulfiram. Table 71–5 shows dosing and monitoring of drug therapy for alcohol dependence.
- Prior to starting disulfiram, obtain baseline liver function tests (LFTs), and repeat at 2 weeks, 3 months, and 6 months, then twice yearly. Wait at least 24 hours after the last drink before starting disulfiram, usually at a dose of 250 mg/day.
- **Naltrexone** reduces craving and the number of drinking days. Do not prescribe it to patients currently dependent on opiates, as it can precipitate severe withdrawal syndrome. A depot formulation allows monthly administration in a usual dose of 380 mg intramuscularly.
- Naltrexone is hepatotoxic and contraindicated in patients with hepatitis, liver failure, or serum aminotransferase levels greater than five times normal. LFTs should be done at baseline and one to 3 months after starting therapy, then annually. Use with caution in patients with moderate to severe renal impairment. Side effects include nausea, headache, dizziness, nervousness, insomnia, and somnolence.
- **Acamprosate**-treated patients have less craving and more success in maintaining abstinence than placebo-treated patients. The most common acamprosate side effect is diarrhea.

Nicotine

- The Agency for Healthcare Research and Quality (AHRQ) released a clinical guideline for smoking cessation in 2008. Every smoker should receive at least minimal treatment at every clinician visit. Every tobacco user should be offered at least brief treatment.
- First-line pharmacotherapies for smoking cessation are **bupropion sustained release, nicotine gum, nicotine inhaler, nicotine lozenge, nicotine nasal spray, nicotine patch**, and **varenicline**. Combinations of these should be considered if a single agent has failed. Second-line pharmacotherapies include **clonidine** and **nortriptyline** and should be considered if first-line therapy fails.
- Interventions are more effective when they last longer than 10 minutes, involve contact with multiple types of clinicians, include at least four sessions, and provide **nicotine-replacement therapy** (NRT). Group and individual counseling is effective, and interventions are more successful when they include social support and training in problem solving, stress management, and relapse prevention.

NICOTINE REPLACEMENT THERAPY

- Dosing and monitoring of pharmacotherapy for smoking cessation is shown in Table 71–6. Use of NRT increases quit rates by 50% to 70%.
- The **2-mg gum** is recommended for those smoking fewer than 25 cigarettes/day, and the 4-mg gum for those smoking 25 or more cigarettes/day. Generally, the gum should be used for up to 12 weeks at no more than 24 pieces per day. It should be chewed slowly until a peppery or minty taste emerges and then parked between the cheek and gums for about 30 minutes or until the taste dissipates. Patients should be given specific dosing instructions, not just as needed.
- The **patch** is available as a prescription and nonprescription medication. It approximately doubles long-term abstinence rates compared to placebo. Treatment of 8 weeks

TABLE 71–5 Dosing and Monitoring of Pharmacologic Agents Used in the Treatment of Alcohol Dependence

Drug	Dosage Range Per Day	Indication	Monitoring	Duration of Dosing	Level of Evidence for Efficacy[a]
Disulfiram (Antabuse)	250–500 mg; used with extreme caution in patients with hepatic cirrhosis or insufficiency	Deterrence	Facial flushing, liver enzymes	Indefinite	B2
Acamprosate (Campral)	999–1998 mg and higher (333 mg tablets) Dosage adjustment necessary in renal impairment	Craving	Patient-reported craving, renal function	Indefinite	A1
Naltrexone (ReVia)	50–100 mg; dosage adjustment may be needed in renal and liver impairment	Craving	Patient-reported craving	Indefinite	A1
Naltrexone (Vivitrol)	380 mg intramuscularly once every 4 weeks Risk of hepatotoxicity lower compared to oral formulation due to lack of first pass effect	Craving	Patient-reported craving	Indefinite	B2
Mood stabilizers (eg, lamotrigine [Lamictal], topiramate [Topamax], carbamazepine [Tegretol], valproic acid [Depakote])	Seizure disorder doses	Craving	Patient-reported craving, plasma drug levels	Indefinite	B2
Antidepressants (eg, clomipramine [Anafranil], bupropion [Wellbutrin], doxepin [Sinequan], fluoxetine [Prozac])	Depression doses	Craving, depression, anxiety	Patient-reported craving	Indefinite	B2

[a]Strength of recommendations: A, B, and C, good, moderate, and poor evidence to support recommendation, respectively.
Quality of evidence: 1, evidence from more than one properly randomized controlled trial; 2, evidence from more than one well-designed clinical trial with randomization, from cohort or case–control analytic studies or multiple time series, or dramatic results from uncontrolled experiments; 3, evidence from opinions of respected authorities, based on clinical experience, descriptive studies, or reports of expert communities.

TABLE 71-6 Dosing and Monitoring of Pharmacologic Agents Used for Smoking Cessation

Drug	Place in Therapy	Dosage Range	Duration	Comments/Monitoring Parameters	LOEE[a]
Bupropion SR[b,c] (Zyban)	First-line	Titrate up to 150 mg orally twice daily. May require reduced initial dose in elderly	3–6 months	Patients receiving both bupropion and a nicotine patch should be monitored for hypertension	A1
Clonidine[c,d] (Catapres)	Second-line	Titrate to response; 0.2–0.75 mg/day. Consider dose reduction in the elderly	6–12 months	Monitor baseline electrolyte and lipid profiles, renal function, uric acid, complete blood count, and blood pressure	B2
Nicotine polacrilex (gum)[b] (Nicorette)	First-line	Initial dose depends on smoking history: 2–4 mg every 1–8 hours	12 weeks (taper down over time)	Heart rate and blood pressure should be monitored periodically during nicotine replacement therapy	A1
Nicotine inhaler[b] (Nicotrol)	First-line	24–64 mg/day (total daily dose)	3–6 months (taper down over time)	Heart rate and blood pressure should be monitored periodically during nicotine replacement therapy	A1
Nicotine nasal spray[b] (Nicotrol NS)	First-line	8–40 mg/day (total daily dose)	14 weeks (taper down over time)	Heart rate and blood pressure should be monitored periodically during nicotine replacement therapy	A1
Nicotine patch[b] (NicoDerm, Nicotrol)	First-line	Initial dose depends on smoking history: 7–21 mg topically once daily	6 weeks (taper down over time)	Heart rate and blood pressure should be monitored periodically during nicotine replacement therapy	A1
Nortriptyline[c,d] (Aventyl)	Second-line	Titrate up to 75–100 mg orally daily	6–12 months	Dry mouth, blurred vision, and constipation are dose-dependent adverse effects	B2
Varenicline[c] (Chantix)	First-line	Titrate up to 1 mg orally twice daily. If CrCl <30 mL/min (0.5 mL/s), 0.5 mg once per day	3–6 months	Monitor renal function, especially in elderly patients. Nausea, headache, insomnia are dose-dependent adverse effects	A1

(LOEE, level of evidence for efficacy)

[a]Strength of recommendations, evidence to support recommendation: A, good; B, moderate; C, poor.
Quality of evidence: 1, evidence from more than one properly randomized controlled trial; 2, evidence from more than one well-designed clinical trial with randomization, from cohort or case–control analytic studies or multiple time series, or dramatic results from uncontrolled experiments; 3, evidence from opinions of respected authorities, based on clinical experience, descriptive studies, or reports of expert communities.
[b]Nicotine replacement therapies can be combined with each other and/or bupropion to increase long-term abstinence rates.
[c]Do not abruptly discontinue. Taper up initially, and taper off once therapy is complete.
[d]Clonidine and nortriptyline are not FDA-approved for smoking cessation.

or less is as effective as longer treatments. The 16- and 24-hour patches have comparable efficacy. A new patch should be placed on a relatively hairless location each morning.

- **Nicotine nasal spray** requires a prescription. It more than doubles long-term abstinence rates compared to placebo spray. Recommended duration of therapy is 3 to 6 months. A dose is one 0.5 mg delivery to each nostril (1 mg total). Initial doses are 1 or 2 doses/h, increasing as needed for symptom relief. The minimum treatment is 8 doses/day, and the maximum is 40 doses/day.
- NRT products have few side effects. Nausea and light-headedness may indicate nicotine overdose. Rotate the patch site to minimize skin irritation. Sleep disturbances are reported in 23% of patients using the patch. Eating or drinking anything except water should be avoided for 15 minutes before and during administration of the lozenge and gum. Long-term NRT may be needed in some patients.

OTHER

- **Bupropion sustained release (SR)** is contraindicated in patients with current or past seizure disorder, current or prior diagnosis of bulimia or anorexia nervosa, and use of a **monoamine oxidase inhibitor within the last 14 days**. Concurrent use of medications that lower the seizure threshold is a concern.
  - ✓ Like other antidepressants, bupropion carries a warning for causing agitation and suicidality in patients aged 24 years or younger. The warnings also highlight the risk of neuropsychiatric symptoms (in adults and pediatric patients), including depression, anxiety, agitation, hostility, suicidal thoughts/behavior, and attempted suicide.
- Bupropion SR should be dosed at 150 mg once daily for 3 days, then twice daily for 7 to 12 weeks or longer, with or without NRT. Patients should stop smoking during the second week of treatment.
- **Varenicline** is a partial agonist that binds selectively to nicotinic acetylcholine receptors with a greater affinity than nicotine, producing a lesser response than nicotine. Prescribe for 12 weeks. A second 12-week treatment can be given if the patient is not abstinent. It may result in a higher rate of cessation than bupropion and than single forms of NRT. It may be equally effective with combination NRT.
- Side effects of varenicline include suicidal thoughts and erratic and aggressive behavior. Screen patients for psychiatric illness or behavior change after starting varenicline. The Food and Drug Administration (FDA) required a boxed warning and updated medication guide. It may be associated with a small increased risk of cardiovascular events. There have also been some reports of seizures, mostly in the first month of treatment.

SECOND-LINE MEDICATIONS

- **Clonidine** is an effective smoking-cessation treatment. Dosing varies from 0.15 to 0.75 mg/day orally and from 0.1 to 0.2 mg/day transdermally. Do not discontinue abruptly, as this may cause nervousness, agitation, headache, tremor, and elevation in blood pressure.
- The most common clonidine side effects include dry mouth, dizziness, hypotension, sedation, and constipation. Monitor blood pressure.
- **Nortriptyline** is initiated 10 to 28 days before the quit date. The dose is initiated at 25 mg/day, gradually increasing to 75 to 100 mg/day. In trials, treatment duration was commonly 12 weeks, and common side effects include sedation, dry mouth, blurred vision, urinary retention, tremor, and light-headedness.

See Chapter 65, Substance-Related Disorders I: Overview and Depressants, Stimulants, and Hallucinogens, authored by Paul L. Doering and Robin Moorman Li, and Chapter 66, Substance-Related Disorders II: Alcohol, Nicotine, and Caffeine, authored by Paul L. Doering and Robin Moorman Li, for a more detailed discussion of the topic.

CHAPTER

72

Acid–Base Disorders

- *Acid–base disorders* are caused by disturbances in hydrogen ion (H^+) homeostasis, which is ordinarily maintained by extracellular buffering, renal regulation of hydrogen ion and bicarbonate excretion, and ventilatory regulation of carbon dioxide (CO_2) elimination.

GENERAL PRINCIPLES

- Buffering refers to the ability of a solution to resist change in pH after the addition of a strong acid or base. The body's principal extracellular buffer system is the carbonic acid/bicarbonate (H_2CO_3/HCO_3^-) system.
- Most of the body's acid production is in the form of CO_2 and is produced from catabolism of carbohydrates, proteins, and lipids.
- There are four primary types of acid–base disturbances, which can occur independently or together as a compensatory response.
- Metabolic acid–base disorders are caused by changes in plasma bicarbonate concentration (HCO_3^-). Metabolic acidosis is characterized by decreased HCO_3^-, and metabolic alkalosis is characterized by increased HCO_3^-.
- Respiratory acid–base disorders are caused by altered alveolar ventilation, producing changes in arterial carbon dioxide tension ($Paco_2$). Respiratory acidosis is characterized by increased $Paco_2$, whereas respiratory alkalosis is characterized by decreased $Paco_2$.

DIAGNOSIS

- Blood gases (Table 72–1), serum electrolytes, medical history, and clinical condition are the primary tools for determining the cause of acid–base disorders and for designing therapy.
- Arterial blood gases (ABGs) are measured to determine oxygenation and acid–base status (Fig. 72–1). Low pH values (<7.35) indicate acidemia, whereas high values (>7.45) indicate alkalemia. The $Paco_2$ value helps determine whether there is a primary respiratory abnormality, whereas the HCO_3^- concentration helps determine whether there is a primary metabolic abnormality. Steps in acid–base diagnosis and interpretation are described in Tables 72–2 and 72–3.

METABOLIC ACIDOSIS

PATHOPHYSIOLOGY

- Metabolic acidosis is characterized by a decrease in pH as a result of a primary decrease in serum HCO_3^- concentration, which can result from the buffering of an exogenous acid (consumption of HCO_3^-), accumulation of an organic acid because of a metabolic disturbance (eg, lactic acid and ketoacids), loss of bicarbonate-rich body fluids (eg, diarrhea), or accumulation of endogenous acids secondary to impaired renal function (eg, phosphates and sulfates). Rapid administration of non-alkali-containing IV fluids can cause dilutional acidosis.

785

TABLE 72–1	**Normal Blood Gas Values**	
	Arterial Blood	**Mixed Venous Blood**
pH	7.40 (7.35–7.45)	7.38 (7.33–7.43)
P_{O_2}	80–100 mm Hg (10.6–13.3 kPa)	35–40 mm Hg (4.7–5.3 kPa)
Sa_{O_2}	95% (0.95)	70–75% (0.70–0.75)
P_{CO_2}	35–45 mm Hg (4.7–6.0 kPa)	45–51 mm Hg (6.0–6.8 kPa)
HCO_3^-	22–26 mEq/L (22–26 mmol/L)	24–28 mEq/L (24–28 mmol/L)

(HCO_3^-, bicarbonate; P_{CO_2}, partial pressure of carbon dioxide; P_{O_2}, partial pressure of oxygen; Sa_{O_2}, saturation of arterial oxygen.)

- Serum anion gap (SAG) can be used to elucidate the cause of metabolic acidosis. SAG is calculated as follows:

$$SAG = [Na^+] - [Cl^-] - [HCO_3^-]$$

  The normal anion gap is approximately 9 mEq/L (9 mmol/L), with a range of 3 to 11 mEq/L (3–11 mmol/L). SAG is a relative rather than an absolute indication of the cause of metabolic acidosis.
- The primary compensatory mechanism for metabolic acidosis is to increase carbon dioxide excretion by increasing the respiratory rate resulting in a decrease in Pa_{CO_2}.

CLINICAL PRESENTATION

- Chronic metabolic acidosis is relatively asymptomatic; major manifestations are bone demineralization with the development of rickets in children and osteomalacia and osteopenia in adults.
- Acute severe metabolic acidemia (pH <7.2) involves the cardiovascular, respiratory, and central nervous systems. Hyperventilation is often the first sign of metabolic acidosis. Respiratory compensation may occur as Kussmaul respirations (ie, deep, rapid respirations characteristic of diabetic ketoacidosis).

TREATMENT

- The primary treatment is to correct the underlying disorder. Additional treatment depends on the severity and onset of acidosis.
- Manage asymptomatic patients with mild to moderate acidemia (HCO_3^- 12–20 mEq/L [12–20 mmol/L]; pH 7.2–7.4) with gradual correction of the acidemia over days to weeks using oral **sodium bicarbonate** or other alkali preparations (Table 72–4). The dose of bicarbonate can be calculated as follows:

  Loading dose (mEq or mmol/L) =
  (Vd HCO_3^- × body weight) × (desired [HCO_3^-] – current [HCO_3^-]),

  where Vd HCO_3^- is the volume of distribution of HCO_3^- (0.5 L/kg).
- Intravenous alkali therapy can be used to treat patients with acute severe metabolic acidosis due to hyperchloremic acidosis, but its role is controversial in patients with lactic acidosis. Therapeutic options include **sodium bicarbonate** and **tromethamine**.
  ✓ Sodium bicarbonate is recommended to raise arterial pH to 7.2. However, no controlled clinical studies have demonstrated reduced morbidity and mortality compared with general supportive care. If IV sodium bicarbonate is administered, the goal is to increase, not normalize, pH to 7.2 and HCO_3^- to 8 to 10 mEq/L (8–10 mmol/L).
  ✓ Tromethamine, a highly alkaline solution, is a sodium-free organic amine that acts as a proton acceptor to prevent or correct acidosis. However, no evidence exists that tromethamine is beneficial or more efficacious than sodium bicarbonate.

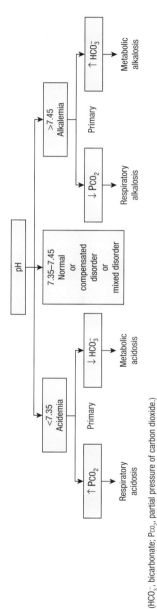

(HCO$_3^-$, bicarbonate; Pco$_2$, partial pressure of carbon dioxide.)

FIGURE 72–1. Analysis of arterial blood gases (ABGs).

TABLE 72–2	Steps in Acid–Base Diagnosis

1. Obtain ABGs and electrolytes simultaneously
2. Compare [HCO_3^-] on ABG and electrolytes to verify accuracy
3. Calculate SAG
4. Is acidemia (pH <7.35) or alkalemia (pH >7.45) present?
5. Is the primary abnormality respiratory (alteration in $Paco_2$) or metabolic (alteration in HCO_3)?
6. Estimate compensatory response
7. Compare change in [Cl^-] with change in [Na^+]

([Cl^-], chloride ion; [HCO_3^-], bicarbonate; [Na^+], sodium ion; $Paco_2$, partial pressure of carbon dioxide from arterial blood; SAG, serum anion gap.)

The usual empiric dosage for tromethamine is 1 to 5 mmol/kg administered IV over 1 hour, and an individualized dose can be calculated as follows:

$$\text{Dose of tromethamine (in mL)} = 1.1 \times \text{body weight (in kg)}$$
$$\times (\text{normal } [HCO_3^-] - \text{current } [HCO_3^-])$$

METABOLIC ALKALOSIS

PATHOPHYSIOLOGY

- Metabolic alkalosis is *initiated* by increased pH and HCO_3^-, which can result from loss of H^+ via the gastrointestinal (GI) tract (eg, nasogastric suctioning, vomiting) or kidneys (eg, diuretics, Cushing syndrome) or from gain of bicarbonate (eg, administration of bicarbonate, acetate, lactate, or citrate).
- Metabolic alkalosis is *maintained* by abnormal renal function that prevents the kidneys from excreting excess bicarbonate.
- The respiratory response is to increase $Paco_2$ by hypoventilation.

TABLE 72–3	Guidelines for Initial Interpretation of Acid–Base Disorders
Acidosis	
Metabolic	$Paco_2$ (in mm Hg) should decrease by 1.3 times the fall in plasma [HCO_3^-] (in mEq/L or mmol/L)
Acute respiratory	The plasma [HCO_3^-] should increase by 0.1 times the increase in $Paco_2$ ± 3 (in mm Hg)
Chronic respiratory	The plasma [HCO_3^-] should increase by 0.35 times the increase in $Paco_2$ ± 4 (in mm Hg)
Alkalosis	
Metabolic	$Paco_2$ (in mm Hg) should increase by 0.4–0.6 times the rise in plasma [HCO_3^-] (in mEq/L or mmol/L)
Acute respiratory	The plasma [HCO_3^-] should decrease by 0.2 times the decrease in $Paco_2$ (in mm Hg), but usually not to < 18 mEq/L (mmol/L)
Chronic respiratory	The plasma [HCO_3^-] should fall by 0.35 times the decrease in $Paco_2$ (in mm Hg), but usually not to < 14 mEq/L (mmol/L)

(HCO_3^-, bicarbonate; $Paco_2$, partial pressure of carbon dioxide from arterial blood.)

TABLE 72–4 Therapeutic Alternatives for Oral Alkali Replacement

Generic Name	Trade Name(s)	Milliequivalents of Alkali	Dosage Form(s)	Comment
Shohl's solution (sodium citrate/citric acid)	Bicitra (Willen)	1 mEq Na/mL, equivalent to 1 mEq bicarbonate	Solution (500 mg Na citrate, 334 mg citric acid/5 mL)	Citrate preparations increase absorption of aluminum
Sodium bicarbonate	Various (eg, Sodamint)	3.9 mEq bicarbonate/tablet (325 mg)	325 mg tablet	Bicarbonate preparations can cause bloating because of carbon dioxide production
		7.8 mEq bicarbonate/tablet (650 mg)	650 mg tablet	
	Baking soda (various)	60 mEq bicarbonate/tsp (5 g/tsp)	Powder	
Potassium citrate	Urocit-K (Mission)	5 mEq citrate/tablet	5 mEq tablet	See above
Potassium bicarbonate/potassium citrate	K-Lyte (Bristol)	25 mEq bicarbonate/tablet	25 mEq tablet (effervescent)	
	K-Lyte DS (Bristol)	50 mEq bicarbonate/tablet (double strength)	50 mEq tablet (effervescent)	See above
Potassium citrate/citric acid	Polycitra-K (Willen)	2 mEq K/mL; equivalent to 2 mEq bicarbonate	Solution (1100 mg K citrate, 334 mg citric acid/5 mL)	See above
		30 mEq bicarbonate/unit dose packet	Crystals for reconstitution (3300 mg K citrate, 1002 mg citric acid/unit dose packet)	
Sodium citrate/potassium citrate/citric acid	Polycitra (Willen) Polycitra-LC (Willen)	1 mEq K, 1 mEq Na/mL; equivalent to 2 mEq bicarbonate	Syrup (Polycitra) solution (Polycitra-LC) (Both contain 550 mg K citrate, 500 mg Na citrate, 334 mg citric acid/5 mL)	See above

CLINICAL PRESENTATION

- No unique signs or symptoms are associated with mild to moderate metabolic alkalosis. Some patients complain of symptoms related to the underlying disorder (eg, muscle weakness with hypokalemia or postural dizziness with volume depletion) or have a history of vomiting, gastric drainage, or diuretic use.
- Severe alkalemia (pH >7.60) can be associated with cardiac arrhythmias and neuromuscular irritability.

TREATMENT

- Aim treatment at correcting the factor(s) responsible for maintaining the alkalosis and depends on whether the disorder is sodium chloride responsive or resistant (**Fig. 72–2**).

RESPIRATORY ALKALOSIS

PATHOPHYSIOLOGY

- Respiratory alkalosis is characterized by a decrease in $Paco_2$ that leads to an increase in pH.
- $Paco_2$ decreases when ventilatory CO_2 excretion exceeds metabolic CO_2 production, usually because of hyperventilation.
- Causes include increases in neurochemical stimulation via central or peripheral mechanisms, or physical increases in ventilation via voluntary or artificial means (eg, mechanical ventilation).
- The earliest compensatory response is to chemically buffer excess bicarbonate by releasing hydrogen ions from intracellular proteins, phosphates, and hemoglobin. If prolonged (>6 hours), the kidneys attempt to further compensate by increasing bicarbonate elimination.

CLINICAL PRESENTATION

- Although usually asymptomatic, respiratory alkalosis can cause adverse neuromuscular, cardiovascular, and GI effects.
- Light-headedness, confusion, decreased intellectual functioning, syncope, and seizures can be caused by decreased cerebral blood flow.
- Nausea and vomiting can occur, probably due to cerebral hypoxia.
- Cardiac arrhythmias can occur in severe respiratory alkalosis.
- Serum electrolytes can be altered; serum chloride is usually increased; serum potassium, phosphorus, and ionized calcium are usually decreased.

TREATMENT

- Treatment is often unnecessary because most patients have few symptoms and only mild pH alterations (ie, pH <7.50).
- Direct measures (eg, treatment of pain, hypovolemia, fever, infection, or salicylate overdose) can be effective. A rebreathing device (eg, paper bag) can help control hyperventilation in patients with anxiety/hyperventilation syndrome.
- Correct respiratory alkalosis associated with mechanical ventilation by decreasing the number of mechanical breaths per minute, using a capnograph and spirometer to adjust ventilator settings more precisely, or increasing dead space in the ventilator circuit.

RESPIRATORY ACIDOSIS

PATHOPHYSIOLOGY

- Respiratory acidosis is characterized by an increase in $Paco_2$ and a decrease in pH.
- Respiratory acidosis results from disorders that restrict ventilation or increase CO_2 production, airway and pulmonary abnormalities, neuromuscular abnormalities, or mechanical ventilator problems.

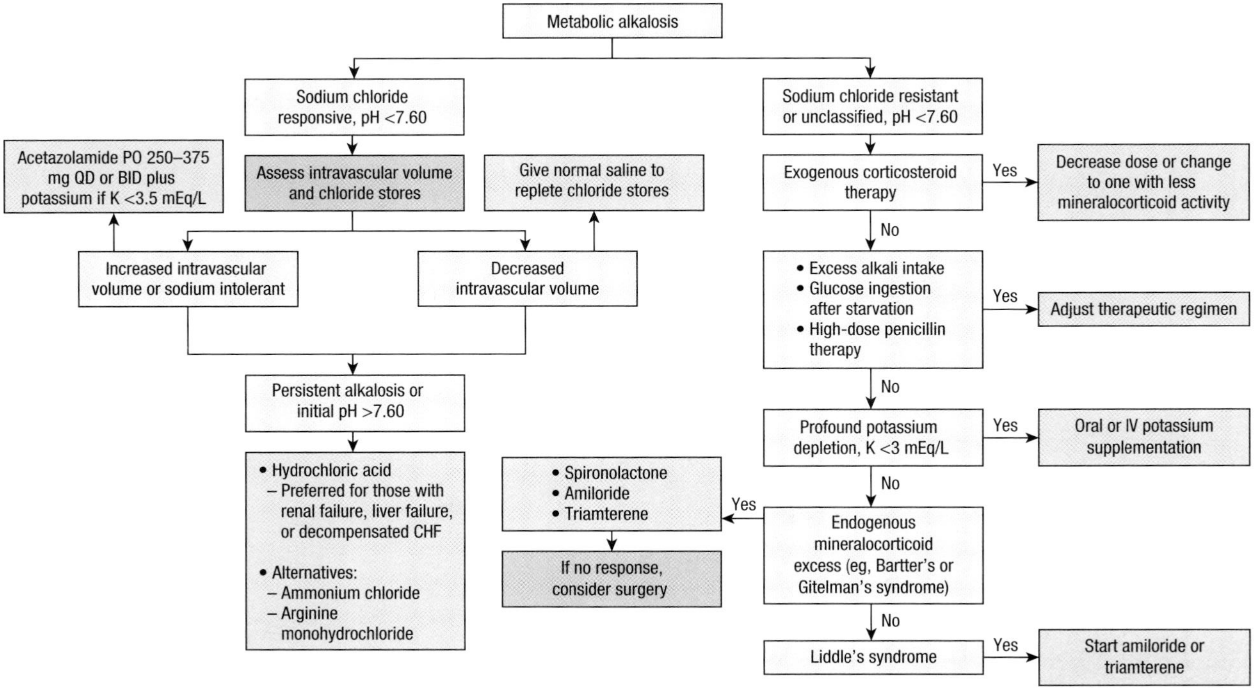

(BID, twice daily; CHF, chronic heart failure; IV, intravenous; K, potassium [serum potassium in mEq/L is numerically equal to mmol/L]; PO, orally; QD, every day.)

FIGURE 72–2. **Treatment algorithm for patients with primary metabolic alkalosis.**

- Early compensatory response to acute respiratory acidosis is chemical buffering. If prolonged (>12–24 hours), proximal tubular HCO_3^- reabsorption, ammoniagenesis, and distal tubular H^+ secretion are enhanced, resulting in an increase in serum HCO_3^- concentration that raises pH to normal.

CLINICAL PRESENTATION

- Neuromuscular symptoms include altered mental status, abnormal behavior, seizures, stupor, and coma. Hypercapnia can mimic a stroke or CNS tumor by producing headache, papilledema, focal paresis, and abnormal reflexes. CNS symptoms are caused by increased cerebral blood flow and are variable, depending in part on the acuity of onset.

TREATMENT

- Provide adequate ventilation if CO_2 excretion is acutely and severely impaired ($Paco_2$ >80 mm Hg [>10.6 kPa]) or if life-threatening hypoxia is present (arterial oxygen tension [Pao_2] <40 mm Hg [<5.3 kPa]). Ventilation can include maintaining a patent airway (eg, emergency tracheostomy, bronchoscopy, or intubation), clearing excessive secretions, administering oxygen, and providing mechanical ventilation.
- Treat underlying cause aggressively (eg, administration of bronchodilators for bronchospasm or discontinuation of respiratory depressants such as narcotics and benzodiazepines). Bicarbonate administration is rarely necessary and is potentially harmful.
- Chronic respiratory acidosis (eg, chronic obstructive pulmonary disease [COPD]) is treated essentially the same as acute respiratory acidosis with a few important exceptions. Oxygen therapy should be initiated carefully and only if the Pao_2 is less than 50 mm Hg (<6.7 kPa) because the drive to breathe depends on hypoxemia rather than hypercarbia.
- For information on chronic respiratory acidosis, see Chap. 78.

MIXED ACID–BASE DISORDERS

PATHOPHYSIOLOGY

- Failure of compensation is responsible for mixed acid–base disorders such as respiratory acidosis and metabolic acidosis, or respiratory alkalosis and metabolic alkalosis. In contrast, excess compensation is responsible for metabolic acidosis and respiratory alkalosis, or metabolic alkalosis and respiratory acidosis.
- Respiratory and metabolic acidosis can develop in patients with cardiorespiratory arrest, with chronic lung disease and shock, and with metabolic acidosis and respiratory failure.
- The most common mixed acid–base disorder is respiratory and metabolic alkalosis, which occurs in critically ill surgical patients with respiratory alkalosis caused by mechanical ventilation, hypoxia, sepsis, hypotension, neurologic damage, pain, or drugs; and with metabolic alkalosis caused by vomiting or nasogastric suctioning and massive blood transfusions.
- Mixed metabolic acidosis and respiratory alkalosis occur in patients with advanced liver disease, salicylate intoxication, and pulmonary-renal syndromes.
- Metabolic alkalosis and respiratory acidosis can occur in patients with COPD and respiratory acidosis who are treated with salt restriction, diuretics, and possibly glucocorticoids.

TREATMENT

- Treat mixed respiratory and metabolic acidosis by initiating oxygen delivery to improve hypercarbia and hypoxia. Mechanical ventilation can be needed to reduce $Paco_2$. During initial therapy, give appropriate amounts of alkali to reverse the metabolic acidosis.

- Correct the metabolic component of mixed respiratory and metabolic alkalosis by administering **sodium** and **potassium chloride solutions**. Readjust the ventilator or treat the underlying disorder causing hyperventilation to treat the respiratory component.
- Treatment of mixed metabolic acidosis and respiratory alkalosis should be directed at the underlying cause.
- In metabolic alkalosis and respiratory acidosis, pH does not usually deviate significantly from normal, but treatment can be required to maintain Pao_2 and $Paco_2$ at acceptable levels. Aim treatment at decreasing plasma bicarbonate with sodium and potassium chloride therapy, allowing renal excretion of retained bicarbonate from diuretic-induced metabolic alkalosis.

EVALUATION OF THERAPEUTIC OUTCOMES

- Patients should be monitored closely because acid–base disorders can be serious and even life threatening.
- ABGs are the primary tools for evaluation of therapeutic outcome.

See Chapter 52, Acid–Base Disorders, authored by John W. Devlin and Gary R. Matzke, for a more detailed discussion of this topic.

Acute Kidney Injury

- *Acute kidney injury* (AKI) is a clinical syndrome generally defined by an abrupt reduction in kidney functions as evidenced by changes in serum creatinine (S_{cr}), blood urea nitrogen (BUN), and urine output.
- RIFLE (Risk, Injury, Failure, Loss of Kidney Function, and End-Stage Renal Disease), AKIN (Acute Kidney Injury Network), and the Kidney Disease: Improving Global Outcomes (KDIGO) Clinical Practice Guidelines are three criteria-based classification systems developed to define and stage AKI in different patient populations (Table 73–1).
- All three staging systems have been validated across different patient populations and their staging correlates closely with hospital mortality, cost, and length of stay.
- S_{cr} and urine output are the main diagnostic criteria for each staging system.

PATHOPHYSIOLOGY

- AKI can be categorized as prerenal (resulting from decreased renal perfusion in the setting of undamaged parenchymal tissue), intrinsic (resulting from structural damage to the kidney, most commonly the tubule from an ischemic or toxic insult), and postrenal (resulting from obstruction of urine flow downstream from the kidney) (Fig. 73–1).

CLINICAL PRESENTATION

- Patient presentation varies widely and depends on the underlying cause. Outpatients often are not in acute distress; hospitalized patients may develop AKI after a catastrophic event.
- Symptoms in the outpatient setting include acute change in urinary habits, sudden weight gain, or severe abdominal or flank pain. Signs include edema, colored or foamy urine, and, in volume-depleted patients, postural hypotension.

DIAGNOSIS

- Thorough medical and medication histories, physical examination, assessment of laboratory values, and, if needed, imaging studies are important in the diagnosis of AKI.
- S_{cr} cannot be used alone to diagnose AKI because it is insensitive to rapid changes in glomerular filtration rate (GFR) lagging behind the GRF's decline by 1 to 2 days leading to a potential delay in diagnosis. The use of BUN in AKI is very limited because urea production and renal clearance are heavily influenced by extrarenal factors such as critical illness, volume status, protein intake, and medications.
- Urine output measured over a specified period of time allows for short-term assessment of renal function, but its utility is limited to cases in which it is significantly decreased.
- In addition to BUN and S_{cr}, selected blood tests, urinary chemistry, and urinary sediment are used to differentiate the cause of AKI and guide patient management (Tables 73–2 and 73–3).
- Simultaneous measurement of urine and serum electrolytes and calculation of the fractional excretion of sodium (FE_{Na}) can help determine the etiology of AKI (see Table 73–2). The FE_{Na} is one of the better diagnostic parameters to differentiate the cause of AKI and is calculated as

$$FE_{Na} = (U_{Na} \times S_{Cr} \times 100)/(U_{Cr} \times S_{Na})$$

where U_{Na} = urine sodium, S_{Cr} = serum creatinine, U_{Cr} = urine creatinine, and S_{Na} = serum sodium.

TABLE 73–1 RIFLE, AKIN, and KDIGO Classification Schemes for Acute Kidney Injury[a]

RIFLE Category	S_{cr} and GFR[b] Criteria	Urine Output Criteria
Risk	S_{cr} increase to 1.5-fold or GFR decrease >25% from baseline	<0.5 mL/kg/h for ≥6 hours
Injury	S_{cr} increase to twofold or GFR decrease >50% from baseline	<0.5 mL/kg/h for ≥12 hours
Failure	S_{cr} increase to threefold or GFR decrease >75% from baseline, or S_{cr} ≥4 mg/dL (≥354 μmol/L) with an acute increase of at least 0.5 mg/dL (44 μmol/L)	Anuria for ≥12 hours
Loss	Complete loss of function (RRT) for >4 weeks	
ESKD	RRT >3 months	

AKIN Criteria	S_{cr} Criteria	Urine Output Criteria
Stage 1	S_{cr} increase ≥0.3 mg/dL (≥27 μmol/L) or 1.5- to 2-fold from baseline	<0.5 mL/kg/h for ≥6 hours
Stage 2	S_{cr} increase >2- to 3-fold from baseline	<0.5 mL/kg/h for ≥12 hours
Stage 3	S_{cr} increase >3-fold from baseline, or S_{cr} ≥4 mg/dL (≥354 μmol/L) with an acute increase of at least 0.5 mg/dL (≥44 μmol/L), or need for RRT	<0.3 mL/kg/h for ≥24 hours or anuria for ≥12 hours

KDIGO Criteria	S_{cr} Criteria	Urine Output Criteria
Stage 1	S_{cr} increase ≥0.3 mg/dL (≥27 μmol/L) or 1.5–1.9 times from baseline	<0.5 mL/kg/h for 6–12 hours
Stage 2	S_{cr} increase 2–2.9 times from baseline	<0.5 mL/kg/h for ≥12 hours
Stage 3	S_{cr} increase three times from baseline, or S_{cr} ≥4 mg/dL (≥354 μmol/L), or need for RRT, or eGFR[c] <35 mL/min/1.73 m² (<0.34 mL/s/m²) in patients <18 years	Anuria for ≥12 hours

(AKIN, Acute Kidney Injury Network; ESKD, end-stage kidney disease; eGFR, estimated glomerular filtration rate; h, hours; KDIGO, Kidney Disease: Improving Global Outcomes; RIFLE, Risk, Injury, Failure, Loss of Kidney Function, and End-Stage Kidney Disease; RRT, renal replacement therapy; S_{cr}, serum creatinine.)

[a]For all staging systems, the criterion that leads to worst possible diagnosis should be used.

[b]GFR calculated using the Modification of Diet in Renal Disease (MDRD) equation.

[c]GFR calculated using the Schwartz formula.

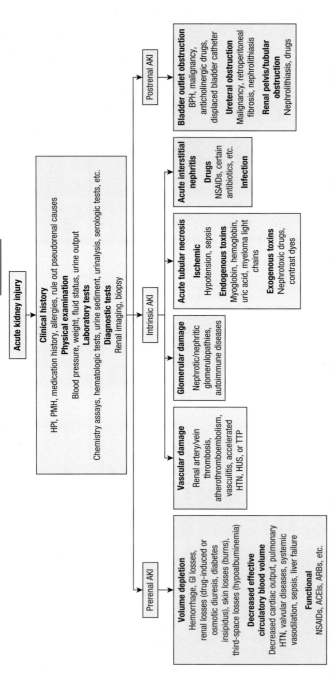

(ACEIs, angiotensin-converting enzyme inhibitors; ARBs, angiotensin receptor blockers; BPH, benign prostatic hyperplasia; GI, gastrointestinal; HPI, history of present illness; HTN, hypertension; HUS, hemolytic uremic syndrome; NSAIDs, nonsteroidal anti-inflammatory drugs; PMH, past medical history; TTP, thrombotic thrombocytopenic purpura.)

FIGURE 73-1. Classification of acute kidney injury (AKI) based on etiology.

TABLE 73–2	Diagnostic Parameters for Differentiating Causes of AKI[a]		
Laboratory Test	**Prerenal AKI**	**Intrinsic AKI**	**Postrenal AKI**
Urine sediment	Hyaline casts, may be normal	Granular casts, cellular debris	Cellular debris
Urinary RBC	None	2–4+	Variable
Urinary WBC	None	2–4+	1+
Urine Na (mEq/L or mmol/L)	<20	>40	>40
FE_{Na} (%)	<1	>2	Variable
Urine/serum osmolality	>1.5	<1.3	<1.5
Urine/S_{cr}	>40:1	<20:1	<20:1
BUN/S_{cr} (urea/S_{cr}, SI)	>20 (>80)	~15 (~60)	~15 (~60)
Urine specific gravity	>1.018	<1.012	Variable

(AKI, acute kidney injury; BUN, blood urea nitrogen; FE_{Na}, fractional excretion of sodium; S_{cr}, serum creatinine; RBC, red blood cell; WBC, white blood cell.)

[a]Common laboratory tests are used to classify the cause of AKI. Functional AKI, which is not included in this table, would have laboratory values similar to those seen in prerenal AKI. However, the urine osmolality-to-plasma osmolality ratios may not exceed 1.5, depending on the circulating levels of antidiuretic hormone. The laboratory results listed under intrinsic AKI are those seen in acute tubular necrosis, the most common cause of intrinsic AKI.

TABLE 73–3	Urinary Findings as a Guide to the Etiology of AKI	
Type of Urinary Evaluation	**Presence of**	**Suggestive of**
Urinalysis	Leukocyte esterases	Pyelonephritis
	Nitrites	Pyelonephritis
	Protein	
	Mild (<0.5 g/day)	Tubular damage
	Moderate (0.5–3 g/day)	Glomerulonephritis, pyelonephritis, tubular damage
	Large (>3 g/day)	Glomerulonephritis, nephrotic syndrome
	Hemoglobin	Glomerulonephritis, pyelonephritis, renal infarction, renal tumors, kidney stones
	Myoglobin	Rhabdomyolysis-associated tubular necrosis
	Urobilinogen	Hemolysis-associated tubular necrosis
Urine sediment Cells	Microorganisms	Pyelonephritis
	Red blood cells	Glomerulonephritis, pyelonephritis, renal infarction, papillary necrosis, renal tumors, kidney stones
	White blood cells	Pyelonephritis, interstitial nephritis
	Eosinophils	Drug-induced interstitial nephritis, renal transplant rejection
	Epithelial cells	Tubular necrosis
Casts	Granular casts	Tubular necrosis
	Hyaline casts	Prerenal azotemia
	White blood cell casts	Pyelonephritis, interstitial nephritis
	Red blood cell casts	Glomerulonephritis, renal infarct, lupus nephritis, vasculitis
Crystals	Urate	Postrenal obstruction
	Calcium phosphate	Postrenal obstruction

- A number of new serum and urinary biomarkers have been investigated to detect and predict the clinical outcomes of AKI.

PREVENTION

- Goals of Prevention: The goals are to screen and identify patients at risk; monitor high-risk patients until the risk subsides; and implement prevention strategies when appropriate.

GENERAL APPROACH TO PREVENTION

Nonpharmacologic Therapies

- Hydration is routinely used to prevent contrast-induced nephropathy (CIN), a common cause of acute tubular necrosis in the inpatient setting. Evidence supports use of isotonic crystalloids over colloids and parenteral over oral administration in high-risk individuals, including those with chronic kidney disease (CKD), diabetes, volume depletion, concurrent nephrotoxic drug therapy, or hemodynamic instability.
- KDIGO guidelines recommend either sodium bicarbonate or isotonic saline infusions. A common sodium bicarbonate regimen is 154 mEq/L (154 mmol/L) infused at 3 mL/kg/h for 1 hour before the procedure and at 1 mL/kg/h for 6 hours after the procedure. One frequently cited normal saline regimen is 1 mL/kg/h for 12 hours pre- and postprocedure.

Pharmacologic Therapies

- **Ascorbic acid** (3 g orally preprocedure and 2 g orally twice daily for two doses post-procedure) and **N-acetylcysteine** (600–1200 mg orally every 12 hours for 2–3 days [first two doses precontrast]) are antioxidant options for prevention of CIN. Study results with these two agents are inconsistent.
- Current KDIGO guidelines suggest that moderate control of blood glucose to levels of 110 to 149 mg/dL (6.1–8.3 mmol/L) with **insulin** therapy is appropriate to prevent hyper- and hypoglycemia in critically ill patients with AKI.

TREATMENT OF ACUTE KIDNEY INJURY

- Goals of Treatment: Short-term goals include minimizing the degree of insult to the kidney, reducing extrarenal complications, and expediting recovery of renal function. Restoration of renal function to pre-AKI baseline is the ultimate goal.

GENERAL APPROACH TO TREATMENT

- Currently, there is no definitive therapy for AKI. Supportive care with a focus on managing fluid overload and acid-base/electrolyte imbalances is the mainstay of AKI management regardless of etiology.

Nonpharmacologic Therapies

- Supportive care goals include maintenance of adequate cardiac output and blood pressure to optimize tissue perfusion while restoring renal function to pre-AKI baseline.
- Discontinue medications associated with diminished renal blood flow. Initiate appropriate fluid and electrolyte management. Avoid use of nephrotoxins. Optimize nutritional status.
- In severe AKI, renal replacement therapy (RRT), such as hemodialysis and peritoneal dialysis, maintains fluid and electrolyte balance while removing waste products. See Table 73–4 for indications for RRT in AKI. Intermittent and continuous options have different advantages (and disadvantages); current KDIGO guidelines suggest using continuous RRT over intermittent hemodialysis in hemodynamically unstable patients. Hybrid approaches (eg, sustained low-efficiency dialysis and slow, extended daily dialysis) have been developed to provide the advantages of both. Knowledge of impact of hybrid approaches on drug removal is very limited.

TABLE 73–4	Common Indications for RRT
Indication for RRT	**Clinical Setting**
A: acid-base abnormalities	Metabolic acidosis (especially if pH <7.2)
E: electrolyte imbalance	Severe hyperkalemia and/or hypermagnesemia
I: intoxications	Salicylates, lithium, methanol, ethylene glycol, theophylline, phenobarbital
O: fluid overload	Fluid overload (especially pulmonary edema unresponsive to diuretics)
U: uremia	Uremia or associated complications (neuropathy, encephalopathy, pericarditis)

(RRT, renal replacement therapy.)

- Intermittent hemodialysis (IHD) is the most frequently used RRT and has the advantage of widespread availability and the convenience of lasting only 3 to 4 hours. Disadvantages include difficult venous dialysis access in hypotensive patients and hypotension due to rapid removal of large amounts of fluid.
- Several continuous RRT (CRRT) variants have been developed including continuous hemofiltration, continuous hemodialysis, or a combination. CRRT gradually removes solute, resulting in better tolerability by critically ill patients. Disadvantages include limited availability of equipment, need for intensive nursing care, and the need to individualize IV replacement, dialysate fluids, and drug therapy adjustments.

Pharmacologic Therapies

- **Mannitol** 20% is typically started at a dose of 12.5 to 25 g IV over 3 to 5 minutes. Disadvantages include IV administration, hyperosmolality risk, and need for monitoring urine output and serum electrolytes and osmolality because mannitol can contribute to AKI.
- Loop diuretics effectively reduce fluid overload but can worsen AKI. Equipotent doses of loop diuretics (**furosemide, bumetanide, torsemide,** and **ethacrynic acid**) have similar efficacy. KDIGO guidelines recommend limiting the use of loop diuretics to the management of fluid overload and avoiding their use for the sole purpose of prevention or treatment of AKI. Continuous infusions of loop diuretics appear to overcome diuretic resistance and to have fewer adverse effects than intermittent boluses.
- Strategies are available to overcome diuretic resistance (Table 73–5). Combination therapy of loop diuretics plus a diuretic from a different pharmacologic class such as diuretics that work at the distal convoluted tubule (thiazides) or the collecting duct (**amiloride, triamterene,** and **spironolactone**), may be synergistic. **Metolazone** is commonly used with a loop diuretic because, unlike other thiazides, it produces effective diuresis at GFR less than 20 mL/min (0.33 mL/s).

ELECTROLYTE MANAGEMENT AND NUTRITION INTERVENTIONS

- Serum electrolytes should be monitored daily. Hyperkalemia is the most common and serious electrolyte abnormality in AKI. Hypernatremia and fluid retention commonly occur, requiring calculation of daily sodium intake, including sodium contained in commonly administered antibiotic and antifungal agents.
- Phosphorus and magnesium should be monitored, especially in patients with significant tissue destruction due to increased amounts of released phosphorus; neither is efficiently removed by dialysis.
- Nutritional management of critically ill patients with AKI is complex due to multiple mechanisms for metabolic derangements. Nutritional requirements are altered by stress, inflammation, and injury that lead to hypermetabolic and hypercatabolic states.

TABLE 73–5 Common Causes of Diuretic Resistance in Patients with Acute Kidney Injury

Causes of Diuretic Resistance	Potential Therapeutic Solutions
Excessive sodium intake (sources may be dietary, IV fluids, and drugs)	Remove sodium from nutritional sources and medications
Inadequate diuretic dose or inappropriate regimen	Increase dose, use continuous infusion or combination therapy
Reduced oral bioavailability (usually furosemide)	Use parenteral therapy, switch to oral torsemide or bumetanide
Nephrotic syndrome (loop diuretic protein binding in tubule lumen)	Increase dose, switch diuretics, use combination therapy
Reduced renal blood flow	
Drugs (NSAIDs, ACEIs, vasodilators)	Discontinue these drugs if possible
Hypotension	Intravascular volume expansion and/or vasopressors
Intravascular depletion	Intravascular volume expansion
Increased sodium resorption	
Nephron adaptation to chronic diuretic therapy	Combination diuretic therapy, sodium restriction
NSAID use	Discontinue NSAID
Heart failure	Treat heart failure, increase diuretic dose, switch to better-absorbed loop diuretic
Cirrhosis	High-volume paracentesis
Acute tubular necrosis	Higher dose of diuretic, diuretic combination therapy; add low-dose dopamine

(ACEIs, angiotensin-converting enzyme inhibitors; IV, intravenous; NSAIDs, nonsteroidal anti-inflammatory drugs.)

DRUG-DOSING CONSIDERATIONS

- Drug therapy optimization in AKI is a challenge. Confounding variables include residual drug clearance, fluid accumulation, and use of RRTs.
- Volume of distribution for water-soluble drugs is significantly increased due to edema. Use of dosing guidelines for CKD does not reflect the clearance and volume of distribution in critically ill patients with AKI.
- Patients with AKI may have a higher residual nonrenal clearance than those with CKD with similar creatinine clearances; this complicates drug-therapy individualization, especially with RRTs.
- The mode of CRRT determines rate of drug removal, further complicating individualization of drug therapy. Rates of ultrafiltration, blood flow, and dialysate flow influence drug clearance during CRRT.

EVALUATION OF THERAPEUTIC OUTCOMES

- Vigilant monitoring of patient status is essential (Table 73–6).
- Therapeutic drug monitoring should be performed for drugs that have a narrow therapeutic index if results can be obtained in a timely manner.

TABLE 73–6	Key Monitoring Parameters for Patients with Established Acute Kidney Injury
Parameter	**Frequency**
Fluid ins/outs	Every shift
Patient weight	Daily
Hemodynamics (blood pressure, heart rate, mean arterial pressure, etc.)	Every shift
Blood chemistries	
Sodium, potassium, chloride, bicarbonate, calcium, phosphate, magnesium	Daily
Blood urea nitrogen/serum creatinine	Daily
Drugs and their dosing regimens	Daily
Nutritional regimen	Daily
Blood glucose	Daily (minimum)
Serum concentration data for drugs	After regimen changes and after renal replacement therapy has been instituted
Times of administered doses	Daily
Doses relative to administration of renal replacement therapy	Daily
Urinalysis	
Calculate measured creatinine clearance	Every time measured urine collection performed
Calculate fractional excretion of sodium	Every time measured urine collection performed
Plans for renal replacement	Daily

See Chapter 43, Acute Kidney Injury, authored by Jenana Halilovic and William Dager, for a more detailed discussion of this topic.

- *Chronic kidney disease* (CKD) is defined as abnormalities in kidney structure or function, present for 3 months or longer, with implications for health.
- CKD is classified by cause of kidney disease, glomerular filtration rate (GFR) category, and albuminuria level based on new recommendations from the Kidney Disease: Improving Global Outcomes (KDIGO) guidelines, referred to as CGA staging (*c*ause, *G*FR, *a*lbuminuria) (Table 74–1).
- A patient is classified with end-stage renal disease (ESRD) when their GFR is below 15 mL/min/1.73 m² (<0.14 mL/s/m²) and either chronic dialysis or kidney transplantation is needed to sustain life. KDIGO classification will be used in this chapter; the term CKD 5D indicates a patient with ESRD requiring dialysis as either hemodialysis (CKD 5HD) or peritoneal dialysis (CKD 5PD).
- Prognosis of CKD depends on cause of kidney disease, GFR at time of diagnosis, degree of albuminuria, and presence of other comorbid conditions.

PATHOPHYSIOLOGY

- *Susceptibility factors* increase the risk for kidney disease but do not directly cause kidney damage. They include advanced age, racial or ethnic minority, low income or education, and exposure to certain chemical and environmental conditions.
- *Initiation factors* directly result in kidney damage and include diabetes mellitus, hypertension, obesity, autoimmune diseases, systemic infections, family history of CKD, reduction in kidney mass, and low birth weight.
- *Progression factors* are associated with further decline in kidney function after initiation of kidney damage. They include diabetes mellitus, hypertension, proteinuria, obesity, and smoking.
- Most progressive nephropathies share a final common pathway to irreversible renal parenchymal damage and ESRD (Fig. 74–1). Key elements of the pathway to ESRD include loss of nephron mass, glomerular capillary hypertension, and proteinuria.

CLINICAL PRESENTATION

- Progression of CKD from category 1 to 5 occurs over decades in the majority of people who are asymptomatic until they reach CKD 4 or 5. Signs and symptoms seen with stages 4 to 5 include fatigue, weakness, shortness of breath, mental confusion, nausea, vomiting, bleeding, anorexia, edema, weight gain, cold intolerance, peripheral neuropathies, changes in urine output, and abdominal distension.

TREATMENT OF CKD

GENERAL APPROACH

- <u>Goal of Treatment</u>: The goal is to delay or prevent the progression of CKD while minimizing the development or severity of complications.
- Use the most current consensus guidelines and the best clinical practices for management of CKD, such as those developed by KDIGO.

NONPHARMACOLOGIC THERAPY

- Restrict protein to 0.8 g/kg/day if GFR is less than 30 mL/min/1.73 m².
- Encourage smoking cessation to slow progression of CKD and reduce the risk of CVD.
- Encourage exercise at least 30 minutes five times per week and achievement of a body mass index (BMI) of 20 to 25 kg/m².

TABLE 74–1	Glomerular Filtration Rate Categories Based on KDIGO Classification	
GFR Category[a]	GFR (mL/min/1.73 m^2 [mL/s/m^2])	Terms
1	>90 (>0.87)	Normal or high
2	60–89 (0.58–0.86)	Mildly decreased
3a	45–59 (0.43–0.57)	Mildly to moderately decreased
3b	30–44 (0.29–0.42)	Moderately to severely decreased
4	15–29 (0.14–0.28)	Severely decreased
5	<15 (<0.14)	Kidney failure

(CKD, chronic kidney disease; GFR, glomerular filtration rate; KDIGO, Kidney Disease: Improving Global Outcomes.)

[a]To meet criteria for CKD there must be a significant reduction in GFR (categories 3a-5) or there must also be evidence of kidney damage (categories 1 and 2) for 3 months or greater.

PHARMACOLOGIC THERAPY

Proteinuria and Hypertension

- Achieving the target blood pressure is the primary goal for CKD patients with hypertension and a secondary goal is to control proteinuria. First-line therapy for patients with diabetic CKD (DCKD) should include an angiotensin-converting enzyme inhibitor (ACEI) or an angiotensin II receptor blocker (ARB) if the patient's urine albumin excretion is in category A2 or greater (albumin-to-creatinine ratio (ACR) between 30 and 300 mg/g (3–30 mg/mmol)). Initiate therapy with the lowest recommended dose and increase dose until albuminuria is reduced by 30% to 50% or side effects such as a greater than 30% decrease in estimated GFR or elevation in serum potassium occur (Fig. 74–2).
- Nondihydropyridine calcium channel blockers are second-line antiproteinuric drugs when an ACEI or ARB is contraindicated or not tolerated.
- KDIGO guidelines recommend a target blood pressure of 140/90 mm Hg or less if urine albumin excretion or equivalent is less than 30 mg/24 h (<3 mg/mmol) (category A1 albuminuria). The target blood pressure for patients with category A2 and higher albuminuria is less than or equal to 130/80 mm Hg and first-line therapy with an ACEI or ARB is recommended. Addition of a thiazide diuretic may be warranted if use of an ACEI or ARB fails to achieve the target blood pressure.
- For more information on hypertension, see Chapter 10.

Diabetes

- Screen patients with diabetes annually for CKD starting at the time of diagnosis of type 2 diabetes and 5 years after diagnosis of type 1 diabetes by ordering serum creatinine, estimated GFR, and ACR.
- Management of diabetes in patients with CKD includes reduction of proteinuria and achievement of target blood pressure and HbA1c.
- For more information on diabetes, see Chap. 19.

TREATMENT OF SECONDARY COMPLICATIONS

Anemia of CKD

- Desired outcomes of anemia management are to increase oxygen-carrying capacity, decrease signs, and symptoms of anemia, and decrease the need for blood transfusions.
- Guide initiation of iron or erythropoiesis-stimulating agent (ESA) therapy by the patient's hemoglobin (Hb), transferrin saturation (TSat), and ferritin (Table 74–2). The risk of mortality and cardiovascular events is higher in CKD patients treated to higher Hb target values with an ESA. The target range for Hb in the CKD population is a topic of much debate.
- Kidney Disease Outcomes Quality Initiative (KDOQI) guidelines suggest a Hb range of 11 to 12 g/DL (110–120 g/L; 6.83–7.45 mmol/L) for all CKD patients, a target

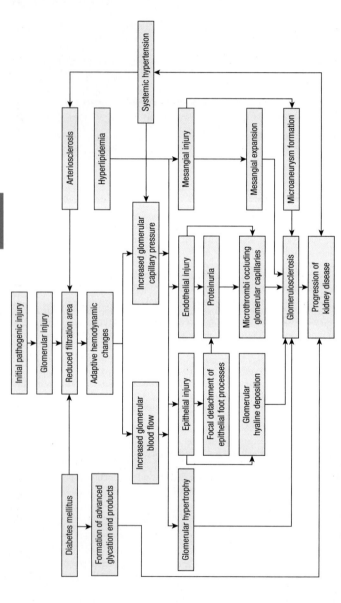

FIGURE 74-1. Proposed mechanisms for progression of renal disease.

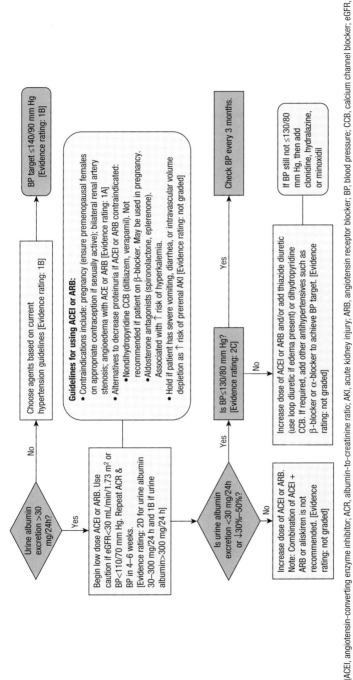

FIGURE 74–2. Treatment of hypertension in chronic kidney disease. *(Data from KDIGO Blood Pressure Work Group. KDIGO Clinical Practice Guideline for the Management of Blood Pressure in Chronic Kidney Disease. Kidney Int Suppl 2012;2:337–414.)*

(ACEI, angiotensin-converting enzyme inhibitor; ACR, albumin-to-creatinine ratio; AKI, acute kidney injury; ARB, angiotensin receptor blocker; BP, blood pressure; CCB, calcium channel blocker; eGFR, estimated glomerular filtration rate.)

TABLE 74–2 KDIGO Recommendations for Initiation of Erythropoiesis Stimulating Agents and Iron in Anemia of Chronic Kidney Disease[a]

	ND-CKD	CKD 5HD and CKD 5PD	Pediatric CKD
ESA initiation	If Hb <10 g/dL (<100 g/L; <6.21 mmol/L). Consider rate of fall of Hb, prior response to iron, risk of needing a transfusion, risk of ESA therapy, and presence of anemia symptoms before initiating an ESA. [2C] Do not initiate if Hb ≥10 g/dL (≥100 g/L; ≥6.21 mmol/L). [2D]	Use ESAs to avoid drop in Hb to <9 g/dL (<90 g/L; <5.59 mmol/L) by starting an ESA when Hb is between 9 and 10 g/dL (90 and 100 g/L; 5.59 and 6.21 mmol/L). [2B]	Selection of Hb concentration at which to initiate ESA therapy should include consideration of potential benefits (eg, improvement in QOL, school attendance, avoidance of blood transfusions) and potential harms. [2D]
Hb level	Do not use ESAs to *intentionally* increase Hb above 13 g/dL (130 g/L, 8.07 mmol/L). [1A] Do not use ESAs to maintain Hb above 11.5 g/dL (115 g/L; 7.14 mmol/L). [2C]	Do not use ESAs to *intentionally* increase Hb above 13 g/dL (130 g/L, 8.07 mmol/L). [1A] Do not use ESAs to maintain Hb above 11.5 g/dL (115 g/L; 7.14 mmol/L). [2C]	Suggest Hb range of 11–12 g/dL (110–120 g/L, 6.83–7.45 mmol/L). [2D]
Iron initiation[b]	If TSat is ≤30% (≤0.30) and ferritin is ≤500 ng/mL (mcg/L; ≤1120 pmol/L). [2C]	If TSat is ≤30% (≤0.30) and ferritin is ≤500 ng/mL (mcg/L; ≤1120 pmol/L). [2C]	If TSat is ≤20% (≤0.20) and ferritin is ≤100 ng/mL (mcg/L; ≤225 pmol/L). [1D]

(CKD, chronic kidney disease; ESA, erythropoiesis stimulating agent; Hb, hemoglobin; ND-CKD, nondialysis CKD patients; QOL, quality of life; TSat, transferrin saturation.)
[a]The Kidney Disease Outcome Quality Initiative (KDOQI) Anemia Guidelines are discussed in the text.
[b]If TSat and serum ferritin are below suggested levels, consider iron supplementation if goal is to increase Hb and/or decrease ESA dose. *Note:* Serum ferritin is an acute-phase reactant-use clinical judgment when above 500 ng/mL (mcg/L; 1120 pmol/L).

TSat of greater than 20% (>0.20), and a serum ferritin of greater than 100 ng/mL (mcg/L; >225pmol/L) for CKD patients not requiring HD and greater than 200 ng/mL (mcg/L; >450 pmol/L) for CKD 5HD patients.

- Oral or IV administration of **iron** supplementation is recommended in non-HD patients (eg, CKD category 3 or higher and PD patients). Supplementation with oral products (see **Table 33–2**) is more convenient but patients are likely to require IV iron supplementation, especially if they are receiving an ESA. Adverse effects of oral iron are primarily GI in nature and include constipation, nausea, and abdominal cramping which may negatively influence adherence.

- IV iron preparations have different pharmacokinetic profiles determined by the size of the iron-containing core and the composition of the surrounding carbohydrate (**Table 74–3**).

- Adverse effects of IV iron include allergic reactions, hypotension, dizziness, dyspnea, headaches, lower back pain, arthralgia, syncope, and arthritis. Some of these reactions can be minimized by decreasing the dose or rate of infusion. Sodium ferric gluconate, iron sucrose, and ferumoxytol have a better safety record than iron dextran products.

- All available ESAs may be administered either IV or subcutaneously (SC) (**Table 74–4**). SQ administration of **epoetin** results in a prolonged absorption phase leading to an extended half-life allowing target Hb to be maintained at doses 15% to 30% lower than IV doses.

- The prolonged half-lives of **darbepoetin alfa** and **methoxy PEG-epoetin beta** allow for less frequent dosing.

- Causes of ESA resistance include iron deficiency, acute illness, inflammation, infection, chronic bleeding, aluminum toxicity, malnutrition, hyperparathyroidism, cancer, and chemotherapy.

- ESAs are well tolerated. Hypertension is the most common adverse event.

Evaluation of Anemia Therapeutic Outcomes

- Evaluate iron indices (TSat; ferritin) before initiating an ESA. Iron status should be reassessed every month during initial ESA treatment and every 3 months for those on a stable ESA regimen.

- Monitor Hb at least monthly after initiation of an ESA or after a dose change until hemoglobin is stable. FDA labeling for ESAs recommends weekly monitoring of Hb until Hb is stable.

- For more information on anemia, see Chap. 33.

CKD-Related Mineral and Bone Disorder

- Disorders of mineral and bone metabolism (CKD-MBD) are common in the CKD population and include abnormalities in parathyroid hormone (PTH), calcium, phosphorus, vitamin D, fibroblast growth factor-23, and bone turnover, as well as soft tissue calcifications.

- Calcium-phosphorus homeostasis is mediated through a complex interplay of hormones and their effects on bone, the gastrointestinal (GI) tract, kidneys, and the parathyroid gland. As kidney function declines, phosphate elimination decreases resulting in hyperphosphatemia and a decrease in serum calcium concentration. Hypocalcemia stimulates secretion of PTH. As renal function declines, serum calcium balance can be maintained only at the expense of increased bone resorption, leading to alterations in structural integrity of bone and other consequences.

- The KDIGO guidelines provide desired ranges of calcium, phosphorus, and intact PTH based on the CKD category (**Table 74–5**).

Treatment

- Dietary phosphorus restriction, dialysis, and parathyroidectomy are nonpharmacologic approaches to management of hyperphosphatemia and CKD-MBD.

PHOSPHATE-BINDING AGENTS

- Phosphate-binding agents decrease phosphorus absorption from the gut and are first-line agents for controlling both serum phosphorus and calcium concentrations (**Table 74–6**).

TABLE 74–3	IV Iron Preparations					
Iron Compounds	Brand Names	Half-Life (Hours)	Molecular Weight (Daltons)	FDA-Approved Indications	FDA-Approved Dosing[a]	Dose Ranges (mg)[b]
Ferric carboxymaltose	Injectafer	7–12	150,000	Adult patients with intolerance to oral iron or who have had an unsatisfactory response to oral iron and in adult patients with CKD not on dialysis	Give 2 doses separated by at least 7 days of 750 mg per dose (if body weight is ≥50 kg) or 15 mg/kg per dose (if body weight is <50 kg) not to exceed 1500 mg per course. Give either IV push (100 mg per min) or diluted in not more than 250 mL of 0.9 NaCl as an infusion over at least 15 minutes	750
Ferumoxytol	Feraheme	15	750,000	Adult patients with iron-deficiency anemia associated with chronic kidney disease	510 mg (17 mL) as a single dose, followed by a second 510 mg dose 3–8 days after the initial dose. Dilute in 50–200 mL of 0.9% NaCl or 5% dextrose and administer as an IV infusion over 15 minutes	510
Iron dextran	INFeD Dexferrum	40–60	96,000 265,000	Patients with iron deficiency in whom oral iron is unsatisfactory or impossible	100 mg over 2 minutes (25-mg test dose required) Note: Equation provided by manufacturer to calculate dose based on desired Hb	25–1000

					Dosing	
Iron sucrose	Venofer	6	43,000	Adult and pediatric CKD 5HD patients aged 2 years and older	Adult: 100 mg over 2–5 minutes or 100 mg in maximum of 100 mL of 0.9% NaCl over 15 minutes per consecutive HD session Pediatric: 0.5 mg/kg not to exceed 100 mg per dose over 5 minutes or diluted in 25 mL of 0.9% NaCl administered over 5–60 minutes (give dose every 2 weeks for 12 weeks)	25–1000
				Adult and pediatric ND-CKD patients aged 2 years and older	Adult: 200 mg over 2–5 minutes on five different occasions within 14-day period. There is limited experience with administration of 500 mg diluted in a maximum of 250 mL of 0.9% NaCl over 3.5 to 4 hours on day 1 and day 14 Pediatric: see pediatric dosing for CKD 5HD (give dose every 4 weeks for 12 weeks)	
				Adult and pediatric CKD 5PD patients aged 2 years and older	Adult: Give 3 divided doses within 28 days as 2 infusions of 300 mg over 1.5 hours 14 days apart followed by one 400 mg infusion over 2.5 hours 14 days later. Dilute in a maximum of 250 mL of 0.9% NaCl Pediatric: see pediatric dosing for CKD 5HD (give dose every 4 weeks for 12 weeks)	
Sodium ferric gluconate	Ferrlecit	1	350,000	Adult and pediatric CKD 5HD patients aged 6 years and older receiving ESA therapy	Adult: 125 mg over 10 minutes or 125 mg in 100 mL of 0.9% NaCl over 60 minutes Pediatric: 1.5 mg/kg in 25 mL of 0.9% NaCl over 60 minutes; maximum dose 125 mg per dose	62.5–1000

(CKD, chronic kidney disease; ESA, erythropoiesis stimulating agent; ND-CKD, non-dialysis CKD patients.)

[a]Monitor for 30 minutes following an infusion; KDIGO guidelines recommend monitoring for 60 minutes (1B recommendation for iron dextran, 2C recommendation for non-dextran products).

[b]With the exception of ferric carboxymaltose and ferumoxytol, small doses (eg, 25–150 mg/wk) are generally used for maintenance regimens. Larger doses (eg, 1 g) should be administered in divided doses.

TABLE 74-4 Erythropoiesis-Stimulating Agents in Chronic Kidney Disease

Drug Name	Brand Name(s)	Starting Dose	Route of Administration	Half-Life (Hours)
Epoetin alfa	Epogen, Procrit	Adults: 50–100 units/kg three times per week Pediatrics: 50 units/kg three times per week	IV or SubQ	8.5 (IV) 24 (SubQ)
Darbepoetin alfa	Aranesp	Adults: ND-CKD: 0.45 mcg/kg once every 4 weeks CKD 5HD or CKD 5PD: 0.45 mcg/kg once per week or 0.75 mcg/kg every 2 weeks Pediatrics: 0.45 mcg/kg once weekly; may give 0.75 mcg/kg once every 2 weeks in ND-CKD patients	IV or SubQ	25 (IV) 48 (SubQ)
Methoxy PEG-epoetin beta	Mircera	All adult CKD patients: 0.6 mcg/kg every 2 weeks; Once Hb stabilizes, double the dose and administer monthly (eg, if administering 0.6 mcg/kg every 2 weeks, give 1.2 mcg/kg every month)	IV or SubQ	134 (IV) 139 (SubQ)

(CKD, chronic kidney disease; ND-CKD, nondialysis CKD patients; PEG, polyethylene glycol; SubQ, subcutaneous.)

TABLE 74-5 KDIGO Monitoring and Goals for Calcium, Phosphorus, and Parathyroid Hormone

Parameter	Chronic Kidney Disease Category[a]			
	3	4	5	ESRD
Corrected calcium[b]				
Monitoring frequency[c]	Every 6–12 months	Every 3–6 months	Every 1–3 months	Every 1–3 months
Goal	Maintain normal range [2D]	Maintain normal range [2D]	Maintain normal range [2D]	Maintain normal range [2D]
Phosphorus				
Monitoring frequency[c]	Every 6–12 months	Every 3–6 months	Every 1–3 months	Every 1–3 months
Goal	Maintain normal range [2C]	Maintain normal range [2C]	Maintain normal range [2C]	"Towards normal" [2C]
Intact PTH				
Monitoring frequency[c]	Based on baseline level and CKD progression	Every 6–12 months	Every 3–6 months	Every 3–6 months
Goal	Normal range[c]	Normal range[c]	Normal range[c]	2–9 times the upper normal limit [2C]

[a]Differences with Kidney Disease Outcome Quality Initiative (KDOQI) guidelines described in text.
[b]Corrected for albumin. Note: CMS finalized a rule that will use an uncorrected calcium level >10.2 mg/dL (>2.55 mmol/L) as a quality measure for the QIP starting in 2016.
[c]Not graded.

TABLE 74–6 Phosphate-Binding Agents for Treatment of Hyperphosphatemia in Chronic Kidney Disease Patients

Category	Drug	Brand Name	Compound Content	Starting Doses	Dose Titration[a]	Comments[b]
Calcium-based binders	Calcium acetate (25% elemental calcium)	PhosLo	25% elemental calcium (169 mg elemental calcium per 667 mg capsule)	1334 mg three times a day with meals	Increase or decrease by 667 mg per meal (169 mg elemental calcium)	Comparable efficacy to calcium carbonate with lower dose of elemental calcium. Approximately 45 mg phosphorus bound per 1 g calcium acetate. Evaluate for drug interactions with calcium
		Phoslyra	667 mg calcium acetate per 5 mL			
	Calcium carbonate[c]	Tums, Os-Cal, Caltrate	40% elemental calcium	0.5–1 g (elemental calcium) three times a day with meals	Increase or decrease by 500 mg per meal (200 mg elemental calcium)	Dissolution characteristics and phosphate binding may vary from product to product. Approximately 39 mg phosphorus bound per 1 g calcium carbonate. Evaluate for drug interactions with calcium
Iron-based binders	Ferric citrate	Auryxia	210 mg tablets (= 1 g ferric citrate)	420 mg ferric iron three times daily with meals	Increase or decrease dose by 1 or 2 tablets per meal	May increase serum iron, ferritin, and TSat. May cause discolored (dark) stools. Evaluate for drug interactions with iron
	Sucroferric oxyhydroxide	Velphoro	500 mg chewable tablets	500 mg three times daily with meals	Increase or decrease by 500 mg per day	May cause discolored (dark) stools. Evaluate for drug interactions with iron

Class	Generic	Brand	Formulation	Dose	Titration	Comments
Resin binders	Sevelamer carbonate	Renvela	800 mg tablet; 0.8 and 2.4 g powder for oral suspension	800–1600 mg three times a day with meals (once-daily dosing also effective)	Increase or decrease by 800 mg per meal	Also lowers low-density lipoprotein cholesterol; Consider in patients at risk for extraskeletal calcification; Risk of metabolic acidosis with sevelamer hydrochloride (less risk with carbonate formulation); May interact with cipro and mycophenolate mofetil
	Sevelamer hydrochloride	Renagel	400 & 800 mg caplets	800–1600 mg three times a day with meals	Increase or decrease by 800 mg per meal	
Other elemental binders	Lanthanum carbonate	Fosrenol	500, 750, and 1000 mg chewable tablets; 750 and 1000 mg oral powder	1500 mg daily in divided doses with meals	Increase or decrease by 750 mg/day	Potential for accumulation of lanthanum due to GI absorption (long-term consequences unknown); Evaluate for drug interactions (eg, cationic antacids, quinolone antibiotics)
	Aluminum hydroxide	AlternaGel	Content varies (range 100–600 mg/unit)	300–600 mg three times a day with meals	Not for long-term use requiring titration	Not a first-line agent; risk of aluminum toxicity; do not use concurrently with citrate-containing products; Reserve for short-term use (4 weeks) in patients with hyperphosphatemia not responding to other binders; Evaluate for drug interactions

(TSat, transferrin saturation.)
a Based on phosphorus levels, titrate every 2 to 3 weeks until phosphorus goal reached.
b GI side effects are possible with all agents (eg, nausea, vomiting, abdominal pain, diarrhea, or constipation).
c Multiple preparations available that are not listed.

TABLE 74-7	Vitamin D Agents					
Nutritional vitamin D						
Generic Name	Brand Name	Form of Vitamin D	Dosage Forms	Initial Dose[a]	Dosage Range	Frequency of Dosing
Ergocalciferol	Drisdol	D_2	po	Varies based on 25(OH) D levels	400–50,000 international units	Daily (doses of 400–2000 international units)
Cholecalciferol[b]	Generic	D_3	po			Weekly or monthly for higher doses (50,000 international units)
Vitamin D and Analogs						
Generic Name	Brand Name	Form of Vitamin D	Dosage Forms	Initial Dose[a,c]	Dosage Range	Dose Titration[d]
Calcitriol	Rocaltrol	D_3	po	0.25 mcg daily	0.25–5 mcg	Increase by 0.25 mcg/day at 4–8 week intervals
	Calcijex		IV	1–2 mcg three times per week	0.5–5 mcg	Increase by 0.5–1 mcg at 2 to 4 week intervals
Doxercalciferol[e]	Hectorol	D_2	po	ND-CKD: 1 mcg daily ESRD: 10 mcg three times per week	5–20 mcg	Increase by 0.5 mcg at 2-week intervals for daily dosing or by 2.5 mcg at 8-week intervals for three times per week dosing
			IV	ESRD: 4 mcg three times per week	2–8 mcg	Increase by 1–2 mcg at 8-week intervals
Paricalcitol	Zemplar	D_2	po	ND-CKD: 1 mcg daily or 2 mcg three times per week if PTH ≤500 pg/mL (ng/L; ≤54 pmol/L); 2 mcg daily or 4 mcg three times per week if PTH >500 pg/mL (ng/L; >54 pmol/L)	1–4 mcg	Increase by 1 mcg (for daily dosing) or 2 mcg (for three times per week dosing) at 2–4 week intervals
			IV	ESRD: 0.04–1 mcg three times per week	2.5–15 mcg	Increase by 2–4 mcg at 2–4 week intervals

(ESRD, end-stage renal disease; ND-CKD, non-dialysis chronic kidney disease; PTH, parathyroid hormone.)

[a]Dose ratios are as follows: 1:1 for IV paricalcitol to oral doxercalciferol, 1.5:1 for IV paricalcitol to IV doxercalciferol, and 1:1 for IV to oral calcitriol.

[b]Multiple preparations are available that are not listed.

[c]Daily orally dosing most common for non-hemodialysis CKD patients, IV dosing three times per week more often used in the hemodialysis population.

[d]Based on PTH, calcium and phosphorus levels. Decreases in dose are necessary if PTH is oversuppressed and/or if calcium and phosphorus are elevated.

[e]Prodrug that requires activation by the liver.

- KDOQI guidelines recommend that elemental calcium from calcium-containing binders should not exceed 1500 mg/day, and the total daily intake from all sources should not exceed 2000 mg. This may necessitate a combination of calcium- and non–calcium-containing products (eg, **sevelamer HCL** and **lanthanum carbonate**).
- Adverse effects of all phosphate binders are generally limited to GI effects, including constipation, diarrhea, nausea, vomiting, and abdominal pain. Risk of hypercalcemia may necessitate restriction of calcium-containing binder use and/or reduction in dietary intake. Aluminum and magnesium binders are not recommended for regular use in CKD because aluminum binders have been associated with CNS toxicity and the worsening of anemia, whereas magnesium binders may lead to hypermagnesemia and hyperkalemia.

VITAMIN D THERAPY

- Serum calcium and phosphorus should be within the normal range before initiation and during continued vitamin D therapy.
- **Calcitriol,** 1,25-dihydroxyvitamin D_3, directly suppresses PTH synthesis and secretion and upregulates vitamin D receptors. The dose depends on the stage of CKD (**Table 74–7**).
- The newer vitamin D analogues **paricalcitol** and **doxercalciferol** may be associated with less hypercalcemia and hyperphosphatemia. Observational studies show all-cause and cardiovascular survival benefit with these agents.

CALCIMIMETICS

- **Cinacalcet** reduces PTH secretion by increasing the sensitivity of the calcium-sensing receptor. The most common adverse events include nausea and vomiting.
- Cinacalcet lowers serum calcium and should not be started if the serum calcium is less than the lower limit of normal. The starting dose is 30 mg daily, which can be titrated to the desired PTH and calcium concentrations every 2 to 4 weeks to a maximum of 180 mg daily.

HYPERLIPIDEMIA

- CKD with or without nephrotic syndrome is frequently accompanied by abnormalities in lipoprotein metabolism. The KDIGO Lipid Guidelines recommend that a complete fasting lipid profile be performed in all adults with newly identified CKD.
- KDIGO Lipid Guidelines recommend:
  1. **Statin** treatment in adults age 18 to 49 years with CKD but not treated with chronic dialysis or kidney transplantation, who have one or more of the following: known coronary disease; diabetes mellitus; prior ischemic stroke; estimated 10-year incidence of coronary death or nonfatal MI greater than 10%.
  2. Statin or statin/**ezetimibe** combination in adults > 50 years with estimated GFR < 60 ml/min/1.73m^2 but not treated with chronic dialysis or kidney transplantation.
  3. Do not initiate statins or statin/ezetimibe combination therapy in adults with dialysis-dependent CKD. Continue these agents if patient is already taking them at the time of dialysis initiation.
- For more information on dyslipidemias, see Chap. 8.

See Chapter 44, Chronic Kidney Disease, authored by Joanna Q. Hudson and Lori D. Wazny, for a more detailed discussion of this topic.

Electrolyte Homeostasis

- *Fluid and electrolyte homeostasis* is maintained by feedback mechanisms, hormones, and many organ systems, and is necessary for the body's normal physiologic functions. Disorders of sodium and water, calcium, phosphorus, potassium, and magnesium homeostasis are addressed separately in this chapter.

DISORDERS OF SODIUM AND WATER HOMEOSTASIS

- Two-thirds (67%) of total body water (TBW) is distributed intracellularly (ICF), and one-third (33%) is contained in the extracellular space.
- Addition of an isotonic solution to the extracellular fluid (ECF) does not change intracellular volume. Adding a hypertonic solution to the ECF decreases cell volume, whereas adding a hypotonic solution increases it. Table 75–1 summarizes the composition of commonly used IV solutions and their respective distribution into the ECF and ICF compartments.
- Hypernatremia and hyponatremia can be associated with conditions of high, low, or normal ECF sodium and volume. Both conditions are most commonly the result of abnormalities of water metabolism.

HYPONATREMIA (SERUM SODIUM <135 mEq/L [<135 mmol/L])

Pathophysiology

- Results from an excess of extracellular water relative to sodium because of impaired water excretion.
- Causes of nonosmotic release of arginine vasopressin (AVP), commonly known as *antidiuretic hormone*, include hypovolemia; decreased effective circulating volume as seen in patients with congestive heart failure (CHF); nephrosis; cirrhosis; and syndrome of inappropriate antidiuretic hormone (SIADH).
- Depending on serum osmolality, hyponatremia is classified as isotonic, hypertonic, or hypotonic (Fig. 75–1).
- Hypotonic hyponatremia, the most common form of hyponatremia, can be further classified as hypovolemic, euvolemic, or hypervolemic.
- Hypovolemic hypotonic hyponatremia is associated with a loss of ECF volume and sodium, with the loss of more sodium than water. It is seen in patients with diarrhea or in those taking **thiazide diuretics**.
- Euvolemic hyponatremia is associated with a normal or slightly decreased ECF sodium content and increased TBW and ECF volume. It is most commonly the result of SIADH release.
- Hypervolemic hyponatremia is associated with an increase in ECF volume in conditions with impaired renal sodium and water excretion, such as cirrhosis, HF, and kidney failure.

Clinical Presentation

- Most patients with hyponatremia are asymptomatic.
- Presence and severity of symptoms are related to the magnitude and rapidity of onset of hyponatremia. Hyponatremia that is severe or develops rapidly is associated with symptoms that progress from nausea and malaise to headache and lethargy and, eventually, to seizures, coma, and death.
- Patients with hypovolemic hyponatremia present with neurologic symptoms and also decreased skin turgor, orthostatic hypotension, tachycardia, and dry mucous membranes.

TABLE 75–1 Composition of Common IV Solutions

Solution	Dextrose	[Na⁺] (mEq/L or mmol/L)	[Cl⁻] (mEq/L or mmol/L)	Osmolality (mOsm/kg or mmol/kg)	Tonicity	% ECF	% ICF	Free water (mL/1000 mL)
Dextrose 5% in water	5 g/dL (50 g/L)	0	0	253	Hypotonic	33	67	1000 mL
0.45% NaCl[a]	0	77	77	154	Hypotonic	67	33	500 mL
Lactated Ringer's	0	130	105	273	Isotonic	97	3	0 mL
0.9% NaCl[b]	0	154	154	308	Isotonic	100	0	0 mL
3% NaCl[c]	0	513	513	1026	Hypertonic	100	0	−2331 mL

(Cl⁻, chloride; ECF, extracellular fluid; ICF, intracellular fluid; IV, intravenous; Na⁺, sodium; NaCl, sodium chloride.)

[a]Also referred to as "half normal saline."

[b]Also referred to as "normal saline."

[c]This hypertonic solution will result in osmotic removal of water from the intracellular space.

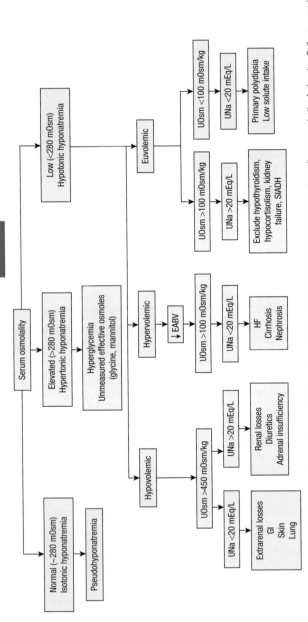

(HF, heart failure; EABV, effective arterial blood volume; GI, gastrointestinal; SIADH, syndrome of inappropriate antidiuretic hormone; UNA, urine sodium concentration [values in mEq/L are numerically equivalent to mmol/L]; Uosm, urine osmolality [values in mOsm/kg are numerically equivalent to mmol/kg].)

FIGURE 75–1. Diagnostic algorithm for the evaluation of hyponatremia.

Treatment

- <u>Goal of Treatment</u>: Resolve underlying cause of the sodium and ECF volume imbalance and safely correct the sodium and water derangements. Too rapid correction of serum sodium concentration can lead to an acute decrease in brain cell volume, contributing to the development of osmotic demyelination syndrome (ODS).

ACUTE OR SEVERELY SYMPTOMATIC HYPOTONIC HYPONATREMIA

- Symptomatic patients, regardless of fluid status, should initially be treated with either a 0.9% or 3% concentrated saline solution until symptoms resolve. Resolution of severe symptoms may require only a 5% increase in serum sodium; some clinicians suggest an initial target serum sodium of ~120 mEq/L (120 mmol/L).
- Treat SIADH with 3% saline plus, if the urine osmolality exceeds 300 mOsm/kg (300 mmol/kg), a loop diuretic (**furosemide**, 20–40 mg IV every 6 hours or **bumetanide**, 0.5–1 mg/dose every 2–3 hours for several doses). Consider a continuous infusion if intermittent doses are not sufficient to manage edema.
- Treat hypovolemic hypotonic hyponatremia with 0.9% saline.
- Treat hypervolemic hypotonic hyponatremia with 3% saline and prompt initiation of fluid restriction. Loop diuretic therapy will also likely be required to facilitate urinary excretion of free water.

NONEMERGENT HYPOTONIC HYPONATREMIA

- Treatment of SIADH involves water restriction and correction of the underlying cause; discontinue drugs that could be a contributing factor. Restrict water intake to approximately 1000 to 1200 mL/day. Treat patients unable to restrict water sufficiently with sodium chloride tablets and a loop diuretic or **demeclocycline** (300 mg orally two to four times daily; onset of action in 3–6 days).
- AVP antagonists or "vaptans" (eg, **conivaptan** [available IV only] and **tolvaptan** [15 mg orally daily]) can be used to treat SIADH as well as other causes of euvolemic and hypervolemic hypotonic hyponatremia that has been nonresponsive to other therapeutic interventions in patients with heart failure and SIADH. Tolvaptan labeling currently includes a warning to NOT use it in patients with liver disease, including cirrhosis. The vaptans have dramatic effects on water excretion and represent a breakthrough in the therapy of hyponatremia and disorders of fluid homeostasis.
- Treatment of asymptomatic hypervolemic hypotonic hyponatremia involves correction of the underlying cause and restriction of water intake to less than 1000 to 1200 mL/day. Dietary intake of sodium chloride should be restricted to 1000 to 2000 mg/day.

HYPERNATREMIA (SERUM SODIUM >145 mEq/L [>145 mmol/L])

Pathophysiology and Clinical Presentation

- Hypernatremia results from either water loss (eg, diabetes insipidus [DI]) or hypotonic fluids, or less commonly from hypertonic fluid administration or excess sodium ingestion.
- Symptoms are primarily caused by decreased neuronal cell volume and can include weakness, lethargy, restlessness, irritability, twitching, and confusion. Symptoms of a more rapidly developing hypernatremia include seizures, coma, and death.

Treatment

- Begin treatment of hypovolemic hypernatremia with 0.9% saline. After hemodynamic stability is restored and intravascular volume is replaced, replace free-water deficit with 5% dextrose or 0.45% saline solution.
- The correction rate should be approximately 1 mEq/L (1 mmol/L) per hour for hypernatremia that developed over a few hours and 0.5 mEq/L (0.5 mmol/L) per hour for hypernatremia that developed more slowly.

TABLE 75–2	Drugs Used to Manage Central and Nephrogenic Diabetes Insipidus	
Drug	**Indication**	**Dose**
Desmopressin acetate	Central and nephrogenic	5–20 mcg intranasally every 12–24 h
Chlorpropamide	Central	125–250 mg orally daily
Carbamazepine	Central	100–300 mg orally twice daily
Clofibrate	Central	500 mg orally 4 times daily
Hydrochlorothiazide	Central and nephrogenic	25 mg orally every 12–24 h
Amiloride	Lithium-related nephrogenic	5–10 mg orally daily
Indomethacin	Central and nephrogenic	50 mg orally every 8–12 h

- Treat central DI with intranasal **desmopressin**, beginning with 10 mcg once daily. Titrate to 20 mcg twice daily based on serum sodium concentration. Oral tablets are available; poor bioavailability contributes to unpredictable response when transitioning between dosage forms.
- Treat nephrogenic DI by decreasing ECF volume with a thiazide diuretic and dietary sodium restriction (2000 mg/day), which can decrease urine volume by as much as 50%. Other treatment options include drugs with antidiuretic properties (Table 75–2).
- Treat sodium overload with loop diuretics (**furosemide**, 20–40 mg IV every 6 hour) and 5% dextrose at a rate that decreases serum sodium by approximately 0.5 mEq/L (0.5 mmol/L) per hour or, if hypernatremia developed rapidly, 1 mEq/L (1 mmol/L) per hour.

EDEMA

Pathophysiology and Clinical Presentation

- Edema, defined as a clinically detectable increase in interstitial fluid volume, develops when excess sodium is retained either as a primary defect in renal sodium excretion or as a response to a decrease in the effective circulating volume despite an already expanded or normal ECF volume.
- Edema occurs in patients with decreased myocardial contractility, nephrotic syndrome, or cirrhosis.
- Edema is initially detected in the feet or pretibial area in ambulatory patients and in the presacral area in bed-bound individuals, and is described as "pitting" when a depression caused by briefly exerting pressure over a bony prominence does not rapidly refill.

Treatment

- Diuretics are the primary pharmacologic therapy for edema. Loop diuretics are the most potent, followed by thiazide diuretics and then potassium-sparing diuretics.
- Severe pulmonary edema requires immediate pharmacologic treatment because it is life threatening. Other forms of edema can be treated gradually with, in addition to diuretic therapy, sodium and water restriction and treatment of the underlying disease state.

DISORDERS OF CALCIUM HOMEOSTASIS

- ECF calcium is moderately bound to plasma proteins (40%), primarily albumin. Ionized or free calcium is the physiologically active form that is homeostatically regulated.
- Each 1 g/dL (10 g/L) drop in serum albumin concentration less than 4 g/dL (40 g/L) decreases total serum calcium concentration by 0.8 mg/dL (0.20 mmol/L).

HYPERCALCEMIA (TOTAL SERUM CALCIUM >10.5 mg/dL [>2.62 mmol/L])

Pathophysiology and Clinical Presentation

- Cancer and hyperparathyroidism are the most common causes of hypercalcemia. Primary mechanisms include increased bone resorption, increased GI absorption, and increased tubular reabsorption by the kidneys.
- Clinical presentation depends on the degree of hypercalcemia and rate of onset. Mild to moderate hypercalcemia (serum calcium concentration <13 mg/dL [<3.25 mmol/L] or ionized calcium concentration <6 mg/dL [<1.50 mmol/L]) can be asymptomatic.
- Hypercalcemia of malignancy develops quickly and is associated with anorexia, nausea and vomiting, constipation, polyuria, polydipsia, and nocturia. Hypercalcemic crisis is characterized by acute elevation of serum calcium to greater than 15 mg/dL (>3.75 mmol/L), acute renal insufficiency, and obtundation. Untreated hypercalcemic crisis can progress to oliguric renal failure, coma, and life-threatening ventricular arrhythmias.
- Chronic hypercalcemia (ie, hyperparathyroidism) is associated with metastatic calcification, nephrolithiasis, and chronic renal insufficiency.
- Electrocardiographic (ECG) changes include shortening of the QT interval and coving of the ST-T wave.

Treatment

- Treatment approach depends on the degree of hypercalcemia, acuity of onset, and presence of symptoms requiring emergent treatment (Fig. 75–2).
- Management of asymptomatic, mild to moderate hypercalcemia begins with attention to the underlying condition and correction of fluid and electrolyte abnormalities.
- Hypercalcemic crisis and acute symptomatic hypercalcemia are medical emergencies requiring immediate treatment. Rehydration with normal saline followed by loop diuretics can be used in patients with normal to moderately impaired renal function. Initiate treatment with **calcitonin** in patients in whom saline hydration is contraindicated (Table 75–3).
- Rehydration with saline and **furosemide** administration may result in normalization of total calcium within 24 to 48 hours.
- **Bisphosphonates** (eg, **pamidronate** and **zoledronic acid**) are indicated for hypercalcemia of malignancy. Total serum calcium decline begins within 2 days and nadirs in 7 days. Duration of normocalcemia varies but usually does not exceed 2 to 3 weeks, depending on treatment response of underlying malignancy.
- **Denosumab** is a monoclonal antibody approved for treatment of hypercalcemia of malignancy. Patients refractory to bisphosphonates were shown to respond to denosumab within 10 days of receiving denosumab on days 1 and 8.
- **Prednisone** or an equivalent agent is usually effective by reducing GI calcium absorption when hypercalcemia results from multiple myeloma, leukemia, lymphoma, sarcoidosis, and hypervitaminoses A and D. Onset of action is relatively slow.
- **Cinacalcet** has been used for the treatment of hypercalcemia secondary to parathyroid carcinoma.

HYPOCALCEMIA (TOTAL SERUM CALCIUM <8.5 mg/dL [<2.13 mmol/L])

Pathophysiology

- Hypocalcemia results from altered effects of parathyroid hormone and vitamin D on the bone, gut, and kidney. Primary causes are postoperative hypoparathyroidism and vitamin D deficiency.
- Hypomagnesemia can be associated with severe symptomatic hypocalcemia that is unresponsive to calcium replacement therapy. Calcium normalization is dependent on magnesium replacement.

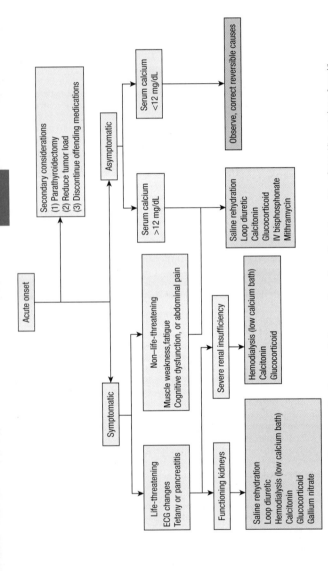

FIGURE 75–2. Pharmacotherapeutic options for the acutely hypercalcemic patient. Serum calcium of 12 mg/dL is equivalent to 3 mmol/L.

TABLE 75–3 Drug Dosing Table for Hypercalcemia

Drug/Brand Name	Starting Dosage	Time Frame to Initial Response	Monitoring and Special Population Considerations
0.9% saline ± electrolytes	200–300 mL/h	24–48 hours	Electrolyte abnormalities; fluid overload CI in renal insufficiency; congestive heart failure
Loop diuretics Furosemide/Lasix® Bumetandide/Bumex® Torsemide/Demadex®	40–80 mg IV q 1–4 h of furosemide or equivalent	N/A	Electrolyte abnormalities (potassium and magnesium) CI in patients with allergy to sulfas (use ethacrynic acid)
Calcitonin/Miacalcin®	4 units/kg q 12 h SC/IM 10–12 units/h IV	1–2 hours	Facial flushing, nausea/vomiting, allergic reaction, CI in patients with allergy to calcitonin
Pamidronate/Aredia®	30–90 mg IV over 2–24 hours	2 days	Fever, fatigue, skeletal pain, CI in renal insufficiency
Zoledronate/Zometa®	4–8 mg IV over 15 minutes	1–2 days	Fever, fatigue, skeletal pain, CI in renal insufficiency
Glucocorticoids	40–60 mg oral prednisone equivalents daily	3–5 days	Diabetes; osteoporosis; infection, CI in patients with serious infections; hypersensitivity

(CI, contraindicated; SC, subcutaneous.)

Clinical Presentation

- Clinical manifestations are variable and depend on the onset of hypocalcemia. Tetany is the hallmark sign of acute hypocalcemia, which manifests as paresthesias around the mouth and in the extremities; muscle spasms and cramps; carpopedal spasms; and, rarely, laryngospasm and bronchospasm.
- Cardiovascular manifestations result in ECG changes characterized by a prolonged QT interval and symptoms of decreased myocardial contractility often associated with CHF.

Treatment

- Acute, symptomatic hypocalcemia requires IV administration of soluble calcium salts (**Fig. 75–3**). Initially, 100 to 300 mg of elemental calcium (eg, 1 g **calcium chloride**, 2–3 g **calcium gluconate**) should be given IV over 10 to 30 minutes (≤60 mg of elemental calcium per minute).
- The initial bolus dose is effective for only 1 to 2 hours and should be followed by a continuous infusion of elemental calcium (0.5–2 mg/kg/h) for 2 to 4 hours and then by a maintenance dose (0.3–0.5 mg/kg/h).
- **Calcium gluconate** is preferred over **calcium chloride** for peripheral administration because the latter is more irritating to veins.
- After acute hypocalcemia is corrected, the underlying cause and other electrolyte problems should be corrected. Magnesium supplementation is indicated for hypomagnesemia.
- Oral calcium supplementation (eg, 1–3 g/day of elemental calcium initially, then 2–8 g/day in divided doses) is indicated for chronic hypocalcemia due to hypoparathyroidism and vitamin D deficiency. If serum calcium does not normalize, add a vitamin D preparation.

DISORDERS OF PHOSPHORUS HOMEOSTASIS

HYPERPHOSPHATEMIA (SERUM PHOSPHORUS >4.5 mg/dL [>1.45 mmol/L])

Pathophysiology

- Most commonly caused by decreased phosphorus excretion, secondary to decreased glomerular filtration rate (GFR).
- Intracellular phosphate release can occur with rhabdomyolysis, hemolysis, and tumor lysis syndrome, a complication of chemotherapy associated with massive cell lysis with highest incidence in patients with acute leukemia and lymphoma.

Clinical Presentation

- Acute symptoms include gastrointestinal (GI) disturbances, lethargy, obstruction of the urinary tract, and, rarely, seizures. Calcium phosphate crystals are likely to form when the product of the serum calcium and phosphate concentrations exceeds 50 to 60 mg^2/dL^2 (4–4.8 mmol^2/L^2).
- The major effect is related to the development of hypocalcemia and damage resulting from calcium phosphate precipitation into soft tissues, intrarenal calcification, nephrolithiasis, or obstructive uropathy.
- For more information on hyperphosphatemia and renal failure, see Chap. 74.

Treatment

- The most effective way to treat nonemergent hyperphosphatemia is to decrease phosphate absorption from the GI tract with phosphate binders (see Chap. 74, **Table 74–6**).
- Severe symptomatic hyperphosphatemia manifesting as hypocalcemia and tetany is treated by the IV administration of calcium salts.

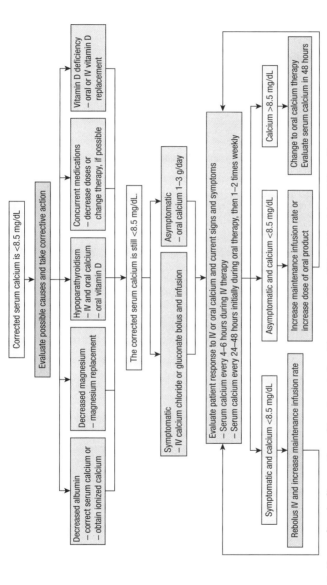

FIGURE 75-3. Hypocalcemia diagnostic and treatment algorithm. Serum calcium of 8.5 mg/dL is equivalent to 2.13 mmol/L.

HYPOPHOSPHATEMIA (SERUM PHOSPHORUS <2 mg/dL [<0.65 mmol/L])

Pathophysiology

- Hypophosphatemia results from decreased GI absorption, reduced tubular reabsorption, or extracellular to intracellular redistribution.
- Hypophosphatemia is associated with chronic alcoholism, parenteral nutrition with inadequate phosphate supplementation, chronic ingestion of antacids, diabetic keto-acidosis, and prolonged hyperventilation.

Clinical Presentation

- Severe hypophosphatemia (serum phosphorus <1 mg/dL [<0.32 mmol/L]) has diverse clinical manifestations that affect many organ systems, including the following:
  - ✓ Neurologic manifestations: Progressive syndrome of irritability, apprehension, weakness, numbness, paresthesias, dysarthria, confusion, obtundation, seizures, and coma.
  - ✓ Skeletal muscle dysfunction: Myalgia, bone pain, weakness, and potentially fatal rhabdomyolysis.
  - ✓ Respiratory muscle weakness and diaphragmatic contractile dysfunction resulting in acute respiratory failure.
  - ✓ Congestive cardiomyopathy, arrhythmias, hemolysis, and increased risk of infection can also occur.
- Chronic hypophosphatemia can cause osteopenia and osteomalacia because of enhanced osteoclastic resorption of bone.

Treatment

- Severe (<1 mg/dL; <0.32 mmol/L) or symptomatic hypophosphatemia should be treated with IV phosphorus replacement. The infusion of 15 mmol of phosphorus in 250 mL of IV fluid over 3 hours is a safe and effective treatment, but the recommended dosage of IV phosphorus (0.08–0.64 mmol/kg) and infusion recommendations (over 4–12 hours) are highly variable.
- Asymptomatic patients or those who exhibit mild to moderate hypophosphatemia can be treated with oral phosphorus supplementation in doses of 1.5 to 2 g (50–60 mmol) daily in divided doses, with the goal of correcting serum phosphorus concentration in 7 to 10 days (Table 75–4).
- Monitor patients with frequent serum phosphorus and calcium determinations, especially if phosphorus is given IV or if renal dysfunction is present.
- Add phosphorus (12–15 mmol/L) routinely to hyperalimentation solutions to prevent hypophosphatemia.

DISORDERS OF POTASSIUM HOMEOSTASIS

HYPOKALEMIA (SERUM POTASSIUM <3.5 mEq/L [<3.5 mmol/L])

Pathophysiology

- Results from a total body potassium deficit or shifting of serum potassium into the intracellular compartment.
- Many drugs can cause hypokalemia (Table 75–5), and it is most commonly seen with use of loop and thiazide diuretics. Other causes of hypokalemia include diarrhea, vomiting, and hypomagnesemia.

Clinical Presentation

- Signs and symptoms are nonspecific and variable and depend on the degree of hypo-kalemia and rapidity of onset. Mild hypokalemia is often asymptomatic.
- Cardiovascular manifestations cardiac arrhythmias (eg, heart block, atrial flutter, par-oxysmal atrial tachycardia, ventricular fibrillation, and digitalis-induced arrhythmias). In severe hypokalemia (serum concentration <2.5 mEq/L; <2.5 mmol/L), ECG changes include ST-segment depression or flattening, T-wave inversion, and U-wave elevation.

TABLE 75–4	Phosphorus Replacement Therapy	
Product (Salt)	**Phosphate Content**	**Initial Dosing Based on Serum K**
Oral Therapy (Potassium Phosphate + Sodium Phosphate)		
Neutra-Phos® (7 mEq/packet each of Na and K)	250 mg (8 mmol)/packet	One packet three times daily[a]
Neutra-Phos-K® (14.25 mEq/packet of K)	250 mg (8 mmol)/packet	Serum K >5.5 mEq/L (>5.5 mmol/L); not recommended
K-Phos Neutral® (13 mEq/tablet Na and 1.1 mEq/tablet K)	250 mg (8 mmol)/tablet	Serum K >5.5 mEq/L (>5.5 mmol/L) one tablet three times daily
Uro-KP-Neutral® (10.9 mEq/tablet Na and 1.27 mEq/tablet K)	250 mg (8 mmol)/tablet	Serum K >5.5 mEq/L (>5.5 mmol/L) one tablet three times daily
Fleets Phospho-soda® (sodium phosphate solution)	4 mmol/mL	Serum K >5.5 mEq/L (>5.5 mmol/L) 2 mL three times daily
IV Therapy		
Sodium PO_4 (4 mEq/mL Na)	3 mmol/mL	Serum K >3.5 mEq/L (>3.5 mmol/L) 15–30 mmol IVPB
Potassium PO_4 (4.4 mEq/mL K)	3 mmol/mL	Serum K <3.5 mEq/L (< 3.5 mmol/L) 15–30 mmol IVPB

(IVPB, IV piggyback; K, potassium; Na, sodium; PO_4, phosphate.)
[a]Monitor serum K closely.

TABLE 75–5	Mechanism of Drug-Induced Hypokalemia	
Transcellular Shift	**Enhanced Renal Excretion**	**Enhanced Fecal Elimination**
β_2-Receptor agonists	Diuretics	Laxatives
Epinephrine	Acetazolamide	Sodium polystyrene sulfonate
Albuterol	Thiazides	Phenolphthalein
Terbutaline	Indapamide	Sorbitol
Fomoterol	Metolazone	Patiromer
Salmeterol	Furosemide	
Isoproterenol	Torsemide	
Ephedrine	Bumetanide	
Pseudoephedrine	Ethacrynic acid	
Tocolytic agents	High-dose penicillins	
Ritodrine	Nafcillin	
Nylidrin	Ampicillin	
Theophylline	Penicillin	
Levothyroxine	Mineralocorticoids	
Decongestants	Miscellaneous	
Caffeine	Aminoglycosides	
Insulin overdose	Amphotericin B	
Verapamil overdose	Cisplatin	
Barium overdose		

- Moderate hypokalemia is associated with muscle weakness, cramping, malaise, and myalgias.

Treatment

- In general, every 1 mEq/L (1 mmol/L) decrease in potassium below 3.5 mEq/L (3.5 mmol/L) corresponds with a total body deficit of 100 to 400 mEq (100–400 mmol). To correct mild deficits, patients receiving chronic loop or thiazide diuretics generally need 40 to 100 mEq (40–100 mmol) of potassium.
- Whenever possible, potassium supplementation should be administered by mouth. Of the available salts, potassium chloride is most commonly used because it is the most effective for common causes of potassium depletion, use of diuretics and with diarrhea.
- Limit IV administration to severe hypokalemia, signs and symptoms of hypokalemia, or inability to tolerate oral therapy. IV supplementation is more dangerous than oral therapy due to the potential for hyperkalemia, phlebitis, and pain at the infusion site. Potassium should be administered in saline because dextrose can stimulate insulin secretion and worsen intracellular shifting of potassium. Generally, 10 to 20 mEq (10–20 mmol) of potassium is diluted in 100 mL of 0.9% saline and administered through a peripheral vein over 1 hour. ECG monitoring to detect cardiac changes is recommended when infusion rates exceed 10 mEq/h (10 mmol/h).
- Evaluate serum potassium following infusion of each 30 to 40 mEq (30–40 mmol) to guide further potassium supplementation.

HYPERKALEMIA (SERUM POTASSIUM >5 mEq/L [>5 mmol/L])

Pathophysiology

- Hyperkalemia develops when potassium intake exceeds excretion or when the transcellular distribution of potassium is disturbed.
- Primary causes of true hyperkalemia include increased potassium intake, decreased potassium excretion, tubular unresponsiveness to aldosterone, and redistribution of potassium to the extracellular space.

Clinical Presentation

- Hyperkalemia is frequently asymptomatic; patients might complain of heart palpitations or skipped heartbeats.
- The earliest ECG change (serum potassium 5.5–6 mEq/L; 5.5–6 mmol/L) is peaked T waves. The sequence of changes with further increases in serum potassium concentration is widening of the PR interval, loss of the P wave, widening of the QRS complex, and merging of the QRS complex with the T wave resulting in a sine-wave pattern.

Treatment

- Treatment depends on the desired rapidity and degree of lowering and the patient's clinical condition (Fig. 75–4, Table 75–6). Dialysis is the most rapid way to lower serum potassium concentration.
- Calcium administration rapidly reverses ECG manifestations and arrhythmias, but it does not lower serum potassium concentrations. Calcium is short acting and therefore must be repeated if signs or symptoms recur.
- Rapid correction of hyperkalemia requires administration of drugs that shift potassium intracellularly (eg, insulin and dextrose, sodium bicarbonate, or albuterol).
- **Sodium polystyrene sulfonate** is a cation-exchange resin suitable for asymptomatic patients with mild to moderate hyperkalemia. Each gram of resin exchanges 1 mEq (1 mmol) of sodium for 1 mEq (1 mmol) of potassium. The sorbitol component promotes excretion of exchanged potassium by inducing diarrhea. The oral route is better tolerated and more effective than the rectal route.

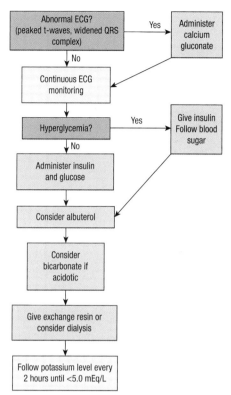

FIGURE 75–4. Treatment approach for hyperkalemia. Serum potassium of 5.5 mEq/L is equivalent to 5.5 mmol/L.

DISORDERS OF MAGNESIUM HOMEOSTASIS

HYPOMAGNESEMIA (SERUM MAGNESIUM <1.4 mEq/L [<1.7 mg/dL; <0.70 mmol/L])

Pathophysiology

- Hypomagnesemia is usually associated with disorders of the intestinal tract or kidneys. Drugs (eg, **aminoglycosides**, **amphotericin B**, **cyclosporine**, diuretics, **digitalis**, and **cisplatin**) or conditions that interfere with intestinal absorption or increase renal excretion of magnesium can cause hypomagnesemia.
- Commonly associated with alcoholism.

Clinical Presentation

- Although typically asymptomatic, the dominant organ systems involved are the neuromuscular and cardiovascular systems. Symptoms include heart palpitations, tetany, twitching, and generalized convulsions.
- Ventricular arrhythmias are the most important and potentially life-threatening cardiovascular effect.
- ECG changes include widened QRS complexes and peaked T waves in mild deficiency. Prolonged PR intervals, progressive widening of the QRS complexes, and flattening of T waves occur in moderate to severe deficiency.

TABLE 75–6	Therapeutic Alternatives for the Management of Hyperkalemia					
Medication	Dose	Route of Administration	Onset/Duration of Action	Acuity	Mechanism of Action	Expected Result
Calcium	1 g	IV over 5–10 minutes	1–2 min/10–30 min	Acute	Raises cardiac threshold potential	Reverses electrocardiographic effects
Furosemide	20–40 mg	IV	5–15 min/4–6 h	Acute	Inhibits renal Na^+ reabsorption	Increased urinary K^+ loss
Regular insulin	5–10 units	IV or SC	30 min/2–6 h	Acute	Stimulates intracellular K^+ uptake	Intracellular K^+ redistribution
Dextrose 10%	1000 mL (100 g)	IV over 1–2 hours	30 min/2–6 h	Acute	Stimulates insulin release	Intracellular K^+ redistribution
Dextrose 50%	50 mL (25 g)	IV over 5 minutes	30 min/2–6 h	Acute	Stimulates insulin release	Intracellular K^+ redistribution
Sodium bicarbonate	50–100 mEq (50–100 mmol)	IV over 2–5 minutes	30 min/2–6 h	Acute	Raises serum pH	Intracellular K^+ redistribution
Albuterol	10–20 mg	Nebulized over 10 minutes	30 min/1–2 h	Acute	Stimulates intracellular K^+ uptake	Intracellular K^+ redistribution
Hemodialysis	4 hours	N/A	Immediate/variable	Acute	Removal from serum	Increased K^+ elimination
Sodium polystyrene sulfonate	15–60 g	Oral or rectal	1 h/variable	Nonacute	Resin exchanges Na^+ for K^+	Increased K^+ elimination
Patiromer	8.4–25.2 g	Oral	Hours/variable	Nonacute	Resin exchanges Ca^{++} for K^+	Increased K^+ elimination

- Many electrolyte disturbances occur with hypomagnesemia, including hypokalemia and hypocalcemia.

Treatment

- The severity of magnesium depletion and the presence of symptoms dictate the route of magnesium supplementation. Intramuscular magnesium is painful and should be reserved for patients with severe hypomagnesemia and limited venous access. IV bolus injection is associated with flushing, sweating, and a sensation of warmth.
- Oral magnesium supplementation is appropriate when the serum magnesium concentration is greater than 1 mEq/L (1.2 mg/dL [0.5 mmol/L]). Sustained release products are preferred due to improved patient compliance and less GI side effects (eg, diarrhea).
- Administer IV magnesium if serum concentrations are less than 1 mEq/L (<1.2 mg/dL [<0.5 mmol/L]) or if signs and symptoms are present regardless of serum concentration. Infuse 4 to 6 g of magnesium over 12 to 24 hours and repeat as needed to maintain serum concentrations above 1 mEq/L (1.2 mg/dL [0.5 mmol/L]). Continue until signs and symptoms resolve. Reduce magnesium dose by 25% to 50% with renal insufficiency.

HYPERMAGNESEMIA (SERUM MAGNESIUM >2 mEq/L [>2.4 mg/dL; >1 mmol/L])

Pathophysiology

- Magnesium concentrations steadily increase as the GFR decreases below 30 mL/min/1.73 m^2 and is generally associated with advanced CKD.
- Other causes include magnesium-containing antacids in patients with renal insufficiency, enteral or parenteral nutrition in patients with multiorgan system failure, magnesium for treatment of eclampsia, lithium therapy, hypothyroidism, and Addison disease.

Clinical Presentation

- Symptoms are rare when the serum magnesium concentration is less than 4 mEq/L (< 4.9 mg/dL [<2 mmol/L]).
- The sequence of neuromuscular signs as serum magnesium increases from 5 to 12 mEq/L (6.1–14.7 mg/dL [2.5–6 mmol/L]) is sedation, hypotonia, hyporeflexia, somnolence, coma, muscular paralysis, and, ultimately, respiratory depression.
- The sequence of cardiovascular signs as serum magnesium increases from 3 to 15 mEq/L (3.7–18.4 mg/dL [1.5–7.5 mmol/L]) is hypotension, cutaneous vasodilation, QT-interval prolongation, bradycardia, primary heart block, nodal rhythms, bundle branch block, QRS- and then PR-interval prolongation, complete heart block, and asystole.

Treatment

- IV calcium (100–200 mg of elemental calcium; eg, calcium gluconate 2 g IV) is indicated to antagonize the neuromuscular and cardiovascular effects of magnesium. Doses should be repeated as often as hourly in life-threatening situations.
- Forced diuresis with 0.45% NaCl and loop diuretics (eg, **furosemide**, 40 mg IV) can promote magnesium elimination in patients with normal renal function or stage 1, 2, or 3 CKD. In dialysis patients, change to a magnesium-free dialysate.

EVALUATION OF THERAPEUTIC OUTCOMES

- The primary end point for monitoring treatment of fluid and electrolyte disorders is the correction of the abnormal serum electrolyte. In general, monitoring is initially performed at frequent intervals and, as homeostasis is restored, subsequently performed at less frequent intervals.

• Monitor all electrolytes as individual electrolyte abnormalities typically coexist with another abnormality (eg, hypomagnesemia with hypokalemia and hypocalcemia, or hyperphosphatemia with hypocalcemia).
• Monitor patients for resolution of clinical manifestations of electrolyte disturbances and for treatment-related complications.

See Chapter 49, Disorders of Sodium and Water Homeostasis, authored by Katherine H. Chessman and Jason Haney; Chapter 50, Disorders of Calcium and Phosphorus Homeostasis, authored by Amy Barton Pai; and Chapter 51, Disorders of Potassium and Magnesium Homeostasis, authored by Rachel W. Flurie and Donald F. Brophy, for a more detailed discussion of this topic.

CHAPTER

76 Allergic Rhinitis

- *Allergic rhinitis* involves inflammation of nasal mucous membranes in sensitized individuals when inhaled allergenic particles contact mucous membranes and elicit a response mediated by immunoglobulin E (IgE). There are two types: seasonal and persistent (formerly called "perennial") allergic rhinitis.

PATHOPHYSIOLOGY

- Airborne allergens enter the nose during inhalation and are processed by lymphocytes, which produce antigen-specific IgE, sensitizing genetically predisposed hosts to those agents. On nasal reexposure, IgE bound to mast cells interacts with airborne allergens, triggering release of inflammatory mediators.
- An immediate reaction occurs within seconds to minutes, resulting in rapid release of preformed and newly generated mediators from the arachidonic acid cascade. Mediators of immediate hypersensitivity include histamine, leukotrienes, prostaglandin, tryptase, and kinins. These mediators cause vasodilation, increased vascular permeability, and production of nasal secretions. Histamine produces rhinorrhea, itching, sneezing, and nasal obstruction.
- A late-phase reaction may occur 4 to 8 hours after initial allergen exposure due to cytokine release from mast cells and thymus-derived helper lymphocytes. This inflammatory response causes persistent chronic symptoms, including nasal congestion.

CLINICAL PRESENTATION

- Seasonal (hay fever) allergic rhinitis occurs in response to specific allergens (pollen from trees, grasses, and weeds) present at predictable times of the year (spring and/or fall) and typically causes more acute symptoms.
- Persistent allergic rhinitis occurs year-round in response to nonseasonal allergens (eg, dust mites, animal dander, and molds) and usually causes more subtle, chronic symptoms.
- Many patients have a combination of both types, with symptoms year-round and seasonal exacerbations.
- Symptoms include clear rhinorrhea, sneezing, nasal congestion, postnasal drip, allergic conjunctivitis, and pruritic eyes, ears, or nose.
- In children, physical examination may reveal dark circles under the eyes (allergic shiners), a transverse nasal crease caused by repeated rubbing of the nose, adenoidal breathing, edematous nasal turbinates coated with clear secretions, tearing, and periorbital swelling.
- Patients may complain of loss of smell or taste, with sinusitis or polyps the underlying cause in many cases. Postnasal drip with cough or hoarseness can be bothersome.
- Untreated rhinitis symptoms may lead to insomnia, malaise, fatigue, and poor work or school performance.
- Allergic rhinitis is associated with asthma; 10% to 40% of allergic rhinitis patients have asthma.
- Complications include recurrent and chronic sinusitis and epistaxis.

DIAGNOSIS

- Medical history includes careful description of symptoms, environmental factors and exposures, results of previous therapy, use of medications, previous nasal injury or surgery, and family history.
- Microscopic examination of nasal scrapings typically reveals numerous eosinophils. Peripheral blood eosinophil count may be elevated, but it is nonspecific and has limited usefulness.
- Allergy testing can help determine whether rhinitis is caused by immune response to allergens. Immediate-type hypersensitivity skin tests are commonly used. Percutaneous testing is safer and more generally accepted than intradermal testing, which is usually reserved for patients requiring confirmation. The radioallergosorbent test (RAST) can detect IgE antibodies in the blood that are specific for a given antigen, but it is less sensitive than percutaneous tests.

TREATMENT

- <u>Goals of Treatment</u>: Minimize or prevent symptoms, prevent long-term complications, minimize or avoid medication side effects, provide economical therapy, and maintain normal lifestyle.
- See Fig. 76–1 for a treatment algorithm for allergic rhinitis.

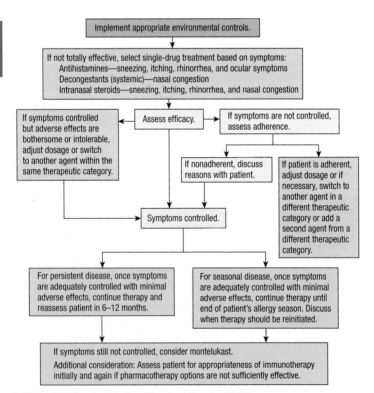

FIGURE 76–1. Treatment algorithm for allergic rhinitis.

NONPHARMACOLOGIC THERAPY

- Avoiding offending allergens is important but difficult to accomplish, especially for perennial allergens. Mold growth can be reduced by keeping household humidity less than 50% and removing obvious growth with bleach or disinfectant.
- Patients sensitive to animals benefit most by removing pets from the home, if feasible. Reducing exposure to dust mites by encasing bedding with impermeable covers and washing bed linens in hot water has little benefit, except perhaps in children.
- Steps to prevent poor air quality in homes include avoiding wall-to-wall carpeting, using moisture control to prevent mold accumulation, and controlling sources of pollution such as cigarette smoke.
- Patients with seasonal allergic rhinitis should keep windows closed and minimize time spent outdoors during pollen seasons. Filter masks can be worn while gardening or mowing the lawn.

PHARMACOLOGIC THERAPY

Antihistamines

- Histamine H_1-receptor antagonists bind to H_1 receptors without activating them, preventing histamine binding and action. They are effective in preventing the histamine response but not in reversing its effects after they have occurred.
- Oral antihistamines are divided into two categories: (1) nonselective (first-generation or sedating antihistamines) and (2) peripherally selective (second-generation or nonsedating antihistamines). However, individual agents should be judged on their specific sedating effects because variation exists among agents within these categories (Table 76–1). The sedating effect may depend on ability to cross the blood–brain barrier. Most older antihistamines are lipid soluble and cross this barrier easily. Peripherally selective agents have little or no central or autonomic nervous system effects.
- Symptom relief is caused in part by an anticholinergic drying effect that reduces nasal, salivary, and lacrimal gland hypersecretion. Antihistamines antagonize increased capillary permeability, wheal-and-flare formation, and itching.
- Drowsiness is the most frequent side effect, and it can interfere with driving ability or adequate functioning. Sedative effects can be beneficial in patients who have difficulty sleeping because of rhinitis symptoms.
- Adverse anticholinergic such as dry mouth, difficulty in voiding urine, constipation, and cardiovascular effects may occur (see Table 76–1). Antihistamines should be used with caution in patients predisposed to urinary retention and in those with increased intraocular pressure, hyperthyroidism, and cardiovascular disease.
- Other side effects include loss of appetite, nausea, vomiting, and epigastric distress. Taking medication with meals or a full glass of water may prevent gastrointestinal (GI) side effects.
- Table 76–2 lists recommended doses of oral agents. Antihistamines are more effective when taken 1 to 2 hours before anticipated exposure to the offending allergen.
- **Azelastine** (Astelin) is an intranasal antihistamine that rapidly relieves symptoms of seasonal allergic rhinitis. However, caution patients about potential for drowsiness because systemic availability is approximately 40%. Patients may also experience drying effects, headache, and diminished effectiveness over time. **Olopatadine** (Patanase) is another intranasal antihistamine that may cause less drowsiness because it is a selective H_1-receptor antagonist.
- **Levocabastine** (Livostin), **olopatadine** (Patanol), and **bepotastine** (Bepreve) are ophthalmic antihistamines that can be used for conjunctivitis associated with allergic rhinitis. Systemic antihistamines are usually also effective for allergic conjunctivitis. Ophthalmic agents are a useful addition to nasal corticosteroids for ocular symptoms. They are also useful for patients whose only symptoms involve the eyes or for patients whose ocular symptoms persist on oral antihistamines.

Decongestants

- Topical and systemic decongestants are sympathomimetic agents that act on adrenergic receptors in nasal mucosa to produce vasoconstriction, shrink swollen mucosa,

TABLE 76-1	Relative Adverse-Effect Profiles of Antihistamines	
Medications	**Relative Sedative Effects**	**Relative Anticholinergic Effects**
Alkylamine class, nonselective		
Brompheniramine maleate	Low	Moderate
Chlorpheniramine maleate	Low	Moderate
Dexchlorpheniramine maleate	Low	Moderate
Ethanolamine class, nonselective		
Carbinoxamine maleate	High	High
Clemastine fumarate	Moderate	High
Diphenhydramine hydrochloride	High	High
Phenothiazine class, nonselective		
Promethazine hydrochloride	High	High
Piperidine class, nonselective		
Cyproheptadine hydrochloride	Low	Moderate
Phthalazinone class, peripherally selective		
Azelastine (nasal only)	Low to none	Low to none
Bepotastine (ophthalmic only)	Low to none	Low to none
Piperazine class, peripherally selective		
Cetirizine	Low to moderate	Low to none
Levocetirizine	Low to moderate	Low to none
Piperidine class, peripherally selective		
Desloratadine	Low to none	Low to none
Fexofenadine	Low to none	Low to none
Loratadine	Low to none	Low to none
Olopatadine (nasal only)	Low to none	Low to none

and improve ventilation. Decongestants work well in combination with antihistamines when nasal congestion is part of the clinical picture.

- Topical decongestants are applied directly to swollen nasal mucosa via drops or sprays (**Table 76–3**). They result in little or no systemic absorption.
- Rhinitis medicamentosa (rebound vasodilation with congestion) may occur with prolonged use of topical agents (>3–5 days). Patients with this condition use more spray more often with less response. Abrupt cessation is an effective treatment, but rebound congestion may last for several days or weeks. Nasal steroids have been used successfully but take several days to work. Weaning off the topical decongestant can be accomplished by decreasing dosing frequency or concentration over several weeks. Combining the weaning process with nasal steroids may be helpful.
- Other adverse effects of topical decongestants are burning, stinging, sneezing, and dryness of the nasal mucosa.
- These products should be used only when absolutely necessary (eg, at bedtime) and in doses that are as small and infrequent as possible. Duration of therapy should be limited to 5 days or less.
- **Pseudoephedrine** (see **Table 76–2**) is an oral decongestant that has a slower onset of action than topical agents but may last longer and cause less local irritation. Rhinitis medicamentosa does not occur with oral decongestants. Doses up to 180 mg produce no

TABLE 76–2 Medication Dosing for Allergic Rhinitis

Drugs	Brand Names	Dosages	Special Population Doses	Other
Antihistamines				
Oral				
Nonselective:				
Chlorpheniramine maleate	Various	Plain: 4 mg every 6 hours Sustained release: 12 mg every 12 hours	Pediatrics: 6–12 years: 2 mg every 6 hours 2–5 years: 1 mg every 6 hours Pediatrics: 6–12 years: 0.67 mg every 12 hours	OTC Available as liquid OTC
Clemastine fumarate	Tavist	1.34 mg every 8 hours		OTC Available as liquid
Diphenhydramine hydrochloride	Benadryl and others	25–50 mg every 8 hours	Pediatrics: 5 mg/kg per day divided every 8 hours (up to 25 mg per dose) Pediatrics: 6–12 years: 10 mg once daily 2–5 years: 5 mg once daily	OTC Available as liquid
Peripherally selective:				
Loratadine	Alavert/Claritin	10 mg once daily	Pediatrics: 2–11 years: 30 mg twice daily	OTC Available as liquid
Fexofenadine	Allegra	60 mg twice daily or 180 mg once daily	Pediatrics: 1–5 years: 2.5 mg daily may increase to twice daily 6–12 months: 2.5 mg once daily	OTC Available as liquid
Cetirizine	Zyrtec	5–10 mg once daily	Pediatrics: 6–11 years: 2.5 mg in the evening 6 months to 5 years: 1.25 mg in the evening	OTC Available as liquid
Levocetirizine	Xyzal	5 mg at bedtime		
Nasal				
Azelastine	Astopro	One to two sprays twice daily	Pediatrics: 5–11 years one spray twice daily	
Olopatadine	Patanase	Two sprays twice daily	Pediatrics: 6–11 years: one spray twice daily	
Ophthalmic				
Bepotastine	Bepreve	One drop twice daily		

(continued)

TABLE 76–2	Medication Dosing for Allergic Rhinitis (*Continued*)			
Drugs	**Brand Names**	**Dosages**	**Special Population Doses**	**Other**
Decongestants				
Oral				
Pseudoephedrine	Various	60 mg every 4–6 hours	Pediatrics: 6–12 years: 30 mg every 4–6 hours	OTC
		Sustained release: 120 mg every 12 hours	4–5 years: 15 mg every 4–6 hours	Available as liquid
		Controlled release: 240 mg once daily		
Phenylephrine	Various	10–20 mg every 4 hours	Pediatrics: 6–12 years: 5 mg every 4 hours	OTC
			4–6 years: 2.5 mg every 4 hours	Available as liquid
Nasal				
Oxymetazoline	Various	Two to three sprays twice daily		OTC
Phenylephrine	Various	Two to three sprays every 4 hours	Pediatrics: >12 years: use 0.25%–0.5% two to three sprays every 4 hours	OTC
			6–12 years: use 0.25% two to three sprays every 4 hours	
			2–6 years: use 0.125% one drop every 2–4 hours	
Nasal steroids				
Beclomethasone	Beconase AQ	One to two inhalations in each nostril twice daily (Beconase AQ)	Pediatric: Beconase AQ: 6–11 years: one inhalation in each nostril twice daily	
	Qnasl	Two inhalations (160 mcg) in each nostril once daily (Qnasl)	Qnasl: 4–11 years: one inhalation (40 mcg) in each nostril once daily	
Budesonide	Rhinocort Aqua	One spray each nostril daily (up to maximum of four sprays each nostril daily)		
Flunisolide	Various	Two sprays in each nostril twice daily	Pediatrics: 6–14 years: two sprays in each nostril twice daily	
Fluticasone	Flonase	Two sprays in each nostril once daily	Pediatrics: >4 years: one spray in each nostril daily (Flonase)	OTC
	Veramyst		2–11 years: one spray in each nostril daily (Veramyst)	
Mometasone	Nasonex	Two sprays in each nostril daily	Pediatrics: 2–11 years: one spray in each nostril daily	
Triamcinolone	Nasacort	Two sprays in each nostril daily (reduce to one spray when symptoms controlled)	Pediatrics: 2–11 years: one spray in each nostril once daily	OTC

Other nasal medications

Cromolyn	Nasalcrom	One spray in each nostril three to four times a day	Pediatrics: >2 years, same as adult dose	OTC
Ipratropium	Atrovent	Two sprays in each nostril two to four times per day	Pediatrics: 5–11 years: two sprays in each nostril two to three times a day	
Montelukast	Singulair	Oral: 10 mg once daily	Pediatrics: 6–23 months: 4 mg (oral granules) once daily 2–5 years: 4 mg once daily (chewable or granules) 6–14 years: 5 mg once daily (chewable)	

TABLE 76–3	Duration of Action of Topical Decongestants
Medications	**Durations of Action (hours)**
Short acting	
Phenylephrine hydrochloride	Up to 4
Intermediate acting	
Naphazoline hydrochloride	2–6
Tetrahydrozoline hydrochloride	
Long acting	
Oxymetazoline hydrochloride	Up to 12
Xylometazoline hydrochloride	

measurable change in blood pressure or heart rate. However, higher doses (210–240 mg) may raise both blood pressure and heart rate. Systemic decongestants should be avoided in hypertensive patients unless absolutely necessary. Severe hypertensive reactions can occur when pseudoephedrine is given with monoamine oxidase inhibitors. Pseudo-ephedrine can cause mild CNS stimulation, even at therapeutic doses. Because of misuse as a component in the illegal manufacture of methamphetamine, pseudoephedrine is restricted to behind-the-counter sale with a limit on monthly purchases.

- **Phenylephrine** has replaced pseudoephedrine in many nonprescription antihistamine–decongestant combination products because of legal restrictions on pseudoephedrine sales.
- Combination oral products containing a decongestant and antihistamine are rational because of different mechanisms of action. Consumers should read product labels carefully to avoid therapeutic duplication and use combination products only for short courses.

Nasal Corticosteroids

- Intranasal corticosteroids relieve sneezing, rhinorrhea, pruritus, and nasal congestion with minimal side effects (see **Table 76–2**). They reduce inflammation by blocking mediator release, suppressing neutrophil chemotaxis, causing mild vasoconstriction, and inhibiting mast cell–mediated, late-phase reactions.
- These agents are an excellent choice for persistent rhinitis and can be useful in seasonal rhinitis, especially if begun in advance of symptoms. Some authorities recommend nasal steroids as initial therapy over antihistamines because of their high degree of efficacy when used properly along with allergen avoidance.
- Side effects include sneezing, stinging, headache, epistaxis, and rare infections with *Candida albicans*.
- Some patients improve within a few days, but peak response may require 2 to 3 weeks. The dosage may be reduced once a response is achieved.
- Blocked nasal passages should be cleared with a decongestant or saline irrigation before administration to ensure adequate penetration of the spray.

Cromolyn Sodium

- **Cromolyn sodium** (Nasalcrom), a mast cell stabilizer, is available as a nonprescription nasal spray for symptomatic prevention and treatment of allergic rhinitis. It prevents antigen-triggered mast cell degranulation and release of mediators, including histamine. The most common side effect is local irritation (sneezing and nasal stinging).
- Dosage for persons at least 2 years of age is one spray in each nostril three or four times daily at regular intervals. Nasal passages should be cleared before administration, and inhaling through the nose during administration enhances distribution to the entire nasal lining.

- For seasonal rhinitis, treatment should be initiated just before the start of the offending allergen's season and continue throughout the season.
- In persistent rhinitis, effects may not be seen for 2 to 4 weeks; antihistamines or decongestants may be needed during this initial phase of therapy.

Ipratropium Bromide

- **Ipratropium bromide** (Atrovent) nasal spray is an anticholinergic agent that may be useful in persistent allergic rhinitis. It exhibits antisecretory properties when applied locally and provides symptomatic relief of rhinorrhea.
- The 0.03% solution is given as two sprays (42 mcg) two or three times daily. Adverse effects are mild and include headache, epistaxis, and nasal dryness.

Montelukast

- **Montelukast** (Singulair) is a leukotriene receptor antagonist approved for treatment of persistent allergic rhinitis in children as young as 6 months and for seasonal allergic rhinitis in children as young as 2 years. It is effective alone or in combination with an antihistamine.
- Dosage for adults and adolescents older than 14 years is one 10-mg tablet daily. Children ages 6 to 14 years may receive one 5-mg chewable tablet daily. Children ages 6 months to 5 years may be given one 4-mg chewable tablet or oral granule packet daily.
- Montelukast is no more effective than antihistamines and less effective than intranasal corticosteroids; therefore, it is considered third-line therapy after those agents.

IMMUNOTHERAPY

- Immunotherapy is the process of administering doses of antigens responsible for eliciting allergic symptoms into a patient with the intent of inducing tolerance to the allergen when natural exposure occurs. Until recently, immunotherapy was only available for subcutaneous injection; sublingual dosage forms are now available for a limited number of allergens.
- Beneficial effects of immunotherapy may result from induction of IgG-blocking antibodies, reduction in specific IgE (long-term), reduced recruitment of effector cells, altered T-cell cytokine balance, T-cell anergy, and alteration of regulatory T cells.
- Good candidates for immunotherapy include patients with a strong history of severe symptoms unsuccessfully controlled by avoidance and pharmacotherapy and patients unable to tolerate adverse effects of drug therapy. Poor candidates include patients with medical conditions that would compromise the ability to tolerate an anaphylactic-type reaction, patients with impaired immune systems, and patients with a history of nonadherence.
- For subcutaneous immunotherapy, very dilute solutions are given initially once or twice weekly. The concentration is increased until the maximum tolerated dose or highest planned dose is achieved. This maintenance dose is continued in slowly increasing intervals over several years, depending on clinical response. Better results are obtained with year-round rather than seasonal injections.
- Sublingual immunotherapy is available for ragweed and certain grass allergies. The products are started 12 weeks before the allergen season and continued throughout the season. The first dose is administered in the physician's office to allow observation of the patient for 30 minutes for hypersensitivity reactions. The patient places the tablet under the tongue where it dissolves; patients should not swallow for at least 1 minute. After the first dose is administered without incident, patients can take immunotherapy at home, but an autoinjectable epinephrine must be prescribed.
- Adverse reactions with subcutaneous immunotherapy include mild local adverse reactions include induration and swelling at the injection site. More severe reactions (generalized urticaria, bronchospasm, laryngospasm, vascular collapse, and death from anaphylaxis) occur rarely. Severe reactions are treated with epinephrine, antihistamines, and systemic corticosteroids. The most common reactions with sublingual immunotherapy are pruritus of the mouth, ears, and tongue; throat irritation; and mouth edema.

EVALUATION OF THERAPEUTIC OUTCOMES

- Monitor patients regularly for reduction in severity of identified target symptoms and presence of side effects.
- Ask patients about their satisfaction with the management of their allergic rhinitis. Management should result in minimal disruption to their normal lifestyle.
- The Medical Outcomes Study 36-Item Short Form Health Survey and the Rhino-conjunctivitis Quality of Life Questionnaire measure symptom improvement and parameters such as sleep quality, nonallergic symptoms (eg, fatigue and poor concentration), emotions, and participation in a variety of activities.

See Chapter 95, Allergic Rhinitis, authored by J. Russell May, for a more detailed discussion of this topic.

CHAPTER 77

Asthma

- *Asthma*, as defined by the Global Initiative for Asthma (GINA), is a heterogeneous disease, usually characterized by chronic airway inflammation. It is defined by a history of respiratory symptoms such as wheezing, shortness of breath, chest tightness, and cough that vary over time and in intensity, together with variable expiratory airflow limitation.

PATHOPHYSIOLOGY

- There is a variable degree of airflow obstruction (related to bronchospasm, edema, and hypersecretion), bronchial hyperresponsiveness (BHR), and airway inflammation.
- In acute inflammation, inhaled allergens in allergic patients causes early-phase allergic reaction with activation of cells bearing allergen-specific immunoglobulin E (IgE) antibodies. After rapid activation, airway mast cells and macrophages release pro-inflammatory mediators such as histamine and eicosanoids that induce contraction of airway smooth muscle, mucus secretion, vasodilation, and exudation of plasma in the airways. Plasma protein leakage induces a thickened, engorged, edematous airway wall and narrowing of lumen with reduced mucus clearance.
- Late-phase inflammatory reaction occurs 6 to 9 hours after allergen provocation and involves recruitment and activation of eosinophils, T lymphocytes, basophils, neutrophils, and macrophages. Eosinophils migrate to airways and release inflammatory mediators.
- T-lymphocyte activation leads to release of cytokines from type 2 T-helper (TH$_2$) cells that mediate allergic inflammation (interleukin [IL]-4, IL-5, and IL-13). Conversely, type 1 T-helper (TH$_1$) cells produce IL-2 and interferon-γ that are essential for cellular defense mechanisms. Allergic asthmatic inflammation may result from imbalance between TH$_1$ and TH$_2$ cells.
- Mast cell degranulation results in release of mediators such as histamine; eosinophil and neutrophil chemotactic factors; leukotrienes C$_4$, D$_4$, and E$_4$; prostaglandins; and platelet-activating factor (PAF). Histamine can induce smooth muscle constriction and bronchospasm and may contribute to mucosal edema and mucus secretion.
- Alveolar macrophages release inflammatory mediators, including proinflammatory and anti-inflammatory cytokines, reactive oxygen species, and eicosanoids. Production of neutrophil chemotactic factor and eosinophil chemotactic factor furthers the inflammatory process. Neutrophils also release mediators (PAFs, prostaglandins, thromboxanes, and leukotrienes) that contribute to BHR and airway inflammation. Leukotrienes C$_4$, D$_4$, and E$_4$ are released during inflammatory processes in the lung and produce bronchospasm, mucus secretion, microvascular permeability, and airway edema.
- Bronchial epithelial cells participate in inflammation by releasing eicosanoids, peptidases, matrix proteins, cytokines, and nitric oxide. Epithelial shedding results in heightened airway responsiveness, altered permeability of airway mucosa, depletion of epithelial-derived relaxant factors, and loss of enzymes responsible for degrading inflammatory neuropeptides. The exudative inflammatory process and sloughing of epithelial cells into the airway lumen impair mucociliary transport. Bronchial glands increase in size, and goblet cells increase in size and number.
- The airway is innervated by parasympathetic, sympathetic, and nonadrenergic inhibitory nerves. Normal resting tone of airway smooth muscle is maintained by vagal efferent activity, and bronchoconstriction can be mediated by vagal stimulation in small bronchi. Airway smooth muscle contains noninnervated β$_2$-adrenergic receptors that produce bronchodilation. The nonadrenergic, noncholinergic nervous system in the trachea and bronchi may amplify inflammation by releasing nitric oxide.

CLINICAL PRESENTATION

CHRONIC ASTHMA

- Symptoms include episodes of shortness of breath, chest tightness, coughing (particularly at night), wheezing, or a whistling sound when breathing. These often occur with exercise but may occur spontaneously or in association with known allergens.
- Signs include expiratory wheezing (rhonchi) on auscultation; dry, hacking cough; and atopy (eg, allergic rhinitis or atopic dermatitis).
- Asthma can vary from chronic daily symptoms to only intermittent symptoms. Intervals between symptoms may be days, weeks, months, or years.
- Severity is determined by lung function, symptoms, nighttime awakenings, and interference with normal activity prior to therapy. Patients can present with mild intermittent symptoms that require no medications or only occasional short-acting inhaled β_2-agonists to severe chronic symptoms despite multiple medications.

ACUTE SEVERE ASTHMA

- Uncontrolled asthma can progress to an acute state in which inflammation, airway edema, mucus accumulation, and severe bronchospasm result in profound airway narrowing that is poorly responsive to bronchodilator therapy.
- Patients may be anxious in acute distress and complain of severe dyspnea, shortness of breath, chest tightness, or burning. They may be able to say only a few words with each breath. Symptoms are unresponsive to usual measures (short-acting inhaled β-agonists).
- Signs include expiratory and inspiratory wheezing on auscultation; dry, hacking cough; tachypnea; tachycardia; pallor or cyanosis; and hyperinflated chest with intercostal and supraclavicular retractions. Breath sounds may be diminished with severe obstruction.

DIAGNOSIS

CHRONIC ASTHMA

- Diagnosis is made primarily by history of recurrent episodes of coughing, wheezing, chest tightness, or shortness of breath and confirmatory spirometry.
- Patients may have family history of allergy or asthma or symptoms of allergic rhinitis or atopic dermatitis. History of exercise or cold air precipitating dyspnea or increased symptoms during specific allergen seasons suggests asthma. Patient may have excessive variability in twice-daily peak expiratory flows (PEF) over 2 weeks.
- Spirometry demonstrates obstruction (forced expiratory volume in 1 second [FEV_1]/forced vital capacity [FVC] <80%) with reversibility after inhaled β_2-agonist administration (at least 12% and 200 mL increase in FEV_1). If baseline spirometry is normal, challenge testing with exercise, histamine, or methacholine can be used to elicit BHR.

ACUTE SEVERE ASTHMA

- PEF and FEV_1 are less than 40% of normal predicted values. Pulse oximetry reveals decreased arterial oxygen and O_2 saturations. The best predictor of outcome is early response to treatment as measured by improvement in FEV_1 at 30 minutes after inhaled β_2-agonists.
- Arterial blood gases may reveal metabolic acidosis and low partial pressure of oxygen (PaO_2).
- History and physical examination should be obtained while initial therapy is provided, assessing for: onset and causes of the exacerbation; severity of symptoms and if associated with anaphylaxis; medication use, adherence, and response to current therapy; and risk factors for asthma-related death (history of near-fatal asthma requiring intubation and mechanical ventilation; hospitalization or emergency care in the past year; recent use of oral corticosteroids; no current use of inhaled

corticosteroids; overuse of short-acting β_2-agonist therapy [more than 1 canister/month; history of psychiatric disease or psychosocial problems; poor medication adherence; lack of a written asthma action plan; and food allergy]. The physical exam will assess vital signs and any complicating factors (eg, pneumonia, anaphylaxis) and comorbid conditions that could be causing acute shortness of breath such as inhaled foreign body, heart failure, pulmonary infection, and pulmonary embolism.

- Lung function testing by PEF or FEV_1 should be measured before treatment if possible and thereafter at 1 hour after start of treatment and then periodically until response is achieved or no further improvement is evident. Oxygen saturation is also monitored closely, preferably by pulse oximetry.
- Arterial blood gases are typically reserved for patients who are poorly responsive to initial treatment or deteriorating.
- Complete blood count may be appropriate for patients with fever or purulent sputum.

TREATMENT

- Goals of Treatment: The GINA long-term goals for asthma management include: (1) achieve good control of symptoms and maintain normal activity levels; and (2) minimize future risk of exacerbations, fixed airflow limitation, and side effects. For acute severe asthma, the primary goal is prevention of life-threatening asthma by early recognition of signs of deterioration and early intervention.

NONPHARMACOLOGIC THERAPY

- Patient education is mandatory to improve medication adherence, self-management skills, and use of healthcare services.
- Objective measurements of airflow obstruction with a home peak flow meter may not improve patient outcomes. NAEPP advocates PEF monitoring only for patients with severe persistent asthma who have difficulty perceiving airway obstruction.
- Avoidance of known allergenic triggers can improve symptoms, reduce medication use, and decrease BHR. Environmental triggers (eg, animals) should be avoided in sensitive patients, and smokers should be encouraged to quit.
- In acute asthma exacerbations, oxygen therapy is initiated to achieve an arterial oxygen saturation of 93% to 95% in adolescents and adults and 94% to 98% in school-aged children and pregnant women or those with cardiac disease.
- Dehydration should be corrected; urine specific gravity may help guide therapy in children when assessment of hydration status is difficult.

PHARMACOTHERAPY

General Approach

- **Figure 77–1** summarizes GINA recommendations for initial controller treatment in adults and adolescents with persistent asthma. Regardless of the long-term therapy, all patients must have a short-acting inhaled β_2-agonist available for quick relief of acute symptoms.
- **Figure 77–2** depicts the GINA stepwise approach for control-based management, which emphasizes three components: (1) ASSESS symptom control and risk factors; (2) ADJUST therapy and treat modifiable risk factors; and (3) REVIEW RESPONSE and optimize control about every 3 months. Step-down of controller treatment may be considered if symptoms have been well controlled and lung function stable for 3 months or longer. While engaging the patient in this effort, monitor symptoms and PEF and schedule follow-up. Stepping down inhaled corticosteroid (ICS) doses by 25% to 50% at 3-month intervals is feasible and safe for most patients.
- The primary therapy of acute exacerbations includes short-acting inhaled β2-agonists and (depending on severity) systemic corticosteroids, inhaled ipratropium, and oxygen. Treatments are typically administered concurrently to facilitate rapid improvement. Initial response is measured one hour after the first three inhaled bronchodilator treatments.

Symptom Presentation	Preferred Treatment (Evidence Level)
Symptoms or need for SABA less than 2×/mo; no waking due to asthma in last month; and no risk factors for exacerbations, including in prior year	No controller
Infrequent symptoms, but patient has one or more risk factors for exacerbation (eg, low lung function, use of OCS in prior year, intensive care treatment for asthma ever)	Low dose ICS
Symptoms or need for SABA between 2×/mo and 2×/week, or patient wakes due to asthma more than once/mo.	Low dose ICS
Symptoms or need for SABA > 2×/week	Low dose ICS*
Troublesome symptoms most days or waking ≥ 1 ×/week, esp. if any risk factors exist	Medium/high dose ICS or low dose ICS/LABA**
Symptoms consistent with severely uncontrolled asthma, or with an acute exacerbation	OCS short course AND start of high-dose ICS or moderate-dose ICS/LABA**

*Less effective options are LTRA or theophylline.
**Not recommended for initial controller treatment in children 6–11 years.
(ICS, inhaled corticosteroids; LABA, long-acting β_2-agonist; LTRA, leukotriene receptor antagonist; OCS, oral corticosteroids; SABA, short-acting β_2-agonist.)

FIGURE 77–1. **GINA recommendations for initial controller treatment in adults and adolescents.**

- Figure 77–3 outlines strategies for self-management of worsening asthma.
- Figure 77–4 is an algorithm for management of acute asthma exacerbations in acute care facilities.

β_2-Agonists

- Short-acting β_2-agonists are the most effective bronchodilators. Aerosol administration enhances bronchoselectivity and provides more rapid response and greater protection against provocations (eg, exercise, allergen challenges) than systemic administration. In adults, administration as either continuous or intermittent (every 20 minutes for 3 doses) administration over 1 hour results in equivalent improvement. In acute severe asthma, continuous nebulization of short-acting β_2-agonists (eg, albuterol) is recommended for patients having unsatisfactory response after three doses (every 20 min) of aerosolized β_2-agonists and potentially for patients presenting initially with PEF or FEV1 values less than 30% of predicted normal.
- **Albuterol** and other inhaled short-acting selective β_2-agonists are indicated for intermittent episodes of bronchospasm and are the treatment of choice for acute severe asthma and EIB. Regular treatment (four times daily) does not improve symptom control over as-needed use.
- Two long-acting β2-agonists (LABA), **formoterol** and **salmeterol**, provide bronchodilation for at least 12 hours. These inhaled LABA are indicated for adjunctive long-term control for patients with symptoms who are already on low to medium doses of inhaled corticosteroids prior to advancing to medium- or high-dose inhaled corticosteroids. Short-acting β2-agonists should be continued for acute exacerbations.
- Three ultra-LABA (**indacaterol, olodaterol,** and **vilanterol**) have a 24-hour bronchodilator duration of effect. Vilanterol in combination with fluticasone furoate is available for once-daily dosing for asthma in adults aged 18 and older in the United States and for children and adults aged 12 and older in Europe. Products containing indacaterol and olodaterol are currently only indicated for COPD but are being evaluated for asthma.

Step	Preferred Option [Evidence Level]	Other Recommended Options [Evidence Level]
1	As-needed SABA	Consider low dose ICS, in addition to as-needed SABA, for patients at risk for exacerbations
2	Low-dose ICS plus as-needed SABA	LTRA Low-dose ICS/LABA ICS started with symptoms of allergic asthma, for seasonal treatment only
3	Low-dose ICS/LABA, plus as-needed SABA for adults/adolescents OR low-dose ICS/formoterol as both maintenance and reliever For children 6–11 years, moderate–dose ICS, plus as-needed SABA	Medium-dose ICS for adults/adolescents Low-dose ICS plus LTRA (A) or low-dose, sustained-release theophylline
4	Medium-dose ICS/LABA, plus as-needed SABA for adults/adolescents OR medium-dose ICS/formoterol as both maintenance and reliever For children 6–11 years, refer child to asthma specialist	Add-on therapy with tiotropium for adults with exacerbation history
5	Referral to specialist and consideration of add-on treatment	Tiotropium if < 18 years of age Omalizumab for moderate–severe allergic asthma Sputum-guided treatment adjusted by eosinophilia >3% Bronchial thermoplasty in some adults with severe asthma Add-on low-dose OCS (≤7.5 mg/day prednisone equivalent)

(ICS, inhaled corticosteroids; LABA, long-acting β$_2$-agonist; LTRA, leukotriene receptor antagonist; OCS, oral corticosteroids; SABA, short-acting β$_2$-agonist.)

FIGURE 77–2. GINA stepwise approach to control symptoms and minimize future risk.

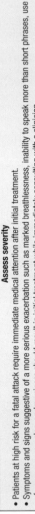

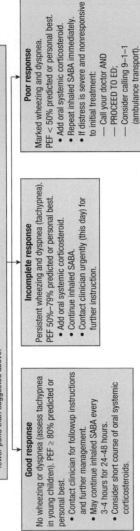

Assess severity

- Patients at high risk for a fatal attack require immediate medical attention after initial treatment.
- Symptoms and signs suggestive of a more serious exacerbation such as marked breathlessness, inability to speak more than short phrases, use of accessory muscles, or drowsiness should result in initial treatment while immediately consulting with a clinician.
- Less severe signs and symptoms can be treated initially with assessment of response to therapy and further steps as listed below.
- If available, measure PEF—values of 50%–79% predicted or personal best indicate the need for quick-relief medication. Depending on the response to treatment, contact with a clinician may also be indicated. Values below 50% indicate the need for immediate medical care.

Initial treatment

- Inhaled SABA: up to two treatments 20 minutes apart of 2–6 puffs by metered-dose inhaler (MDI) or nebulizer treatments.
- Note: Medication delivery is highly variable. Children and individuals who have exacerbations of lesser severity may need fewer puffs than suggested above.

Good response

No wheezing or dyspnea (assess tachypnea in young children). PEF ≥ 80% predicted or personal best.
- Contact clinician for followup instructions and further management.
- May continue inhaled SABA every 3–4 hours for 24–48 hours.
- Consider short course of oral systemic corticosteroids.

Incomplete response

Persistent wheezing and dyspnea (tachypnea). PEF 50%–79% predicted or personal best.
- Add oral systemic corticosteroid.
- Continue inhaled SABA.
- Contact clinician urgently (this day) for further instruction.

Poor response

Marked wheezing and dyspnea. PEF < 50% predicted or personal best.
- Add oral systemic corticosteroid.
- Repeat inhaled SABA immediately.
- If distress is severe and nonresponsive to initial treatment:
  — Call your doctor AND
  — PROCEED TO ED;
  — Consider calling 9–1–1 (ambulance transport).

- To ED.

(ED, emergency department; MDI, metered-dose inhaler; PEF, peak expiratory flow; SABA, short-acting β₂-agonist (quick-relief inhaler).)

FIGURE 77–3. Self-management of worsening asthma in adults and adolescents with a written asthma action plan. *(Adapted from Global Initiative for Asthma. Global strategy for asthma management and prevention, 2015. Source: www.ginasthma.org.)*

- Table 77–1 contains dosing guidelines for acute severe asthma exacerbations.
- Inhaled β_2-agonists are the treatment of choice for EIB. Short-acting agents provide complete protection for at least 2 hours; long-acting agents provide significant protection for 8 to 12 hours initially, but duration decreases with chronic regular use.
- In nocturnal asthma, long-acting inhaled β_2-agonists are preferred over oral sustained-release β_2-agonists or sustained-release theophylline. However, nocturnal asthma may be an indicator of inadequate antiinflammatory treatment.

Corticosteroids

- Inhaled corticosteroids (ICS) are the preferred long-term control therapy for persistent asthma because of potency and consistent effectiveness; they are the only therapy shown to reduce risk of dying from asthma. See Table 77–2 for comparative ICS doss. Most patients with moderate disease can be controlled with twice-daily dosing; some products have once-daily dosing indications. Patients with more severe disease require multiple daily dosing. Because inflammation inhibits steroid receptor binding, patients should be started on higher and more frequent doses and then tapered down once control has been achieved. Response to inhaled corticosteroids is delayed; symptoms improve in most patients within the first 1 to 2 weeks and reach maximum improvement in 4 to 8 weeks. Maximum improvement in FEV_1 and PEF rates may require 3 to 6 weeks.
- Systemic toxicity of inhaled corticosteroids is minimal with low to moderate doses, but risk of systemic effects increases with high doses. Local adverse effects include dose-dependent oropharyngeal candidiasis and dysphonia, which can be reduced by using a spacer device.
- Systemic corticosteroids (Table 77–3) are indicated in all patients with acute severe asthma not responding completely to initial inhaled β_2-agonist administration (every 20 min for 3 or 4 doses) and should be administered within one hour of presentation. IV therapy offers no advantage over oral administration except in patients unable to take oral medications. Adults are treated effectively with a 5 to 7 day course of prednisone (or equivalent), but children may require only 3 to 5 days. Dexamethasone as 1 or 2 doses is an option for children and has the benefit of less vomiting. Full doses should be continued until the PEF reaches 70% of predicted normal or personal best. Tapering the dose after discharge is unnecessary if patients are prescribed an ICS for outpatient therapy.
- In patients who require chronic systemic corticosteroids for asthma control, the lowest possible dose should be used. Toxicities may be decreased by alternate-day therapy or high-dose inhaled corticosteroids.

Methylxanthines

- **Theophylline** appears to produce bronchodilation through nonselective phosphodiesterase inhibition. Methylxanthines are ineffective by aerosol and must be taken systemically (orally or IV). Sustained-release theophylline is the preferred oral preparation, whereas its complex with ethylenediamine (**aminophylline**) is the preferred parenteral product due to increased solubility. IV theophylline is also available.
- Theophylline is eliminated primarily by metabolism via hepatic CYP P450 enzymes (primarily CYP1A2 and CYP3A4) with 10% or less excreted unchanged in urine. CYP P450 enzymes are susceptible to induction and inhibition by environmental factors and drugs. Significant reductions in clearance can result from cotherapy with cimetidine, erythromycin, clarithromycin, allopurinol, propranolol, ciprofloxacin, interferon, ticlopidine, zileuton, and other drugs. Some substances that enhance clearance are rifampin, carbamazepine, phenobarbital, phenytoin, charcoal-broiled meat, and cigarette smoking.
- Because of large interpatient variability in theophylline clearance, routine monitoring of serum theophylline concentrations is essential for safe and effective use. A steady-state range of 5 to 15 mcg/mL (27.75–83.25 μmol/L) is effective and safe for most patients.

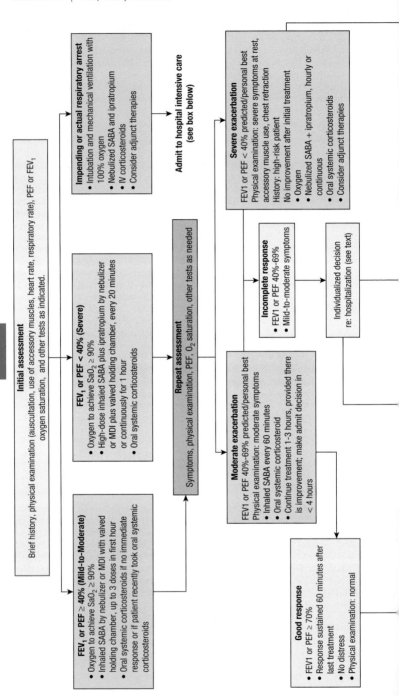

Initial assessment

Brief history, physical examination (auscultation, use of accessory muscles, heart rate, respiratory rate), PEF or FEV₁ oxygen saturation, and other tests as indicated.

FEV₁ or PEF ≥ 40% (Mild-to-Moderate)
- Oxygen to achieve SaO₂ ≥ 90%
- Inhaled SABA by nebulizer or MDI with valved holding chamber, up to 3 doses in first hour
- Oral systemic corticosteroids if no immediate response or if patient recently took oral systemic corticosteroids

FEV₁ or PEF < 40% (Severe)
- Oxygen to achieve SaO₂ ≥ 90%
- High-dose inhaled SABA plus ipratropium by nebulizer or MDI plus valved holding chamber, every 20 minutes or continuously for 1 hour
- Oral systemic corticosteroids

Impending or actual respiratory arrest
- Intubation and mechanical ventilation with 100% oxygen
- Nebulized SABA and ipratropium
- IV corticosteroids
- Consider adjunct therapies

Admit to hospital intensive care (see box below)

Repeat assessment

Symptoms, physical examination, PEF, O₂ saturation, other tests as needed

Moderate exacerbation
FEV1 or PEF 40%-69% predicted/personal best
Physical examination: moderate symptoms
- Inhaled SABA every 60 minutes
- Oral systemic corticosteroid
- Continue treatment 1-3 hours, provided there is improvement; make admit decision in < 4 hours

Severe exacerbation
FEV1 or PEF < 40% predicted/personal best
Physical examination: severe symptoms at rest, accessory muscle use, chest retraction
History: high-risk patient
No improvement after initial treatment
- Oxygen
- Nebulized SABA + ipratropium, hourly or continuous
- Oral systemic corticosteroids
- Consider adjunct therapies

Incomplete response
- FEV1 or PEF 40%-69%
- Mild-to-moderate symptoms

Individualized decision re: hospitalization (see text)

Good response
- FEV1 or PEF ≥ 70%
- Response sustained 60 minutes after last treatment
- No distress
- Physical examination: normal

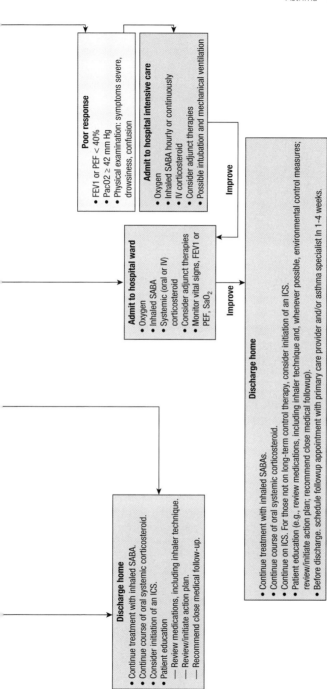

Poor response
- FEV1 or PEF < 40%
- PacO2 ≥ 42 mm Hg
- Physical examination: symptoms severe, drowsiness, confusion

Admit to hospital intensive care
- Oxygen
- Inhaled SABA hourly or continuously
- IV corticosteroid
- Consider adjunct therapies
- Possible intubation and mechanical ventilation

Improve

Admit to hospital ward
- Oxygen
- Inhaled SABA
- Systemic (oral or IV) corticosteroid
- Consider adjunct therapies
- Monitor vital signs, FEV1 or PEF, SaO₂

Improve

Discharge home
- Continue treatment with inhaled SABA.
- Continue course of oral systemic corticosteroid.
- Consider initiation of an ICS.
- Patient education
  — Review medications, including inhaler technique.
  — Review/initiate action plan.
  — Recommend close medical follow-up.

Discharge home
- Continue treatment with inhaled SABAs.
- Continue course of oral systemic corticosteroid.
- Continue on ICS. For those not on long-term control therapy, consider initiation of an ICS.
- Patient education (e.g., review medications, including inhaler technique and, whenever possible, environmental control measures; review/initiate action plan; recommend close medical followup).
- Before discharge, schedule followup appointment with primary care provider and/or asthma specialist In 1-4 weeks.

FEV₁, forced expiratory volume in 1 second; ICS, inhaled corticosteroid; MDI, metered-dose inhaler; PacO₂, partial pressure carbon dioxide; PEF, peak expiratory flow; SABA, short-acting β₂-agonist; SaO₂, oxygen saturation.

FIGURE 77–4. Management of asthma exacerbations in acute care facility (e.g., emergency department).

TABLE 77–1 Drug Dosages for Acute Severe Exacerbations of Asthma in the Emergency Department or Hospital

Medications	≥12 Years Old	<12 Years Old	Comments
Inhaled β-agonists			
Albuterol nebulizer solution (5 mg/mL, 0.63 mg/3 mL, 1.25 mg/3 mL, 2.5 mg/3 mL)	2.5–5 mg every 20 minutes for three doses, and then 2.5–10 mg every 1–4 hours as needed, or 10–15 mg/h continuously	0.15 mg/kg (minimum dose 2.5 mg) every 20 minutes for three doses, and then 0.15–0.3 mg/kg up to 10 mg every 1–4 hours as needed, or 0.5 mg/kg/h by continuous nebulization	Only selective β₂-agonists are recommended. For optimal delivery, dilute aerosols to minimum of 4 mL at gas flow of 6–8 L/min. Use face mask if <4 years of age
Albuterol MDI (90 mcg/puff)	4–8 puffs every 30 minutes up to 4 hours, and then every 1–4 hours as needed	4–8 puffs every 20 minutes for three doses, and then every 1–4 hours as needed	In patients in severe distress, nebulization is preferred; use VHC-type spacer with face mask if <4 years old
Levalbuterol nebulizer solution (0.31 mg/3 mL, 0.63 mg/3 mL, 2.5 mg/1 mL, 1.25 mg/3 mL)	Give at one half the milligram dose of albuterol above	Give at one half the milligram dose of albuterol above	The single isomer of albuterol is twice as potent on a milligram basis Not recommended
Levalbuterol MDI (45 mcg/puff)	See albuterol MDI dose	See albuterol MDI dose above	See albuterol MDI dose; one half as potent as albuterol on a microgram basis Not recommended

Anticholinergics

Ipratropium bromide nebulizer solution (0.25 mg/mL)	500 mcg every 30 minutes for three doses, and then every 2–4 hours as needed	250 mcg every 20 minutes for three doses, and then 250 mcg every 2–4 hours
		May mix in same nebulizer with albuterol; only add to β_2-agonist therapy
Ipratropium bromide MDI (18 mcg/puff)	8 puffs every 20 minutes as needed for up to 3 hours	4–8 puffs as needed every 2–4 hours
		Not to be continued once hospitalized

Corticosteroids

Prednisone, methylprednisolone, prednisolone	50 mg in one or two divided doses (prednisone equivalent)	1 mg/kg (maximum 40 mg/day) in two divided doses (prednisone equivalent)
		For outpatient "burst" use 1–2 mg/kg/day, maximum 60 mg, for 3–5 days in children and 40–60 mg/day in one or two divided doses for 5–7 days in adults

Note: No advantage has been found for very-high-dose corticosteroids in acute severe asthma, nor is there any advantage for IV administration over oral therapy. The usual regimen is to continue the oral corticosteroid for the duration of hospitalization. The final duration of therapy following a hospitalization or emergency department visit may be from 3 to 10 days. If patients are then started on an ICS, there is no need to taper the systemic corticosteroid dose. An ICS can be started at any time during the exacerbation.

TABLE 77–2 Available Inhaled Corticosteroid Products, Lung Delivery, and Comparative Daily Dosages

ICS	Product	Lung Delivery[a]
Beclomethasone dipropionate (BDP)	40 and 80 mcg/actuation HFA MDI	50%–60%
Budesonide (BUD)	90 or 180 mcg/dose DPI, Flexhaler	15%–30%
	200 and 500 mcg ampules, 1 mg	5%–8%
Ciclesonide (CIC)	80 or 160 mcg/actuation HFA MDI	50%
Flunisolide (FLU)	80 mcg/actuation HFA MDI	68%
Fluticasone furoate (FF)	100, 200 mcg/actuation DPI, Ellipta	80%–85%
Fluticasone propionate (FP)	44, 110, and 220 mcg/actuation HFA MDI	20%
	50, 100, and 250 mcg/dose DPI, Diskus	15%
Mometasone furoate (MF)	110 and 220 mcg/dose DPI, Twisthaler; 100 mcg and 200 mcg/actuation HFA MDI	11%

Comparative Daily Dosages (mcg) of Inhaled Corticosteroids

	Low Daily Dose Child[a]/Adult	Medium Daily Dose Child[a]/Adult	High Daily Dose Child[a]/Adult
BDP			
HFA MDI	80–160/80–240	>160–320/>240–480	>320/>480
BUD			
DPI	180–360/180–540	>360–720/>540–1080	>720/>1080
Nebules	500/UK	1000/UK	2000/UK
CIC HFA MDI	80–160/160–320	>160–320/>320–640	>320/>640
FLU			
HFA MDI	160/320	320/320–640	≥640/>640
FFDPI		UK/100	UK/200
FP			
HFA MDI	88–176/88–264	176–352/264–440	>352/>440
DPIs	100–200/100–300	200–400/300–500	>400/>500
MF, DPI	110/110–220	220–440/>220–440	>440/>440

[a]5–11 years of age, except for BUD Nebules, which is 2–11 years of age. UK, unknown.

TABLE 77–3	Comparison of Systemic Corticosteroids			
Systemic	Anti-inflammatory Potency	Mineralocorticoid Potency	Duration of Biologic Activity (Hours)	Elimination Half-Life (Hours)
Hydrocortisone	1	1	8–12	1.5–2
Prednisone	4	0.8	12–36	2.5–3.5
Methylprednisolone	5	0.5	12–36	3.3
Dexamethasone	25	0	36–72	3.4–4

- **Figure** 77–5 gives recommended dosages, monitoring schedules, and dosage adjustments for theophylline.
- Sustained-release oral preparations are preferred for outpatients, but each product has different release characteristics. Preparations unaffected by food that can be administered every 12 or 24 hours are preferable.
- Adverse effects include nausea, vomiting, tachycardia, jitteriness, and difficulty sleeping; more severe toxicities include cardiac tachyarrhythmias and seizures.
- Sustained-release theophylline is less effective than inhaled corticosteroids and no more effective than oral sustained-release β_2-agonists, cromolyn, or leukotriene antagonists.
- Addition of theophylline to optimal inhaled corticosteroids is similar to doubling the dose of the inhaled corticosteroid and is less effective overall than long-acting β_2-agonists as adjunctive therapy.

Anticholinergics

- **Ipratropium bromide** and **tiotropium bromide** produce bronchodilation only in cholinergic-mediated bronchoconstriction. Anticholinergics are effective bronchodilators but are not as effective as β_2-agonists. They attenuate but do not block allergen- or exercise-induced asthma in a dose-dependent fashion.
  Time to reach maximum bronchodilation from aerosolized ipratropium is longer than from aerosolized short-acting β_2-agonists (30–60 min vs 5–10 min). However, some bronchodilation is seen within 30 seconds, and 50% of maximum response occurs within 3 minutes. Ipratropium bromide has a duration of action of 4 to 8 hours; tiotropium bromide has a duration of 24 hours.

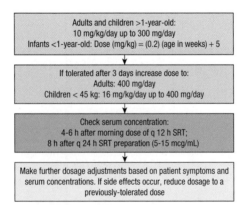

FIGURE 77–5. **Algorithm for slow titration of theophylline dosage and guide for final dosage adjustment based on serum theophylline concentration measurement.**

- In acute exacerbations, inhaled ipratropium bromide produces a further improvement in lung function of 10% to 15% over inhaled β2-agonists alone. When added to initial therapy, ipratropium bromide reduces the hospitalization rate in patients with moderate to severe exacerbations.
- Inhaled ipratropium bromide is only indicated as adjunctive therapy in severe acute asthma not completely responsive to β_2-agonists alone.

Magnesium Sulfate

- Magnesium sulfate is a moderately potent bronchodilator, producing relaxation of smooth muscle by blocking calcium ion influx into smooth muscles; it may also have antiinflammatory effects.
- For patients with severe asthma exacerbations, a single 2-gram IV infusion may reduce hospital admissions in adults who have an FEV_1 <25% to 30% predicted upon arrival in the emergency department, children and adults who have persistent hypoxemia after standard treatment, and children whose FEV_1 remains below 60% predicted after 1 hour of standard treatment. Adverse effects include hypotension, facial flushing, sweating, depressed deep tendon reflexes, hypothermia, and CNS and respiratory depression.

Leukotriene Modifiers

- **Zafirlukast** (Accolate) and **montelukast** (Singulair) are oral leukotriene receptor antagonists that reduce the proinflammatory (increased microvascular permeability and airway edema) and bronchoconstriction effects of leukotriene D_4. In persistent asthma, they improve pulmonary function tests, decrease nocturnal awakenings and β_2-agonist use, and improve symptoms. However, they are less effective than low-dose inhaled corticosteroids. They are not used to treat acute exacerbations and must be taken on a regular basis, even during symptom-free periods. Adult zafirlukast dose is 20 mg twice daily, taken at least 1 hour before or 2 hours after meals; dose for children ages 5 through 11 years is 10 mg twice daily. Montelukast adult dose is 10 mg once daily, taken in the evening without regard to food; dose for children ages 6 to 14 years is one 5-mg chewable tablet daily in the evening.
- Rare elevations in serum aminotransferase concentrations and clinical hepatitis have been reported. An idiosyncratic syndrome similar to the Churg–Strauss syndrome, with marked circulating eosinophilia, heart failure, and associated eosinophilic vasculitis, has been reported rarely; a direct causal association has not been established.
- **Zileuton** (Zyflo) is a 5-lipoxygenase inhibitor; use is limited due to potential for elevated hepatic enzymes, especially in first 3 months of therapy, and inhibition of metabolism of some drugs metabolized by CYP3A4 (eg, theophylline and warfarin). Dose of zileuton tablets is 600 mg four times daily with meals and at bedtime. Dose of zileuton extended-release tablets is two 600-mg tablets twice daily, within 1 hour after morning and evening meals (total daily dose 2400 mg).

Omalizumab

- **Omalizumab** (Xolair) is an anti-IgE antibody approved for treatment of allergic asthma not well controlled by oral or inhaled corticosteroids. Dosage is determined by baseline total serum IgE (international units/mL) and body weight (kg). Doses range from 150 to 375 mg subcutaneously at either 2- or 4-week intervals.
- Because of high cost, omalizumab is only indicated as step 5 or 6 care for patients with allergies and severe persistent asthma inadequately controlled with combination of high-dose inhaled corticosteroids and long-acting β_2-agonists and at risk for severe exacerbations.
- Because of 0.2% incidence of anaphylaxis, observe patients for a reasonable period after injection because 70% of reactions occur within 2 hours. Some reactions have occurred up to 24 hours after injection.

EVALUATION OF THERAPEUTIC OUTCOMES

CHRONIC ASTHMA

- The two domains of asthma control are "symptom control" and "future risk of adverse outcomes." Symptom control is assessed by frequency of daytime and nighttime asthma symptoms, reliever medication use, and activity limitations; poor symptom control is an indicator of future risk for exacerbations.
- Future risk of adverse outcomes includes assessment of risks for future exacerbations, fixed airflow limitation (and thus diminished response to therapy), and medication adverse effects. To assess the risk for future exacerbations, lung function should be measured before the start of treatment and then 2 months later when maximum response to controller medications is likely attained.
- During ongoing care, measure spirometry yearly but reserve long-term PEF monitoring for patients with severe asthma.
- Validated questionnaires can be administered regularly, such as the Asthma Control Test, Asthma Therapy Assessment Questionnaire, and Asthma Control Questionnaire.
- Ask patients about exercise tolerance because perceived good exercise tolerance may be biased by a sedentary lifestyle adapted to the frequency of bothersome symptoms.
- All patients on inhaled drugs should have their inhalation technique evaluated monthly initially and then every 3 to 6 months.
- After initiation of antiinflammatory therapy or increase in dosage, most patients should experience decreased symptoms within 1 to 2 weeks and achieve maximum improvement within 4 to 8 weeks. Improvement in baseline FEV_1 or PEF should follow a similar time course, but decrease in BHR as measured by morning PEF, PEF variability, and exercise tolerance may take longer and improve over 1 to 3 months.

ACUTE SEVERE ASTHMA

- Patients at risk for acute severe exacerbations should monitor morning peak flows at home.
- Monitor lung function, either spirometry or peak flows, 5 to 10 minutes after each treatment. Monitoring of pulse oximetry, lung auscultation, and observation for supraclavicular retractions are useful.
- Most patients respond within the first hour of initial inhaled β-agonists. Monitor patients not achieving initial response every 0.5 to 1 hour.

See Chapter 26, Asthma, authored by Christine A. Sorkness and Kathryn Blake, for a more detailed discussion of this topic.

CHAPTER 78

Chronic Obstructive Pulmonary Disease

- Chronic obstructive pulmonary disease (COPD) is characterized by progressive airflow limitation that is not fully reversible. Two principal conditions (referred to as phenotypes) include:
  - ✓ *Chronic bronchitis*: chronic or recurrent excess mucus secretion with cough that occurs on most days for at least 3 months of the year for at least 2 consecutive years.
  - ✓ *Emphysema*: abnormal, permanent enlargement of the airspaces distal to the terminal bronchioles, accompanied by destruction of their walls, without fibrosis.

PATHOPHYSIOLOGY

- Chronic inflammatory changes lead to destructive changes and chronic airflow limitation. The most common cause is exposure to tobacco smoke.
- Inhalation of noxious particles and gases activates neutrophils, macrophages, and CD8$^+$ lymphocytes, which release chemical mediators, including tumor necrosis factor-α, interleukin-8, and leukotriene B$_4$. Inflammatory cells and mediators lead to widespread destructive changes in airways, pulmonary vasculature, and lung parenchyma.
- Oxidative stress and imbalance between aggressive and protective defense systems in the lungs (proteases and antiproteases) may also occur. Oxidants generated by cigarette smoke react with and damage proteins and lipids, contributing to tissue damage. Oxidants also promote inflammation and exacerbate protease–antiprotease imbalance by inhibiting antiprotease activity.
- The protective antiprotease α$_1$-antitrypsin (AAT) inhibits protease enzymes, including neutrophil elastase. In presence of unopposed AAT activity, elastase attacks elastin, a major component of alveolar walls. Hereditary AAT deficiency increases risk for premature emphysema. In emphysema from cigarette smoking, imbalance is associated with increased protease activity or reduced antiprotease activity.
- Inflammatory exudate in airways leads to increased number and size of goblet cells and mucus glands. Mucus secretion increases and ciliary motility is impaired. There is thickening of the smooth muscle and connective tissue in airways. Chronic inflammation leads to scarring and fibrosis. Diffuse airway narrowing occurs and is more prominent in small peripheral airways.
- Smoking-related COPD usually results in centrilobular emphysema that primarily affects respiratory bronchioles. Panlobular emphysema is seen in AAT deficiency and extends to the alveolar ducts and sacs.
- Vascular changes include thickening of pulmonary vessels that may lead to endothelial dysfunction of pulmonary arteries. Later, structural changes increase pulmonary pressures, especially during exercise. In severe COPD, secondary pulmonary hypertension leads to right-sided heart failure (cor pulmonale).

CLINICAL PRESENTATION

- Initial symptoms include chronic cough and sputum production; patients may experience cough for several years before dyspnea develops.
- Physical examination is normal in most patients in milder stages. When airflow limitation becomes severe, patients may have cyanosis of mucosal membranes, development of a "barrel chest" due to hyperinflation of the lungs, increased resting respiratory rate, shallow breathing, pursing of lips during expiration, and use of accessory respiratory muscles.
- Patients experiencing COPD exacerbation may have worsening dyspnea, increased sputum volume, or increased sputum purulence. Other features of exacerbation include chest tightness, increased need for bronchodilators, malaise, fatigue, and decreased exercise tolerance.

DIAGNOSIS

- Diagnosis is based in part on patient symptoms and history of exposure to risk factors such as tobacco smoke and occupational substances.
- Classification of disease severity is based on assessment of airflow limitation by spirometry, measurement of symptom severity, and assessment of exacerbation frequency. Symptom severity should be measured at baseline and then during routine visits using the COPD Assessment Test (CAT), the modified Medical Research Council (mMRC) scale, or the Clinical COPD Questionnaire (CCQ). Patients are first classified according to severity of airflow obstruction (Grades 1–4) and then placed into a group (Patient Category A, B, C, or D) based on the impact of symptoms and risk for future exacerbations.

SPIROMETRY

- The presence of airflow limitation should be confirmed with spirometry. The forced expiratory volume after 1 second (FEV_1) is reduced except in very mild disease. The forced vital capacity (FVC) may also be decreased. The hallmark of COPD is reduced FEV_1:FVC ratio to less than 70%. It is no longer recommended to obtain prebronchodilator values or to calculate the degree of reversibility after bronchodilator administration in order to diagnose COPD. Postbronchodilator spirometry results should be used in assessing lung function in patients with COPD.

ARTERIAL BLOOD GASES

- Significant changes in arterial blood gases (ABG) are not usually present until FEV_1 is less than 1 L. At this stage, hypoxemia and hypercapnia may become chronic. Hypoxemia usually occurs initially with exertion but develops at rest as the disease progresses.
- Patients with severe COPD can have low arterial oxygen tension (partial pressure of O_2 [Pao_2] 45–60 mm Hg) and elevated arterial carbon dioxide tension (partial pressure of CO_2 [$Paco_2$] 50–60 mm Hg). Hypoxemia results from hypoventilation (V) of lung tissue relative to perfusion (Q). The low V:Q ratio progresses over several years, resulting in a decline in Pao_2.
- Some patients lose ability to increase rate or depth of respiration in response to persistent hypoxemia. As COPD progresses and lung function and gas exchange worsen, some patients exhibit chronic hypercapnia and are referred to as carbon dioxide retainers. In these patients, the central respiratory response to chronically increased $Paco_2$ can be blunted. Because changes in Pao_2 and $Paco_2$ are subtle and progress over many years, the pH is usually near normal because the kidneys compensate by retaining bicarbonate.
- If acute respiratory distress develops (eg, due to pneumonia or COPD exacerbation), $Paco_2$ may rise sharply, resulting worsening respiratory acidosis.

DIAGNOSIS OF ACUTE RESPIRATORY FAILURE IN COPD

- Diagnosis of acute respiratory failure is based on acute drop in Pao_2 of 10–15 mm Hg or any acute increase in $Paco_2$ that decreases serum pH to 7.3 or less.
- Acute manifestations include restlessness, confusion, tachycardia, diaphoresis, cyanosis, hypotension, irregular breathing, miosis, and unconsciousness.
- The most common cause of acute respiratory failure is acute exacerbation of bronchitis with increased sputum volume and viscosity. This worsens obstruction and further impairs alveolar ventilation, thereby worsening hypoxemia and hypercapnia.

TREATMENT

- <u>Goals of Treatment</u>: Prevent or minimize disease progression, relieve symptoms, improve exercise tolerance, improve health status, prevent and treat exacerbations, prevent and treat complications, and reduce morbidity and mortality.

NONPHARMACOLOGIC THERAPY

- Patients should receive education about their disease, treatment plans, and strategies to slow progression and prevent complications.
- Smoking cessation is the most important intervention to prevent development and progression of COPD. Reducing exposure to occupational dust and fumes as well as other environmental toxins is also important.
- Pulmonary rehabilitation programs include exercise training, breathing exercises, optimal medical treatment, psychosocial support, and health education.
- Administer the influenza vaccine annually during influenza season. The CDC recommends giving the 23-valent pneumococcal polysaccharide vaccine (PPSV23) for people from ages 2 to 64 who have chronic lung disease, smokers over the age of 18, and all people older than 65 years. The GOLD guidelines recommend the pneumococcal vaccine for COPD patients less than age 65 only if the FEV_1 is less than 40% predicted.
- Once patients are stabilized as outpatients and pharmacotherapy is optimized, institute long-term oxygen therapy if either (1) resting Pao_2 less than 55 mm Hg or Sao_2 less than 88% with or without hypercapnia, or (2) resting Pao_2 55 to 60 mm Hg or Sao_2 less than 88% with evidence of right-sided heart failure, polycythemia, or pulmonary hypertension. The goal is to raise Pao_2 above 60 mm Hg.

PHARMACOLOGIC THERAPY

- An approach to initial pharmacotherapy of stable COPD based on combined assessment of airflow limitation, symptom severity, and risk of exacerbations is shown in Table 78–1. Treat patients with intermittent symptoms and low risk for exacerbations (Group A) with short-acting inhaled bronchodilators as needed. When symptoms become more persistent (Group B), initiate long-acting inhaled bronchodilators. For patients at high risk for exacerbations (Groups C and D), consider inhaled corticosteroids (ICS) combined with long-acting bronchodilators.
- Short-acting inhaled bronchodilators (β_2-agonists or anticholinergics) are initial therapy for patients with intermittent symptoms; they relieve symptoms and increase exercise tolerance.
- Long-acting inhaled β_2-agonists or anticholinergics relieve symptoms, reduce exacerbation frequency, and improve quality of life and health status. They are recommended for moderate to severe COPD when symptoms occur on a regular and consistent basis, when short-acting agents provide inadequate relief, and for patients at risk for exacerbation (Category C and D).

TABLE 78–1	Recommended Pharmacologic Therapy for Stable COPD		
Patient Category	**First Choice**	**Second Choice**	**Alternate Therapy**
A (less symptoms, less risk)	SABA prn or SAMA prn	LAMA or LABA or SAMA and SABA	Theophylline
B (more symptoms, less risk)	LAMA or LABA	LAMA and LABA	SABA and/or SAMA theophylline
C (less symptoms, more risk)	ICS and LABA or LAMA	LAMA and LABA or LAMA and PDE4I or LABA and PDE4I	SABA and/or SAMA theophylline
D (more symptoms, more risk)	ICS and LABA and/or LAMA	ICS and LABA and LAMA or ICS and LABA and PDE4I or LAMA and LABA or LAMA and PDE4I	SABA and/or SAMA Theophylline

(ICS, inhaled corticosteroids; LABA, long acting beta agonist; LAMA, long-acting muscarinic antagonists; PDE4I, phosphodiesterase type 4 inhibitor (roflumilast); SABA, short acting beta-agonist; SAMA, short-acting muscarinic antagonists.)

SECTION 15 | Respiratory Disorders

Sympathomimetics (β₂-Selective Agonists)

- β₂-Selective agonists cause relaxation of bronchial smooth muscle and bronchodilation and may also improve mucociliary clearance. Administration via metered-dose inhaler (MDI) or dry-powder inhaler (DPI) is at least as effective as nebulization therapy and is usually favored because of cost and convenience.
- **Short-acting β₂-agonists (SABA)** are preferred over other short-acting sympathomimetics (isoproterenol, metaproterenol, isoetharine) because they have greater β₂ selectivity and longer durations of action (4–6 hours). Inhalation is preferred over oral and parenteral administration in terms of efficacy and adverse effects. SABA can be used for acute relief of symptoms or on a scheduled basis to prevent or reduce symptoms. If patients do not achieve adequate control with a SABA alone, it is reasonable to add ipratropium bromide. Recommended doses of SABA are as follows:
  ✓ **Albuterol** inhalation aerosol (Proventil HFA, Ventolin HFA, ProAir HFA) and inhalation powder (ProAir RespiClick) 1 to 2 inhalations every 4 to 6 hours
  ✓ **Levalbuterol** inhalation aerosol (Xopenex HFA) 1 to 2 inhalations every 4 to 6 hours
  ✓ **Terbutaline** oral tablets 2.5 to 5 mg 3 times daily, 6 hours apart (maximum 15 mg/day)
- **Long-acting β₂-agonists (LABA)** are dosed every 12 to 24 hours on a scheduled basis and provide bronchodilation throughout the dosing interval. In addition to providing greater convenience than SABA for patients with persistent symptoms, LABA produce similar or superior improvements in lung function, symptom relief, reduced exacerbation frequency, and need for hospitalization. These agents are not recommended for acute relief of symptoms. Recommended doses by inhalation for maintenance therapy are as follows:
  ✓ **Salmeterol** inhalation powder (Serevent) 1 inhalation every 12 hours
  ✓ **Formoterol** inhalation powder (Foradil) 1 inhalation every 12 hours
  ✓ **Arformoterol** inhalation solution (Brovana) 1 × 15 mcg/2 mL vial by nebulization every 12 hours
  ✓ **Indacaterol** inhalation powder (Arcapta) 1 inhalation once daily
  ✓ **Olodaterol** inhalation spray (Striverdi Respimat) 2 inhalations once daily
  ✓ **Vilanterol** is available in the U.S. only as a combination product with fluticasone (Breo Ellipta, see *Corticosteroids* section later) or the anticholinergic umeclidinium (Anoro Ellipta, see *Combination* section later)

Anticholinergics

- When given by inhalation, anticholinergics (also known as muscarinic antagonists) produce bronchodilation by competitively inhibiting cholinergic receptors in bronchial smooth muscle.
- **Short-acting muscarinic antagonists (SAMA)** for COPD include primarily ipratropium bromide. It has a slower onset of action than SABA (15–20 min vs 5 min for albuterol). It may be less suitable for as-needed use but is often prescribed in this manner. Ipratropium has a more prolonged effect than SABA, with the peak effect occurring in 1.5 to 2 hours and the duration up to 8 hours. If patients do not achieve adequate control with ipratropium alone, it is reasonable to combine it with an SABA. The most frequent patient complaints are dry mouth, nausea, and, occasionally, metallic taste. Because it is poorly absorbed systemically, anticholinergic side effects are uncommon (eg, blurred vision, urinary retention, nausea, and tachycardia). The recommended doses for maintenance COPD treatment are as follows:
  ✓ **Ipratropium bromide** inhalation aerosol (Atrovent HFA) 2 inhalations four times per day (maximum 12 inhalations/day). Doses are often titrated upward to 24 inhalations per day.
  ✓ **Ipratropium bromide** nebulization solution 500 mcg every 6 to 8 hours
- **Long-acting muscarinic antagonists (LAMA)** available in the United States and recommended doses for maintenance treatment are as follows:
  ✓ **Tiotropium bromide** inhalation spray (Spiriva Respimat) 2 inhalations once daily or inhalation powder (Spiriva HandiHaler) one capsule (with 2 inhalations) once daily

✓ **Umeclidinium** inhalation powder (Incruse Ellipta) 1 inhalation once daily
✓ **Aclidinium bromide** inhalation powder (Tudorza Pressair) 1 inhalation twice daily
✓ **Glycopyrrolate** inhalation powder (Seebri Neohaler) 1 inhalation twice daily

Combination Anticholinergics and Sympathomimetics

- Combination of an inhaled anticholinergic and β_2-agonist is often used, especially as the disease progresses and symptoms worsen. Combinations allow the lowest effective doses to be used and reduce adverse effects from individual agents. Combination of both short- and long-acting β_2-agonists with anticholinergics provides added symptomatic relief and improvements in pulmonary function. Recommended doses for COPD maintenance therapy include:
  ✓ **Ipratropium plus albuterol** inhalation spray (Combivent Respimat) 1 inhalation four to six times per day
  ✓ **Ipratropium plus albuterol** nebulization solution (DuoNeb) one 3-mL vial four times per day by nebulization with up to two additional 3-mL doses allowed per day, if needed.
- Several combination products containing a LABA and LAMA are available. Clinical trials have demonstrated improvement in lung function and symptom scores with combination long-acting bronchodilators compared to single-agent therapy, but additional benefit in exacerbation reduction needs to be evaluated. Recommended doses for maintenance treatment are as follows:
  ✓ **Vilanterol/umeclidinium** inhalation powder (Anoro Ellipta) 1 inhalation once daily
  ✓ **Olodaterol/tiotropium bromide** inhalation spray (Stiolto Respimat) 2 inhalations once daily
  ✓ **Indacaterol/glycopyrrolate** inhalation powder (Utibron Neohaler) 1 inhalation twice daily

Methylxanthines

- **Theophylline** and **aminophylline** produce bronchodilation by inhibiting phosphodiesterase and other mechanisms.
- Chronic theophylline use in COPD may improve lung function, including vital capacity and FEV_1. Subjectively, theophylline reduces dyspnea, increases exercise tolerance, and improves respiratory drive.
- Methylxanthines have a very limited role in COPD therapy because of drug interactions and interpatient variability in dosage requirements. Theophylline may be considered in patients intolerant of or unable to use inhaled bronchodilators. It may also be added to the regimen of patients not achieving optimal response to inhaled bronchodilators.
- Subjective parameters, such as perceived improvements in dyspnea and exercise tolerance, are important in assessing acceptability of methylxanthines for COPD patients.
- Sustained-release theophylline preparations improve adherence and achieve more consistent serum concentrations than rapid-release products. Caution should be used in switching from one sustained-release preparation to another because of variations in sustained-release characteristics.
- Initiate therapy with 200 mg twice daily and titrated upward every 3 to 5 days to the target dose; most patients require 400 to 900 mg daily.
- Make dose adjustments based on trough serum concentrations. A therapeutic range of 8 to 15 mcg/mL (44.4–83.3 µmol/L) is often targeted to minimize risk of toxicity. Once a dose is established, monitor concentrations once or twice a year unless the disease worsens, medications that interfere with theophylline metabolism are added, or toxicity is suspected.
- Common theophylline side effects include dyspepsia, nausea, vomiting, diarrhea, headache, dizziness, and tachycardia. Arrhythmias and seizures may occur, especially at toxic concentrations.

- Factors that may decrease theophylline clearance and lead to reduced dosage requirements include advanced age, bacterial or viral pneumonia, heart failure, liver dysfunction, hypoxemia from acute decompensation, and drugs such as cimetidine, macrolides, and fluoroquinolone antibiotics.
- Factors that may enhance theophylline clearance and result in need for higher doses include tobacco and marijuana smoking, hyperthyroidism, and drugs such as phenytoin, phenobarbital, and rifampin.

Corticosteroids

- Corticosteroids reduce capillary permeability to decrease mucus, inhibit release of proteolytic enzymes from leukocytes, and inhibit prostaglandins.
- Appropriate situations for corticosteroids in COPD include (1) short-term systemic use for acute exacerbations and (2) inhalation therapy for chronic stable COPD in select patients. Chronic systemic corticosteroids should be avoided in COPD management because of questionable benefits and high risk of toxicity.
- Inhaled corticosteroid therapy may be beneficial in patients with severe COPD and at high risk of exacerbation (Groups C and D) who are not controlled with inhaled bronchodilators.
- Side effects of inhaled corticosteroids are mild and include hoarseness, sore throat, oral candidiasis, and skin bruising. Severe side effects such as adrenal suppression, osteoporosis, and cataract formation occur less frequently than with systemic corticosteroids, but clinicians should monitor patients receiving high-dose chronic inhaled therapy.
- Combination of inhaled corticosteroids and long-acting bronchodilators is associated with greater improvements in FEV_1, health status, and exacerbation frequency than either agent alone. Availability of combination inhalers makes administration of both drugs convenient and decreases the total number of inhalations needed daily. Recommended doses for COPD maintenance include:
  ✓ **Budesonide plus formoterol** inhalation aerosol (Symbicort) 160 mcg/4.5 mcg, 2 inhalations twice daily
  ✓ **Fluticasone plus salmeterol** inhalation powder (Advair Diskus DPI) 250 mcg/50 mcg, 1 inhalation twice daily
  ✓ **Fluticasone plus vilanterol** (Breo Ellipta) inhalation powder 100 mcg/25 mcg, 1 inhalation once daily)
- For patients with more symptoms and at high risk of exacerbation (category D), triple therapy (LABA plus LAMA plus inhaled corticosteroid) may be considered as a first or second choice.

Phosphodiesterase Inhibitors

- **Roflumilast** (Daliresp) is a phosphodiesterase 4 (PDE4) indicated to reduce risk of exacerbations in patients with severe COPD associated with chronic bronchitis and a history of exacerbations.
- The dose is 500 mcg orally once daily, with or without food. Major adverse effects include weight loss and neuropsychiatric effects such as suicidal thoughts, insomnia, anxiety, and new or worsened depression.
- Roflumilast is metabolized by CYP3A4 and 1A2; coadministration with strong CYP P450 inducers is not recommended due to potential for subtherapeutic plasma concentrations. Use caution when administering roflumilast with strong CYP P450 inhibitors due to potential for adverse effects.
- Roflumilast may be beneficial in patients with severe or very severe COPD who are at high risk of exacerbation (Group C and D) and are not controlled by inhaled bronchodilators. It may also be considered for patients who are intolerant or unable to use inhaled bronchodilators or corticosteroids. Roflumilast is not recommended for use with theophylline because the drugs share similar mechanisms.

TREATMENT OF COPD EXACERBATIONS

- <u>Goals of Treatment</u>: The goals are to: (1) prevent hospitalization or reduce length of hospital stay, (2) prevent acute respiratory failure and death, (3) resolve symptoms, and (4) return to baseline clinical status and quality of life.

NONPHARMACOLOGIC THERAPY

- Provide oxygen therapy for patients with significant hypoxemia (eg, oxygen saturation less than 90%). Use caution because many COPD patients rely on mild hypoxemia to trigger their drive to breathe. Overly aggressive oxygen administration to patients with chronic hypercapnia may result in respiratory depression and respiratory failure. Adjust oxygen to achieve Pao_2 greater than 60 mm Hg or oxygen saturation (Sao_2) greater than 90%. Obtain ABG after oxygen initiation to monitor CO_2 retention resulting from hypoventilation.
- Noninvasive positive-pressure ventilation (NPPV) provides ventilatory support with oxygen and pressurized airflow using a face or nasal mask without endotracheal intubation. NPPV is not appropriate for patients with altered mental status, severe acidosis, respiratory arrest, or cardiovascular instability. Intubation and mechanical ventilation may be needed in patients failing NPPV or who are poor candidates for NPPV.

PHARMACOLOGIC THERAPY

Bronchodilators

- Dose and frequency of bronchodilators are increased during acute exacerbations to provide symptomatic relief. Short-acting β2-agonists are preferred because of rapid onset of action. Anticholinergic agents may be added if symptoms persist despite increased doses of β2-agonists.
- Bronchodilators may be administered via MDI, DPI, or nebulization with equal efficacy. Nebulization may be considered for patients with severe dyspnea who are unable to hold their breath after actuation of an MDI.
- Theophylline should generally be avoided due to lack of evidence documenting benefit. It may be considered for patients not responding to other therapies.

Corticosteroids

- Clinical trial results suggest that patients with acute COPD exacerbations should receive a short course of IV or oral corticosteroids. Although optimal dose and duration are unknown, prednisone 40 mg orally daily (or equivalent) for 10 to 14 days can be effective for most patients.
- If treatment is continued for longer than 2 weeks, employ a tapering oral schedule because of hypothalamic-pituitary-adrenal axis suppression.

Antimicrobial Therapy

- Antibiotics are of most benefit and should be initiated if at least two of the following three symptoms are present: (1) increased dyspnea, (2) increased sputum volume, and (3) increased sputum purulence. Utility of sputum Gram stain and culture is questionable because some patients have chronic bacterial colonization of the bronchial tree between exacerbations.
- Selection of empiric antimicrobial therapy should be based on the most likely organisms: *Haemophilus influenzae, Moraxella catarrhalis, Streptococcus pneumoniae,* and *Haemophilus parainfluenzae.* Site-specific sensitivities should also be considered in drug selection.
- Initiate therapy within 24 hours of symptoms to prevent unnecessary hospitalization and generally continue for at least 7 to 10 days. Five-day courses with some agents may produce comparable efficacy.

- In uncomplicated exacerbations, recommended therapy includes a **macrolide** (**azithromycin** or **clarithromycin**), **second- or third-generation cephalosporin**, or **doxycycline**. Avoid trimethoprim–sulfamethoxazole because of increasing pneumococcal resistance. Amoxicillin and first-generation cephalosporins are not recommended because of β-lactamase susceptibility. Erythromycin is not recommended because of insufficient activity against *H. influenzae*.
- In complicated exacerbations where drug-resistant pneumococci, β-lactamase-producing *H. influenzae* and *M. catarrhalis*, and some enteric gram-negative organisms may be present, recommended therapy includes **amoxicillin/clavulanate** or a fluoroquinolone with enhanced pneumococcal activity (**levofloxacin, gemifloxacin,** or **moxifloxacin**).
- In complicated exacerbations with risk of *Pseudomonas aeruginosa*, recommended therapy includes a fluoroquinolone with enhanced pneumococcal and *P. aeruginosa* activity (**levofloxacin**). If IV therapy is required, a β-lactamase-resistant penicillin with antipseudomonal activity or a third- or fourth-generation cephalosporin with antipseudomonal activity should be used.

EVALUATION OF THERAPEUTIC OUTCOMES

- In chronic stable COPD, assess pulmonary function tests with any therapy addition, change in dose, or deletion of therapy. Other outcome measures are dyspnea score, quality-of-life assessments, and exacerbation rates (including emergency department visits and hospitalizations).
- In acute exacerbations of COPD, assess white blood cell count, vital signs, chest radiograph, and changes in frequency of dyspnea, sputum volume, and sputum purulence at the onset and throughout the exacerbation. In more severe exacerbations, ABG and Sao_2 should also be monitored.
- Evaluate patient medication adherence, side effects, potential drug interactions, and subjective measures of quality of life.

See Chapter 27, Chronic Obstructive Pulmonary Disease, authored by Sharya V. Bourdet and Dennis M. Williams, for a more detailed discussion of this topic.

CHAPTER 79

Benign Prostatic Hyperplasia

- *Benign prostatic hyperplasia* (BPH), a nearly ubiquitous condition, is the most common benign neoplasm of American men.

PATHOPHYSIOLOGY

- Three types of prostate gland tissue: epithelial or glandular, stromal or smooth muscle, and capsule. Both stromal tissue and capsule are embedded with α_1-adrenergic receptors.
- The precise pathophysiologic mechanisms that cause BPH are not clear. Both intraprostatic dihydrotestosterone (DHT) and type II 5α-reductase are thought to be involved.
- BPH commonly results from both static (gradual enlargement of the prostate) and dynamic (agents or situations that increase α-adrenergic tone and constrict the gland's smooth muscle) factors. Examples of drugs that can exacerbate symptoms include testosterone, α-adrenergic agonists (eg, decongestants), and those with significant anticholinergic effects (eg, antihistamines, phenothiazines, tricyclic antidepressants, antispasmodics, and antiparkinsonian agents).

CLINICAL PRESENTATION

- Patients present with a variety of signs and symptoms categorized as obstructive or irritative. Symptoms vary over time.
- Obstructive signs and symptoms result when dynamic and/or static factors reduce bladder emptying. Patients experience urinary hesitancy, urine dribbles out of the penis, and the bladder feels full even after voiding.
- Irritative signs and symptoms are common and result from long-standing obstruction at the bladder neck. Patients experience urinary frequency, urgency, and nocturia.
- BPH progression may produce complications including chronic kidney disease, gross hematuria, urinary incontinence, recurrent urinary tract infection, bladder diverticula, and bladder stones.

DIAGNOSIS

- Includes careful medical history, physical examination, objective measures of bladder emptying (eg, peak and average urinary flow rate and postvoid residual [PVR] urine volume), and laboratory tests (eg, urinalysis and prostate-specific antigen [PSA]).
- On digital rectal examination, the prostate is usually but not always enlarged (>20 g), soft, smooth, and symmetric.

TREATMENT

- <u>Goals of Treatment</u>: The goals are to control symptoms, prevent progression of complications, and delay need for surgical intervention.
- Management options include watchful waiting, drug therapy, and surgical intervention. The choice depends on severity of signs and symptoms (**Table 79–1**).

TABLE 79-1	Categories of BPH Disease Severity Based on Symptoms and Signs	
Disease Severity	AUA Symptom Score	Typical Symptoms and Signs
Mild	≤7	Asymptomatic Peak urinary flow rate <10 mL/s PVR urine volume >25–50 mL
Moderate	8–19	All of the above signs plus obstructive voiding symptoms and irritative voiding symptoms (signs of detrusor instability)
Severe	≥20	All of the above plus one or more complications of BPH

(AUA, American Urological Association; BPH, benign prostatic hyperplasia; PVR, postvoid residual.)

- Watchful waiting is appropriate for patients with mild disease (Fig. 79–1). Patients are reassessed at 6 to 12 month intervals and educated about behavior modification, such as fluid restriction before bedtime, minimizing caffeine and alcohol intake, frequent emptying of the bladder, and avoiding drugs that exacerbate voiding symptoms.

PHARMACOLOGIC THERAPY

- Pharmacologic therapy is appropriate for patients with moderate BPH symptoms and as an interim measure for patients with severe BPH.
- Pharmacologic therapy interferes with the stimulatory effect of testosterone on prostate gland enlargement (reduces the static factor), relaxes prostatic smooth muscle (reduces the dynamic factor), or relaxes bladder detrusor muscle (Table 79–2).
- Initiate therapy with an α_1-adrenergic antagonist for faster onset of symptom relief. Select a 5α-reductase inhibitor in patients with a prostate gland more than 40 g who cannot tolerate the cardiovascular adverse effects of α_1-adrenergic antagonists. Consider combination therapy for symptomatic patients with a prostate gland more than 40 g and PSA of 1.4 ng/mL or more (1.4 mcg/L).
- Consider monotherapy with a phosphodiesterase inhibitor or use in combination with an α-adrenergic antagonist when erectile dysfunction and BPH are present.

α-Adrenergic Antagonists

- α-Adrenergic antagonists relax smooth muscle in the prostate and bladder neck, increasing urinary flow rates by 2 to 3 mL/sec in 60% to 70% of patients and reducing PVR urine volumes. These agents do not decrease prostate volume or PSA levels.
- **Prazosin, terazosin, doxazosin**, and **alfuzosin** are second-generation α_1-adrenergic antagonists. They antagonize peripheral vascular α_1-adrenergic receptors in addition to those in the prostate. Adverse effects include first-dose syncope, orthostatic hypotension, and dizziness. Current practice guidelines do not recommend Prazosin due to multiple doses/day and significant cardiovascular adverse effects. Alfuzosin is less likely to cause cardiovascular adverse effects than other second-generation agents and is considered functionally and clinically uroselective.
- **Tamsulosin** and **silodosin**, third-generation α_1-adrenergic antagonists, are selective for prostatic α_{1A}-receptors. Therefore, they do not cause peripheral vascular smooth muscle relaxation and associated hypotension. Dose titration is minimal and the onset of peak action is seen within a week.
- Potential drug interactions include decreased metabolism of α_1-adrenergic antagonists with CYP 3A4 inhibitors (eg, **cimetidine** and **diltiazem**) and increased catabolism of α_1-adrenergic antagonists with concurrent use of CYP 3A4 stimulators (eg, **carbamazepine** and **phenytoin**).
- Reduce the dose of silodosin in patients with moderate renal impairment or hepatic dysfunction.

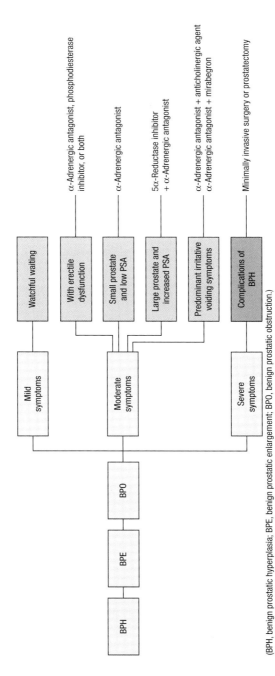

FIGURE 79-1. Management algorithm for benign prostatic hyperplasia (BPH).

(BPH, benign prostatic hyperplasia; BPE, benign prostatic enlargement; BPO, benign prostatic obstruction.)

TABLE 79-2	Dosing of Drugs Used in Treatment of Benign Prostatic Hyperplasia		
Drug	Brand Name	Initial Dose	Usual Dose	Special Population Dose
α-Adrenergic antagonists			
Prazosin	Minipress	0.5 mg twice a day orally	1–5 mg twice a day orally	For uptitrating the dose, double the dose every 2 weeks
Terazosin	Hytrin	1 mg at bedtime orally	10–20 mg daily orally	For uptitrating the dose, increase slowly to 2 mg, 5 mg, and then 10 mg daily in a stepwise fashion. Take extra care if the patient is taking other drugs that lower blood pressure
Doxazosin	Cardura Cardura XL	1 mg daily orally 4 mg daily orally	8 mg daily orally 4–8 mg daily	For the immediate-release formulation, doses of 16 mg daily have been used for hypertension. For the XL formulation, increase from 4 to 8 mg daily after a 3- to 4-week interval. When switching from the immediate- to the extended-release formulation, start at 4 mg of the extended-release formulation no matter what maintenance dose of immediate-release doxazosin the patient is taking
Alfuzosin	Uroxatral	10 mg daily orally	10 mg daily orally (no dose titration)	This is an extended-release formulation, and it should not be chewed or crushed. The drug should be taken after meals and used cautiously in patients with creatinine clearance is less than 30 mL/min (0.5 mL/s)
Tamsulosin	Flomax	0.4 mg daily orally	0.4–0.8 mg daily orally	This is an extended-release formulation, and it should not be chewed or crushed. The drug should be taken after meals. No dosage adjustment is needed in patients with renal or liver dysfunction. Allow several weeks after starting a dose before increasing to a higher dose
Silodosin	Rapaflo	8 mg daily orally	8 mg daily orally (no dose titration)	This drug is contraindicated when creatinine clearance is less than 30 mL/min (0.5 mL/s). If creatinine clearance is 30–50 mL/min (0.5–0.83 mL/s), use 4 mg daily orally, preferably after the same meal each day. Should not be given to patients on potent CYP 3A4 inhibitors or to patients known to be poor metabolizers of CYP 2D6.

5α-Reductase inhibitors

Finasteride	Proscar	5 mg daily orally	No dosage adjustment in patients with renal impairment. Use cautiously in patients with hepatic impairment
Dutasteride	Avodart	0.5 mg daily orally	No dosage adjustment in patients with renal impairment. Use cautiously in patients with hepatic impairment
Dutasteride + tamsulosin	Jalyn	1 tablet (equivalent to 0.5 mg dutasteride + 0.4 mg tamsulosin) daily orally	No dosage adjustment needed in patients with renal or hepatic impairment

Phosphodiesterase inhibitor

Tadalafil	Cialis	5 mg daily orally	If creatinine clearance is 30–50 mL/min (0.5–0.83 mL/s), use 2.5 mg daily orally. Do not use if creatinine clearance is less than 30 mL/min (0.5 mL/s)

Anticholinergic agents

Darifenacin	Enablex	7.5–15 mg daily orally	For uptitrating the dose, double the dose after 2 weeks. If the patient is taking a potent CYP3A4 inhibitor (eg, ketoconazole, itraconazole, ritonavir, nelfinavir, and clarithromycin), do not exceed 7.5 mg daily orally
Fesoterodine	Toviaz	4–8 mg daily orally	This is an extended-release formulation, and it should not be chewed or crushed. If the patient is taking a potent CYP3A4 inhibitor (eg, ketoconazole, itraconazole, ritonavir, nelfinavir, and clarithromycin), do not exceed 4 mg daily orally. If the creatinine clearance is less than 30 mL/min (0.5 mL/s), do not exceed 4 mg daily orally

(continued)

TABLE 79–2 Dosing of Drugs Used in Treatment of Benign Prostatic Hyperplasia (*Continued*)

Drug	Brand Name	Initial Dose	Usual Dose	Special Population Dose
Anticholinergic agents				
Oxybutynin	Ditropan	5 mg two to three times a day orally	5–10 mg two to three times a day orally	Increase daily dose at 5-mg increments at weekly intervals. No specific dosing modifications available for patients with renal impairment, however use cautiously in these patients.
	Ditropan XL	5 mg daily orally	5–30 mg daily orally	This is an extended release formulation, and it should not be crushed or chewed. Increase daily dose at 5-mg increments at weekly intervals. No specific dosing modifications available for patients with renal impairment, but use cautiously in these patients.
	Oxytrol TDS	1 patch (3.9 mg oxybutynin) twice weekly	1 patch (3.9 mg) twice weekly	This is a transdermal patch. Apply to abdomen, hip, or buttock. Rotate application site. Do not expose patch to sunlight. No specific dosing modifications available for patients with renal impairment, however use cautiously in these patients.
	Gelnique 10% gel	1 g gel (100 mg oxybutynin) daily	1 g gel (100 mg oxybutynin) daily	This is available as premeasured dose packets. Apply to abdomen, thighs, upper arms or shoulders. Wash hands after application. Do not bathe, shower, or swim for 1 hour after application. Cover application site with clothing until medication dries on skin. Rotate application site daily. No specific dosing modifications available for patients with renal impairment, but use cautiously in these patients.
Solifenacin	Vesicare	5 mg daily orally	5–10 mg daily orally	If the creatinine clearance is less than 30 mL/min (0.5 mL/s) or the patient has moderate hepatic impairment, do not exceed 5 mg daily orally. If the patient is taking a potent CYP3A4 inhibitor (eg, ketoconazole, itraconazole, ritonavir, nelfinavir, and clarithromycin), do not exceed 5 mg daily orally
Tolterodine	Detrol	2 mg twice daily orally	2 mg twice daily orally	If the patient has significant renal impairment, limit dose to 1 mg twice a day
	Detrol LA	4 mg daily orally	4 mg daily orally	The LA formulation is an extended-release formulation, and it should not be chewed or crushed. If the creatinine clearance is 10–30 mL/min (0.17–0.5 mL/s) or the patient has mild/moderate hepatic impairment, do not exceed 2 mg daily orally. If the creatinine clearance is less than 10 mL/min (0.17 mL/s), do not use Detrol LA

Trospium	Sanctura	20 mg twice daily orally	20 mg twice daily orally	Avoid alcohol ingestion for 2 hours after a dose. Use cautiously in patients with moderate or severe hepatic impairment. In patients older than 75 years, use the immediate-release formulation and start with 20 mg daily orally. If the creatinine clearance is less than 30 mL/min (0.5 mL/s), use 20-mg immediate-release formulation
	Sanctura XR	60 mg daily orally	60 mg daily orally	The XR is an extended-release formulation, and it should not be chewed or crushed. This is not recommended in patients with creatinine clearance less than 30 mL/min (0.5 mL/s)
β₃-Adrenergic agonist				
Mirabegron	Myrbetriq	25 mg daily orally	25–50 mg daily orally	This is an extended-release formulation. Do not chew, crush, or divide tablet. In patients with a creatinine clearance of 15–29 mL/min (0.25–0.48 mL/s) or those with moderate hepatic impairment, the maximum daily dose should be 25 mg daily. This drug is not recommended in patients with creatinine clearance less than 15 mL/min (0.25 mL/s).

5α-Reductase Inhibitors

- 5α-Reductase inhibitors interfere with the stimulatory effect of testosterone. These agents slow disease progression and decrease the risk of complications.
- Compared with α_1-adrenergic antagonists, disadvantages of 5α-reductase inhibitors include 6 to 12 months of use to maximally shrink prostate, less likely to induce objective improvement and more sexual dysfunction. They are considered second-line therapy in sexually active males.
- **Dutasteride** inhibits types I and II 5α-reductase, whereas **finasteride** inhibits only type II.
- 5α-Reductase inhibitors may be preferred in patients with uncontrolled arrhythmias, poorly controlled angina, take multiple antihypertensives, or cannot tolerate hypotensive effects of α_1-adrenergic antagonists.
- Measure PSA at baseline and again after 6 months of therapy. If PSA does not decrease by 50% after 6 months of therapy in an adherentpatient, evaluate the patient for prostate cancer.
- 5α-Reductase inhibitors are in FDA pregnancy category X and are therefore contraindicated in pregnant women. Women who are pregnant or of childbearing age should not handle the tablets or have contact with semen from men taking 5α-reductase inhibitors.

Phosphodiesterase Inhibitors

- Increase in cyclic GMP by phosphodiesterase inhibitors (PI) relaxes smooth muscle in the prostate and bladder neck.
- **Tadalafil** 5 mg daily improves voiding symptoms but does not increase urinary flow rate or reduce PVR urine volume. Combination therapy with α-adrenergic antagonist results in significant improvement in lower urinary tract symptoms (LUTS), increased urinary flow rates, and decreased PVR volume.

Anticholinergic Agents

- Addition of **oxybutynin** and **tolterodine** to α-adrenergic antagonists relieves irritative voiding symptoms including urinary frequency, urgency, and nocturia. Start with lowest effective dose to determine tolerance of CNS adverse effects and dry mouth. Measure PVR urine volume before initiating treatment (should be less than 150 mL).
- Consider transdermal (eg, oxybutynin) or extended-release formulations (eg, tolterodine) or uroselective agents (eg, **darifenacin** or **solifenacin**) if systemic anticholinergic adverse effects are poorly tolerated.

B₃-Adrenergic Agonist

- **Miragegron** is a β_3-adrenergic agonist that relaxes the detrusor muscle reducing irritative voiding systems, increases urinary bladder capacity, and increases the interval between voidings. It does not cause anticholinergic adverse effects and is an alternative to anticholinergic agents in patients with LUTS.

SURGICAL INTERVENTION

- Prostatectomy, performed transurethrally or suprapubically, is the gold standard for treatment of patients with moderate or severe symptoms of BPH and for all patients with complications.
- Retrograde ejaculation complicates up to 75% of transurethral prostatectomy procedures. Other complications seen in 2% to 15% of patients are bleeding, urinary incontinence, and erectile dysfunction.

PHYTOTHERAPY

- Although widely used in Europe for BPH, phytotherapy with products such as saw palmetto berry (*Serenoa repens*), stinging nettle (*Urtica dioica*), and African plum (*Pygeum africanum*) should be avoided. Studies are inconclusive, and the purity of available products is questionable.

EVALUATION OF THERAPEUTIC OUTCOMES

- The primary therapeutic outcome of BPH therapy is restoring adequate urinary flow with minimal treatment-related adverse effects.
- Outcome depends on the patient's perception of effectiveness and acceptability of therapy. The American Urological Association Symptom Score is a validated standardized instrument that can be used to assess patient quality of life.
- Objective measures of bladder emptying (eg, urinary flow rate and PVR urine volume) are useful measures in patients considering surgery.
- Monitor laboratory tests (eg, blood urea nitrogen, creatinine, and PSA) and urinalysis regularly. An annual digital rectal examination is recommended if life expectancy is at least 10 years.

See Chapter 84, Benign Prostatic Hyperplasia, authored by Mary Lee and Roohollah Sharifi, for a more detailed discussion of this topic.

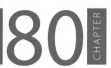
- *Erectile dysfunction* (ED) is the persistent failure (minimum of 3 months) to achieve a penile erection suitable for sexual intercourse. Patients often refer to it as impotence.

PATHOPHYSIOLOGY

- ED can result from any single abnormality or combination of abnormalities of the four systems necessary for a normal penile erection. Vascular, neurologic, or hormonal etiologies of ED are referred to as *organic ED*. Patients who do not respond to psychogenic stimuli and have no organic cause for dysfunction have *psychogenic ED*.
- The penis has two corpora cavernosa and one corpus spongiosum, which contain interconnected sinuses that fill with blood to produce an erection.
- Acetylcholine works with other neurotransmitters (ie, cyclic guanylate monophosphate, cyclic adenosine monophosphate, and vasoactive intestinal polypeptide) to produce penile arterial vasodilation and ultimately an erection.
- Organic ED is associated with diseases that compromise vascular flow to the corpora cavernosum (eg, peripheral vascular disease, arteriosclerosis, and essential hypertension), impair nerve conduction to the brain (eg, spinal cord injury and stroke), or impair peripheral nerve conduction (eg, diabetes mellitus). Secondary ED is associated with hypogonadism.
- Psychogenic ED is associated with malaise, reactive depression or performance anxiety, sedation, Alzheimer disease, hypothyroidism, and mental disorders. Patients with psychogenic ED generally have a higher response rate to interventions than those with organic ED.
- Social habits (eg, cigarette smoking and excessive ethanol intake) and medications (**Table 80–1**) can also cause ED.

CLINICAL PRESENTATION

- Signs and symptoms of ED can be difficult to detect. The patient's partner is often the first to report ED to the healthcare provider.
- Nonadherence to drugs thought to cause ED can be a sign of ED.

DIAGNOSIS

- Key diagnostic assessments include description of ED severity, medical, psychological, and surgical histories, review of concurrent medications, physical examination, and laboratory tests (ie, serum blood glucose, lipid profile, and testosterone level).
- Assess the severity of ED with a standardized questionnaire.
- Complete a cardiovascular risk assessment before initiating ED therapy in older men and in those at intermediate and high risk for cardiovascular disease.

TREATMENT

- <u>Goal of Treatment</u>: The goal is to improve the quantity and quality of penile erections suitable for intercourse.
- The first step in management of ED is to identify and, if possible, reverse underlying causes. Psychotherapy can be used as monotherapy for psychogenic ED or as an adjunct to specific treatments.
- Treatment options include vacuum erection devices (VEDs), drugs (**Table 80–2**), and surgery. Although no option is ideal, the least invasive options are chosen first (**Fig. 80–1**).

TABLE 80–1 Medication Classes That Can Cause Erectile Dysfunction

Drug Class	Proposed Mechanism by Which Drug Causes Erectile Dysfunction	Special Notes
Anticholinergic agents (antihistamines, antiparkinsonian agents, tricyclic antidepressants, phenothiazines)	Anticholinergic activity	• Second-generation nonsedating antihistamines (eg, loratadine, fexofenadine, or cetirizine) are associated with less erectile dysfunction (ED) than first-generation agents. • Selective serotonin reuptake inhibitor (SSRI) antidepressants cause less ED than tricyclic antidepressants. Of the SSRIs, paroxetine, sertraline, and fluoxetine cause ED more commonly than venlafaxine, nefazodone, trazodone, or mirtazapine. • Phenothiazines with less anticholinergic effect (eg, chlorpromazine) can be substituted in some patients if ED is a problem.
Dopamine antagonists (eg, metoclopramide, phenothiazines)	Inhibit prolactin inhibitory factor, thereby increasing prolactin levels	• Increased prolactin levels inhibit testicular testosterone production; depressed libido results.
Estrogens, antiandrogens (eg, luteinizing hormone–releasing hormone superagonists, digoxin, spironolactone, ketoconazole, cimetidine)	Suppress testosteronemediated stimulation of libido	• In the face of a decreased libido, a secondary ED develops because of diminished sexual drive.
Central nervous system depressants (eg, barbiturates, narcotics, benzodiazepines, short-term use of large doses of alcohol, anticonvulsants)	Suppress perception of psychogenic stimuli	

(continued)

TABLE 80–1   Medication Classes That Can Cause Erectile Dysfunction (Continued)

Drug Class	Proposed Mechanism by Which Drug Causes Erectile Dysfunction	Special Notes
Agents that decrease penile blood flow (eg, diuretics, peripheral β-adrenergic antagonists, or central sympatholytics [methyldopa, clonidine, guanethidine])	Reduce arteriolar flow to corpora	• Any diuretic that produces a significant decrease in intravascular volume can decrease penile arteriolar flow. • Safer antihypertensives include angiotensin-converting enzyme inhibitors, postsynaptic α_1-adrenergic antagonists (terazosin, doxazosin), calcium channel blockers, and angiotensin II receptor antagonists.
Miscellaneous • Finasteride, dutasteride • Lithium carbonate • Gemfibrozil • Interferon • Clofibrate • Monoamine oxidase inhibitors	Unknown mechanism	

TABLE 80–2 Dosing Regimens for Selected Drug Treatments for Erectile Dysfunction

Drug	Brand Name	Initial Dose	Usual Range	Special Population Dose	Other
Phosphodiesterase inhibitor					
Sildenafil	Viagra	50 mg orally 1 hour before intercourse	25–100 mg 1 hour before intercourse. Limit to one dose per day	In patients age 65 years and older, start with 25 mg dose. In patients with creatinine clearance less than 30 mL/min (0.5 mL/s) or severe hepatic impairment, limit starting dose to 25 mg. In patients taking potent P450 CYP3A4 inhibitors, limit starting dose to 25 mg every 48 hours.	Titrate dose so that erection lasts no more than 1 hour. Food decreases absorption by 1 hour. Contraindicated with nitrates by any route of administration.
Vardenafil	Levitra	5–10 mg orally 1 hour before intercourse	5–20 mg 1 hour before intercourse. Limit to one dose per day	In patients age 65 years and older, start with 5 mg Levitra. No dosage adjustment is required in patients with decreased creatinine clearance. In patients with moderate hepatic impairment, start with 5 mg Levitra. In patients taking potent P450 CYP3A4 inhibitors, limit starting dose to 2.5–5 mg every 24–72 hours. Not recommended in patients with congenital prolonged QT interval or in patients taking Type 1A or Type 3 antiarrhythmics.	Titrate dose so that erection lasts no more than 1 hour. Food decreases absorption by 1 hour. Contraindicated with nitrates by any route of administration.

(continued)

TABLE 80–2 Dosing Regimens for Selected Drug Treatments for Erectile Dysfunction (*Continued*)

Drug	Brand Name	Initial Dose	Usual Range	Special Population Dose	Other
	Staxyn	10 mg tablet to dissolve on the tongue 1 hour before intercourse	10 mg tablet to dissolve on the tongue 1 hour before intercourse. Limit to one dose per day.	Dose of Staxyn requires no adjustment in patients 65 years or older or in patients with creatinine clearance less than 30 mL/min (0.5 mL/s). Do not use in patients with moderate or severe hepatic impairment or those taking moderately or highly potent P450 CYP3A4 inhibitors. Do not initiate Staxyn in patients taking α-adrenergic antagonists.	Staxyn should be taken without any liquid or food. The tablet should be placed on the tongue where it will dissolve. No up-titration of dose is recommended. Do not substitute Staxyn for Levitra, or vice versa.
Tadalafil	Cialis	5–10 mg orally at least 30 minutes before intercourse OR 2.5–5 mg orally once daily	10–20 mg at least 30 minutes before intercourse. Limit to one dose per day; the drug improves erectile function for up to 36 hours 2.5–5 mg once daily. Limit to one dose per day	Dose of tadalafil requires no dosage adjustment in patients 65 years or older. In patients with creatinine clearance of 30–50 mL/min (0.5–0.83 mL/s), limit starting dose to 10 mg every 48 hours; if less than 30 mL/min (0.5 mL/s), limit starting dose to 5 mg every 72 hours. In patients with mild–moderate hepatic impairment, limit starting dose to 10 mg every 24 hours. Do not use in patients with severe hepatic impairment. In patients taking potent P450 CYP3A4 inhibitors, limit starting dose to 10 mg every 72 hours (if using it on demand) or 2.5 mg daily (if using a continuous daily regimen).	Titrate dose so that erection lasts not more than 1 hour. Food does not affect rate or extent of drug absorption. Contraindicated with nitrates by any route of administration. When taken with large amounts of ethanol, tadalafil may cause orthostatic hypotension.

Avanafil	Stendra	100 mg orally 15–30 minutes before intercourse	50–200 mg orally 15–30 minutes before intercourse	In patients with creatinine clearance of 30–89 mL/min (0.5–1.49 mL/s), no dosage adjustment is needed. Do not use if creatinine clearance is less than 30 mL/min (0.5 mL/s), if the patient has severe hepatic disease, or if the patient is taking P450 CYP3A4 inhibitors.	May be taken with food. When taken with large amounts of ethanol, avanafil may cause orthostatic hypotension.
Prostaglandin E1					
Alprostadil intracavernosal injection	Caverject, Edex	2.5 mcg intracavernosally 5–10 minutes before intercourse	10–20 mcg 5–10 minutes before intercourse. Maximum recommended dose is 60 mcg. Limit to not more than one injection per day and not more than three injections per week with a 24 hour interval between doses.	None	Titrate dose to achieve an erection that lasts 1 hour. Patient will require training on aseptic intracavernosal injection technique. Avoid intracavernosal injections in patients with sickle cell anemia, multiple myeloma, leukemia, severe coagulopathy, schizophrenia, poor manual dexterity, severe venous incompetence, severe cardiovascular disease, or Peyronie's disease.
Alprostadil intraurethral pellet	Muse	125–250 mcg intraurethrally 5–10 minutes before intercourse	250–1000 mcg just before intercourse. Limit to not more than two doses per day	None	Patient will require training on proper intraurethral administration techniques. Use applicator provided to administer medications to avoid urethral injury.

(continued)

TABLE 80–2   Dosing Regimens for Selected Drug Treatments for Erectile Dysfunction (Continued)

Drug	Brand Name	Initial Dose	Usual Range	Special Population Dose	Other
Testosterone supplements					
Methyltestosterone	Android, Testred, Methitest	10 mg once daily	10–50 mg once daily	Will likely cause fluid retention in patients with renal or hepatic disease	Not recommended for use due to extensive first-pass hepatic catabolism and because it is associated with hepatotoxicity.
Fluoxymesterone	Androxy	5 mg once daily	5–20 mg once daily	Contraindicated in patients with severe renal or hepatic impairment	Not recommended because it is associated with hepatotoxicity. This is a 17α-alkylated androgen.
Testosterone buccal system	Striant	30 mg every 12 hours, morning and evening	30 mg every 12 hours, morning and evening		Time the dose so that buccal system is removed before every morning and evening toothbrushing. Place buccal system just above incisor tooth on both sides of the mouth, and hold in place for 30 seconds to adhere. To remove, slide buccal system down toward the tooth. Buccal tablet may become detached during eating. If this occurs, discard and replace with new buccal system. Do not chew or swallow buccal system.
Testosterone cypionate intramuscular injection	Depo-Testosterone	200–400 mg every 2–4 weeks	200–400 mg every 2–4 weeks (up to 6 weeks)	Contraindicated in patients with severe hepatic or renal impairment	During the dosing interval, supraphysiologic serum concentrations of testosterone are produced during a portion of the dosing interval. This has been linked to mood swings.
Testosterone enanthate intramuscular injection	Delatestryl	200–400 mg every 2–4 weeks	200–400 mg every 2–4 weeks (up to 6 weeks)	Although not so labeled, it should probably not be used in patients with severe hepatic or renal impairment	During the dosing interval, supraphysiologic serum concentrations of testosterone are produced during a portion of the dosing interval. This has been linked to mood swings.

Testosterone undecanoate intramuscular injection	Aveed	750 mg as a single dose	750 mg as a single dose on day 0, week 4, and then 750 mg every 10 weeks		Only available in facilities certified through a Risk Evaluation and Mitigation Strategy Program.
Testosterone transdermal patch	Androderm	4 mg as a single dose at bedtime	2–6 mg as a single dose at bedtime	Safety in patients with hepatic or renal dysfunction has not been evaluated	When administered at bedtime, serum concentrations of testosterone in the usual circadian pattern are produced. Apply to those sites recommended in the package labeling: upper arm, back, abdomen, and thigh. Rotate application sites every 7 days. May have to apply multiple patches at one time to achieve appropriate serum testosterone level. Avoid swimming, showering, or washing administration site for 3 hours after patch application.
Testosterone gel	Androgel 1%, Testim 1%	5–10 g of gel (equivalent to 50–100 mg testosterone, respectively) as a single dose in the morning	5–10 g of gel (equivalent to 50–100 mg testosterone, respectively) as a single dose in the morning. Titrate dose up at 14-day intervals	None	Cover application site to avoid inadvertent transfer to others. Avoid swimming, showering, or washing administration site for 2 hours after gel application. Apply to those sites recommended in the product labeling: shoulders, upper arms, or abdomen. Children and women should avoid contact with unclothed or unwashed application sites. Patients should wash hands with soap and water after administration of transdermal testosterone product. For patients who have difficulty measuring the appropriate dose using tubes of gel, it is also available in premeasured dose packets or from a pump dispenser.

(continued)

TABLE 80–2	Dosing Regimens for Selected Drug Treatments for Erectile Dysfunction (*Continued*)				
Drug	Brand Name	Initial Dose	Usual Range	Special Population Dose	Other
	Androgel 1.6%	2 pumps (equivalent to 40.5 mg testosterone) as a single dose in the morning	2–4 pumps (equivalent to 40.5–81 mg) as a single dose in the morning		Apply to shoulders and upper arms. Avoid swimming, showering, or washing administration site for 2 hours after application. Titrate dose 14–28 days after starting treatment.
Testosterone transdermal spray	Fortesta	Four sprays (equivalent to 40 mg testosterone) once daily	Four to seven sprays (equivalent to 40–70 mg testosterone) once daily. Titrate dose up at 14- to 35-day intervals.		Cover application site to avoid inadvertent transfer to others. Avoid swimming, showering, or washing administration site for 2 hours after spray application. Apply to those sites recommended in the product labeling: front and inner thighs. Children and women should avoid contact with unclothed or unwashed application sites. Patients should wash hands with soap and water after administration of transdermal testosterone product.
Testosterone transdermal solution	Axiron	Two pump sprays (equivalent to 60 mg testosterone) to left or right axilla daily	One to four pump sprays (equivalent to 30–120 mg testosterone, respectively) to left or right axilla daily. Titrate dose up at 14- to 35-day intervals		Limit application to axilla. Apply antiperspirant or deodorant before Axiron. Avoid swimming, showering, or washing administration site for 2 hours after application.

| Testosterone subcutaneous implant pellet | Testopel | 150–450 (equivalent to 2–6 pellets) mg as a single dose every 3–6 months. Administration of the dose requires a forearm incision and subcutaneous dose implant under local anesthesia | 150–450 mg as a single dose every 3–6 months | Trained health professional is required to administer the dose. Should use sterile implanter kit. Clinical onset is delayed for 3–4 months after initial dose. Generic formulations are available in higher strengths: 100 mg or 200 mg per pellet. |

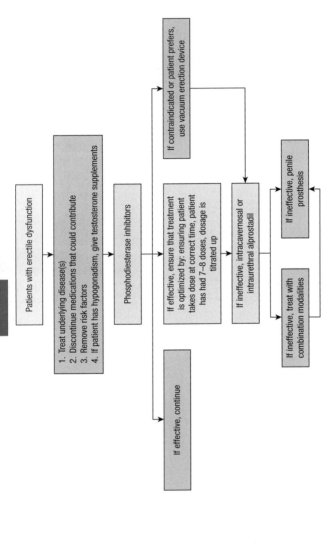

FIGURE 80–1. Algorithm for selecting treatment for erectile dysfunction (ED).

NONPHARMACOLOGIC TREATMENT

Vacuum Erection Device

- First-line therapy for older patients in stable relationships. Onset of action is slow (ie, 3–20 minutes). An erection can be prolonged through use of constriction bands or tension rings.
- Consider VEDs as second-line therapy after failure of oral or injectable drugs. Response rate improves with addition of **alprostadil** or a phosphodiesterase inhibitor (PI).
- VEDs are contraindicated in patients with sickle cell disease or a history of prolonged erections. Use cautiously in patients taking warfarin because, through a poorly understood and idiosyncratic mechanism, it can cause priapism.

Surgery

- Surgical insertion of a penile prosthesis, the most invasive treatment for ED, is used after failure of less invasive treatments and for patients who are not candidates for other treatments.

PHARMACOLOGIC TREATMENTS

Phosphodiesterase Inhibitors

- Phosphodiesterase mediates catabolism of cyclic guanylate monophosphate, a vasodilatory neurotransmitter in the corporal tissue.
- PIs are selective for isoenzyme type 5 in genital tissue. Inhibition of this isoenzyme in nongenital tissues (eg, peripheral vascular tissue, tracheal smooth muscle, and platelets) can produce adverse effects.
- Available agents (**avanafil, sildenafil, tadalafil,** and **vardenafil**) have different pharmacokinetic profiles (**Table 80–3**), drug–food interactions, and adverse effects. They are considered equally effective despite no comparative clinical trial data.
- PIs are first-line therapy for younger patients. Effectiveness appears to be dose related; nonresponse rate is 30% to 40%. Patient education is critical for clinical success.
- Hepatic metabolism of all four PIs can be inhibited by enzyme inhibitors of CYP 3A4. Use a lower starting dose to minimize dose-related adverse effects.
- Avoid exceeding prescribed doses due to increased frequency of adverse effects and inconsistent erectile responses.
- In usual doses, the most common adverse effects include headache, facial flushing, dyspepsia, nasal congestion, and dizziness that are all dose related.
- Sildenafil and vardenafil decrease systolic/diastolic blood pressure by 8 to 10/5 to 6 mm Hg for 1 to 4 hours after a dose. Although most patients are asymptomatic, multiple antihypertensives, **nitrates**, and baseline hypotension increase the risk of developing adverse effects. Avanafil is associated with similar decreases in blood pressure. Tadalafil is not associated with blood pressure decreases, but use with caution in patients with cardiovascular disease because of the inherent cardiac risk associated with sexual activity.
- Guidelines are available for stratifying patients on the basis of their cardiovascular risk (**Table 80–4**).
- Use PIs cautiously in patients at risk for retinitis pigmentosa and by pilots who rely on blue and green lights to land airplanes. Evaluate patients with sudden vision loss before continuing treatment.
- Tadalafil inhibits type 11 phosphodiesterase, which is thought to account for the dose-related back and muscle pain seen in 7% to 30% of patients.
- PIs are contraindicated in patients taking nitrates. Use cautiously in patients taking α-adrenergic antagonists.

Testosterone-Replacement Regimens

- **Testosterone**-replacement regimens restore serum testosterone levels to the normal range (300–1100 ng/dL; 10.4–38.2 nmol/L). These regimens are indicated for symptomatic patients with hypogonadism as confirmed by both a decreased libido and low serum testosterone concentrations.

TABLE 80-3	Pharmacodynamics and Pharmacokinetics of Phosphodiesterase Inhibitors			
	Sildenafil (Viagra)	Vardenafil (Levitra/Staxyn)	Tadalafil (Cialis)	Avanafil (Stendra)
Inhibits PDE-5	Yes	Yes	Yes	Yes
Inhibits PDE-6	Yes	Minimally	No	Minimally
Inhibits PDE-11	No	No	Yes	Minimally
Time to peak plasma level (hours)	0.5–1	0.7–0.9/1.5	2	0.5–0.8
Oral bioavailability (%)	40	15/21–44	36	15
Fatty meal decreases rate of oral absorption?	Yes	Yes/No[a]	No	No
Mean plasma half-life (hours)	3.7	4.4–4.8/4–6	18	4–5
Active metabolite	Yes	Yes/Yes	No	Yes
Is CYP 3A4 principally responsible for metabolism?	Yes	Yes	Yes	Yes
Other CYP enzymes responsible for metabolism	CYP 2C9	CYP 3A5, CYP 2C9		CYP 2C
Percentage of dose excreted in feces	80	91–95/91–95	61	62
Percentage of dose excreted in urine	13	2–6/2–6	36	21
Clinical onset (minutes)	30	30/60	45	25–40
Duration (hours)	4	4–5/4–6	24–36	6+

(PDE, phosphodiesterase.)
[a]When Staxyn is taken with water, the area under the curve decreases by 29%.
Used with permission from Nehra A, Jackson G, Miner M, et al. The Princeton III Consensus Recommendations for the Management of Erectile Dysfunction and Cardiovascular Disease. Mayo Clin Proc 2012;87(8):766–778.

- Testosterone-replacement regimens correct secondary ED by improving libido. Improved muscle strength, sexual drive, and mood are observed within days or weeks of initiating treatment.
- Oral, buccal, parenteral, and transdermal products are available (see Table 80-2). Injectable regimens are preferred because they are effective, inexpensive, and do not have the bioavailability problems or adverse hepatotoxic effects of oral regimens. Testosterone patches, gels, and sprays are more expensive than other forms and should be reserved for patients who refuse injections.
- Screen patients 40 years and older for breast cancer, benign prostatic hyperplasia (BPH) and prostate cancer before starting therapy. Continue treatment for 2 to 3 months before an increase in dosage is considered.
- Testosterone replacement can cause sodium retention, which can result in weight gain or exacerbate hypertension, congestive heart failure, and edema; gynecomastia; serum lipoprotein changes; and polycythemia.
- Oral testosterone-replacement regimens can cause hepatotoxicity, ranging from mildly elevated hepatic transaminases to serious liver diseases (eg, peliosis hepatitis, hepatocellular and intrahepatic cholestasis, and benign or malignant tumors).
- Topical testosterone patches may cause contact dermatitis that responds to topical corticosteroids.

TABLE 80–4 Recommendations of the Third Princeton Consensus Conference for Cardiovascular Risk Stratification of Patients Being Considered for Phosphodiesterase Inhibitor Therapy

Risk Category	Description of Patient's Condition	Management Approach
Low risk	Has asymptomatic cardiovascular disease with <3 risk factors for cardiovascular disease Has well-controlled hypertension Has mild congestive heart failure (NYHA class I or II) Has mild valvular heart disease Had a myocardial infarction >8 weeks ago	Patient can be started on phosphodiesterase inhibitor
Intermediate risk	Has ≥3 risk factors for cardiovascular disease Has mild or moderate, stable angina Had a recent myocardial infarction or stroke within the past 2-8 weeks Has moderate congestive heart failure (NYHA class III) History of stroke, transient ischemic attack, or peripheral artery disease	Patient should undergo complete cardiovascular workup and treadmill stress test to determine tolerance to increased myocardial energy consumption associated with increased sexual activity. Reclassify in low or high risk category
High risk	Has unstable or refractory angina, despite treatment Has uncontrolled hypertension Has severe congestive heart failure (NYHA class IV) Had a recent myocardial infarction or stroke within past 2 weeks Has moderate or severe valvular heart disease Has high-risk cardiac arrhythmias Has obstructive hypertrophic cardiomyopathy	Phosphodiesterase inhibitor is contraindicated; sexual intercourse should be deferred

(NYHA, New York Heart Association.)

Alprostadil

- **Alprostadil**, or prostaglandin E_1, stimulates adenyl cyclase to increase production of cyclic adenosine monophosphate, a neurotransmitter that ultimately enhances blood flow to and blood filling of the corpora.
- Alprostadil is approved as monotherapy for the management of ED. It is generally prescribed after failure of VEDs and PIs and for patients who cannot use these therapies. The intracavernosal route is more effective than the intraurethral route.

INTRACAVERNOSAL INJECTION

- Intracavernosal alprostadil is effective in 70% to 90% of patients, but 30% to 50% discontinue therapy during first 6 to 12 months. Perceived ineffectiveness, inconvenience of administration, unnatural, nonspontaneous erection, needle phobia, loss of interest, and cost of therapy are reasons given for discontinuation.
- Intracavernosal alprostadil is used successfully in combination with VEDs or vasoactive agents (eg, papaverine and phentolamine) that act by different mechanisms.
- Intracavernosal alprostadil acts rapidly, with an onset of 5 to 15 minutes. Duration of action is dose related and, within the usual dosage range, lasts less than 1 hour. To avoid adverse effects, the maximum number of injections is one daily and three weekly, with at least 24 hours between doses.
- Usual dose is 10 to 20 mcg up to a maximum of 60 mcg. The manufacturer recommends slow dose titration, but in clinical practice, most patients start with 10 mcg and titrate quickly.
- Local adverse effects occur during the first year of therapy, including cavernosal plaques or fibrosis at the injection site (2%–12% of patients), penile pain (10%–44%), and priapism (1%–15%). Penile pain is usually mild and self-limiting, but priapism (ie, painful, drug-induced erection lasting >1 hours) necessitates immediate medical attention.
- Use cautiously in patients at risk of priapism (eg, sickle cell disease or lymphoproliferative disorders) and bleeding complications secondary to injections.

INTRAURETHRAL ADMINISTRATION

- Instill intraurethral alprostadil, 125 to 1000 mcg 5 to 10 minutes before intercourse after emptying the bladder. No more than two doses daily are recommended.
- Intraurethral administration is associated with mild pain in 24% to 32% of patients. Prolonged painful erections are rare.
- Female partners may experience vaginal burning, itching, or pain, which is probably related to transfer of alprostadil during intercourse.

Unapproved Agents

- A variety of commercially available and investigational agents have been used for management of ED. Examples include **yohimbine** (6 mg three times daily), **papaverine** (7.5–60 mg [single-agent therapy] or 0.5–20 mg [combination therapy] intracavernosal injection), and **phentolamine** (0.5–1 mg in combination with 30 mg papaverine; dose administered ranges from 0.1 to 1 mL of the mixture as an intracavernosal injection).

EVALUATION OF THERAPEUTIC OUTCOMES

- The primary therapeutic outcomes for ED are improving the quantity and quality of penile erections suitable for intercourse and avoiding adverse drug reactions and interactions.
- Assess the patient at baseline and after a treatment trial period of 1 to 3 weeks.
- Identify patients with unrealistic expectations and counsel accordingly to avoid adverse effects due to excessive use of erectogenic agents.

See Chapter 83, Erectile Dysfunction, authored by Mary Lee and Roohollah Sharifi, for a more detailed discussion of this topic.

- *Urinary incontinence* (UI) is the complaint of involuntary leakage of urine.

PATHOPHYSIOLOGY

- The urethral sphincter, a combination of smooth and striated muscles within and external to the urethra, maintains adequate resistance to the flow of urine from the bladder until voluntary voiding is initiated.
- Volitional and involuntary bladder contractions are mediated by activation of postsynaptic muscarinic receptors by acetylcholine. Bladder smooth muscle cholinergic receptors are mainly of the M_2 variety; however, M_3 receptors are responsible for both emptying contraction of normal micturition and involuntary bladder contractions, which can result in UI. Therefore, most pharmacologic antimuscarinic therapy is anti-M_3 based.
- UI occurs as a result of overactivity or underactivity of the urethra, bladder, or both.
- Urethral underactivity is known as *stress UI* (SUI) and occurs during activities such as exercise, running, lifting, coughing, and sneezing. The urethral sphincter no longer resists the flow of urine from the bladder during periods of physical activity.
- Bladder overactivity is known as *urge UI* (UUI) and is associated with increased urinary frequency and urgency, with or without urge incontinence. The detrusor muscle is overactive and contracts inappropriately during the filling phase.
- Urethral overactivity and/or bladder underactivity is known as overflow incontinence. The bladder is filled to capacity but is unable to empty, causing urine to leak from a distended bladder past a normal outlet and sphincter. Common causes of urethral overactivity include benign prostatic hyperplasia (see Chap. 79); prostate cancer (see Chap. 64); and, in women, cystocele formation or surgical overcorrection after SUI surgery.
- Mixed incontinence includes the combination of bladder overactivity and urethral underactivity.
- Functional incontinence is not caused by bladder- or urethra-specific factors but rather occurs in patients with conditions such as cognitive or mobility deficits.
- Many medications may precipitate or aggravate voiding dysfunction and UI (Table 81–1).

CINICAL PRESENTATION

- Signs and symptoms of UI depend on the underlying pathophysiology (Table 81–2). Patients with SUI generally complain of urine leakage with physical activity, whereas those with UUI complain of frequency, urgency, high-volume incontinence, and nocturia and nocturnal incontinence.
- Urethral overactivity and/or bladder underactivity is a rare but important cause of UI. Patients complain of lower abdominal fullness, hesitancy, straining to void, decreased force of stream, interrupted stream, and sense of incomplete bladder emptying. Patients can also have urinary frequency, urgency, and abdominal pain.

DIAGNOSIS

- A complete medical history, physical examination (ie, abdominal examination to exclude distended bladder, pelvic examination in women looking for evidence of prolapse or hormonal deficiency, and genital and prostate examination in men), and brief neurologic assessment of the perineum and lower extremities are recommended.
- For SUI, the preferred diagnostic test is observation of urethral meatus while the patient coughs or strains.

891

TABLE 81–1	Medications That Influence Lower Urinary Tract Function
Medication	**Effect**
Diuretics, acetylcholinesterase inhibitors	Polyuria resulting in urinary frequency, urgency
α-Receptor antagonists	Urethral muscle relaxation and stress urinary incontinence
α-Receptor agonists	Urethral muscle contraction (increased urethral closure forces) resulting in urinary retention (more common in men)
Calcium channel blockers	Urinary retention due to reduced bladder contractility
Narcotic analgesics	Urinary retention due to reduced bladder contractility
Sedative hypnotics	Functional incontinence caused by delirium, immobility
Antipsychotic agents	Anticholinergic effects resulting in reduced bladder contractility and urinary retention
Anticholinergics	Urinary retention due to reduced bladder contractility
Antidepressants, tricyclic	Anticholinergic effects resulting in reduced bladder contractility, and α-antagonist effects resulting in urethral smooth muscle contraction (increased urethral closure forces) both contributing to urinary retention
Alcohol	Polyuria resulting in urinary frequency, urgency
ACEIs	Cough as a result of ACEIs may aggravate stress urinary incontinence

(ACEIs, angiotensin-converting enzyme inhibitors.)

- For UUI, the preferred diagnostic tests are urodynamic studies. Perform urinalysis and urine culture to rule out urinary tract infection.
- For urethral overactivity and/or bladder underactivity, perform digital rectal examination or transrectal ultrasound to rule out prostate enlargement. Perform renal function tests to rule out renal failure.

TREATMENT

- <u>Goals of Treatment</u>: Restoration of continence, reduction in the number of UI episodes, and prevention of complications.

NONPHARMACOLOGIC TREATMENT

- Nonpharmacologic, nonsurgical treatment (eg, lifestyle modifications, toilet scheduling regimens, and pelvic floor muscle rehabilitation) is first-line treatment for UI.
- Surgery rarely plays a role in initial management of UI but can be required for secondary complications (eg, skin breakdown or infection). The decision to surgically treat symptomatic UI requires that lifestyle compromise warrant an elective operation and that nonoperative therapy be proven undesirable or ineffective.

TABLE 81-2	Differentiating Bladder Overactivity from Urethral Underactivity-Related UI	
Symptoms	Bladder Overactivity (UUI)	Urethral Underactivity (SUI)
Urgency (strong, sudden desire to void)	Yes	Sometimes
Frequency with urgency	Yes	Rarely
Leaking during physical activity (eg, coughing, sneezing, lifting)	No	Yes
Amount of urinary leakage with each episode of incontinence	Large if present	Usually small
Ability to reach the toilet in time following an urge to void	No or just barely	Yes
Nocturnal incontinence (presence of wet pads or undergarments in bed)	Yes	Rare
Nocturia (waking to pass urine at night)	Usually	Seldom

PHARMACOLOGIC TREATMENT

Bladder Overactivity: Urge Urinary Incontinence

- The pharmacotherapy of first choice for UUI is anticholinergic/antispasmodic drugs, which antagonize muscarinic cholinergic receptors (Table 81–3).

OXYBUTYNIN

- **Oxybutynin immediate-release** (IR) is the drug of first choice for UUI and the "gold standard" against which other drugs are compared. Financial considerations favor generic oxybutynin IR.
- Many patients discontinue oxybutynin IR because of adverse effects due to antimuscarinic effects (eg, dry mouth, constipation, vision impairment, confusion, cognitive dysfunction, and tachycardia), α-adrenergic inhibition (eg, orthostatic hypotension), and histamine H_1 inhibition (eg, sedation and weight gain).
- **Oxybutynin extended-release** (XL) is better tolerated than oxybutynin IR. Maximum benefits may take up to 4 weeks after starting therapy or dose escalation.
- **Oxybutynin transdermal system** (TDS) has similar efficacy but is better tolerated than oxybutynin IR presumably because this route avoids first-pass metabolism in the liver, which generates the metabolite thought to cause adverse events, especially dry mouth.
- **Oxybutynin gel** is also available for daily use. No data are available comparing it with an active control.

TOLTERODINE

- **Tolterodine**, a competitive muscarinic receptor antagonist, is considered first-line therapy in patients with urinary frequency, urgency, or urge incontinence.
- Controlled studies demonstrate that tolterodine is more effective than placebo and as effective as oxybutynin IR in efficacy outcomes with lower drug discontinuation rates.
- Tolterodine undergoes hepatic metabolism involving cytochrome (CYP) 2D6 and 3A4 isoenzymes. Therefore, elimination may be impaired by CYP 3A4 inhibitors, including **fluoxetine, sertraline, fluvoxamine**, macrolide antibiotics, azole antifungals, and grapefruit juice.
- Tolterodine's most common adverse effects include dry mouth, dyspepsia, headache, constipation, and dry eyes. The maximum benefit of tolterodine is not realized for up to 8 weeks after starting therapy or dose escalation.
- **Tolterodine long acting** (LA) offers once-daily dosing and may also take up to 8 weeks after starting therapy or dose escalation to see maximum benefit.
- Fesoterodine fumarate is a prodrug for tolterodine and is considered an alternative first-line therapy for UI in patients with urinary frequency, urgency, or urge incontinence.

TABLE 81–3 Dosing of Medications Approved for OAB or UUI

Drug	Brand Name	Initial Dose	Usual Range	Special Population Dose	Comments
Anticholinergics/Antimuscarinics					
Oxybutynin IR	Ditropan	2.5 mg twice daily	2.5–5 mg two to four times daily		Titrate in increments of 2.5 mg/day every 1–2 months; available in oral solution
Oxybutynin XL	Ditropan XL	5–10 mg once daily	5–30 mg once daily		Adjust dose in 5-mg increments at weekly interval; swallow whole
Oxybutynin TDS	Oxytrol		3.9 mg/day apply one patch twice weekly		Apply every 3–4 days; rotate application site
Oxybutynin gel 10%	Gelnique		One sachet (100 mg) topically daily		Apply to clean and dry, intact skin on abdomen, thighs or upper arms/shoulders; contains alcohol
Oxybutynin gel 3%	Gelnique 3%		Three pumps (84 mg) topically daily		Same as above
Tolterodine IR	Detrol		1–2 mg twice daily	1 mg twice daily if patient is taking CYP3A4 inhibitors, or with renal/hepatic impairment	
Tolterodine LA	Detrol LA		2–4 mg once daily	2 mg once daily in those who are taking CYP3A4 inhibitors, or with renal/hepatic impairment	Swallow whole; avoid in patients with creatinine clearance ≤10 mL/min (≤0.17 mL/s)
Trospium chloride IR	Sanctura		20 mg twice daily	20 mg once daily in patient age ≥75 years or creatinine clearance ≤30 mL/min (≤0.5 mL/s)	Take 1 hour before meals or on empty stomach; patient age ≥75 years should take at bedtime
Trospium chloride ER	Sanctura XR		60 mg once daily	Avoid in patient age ≥75 years or creatinine clearance ≤30 mL/min (≤0.5 mL/s)	Take 1 hour before meals or on empty stomach; swallow whole

Solifenacin	VESIcare	5 mg daily	5–10 mg once daily	5 mg daily if patient is taking CYP3A4 inhibitors or with creatinine clearance ≤30 mL/min (≤0.5 mL/s) or moderate hepatic impairment; avoid in severe hepatic impairment	Swallow whole
Darifenacin ER	Enablex	7.5 mg once daily	7.5–15 mg once daily	7.5 mg daily if patient is taking potent CYP3A4 inhibitors or with moderate hepatic impairment; avoid in severe hepatic impairment	Titrate dose after at least 2 weeks; swallow whole
Fesoterodine ER	Toviaz	4 mg once daily	4–8 mg once daily	4 mg daily if patient is taking potent CYP3A4 inhibitors or with creatinine clearance ≤30 mL/min (≤0.5 mL/s); avoid in severe hepatic impairment	Prodrug (metabolized to 5-hydroxymethyl tolterodine); swallow whole
β_3-Adrenergic Agonist					
Mirabegron ER	Myrbetriq	25 mg once daily	25–50 mg once daily	25 mg once daily if creatinine clearance 15–29 mL/min (0.25–0.49 mL/s) or moderate hepatic impairment; avoid in patients with ESRD or severe hepatic impairment	Swallow whole

(CYP, cytochrome P450 enzyme; ER, extended release; ESRD, end-stage renal disease; IR, immediate-release; LA, long-acting; OAB, overactive bladder; TDS, transdermal system; UUI, urge urinary incontinence; XL, extended-release.)

OTHER PHARMACOLOGIC THERAPIES
FOR URGE URINARY INCONTINENCE

- **Trospium chloride IR**, a quaternary ammonium anticholinergic, is superior to placebo and is equivalent to oxybutynin IR and tolterodine IR. It causes the expected anticholinergic adverse effects with increased frequency in patients 75 years or older. An extended-release product is also available.
- **Solifenacin succinate** and **darifenacin** are second-generation antimuscarinic agents. Both have been shown to improve quality-of-life domains. Drug interactions are possible if CYP 3A4 inhibitors are given with solifenacin succinate or CYP 2D6 or 3A4 inhibitors with darifenacin.
- **Mirabegron** is a β_3-adrenergic agonist alternative to anticholinergic/antimuscarinic drugs for managing UUI. It has modest efficacy as compared with placebo. Hypertension, nasopharyngitis, urinary tract infection, and headache were the most common adverse effects reported. It is a moderate inhibitor of CYP2D6.
- Use of other agents, including tricyclic antidepressants, **propantheline, flavoxate, hyoscyamine**, and **dicyclomine hydrochloride**, is not recommended. They are less effective, not safer, or have not been adequately studied.
- Selection of initial drug therapy depends on side-effect profile, comorbidities, concurrent drug therapy, and patient preference in drug delivery methods (Table 81–4).
- **Botulinum toxin A** temporarily paralyzes smooth or striated muscle. It is indicated for the treatment of detrusor overactivity associated with neurologic condition and overactive bladder (OAB).
- Adverse effects of botulinum toxin A include dysuria, hematuria, urinary tract infection, and urinary retention (up to 20%). Therapeutic and adverse effects are seen 3 to 7 days after injection and subside after 6 to 8 months.

Urethral Underactivity: Stress Urinary Incontinence

- Treatment of SUI is aimed at improving urethral closure by stimulating α-adrenergic receptors in smooth muscle of the bladder neck and proximal urethra, enhancing supportive structures underlying the urethral epithelium, or enhancing serotonin and norepinephrine effects in the micturition reflex pathways.

TABLE 81–4	Adverse Event Incidence Rates with Approved Drugs for Bladder Overactivity[a]			
Drug	**Dry Mouth**	**Constipation**	**Dizziness**	**Vision Disturbance**
Oxybutynin IR	71	15	17	10
Oxybutynin XL	61	13	6	14
Oxybutynin TDS	7	3	NR	3
Oxybutynin gel	10	1	3	3
Tolterodine	35	7	5	3
Tolterodine LA	23	6	2	4
Trospium chloride IR	20	10	NR	1
Trospium chloride XR	11	9	NR	2
Solifenacin	20	9	2	5
Darifenacin ER	24	18	2	2
Fesoterodine ER	27	5	NR	3
Mirabegron ER	3	3	3	NR

(IR, immediate-release; LA, long-acting; NR, not reported; TDS, transdermal system; XL, extended-release; XR/ER, extended-release.)
[a]All values constitute mean data, predominantly using product information from the manufacturers.

ESTROGENS

- Historically, local and systemic **estrogens** have been the mainstays of pharmacologic management of SUI.
- A meta-analysis of 34 trials evaluating the use of local or systemic estrogen therapy on UI in postmenopausal women found that systemic administration of estrogen alone or in combination with progesterone resulted in UI worsening. There was some evidence that vaginal estrogen may improve UI, and reduce urgency and frequency.
- A meta-analysis of 17 trials of local estrogen compared to placebo or no treatment found beneficial effects on UI and OAB symptoms and some urodynamic parameters.
- Based on the results of these analyses, only topical estrogen products should be used for treatment of UI or OAB in postmenopausal women.

α-ADRENERGIC RECEPTOR AGONISTS

- Many open trials support the use of a variety of α-adrenergic receptor agonists in SUI. Combining an α-adrenergic receptor agonist with an estrogen yields somewhat superior clinical and urodynamic responses compared with monotherapy.
- Contraindications to these agents include hypertension, tachyarrhythmias, coronary artery disease, myocardial infarction, cor pulmonale, hyperthyroidism, renal failure, and narrow-angle glaucoma.

DULOXETINE

- **Duloxetine**, a dual inhibitor of serotonin and norepinephrine reuptake indicated for depression and painful diabetic neuropathy, is approved in many countries for the treatment of SUI, but not in the United States. Duloxetine is thought to facilitate the bladder-to-sympathetic reflex pathway, increasing urethral and external urethral sphincter muscle tone during the storage phase.
- Six placebo-controlled studies showed that duloxetine reduces incontinent episode frequency and the number of daily micturitions, increases micturition interval, and improves quality-of-life scores. These benefits were statistically significant but clinically modest.
- Monitor patients taking concurrent CYP 2D6 and 1A2 substrates or inhibitors closely.
- The adverse event profile might make adherence problematic. Adverse events include nausea, headache, insomnia, constipation, dry mouth, dizziness, fatigue, somnolence, vomiting, and diarrhea.

OVERFLOW INCONTINENCE

- Overflow incontinence secondary to benign or malignant prostatic hyperplasia may be amenable to pharmacotherapy (see Chaps. 64 and 79).

EVALUATION OF THERAPEUTIC OUTCOMES

- Total elimination of UI signs and symptoms may not be possible. Therefore, realistic goals should be established for therapy.
- In the long-term management of UI, the clinical symptoms of most distress to the individual patient need to be monitored.
- Survey instruments used in UI research along with quantitating the use of ancillary supplies (eg, pads) can be used in clinical monitoring.
- Therapies for UI frequently have nuisance adverse effects, which need to be carefully elicited. Adverse effects can necessitate drug dosage adjustments, use of alternative strategies (eg, chewing sugarless gum, sucking on hard sugarless candy, or use of saliva substitutes for xerostomia), or even drug discontinuation.

See Chapter 85, Urinary Incontinence, authored by Eric S. Rovner, Jean Wyman, and Sum Lam, for a more detailed discussion of this topic.

1

Drug Allergy

TABLE A1–1 Classification of Allergic Drug Reactions

Type	Descriptor	Characteristics	Typical Onset	Drug Causes
I	Immediate (IgE mediated)	Allergen binds to IgE on basophils or mast cells, resulting in release of inflammatory mediators	Within 1 hour (may be within 1–6 hours)	Penicillin anaphylaxis, angioedema Blood products Polypeptide hormones Vaccines Dextran
II	Delayed; Cytotoxic	Cell destruction occurs because of cell-associated antigen that initiates cytolysis by antigen-specific antibody (IgG) and complement. Most often involves blood elements.	Typically >72 hours to weeks	Penicillin, quinidine, quinine, heparin, thiouracils, sulfonamides, methyldopa
III	Delayed; Immune complex	Antigen–antibody (IgG or IgM) complexes form and deposit on blood vessel walls and activate complement. Result is a serum sickness-like syndrome or vasculitis.	>72 hours to weeks	May be caused by penicillins, sulfonamides, minocycline, hydantoins
IV	Delayed; T Cell-mediated	Antigens cause activation of T lymphocytes, which release cytokines and recruit effector cells	>72 hours	
	IVa	Th1 cells and interferon-γ, monocytes and eosinophils respond to the antigen	1–21 days	Tuberculin reaction, contact dermatitis
	IVb	Th2 cells, interleukin-4 and interleukin-5 respond to the antigen	1–6 weeks	Maculopapular rashes with eosinophilia
	IVc	Cytotoxic T cells, perforin, granzyme B, FasL respond to the antigen	4–28 days	Bullous exanthems; fixed drug eruptions
	IVd	T cells and interleukin-8 respond to the antigen	>72 hours	Acute generalized exanthematous pustulosis

TABLE A1–2	Top 10 Drugs and Agents Reported to Cause Skin Reactions
	Reactions per 1000 Recipients
Amoxicillin	51.4
Trimethoprim–sulfamethoxazole	33.8
Ampicillin	33.2
Iopodate	27.8
Blood	21.6
Cephalosporins	21.1
Erythromycin	20.4
Dihydralazine hydrochloride	19.1
Penicillin G	18.5
Cyanocobalamin	17.9

Data from Roujeau JC, Stern RS. Severe adverse cutaneous reactions to drugs. N Engl J Med 1994;331:1272-1285.

TABLE A1–3	Treatment of Anaphylaxis

1. Remove the inciting allergen, if possible.
2. Assess airway, breathing, circulation, and orientation. Support the airway.
3. Cardiopulmonary resuscitation: Start chest compressions (100/min) if cardiovascular arrest occurs at any time.
4. Administer epinephrine 1:1000 (adults: 0.3–0.5 mg; children: 0.01 mg/kg) IM in the lateral aspect of the thigh.
5. Place patient in recumbent position.
6. Administer oxygen 8–10 L/min through facemask or up to 100% oxygen as needed; monitor by pulse oximetry, if available.
7. Repeat IM epinephrine every 5–15 minutes for up to 3 injections if the patient is not responding.
8. Establish IV line for venous access. Keep line open with 0.9% saline solution. For hypotension or failure to respond to epinephrine, administer 1–2 L at a rate of 5–10 mL/kg in the first 5–10 minutes. Children should receive up to 30 mL/kg in the first hour.
9. Consider nebulized albuterol 2.5–5 mg in 3 mL of saline for lower airway obstruction; repeat as necessary.
10. In cases of refractory bronchospasm or hypotension not responding to epinephrine because a β-adrenergic blocker is complicating management, glucagon 1–5 mg IV (20–30 mcg/kg; maximum, 1 mg in children) given IV over 5 minutes.
11. Give epinephrine by continuous IV infusion for patients with inadequate response to IM epinephrine and IV saline. Add 1 mg (1 mL of 1:1000) of epinephrine to 1000 mL of 0.9% saline solution; Start infusion at 2 mcg/min and increase up to 10 mcg/min based on blood pressure, heart rate, and cardiac function.
12. Consider intraosseous access for either adults or children if attempts at IV access are unsuccessful.
13. Consider the antihistamine diphenhydramine (adults 25–50 mg; children 1 mg/kg, up to 50 mg) IM or by slow IV infusion.
14. Consider ranitidine 50 mg in adults and 12.5–50 mg (1 mg/kg) in children. The dose may be diluted in 5% dextrose in water to a volume of 20 mL and injected over 5 minutes.
15. Consider methylprednisolone 1–2 mg/kg/dose up to 125 mg (or an equivalent steroid) to reduce the risk of recurring or protracted anaphylaxis. Prednisone 20 mg orally can be given in mild cases. These doses can be repeated every 6 hours as required.

(IM, intramuscular.)
Adapted from Lieberman P, Nicklas RA, Randolph C, et al. Anaphylaxis - a practice parameter update 2015. Ann Allergy Asthma Immunol 2015;115:341-384. Copyright © 2015 Elsevier.

TABLE A1–4	Procedure for Performing Penicillin Skin Testing

A. Percutaneous (Prick) Skin Testing (Using a 22- to 28-Gauge Needle)

Materials	Volume (Drop)
Pre-Pen 6×10^6 M	1
Penicillin G 10,000 units/mL	1
β-Lactam drug (amoxicillin) 2 mg/mL	1
Saline control	1
Histamine control (1 mg/mL)	1

1. Place a drop of each test material on the volar surface of the forearm.
2. Prick the skin with the needle to make a single shallow puncture of the epidermis through the drop.
3. Interpret skin responses during the next 15 minutes. Observe for a wheal or erythema and the occurrence of itching.
4. A wheal in diameter of 5 mm or greater surrounding the puncture site is considered a positive test result.
5. Wipe off the solution near the puncture site.
6. If the prick test result is negative or equivocal (wheal <5 mm in diameter with no itching or erythema), proceed to the intradermal test.
7. If the histamine control is nonreactive, the test is considered uninterpretable. Ensure no interference by antihistamines.

B. Intradermal Skin Testing[a]

Materials	Volume (mL)
Pre-Pen 6×10^6 M	0.02
Penicillin G 10,000 units/mL	0.02
β-Lactam drug (amoxicillin) 2 mg/mL	0.02
Saline control	0.02
Histamine control (0.1 mg/mL)	0.02

1. Inject 0.02—0.03 mL of Pre-Pen intradermally (amount sufficient to produce a small bleb of about 3 mm in diameter) in duplicate at least 2 cm apart.
2. Inject 0.02—0.03 mL of the other materials at least 5 cm from the Pre-Pen sites.
3. Interpret skin responses after 20 minutes.
4. Itching or a significant increase in the size of the original bleb to at least 5 cm is considered a positive result. An ambiguous response is a wheal only slightly larger than the original bleb or discordance between the duplicates. The control site should show no increase in the original bleb.
5. If the histamine control is nonreactive, the test is considered uninterpretable. Antihistamines may blunt the response and cause false-negative results.

[a]Using a 0.5- to 1-cc syringe with a 3/8- to 5/8-inch long (1–1.6 cm), 26- to 30-gauge short-bevel needle.
Pre-Pen (benzylpenicilloyl polylysine injection, solution) Product Information, AllerQuest LLC and ALK-Abello, Inc., Round Rock TX, 2009.

(See e/Chapter 88, Drug Allergy, authored by Lynne M. Sylvia, for a more detailed discussion of this topic.)

Geriatrics

APPENDIX

2

TABLE A2–1	Physiologic Changes with Aging
Organ System	**Manifestation**
Balance and gait	↓ Stride length and slower gait ↓ Arm swing ↑ Body sway when standing
Body composition	↓ Total body water ↓ Lean body mass ↑ Body fat ↔ or ↓ Serum albumin ↑ α_1-Acid glycoprotein (↔ or ↑ by several disease states)
Cardiovascular	↓ Cardiovascular response to stress ↓ Baroreceptor activity leading to ↑ orthostatic hypotension ↓ Cardiac output ↑ Systemic vascular resistance with loss of arterial elasticity and dysfunction of systems maintaining vascular tone ↓ Resting and maximal heart rate
Central nervous system	↓ Size of the hippocampus and frontal and temporal lobes ↓ Number of receptors of all types and ↑ sensitivity of remaining receptors ↓ Short-term memory, coding and retrieval, and executive function Altered sleep patterns
Endocrine	↓ Estrogen, testosterone, TSH, and DHEA-S levels Altered insulin signaling
Gastrointestinal	↓ Motility of the large intestine ↓ Vitamin absorption by active transport mechanisms ↓ Splanchnic blood flow ↓ Bowel surface area
Genitourinary	Atrophy of the vagina with decreased estrogen Prostatic hypertrophy with androgenic hormonal changes Detrusor hyperactivity may predispose to incontinence
Hepatic	↓ Hepatic size ↓ Hepatic blood flow ↓ Phase I (oxidation, reduction, hydrolysis) metabolism
Immune	↓ Antibody production in response to antigen ↑ Autoimmunity
Oral	Altered dentition ↓ Ability to taste salt, bitter, sweet, and sour
Pulmonary	↓ Respiratory muscle strength ↓ Chest wall compliance ↓ Arterial oxygenation and impaired carbon dioxide elimination ↓ Vital capacity ↓ Maximal breathing capacity ↑ Residual volume

(continued)

TABLE A2–1	Physiologic Changes with Aging (Continued)
Organ System	**Manifestation**
Renal	↓ GFR
	↓ Renal blood flow
	↓ Filtration fraction
	↓ Tubular secretory function
	↓ Renal mass
Sensory	Presbyopia (diminished ability to focus on near objects)
	↓ Night vision
	Presbycusis (high-pitch, high-frequency hearing loss)
	↓ Sensation of smell and taste
Skeletal	↓ Skeletal bone mass (osteopenia)
	Joint stiffening caused by reduced water content in tendons, ligaments, and cartilage
Skin/hair	Thinning of stratum corneum
	↓ Langerhans cells, melanocytes, and mast cells
	↓ Depth and extent of the subcutaneous fat layer
	Thinning and graying of hair caused by more hairs in the resting phase and shortening of the growth phase as well as changes in follicular melanocytes

(DHEA-S, dehydroepiandrosterone-S; GFR, glomerular filtration rate; TSH, thyroid-stimulating hormone.)

TABLE A2–2	Age-Related Changes in Drug Pharmacokinetics
Pharmacokinetic Phase	**Pharmacokinetic Parameters**
Gastrointestinal absorption	Unchanged passive diffusion and no change in bioavailability for most drugs
	↓ Active transport and ↓ bioavailability for some drugs
	↓ First-pass metabolism, ↑ bioavailability for some drugs, and ↓ bioavailability for some prodrugs
Distribution	↓ Volume of distribution and ↑ plasma concentration of water-soluble drugs
	↑ Volume of distribution and ↑ terminal disposition half-life ($t_{1/2}$) for lipid-soluble drugs
Hepatic metabolism	↓ Clearance and ↑ $t_{1/2}$ for some drugs with poor hepatic extraction (capacity-limited metabolism); phase I metabolism may be affected more than phase II
	↓ Clearance and ↑ $t_{1/2}$ for drugs with high hepatic extraction ratios (flow-limited metabolism)
Renal excretion	↓ Clearance and ↑ $t_{1/2}$ for renally eliminated drugs and active metabolites

TABLE A2–3	Atypical Disease Presentation in Older Adults
Disease	**Presentation**
Acute myocardial infarction	Only ~50% present with chest pain. In general, older adults present with weakness, confusion, syncope, and abdominal pain; however, electrocardiographic findings are similar to those in younger patients.
Congestive heart failure	Instead of dyspnea, older patients may present with hypoxic symptoms, lethargy, restlessness, and confusion.
Gastrointestinal bleed	Although the mortality rate is ~10%, presenting symptoms are nonspecific, ranging from altered mental status to syncope with hemodynamic collapse. Abdominal pain often is absent.
Upper respiratory infection	Older patients typically present with lethargy, confusion, anorexia, and decompensation of a preexisting medical condition. Fever, chills, and a productive cough may or may not be present.
Urinary tract infection	Dysuria, fever, and flank pain may be absent. More commonly, older adults present with incontinence, confusion, abdominal pain, nausea or vomiting, and azotemia.

TABLE A2–4	Examples for Monitoring of Medication Use in Older Long-Term Care Facility Patients	
Drug	**Monitoring**	**Monitoring Interval (in mo)**
Amiodarone	Hepatic function tests, TSH level	6
Antiepileptic agents (carbamazepine, phenobarbital, phenytoin, primidone, and valproate)	Drug levels	3–6
Angiotensin-converting enzyme inhibitors or angiotensin I receptor blockers	Potassium levels	6
Antipsychotic agents	Extrapyramidal side effects, fasting serum glucose, serum lipid panel	6
Appetite stimulants	Weight, appetite	a
Digoxin	Serum blood urea nitrogen, creatinine, trough drug level	6
Diuretics	Serum sodium and potassium levels	3
Erythropoiesis stimulants	Blood pressure, iron and ferritin levels, CBC	1
Fibrates	Hepatic function test, CBC	6
Hypoglycemic agents	Fasting serum glucose level or glycated hemoglobin level	6
Iron	Iron and ferritin levels, CBC	a
Lithium	Trough serum drug levels	3
Niacin	Blood sugar levels, hepatic function tests	6
Theophylline	Trough serum drug levels	3
Thyroid replacement	TSH level	6
Warfarin	Prothrombin time or international normalized ratio	1

(CBC, complete blood count; TSH, thyroid-stimulating hormone.)
aConsensus agreement about interval could not be reached.

TABLE A2–5	Medication Appropriateness Index

Questions to Ask About Each Individual Medication

1. Is there an indication for the medication?
2. Is the medication effective for the condition?
3. Is the dosage correct?
4. Are the directions correct?
5. Are the directions practical?
6. Are there clinically significant drug–drug interactions?
7. Are there clinically significant drug–disease or drug–condition interactions?
8. Is there unnecessary duplication with other medication(s)?
9. Is the duration of therapy acceptable?
10. Is this medication the least expensive alternative compared with others of equal utility?

(Used with permission from J Clin Epidemiol, Vol. 45, Hanlon JT, Schmader KE, Samsa GP, et al. A method for assessing drug therapy appropriateness, Pages 1045–1051, Copyright © 1992 Elsevier.)

(See e/Chapter 7, Geriatrics, authored by Emily R. Hajjar, Shelly L. Gray, Patricia W. Slattum, Lauren R. Hersh, Jennifer G. Naples, and Joseph T. Hanlon, for a more detailed discussion of this topic.)

Drug-Induced Hematologic Disorders

APPENDIX 3

TABLE A3–1	Drugs Associated with Aplastic Anemias

Observational study evidence
Carbamazepine
Furosemide
Gold salts
Mebendazole
Methimazole
NSAIDs
Oxyphenbutazone
Penicillamine
Phenobarbital
Phenothiazines
Phenytoin
Propylthiouracil
Sulfonamides
Thiazides
Tocainide

Case report evidence (*probable* or *definite* causality rating)
Acetazolamide
Aspirin
Captopril
Chloramphenicol
Chloroquine
Chlorothiazide
Chlorpromazine
Dapsone
Felbamate
Interferon alfa
Lisinopril
Lithium
Nizatidine
Pentoxifylline
Quinidine
Sulindac
Ticlopidine

MedWatch postmarketing reports 2009–2015
Adalimumab
Aliskirin
Amlodipine
Carvedilol
Dantrolene
Etanercept
Oxcarbazepine
Valsartan

(NSAID, nonsteroidal anti-inflammatory drug.)

TABLE A3–2	Drugs Associated with Agranulocytosis		
Observational Study Evidence	**Case Report Evidence** (*Probable* or *Definite* Causality Rating)		**MedWatch Postmarketing Reports 2009–2015**
β-Lactam antibiotics	Acetaminophen	Levodopa	Amlodipine
Carbamazepine	Acetazolamide	Meprobamate	Aripiprazole
Carbimazole	Ampicillin	Methazolamide	Benazapril
Clomipramine	Captopril	Methyldopa	Bocepravir
Digoxin	Carbenicillin	Metronidazole	Clozapine
Dipyridamole	Cefotaxime	Nafcillin	Defarasirox
Ganciclovir	Cefuroxime	NSAIDs	Fluoxetine
Glyburide	Chloramphenicol	Olanzapine	Haloperidol
Gold salts	Chlorpromazine	Oxacillin	Hydrochlorothiazide
Imipenem–cilastatin	Chlorpropamide	Penicillamine	lacosamide
Indomethacin	Chlorpheniramine	Penicillin G	Leflunomide
Macrolide antibiotics	Clindamycin	Pentazocine	Levitiracetam
Methimazole	Clozapine	Phenytoin	Memantine
Mirtazapine	Colchicine	Primidone	Molindone
Phenobarbital	Doxepin	Procainamide	Olanzapine
Phenothiazines	Dapsone	Propylthiouracil	Oxcarbazepine
Prednisone	Desipramine	Pyrimethamine	Paliperidone
Propranolol	Ethacrynic acid	Quinidine	Pantoprazole
Spironolactone	Ethosuximide	Quinine	Pimozide
Sulfonamides	Flucytosine	Rifampin	Propafenone
Sulfonylureas	Gentamicin	Streptomycin	Quetiapine
Ticlopidine	Griseofulvin	Terbinafine	Rifabutin
Valproic acid	Hydralazine	Ticarcillin	Risperidone
Zidovudine	Hydroxychloroquine	Tocainide	Sulfasalazide
	Imipenem–cilastatin	Tolbutamide	Thiothixene
	Imipramine	Vancomycin	Trandolapril
	Lamotrigine		Ziprasidone

(NSAID, nonsteroidal anti-inflammatory drug.)

TABLE A3–3	Drugs Associated with Hemolytic Anemia

Observational study evidence
Phenobarbital
Phenytoin
Ribavirin

Case report evidence (*probable* or *definite* causality rating)
Acetaminophen
Angiotensin-converting enzyme inhibitors
β-Lactam antibiotics
Cephalosporins
Ciprofloxacin
Clavulanate
Erythromycin
Hydrochlorothiazide
Indinavir
Interferon alfa
Ketoconazole
Lansoprazole
Levodopa
Levofloxacin
Methyldopa
Minocycline
NSAIDs
Omeprazole
p-Aminosalicylic acid
Phenazopyridine
Probenecid
Procainamide
Quinidine
Rifabutin
Rifampin
Streptomycin
Sulbactam
Sulfonamides
Sulfonylureas
Tacrolimus
Tazobactam
Teicoplanin
Tolbutamide
Tolmetin
Triamterene

MedWatch postmarketing reports 2009–2015
Amlodipine
Bevacizumab
Chlorpropamide
Pegademase
Pioglitazone
Rosiglitazone

(NSAID, nonsteroidal anti-inflammatory drug.)

TABLE A3–4	Drugs Associated with Metabolic Hemolytic Anemia

Observational study evidence
Dapsone
Rasburicase

Case report evidence (*probable* or *definite* causality rating)
Ascorbic acid
Metformin
Methylene blue
Nalidixic acid
Nitrofurantoin
Phenazopyridine
Primaquine
Sulfacetamide
Sulfamethoxazole
Sulfanilamide

TABLE A3–5	Drugs Associated with Megaloblastic Anemia

Case report evidence (*probable* or *definite* causality rating)
Azathioprine
Chloramphenicol
Colchicine
Cotrimoxazole
Cyclophosphamide
Cytarabine
5-Fluorodeoxyuridine
5-Fluorouracil
Hydroxyurea
6-Mercaptopurine
Methotrexate
Oral contraceptives
p-Aminosalicylate
Phenobarbital
Phenytoin
Primidone
Pyrimethamine
Sulfasalazine
Tetracycline
Vinblastine

TABLE A3–6	Drugs Associated with Thrombocytopenia

Observational study evidence
Carbamazepine
Phenobarbital
Phenytoin
Valproic acid

Case report evidence (*probable* or *definite* causality rating)
Abciximab
Acetaminophen
Acyclovir
Albendazole
Aminoglutethimide
Aminosalicylic acid
Amiodarone
Amphotericin B
Ampicillin
Aspirin
Atorvastatin
Captopril
Chlorothiazide
Chlorpromazine
Chlorpropamide
Cimetidine
Ciprofloxacin
Clarithromycin
Clopidogrel
Danazol
Deferoxamine
Diazepam
Diazoxide
Diclofenac
Diethylstilbestrol
Digoxin
Ethambutol
Felbamate
Fluconazole
Gold salts
Haloperidol
Heparin
Hydrochlorothiazide
Ibuprofen
Inamrinone
Indinavir
Indomethacin
Interferon alfa-2b
Isoniazid
Isotretinoin
Itraconazole

Levamisole
Linezolid
Lithium
Low-molecular-weight heparins
Measles, mumps, and rubella vaccine
Meclofenamate
Mesalamine
Methyldopa
Minoxidil
Morphine
Nalidixic acid
Naphazoline
Naproxen
Nitroglycerin
Octreotide
Oxacillin
p-Aminosalicylic acid
Penicillamine
Pentamidine
Pentoxifylline
Piperacillin
Primidone
Procainamide
Pyrazinamide
Quinidine
Quinine
Ranitidine
Recombinant hepatitis B vaccine
Rifampin
Simvastatin
Sirolimus
Sulfasalazine
Sulfonamides
Sulindac
Tamoxifen
Tolmetin
Trimethoprim
Vancomycin

MedWatch postmarketing reports 2009–2015
Acarbose
Adalimumab
Ado-trastuzumab
Alfuzosin
Aliskiren
Amlodipine
Benazepril
Bevacizumab
Boceprevir

Bortezomib
Chlorambucil
Cladribine
Cotrimoxazole
Dabigatran
Dalteparin
Dantrolene
Deferasirox
Didanosine
Drotecogin alfa
Efalizumab
Eltrombopag
Enoxaparin
Epirubicin
Epoprostenol
Eptifibatide
Ethionamid
Filgrastim
Fondaparinux
Glimepiride
Heparin
Hydrochlorothiazide
Indomethacin
Iloprost
Interferon beta 1a
Leflunomide
Linezolid
Losartan
Montelukast
Morphine
Obinutuzumab
Octreotide
Oxcarbazepine
Palivizumab
Pamidronate
Pemetrexed
Pioglitazone
Pomalidomide
Propylthiouracil
Quinine
Raltegravir
Rivaroxaban
Rosiglitazone
Rosuvastatin
Spironolactone
Sunitinib
Telmisartan
Torsemide
Trepostinil
Ursodiol

(See e/Chapter 103, Drug-Induced Hematologic Disorders, authored by Elisa M. Greene and Tracy M. Hagemann, for a more detailed discussion of this topic.)

Drug-Induced Liver Disease

TABLE A4–1 An Approach to Evaluating a Suspected Hepatotoxic Reaction

Points	−3	−1	0	+1	+2	+3
What is the temporal relationship? (days)						
From the start of therapy	—	—	??	<5	>90	5–90
From the end of therapy	>30	—	??	—	—	<30
Is there evidence of the concurrent use of a hepatotoxin^a?	Yes	Maybe	??	—	—	No
Is there an alternate cause, such as viral hepatitis?	Yes	Most likely—Yes	??	Most likely—No		No
Are there extrahepatic signs or symptoms?						
Dermatologic: rash, palmar erythema, cutaneous vasculitis	—	—	No	Yes (+1 for each)	—	—
Dermatologic: spider nevi, white nails (aka Terry's nails)	—	—	No	Yes (+1 for each)	—	—
Hematologic: coagulation disorders	—	—	No	Yes (+1 for each)	—	—
Endocrine: insulin resistance, thyroid dysfunction	—	—	No	Yes (+1 for each)	—	—
Endocrine: adrenal insufficiency, hypogonadism	—	—	No	Yes (+1 for each)	—	—
Skeletal muscular: arthralgias, arthritis	—	—	No	Yes (+1 for each)	—	—
Neurologic: encephalopathy	—	—	No	Yes (+1 for each)	—	—
Portopulmonary hypertension	—	—	No	Yes (+1 for each)	—	—
Does the literature support a connection with this drug?						
Listed in the product labeling	—	—	—	—	—	Yes
Published reports in the literature	—	—	—	—	Yes	—
No information available, reaction is undocumented	—	—	Yes	—	—	—
Results from a rechallenge with the drug	Negative	—	—	Inconclusive	—	Positive

(??, Uncertain.)
A total score <7 makes it unlikely that this is a hepatotoxic reaction.
As the score approaches 14; the possibility that this is a hepatotoxic reaction increases toward certainty.
^a Drug, herbal remedy, or other occupational exposure known to be potentially hepatotoxic.

TABLE A4-2	Environmental Hepatotoxins and Associated Occupations at Risk for Exposure
Hepatotoxin	**Associated Occupations at Risk for Exposure**
Arsenic	Chemical plant, agricultural workers
Carbon tetrachloride	Chemical plant workers, laboratory technicians
Copper	Plumbers, sculpture artists, foundry workers
Dimethylformamide	Chemical plant workers, laboratory technicians
2,4-Dichlorophenoxyacetic acid	Horticulturists
Fluorine	Chemical plant workers, laboratory technicians
Toluene	Chemical plant, agricultural workers, laboratory tech
Trichloroethylene	Printers, dye workers, cleaners, laboratory technicians
Vinyl chloride	Plastics plant workers; also found as a river pollutant

TABLE A4-3		Relative Patterns of Hepatic Enzyme Elevation in Liver Injury. R = (Measured ALT/ Upper Normal Limit of ALT) ÷ (Measured Alk Phos/Upper Normal Limit of Alk Phos)			
Enzyme		**Hepatocellular**	**Cholestatic**	**Mixed Injury**	**Chronic**
R-Values		5	2	3–4	—
Alkaline phosphatase	Alk Phos	↑	↑↑↑	↑↑↑	↑
5'-Nucleotidase	5-NC, 5NC	↑	↑↑↑	↑↑↑	↑
γ-Glutamyltransferase	GGT, GGTP	↑	↑↑↑	↑↑↑	↑↑
Aspartate aminotransferase	AST	↑↑↑	↑	↑↑↑	↑↑
Alanine aminotransferase	ALT	↑↑↑	↑	↑↑↑	↑↑
Lactate dehydrogenase	LDH	↑↑↑	↑	↑↑↑	↑

(↑, <100% of normal; ↑↑, >100% of normal; ↑↑↑, >300% of normal.)

(See e/Chapter 38, Drug-Induced Liver Disease, authored by William R. Kirchain, for a more detailed discussion of this topic.)

Drug-Induced Pulmonary Disease

TABLE A5–1	Drugs That Induce Apnea	
		Relative Frequency of Reactions
Central nervous system depression		
Narcotic analgesics		F
Barbiturates		F
Benzodiazepines		F
Other sedatives and hypnotics		I
Tricyclic antidepressants		R
Phenothiazines		R
Ketamine		R
Promazine		R
Anesthetics		R
Antihistamines		R
Alcohol		R
Fenfluramine		I
L-Dopa		R
Oxygen		R
Respiratory muscle dysfunction		
Aminoglycoside antibiotics		I
Polymyxin antibiotics		I
Neuromuscular blockers		I
Quinine		R
Digitalis		R
Myopathy		
Corticosteroids		F
Diuretics		I
Aminocaproic acid		R
Clofibrate		R

(F, frequent; I, infrequent; R, rare.)

TABLE A5–2 Drugs That Induce Bronchospasm	
	Relative Frequency of Reactions
Anaphylaxis (IgE-mediated)	
Penicillins	F
Sulfonamides	F
Serum	F
Cephalosporins	F
Bromelin	R
Cimetidine	R
Papain	F
Pancreatic extract	I
Psyllium	I
Subtilase	I
Tetracyclines	I
Allergen extracts	I
Ll-Asparaginase	F
Pyrazolone analgesics	
Direct airway irritation	
Acetate	R
Bisulfite	F
Cromolyn	R
Smoke	F
N-acetylcysteine	F
Inhaled steroids	I
Precipitating IgG antibodies	
β-Methyldopa	R
Carbamazepine	R
Spiramycin	R
Cyclooxygenase inhibition	
Aspirin/NSAIDs	F
Phenylbutazone	I
Acetaminophen	R
Anaphylactoid mast-cell degranulation	
Narcotic analgesics	I
Ethylenediamine	R
Iodinated-radiocontrast media	F
Platinum	R
Local anesthetics	I
Steroidal anesthetics	I
Iron–dextran complex	I
Pancuronium bromide	R
Benzalkonium chloride	I

(continued)

TABLE A5–2 Drugs That Induce Bronchospasm (*Continued*)	Relative Frequency of Reactions
Pharmacologic effects	
α-Adrenergic receptor blockers	I-F
Cholinergic stimulants	I
Anticholinesterases	R
β-Adrenergic agonists	R
Ethylenediamine tetraacetic acid	R
Unknown mechanisms	
ACE inhibitors	I
Anticholinergics	R
Hydrocortisone	R
Isoproterenol	R
Monosodium glutamate	I
Piperazine	R
Tartrazine	R
Sulfinpyrazone	R
Zinostatin	R
Losartan	R

(ACE, angiotensin-converting enzyme; F, frequent; I, infrequent; Ig, immunoglobulin; NSAIDs, nonsteroidal anti-inflammatory drugs; R, rare.)

TABLE A5–3 Tolerance of Anti-inflammatory and Analgesic Drugs in Aspirin-Induced Asthma	
Cross-Reactive Drugs	**Drugs with No Cross-Reactivity**
Diclofenac	Acetaminophen[a]
Diflunisal	Benzydamine
Fenoprofen	Chloroquine
Flufenamic acid	Choline salicylate
Flurbiprofen	Corticosteroids
Hydrocortisone hemisuccinate	Dextropropoxyphene
Ibuprofen	Phenacetin[a]
Indomethacin	Salicylamide
Ketoprofen	Sodium salicylate
Mefenamic acid	
Naproxen	
Noramidopyrine	
Oxyphenbutazone	
Phenylbutazone	
Piroxicam	
Sulindac	
Sulfinpyrazone	
Tartrazine	
Tolmetin	

[a]A very small percentage (5%) of aspirin-sensitive patients react to acetaminophen and phenacetin.

TABLE A5–4	Drugs That Induce Pulmonary Edema	
	Relative Frequency of Reactions	
Cardiogenic pulmonary edema		
Excessive intravenous fluids	F	
Blood and plasma transfusions	F	
Corticosteroids	F	
Phenylbutazone	R	
Sodium diatrizoate	R	
Hypertonic intrathecal saline	R	
β_2-Adrenergic agonists	I	
Noncardiogenic pulmonary edema		
Heroin	F	
Methadone	I	
Morphine	I	
Oxygen	I	
Propoxyphene	R	
Ethchlorvynol	R	
Chlordiazepoxide	R	
Salicylate	R	
Hydrochlorothiazide	R	
Triamterene + hydrochlorothiazide	R	
Leukoagglutinin reactions	R	
Iron–dextran complex	R	
Methotrexate	R	
Cytosine arabinoside	R	
Nitrofurantoin	R	
Dextran 40	R	
Fluorescein	R	
Amitriptyline	R	
Colchicine	R	
Nitrogen mustard	R	
Epinephrine	R	
Metaraminol	R	
Bleomycin	R	
Iodide	R	
Cyclophosphamide	R	
VM-26	R	

(F, frequent; I, infrequent; R, rare.)

TABLE A5–5	Drugs That Induce Pulmonary Infiltrates with Eosinophilia (Loeffler's Syndrome)
Drug	**Relative Frequency of Reactions**
Nitrofurantoin	F
para-Aminosalicylic acid	F
Amiodarone	F
Iodine	F
Captopril	F
Bleomycin	F
L-tryptophan	F
Methotrexate	F
Phenytoin	F
Gold salts	F
Sulfonamides	I
Penicillins	I
Carbamazepine	I
Granulocyte-macrophage colony stimulating factor	I
Imipramine	I
Minocycline	I
Nilutamide	I
Propylthiouracil	I
Sulfasalazine	I
Tetracycline	R
Procarbazine	R
Cromolyn	R
Niridazole	R
Chlorpromazine	R
Naproxen	R
Sulindac	R
Ibuprofen	R
Chlorpropamide	R
Mephenesin	R

(F, frequent; I, infrequent; R, rare.)

TABLE A5–6	Drugs That Induce Pneumonitis and/or Fibrosis
Drug	**Relative Frequency of Reactions**
Oxygen	F
Radiation	F
Bleomycin	F
Busulfan	F
Carmustine	F
Hexamethonium	F
Paraquat	F
Amiodarone	F
Mecamylamine	I
Pentolinium	I
Cyclophosphamide	I
Practolol	I
Methotrexate	I
Mitomycin	I
Nitrofurantoin	I
Methysergide	I
Sirolimus	I
Azathioprine, 6-mercaptopurine	R
Chlorambucil	R
Melphalan	R
Lomustine and semustine	R
Zinostatin	R
Procarbazine	R
Teniposide	R
Sulfasalazine	R
Phenytoin	R
Gold salts	R
Pindolol	R
Imipramine	R
Penicillamine	R
Phenylbutazone	R
Chlorphentermine	R
Fenfluramine	R
Leflunomide	R
Mefloquine	R
Pergolide	R

(F, frequent; I, infrequent; R, rare.)

TABLE A5-7 Possible Causes of Pulmonary Fibrosis

Idiopathic pulmonary fibrosis (fibrosing alveolitis)

Pneumoconiosis (asbestosis, silicosis, coal dust, talc berylliosis)

Hypersensitivity pneumonitis (molds, bacteria, animal proteins, toluene diisocyanate, epoxy resins)

Smoking

Sarcoidosis

Tuberculosis

Lipoid pneumonia

Systemic lupus erythematosus

Rheumatoid arthritis

Systemic sclerosis

Polymyositis/dermatomyositis

Sjögren syndrome

Polyarteritis nodosa

Wegener granuloma

Byssinosis (cotton workers)

Siderosis (arc welders' lung)

Radiation

Oxygen

Chemicals (thioureas, trialkylphosphorothioates, furans)

Drugs (see Tables e30-5, e30-6, and e30-8)

TABLE A5–8	Drugs That May Induce Pleural Effusions and Fibrosis
	Relative Frequency of Reactions
Idiopathic	
Methysergide	F
Practolol	F
Pindolol	R
Methotrexate	R
Nitrofurantoin	R
Drug-induced lupus syndrome	
Procainamide	F
Hydralazine	F
Isoniazid	R
Phenytoin	R
Mephenytoin	R
Griseofulvin	R
Trimethadione	R
Sulfonamides	R
Phenylbutazone	R
Streptomycin	R
Ethosuximide	R
Tetracycline	R
Pseudolymphoma syndrome	
Cyclosporine	R
Phenytoin	R

(F, frequent; I, infrequent; R, rare.)

(See e/Chapter 30, Drug-Induced Pulmonary Diseases, authored by Hengameh H. Raissy and Michelle Harkins, for a more detailed discussion of this topic.)

Drug-Induced Kidney Disease

TABLE A6–1 Drug-Induced Kidney Structural–Functional Alterations

Tubular epithelial cell damage

Acute tubular necrosis
- Aminoglycoside antibiotics
- Radiographic contrast media
- Cisplatin, carboplatin
- Amphotericin B
- Cyclosporine, tacrolimus
- Adefovir, cidofovir, tenofovir
- Pentamidine
- Foscarnet
- Zoledronate

Osmotic nephrosis
- Mannitol
- Dextran
- IV immunoglobulin

Hemodynamically mediated kidney injury

- Angiotensin-converting enzyme inhibitors
- Angiotensin II receptor blockers
- Nonsteroidal anti-inflammatory drugs (NSAIDs)
- Cyclosporine, tacrolimus
- OKT3

Obstructive nephropathy

Crystal nephropathy
- Acyclovir
- Sulfonamides
- Indinavir
- Foscarnet
- Methotrexate

Nephrolithiasis
- Sulfonamides
- Triamterene
- Indinavir

Nephrocalcinosis
- Oral sodium phosphate solution

Glomerular disease

Minimal change disease
- NSAIDs, COX-2 inhibitors
- Lithium
- Pamidronate
- Interferon-α and -β

Membranous disease
- NSAIDs
- Penicillamine
- Captopril

Focal Segmental Glomerulosclerosis
- Pamidronate
- Interferon-α and -β
- Lithium
- Sirolimus
- Anabolic steroids

Tubulointerstitial disease

Acute allergic interstitial nephritis
- Penicillins
- Ciprofloxacin
- NSAIDs, cyclooxygenase-2 inhibitors
- Proton pump inhibitors
- Loop diuretics

Chronic interstitial nephritis
- Cyclosporine
- Lithium
- Aristolochic acid

Papillary necrosis
- NSAIDs, combined phenacetin, aspirin, and caffeine analgesics

Renal vasculitis, thrombosis, and cholesterol emboli

Vasculitis and thrombosis
- Hydralazine
- Propylthiouracil
- Allopurinol
- Penicillamine
- Gemcitabine
- Mitomycin C
- Methamphetamines
- Cyclosporine, tacrolimus
- Adalimumab
- Bevacizumab

Cholesterol emboli
- Warfarin
- Thrombolytic agents

TABLE A6–2	Potential Risk Factors for Aminoglycoside Nephrotoxicity

(A) Related to aminoglycoside dosing:
Large total cumulative dose
Prolonged therapy
Trough concentration exceeding 2 mg/L[a]
Recent previous aminoglycoside therapy

(B) Related to synergistic nephrotoxicity. Aminoglycosides in combination with
Cyclosporine
Amphotericin B
Vancomycin
Diuretics
Iodinated radiographic contrast agents
Cisplatin
NSAIDs

(C) Related to predisposing conditions in the patient
Preexisting kidney disease
Diabetes
Increased age
Poor nutrition
Shock
Gram-negative bacteremia
Liver disease
Hypoalbuminemia
Obstructive jaundice
Dehydration
Hypotension
Potassium or magnesium deficiencies

[a]The equivalent concentration in SI molar units are 4.3 µmol/L for tobramycin and 4.2 µmol/L for gentamicin.

TABLE A6–3 Recommended Interventions for Prevention of Contrast Nephrotoxicity

Intervention	Recommendation	Recommendation Grade[a]
Contrast	• Minimize contrast volume/dose	A-1
	• Use noniodinated contrast studies	A-2
	• Use low- or iso-osmolar contrast agents	A-2
Medications	• Avoid concurrent use of potentially nephrotoxic drugs, eg, NSAIDs, aminoglycosides	A-2
Isotonic sodium chloride (0.9%)	• Initiate infusion 3–12 hours prior to contrast exposure and continue 6–24 hours postexposure	A-1
	• Infuse at 1–1.5 mL/kg/h adjusting postexposure as needed to maintain a urine flow rate of 150 mL/h	
	• Alternatively, in urgent cases, initiate infusion at 3 mL/kg/h, beginning 1 hour prior to contrast exposure, then continue at 1 mL/kg/h for 6 hours postexposure	
N-acetylcysteine	• Administer 600–1200 mg by mouth (PO) every 12 hours, 4 doses beginning prior to contrast exposure (ie, 1 dose prior to exposure and 3 doses postexposure)	B-1

[a]*Strength of recommendations*: A, B, and C are good, moderate, and poor evidence to support recommendation, respectively. *Quality of evidence*: 1, evidence from more than 1 properly randomized, controlled trial; 2, evidence from more than 1 well-designed clinical trial with randomization, from cohort or case-controlled analytic studies or multiple time series, or dramatic results from uncontrolled experiments; 3, evidence from opinions of respected authorities, based on clinical experience, descriptive studies, or reports of expert communities.

TABLE A6–4	Drugs Associated with Allergic Interstitial Nephritis

Antimicrobials

Acyclovir	Indinavir
Aminoglycosides	Rifampin
Amphotericin B	Sulfonamides
β-Lactams	Tetracyclines
Erythromycin	Trimethoprim–sulfamethoxazole
Ethambutol	Vancomycin

Diuretics

Acetazolamide	Loop diuretics
Amiloride	Triamterene
Chlorthalidone	Thiazide diuretics

Neuropsychiatric

Carbamazepine	Phenytoin
Lithium	Valproic acid
Phenobarbital	

Nonsteroidal anti-inflammatory drugs

Aspirin	Ketoprofen
Indomethacin	Phenylbutazone
Naproxen	Diclofenac
Ibuprofen	Zomepirac
Diflunisal	Cyclooxygenase-2 inhibitors
Piroxicam	

Miscellaneous

Acetaminophen	Lansoprazole
Allopurinol	Methyldopa
Interferon-α	Omeprazole
Aspirin	P-aminosalicylic acid
Azathioprine	Phenylpropanolamine
Captopril	Propylthiouracil
Cimetidine	Radiographic contrast media
Clofibrate	Ranitidine
Cyclosporine	Sulfinpyrazone
Glyburide	Warfarin sodium
Gold	

(See Chapter 46, Drug-Induced Kidney Disease, authored by Thomas D. Nolin, for a more detailed discussion of this topic.)

Index

Note: Page numbers followed by *f* or *t* indicate figures or tables, respectively.

Index

Index

Index

Index